Prescription &
Over-the-Counter
DRUGS

READER'S DIGEST

▼

Prescription &
Over-the-Counter
DRUGS

The Reader's Digest Association, Inc.
Pleasantville, New York • Montreal

Reader's Digest Project Staff

Project Editor	Marianne Wait
Production Technology Manager	Douglas A. Croll
Editorial Manager	Christine R. Guido
Contributing Editor	Bridget A. Maron

Reader's Digest Illustrated Reference Books

Editor-in-Chief	Christopher Cavanaugh
Art Director	Joan Mazzeo
Operations Manager	William J. Cassidy

A Reader's Digest Book Produced by Rebus, Inc.

Publisher	Rodney Friedman
Editorial Director	Evan Hansen
Associate Editor	Jeremy D. Birch
Chief of Information Resources	Tom Damrauer
Production Database Manager	Carney W. Mimms III
Art Director	Timothy Jeffs

Writers

Edward Edelson

Maureen O'Sullivan

Steven B. Abrams, M.D.

Illustrator

Enid Hatton

Address any comments about Prescription & Over-the-Counter Drugs to:
Reader's Digest
Editor-in-Chief, Illustrated Reference Books
Reader's Digest Road, Pleasantville, NY 10570

To order additional copies of Prescription & Over-the-Counter Drugs,
call 1-800-846-2100.

Visit our website at
www.readersdigest.com.

Library of Congress has cataloged the original version as follows:
Prescription & over-the-counter drugs / Reader's Digest.
          p.   cm.
     Includes index.
     ISBN 0-7621-0053-2
1. Drugs—Handbooks, manuals, etc.   2. Drugs, Nonprescription—
Handbooks, manuals, etc.   3. Drugs—Popular works.   4. Drugs,
Nonprescription—Popular works.   I. Reader's Digest Association.
RM301.12.P74   1998
615'.1—dc21   97-31756
ISBN 0-7621-0323-X   Updated Edition April 2001

CONTENTS

▼

HOW TO USE THIS BOOK

▼

This book presents the essential facts on thousands of the most common generic and brand name drugs in use today. With all the prescription and nonprescription drugs that are now available, it's more important than ever to be well informed on the safe and proper use of medications—whether for yourself, an aging parent, or a sick child. This book will help you to do that. It presents the facts in clear, easy-to-understand language, and in a context that will help you to make the best decisions and to use your medicines in the safest and most effective way possible.

THE BOOK CONSISTS OF THREE MAIN SECTIONS:

A General Medication Overview. The introductory portion of the book contains essential information to help you use medicines wisely, including (1) advice on *Understanding Your Medications*, with useful tips on drug safety, traveling with medications, proper storage, and dozens of other topics; (2) an illustrated tour of *Drugs and Your Body* that covers the body's major organ systems, disorders that can affect them, and the many classes of drugs used to treat them; (3) a comprehensive listing of *Common Disorders and the Drugs Prescribed for Them*; and (4) a *Color Pill Locator*, with actual-size photographs, arranged by color, to help you quickly identify a particular drug by sight.

A-to-Z Individual Drug Profiles. The core of **PRESCRIPTION & OVER-THE-COUNTER DRUGS** is an A-to-Z resource of more than 750 individual drug profiles, covering thousands of generic and brand name medications. Here you'll find the information you need about a particular drug and its proper use, including why it's prescribed, how it works, dosage guidelines, precautions, side effects, what to do in the case of an overdose, and food and drug interactions. Each drug profile is clearly organized in a one- to two-page format for quick, easy lookup.

A Glossary, Directories, and General Index. The back pages of the book contain a comprehensive *Glossary of Drug Terms*, a state-by-state directory of *Certified Poison Control Centers*, a *Directory of Health Information Organizations*, and a *General Index* to help you quickly and easily find the appropriate drug profile.

Remember, you are part of a health-care team. This book will help you to become better informed about your drugs and medications. Use it to work closely with your doctor, pharmacist, and other trusted health-care professionals, to help answer any questions you may have about getting the most out of your medications and to obtain the best possible medical care and advice.

UNDERSTANDING YOUR MEDICATIONS

▼ THE DRUG PROFILE

Each of the medications covered in this book is given a drug profile, which contains the essential facts about it in an easy-to-follow, standardized, one- to two-page format. The profile will tell you the various names and formulations for a drug, information on its proper use or uses, guidelines for taking the drug, side effects and precautions associated with the drug, any potentially dangerous interactions with food or other medicines, and additional facts that you need to know to manage your medications. The individual components of each drug profile are discussed below, with a brief description of the topics covered under each heading. General tips and suggestions for using your medicines safely and effectively are provided here as well. You can use this overview to get acquainted with how the profiles are organized and to obtain important general advice about your medications. Refer to it again to answer any questions you may have about general drug safety after consulting a specific drug profile, or whenever you begin a new course of medication.

◆ Generic and Brand Names

The drug profile identifies each drug in large, bold type at the top of the page by its generic name—a unique and standardized scientific designation that is recognized worldwide. In addition, many drugs are commonly known by one or more brand names—the name that the drug manufacturer selects to market its product. For example, ibuprofen is the generic designation for a commonly used pain reliever; Motrin, Nuprin, Medipren, and Advil are four of the brand names for ibuprofen. The drug profile includes brand names that are commonly available in the United States. Unlike generic designations, brand names (also referred to as trade names) may vary from country to country.

Generic drug names are listed alphabetically in the main portion of the book. If you know the generic name of a drug, you can use this A-to-Z resource to quickly locate the relevant information. Note that some profiles cover combinations of two or more generic drugs, formulated as a single preparation. Also, terms such as "hydrochloride" or "sodium" are sometimes included in a generic

 GENERIC VERSUS BRAND NAME: WHICH IS BETTER?

Generic drugs have become increasingly popular since the 1980s, when the generic drug approval process was expanded and safety guidelines were issued by the Food and Drug Administration (FDA). About 250 new generic drugs are approved by the FDA each year. Generics are less expensive than brand name drugs. But are they as effective?

Ongoing supervision by the FDA helps to assure that generics sold in this country *are* as safe and effective as their brand name counterparts. The FDA requires that all generic drugs be bioequivalent to their brand name counterparts—that is, they must deliver the same amount of active drug ingredient to the body in a similar time frame. Furthermore, they must have similar chemical stability, so that they maintain their potency for an equivalent period of time. In addition, all drugs, including generics, must meet specifications set by the U.S. Pharmacopeial Convention, a private scientific organization that sets standards for drugs and drug products in the United States. Although there are stories in the media from time to time about the sale of substandard generic drugs, such occurrences are rare. The FDA maintains strict standards and inspection practices as well as extensive testing and monitoring of all drug manufacturing processes. About 80 percent of generic drugs sold in this country are manufactured by brand name firms in state-of-the-art plants.

You and your doctor can discuss whether generic or brand name drugs are right for you. Once you have started on a new drug therapy, it's best to stick with what you've been using—be it generic or name brand—unless your doctor says its okay to change. There are subtle variations between some generic and brand name drugs that may make one type preferable for your situation. Switching from one form to the other could, for example, slightly alter the dose that your doctor has determined to be most suitable for your needs.

drug's name. In many instances the modified formulation (sometimes called a "salt") is not important, because the drug will break down into a single active ingredient in the body. The pain reliever naproxen, for example, is sold by prescription simply as naproxen, whereas the version of the drug that has been approved for non-prescription use is formulated as naproxen sodium; both versions act identically once the common active ingredient (naproxen) is released in the body, and hence both are combined in a single drug profile. In other cases, though, a chemical modification is significant. Magnesium citrate, magnesium oxide, and magnesium sulfate, for example, act differently enough in the body to qualify as separate drugs, and each has its own profile.

If you know a drug by its brand name, you can find its profile quickly by consulting the main index at the back of the book, which lists both generic and brand names for drugs and the appropriate page number for their profiles. (The main index also indicates if a color picture of the drug is available in the *Color Pill Locator*. A picture is indicated by the letter "C" followed by the page number.) Of course, due to space constraints, not every single medication sold around the world is included in this book. We have selected the several thousand generic and brand name drugs that are used most commonly in the United States.

◆ Available Forms

The drug profile lists the available forms of a drug, such as tablet, capsule, liquid, or inhalant. Each form has certain properties that may make it preferable for your condition or that can make taking your medications

 TIPS FOR TAKING YOUR MEDICATIONS

TABLETS AND CAPSULES

Tablets come in many forms besides the standard round pill. Capsules and caplets (oblong-shaped tablets) are preferred by some people because they are easier to swallow than most round tablets. Chewable tablets are good for those who have trouble swallowing any type of pill; they should be chewed thoroughly to avoid stomach upset and should not be given to children younger than two (who can't chew them properly).

Some people prefer crushing tablets and mixing them with juice, water, or soft foods like applesauce to make them easier to swallow. This may be okay for some drugs, but certain medications are not designed for this. Enteric-coated tablets, for example, have a protective layer that allows the pill to dissolve in the intestine rather than the stomach. Crushing the tablet could cause stomach irritation. Similarly, pills that have a sustained-release, timed-release, or extended-release formulation are designed to disintegrate slowly within the body and should be swallowed whole. Capsules, too, are not supposed to be broken up or cut into pieces. Check with your doctor or pharmacist before crushing any pills or tablets.

Additional Tips

• To make a pill easier to swallow, it may be helpful to drink some water before taking it and a glass of water after. It's also a good idea to stand up while swallowing.

• If a pill gets stuck in your throat, try eating a soft food such as a banana. Swallowing the food may help to carry the pill down.

EYE AND EAR MEDICATIONS

Always wash your hands before and after administering eye (ophthalmic) or ear (otic) medications. In addition, be careful not to touch the tip of the dropper or applicator to any surface, including the ear canal or eye lids, to avoid contamination. Following are additional tips for applying these medications.

Using an Eyedropper
• Tilt the head back.

• Pull the lower eyelid downward using a finger or by pinching and pulling with the thumb and index finger, creating a pocket between the eye and lower lid.

• Drop the medication into this eyelid pocket.

Applying Eye Ointments
• Pull the lower eyelid down using a finger or by pinching and pulling with the thumb and index finger to create a pocket.

• Squeeze the tube and apply a thin strip (about a third of an inch) of ointment into the eyelid pouch.

Administering Ear Drops
• Lie down or tilt the head so that the affected ear faces up.

• For adults, pull the ear lobe up and back to straighten the ear canal. In young children, pull the ear lobe down and back.

• Drop the medication into the ear canal, but don't insert the tip of the dropper any deeper than the outer ear.

• Keep ear facing up for a few minutes so the medication can reach the bottom of the ear canal.

RECTAL SUPPOSITORIES

A rectal suppository is a relatively large, bullet-shaped drug preparation that is designed to be inserted into the rectum. Once inside, it melts with body heat and the drug is released. Suppositories may be useful for very ill patients, young children, or for others who cannot take oral medications. Lubricant suppositories may also be helpful for the treatment of constipation.

Inserting a Rectal Suppository

• The suppository should not be too soft or it will be difficult to insert. If necessary, before removing the foil wrapper, run the suppository under cold water or chill in the refrigerator for about a half hour, until it is firm.

• Wearing a latex glove, unwrap the suppository and moisten it with water. Lie on your side and gently push the suppository, rounded end first, well up into the rectum with your finger.

• In children, gently insert the suppository no more than 3 inches into the rectum.

• Lie still and try to retain the suppository for at least 20 minutes so that the drug is absorbed.

VAGINAL MEDICATIONS

Use the special applicator that comes with your medicine and follow the directions carefully. To administer the medicine, lie on your back with your knees pulled up. Insert the applicator into the vagina as far as you can without forcing it, then press the plunger to release the medicine. Withdraw the applicator; wash it with soap and warm water.

INHALERS AND SPACERS

Many people who have asthma or related respiratory disorders need to use a metered-dose inhaler (also known as a nebulizer)—a pressurized container that propels aerosolized medication into the mouth and down the throat where it can be delivered to the airways. The inhaler must be used properly to assure that enough of the medication is delivered to the airways, where it will exert its therapeutic effect, rather than to the sides of the mouth and throat.

Using an Inhaler Correctly

• Shake the inhaler well before use.

• Tilt the head back slightly and hold the mouthpiece a half an inch from the mouth. The bottom of the nebulizer bottle should be pointing up.

• Exhale normally. At the end of the exhale, inhale slowly over five seconds while firmly pressing the bottle against the mouthpiece, which releases the drug. Slow inhalation is the key to getting an effective dose. Hold your breath for 5 to 10 seconds.

• If your doctor wants you to receive more than one dose of the drug, wait a few minutes and then repeat the steps above.

A spacer—a plastic chamber or holding bag that attaches to the inhaler and that acts as a reservoir to hold the mist—may make the job easier by allowing you to inhale at a comfortable rate. Follow the doctor's instructions for how much drug to take and how often, and have the doctor check your technique from time to time to be sure it is correct.

NASAL MEDICATIONS

Blow the nose gently before administering nasal medications. After use, rinse the tip of the applicator with hot water and dry with a clean tissue. To avoid spreading infection, don't share medications with others.

Administering Nose Drops

• Tilt the head back and place the recommended number of drops in each nostril. Keep the head back for several minutes to allow the medicine to spread through the nasal passages.

Administering Nasal Sprays

• Keep the head upright and squeeze bottle firmly to spray medicine into each nostril while sniffing in briskly. Hold the breath for a few seconds, then breath out through the mouth.

LIQUID MEDICATIONS

Measure the liquid carefully. Don't use ordinary kitchen spoons to measure out a dose; instead, use any measuring device that comes with the drug or a specially marked measuring spoon.

INJECTIONS

Some drugs, for example, insulin for diabetes or an anaphylaxis medicine for life-threatening allergic reactions, are best administered by injection. Injections are given intravenously (into a vein), intramuscularly (into a muscle), or subcutaneously (under the skin). If you need to give yourself or a partner home injections, carefully review the correct procedure with your doctor or other health educator. Don't be reluctant to ask questions, and return for periodic reviews.

easier, safer, or more effective. If you have a skin infection, for example, you may need an antibiotic skin cream; an eye or ear infection, on the other hand, may call for ophthalmic or otic drops or ointment.

A distinction is sometimes made between local and systemic drugs. Local drugs, including topical preparations—which are applied to the skin, eyes, ears, hair, or mucous membranes (lips, nasal passages, vagina, rectum, for example)—and certain types of injections into the skin, muscles, or joints, tend to exert their effects over a limited area of the body. This contrasts with systemic drugs—a category that includes oral preparations that are taken by mouth (such as tablets, capsules, or liquids) as well as injections into a vein—which are absorbed by the bloodstream and circulated widely through many of the body's organ systems. Locally acting formulations tend to cause fewer and less serious side effects (for example, a limited skin rash) than systemic drugs, though they do sometimes cause widespread reactions.

Formulations can also affect how rapidly a drug is absorbed, how much of the drug is absorbed, or how quickly it can take effect. An injection of a medication directly into a vein takes nearly immediate effect and can be critical during emergency situations. At the other end of the spectrum are so-called controlled-release, timed-release, sustained-release, or prolonged-action preparations, including specially formulated capsules or transdermal skin patches. These are made specifically to provide slow, uniform absorption of a drug over a period of 8 hours or longer. Enteric-coated oral preparations are designed to keep the drug from being dissolved by stomach

DRUG NAMES **THAT LOOK OR SOUND ALIKE**

Marketers continue to think up new brand names for drugs, and a certain number of these are rejected every year by regulators on the basis that the proposed brand name looks or sounds too similar to existing names and may lead to errors when a drug prescription is filled. But prescription mix-ups continue to occur, in part because prescriptions are all too often scribbled in semilegible script or quickly called in to a pharmacy. Review the common name-related errors below (brand names are in upper case), which are based on reporting to the Food and Drug Administration (FDA). This is only a small sample—so be on guard the next time you have a prescription filled!

Accutane (for acne) ....Accupril (for hypertension)

acetazolamide (for glaucoma, ...acetohexamide (for diabetes)
   seizures, heart failure)

Altace (for hypertension).........................Artane (for Parkinson's disease)

Ambien (for insomnia)..............................Amen (for menstrual disorders)

Asacol (for bowel disease).........................Os-Cal (calcium supplement)

Ativan (for anxiety)...................................Atarax (for allergies, anxiety)

Cardene (for angina).................................codeine (for pain relief)

Cardura (for hypertension, ...Coumadin (for blood clots)
   prostate enlargement)

Cardene SR (for angina) ....Cardizem SR (for heart disease)

Celebrex (for pain relief) ....Celexa (for depression)

codeine (for pain relief).............................Lodine (for pain relief)

cycloserine (for tuberculosis) ....cyclosporine (for organ transplants)

Darvon (for pain relief)..............................Diovan (for hypertension)

Levoxine (for thyroid disease) ....Lanoxin (for heart disease)

Lorabid (for infections) ....Lortab (for infections)

Luvox (for obsessive-...............................Lasix (for heart disease)
   compulsive disorder)

Naprosyn (for pain relief).........................Naprelan (for pain relief)

Ocuflox (for eye infections) ....Ocufen (for eye disorders)

penicillamine (for arthritis) ....penicillin (for infections)

pindolol (for hypertension) ....Plendil (for hypertension)

Plendil (for hypertension).........................Prinivil (for heart disease)

Prilosec (for ulcer, heartburn) ....Prozac (for depression)

Prozac (for depression)............................Proscar (for prostate enlargement)

Verelan (for heart disease) ....Virilon (for homone disorders)

Zantac (for digestive disorders)...............Xanax (for anxiety)

acids, lessening the likelihood of gastrointestinal side effects.

Other drug formulations include sublingual preparations (which are rapidly absorbed under the tongue), nasal and inhalant preparations (breathed in through the nose or mouth), rectal suppositories, and vaginal creams or suppositories. Many additional drug preparations are available. Your doctor can determine which form of medication is best for you.

SELECTING **OVER-THE-COUNTER DRUGS**

Over-the-counter (OTC) drugs should not be taken lightly. All drugs have side effects and must be taken as directed—whether that direction comes from your doctor, pharmacist, or the back of the package. To help avoid mishaps, take the following steps when choosing an OTC preparation.

1. Read the label. All OTC drugs sold in the United States must meet strict labeling requirements. Follow all directions carefully.

2. Check for ingredients. Many products with similar sounding brand names actually contain different active ingredients. A non-drowsy formula, for example, may contain a different drug than the regular formula. Check inactive ingredients as well. Some products contain dyes or fillers that can cause allergic reactions. People who are allergic to aspirin, for example, will also be allergic to the dye, Yellow No. 5.

3. Be aware of combination products. Many OTC products contain multiple active ingredients, some of which may not be appropriate for you. Patients with liver disease, for example, should be wary of products that contain acetaminophen, a common ingredient in many OTC preparations.

4. Protect against tampering. Learn about the product's tamper-evident features from the label and look at the package for signs of tampering, such as broken seals, puncture holes, or open or damaged wrapping. Never take medicine that is discolored, has an unusual odor, or seems suspicious in some other way. Return suspicious medicine to the store manager or pharmacist.

5. Save money by buying generics. They are as safe and effective as their brand-name counterparts and are much less costly.

6. Be cautious when shopping overseas. Many foreign countries do not have the strict guidelines required in the U.S. for ensuring drug quality.

7. Check the expiration date. You do not want to buy a product that will soon expire, though you can safely use some OTC drugs past their expiration date. If stored under good conditions, most OTC drugs retain 70 to 80 percent of their potency for one or two years after the expiration date, even if the package has been opened. (Prescription drugs should never be used past their expiration date.)

8. Buy the right strength. Many OTC medications are available in multiple strengths or concentrations. Check with your doctor for advice on the potency that's right for you.

9. Watch for product reformulations. Brand-name OTC drugs occasionally are reformulated with different ingredients but retain their popular name. If you are used to taking a particular OTC drug, check the ingredients when restocking to be sure you are getting the same medication.

10. Don't confuse products. In addition to producing different products that have similar sounding brand names, some drug manufacturers also wrap their products in similar packaging. Double check the label when you buy a product and again when you take it, to make sure you are getting the right medication.

◆*Available OTC?*
Each drug profile indicates whether or not a drug is available over-the-counter (OTC)–that is, obtainable without a prescription in a drug store, supermarket, or other convenience store. Common OTC drugs include laxatives; diet pills; vitamins; cold medicine; aspirin or other pain, headache, or fever medicine; cough medicine; allergy relief medicine; antacids; and sleeping pills.

Most new drugs are available only by prescription initially and later become available OTC. A drug is granted OTC status by the FDA after a panel of experts determines that it can be used safely and effectively without a doctor's supervision, although all drugs carry at least a few risks. Many medications continue as prescription drugs even after an OTC version becomes available. Typically, the OTC form has a different brand name, a lower dosage, and more limited uses. OTC drugs must be taken with the same caution as prescriptions. Pay careful attention to the labels, including proper dosing and any food or drug interactions.

◆*Available as Generic?*
The drug profile tells you whether or not a drug is available in a generic form. A generic drug is a copycat version of a brand-name drug–it should not be confused with the generic name for a drug (see page 7). All drugs have a scientific, or generic, name, but only certain drugs are available in generic versions. Typically, a pharmaceutical company will

conduct exhaustive research and testing to launch a pioneer drug, or the first version of a new drug. In return, the company usually has patents and an exclusive license to sell that new drug for a set period of time, normally about 20 years from the time testing begins. The drug is usually marketed under a brand name. However, once that license expires, other drug companies are free to make generic versions of that drug—provided the copy is as safe and effective as the original.

The FDA estimates that about three-fourths of generic drugs are made by the same manufacturers who make the brand name drug. Generic drugs are usually sold under their generic, or scientific, name, often at half the price of the brand name version. Commonly, there are many generic versions of a popular parent drug, and generics are available for both prescription and OTC drugs.

◆ Drug Class

Each drug is classified according to its drug class—a group of drugs that have similar chemical structures or similar actions on the body. For example, a drug that reduces hypertension falls into the antihypertensive class; one that kills infectious bacteria belongs in the antibiotic class. Some drugs have multiple functions and may therefore belong to more than one drug class. In general, drugs with similar chemical structures have somewhat similar actions.

Additional information about drug classes is covered in "Drugs and Your Body" (see page 21). You can review that section to educate yourself about the many different groups of drugs and how they work. There, you will also find listings of drugs from the most common drug classes; if you're

having problems with one medication, an alternative from the same drug group may be an appropriate option to discuss with your doctor.

▼ USAGE INFORMATION

◆ Why It's Prescribed

The specific conditions, disorders, diseases, or symptoms for which a drug is prescribed are known as its indications. All drugs—prescription and OTC—must be approved specifically for one or more indications before the drug is brought to market; additional indications may later be approved by the FDA after appropriate studies have been conducted.

For OTC drugs, all indications listed on the drug's label must be approved by the FDA. Hence, you will sometimes see OTC indications referred to as "FDA approved uses" or simply "approved uses."

The situation is slightly different for prescription drugs. Once a drug has been approved for at least one indication, doctors are free to prescribe it for any purpose they deem appropriate—a common practice known as "off-label use." For example, various antibiotics that are not specifically approved for Lyme disease are often used to treat it and other infectious diseases. Indeed, about half of all prescriptions are written for off-label purposes.

Approved indications for specific drugs are included in each drug profile under the heading "Why It's Prescribed." In addition, beginning on page 63 you will find a listing of "Common Disorders and the Drugs Prescribed for Them." Here you can look up a disease or ailment and find a list of drugs that have been specifically approved by the FDA for that condi-

tion. Off-label uses are not noted in either location because their use is unofficial. If you're taking a particular drug but don't see its indication listed, you may be following an off-label prescription. You should discuss any concerns you may have about this with your doctor or pharmacist.

◆ How It Works

This section of the drug profile briefly describes how a drug acts on or within your body to achieve its desired therapeutic effect. Some drug actions are well understood. For many drugs, however, the precise mechanism of action is unknown. More information on how drugs work is included in the discussion of "Drugs and Your Body" that begins on page 21.

▼ DOSAGE GUIDELINES

The first safety rule for any medicine—be it prescription or OTC—is to take the correct dose at the right intervals. You should take great care to follow the dosage instructions of your doctor, pharmacist, or labels on prescription or OTC drugs precisely. Never take more or less of a drug without talking to your doctor first.

◆ Range and Frequency

The drug profile lists the usual dosage ranges for each drug. Use these figures as general guidelines, but don't be needlessly alarmed if your dosage is slightly above or below the range given. The correct dosage will vary from person to person and will depend on many factors, including age, weight, state of health, kidney and liver function, and use of other medications. All these factors can affect how much drug your body absorbs, how it is distributed in your body, how long it stays there, and the amount needed for a response. Your doctor will determine the right dosage for you. If you have any questions or concerns, or suspect a dosing error, do not hesitate to contact your doctor or other health-care professional.

Note that drug dosages are often given in metric units of weight, such as grams (g; there are about 454 g in a pound); milligrams (mg, or one thousandth of a gram); or micrograms (mcg, or one millionth of a gram). Dosages for some drugs, including vitamins, may be given in milliequivalents (mEq), a standard chemical unit of measure. Sometimes drug dosages are allocated per pound of body weight; this is especially useful in determining the optimal dosage for children.

◆ Onset of Effect

Many drugs exert their effects within minutes. Common analgesics such as aspirin or acetaminophen, for example, begin to relieve pain within an hour. Often, though, you must take multiple doses of a drug before levels have built up in your body sufficiently to be effective. Usually this will occur within a day or two; however, for certain drugs such as some antidepressants, it may take several weeks for the drug to exert a noticeable effect.

◆ Duration of Effect

How long a drug exerts its effects depends on the individual medication. Some can stay in your system for days, or even much longer; others will last only a few hours. The body metabolizes different drugs at different rates. In general, the faster a drug is metabolized, the more frequently you will need to take another dose. The drug profile indicates how long, on average,

 AVOIDING **PRESCRIPTION ERRORS**

Prescription errors can—and do—occur. There are a number of easy steps you can take to help avoid these errors. First, make sure you understand the prescription fully, including what it has been prescribed for as well as its generic and, if applicable, brand names. Ask your doctor to write legibly and carefully check prescription refills and renewals. Many doctors use Latin abbreviations and other notations when writing out a drug prescription; below is a list of some commonly used terms. It may also be a good idea to have the doctor include the intended use of the drug (for example, by indicating that it is for diabetes or hypertension) on the prescription.

READING A PRESCRIPTION

TERM	ABBREVIATION	MEANING
ante cibum	ac	before meals
bis in die	bid	twice a day
gutta	gt	drop
hora somni	hs	at bedtime
milligrams	mg	
milliliters	ml	
oculus dexter	od	right eye
oculus sinister	os	left eye
per os	po	by mouth
post cibum	pc	after meals
pro re nata	prn	as needed
quaque 3 hora	q3h	every 3 hours
quaque die	qd	every day
quattuor in die	qid	4 times a day
ter in die	tid	3 times a day

The Brown Bag Review

Another measure to help avoid prescription errors, especially if you're taking several drugs on a regular basis, is to have an annual "brown bag review." Once a year, bring in all the medications you are taking, both prescription and over-the-counter, so that your doctor can evaluate them and, if needed, modify your regimen. In addition, keep thorough records, and clearly indicate any medications you are taking to any new doctors who may be prescribing additional drugs. Finally, check refills and renewals carefully. A refill or renewal of a generic drug may be a different color, shape, or size because the drug comes from a different manufacturer, but it can also mean an error has been made. If you have any doubts, don't hesitate to ask your doctor or pharmacist.

a drug may remain in your system. Various factors, including general health, kidney or liver function, and food or drug interactions, can significantly increase or decrease a drug's duration of action.

◆ Dietary Advice

The drug profile tells you if a medication should be taken with or without food. Food can affect how much of the drug will enter your system, and how quickly.

Many drugs should be taken with a meal, especially with foods that contain some protein and fat. Food delays emptying of stomach contents, allowing more time for a pill or capsule to be dissolved before entering the intestines, where many drugs are absorbed. In addition, some drugs can irritate the stomach's lining if taken on an empty stomach. Taking them with food, or even a glass of milk, can help minimize the likelihood of stomach upset or other gastrointestinal disturbances. Avoid taking drugs with coffee, tea, or other hot beverages, however, because heat can inactivate or alter some medications.

Other drugs should be taken on an empty stomach—which means at least an hour before or two hours after a meal. In general, such drugs are poorly absorbed if they're taken with food. They should, however, be taken with a glass of water.

Specific foods and drinks, including alcohol, can also interact with individual drugs. These effects are discussed under "Precautions" (see page 16) and "Food Interactions" (see page 20).

◆ Storage

Requirements for storing your medicines should be clearly indicated on the label. In general, it is recommended that most medications be kept in a cool and dry place. This usually precludes the bathroom medicine cabinet, because bathrooms tend to be humid. Similarly, drugs should not be kept near a hot kitchen stove. A bedroom or kitchen closet, which tends to be cooler and drier, may be preferable.

Some liquid medicines, such as insulin or antibiotics for children's use, may need to be refrigerated. Unless your doctor or pharmacist tells you otherwise, though, it is not necessary

TRAVELING **WITH YOUR MEDICATIONS**

• Make sure you bring enough medications to last your entire trip, plus an extra supply to cover unexpected travel delays. Don't pack medications in suitcases that you plan to check; the luggage might be delayed or lost. If you carry syringes or certain drugs like narcotic pain relievers, it's wise to carry a note from your doctor that clearly explains your health history and medication requirements; in some countries, these belongings may otherwise be confiscated at customs.

• Keep drugs in their original, labeled containers. Pill bottles should be stuffed with cotton to prevent damage during transit; liquid medications should be stored in self-sealing plastic bags.

• Carry extra copies of any prescriptions, in case you need to obtain additional medicine during your trip. Prescriptions should be typed, with the generic drug name included, since drugs may be known by different brand names outside of the United States.

• Be up to date on your immunizations. You may also need additional shots or medications for travel to certain exotic locales. Consult your doctor, or a doctor who specializes in travel medicine, at least six weeks prior to your trip about the need for any new vaccinations or drugs. You may also want to check beforehand about where to obtain emergency medical help while traveling.

• Be aware that a change in climate may bring on untoward drug side effects. In hot climates, for example, diuretics may cause some dizziness at first, but such side effects are usually fleeting. Other drugs, such as antihistamines, cold preparations, and tranquilizers, can decrease your ability to perspire.

• If you are crossing several time zones and are on a fixed dosage schedule (for example, for insulin injections), you may have to make dosing adjustments. Discuss these and any other concerns with your doctor before you depart.

to refrigerate most medications.

It's always a good idea to store drugs in their original containers. Discard the cotton at the top of pill bottles; it can quickly become contaminated with the bacteria on your skin once it is touched. If you need to use a pill organizer, check with your doctor or pharmacist to make sure that the amount of light or moisture it lets through will not adversely affect any of your medicines.

If young children are around the house, be sure to store medicines in containers with childproof caps and well out of a child's reach. In addition,

don't store medicines near any dangerous substances that might be taken by mistake.

◆ Missed Dose

Everyone misses a dose of medication now and then. The drug profile tells you what to do when this occurs. For some drugs, the missed dose should be taken right away. For others, you can modify your schedule or wait until the next scheduled dose. In general, it's better not to simply double up on missed doses because you run the risk of raising the drug concentrations in your body to dangerously high levels.

TRAVELER'S **MEDICAL KIT**

Wherever you plan to travel, it's a good idea to pack certain essential items. What goes into a medical travel kit will obviously depend on where you're going, for how long, and the general health condition and ages of those traveling. But there are certain basic items that it's prudent for virtually any traveler to have. The list below outlines some items that might be included in a basic medical kit. Review these and decide which might be appropriate for you to bring along. It's best to be prepared so that an unexpected injury or ailment doesn't spoil a much-anticipated trip.

HEALTH CONCERN	WHAT TO PACK
Allergies and allergic reactions	An antihistamine, such as diphenhydramine hydrochloride.
Children's and infants' special needs	Syrup of ipecac, activated charcoal (antidotes for some cases of accidental poisoning); fluid replacement formula; ear drops and antibiotics, in case of bacterial infection. Keep any medications in childproof containers and out of reach.
Constipation	A laxative.
Colds, cough, or sinus congestion	Throat lozenges; gargle; cough syrup. For air travel, a decongestant, taken a half hour before takeoff and landing, can help to ease sinus and ear discomfort.
Cuts and scrapes/ skin infections	Topical antibiotic ointment, such as iodine antiseptic, chlorhexidine gluconate solution, or bacitracin.
Diarrhea, indigestion	Bismuth subsalicylate, loperamide hydrochloride, antacids, and/or antigas preparations.
Eye care	Spare pair of eyeglasses and/or contact lenses along with cleaning supplies, and a copy of your lens prescription.
Fever, headache, minor aches and pains	Aspirin, acetaminophen, naproxen, or ibuprofen.
First aid supplies	Bandages, gauze, tape, scissors, tweezers, pocket knife, safety pins, alcohol wipes, fever thermometer—stored in a waterproof case. Don't forget to bring along any health insurance or Medical Alert cards.
Insects	Insect repellent containing DEET or permethrin.
Itches, bites, skin rashes	A topical corticosteroid cream, such as hydrocortisone 1%; an antihistamine.
Motion sickness	An over-the-counter antihistamine, such as dimenhydrinate or meclizine, or a prescription scopolamine skin patch.
Nasal congestion due to colds or allergies	A decongestant, such as pseudoephedrine, and/or an antihistamine.
Sprains and strains	An elastic bandage along with an anti-inflammatory pain reliever, such as aspirin or ibuprofen.
Sun protection	Sunscreen and lip balm with an SPF of 15 or higher.
Water impurities	Water purification tablets may be needed in certain areas.

Products are available that help remind you to take your medicines on a proper schedule. These items, sometimes called compliance aids, include check-off calendars, containers with sections for daily doses, electronic devices that beep when it's time for a dose, and computerized pill dispensers. If you need help in selecting a compliance aid, check with your doctor or pharmacist.

◆ Stopping the Drug

Never stop taking a prescribed drug, even if you're feeling better, without consulting your doctor. Even a minor infection that appears to have cleared up with a few days' worth of antibiotics usually requires a full course of therapy (often 10 days to 2 weeks). If you stop taking the antibiotic too soon, resistant bacteria can multiply and cause an even more serious infection. Abrupt changes in dosage of some drugs can also be dangerous. For example, a narcotic pain reliever may have to be reduced gradually to avoid withdrawal symptoms. Or if a hypertensive medicine is stopped suddenly, blood pressure may soar.

For all drugs, it's important that you follow through with the recommended course of therapy. Some drugs may take months to produce full benefit. Others should be continued indefinitely on a long-term basis. If you experience bothersome side effects or don't feel that a drug is having the intended effect, talk with your doctor or pharmacist, but don't change your medication schedule on your own.

◆ Prolonged Use

If you require a drug for a chronic condition, you may need to take it for extended periods, or even a lifetime. Regular checkups or periodic testing or monitoring may be required to make sure the drug is not causing any insidious adverse effects.

▼ SIDE EFFECTS

Along with their desired therapeutic actions, drugs typically exert other side effects on the body, many of which are undesirable. Side effects can occur with virtually all prescription and over-the-counter drugs, even when they're taken properly. It's important to remember, though, that only a small percentage of patients who are taking a drug actually experience side effects, even the relatively common ones.

The drug profile groups the side effects as serious, common, and less common. Serious side effects are those that may be life-threatening or otherwise have a significant impact on well being. You should seek immediate medical assistance if you experience a serious side effect from a drug. Of course, even a mild one is significant if it has a negative impact on your quality of life. It's a good idea to call your doctor if you are concerned about any side effect, even a seemingly minor one. Write down any problems you have with your medicine so you'll remember them when you talk with your doctor or pharmacist, and don't be afraid to ask questions.

▼ PRECAUTIONS

◆ Over 60

Drugs should be used with special caution by people older than 60. Physiologic changes brought on by aging—including diminishing kidney and liver function, an increase in the ratio of fat to muscle, and a decrease in the amount of water in body tissues—all act to concentrate medications and prevent them from being eliminated quickly. Consequently, older adults may require lower dosages than the standard amounts usually recommended.

According to the FDA, 17 percent of all hospitalizations among older adults are caused by the side effects of prescription drugs—six times more than for the general population. Drug side effects, as well as drug and food interactions and overdose, are more common in older patients in part because they are much more likely than younger people to be taking medications in the first place. The problem is compounded when multiple medications are involved, particularly when drugs are prescribed by different doctors, who are not always aware of other medications the patient is taking. In addition, studies have shown that a surprisingly sizeable percentage of elderly patients are prescribed drugs that are contraindicated for those in their age group.

It's important to let all of your doctors know of any medications you are taking—whether prescription or OTC—and to know as much about the drugs you are taking as possible. As a general rule, don't attribute any changes in mood or any new or unusual reactions or physical changes simply to old age; they may actually be drug side effects or dangerous interactions.

◆ Driving and Hazardous Work

Because some medications may cause drowsiness or confusion, they should not be used when driving, working with dangerous tools or machinery, or in other situations where a lapse in concentration could cause serious injury. If a drug makes you drowsy, talk to your doctor about scheduling doses near your bedtime, or ask about other drugs that might be substituted. Always check to see if a drug may affect alertness and concentration before driving or engaging in a potentially hazardous activity.

◆ *Alcohol*

Certain medications, including many OTC drugs, can be dangerous if they are taken with alcohol. It's important for you to know whether or not alcohol should be avoided whenever you begin taking a new drug. Common signs of alcohol-drug interactions include excessive sleepiness, difficulty breathing, and stomach irritation. If in doubt, it's always a good idea to avoid alcoholic beverages while taking a medication. According to the FDA, "of the 100 medicines most commonly prescribed, more than half contain at least one substance that reacts badly with alcohol."

◆ *Pregnancy*

Some drugs are known to be harmful during pregnancy and should unequivocally be avoided during that time. A few have been shown to be safe. But for most drugs, not enough studies have been conducted for researchers to know for sure if the drug is truly dangerous to the fetus.

In general, it's a good idea to minimize the use of prescription and OTC drugs during pregnancy (though certain medications, such as vitamin supplements, may be recommended by your doctor). This includes the use of alcohol (present in some drug preparations), which most experts recommend avoiding. Your medical needs—as assessed by your doctor—will determine whether a drug is absolute-

BASIC MEDICINE SAFETY TIPS

1. Follow instructions carefully. It's essential that you take the correct dose at the proper time intervals, and avoid potential food and drug interactions.

2. Keep a log of your medicines and let your doctor know your drug and medical history. It's a good idea to review your medications with your primary-care doctor annually, including both prescription and OTC drugs.

3. Try to have prescriptions filled at one pharmacy. The pharmacist will get to know you and your medicines, and will be more likely to detect any possible prescription errors.

4. Store medicines properly, away from sunlight, heat, and humidity. The bathroom medicine cabinet, because of the humidity, is not a good location. A locked closet—away from the reach and sight of children—is ideal.

5. Discard outdated medicines. Prescription drugs should not be used past their expiration date. Some drugs lose their potency with time; other outdated medicines, such as the tetracycline antibiotics, may have dangerous side effects. Ask your pharmacist to label your prescription container with an expiration date, and regularly discard old medicines down the toilet.

6. Don't share prescription drugs or borrow them from others. What's good for one person may be harmful to another.

7. Don't take medicines in the dark. You could take the wrong pill by accident. Read the label carefully each time you take a drug to be sure you are getting the right medicine.

8. Keep emergency phone numbers handy. You should have the numbers of your doctor, emergency medical services, and the nearest poison control center readily available in case a medical emergency arises.

9. Don't be afraid to ask questions. Understand your medicines as thoroughly as possible: why you are taking them, how and when they should be taken, things to look out for. People who ask questions are more satisfied with their medical care.

10. Alert your doctor to any side effects or changes in your condition. He or she may be able to adjust your dosage or give you a substitute medication.

ly necessary. Remember that the benefits of many drugs, when indicated, far outweigh the slight possible risk to mother or fetus.

◆ *Breast-Feeding*

Check with your doctor before taking any prescription or OTC medicine if you are nursing. Most drugs—including vitamins and herbal supplements—pass into breast milk to some extent, though some do so more readily than others. And while most medications have little or no apparent effect on the nursing infant, some—such as anti-cancer drugs or lithium—are known to be dangerous.

The drug profile indicates if a specific drug should be avoided by nursing mothers. In general, as for pregnancy, it's a good idea to minimize the use of medications during this time.

Most experts recommend avoiding or strictly limiting alcohol intake as well. For mild pain relief, ibuprofen may be preferable to aspirin or other analgesics, although most analgesics can be used relatively safely while breast-feeding; check with your doctor about the best choice for you.

Of course, your medical condition may require that you take certain medications while breast-feeding. Your doctor can help you to weigh the risks and benefits of drug therapy. In some cases, a drug regimen can be suspended during the nursing period, breast-feeding can be temporarily suspended if a drug is needed for only a short time, the dosing regimen can be modified, or a substitute drug can be used.

◆ *Infants and Children*

Children are more sensitive than adults to many drugs. If a drug is indicated for use by children, be especially attentive to adverse reactions. If you have any concerns, talk to your doctor, pediatrician, or pharmacist.

OTC drugs, like all medications, should be used judiciously by children. Study the label of an OTC medicine thoroughly to make sure the drug is safe for them. If the label does not have a pediatric dose listed, don't just assume it is safe for anyone under age 12. OTC drugs should not be used by any child younger than two years without talking to the doctor or pharmacist first. In addition, avoid combining OTC remedies. Many preparations contain more than one active ingredient, and giving your child two or more different remedies can more easily lead to side effects or overdose.

Important note: Aspirin and other salicylates should not be given to children under 16 unless your doctor instructs otherwise. These drugs have

been associated with Reye's syndrome, a rare but potentially fatal liver disorder, when used to treat chicken pox or flu. Use acetaminophen or ibuprofen instead.

It's also important to remember that many OTC medications contain alcohol, which can be dangerous to small children.

◆ *Special Concerns*

The drug profile also notes any additional special concerns that you should be aware of. One such possibility is an allergic reaction, which occurs when the immune system mounts a response against a particular drug. Allergic reactions can occur with virtually any drug, though they are most common with penicillin and related antibiotics. Other common allergens include sulfa drugs, barbiturates, anticonvulsants, certain insulin preparations, and local anesthetics.

Common signs of an allergic drug reaction include a skin rash, hives, and itching. Severe reactions, known by the medical term anaphylaxis, can result in swelling of the face, tongue, lips, arms, or legs; swelling can also extend to the airways, making breathing difficult—a life-threatening emergency that requires immediate medical attention.

Call the doctor if you develop any signs of an allergic reaction. Most drug allergies respond readily to treatment. Antihistamines or topical corticosteroids may be advised for skin rashes, hives, or itching. Bronchodilators can make breathing easier. Epinephrine relieves severe reactions. In some cases, a doctor may improve tolerance to a drug, such as penicillin, by giving a series of slightly increasing doses of the drug—a treatment process known medically as desensitization.

Take note of the drug that caused the reaction and let doctors, dentists, and other health-care personnel know of it in the future. You should be careful to avoid taking that drug again, since the allergic reaction may be more serious with subsequent doses. A medical alert tag, worn as a bracelet or necklace or carried as a card, may also be helpful. The tag states the medical concern and sometimes includes a phone number that can be dialed for a detailed medical history; you can discuss this option with your doctor. In addition, be sure to read OTC drug labels carefully for any ingredients that may precipitate an allergic reaction in you or a child.

◆ *Overdose: Symptoms and What to Do*

Virtually any drug can be toxic if taken in high enough doses, but the seriousness will depend on the individual and the particular drug taken. Every profile includes discussion of the symptoms that are typical of an overdose and what to do in the event of one.

Accidental poisonings are of particular concern in infants and children. Supplements that contain iron are a leading cause of death in young children, who cannot metabolize the mineral well. Prescription or OTC diet pills, stimulants, decongestants, and antidepressants are also common causes of childhood poisoning. With certain drugs, even a single tablet can be life-threatening to a small child. Properly store all medications in child-resistant containers out of the reach—and sight—of children. Remember that a child-resistant container is designed so that it takes longer than 5 minutes for 80 percent of 5-year-olds to open; it is not child-proof!

The elderly are also at increased risk for overdose. They are more sensitive to some drugs or may forget when they took their last dose.

Intentional overdose, commonly associated with suicide attempts, is a concern in depressed patients of any age, who may have access to large quantities of potentially lethal antidepressant medications.

Most drug poisonings work fairly quickly, though some overdose effects can take weeks to appear. Signs and symptoms of overdose vary widely and may include listlessness, confusion, rolling eyes, breathing difficulties, unusual sleepiness, or stomach upset. If a child is involved, look for open drug containers, stains around the mouth, or a strange breath odor.

If you suspect an overdose, don't panic. Call your doctor or poison control center right away. Depending on the drug, an antidote such as ipecac syrup may be recommended. It's a good idea to keep a bottle of ipecac on hand (safely stored)—it induces vomiting and helps rid the body of the drug. Some experts also recommend activated charcoal (available in drugstores, usually in liquid form), which acts to absorb the poison, preventing it from spreading through the body. (Activated charcoal should not be given with ipecac syrup, since the charcoal will absorb it.) For both antidotes, the patient must be conscious. Unconscious victims need immediate professional attention. Neither antidote should be used until you have talked with a doctor or poison control center, because in some cases, ipecac or charcoal can make a patient worse.

DRUGS AND CHILDREN: **SPECIAL SAFETY MEASURES**

• Keep all prescription and over-the-counter medications out of the reach of children. Some medicines, such as iron supplements, are very toxic to youngsters.

• Use child-resistant caps, and never leave containers uncapped.

• Never give medicine to children unless it is recommended for them on the label or by a doctor.

• Check with the doctor or pharmacist before giving a child more than one medicine at a time.

• Examine dose cups carefully. Cups may be marked with various standard abbreviations. Follow label directions.

• When using a dosing syringe that has a cap, discard the cap before using the syringe.

• Never guess when converting measuring units—from teaspoons or tablespoons to ounces, for example. Consult a reliable source, such as a pharmacist.

• Don't try to remember the dose used during previous illnesses; read the label each time.

• Never use medicine for purposes not mentioned on the label, unless so directed by a doctor.

• Check with the doctor before giving a child aspirin products. Never give aspirin to a child or teenager who has or is recovering from chicken pox, flu symptoms (nausea, vomiting, or fever), or flu. Aspirin may be associated in such patients with an increased risk of Reye's syndrome, a rare but serious illness.
FDA Consumer

▼ INTERACTIONS

Drugs can interact with other drugs or particular foods or be affected by certain diseases. The drug profile indicates specific interactions to watch for. Effects can range from mild to life-threatening. Elderly patients are especially prone to these interactions and should exercise special caution.

◆ *Drug Interactions*

Drug interactions occur when two or more medications react with one another, causing adverse effects. Some drugs diminish the effectiveness of another one; others can bolster another medication's actions. Drug interactions may be felt almost immediately, or they can take days, weeks, or even months to develop. It's important to note that the effects of drug interactions vary from person to person. Most patients who receive drugs that could interact do not develop notable adverse effects. On the other hand, a few patients experience life-threatening reactions. Special care should be taken by anyone who is taking multiple medications, especially if they are prescribed by different doctors. In some cases, however, a doctor will knowingly prescribe two potentially interacting drugs after determining that the benefits they provide will sufficiently outweigh the drawbacks of a possible interaction.

Check with your doctor if you are concerned about possible drug interactions or notice unusual symptoms. Take care with OTC drugs as well; they may interact with prescription drugs or with other OTC preparations. For example, don't automatically take an OTC antacid if another drug causes stomach upset, since antacids can alter the effectiveness of certain drugs.

Similarly, some vitamin or mineral supplements can interact with drugs (see box at right).

◆ Food Interactions

Certain drugs should be taken on an empty stomach, whereas others should be taken with food. For still others, it doesn't really make a great deal of difference whether you take it with food or not. These general dietary recommendations are covered in the drug profile under "Dietary Advice" (see page 13).

Listed in this section are specific foods or drinks that can interact with a particular drug. For example, dairy products can inactivate certain antibiotics. Peculiar interactions have likewise been noted between certain drugs and specific foods such as grapefruit juice (but not orange juice). The list of potential food interactions is long and drug specific. Pay close attention to the food or drink interactions for your medications to help assure you're not interfering with the proper course of drug therapy.

◆ Disease Interactions

The final section of each drug profile details specific diseases that can have a significant impact on a particular medication. Kidney or liver disease, for example, can dramatically affect drug levels in your system. Many drugs are metabolized in the liver and excreted by way of the kidneys. If either of these organs is impaired, an excess of a drug may build up in your body. Many other disorders, such as diabetes mellitus or heart disease, may also affect your course of medication. It's important to tell your doctor about all diseases or conditions that you have, even if they are not related to your immediate medical concerns.

DRUGS & HERBAL SUPPLEMENTS: **SOME CAVEATS**

Herb–Drug Interactions

While there are entire databases documenting how drugs may interact with other drugs, few studies have been done on how drugs interact with herbal supplements. Furthermore, unlike prescription and over-the-counter drugs, herbal products are not regulated by the FDA. Thus many consumers are unaware of the potentially serious risks of mixing botanicals with pharmaceuticals.

The main drugs to worry about are known as narrow therapeutic index (NTI) agents. These drugs require precise dosages in order to be effective without being toxic. The anticoagulant drug warfarin (Coumadin) is one example: Too little is ineffective; too much can cause life-threatening bleeding episodes. Supplements like feverfew, fish oil, garlic, pau d'arco, devil's claw, dong quai, papaya, and vitamins E and K can dangerously alter blood levels of anticoagulants.

Other Significant Examples

Chili pepper (capsaicin) can increase the risk of side effects from ACE inhibitors (taken for high blood pressure), as well as boost theophylline (an asthma drug) to dangerous levels in the blood. Ginkgo biloba—when taken with aspirin, acetaminophen, or caffeine-containing pain relievers or with anticoagulants—may lead to hyphema (bleeding into the front chamber of the eye) or hemorrhagic stroke (bleeding into the brain). Licorice may interfere with corticosteroids and cause serious complications in women taking oral contraceptives. Ginseng may interact adversely with MAO inhibitors (a variety of antidepressant) and

digoxin (a heart drug). St. John's wort may be hazardous to people taking selective serotonin reuptake inhibitors (SSRIs) for depression, and it may interfere with warfarin, digoxin, oral contraceptives, and cyclosporine (an immunosuppressant taken for organ transplants).

Some supplements pose such significant risks that they should be avoided altogether. These include comfrey, coltsfoot, chaparral, ephedra (ephedrine or ma huang), sassafras, and yohimbe.

Avoiding Problems

• Tell your doctor about any supplements you take, and ask your doctor or pharmacist about risks of herb–drug interactions. People taking medication for chronic conditions like diabetes, heart disease, or hypertension should be especially cautious.

• Avoid herbal supplements if you are pregnant, may be pregnant, or are breast-feeding. Check with your doctor before giving herbal preparations to children.

• Discontinue herbal supplements two to three weeks prior to surgery, as they may promote bleeding during and after the operation.

• Don't use an herb and a drug for the same condition—for example, taking St. John's wort and Prozac simultaneously for depression. Such combinations may heighten side effects.

• Don't suddenly start and stop taking herbs or drugs, as this may produce unpredictable and potentially harmful fluctuations in blood levels of your medications.

• Stop taking supplements right away if you experience side effects.

The Heart and Cardiovascular System

The heart, beating 60 to 80 times each minute, is a marvelous pump that continuously propels blood through your lungs and then throughout your body to supply all the cells with oxygen and essential nutrients. Weighing 7 to 10 ounces, the heart is a muscular organ that has four chambers: the left and right atria and the left and right ventricles. The movement of blood in the heart is controlled by valves, which ensure that the blood always flows in the correct direction.

As the heart contracts with each beat, the left ventricle pumps about three ounces of oxygen-rich blood into the aorta, the largest artery in the body. From the aorta the blood is carried to all parts of your body through an intricate network of arteries, arterioles, and capillaries. As blood flows through your tissues, it releases oxygen and picks up carbon dioxide and other waste products. A system of veins then transports this blood, now depleted of oxygen, back to your heart. The returning stream of blood enters the right atrium through a very large vein, the superior vena cava, is then pumped into the right ventricle, and from there goes into the lungs, where it is again enriched with oxygen. This oxygen-rich blood now reenters the left atrium through the pulmonary vein and passes through the mitral valve into the left ventricle, where it is now ready to resume its journey. Each day, the average heart accomplishes an incredible feat, pumping more than 2,000 gallons of blood through a total of about 60,000 miles of blood vessels.

To carry out its constant pumping action, the heart itself requires a steady flow of oxygen-rich blood. The coronary arteries, which encircle the heart, fulfill this function. Branching off at the root of the aorta, these small blood vessels provide blood and oxygen to all parts of the heart muscle.

▼ CARDIOVASCULAR DRUGS

As might be expected, there are many things that can go wrong with a dynamic organ such as the heart, which contracts and expands virtually every second of every day. Two of the most common disorders affecting the heart and blood vessels are high blood pressure, or hypertension, and coronary artery disease. High blood pressure is an important risk factor for heart attacks and is the leading cause of stroke. Coronary artery disease, which is the primary cause of heart attacks, results from atherosclerosis—the build-up of fatty deposits in and under the lining of the artery walls. People with diseased coronary arteries may also experience a type of crushing chest pain called angina pectoris. A heart attack, or myocardial infarction, occurs when a clot lodges in a narrowed coronary artery and obstructs the flow of blood to a portion of the heart muscle, causing it to die. Other major cardiovascular problems

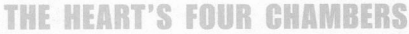

THE HEART'S FOUR CHAMBERS

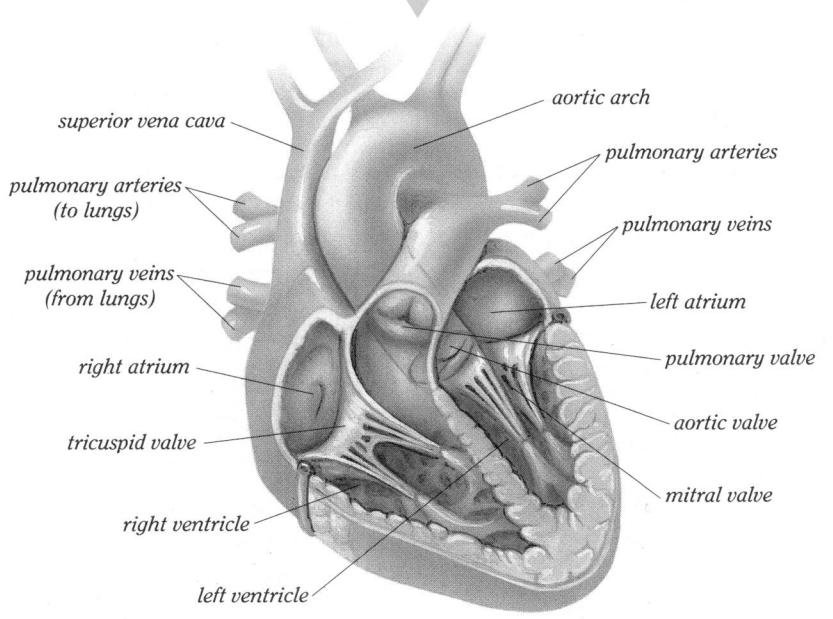

superior vena cava

pulmonary arteries (to lungs)

pulmonary veins (from lungs)

right atrium

tricuspid valve

right ventricle

left ventricle

aortic arch

pulmonary arteries

pulmonary veins

left atrium

pulmonary valve

aortic valve

mitral valve

include arrhythmias, or disturbances in the heart's rhythm, and congestive heart failure (commonly called "heart failure"), in which the heart muscle is damaged and unable to pump enough blood to meet the body's needs. Various classes of drugs may be prescribed if lifestyle changes fail to control a cardiovascular condition.

◆ Diuretics

Diuretics act on the kidneys to promote the excretion of more than normal amounts of water. This reduction in body water decreases the total volume of blood circulating in your system, thus lowering the pressure within your blood vessels.

Three classes of diuretics—loop diuretics, the thiazides, and potassium-sparing diuretics—are commonly prescribed for the treatment of high blood pressure. All three types block the reabsorption of sodium and water by the bloodstream, leading to an increase in the volume of urine. Because the thiazides and loop diuretics may cause your body to lose excessive amounts of potassium, which can lead to weakness and confusion or abnormal heart rhythms, you may be advised to take a potassium supplement. Alternatively, your doctor may prescribe a potassium-sparing diuretic, which is a mild diuretic that prevents excessive potassium loss, together with a thiazide or loop diuretic.

Diuretics are also prescribed for the treatment of congestive heart failure because they help to remove the buildup of excess fluid in the tissues and reduce the work of the heart.

◆ Beta-Blockers

Beta-blockers are commonly prescribed to lower blood pressure in those with hypertension because they slow the heart rate and reduce the force of the heartbeat. Beta-blockers are also given to relieve or prevent angina, to treat a variety of arrhythmias, and to prevent second heart attacks. These drugs bind to specific cellular structures termed beta receptors that are located in the heart, blood vessels, and airways. In addition to their effect on the heart, beta-blockers can cause constriction of the airways. Hence, they are prescribed cautiously for people with asthma, bronchitis, or other respiratory problems. A beta-blocker may be given alone or in combination with another drug, usually a thiazide diuretic.

◆ Calcium Channel Blockers

Calcium channel blockers, which are commonly prescribed to treat hypertension, are powerful vasodilators that induce the muscles surrounding your blood vessels to relax. Before arterial smooth muscles can contract and reduce the diameter of your blood vessels, a small amount of calcium must pass through special channels in the membranes of the muscle cells. These drugs work by decreasing the movement of calcium into the muscles of the blood vessels, thereby reducing their constriction. As a result, the blood vessels dilate, leading to a fall in blood pressure. Because calcium channel blockers can reduce the strain on the heart muscle and slow conduction of electrical impulses in the heart, they are used to treat some cases of angina or arrhythmias as well.

◆ ACE Inhibitors

ACE (angiotensin converting enzyme) inhibitors prevent the formation of a naturally occurring substance termed angiotensin II that constricts the blood vessels. They accomplish this by blocking the enzyme (ACE) that converts angiotensin I, an inactive compound, into angiotensin II. Angiotensin II acts directly on the arteries, causing them to constrict and raising the blood pressure. In the absence of angiotensin II, the blood vessels dilate, and blood pressure drops quickly. ACE inhibitors are prescribed to treat congestive heart failure as well as high blood pressure.

◆ Miscellaneous Antihypertensive Drugs

Other categories of drugs for high blood pressure include centrally acting antihypertensives and peripherally acting antihypertensives. The centrally acting forms, such as clonidine, work in the brain to decrease the activity of the sympathetic nervous system. They reduce blood pressure by decreasing the heart rate and lowering the amount of blood that is pumped with each beat. Clonidine has also proved effective in helping people to quit smoking, and so it may be a good choice if you are a hypertensive smoker trying to kick the habit.

Peripherally acting antihypertensives, also termed sympatholytics, interfere with the nerve signals that trigger constriction of blood vessels. As a result, the blood vessels dilate, leading to a decline in blood pressure. Sympatholytics may also help to alleviate the symptoms of congestive heart failure.

◆ Nitrates

Nitrates relieve angina by dilating the blood vessels, making it easier for the overtaxed heart to pump a sufficient amount of blood through

MAJOR CLASSES OF HEART AND CARDIOVASCULAR DRUGS

DIURETICS

Thiazide Diuretics
Chlorthalidone
Chlorothiazide
Hydrochlorothiazide
Indapamide
Metolazone

Loop Diuretics
Bumetanide
Ethacrynic Acid (Ethacrynate)
Furosemide
Torsemide

Potassium-Sparing Diuretics
Amiloride Hydrochloride
Spironolactone
Triamterene

LIPID-LOWERING DRUGS

Statins
Atorvastatin
Cerivastatin
Fluvastatin
Lovastatin
Pravastatin
Simvastatin

Others
Cholestyramine
Colestipol Hydrochloride
Gemfibrozil

CENTRALLY ACTING ANTIHYPERTENSIVES
Clonidine Hydrochloride
Guanabenz Acetate
Guanfacine Hydrochloride
Methyldopa
Phenoxybenzamine Hydrochloride

PERIPHERALLY ACTING ANTIHYPERTENSIVES
Guanadrel Sulfate
Guanethidine Monosulfate
Prazosin

DIGITALIS DRUGS
Digitoxin
Digoxin

ACE INHIBITORS
Benazepril Hydrochloride
Captopril
Enalapril Maleate
Fosinopril Sodium
Lisinopril
Moexipril Hydrochloride
Perindopril Erbumine
Quinapril Hydrochloride
Ramipril
Trandolapril

CALCIUM CHANNEL BLOCKERS
Amlodipine
Diltiazem Hydrochloride
Felodipine
Isradipine
Nicardipine Hydrochloride Oral
Nifedipine
Nimodipine
Verapamil

NITRATES (ANTI-ANGINALS)
Amyl Nitrite
Isosorbide Dinitrate
Isosorbide Mononitrate
Nitroglycerin

BETA-BLOCKERS
Acebutolol Hydrochloride
Atenolol
Betaxolol Oral
Bisoprolol Fumarate
Carteolol Hydrochloride Oral
Labetalol Hydrochloride
Metoprolol
Nadolol
Penbutolol Sulfate
Pindolol
Propranolol Hydrochloride
Sotalol Hydrochloride
Timolol Maleate Oral

the circulatory system. A rapid-acting nitrate such as nitroglycerin may be taken sublingually (placed under the tongue) to relieve an individual episode of angina. Other longer-acting nitrates, such as isosorbide dinitrate, are available in a sustained-release form and can be taken by mouth to prevent angina attacks.

A slow-release type of nitroglycerin that is available in an adhesive transdermal patch can also provide prolonged relief from angina pain. Nitrates are sometimes given also to help alleviate the symptoms of congestive heart failure.

◆ Lipid-Lowering Drugs
A high level of fats, or lipids, in the blood is a primary risk factor for atherosclerosis. Your physician may prescribe a lipid-lowering drug (sometimes called a cholesterol-lowering drug) to bring your lipid levels within the normal range.

Some lipid-lowering drugs, such as cholestyramine and colestipol hydrochloride, combine with cholesterol-carrying substances called bile salts in the intestine and prevent their reabsorption into the bloodstream. This action causes the liver to compensate by converting more cholesterol into

bile salts, thereby lowering the level of cholesterol in the blood.

Other lipid-lowering drugs, such as the statins, lower lipid levels by interfering with the conversion of fatty acids to lipids in the liver.

The choice of drug depends to a certain extent on what specific lipid abnormalities are present and how severe they are.

◆ Digitalis Drugs
Digitalis drugs (also called cardiac glycosides) cause the heart to beat more slowly by reducing the flow of electrical impulses in the heart. They also pro-

mote chemical changes that increase the force with which the heart beats. By strengthening the heartbeat, digitalis drugs increase blood flow to the kidneys, enabling them to remove excess fluid from the tissues of people who have congestive heart failure. The drugs are also prescribed to decrease the ventricular rate in certain cases of arrhythmia.

◆ Anti-Clotting Drugs

Two general classes of drugs are used to prevent a potentially dangerous blood clot or embolus (a portion of a blood clot that breaks off and is carried away in the bloodstream): antiplatelet agents and anticoagulants.

Antiplatelet agents, such as aspirin (usually taken in low doses), reduce the tendency of small blood cells termed platelets to clump together and form clots in areas where normal blood flow is disrupted, such as around fatty deposits in diseased coronary arteries.

Anticoagulants, such as heparin or warfarin, block the activity of certain clotting factors and can either impede the formation of a clot or prevent an already formed clot from breaking away and stopping the circulation in a critical organ.

A third class of anti-clotting drugs, termed fibrinolytic agents, are typically administered in a hospital by intravenous injection to dissolve clots that have already formed, such as a blood clot blocking a coronary artery during the onset of a heart attack.

𝒯he 𝓑ones, 𝒥oints, and 𝓜uscles

Your body contains 206 bones, which make up about one tenth of your body weight. The bones provide a framework that encases and protects your body's vital internal organs. For example, ribs surround and protect your lungs, heart, liver, and kidneys, while your skull encases the delicate tissue of the brain. The spinal column—33 bony blocks, or vertebrae—shields the spinal cord, the main pathway for nervous impulses to and from the brain. Bones in the pelvic girdle protect the bladder as well as the reproductive organs in women.

Although we usually think of bones as solid and inert, they are actually living, changing tissues that are constantly being remodeled. Bone also serves as a repository for vital minerals such as calcium and phosphate, while the marrow, a spongy core of tissue located in the center of certain bones, manufactures new blood cells.

The bones in your body are connected to each other at junctions termed joints. Some joints, such as your elbow, are basically hinges that permit movement in only a single plane. By contrast, ball and socket joints, such as your hip and shoulder, allow a much wider range of motion.

More than 600 muscles cover the skeleton and give the human body its distinctive shape. There are three types: smooth muscle, which is found in such internal organs as the stomach, intestines, and bladder, and within the walls of blood vessels; cardiac muscle, which occurs only in the heart; and skeletal (or striated) muscle. Skeletal muscles control voluntary movement and are connected to your bones by strong fibrous bands of tissue called tendons. The elastic fibers in skeletal muscles can shorten and lengthen and thus produce movement at your joints. Only the skeletal muscles are under voluntary control—that is, they are the only muscles in the body that can be consciously flexed and relaxed.

▼ MUSCULOSKELETAL DRUGS

Musculoskeletal disorders—those affecting the skeleton and its system of muscles and joints—are common and have a tremendous impact on the normal quality of life. Bone disorders such as osteoporosis, osteomalacia (called rickets when it occurs in children), and Paget's disease are often marked by brittle or deformed bones that are prone to fracture. Joint disorders such as osteoarthritis, rheumatoid arthritis, and gout can lead to painful, swollen, or inflamed joints. Muscle disorders such as sprains, pulled muscles, and muscle spasms can bring on sudden intense pain or stiffness, whereas myasthenia gravis, an autoimmune disorder that interferes with the transmission of nerve impulses to voluntary muscles, can cause severe muscle weakness.

To help maintain musculoskeletal health, physicians stress the importance of eating foods rich in calcium and vitamin D, following a program that includes weight-bearing exercises such as walking, and avoiding smoking. In addition to these lifestyle measures, medications are often required for those with conditions that impair daily functioning.

◆ Drugs for Bone Disorders

Estrogen Supplements. Estrogen replacement therapy is the most effective approach for preventing or treating the increased bone loss that occurs during and after menopause. Normal bone metabolism is regulated by various hormones, including estrogen. The decline in estrogen levels during menopause accelerates bone demineralization, causing the bones to become less dense and more fragile. Replacement therapy—with conjugated estrogens (estrogen combined with progestin), estradiol, or estropipate—can prevent further bone loss and help to avoid the potentially serious complications of osteoporosis.

Bone Resorption Inhibitors. Drugs that inhibit the resorption of bone can be very effective in the treatment of osteoporosis. Alendronate, a newer drug that binds to a compound in bone and specifically inhibits the activity of osteoclasts, the cells that resorb bone, can produce significant increases in bone mass and a reduced incidence of vertebral fractures, one of

MAJOR BONES AND MUSCLES IN THE HUMAN BODY

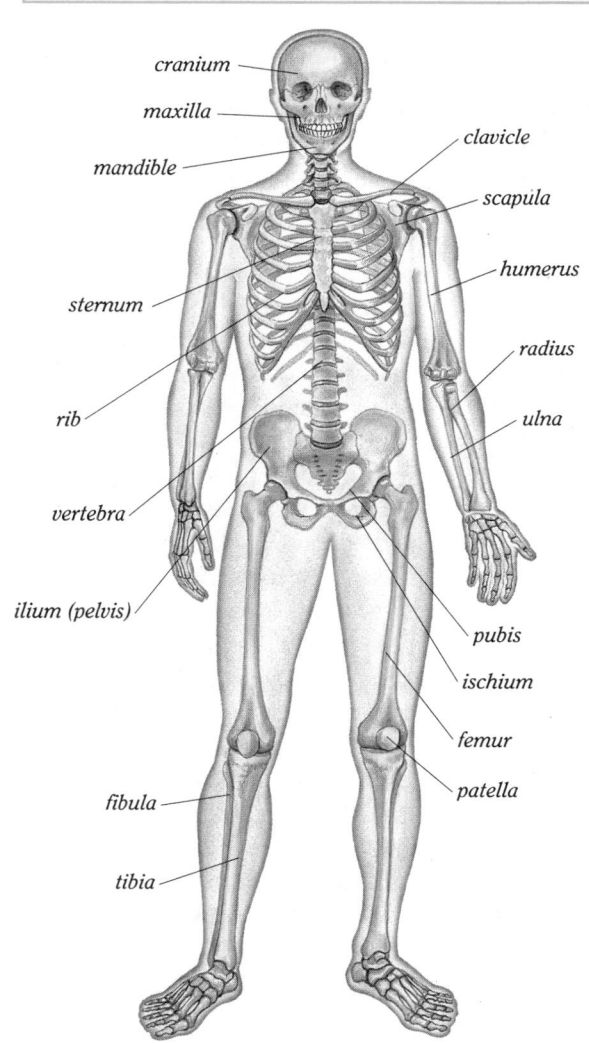

cranium
maxilla
mandible
clavicle
scapula
humerus
sternum
radius
ulna
rib
vertebra
ilium (pelvis)
pubis
ischium
femur
patella
fibula
tibia

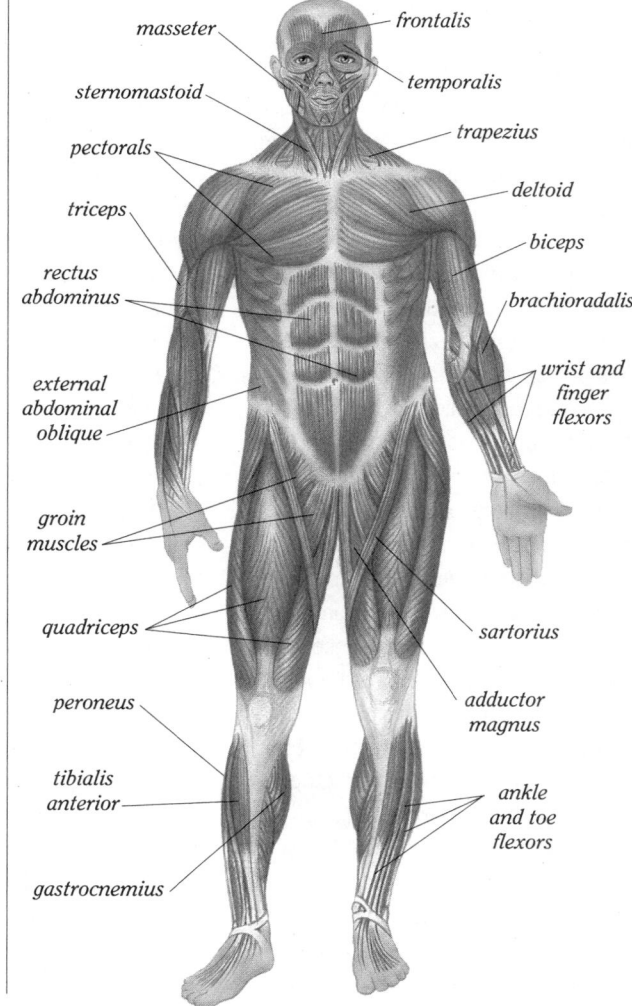

masseter
frontalis
sternomastoid
temporalis
pectorals
trapezius
triceps
deltoid
rectus abdominus
biceps
brachioradalis
external abdominal oblique
wrist and finger flexors
groin muscles
quadriceps
sartorius
peroneus
adductor magnus
tibialis anterior
ankle and toe flexors
gastrocnemius

the more serious complications of osteoporosis. This condition is also treated with hormones such as etidronate or a synthetic form of calcitonin, a hormone produced by the thyroid gland that helps control the level of calcium in the blood by inhibiting bone resorption. Bone resorption inhibitors are also used to slow the accelerated turnover of bone that occurs in Paget's disease.

Vitamin and Mineral Supplements. Calcium and Vitamin D may be combined with calcitonin or other drugs to prevent the progressive loss of bone mass in osteoporosis. Treatment of osteomalacia, which results from a deficiency of vitamin D caused by an intestinal problem, a kidney defect, or a lack of vitamin D in the diet, focuses on correcting the underlying problem plus the use of calcium and vitamin D supplements if necessary.

◆ Drugs for Joint Disorders

NSAIDs. Nonsteroidal anti-inflammatory drugs (NSAIDs) are often the first line of treatment for rheumatoid arthritis. These medications do not alter the progress of disease, but they do reduce inflammation and thus alleviate joint pain and swelling. There are numerous drugs in this group, including aspirin, ibuprofen, indomethacin, naproxen, oxaprozin, piroxicam, and sulindac. Because the response to a particular NSAID varies from one individual to another, a physician must sometimes prescribe several different NSAIDs in turn before finding the one that works best for a person.

Prostaglandins, hormone-like substances that are released at the site of an injury, are thought to play a critical role in causing both pain and inflammation in affected joints. All NSAIDs

COMMON NSAIDS AND CORTICOSTEROIDS

NONSTEROIDAL ANTI-INFLAMMATORY DRUGS (NSAIDs)

Aspirin	Indomethacin	Naproxen
Celecoxib	Ketoprofen	Oxaprozin
Diclofenac Systemic	Ketorolac Tromethamine Systemic	Piroxicam
Diflunisal		Rofecoxib
Etodolac	Meclofenamate Sodium	Salsalate
Fenoprofen Calcium		Sulindac
Flurbiprofen Oral	Mefenamic Acid	Tolmetin Sodium
Ibuprofen	Nabumetone	

SYSTEMIC CORTICOSTEROIDS

Betamethasone Systemic	Methylprednisolone
Cortisone Oral	Prednisolone Systemic
Dexamethasone Systemic	Prednisone
Hydrocortisone Systemic	Triamcinolone Systemic

achieve their effect by blocking the production of prostaglandins, thereby reducing pain and inflammation. Most NSAIDs start to relieve symptoms within an hour after they are taken. Relief is temporary, and most of these agents must be taken several times a day to achieve their optimal effect. Some of the newer NSAIDs, however, are effective when taken only once or twice daily. Treatment with an NSAID does not repair damage to the joint, and symptoms are likely to reappear if the drug is stopped.

NSAIDs are also used to treat mild to moderate pain and inflammation caused by tendinitis, osteoarthritis, bursitis, gout, soft tissue injuries, migraine and vascular headaches, menstrual cramps, and other conditions.

The pain reliever acetaminophen (not an NSAID) is sometimes chosen instead of aspirin or other NSAIDs to treat mild arthritis, muscle aches, headaches, and similar conditions.

Cyclooxygenase-2 (COX-2) Inhibitors. A new variety of NSAID, COX-2s are prescribed for arthritis as well as menstrual pain and other types of general pain. They are less likely to produce gastrointestinal side effects, such as bleeding or stomach ulcers, common to aspirin and other NSAIDs.

Corticosteroids. Corticosteroids (often simply termed steroids) are used in the treatment of rheumatoid arthritis and many other disorders. They are derived from or are synthetic variants of natural hormones produced by the adrenal cortex. Corticosteroids suppress inflammation in two ways: they dampen the activity of the white blood cells that produce inflammation, and they block the synthesis of prostaglandins, which can trigger the inflammatory response. To be effective against arthritis, steroids may be administered either systemically (by mouth) or locally, by injection directly into an inflamed joint. When given systemically, steroids can dramatically relieve the pain, swelling, and inflammation associated with rheumatoid arthritis. The beneficial effects of steroids, however, tend to be temporary, and long-term therapy can lead to a variety of side effects, some of them serious.

Local injections of corticosteroids typically do not produce any of the serious adverse effects seen with oral therapy, because the drugs tend to be concentrated in the affected area. Often a single injection into an inflamed joint, such as the knee, shoulder, or finger joint, can dramatically relieve both pain and swelling and enhance a patient's mobility.

Antirheumatics. Gold-based drugs such as auranofin and gold sodium thiomalate are often highly effective against rheumatoid arthritis. Precisely how gold works is not known, but it appears to suppress the disease process at a very fundamental level. Typically, gold salts must be given for 3 to 4 months before a beneficial effect is seen. Once this occurs, doctors usually start their patients on maintenance therapy with an injection every 3 or 4 weeks for an indefinite period to preserve the improvement.

Penicillamine, which like gold is a slow-acting drug, may also be used to treat arthritis that is progressing rapidly. When gold has become ineffective or is no longer tolerated, penicillamine can be used as an alternative.

Immunosuppressant drugs (those that suppress the immune system), such as methotrexate and azathioprine, which are normally used in cancer chemotherapy, can be highly effective for treating rheumatoid arthritis. Methotrexate appears to act primarily as an anti-inflammatory agent. Because a major flare-up of arthritis typically occurs when methotrexate is discontinued, this drug has to be taken indefinitely.

Antigout Drugs. Gout is caused by excessive levels of uric acid in the blood. If you experience an acute attack of gout, your doctor may pre-

scribe colchicine or an NSAID (see page 26) to relieve the associated pain and inflammation. If you are suffering frequent, recurrent attacks of gout, your physician will probably start you on preventive therapy with a uricosuric drug or allopurinol.

Colchicine is a highly specific drug for gout. In fact, doctors often administer this medication to confirm their diagnosis: if colchicine dramatically relieves an acute attack of joint pain, the disorder is almost certainly gouty arthritis. Precisely how colchicine works to ease the symptoms of gout is still unknown.

Uricosuric drugs such as probenecid and sulfinpyrazone promote the excretion of uric acid in the urine by blocking the reabsorption of uric acid from the kidney tubules. By lowering the level of uric acid in the blood, these drugs can prevent gout from recurring. If you are taking a uricosuric drug, you should regularly drink plenty of fluids so that uric acid crystals will not form in your kidneys.

Allopurinol reduces the level of uric acid in the blood by interfering with an enzyme involved in the production of uric acid. This drug is sometimes preferred for the treatment of persons with concomitant kidney problems who cannot take one of the uricosuric agents. Some people, however, will have to take both allopurinol and a uricosuric drug in order to normalize their blood uric acid level.

◆ *Drugs for Muscle Disorders*

Muscle Relaxants. When analgesics and NSAIDs fail to relieve muscular discomfort or muscle spasm resulting from a sprain, strain, or other form of physical injury, a muscle relaxant may be prescribed for a brief period to

alleviate the symptoms. There are two main types of muscle relaxants: centrally acting drugs and those such as dantrolene that act directly on the muscle itself.

Centrally acting muscle relaxants, such as diazepam, chlorzoxazone, and methocarbamol, retard the passage of the nerve signals from the central nervous system to the muscles, thus reducing excessive stimulation and allowing the muscles to relax.

Dantrolene produces muscle relaxation by affecting the contractile response of the muscles themselves. It reduces the sensitivity of muscles to nerve signals, probably by interfering with the release of calcium, which is essential for muscle contraction, from muscle cells. Dantrolene is used to treat the chronic spasticity that commonly occurs in such neurological disorders as multiple sclerosis, stroke, and cerebral palsy.

Muscle Stimulants. In myasthenia gravis, abnormal immune system activity destroys many receptors on muscle cells, thereby disrupting the transmission of signals between nerve endings and muscle cells and causing muscle weakness. The disease is usually treated with muscle stimulants such as neostigmine and pyridostigmine that raise levels of acetylcholine, a neurotransmitter that binds to receptors on muscle cells and causes them to contract. Because the concentration of acetylcholine is increased, the remaining receptors can function more efficiently, and muscle function can be restored to near-normal levels. These agents are sometimes combined with drugs that depress immune function, such as azathioprine and corticosteroids (see page 26).

The Digestive System

All the food you ingest must first be broken down into its most basic constituents, or molecules, before it can be absorbed and converted into the energy your body needs to function. The process of digestion is carried out in the gastrointestinal (GI) tract, which is essentially a 25-foot-long food-processing tube consisting of the mouth, esophagus, stomach, and small and large intestines. Other organs, such as the salivary glands, liver, pancreas, and gallbladder, are connected to the digestive tract and supply critical enzymes and other substances that are required for healthy digestion.

Digestion begins in the mouth as you chew your food and grind it into smaller, more easily digestible pieces. As food mingles with the saliva secreted by your salivary glands, the enzyme ptyalin starts to break down starches into the simple sugars your body uses for fuel. After you swallow a mouthful of food, it passes through your pharynx (or throat) into the esophagus, a thick-walled muscular tube that is about 10 inches long. A series of wavelike muscular contractions termed peristalsis then propel the food down the esophagus. As the food approaches the esophageal sphincter, a muscle that encircles the lower portion of the esophagus, the sphincter opens and allows the food to pass through to your stomach. It then contracts to prevent any food from flowing back, or regurgitating, into your esophagus and damaging its sensitive lining.

After the food enters your stomach, powerful stomach muscles contract to produce a churning action that pulverizes the food and mixes it with gastric juices containing digestive enzymes.

Hydrochloric acid, released by cells in the stomach lining, kills most of the bacteria present in food and also facilitates the action of pepsin, an enzyme that breaks down proteins. The partially processed food, termed chyme, then exits the stomach through the valvelike pyloric sphincter and moves into your small intestine, a coiled tube 12 to 22 feet in length. There, the digestive process is completed and most of the nutrients contained in your food are absorbed.

The small intestine is divided into three sections—the duodenum, the jejunum, and the ileum. In the duodenum, food is broken down into smaller particles and digested further by various pancreatic enzymes. Bile from the liver and gallbladder also empties into the duodenum, where it enhances the solubility of fat molecules so that they can be absorbed into the bloodstream. As the food moves through the jejunum, all of its components are broken down further into less complex units—for example, simple sugars, amino acids, and glycerol and fatty acids. These molecules, as well as vitamins, minerals such as sodium and calcium, and water, are then absorbed into the bloodstream through the villi,

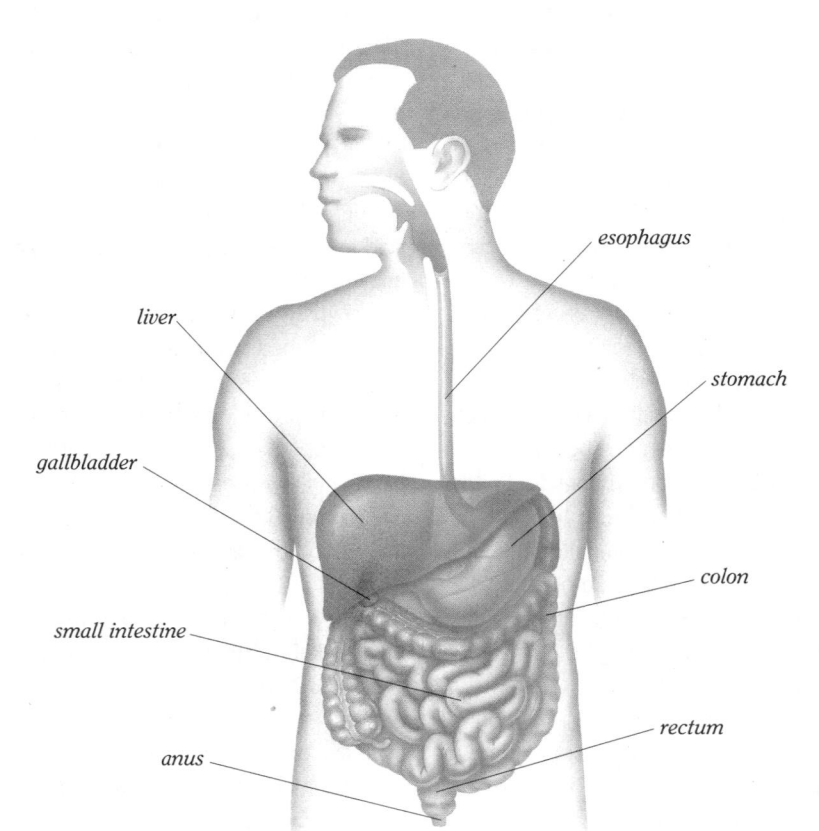

ORGANS OF THE DIGESTIVE SYSTEM

esophagus

liver

stomach

gallbladder

colon

small intestine

rectum

anus

which are tiny fingerlike projections on the surface of the small intestine.

By the time the digested food, in the form of liquid chyme, passes from the ileum into your large intestine, or colon, the nutrients required for bodily functions have already been extracted. Water and salt are then absorbed through the lining of the colon into the circulation, transforming the liquid mass into more solid feces. As the waste material travels through the colon, it is broken down further by bacteria that live in the intestine. Peristaltic waves then move the fecal material into the rectum, and it is eventually excreted through the anus.

In addition to its role in digesting food, the GI tract plays a pivotal part in controlling drug absorption. Any drug taken orally—as a tablet or capsule or in solution—must be absorbed from the digestive tract into the bloodstream before it can exert its therapeutic effect. Certain weakly acidic, lipid-soluble drugs may be absorbed in the stomach, but most drug absorption occurs in the small intestine. Some drugs should be taken on an empty stomach because food can slow the rate of gastric emptying and delay drug absorption from the small intestine.

Three other organs—the liver, the gallbladder, and the pancreas—also play critical roles in digestion and other bodily processes. The liver produces cholesterol and bile, clotting factors and other complex proteins, and vitamin A, while it stores iron, fat-soluble vitamins, and glycogen. Your liver also detoxifies alcohol and other potentially harmful chemicals, including drugs. In addition, it metabolizes medications that cannot be excreted directly in the urine and they are then excreted in the stool.

The gallbladder, a small sac that sits beneath the liver, concentrates and stores bile and then discharges it by way of the cystic and common bile ducts into the duodenum to aid in the digestion of fats.

The pancreas, which extends from the duodenum to the spleen, produces pancreatic juice and secretes it into the duodenum via the pancreatic duct. Pancreatic juice is rich in enzymes that break down proteins, fats, and carbohydrates. The pancreas also manufactures insulin and glucagon, both of which help to regulate the metabolism of sugar and protein in the liver and other tissues.

▼ DRUG THERAPY FOR COMMON DIGESTIVE DISORDERS

Because the gastrointestinal tract has a variety of components and is structurally complex, it is not surprising that many different types of disorders can impede its normal function. The most common include ulcers (ulcerations of the mucous membrane of the stomach or duodenum), heartburn and acid indigestion, nausea and vomiting, diarrhea, and constipation. Other gastrointestinal complaints are diveriticulosis, or the appearance of small pouches in the intestinal wall; hemorrhoids, which are swollen veins in the lower rectum; and inflammatory bowel disease, characterized by persistent diarrhea, rectal bleeding, cramps, fever, and weight loss. Viral hepatitis, an inflammation of the liver caused by viral infection, and gallstones, or small hard pellets that can block the ducts of the gallbladder, are among the other disorders that can affect the digestive system. Medical problems affecting the gas-

trointestinal tract that can often be effectively managed with drug therapy include peptic ulcers, heartburn, inflammatory bowel disease, diarrhea, and constipation.

◆ Drugs for Peptic Ulcer
A number of different medications are currently used in ulcer therapy.
Antibiotics/Acid Inhibitors. Several regimens are now being prescribed in an effort to eradicate the *Helicobacter pylori* infection that underlies most cases of peptic ulcer. In these regimens, either one or two antibiotics are given in combination with a drug that coats the stomach lesions (bismuth subsalicylate) or one that inhibits the secretion of stomach acid (omeprazole, lansoprazole, or rabeprazole). The regimens have proved to be highly effective, eliminating the organism in more than 90 percent of patients and preventing the recurrence of peptic ulcers.
Antacids. Peptic ulcers result from damage to the mucous lining of the stomach or duodenum that leads to erosion when stomach acid comes into contact with the exposed underlying tissue. Antacids react with and neutralize the stomach acid, thus helping to relieve the pain and inflammation associated with ulcers and promote healing of the mucous lining.
Histamine (H2) Blockers. Histamine, a compound produced by immune system cells, has numerous effects, including stimulating certain cells in the stomach wall to secrete acid when it binds to a specialized receptor called an H2 receptor. Drugs termed H2 blockers, such as cimetidine, famotidine, nizatidine, and ranitidine, bind to the H2 receptors and prevent histamine from triggering acid secretion, thus promoting ulcer healing.

◆ Antireflux Agents

Heartburn, or reflux esophagitis, may be treated with antacids, H2 blockers, or an acid inhibitor. Sucralfate, a drug that coats the lining of the esophagus and helps protect it from attack by gastric acid, may also be prescribed.

◆ Gastrointestinal Anti-Inflammatories

Inflammatory bowel disorders such as Crohn's disease and ulcerative colitis are often treated with systemic corticosteroids (see page 26), which help suppress inflammation by inhibiting the movement of white blood cells into the intestinal wall. Sulfasalazine, which inhibits the formation of prostaglandins around the damaged tissue in the intestinal wall, has also proved effective.

◆ Antidiarrheal Drugs

Many episodes of diarrhea resolve rapidly and do not require any drug therapy. If simple remedies are not effective in relieving diarrhea and your physician has determined that the diarrhea is not caused by an infection or toxin, he or she may prescribe an antidiarrheal drug such as a narcotic. Narcotics (for example, loperamide, diphenoxylate hydrochloride, and atropine sulfate) decrease the contraction of intestinal muscles by reducing the transmission of nerve signals to these muscles. Because bowel contraction is slowed, more water can be absorbed from food residue, and fecal matter passes more slowly through the intestine, relieving the diarrhea. The popular OTC drug bismuth subsalicylate can also be effective, though another popular OTC product, kaolin with pectin, has no proven benefit against diarrhea. If severe pain is present, an antispasmodic agent such as belladonna may also be prescribed.

◆ Laxatives

Constipation can often be managed effectively by ingesting more fluid and fiber—fruits, vegetables, and whole grain breads and cereals—and by increasing your level of exercise. If such remedies are unsuccessful, your physician may prescribe a laxative to relieve the constipation. There are various classes of laxatives. Stimulant laxatives cause increased contraction of the intestinal muscles, speeding the movement of fecal matter through the large intestine. Because there is less time for water to be absorbed, bowel movements become more fluid and occur more frequently. Bulk-forming laxatives absorb large quantities of water in the intestine, increasing the volume of fecal matter and making bowel movements easier to pass. Laxative salts, or osmotics, draw water into the intestine, making bowel movements more fluid, whereas lubricant laxatives make the intestinal wall and fecal matter more slippery. Finally, stool softeners combine with fecal matter in the digestive tract to soften its consistency.

The Kidneys and Urinary Tract

The kidneys and urinary tract form an intricate system designed to remove excess fluid and waste material from the blood and thereby control your body's delicate fluid and chemical balance. The main components of this system are the kidneys, ureters, urinary bladder, and urethra. The kidneys are a pair of bean-shaped organs located at the back of the abdominal cavity on either side of the spine at the lower end of the rib cage. Each adult kidney measures approximately 4 inches long by 2 inches wide and weighs 5 to 6 ounces. Your blood is filtered as it passes through the kidneys, and the urine formed in them descends to the bladder through long, slender muscular tubes termed ureters. After urine reaches your bladder, it is stored there until the bladder is approximately half full. At this point, nerves in the bladder will signal a feeling of fullness, muscles at the bladder outlet will relax, and the urine will be expelled through the urethra.

All critical filtering operations take place in the kidneys: these complex structures clear out toxic wastes and excess fluid and maintain a critical balance of salt, potassium, and acid. Almost one fourth of the blood pumped with each heartbeat passes through your kidneys. It enters each kidney via the renal artery, which branches directly from the aorta, the body's main artery. Once inside the kidney, blood passes through a series of complex filtering units termed nephrons; each kidney contains more than 1 million nephrons. A nephron is composed of a glomerulus, a rounded tuft of tiny capillary blood vessels, and a long thin renal tubule. As blood passes through the glomerulus, it is filtered under pressure. Blood cells, proteins, other large particles, and some of the water remain in the blood that is flowing through the capillaries. The rest of the fluid, which contains a large volume of water, sodium, potassium, glucose, urea, and uric acid, is filtered out and passes into the renal tubule. As this filtrate travels down the coiled renal tubules, about 99 percent of the water, salts, and vital nutrients that were initially filtered in the glomerulus will be reabsorbed. These substances are then returned to the bloodstream, while waste products such as urea and uric acid and excess salts, water, and calcium remain in the

tubule and are eventually eliminated as urine. The average adult excretes about 1.5 quarts of urine each day.

Your kidneys (together with the liver) also play a primary role in eliminating drugs from the body. In the kidneys, drugs are filtered by the glomerulus and may also be secreted in a portion of the renal tubule. As the drug passes through the nephron, its chances of being reabsorbed depend on two factors: its solubility in lipid (fat) and its charge (whether or not it is ionized). Drugs that are lipid-soluble and nonionized are almost completely reabsorbed, while water-soluble, ionized drugs are more likely to be eliminated in the urine. Many lipid-soluble drugs are first converted in the liver to more water-soluble metabolites, which

are then excreted in the urine. The rate at which a drug is eliminated depends on the adequacy of kidney function. Thus, physicians must adjust drug dosages in persons with impaired kidney function, or chronic renal failure, to prevent drugs from reaching toxic levels in the blood.

In addition to cleansing your body of toxic wastes, your kidneys also synthesize important hormones such as erythropoietin, which stimulates red blood cell production, as well as substances that help regulate blood pressure and bone formation.

▼ TREATMENT OF KIDNEY AND URINARY TRACT DISORDERS

Some of the disorders affecting the kidney and urinary tract respond to drug therapy, others require a surgical approach, and the most serious—kidney failure—is often managed successfully with dialysis or transplantation.

◆ *Vesicoureteral Reflux*
Mild cases of vesicoureteral reflux, the most common urinary tract problem in children, often resolve as a child matures. The condition is marked by a backup of urine from the bladder. Prophylactic antibiotics may be given to ward off infection in the meantime and prevent any permanent renal damage. More severe cases of reflux may have to be corrected surgically.

◆ *Polycystic Kidney Disease*
Almost half of patients with this hereditary disorder, in which clusters of fluid-filled cysts form in the kidney, develop chronic kidney failure, usually after age 50. No cure is currently available, but appropriate medication

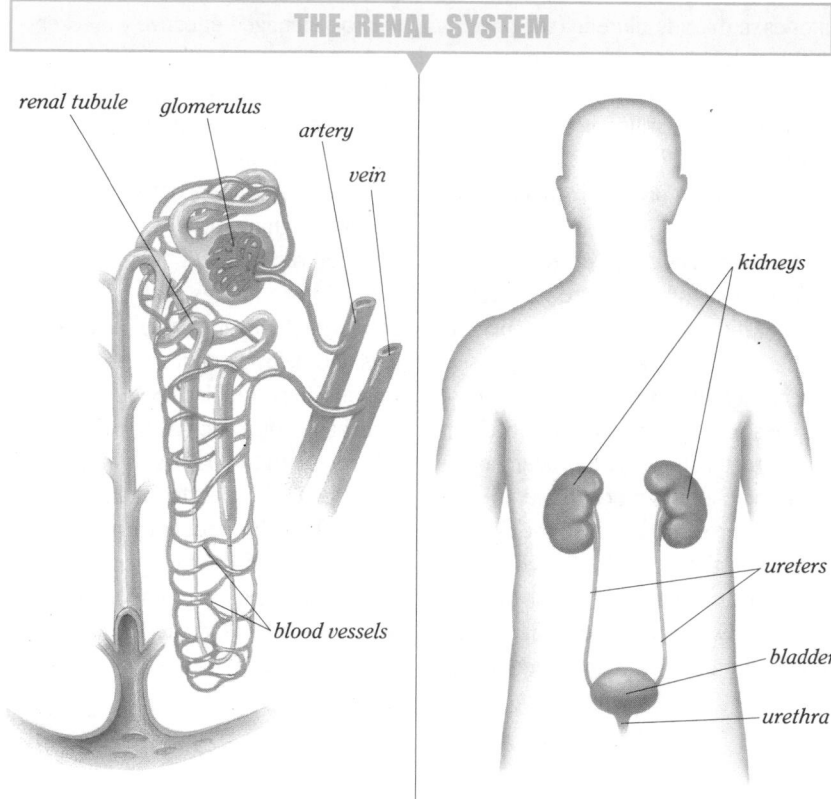

THE RENAL SYSTEM

renal tubule
glomerulus
artery
vein
blood vessels

kidneys
ureters
bladder
urethra

for high blood pressure and prompt antibiotic therapy for bladder or kidney infections can help prolong life.

Glomerulonephritis

Glomerulonephritis is marked by inflammation of the glomerulus, the filtering apparatus of the kidney. If an active infection is causing acute (sudden onset) glomerulonephritis, your physician will prescribe an appropriate antibiotic. Diuretics (see page 22) may also be given for fluid retention and antihypertensive therapy for high blood pressure. If you are suffering from chronic glomerulonephritis, your physician may recommend a diet low in protein and phosphate. People with certain types of glomerular lesions may respond to systemic corticosteroid therapy (see page 26). If you are diabetic, your physician may also prescribe captopril, an ACE inhibitor (see page 22), because there is evidence that captopril can slow or prevent the progression of kidney disease that is caused by diabetes.

Nephrotic Syndrome

Nephrotic syndrome is marked by the excretion of excessive amounts of protein in the urine, a low level of protein in the blood, and fluid retention. Systemic corticosteroids (see page 26) are usually prescribed to reduce the excessive protein excretion in the urine and increase the chances of a remission. If the condition does not respond to corticosteroids, diuretics will likely be given to control high blood pressure and the swelling that is caused by fluid retention.

Kidney Stones

Kidney stones, a relatively common disorder, develop when concentrated chemicals in the urine precipitate to form stones in the kidney tubules, ureter, or bladder. Because about 90 percent of stones will eventually pass naturally, treatment usually entails drinking large quantities of liquid to promote their excretion. Antibiotics may be prescribed if an infection is present, and analgesics may be given to control the severe pain that typically occurs. Larger stones can be removed by laser surgery, percutaneous surgery (surgery performed through a small incision in the skin), or lithotripsy (the use of sound waves to break the stone into small fragments). Therapies to prevent new stone formation depend on the composition of the stone. For calcium stones, a thiazide diuretic (see page 22) may be given to decrease the amount of calcium excreted in the urine, while the antigout drug allopurinol (see page 27) may be prescribed to help prevent uric acid stones.

Urinary Tract Infections

Urinary tract infections are very common and most often affect the bladder (cystitis) or urethra (urethritis). Most are caused by *Escherichia coli*, a species of bacteria commonly present in the rectal area. The frequency of such infections is much higher in women, probably because the short female urethra—about 1.5 inches compared with about 8 inches for the male—allows bacteria from the vagina and rectum to invade the bladder more readily. Chlamydia, a sexually transmitted organism, is also responsible for some cases of cystitis. The disorder is usually treated with a short course (7 to 10 days) of an appropriate antibiotic. Physicians sometimes recommend that women with recurrent bladder infections take a low dose of an antibiotic on a continuing basis for prevention. Sometimes, infection can travel up the ureters to involve the kidneys (pyelonephritis), a potentially life-threatening condition in an elderly or weakened person. This infection requires prompt treatment and, in some cases, hospitalization. A combination of antibiotics are usually given for several weeks to prevent a recurrence of infection.

Urinary Incontinence

Some forms of urinary incontinence may be managed effectively by exercises that can strengthen the pelvic floor muscles or by surgery to tighten stretched ligaments. So-called stress incontinence, the involuntary loss of urine during physical activity, sneezing, or coughing, may respond to estrogen replacement therapy (see page 25) or to drugs such as ephedrine that stimulative nerve endings and help to constrict the sphincter muscle at the bladder outlet. Antispasmodics such as flavoxate that interfere with the passage of nerve impulses to the bladder muscle may help reduce the frequency of urination in persons with another type of incontinence—so-called urge incontinence, which is marked by a sudden and irresistible desire to urinate.

The Lungs and Respiratory System

The oxygen you breathe is an absolute requirement for sustaining life. Your body can endure being deprived of food and water for prolonged periods and still survive, but once the normal flow of oxygen is disrupted, your cells will begin to die within minutes.

Your respiratory system maintains this lifeline to your body, continuously replenishing your blood with oxygen and expelling the carbon dioxide formed as a waste product of body processes. The principal organs of respiration are your lungs, cone-shaped structures located in your chest cavity. Your right lung is divided into three lobes, your left lung has only two, leaving room for the heart. In addition to the lungs, the primary components of your respiratory system are the air passages, which convey air from your mouth and nose to your lungs, and the diaphragm and other chest muscles that help to control the breathing process.

When you inhale, the air you take in is filtered, heated, and moistened as it travels through the nasal passages to your throat and larynx and then down your trachea, which is the main airway to your lungs. The trachea divides into two primary bronchi, one on either side of the lung. These bronchi branch into smaller airways that then subdivide further into increasingly finer branches until they form small tubes, or bronchioles, that end in tiny elastic air sacs called alveoli. The structure of the respiratory system resembles that of an inverted tree, with the trachea forming the trunk, the bronchi and bronchioles making up the branches, and the alveoli representing the buds at the ends of the twigs.

Your lungs contain several hundred million alveoli, which the respiratory bronchioles fill with oxygen-rich air. These tiny air sacs are encircled by capillaries that are so small your blood cells often move through them in single file. It is within these alveoli that the critical exchange of oxygen and carbon dioxide takes place. The oxygen in the air you inhale flows through the membranes of the alveoli and is taken up by the red blood cells circulating through the capillaries. Carbon dioxide moves in the opposite direction, diffusing from the blood into the alveoli and then passing up the bronchial tree until it is exhaled. Scavenger cells called macrophages line the interior of each alveolus and purify the incoming air by gobbling up and destroying airborne irritants such as bacteria, chemicals, and dust.

Normal breathing is controlled by the muscles that enclose your chest cavity. The volume of the chest cavity increases when your diaphragm contracts and pushes down on your abdomen. At the same time, muscles that lie between your ribs also contract, causing the ribs to pull together and rise, expanding your rib cage. Both of these actions create negative pressure within the chest cavity, pulling air into your lungs. When your diaphragm and rib muscles relax, the

COMPONENTS OF THE RESPIRATORY SYSTEM

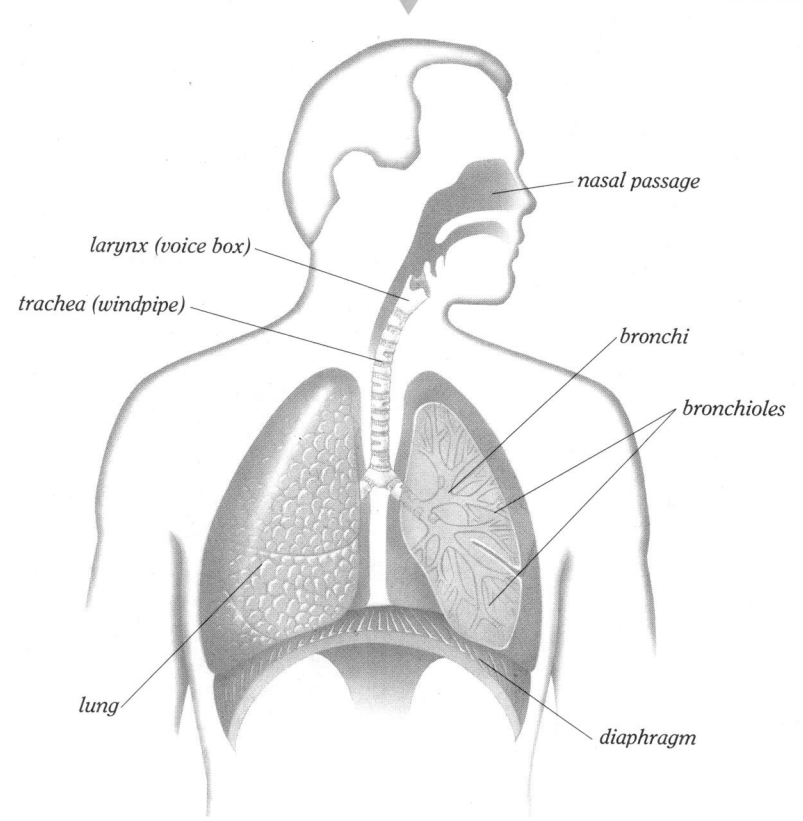

- nasal passage
- larynx (voice box)
- trachea (windpipe)
- bronchi
- bronchioles
- lung
- diaphragm

volume of your chest cavity decreases, compressing your lungs and pushing carbon dioxide–laden air out of your body. A lubricating fluid, secreted by the pleural membranes enclosing your lungs, allows them to move easily as they expand and contract during respiration. An adult typically breathes from 12 to 17 times a minute and inhales about one pint of air with each breath. Breathing, normally an involuntary process, is controlled by the respiratory centers in the brain stem.

Air passages are equipped with several defense mechanisms that help prevent airborne impurities from entering your lungs. The first line of defense consists of nasal hairs and mucous membranes in the nasal cavity that trap and filter out large inhaled particles. Inhaled air is also cleansed of infectious agents as it moves past your tonsils and adenoids on its way to your throat. In addition, cells lining your airways secrete mucus, a sticky fluid that traps bacteria, dust, and other airborne impurities. The mucus also moistens and lubricates the airways and helps prevent drying of the delicate lung tissue. Finally, tiny hairs, or cilia, that project from the mucous lining of the respiratory tract beat continuously to prevent airborne particles from entering your lungs. This rhythmic movement of the cilia also helps to clear your lungs of mucus by propelling it upward toward your throat, where the mucus will either be coughed up or swallowed.

Many drugs used to treat respiratory disorders are given by inhalation. The advantage of inhalants is that they deliver the drug directly into the lungs so that it can have maximum therapeutic effect on bronchial mucosa without causing excessive side effects.

Other respiratory system drugs are administered intranasally, either by nasal spray or nose drops, so that they can exert their primary effect locally, on the nasal mucosa.

▼ DRUG THERAPY FOR COMMON RESPIRATORY DISORDERS

Certain disorders of the respiratory tract may need to be treated surgically (lung cancer is one) or with supplemental oxygen (for example, chronic obstructive pulmonary disease), however, many common problems can be managed effectively with drugs. These disorders include those caused by infections (such as influenza, pneumonia, and tuberculosis) and those characterized by inflammation (such as asthma and chronic bronchitis).

◆ *Drugs for Asthma*
Asthmatic attacks are often triggered by exposure to a specific allergen, which causes inflammation, increased secretion of mucus, and constriction of the bronchiolar walls, leading to airway obstruction. Asthma is usually treated by eliminating or reducing exposure to the suspected allergen and by administering one or more of the following agents: bronchodilators, corticosteroids, and mast-cell stabilizers.

Bronchodilators. Bronchodilators are given to relieve the symptoms of airflow obstruction. There are three types of bronchodilators—sympathomimetics, anticholinergics, and

MAJOR CLASSES OF RESPIRATORY DRUGS

SYMPATHOMIMETIC BRONCHODILATORS
Albuterol
Bitolterol Mesylate
Epinephrine Hydrochloride
Isoetharine
Isoproterenol
Metaproterenol Sulfate
Pirbuterol Acetate
Salmeterol Xinafoate
Terbutaline Sulfate

BRONCHODILATORS/ XANTHINES
Aminophylline
Dyphylline
Theophylline

LEUKOTRIENE RECEPTOR ANTAGONISTS
Montelukast
Zafirlukast

DECONGESTANTS/ DRUGS FOR COUGHS
Acetylcysteine
Phenylephrine HCl Systemic
Phenylpropanolamine HCl
Phenylpropanolamine HCl/ Guaifenesin
Pseudoephedrine
Pseudoephedrine/Guaifenesin

RESPIRATORY CORTICOSTEROIDS
Beclomethasone Inhalant/Nasal
Budesonide
Dexamethasone Inhalant/Nasal
Flunisolide
Fluticasone
Triamcinolone Inhalant/Nasal

RESPIRATORY INHALANTS/ MISCELLANEOUS BRONCHODILATORS
Cromolyn Sodium Inhalant/Nasal
Ipratropium Bromide
Nedocromil Sodium Inhalant

xanthines—all of which act to relax the muscles surrounding the bronchioles and thereby open the airways. The sympathomimetic drugs are primarily used to provide rapid relief for an acute asthmatic attack, while the anticholinergic and xanthine agents are more frequently used for long-term prevention. The sympathomimetic bronchodilators, which are administered by inhalation, enhance the transmission of nerve signals that promote the relaxation of bronchiolar muscles. Anticholinergic bronchodilators, such as atropine, achieve their effect by blocking the neurotransmitters that stimulate the contraction of bronchiolar muscles. Xanthines, such as theophylline or aminophylline, directly relax the bronchiolar smooth muscle, but their exact mode of action has not been determined.

Corticosteroids. Although bronchodilators open the airways, they do not reduce inflammation in the mucous lining of the bronchioles. Corticosteroids are used as long-term therapy to prevent the underlying process that leads to airway obstruction. Inhaled corticosteroids such as triamcinolone and flunisolide widen the bronchioles by decreasing inflammation. These agents are thought to produce their effect by blocking the synthesis of certain inflammation-causing substances.

Mast-Cell Stabilizers. Mast cells in the bronchioles play a critical role in the allergic response that underlies most asthmatic attacks. Allergens attach to these cells, prompting them to release histamine. Mast-cell stabilizers such as cromolyn sodium prevent the release of histamine by bronchiolar mast cells, thus reducing inflammation of the airways. Like inhaled corticosteroids, mast-cell stabilizers are used for long-term maintenance therapy to prevent recurrences of asthma.

◆ *Drugs for Respiratory Infections*

Common colds, influenza ("flu"), and most cases of acute bronchitis are caused by viral infections and are usually associated with such symptoms as nasal congestion and cough. Decongestants and cough medications are commonly prescribed to treat these symptoms.

Decongestants. Virus-induced inflammation of the delicate mucous membrane lining the nasal passages causes the blood vessels supplying the membrane to become enlarged. As a result, additional amounts of fluid pass into the mucous membrane, causing swelling and excessive production of mucus. Decongestants such as pseudoephedrine stimulate constriction of the blood vessels in the nasal mucosa, reducing swelling and decreasing mucus production.

Cough Medications. The type of cough medication you should take will probably depend on whether your cough is dry or productive, that is, producing phlegm. A productive cough usually helps clear excess phlegm from the body and may help speed your recovery from the respiratory infection. In such cases, a mucolytic or expectorant is usually preferred to assist you in coughing up phlegm. Dry, hacking coughs, on the other hand, may sometimes increase irritation of the air passages, and your physician may recommend a suppressant to ease the cough.

Mucolytic agents, which are usually given by inhalation, act directly on the airways to alter the consistency of the phlegm, reducing its viscosity and making it easier to cough up. Expectorants help promote coughing by decreasing the adherence of pulmonary secretions in the lower respiratory tract. Agents used to suppress a dry cough may be either narcotic (for example, codeine) or non-narcotic (such as dextromethorphan or antihistamines). Cough suppressants act on the coughing center in the brain to suppress the cough reflex. Antihistamines (see page 52) have a sedating effect on the cough mechanism and are often given for mild coughs, especially in children. Mild narcotics such as codeine are prescribed for more persistent coughs.

Anti-Infectives. Numerous infectious agents can attack the pulmonary system, producing such diseases as histoplasmosis, Legionnaires' disease, and various forms of bacterial and viral pneumonia. Appropriate antibiotic therapy (see page 51) may be prescribed to treat these disorders.

Tuberculosis (TB), a chronic infection that usually affects the lungs, is typically treated with a combination of several antitubercular agents, such as isoniazid, rifampin, streptomycin, aminosalicylate sodium, cycloserine, rifabutin, or pyrazinamide. Drug therapy aims at treating active infection or preventing the onset of active disease in those who have been infected with the TB bacteria.

To prevent flu, the influenza virus vaccine is often recommended before the start of the flu season. Flu is also sometimes treated with the antiviral drugs amantadine hydrochloride or rimantadine hydrochloride. Most antibiotics, however, are not effective against colds, flu, and other viral infections (see page 51).

Hormones and the Endocrine System

Hormones (derived from a Greek word meaning "to spur on") act as chemical messengers in your body's internal communications system. These powerful compounds control and coordinate the function of virtually all of your body's cells and tissues. The endocrine system, a complex assortment of glands distributed throughout the body, produces hormones and releases them into the bloodstream. Working in conjunction with the nervous system, hormones regulate such functions as the growth and repair of tissues, metabolism, blood pressure, sexual development and reproduction, and the body's response to stress. By their actions, hormones enable your body to respond efficiently to changes in your internal and external environment.

The endocrine glands include the pituitary, thyroid, parathyroid, adrenal, thymus, and pineal glands as well as the pancreas, ovaries (in women), and testes (in men). Specialized cells in other organs, such as the kidneys, heart, lungs, and gastrointestinal tract, also secrete hormones. After they are released into your bloodstream, hormones travel to their target tissues, where they elicit specific reactions. Two basic types have been identified: steroid hormones, such as the adrenal steroids; and protein or peptide hormones, such as insulin. Because steroid hormones are small enough to pass through the membrane of the target cell, they can act directly on the cell's genetic material to obtain the desired effect. Protein hormones, by contrast, do not enter the target cells. Instead, they attach to specific cell membrane receptors that then induce the sought-after response.

Each endocrine gland releases hormones that trigger reactions in specific target tissues. For example, the thyroid gland, which is located at the front of the throat, secretes the hormones thyroxine and triiodothyronine, which stimulate metabolism and protein synthesis. The thyroid also produces calcitonin, a hormone that lowers calcium levels in the blood. By contrast, the four parathyroid glands, which lie adjacent to the thyroid, make a hormone that increases blood calcium levels. The tiny pineal gland, located in the brain, secretes melatonin, a hormone that controls such body rhythms as the sleeping and waking cycle. The thymus, a lymph gland situated in the middle of the chest cavity, secretes thymosin, a hormone that influences the development of the body's immune defenses.

The pancreas, a gland that stretches across the abdomen behind the stomach, secretes insulin and glucagon, hormones that control your body's metabolism of glucose. The adrenal glands lie atop the kidneys. The inner core, or medulla, of the adrenal gland manufactures epineph-

ENDOCRINE GLANDS

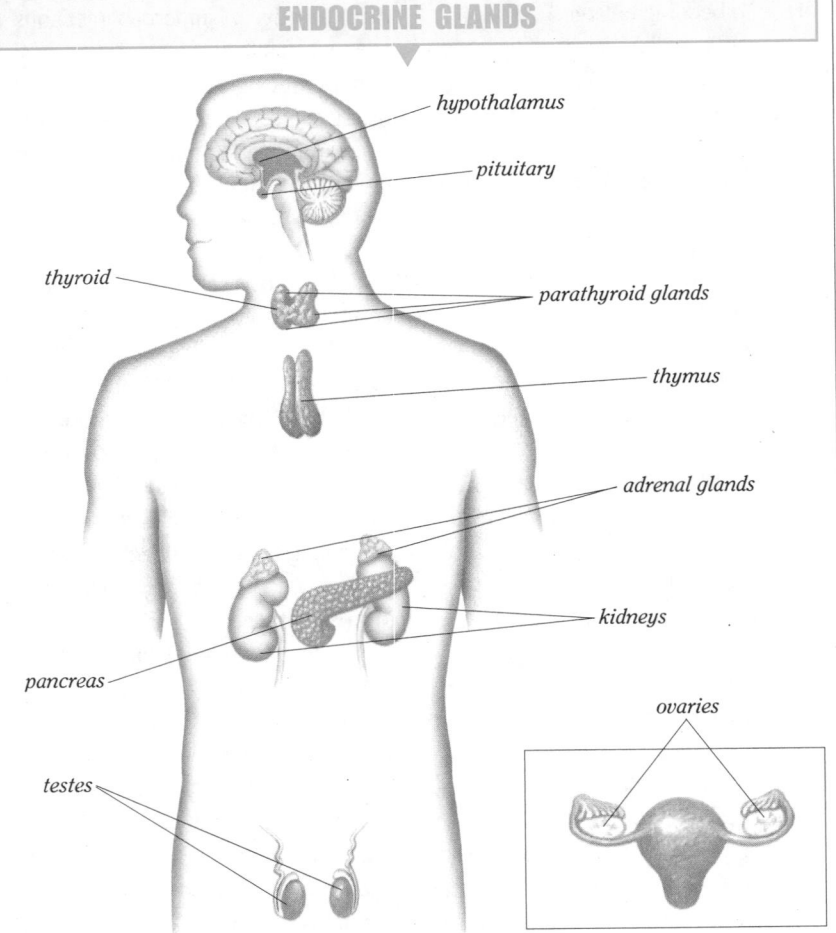

- hypothalamus
- pituitary
- thyroid
- parathyroid glands
- thymus
- adrenal glands
- kidneys
- pancreas
- ovaries
- testes

rine and norepinephrine, hormones that affect your body's response to stress. The outer layer, or cortex, produces corticosteroids, including the sex hormones; the glucocorticoids, which help to control the metabolism of fat, protein, and carbohydrates and to reduce inflammation; and aldosterone, which regulates the body's water and mineral content. The testes, located in the scrotum, produce male sex hormones such as testosterone, which controls the development of male sexual and physical characteristics. The ovaries, positioned on either side of the uterus, produce estrogen and progesterone, which help regulate female sexual development and prepare the uterus for pregnancy.

The pituitary gland, positioned at the base of the brain, secretes a large number of hormones with varying functions, including prolactin, growth hormone, adrenocorticotropic hormone (ACTH), antidiuretic hormone, oxytocin, melanocyte-stimulating hormone, and gonadotropins. Some pituitary hormones act directly on their target tissue to produce the desired effect. For example, prolactin stimulates breast tissue to produce milk after childbirth. Other pituitary hormones, such as thyroid-stimulating hormone, act indirectly by stimulating a target gland (in this case, the thyroid) to release other hormones.

The pituitary has been termed the master gland because it plays a critical role in the finely tuned operation of the endocrine system. A complex feedback mechanism directed by the hypothalamus, located at the base of the brain, coordinates hormone production by secreting so-called releasing hormones. The releasing hormones, in turn, affect the secretion of certain pituitary hormones that control the activities of other endocrine glands. If, for instance, thyroid hormone levels are too high, negative feedback signals the hypothalamus to produce less of thyrotropin-releasing hormone (TRH). The reduction in TRH causes the pituitary to lower its production of thyroid-stimulating hormone (TSH), and the thyroid responds by secreting less thyroid hormone. Conversely, if thyroid hormone levels fall too low, the feedback mechanism operates to correct the deficiency. In this way, the hypothalamus and pituitary work together to orchestrate the proper functioning of all the other major endocrine glands, thereby ensuring that hormone levels remain within the proper range.

▼ DRUG THERAPY FOR ENDOCRINE DISORDERS

Endocrine disorders are typically caused by the production of too much or too little of a specific hormone. Hyperthyroidism, for example, results from overproduction of the thyroid hormone thyroxine, whereas hypothyroidism stems from too little hormone. Because the influence of the endocrine system on bodily processes is so widespread, a disorder that affects any of the endocrine glands may disrupt numerous body functions. Diabetes mellitus, for example, characterized by an abnormal increase in blood glucose levels, is caused by either a deficiency of the pancreatic hormone insulin (Type 1) or the inability of the body to properly use insulin (Type 2). It exhibits such varied symptoms as thirst, fatigue, weight loss, infections, blurred vision, numbness in the hands and feet, and, over the long term, heart and kidney disease.

In general, endocrine disorders marked by hormone deficiency are managed by hormone replacement therapy, whereas disorders that result from overproduction of a particular hormone may be treated by surgery, radiation, or drug therapy to reduce the activity of the endocrine gland.

Various drugs contain hormones as their active ingredients. Some come from natural sources and mimic the actions of hormones in the body. Others are synthesized in a laboratory, their chemical structures often modified, or improved upon, to make the hormone more potent or to adapt it for use in a specific form (for example, as a pill to be swallowed, rather than a liquid injection). Still other drugs act to block or diminish the effects of hormones or adjust their levels. Which particular drug will be given depends on the condition being treated.

◆ *Drugs for Diabetes Mellitus*
The management of diabetes involves a combination of lifestyle measures—dietary changes, weight loss (if necessary), and a program of physical activity. For some Type 2 diabetics, such changes can reduce the body's insulin requirements sufficiently to restore normal blood glucose levels. For all Type 1 diabetics and for those people with Type 2 disease that is not adequately controlled by diet and exercise, some form of drug therapy is also necessary.

Insulin. Insulin must be administered by injection to replace the hormone that is lacking in people with Type 1 diabetes, and such treatment must be continued for life. Insulin may also be given to Type 2 diabetics if oral antidiabetic therapy fails to control their blood sugar levels. Various forms of insulin with different durations of action—short, medium, and long—are available, and sometimes they are combined to provide more precise control of daily blood glucose levels.

Sulfonylureas. Sulfonylurea drugs are the most commonly administered oral antidiabetic agents. These drugs stimulate the islet cells of the pancreas to produce increased amounts of insulin to meet the body's needs. Such agents are effective only when some insulin-secreting cells remain active, as occurs in Type 2 disease. By increasing insulin levels in the blood, the sulfonylurea drugs encourage the uptake of glucose by the body's tissues and thus help to restore normal blood glucose levels.

◆ Thyroid Drugs
Drugs for Hypothyroidism (Underactive Thyroid). This disorder requires lifelong therapy with synthetic thyroid hormone preparations. Such supplements restore thyroid hormone levels to normal and eliminate symptoms of hypothyroidism. Because symptoms of hyperthyroidism (for example, weight loss, high blood pressure, nervousness, and tremors) may develop if the dose of replacement hormone is too high, your doctor will probably order routine blood tests to ensure that you are taking the correct dose.

Drugs for Hyperthyroidism (Overactive Thyroid). This condition may be treated with surgery, radiation (in the form of radioactive iodine), or antithyroid drugs. In the thyroid gland, iodine combines with the amino acid tyrosine to form thyroid hormones. Antithyroid medications decrease the production of thyroid hormones by preventing

DRUG TREATMENT OF DIABETES MELLITUS

INSULINS
Insulin (regular)
Insulin (NPH)
Insulin (Ultralente)
Insulin (Lispro rDNA origin)
Insulin Glargine (rDNA origin)

SULFONYLUREAS
Acetohexamide
Chlorpropamide
Glimepiride

Glipizide
Glyburide
Tolazamide
Tolbutamide

OTHER DIABETES DRUGS
Acarbose
Glucagon
Metformin
Pioglitazone
Rosiglitazone

iodine from combining with tyrosine. If these medications do not provide sufficient benefit, your physician may recommend radioactive iodine therapy or surgery to help restore thyroid hormone levels to normal.

◆ Corticosteroids
Replacement therapy with oral corticosteroids, taken on a regular basis, is the typical treatment for Addison's disease, which is caused by a severe deficiency of adrenal steroids due to gradual destruction of the adrenal glands. Typically, therapy consists of a glucocorticoid drug, such as prednisone, and a mineralocorticoid drug, such as fludrocortisone, that replaces aldosterone. The glucocorticoid agent helps maintain normal blood sugar levels and promotes recovery from injury and stress. The mineralocorticoid helps control the balance of sodium and potassium and the water content of the body. When given in low doses by mouth for the treatment of Addison's disease, these drugs produce few adverse effects.

Systemic corticosteroids are also used to suppress inflammation in a variety of other disorders, including various forms of cancer, asthma, and

rheumatoid arthritis (see page 26). Taken in higher doses and for long periods of time, corticosteroids can cause debilitating side effects.

◆ Growth Hormones
A deficiency of growth hormone can impair normal growth in children. This condition can be remedied by the administration of synthetic forms of a growth hormone developed by recombinant DNA technology (somatrem or somatropin). The replacement hormone is given by regular injections, starting during early childhood and continuing until the end of adolescence.

◆ Drugs for Diabetes Insipidus
The kidneys of people who have diabetes insipidus are unable to retain water and excrete large quantities in the urine. The disorder, which can be caused by a pituitary tumor, is due to a lack of antidiuretic hormone (also termed ADH or vasopressin). Diabetes insipidus is treated by administering a synthetic form of ADH such as desmopressin. The replacement hormone can be administered orally, intranasally, or by injection.

The Reproductive System

The reproductive organs of men and women are designed to serve one of the primal functions of the human body—replicating itself.

▼ MALE REPRODUCTIVE ORGANS

Male genital organs produce, store, and release sperm, the reproductive cell of the male. Major reproductive organs include the testicles (or testes), penis, epididymis, vas deferens, seminal vesicles, and prostate. The testicles carry out two important functions: they manufacture sperm cells required for reproduction, and secrete male sex hormones such as testosterone, which foster the development of masculine physical characteristics. Located outside the abdominal cavity in a pouch called the scrotum, the testicles are maintained at a temperature slightly cooler than normal body temperature, which is essential for the satisfactory production of viable sperm.

After puberty, sperm cells are made continuously in the testicles within tiny, threadlike tubes termed seminiferous tubules; over an average lifetime, a man typically produces about 12 trillion sperm. Newly produced sperm cells pass into the epididymis, a tightly coiled tube that lies on top of the testicle, where they mature for two to four weeks. A long, thin duct called the vas deferens ferries sperm cells from the epididymis to the seminal vesicles, where they are stored until ejaculation. Semen that is ejaculated through the urethra during sexual activity is composed of sperm cells mixed with fluids secreted by the seminal glands and prostate.

▼ FEMALE REPRODUCTIVE ORGANS

The major reproductive organs in women are the uterus, ovaries, fallopian tubes, cervix, and vagina. The uterus, a hollow organ with muscular walls, is located in the center of the pelvic cavity. The ovaries are small, oval-shaped organs that lie on either side of the uterus. Each ovary is attached to the uterus by a short supportive ligament. The fallopian tubes, each about four inches long, extend from either side of the upper portion of the uterus and end in fringelike projections that lie adjacent to the ovaries. The cervix, the lower, narrow end of the uterus, has a very small central opening that dilates greatly during childbirth to allow passage of the baby. The cervix extends into the vaginal canal, which has an inner mucous membrane and an outer muscular wall. The vagina normally has an acidic environment, which acts as a natural barrier to infection. Many drugs are administered directly into the vagina to treat vaginal infections. Because such drugs typically are not absorbed substantially from the vaginal mucosa, they can be given in relatively high doses without producing any significant systemic toxicity.

THE MALE AND FEMALE REPRODUCTIVE SYSTEMS

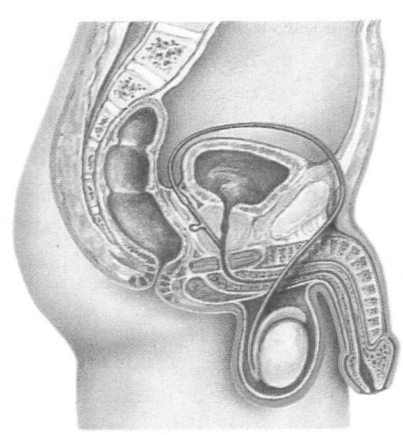

vas deferens

bladder

prostate gland

penis

urethra

epididymis

testis

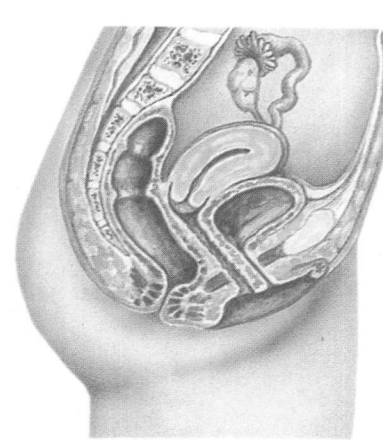

fallopian tube

ovary

uterus

bladder

cervix

vagina

rectum

During puberty, the ovaries start to synthesize the sex hormones estrogen and progesterone, which influence the development of female physical characteristics, including breast enlargement and menstrual cycles. At this time, the pituitary gland also begins to secrete two hormones—luteinizing hormone (LH) and follicle-stimulating hormone (FSH)—that stimulate the ovaries to release one, or occasionally two or three, eggs each month at the midpoint of the menstrual cycle (ovulation). The ovaries, which contain a supply of more than 500,000 immature eggs at birth, will release a total of about 400 mature eggs between puberty and menopause. Once an egg has been released, it travels down one of the fallopian tubes to the uterus. Endometrial tissue lining the uterus thickens to prepare the uterus for implantation of a fertilized egg. If fertilization fails to occur, the endometrium is shed during menstruation.

▼ FERTILIZATION

The two days after ovulation define the fertile period, that interval during which conception can take place. Conception occurs when sperm that have been ejaculated into the vagina during intercourse swim up through the uterus and fertilize the egg in the fallopian tube. Although a single ejaculation typically contains from 250 to 500 million sperm, only about 200 or so sperm cells ultimately reach the region of the egg in the fallopian tube. Once a single sperm has succeeded in penetrating and fertilizing the egg, the fertilized egg then divides continually as it passes down the fallopian tube. After several days, the fertilized egg implants itself in the endometrial lining of the uterine wall and proceeds to develop into an embryo.

▼ DRUG THERAPY FOR COMMON REPRODUCTIVE CONDITIONS AND DISORDERS

Many disorders that affect the reproductive organs are treated most effectively by surgery, including fibroids (benign tumors of the uterine wall), varicocele (a swelling in the scrotum caused by an abnormally distended vein), ovarian cysts, and various cancers, such as those affecting the breast, ovaries, uterus, cervix, testes, and prostate (though drugs are often used along with surgery).

Drugs are commonly used to prevent conception and to treat such reproductive system disorders as infertility, endometriosis, benign (noncancerous) prostate enlargement, and sexually transmitted diseases.

◆ *Oral Contraceptives*

The oral contraceptive has proved to be the most reliable method for avoiding pregnancy for most women. Three forms of oral contraceptives are currently available: a combined pill, a progestin-only pill, and a phased pill. All of these contain progestin, a synthetic form of progesterone, while the combined and phased pills also contain estrogen. The combined pills contain a fixed dose of estrogen and progestin. In the phased pills, the proportion of estrogen and progestin in the pills varies at different times, or phases, of the month, mimicking the fluctuations of a normal menstrual cycle. All three types are taken on a monthly cycle.

The estrogen and progesterone in both the combined and phased pills work primarily by inhibiting the secretion of FSH and LH by the pituitary, thereby preventing ovulation. Although the progestin-only pills may also suppress ovulation in some women, they are believed to produce their contraceptive effect mainly by causing the cervical mucus to thicken so that it becomes impervious to sperm and by changing the endometrium in such a way as to reduce the likelihood of implantation. These effects may also occur to a lesser extent with the combined and phased pills.

◆ *Fertility Drugs*

Infertility is not diagnosed until a couple trying to have a child has failed to conceive after having sexual intercourse on a regular basis for more

---

SOME REPRODUCTIVE SYSTEM DRUGS

ESTROGENS
Chlorotrianisene
Estradiol
Estrogens, Conjugated
Estropipate
Ethinyl Estradiol

CONTRACEPTIVES
Contraceptives, Oral
   (Combination Products)
Contraceptives, Oral (Progestin)
Levonorgestrel Implants
Progesterone Intrauterine
   System

than one year. If a defect in sperm production has been ruled out and the woman has been found to have a hormonal abnormality that inhibits ovulation, treatment with one of the fertility drugs may be recommended.

The choice of drug depends on the presumed cause of infertility. For women who fail to ovulate because of excessive secretion of prolactin, the pituitary hormone that stimulates milk production after childbirth, bromocriptine mesylate is preferred because it interacts with dopamine receptors to inhibit prolactin secretion. For other women, such as those with polycystic ovary syndrome, who do not ovulate because they are producing inadequate amounts of the pituitary hormones FSH and LH, treatment is with clomiphene citrate. This drug opposes the action of estrogen, which usually inhibits the output of FSH and LH, and thus restores normal production of these two hormones so that ovulation is induced.

Various additional hormone-type drugs are also available. If clomiphene citrate therapy is unsuccessful, treatment with menotropins and human chorionic gonadotropin (HCG) may be tried. Menotropins, which contain FSH and LH, stimulate growth and maturation of the ovarian follicles. After the follicle has ripened, HCG, which mimics the action of LH, is given to stimulate ovulation and spur the production of progesterone by the ovaries.

Women who fail to ovulate because of a hypothalamic disorder may respond to treatment with gonadorelin, a synthetic form of the hypothalamic hormone GnRH. Gonadorelin stimulates the pituitary release of FSH and LH in a normal manner, thereby inducing ovulation. You can discuss these drugs with your doctor.

◆ Drugs for Endometriosis

Endometriosis, which can cause painful menstruation and infertility, occurs when fragments of endometrial tissue migrate outside the uterus and become implanted on other pelvic organs, including the ovaries, fallopian tubes, and on the outside of the uterus or its supporting ligaments. In such cases, drugs that suppress ovarian function and the growth of endometrial tissue may be given for extended periods to induce the abnormal tissue to wither away. Such agents include danazol, a synthetic androgen that suppresses ovulation, and gonadotropin-releasing hormone (GnRH) agonists, such as nafarelin acetate and leuprolide acetate, which inhibit estrogen production by the ovaries and curb the growth of endometrial tissue.

◆ Drugs for Prostate Enlargement

Many men older than 50 experience a benign enlargement of the prostate, a condition known as benign prostatic hypertrophy, that leads to compression of the urethra and obstruction of normal urine flow.

Alpha Blockers. An increase in smooth muscle tone in the prostate and neck of the bladder contributes to the reduced urinary flow and other symptoms of benign prostatic hypertrophy. Agents such as doxazosin mesylate and terazosin block the alpha adrenergic nerve receptors that regulate the increase in muscle tone. Such drugs may thus relieve the urethral obstruction and alleviate the symptoms of this disorder.

Androgen Antagonists. The potent hormone dihydrotestosterone stimulates the enlargement of the prostate gland. Administration of the androgen antagonist finasteride inhibits the formation of dihydrotestosterone, shrinking the enlarged prostate and increasing urinary flow.

◆ Drugs for Erectile Dysfunction (Impotence)

Treatment of erectile dysfunction, or a persistent inability to achieve or maintain an erection, depends on the underlying cause and may include psychological counseling, surgery, lifestyle measures, or drugs. Medications that dilate blood vessels in the penis, such as sildenafil (Viagra), papaverine (given by self injection) or alprostadil, may be helpful. Hormone imbalances are a cause of erectile dysfunction; testosterone injections may be given if testosterone levels are low, or bromocriptine mesylate may be prescribed to correct elevated prolactin levels. Yohimbine, a drug that is believed to bolster nervous system signals, is also sometimes given. It's important to remember that erectile dysfunction is also a side effect of many drugs.

◆ Drugs for Sexually Transmitted Diseases

Common sexually transmitted diseases include bacterial infections (gonorrhea, syphilis, and chlamydial infection), viral infections (genital herpes, genital warts, and the acquired immunodeficiency syndrome, AIDS), protozoan infections such as trichomoniasis, and certain types of fungal infections. Bacterial, protozoan, and fungal infections can usually be cured with timely and appropriate anti-infective therapy. Viral infections such as herpes and AIDS can often be effectively managed, though not cured, with currently available antiviral drugs (see page 52).

Skin, Hair, and Nails

The skin, the largest organ in the human body, covers a total area of about 20 square feet in an average-sized adult. Forming the outer boundary of your body, skin carries out several essential functions: it acts as a barrier to protect vital internal organs against infection and injury; it helps to dissipate heat and regulate body temperature; and it synthesizes vitamin D when exposed to ultraviolet light. In addition, the various sensory receptors present throughout your skin enable it to respond to such sensations as heat, cold, pain, and pressure.

Each square inch of your skin contains millions of cells, numerous specialized nerve endings, hair follicles, muscles, sweat glands to cool the body, and sebaceous glands that release oil to lubricate skin. These diverse structures and glands are nourished by a permeating, elaborate network of blood vessels. The thickness of human skin varies markedly on different parts of your body, ranging from fairly thin over protected areas such as the eyelids to very thick over areas subject to abrasion such as your palms and soles.

Skin is composed of three layers: the epidermis, a thin uppermost layer; the dermis, a thicker layer that lies beneath the epidermis and makes up about 90 percent of skin mass; and the subcutaneous layer, which is composed primarily of fatty tissue. New skin cells called keratinocytes are formed in the basal cell layer of the epidermis and migrate upward over a period of about four weeks. As the cells move toward the surface, they grow flatter and more scaly, eventually losing their nuclei and changing into dead skin cells that contain an inert protein called keratin. Keratin, which constitutes the outermost layer of the epidermis, forms a protective barrier that helps control water loss from the body. Ultimately, the outermost keratin layer sloughs off as a result of washing and friction. Hair and nails, which are composed of keratin, are also products of the epidermis.

About 95 percent of the cells in the epidermis are keratinocytes. The other 5 percent of epidermal cells are pigment cells, or melanocytes, that manufacture melanin, a protein that gives coloring to your skin and protects your body from ultraviolet light. Skin coloring is determined not by the total number of melanocytes—which is relatively constant for all races—but rather by the rate at which these cells produce melanin.

The underlying dermis contains fibers such as collagen and elastin as well as water and jellylike materials that make the skin compressible. Collagen fibers help to prevent tearing of the skin, while elastin, a flexible fiber, is what makes the skin resilient. Distributed throughout the dermis are such structures as blood vessels, lymph channels, nerve fibers, muscle cells, hair follicles, and sebaceous and sweat glands.

The subcutaneous layer, which manufactures fat, provides insulation and serves as a depository for reserve calories. Subcutaneous tissue is unevenly distributed, and as you age, this layer thins considerably.

The skin is also an important route of administration for drugs. Many topical drugs are applied to the skin as a cream, ointment, or liquid. Most do not significantly penetrate the skin layers, and hence tend to cause fewer side effects than systemic drugs (those taken orally or intravenously injected). The latter are taken up by the circulation and widely distributed through the body. Also available are

LAYERS OF THE SKIN

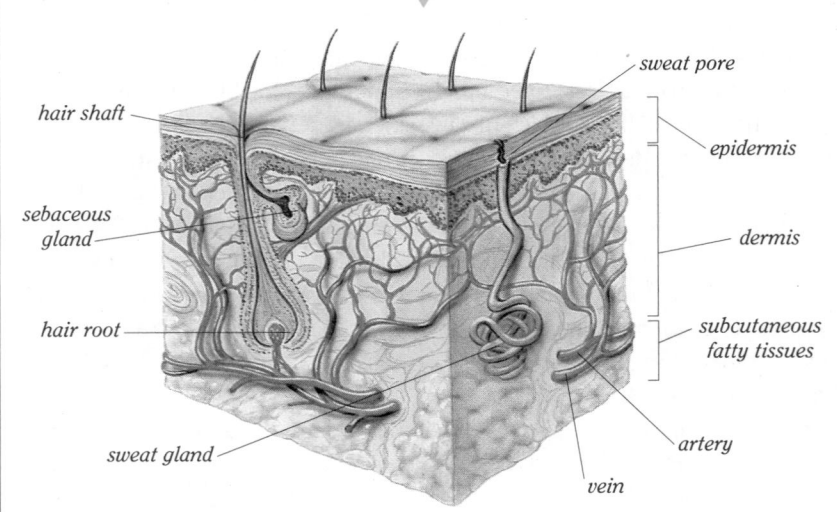

hair shaft
sebaceous gland
hair root
sweat gland
sweat pore
epidermis
dermis
subcutaneous fatty tissues
artery
vein

transdermal skin patches, worn on the chest or behind the ear, for example, which release controlled amounts of drug. Subcutaneous injections of certain drugs are given to deeper layers of skin, where they may be absorbed by the circulation. Finally, solid pellets containing hormones or other agents are sometimes implanted under the skin, where the drug is absorbed slowly over weeks or months.

▼ DRUG THERAPY FOR DERMATOLOGIC DISORDERS

Your skin, which is continuously exposed to the environment, may be affected by a wide range of disorders, including inflammation, allergic reactions, infections, and tumors. Some rashes represent an allergic reaction to a particular medication and usually occur during the first few days after taking it. Hives, or raised, pink or red itchy bumps on the skin, typically are caused by allergies to such foods as shellfish, chocolate, and nuts, but they may also develop in response to certain drugs, such as penicillin or aspirin. Many skin disorders resolve spontaneously, others can be managed with drug therapy, and still others, such as skin tumors, large cysts, or moles, may require surgery.

◆ *Drugs for Acne*
Acne, a very common skin disorder marked by whiteheads, blackheads, pimples, and cysts on the face, back, and chest, is sometimes treated with topical keratolytic (or peeling) agents, topical or systemic antibiotics, or vitamin A derivatives.

Keratolytic Agents. Topical preparations of benzoyl peroxide, resorcinol, or sulfur all have a keratolytic effect. (Benzoyl peroxide and sulfur also have antibacterial properties.) Application of these ointments causes the layer of dead skin cells on the surface to peel off, thereby clearing the blocked hair follicles that are apparently a factor in the formation of blemishes.

Antibiotics. An antibiotic such as erythromycin or clindamycin is sometimes administered in a topical cream for cases of persistent acne. If acne does not respond to topical treatment, a long course of an oral antibiotic such as tetracycline may be prescribed.

Vitamin A Derivatives. If you have severe acne, your physician may prescribe one of the powerful vitamin A derivatives (retinoids)—tretinoin or isotretinoin. Tretinoin, which is available as a gel, cream, or liquid, is applied topically. Isotretinoin is given orally and is usually reserved for cases of severe, disfiguring cystic acne. It works by decreasing the secretion of the fatty oil termed sebum, produced in excessive amounts by the sebaceous glands and a contributing cause of acne. Women must use effective contraception during treatment with isotretinoin because use of this drug during pregnancy has been associated with severe birth defects.

◆ *Topical Anti-Infectives*
Your skin is prey to various infections, and various topical (and sometimes systemic) anti-infectives may be given to kill the infectious microorganism. Antibiotics may be useful for acne (see above) or impetigo, a common bacterial infection in children characterized by the appearance of itchy, red sores with honey-colored crusts on the face, arms, or legs. Antifungals help to combat fungal nail or skin infections such as Athlete's foot, jock itch, or ringworm (a superficial infection that commonly causes severe itching and scaling of the scalp in children). Viral infections account for such common skin disorders as cold sores, shingles, and warts and may be treated with various antiviral agents. Parasites, responsible for skin infestations such as head lice and scabies, are treated with antiparasitics.

◆ *Topical Corticosteroids*
Scaling, rashes, or itching characterize dermatitis, or eczema, a general term for any inflammation of the skin. This condition usually responds to topical corticosteroid therapy. When contact with an allergen or another irritant causes inflammation, white blood cells release substances that dilate the blood vessels, causing tissue swelling. Corticosteroid creams or ointments that are applied directly to the skin surface can counteract the action of the chemicals that trigger inflammation. Topical corticosteroids typically do not cause the serious adverse effects associated with systemic corticosteroids. Prolonged use, however, may produce thinning of the skin, leading to stretch marks and increasing the visibility of tiny blood vessels located close to the skin surface.

◆ *Antipsoriasis Drugs*
Psoriasis is a common skin disorder characterized by dry, red patches of skin covered with silvery scales. Genetic factors favoring the overproduction of skin cells are thought to be at the root of the disorder. Exposing skin areas affected by psoriasis to sunlight or an ultraviolet lamp and using an emollient cream to lubricate the skin may help clear up mild cases of

the disease. If such measures are not effective, topical preparations such as coal-tar ointments may be beneficial. If scaling persists, topical corticosteroids (see page 43) may be prescribed. The immunosuppressant drug methotrexate or the vitamin A derivative acitretin may prove helpful in controlling more severe cases of the condition. Severe psoriasis that fails to improve with other treatments may respond to PUVA, a form of therapy that combines a drug with ultraviolet A light.

◆ *Hair Regrowth Agents*

A side effect of minoxidil, originally prescribed orally to treat moderate to severe hypertension, is increased hair growth. Minoxidil has since been formulated and approved as a topical solution to be applied directly to the scalp. It stimulates hair growth in some men and women who have certain types of baldness (alopecia), including male pattern baldness—marked by a receding hairline and partial to total loss of hair on the scalp, especially on the crown. The drug's mechanism of action in promoting hair regrowth is not well understood.

The Senses: Eyes, Ears, and Nose

Our senses—sight, hearing, smell, taste, and touch—link us with our surroundings, helping us to glean essential information that our brains then process and interpret to provide us with information about the world.

▼ THE EYES

Of the five senses, vision is by far the most complex, and this complexity is mirrored in the anatomic structure of the eye itself. Each of the eyes is composed of several layers of tissue. A mucous membrane called the conjunctiva covers and moistens the inner surface of the eyelid as well as the sclera, the tough white layer that coats most of the eyeball and helps maintain its shape. At the front center of the eye lies the cornea, a transparent, curved membrane that refracts incoming light before it passes through the lens. Directly behind the cornea lies the anterior chamber, an area that is filled with a clear, watery fluid called the aqueous humor.

A layer behind the anterior chamber contains the iris (the colored part of the eye) and the pupil, the opening in the center of the iris that allows light to pass through to the back of the eye. The pupil can dilate or contract, allowing more or less light to enter. The lens, located directly behind the iris, is a curved, crystalline structure that expands and contracts to focus incoming light rays on the retina. Situated behind the lens is the largest portion of the eye—the vitreous chamber, a round cavity filled with a clear gel called the vitreous humor.

In back of the vitreous chamber lies the retina, a membrane of nervous tissue containing light-sensitive cells called rods and cones that convert the incoming light rays into electrical impulses. The optic nerve then transmits these impulses from each retina to the brain, where the signals are merged to create the colored, three-dimensional images that you perceive.

▼ THE EARS

The ear performs two essential functions—it enables you to hear, and it helps you maintain your balance. This hearing organ is divided into three parts: outer ear, middle ear, and inner ear. The outer ear, which consists of the external cartilage and skin and the outer ear canal, serves to channel sound to the middle ear. The middle ear is a cavity that lies between the eardrum and the inner ear. Three tiny bones, or ossicles, in the middle ear—the malleus, incus, and stapes—transfer sound vibrations from the eardrum to the inner ear. The eustachian tube, a narrow channel connecting the middle ear with the back of the nasal cavity, provides a way of equalizing the air pressure in your middle ear with that on the outside.

The structures for hearing and balance are located in separate areas of the inner ear. Specialized receptors in three semicircular canals respond to movement and are responsible for your sense of balance. Sound vibrations are conveyed from the middle ear to the cochlea, a snail-shaped organ lined with tiny hairs that convert the vibrations into electrical impulses. These impulses, when transmitted by the auditory nerve to your brain, are then perceived as sound.

▼ THE NOSE

Your nose is the main portal by which air enters your respiratory system. Hairlike cilia and mucus in your nasal passages filter, warm, and moisten the air you breathe before it passes down the throat and on into the lungs. The nose is divided into two chambers by a wall, or septum, composed of cartilage and bone. The sinuses, cavities surrounding the nose, are lined with sticky mucus. The mucous lining of the nose and surrounding sinuses helps cleanse incoming air by trapping bacteria and airborne particles of dirt.

A multipurpose organ, your nose is also responsible for your sense of smell and, to a large extent, sense of taste. Fine, hairlike fibers, or cilia, project from the end of the olfactory nerve, located high in the nasal cavity, and detect odor molecules dissolved in nasal mucus. When stimulated, the cilia generate a nerve impulse that is transmitted to your brain, allowing you to perceive and identify more than 10,000 distinct odors.

▼ DRUG THERAPY FOR DISORDERS OF THE EYES, EARS, AND NOSE

The eyes, ears, and nose are vulnerable to numerous disorders. Although seldom fatal, many of these illnesses can be extremely debilitating. Some do not require drugs (nosebleeds) or can be treated surgically (cataracts), but many respond to pharmacologic therapy. Various drugs come as ophthalmic (eye), otic (ear), or nasal drops, ointments, sprays, or solutions. Many of these preparations act locally (on a restricted area of the body) and thus generally do not cause systemic side effects, although they sometimes are absorbed in high enough concentrations to cause systemic reactions. Some nasal preparations (hormones) are actually intended to be absorbed into the general circulation. Oral or injectable systemic drugs are also

ANATOMY OF THE EYE, EAR, AND NOSE

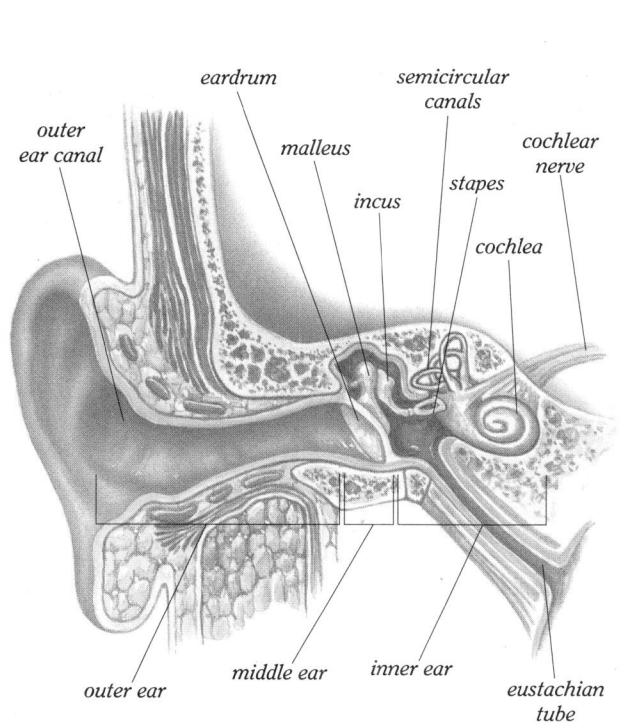

outer ear canal • eardrum • malleus • incus • semicircular canals • stapes • cochlear nerve • cochlea • outer ear • middle ear • inner ear • eustachian tube

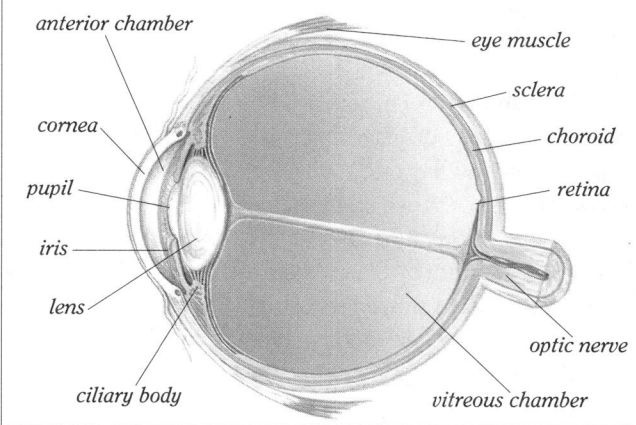

anterior chamber • cornea • pupil • iris • lens • ciliary body • eye muscle • sclera • choroid • retina • optic nerve • vitreous chamber

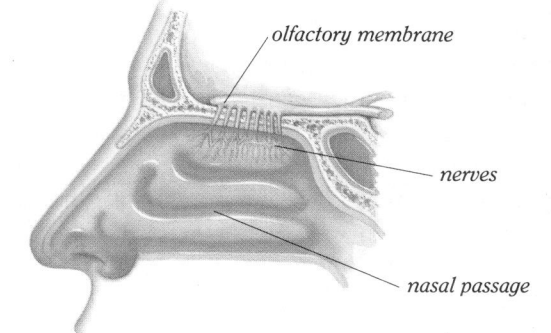

olfactory membrane • nerves • nasal passage

sometimes used to treat these disorders. Common classes of drugs used to treat disorders of the eyes, ears, and nose are discussed below.

◆ *Antiglaucoma Drugs*

Glaucoma, caused by the buildup of pressure in the aqueous humor, can cause progressive damage to the optic nerve, resulting in blindness. Three main classes of drugs are used to reduce ocular pressure: beta-blockers, miotics, and carbonic anhydrase inhibitors. Signals transmitted through specialized nerve receptors (beta receptors) stimulate cells within the ciliary body to secrete fluid into the aqueous humor. Beta-blockers such as timolol maleate prevent the transmission of these signals, thereby reducing the output of aqueous humor and lowering the pressure of fluid in the eye. Miotics such as pilocarpine cause constriction of the pupils (miosis) and reduce pressure within the eye by increasing the outflow of aqueous humor through its drainage channel. These pupil-enlarging drugs are also sometimes used for eye examinations. Carbonic anhydrase inhibitors such as acetazolamide work by blocking the activity of carbonic anhydrase, an enzyme that is involved in the production of aqueous humor.

◆ *Anti-Infectives/ Anti-Inflammatories*

Various groups of drugs are employed to treat infections or inflammations of the eyes, ears, or nose. Conjunctivitis, marked by redness and itching of the eye, is an inflammation of the conjunctiva that can result from a bacterial or viral infection or an allergic reaction. Your physician may prescribe antibiotic eye drops if a bacterial infection is responsible for the conjunctivitis. Allergic conjunctivitis may be treated with an antihistamine (see page 52) and with corticosteroid eye drops to reduce inflammation.

External otitis, or swimmer's ear, is marked by itching and pain in the outer ear canal. The condition can be caused by eczema or it may develop when water becomes trapped in the external ear canal, predisposing it to a fungal or bacterial infection. If eczema is the only contributing factor, the condition is treated with corticosteroid ear drops to reduce inflammation. If both infection and inflammation are present, your physician will probably prescribe ear drops containing a corticosteroid as well as antibiotics, typically neomycin combined with either polymyxin B or colistin.

Otitis media is an infection of the middle ear that usually produces a severe earache, fever, a feeling of fullness or blockage in the ear, and muffled hearing. Because of the position and small size of their eustachian tubes, children are particularly vulnerable to otitis media. Bacterial infections of the middle ear frequently block the eustachian tube, causing a buildup of pus and mucus behind the ear, which carries the risk of perforation. Your doctor may prescribe a decongestant (see page 35) or an antihistamine (see page 52) to relieve swelling in the eustachian tube and an oral antibiotic to eradicate the infection.

Sinusitis refers to any infection or allergic reaction that causes an inflammation of the lining of the sinus cavities. Sinusitis can produce such symptoms as pain around your eyes or cheeks, fever, and difficulty breathing through your nose. Most forms of acute sinusitis are caused by bacterial infection and are treated with oral antibiotics. Your physician may also recommend the use of decongestants (see page 35) in the form of drops, sprays, or tablets to open the nasal passages and promote the drainage of secretions from your sinuses.

Chronic rhinitis, an inflammation of the membranes lining the nose, may be associated with excessive production of mucus, a stuffy nose, and postnasal drip. The condition may develop as a result of exposure to certain irritating chemicals or it may be due to an allergic response. Corticosteroids or antihistamines may be given to ease allergic reactions.

◆ *Drugs for Nausea or Dizziness*

Ménière's disease is marked by episodes of vertigo accompanied by nausea and vomiting, ringing or buzzing in the ears (tinnitus), and muffled hearing. Thought to be caused by increased fluid in the semicircular canals of the inner ear, this disorder disrupts both the sense of balance and hearing. Ménière's disease, and other causes of nausea and dizziness, may be treated with an antihistamine (see page 52) or a sedative (see page 49) to relieve the vertigo. A diuretic (see page 22) may also be given to reduce the excess fluid in the inner ear.

The Brain, Nervous System, and Emotions

Functioning as an elaborate central processing unit, your brain constantly receives input in the form of billions of electrical and chemical impulses that keep it informed about the state of affairs both inside and outside your body. Your brain then analyzes this information and transmits messages to your body's various organs, glands, and muscles, enabling them to respond appropriately. Your brain, and specifically that portion termed the cerebrum, is also the source of consciousness, emotions, memory, language, creativity, and thought.

Emerging from the base of the brain is a cable of nerve tissue termed the spinal cord, which extends about 17 inches from the brain stem to the lower part of the back. Together, your brain and spinal cord comprise the central nervous system. Both components are encased in bone for protection: the skull encloses the brain, while the vertebral canal surrounds the spinal cord.

Extending outward from your brain and spinal cord is the peripheral nervous system, which consists of three main components: peripheral spinal nerves, cranial nerves, and the autonomic nervous system.

The spinal nerves, which transmit information to and from your brain, emerge from the spinal cord and exit through openings between the vertebrae. Sensory fibers in the spinal nerves receive stimuli from the skin and internal organs, while motor fibers in the spinal nerves trigger the contraction of skeletal muscles.

Cranial nerves, which arise from the underside of your brain, relay sensory information and control muscles primarily in the head and neck region.

The autonomic nervous system plays the key role in functions that are involuntary. For example, it regulates breathing, heartbeat, sweating, circulation, and digestion. It also controls the actions of muscles in blood vessels and internal organs and governs the activities of various glands. This system has two components: the sympathetic and parasympathetic. The sympathetic nervous system prompts various body functions: for example, it speeds up your heart rate, constricts blood vessels, and widens the airways. The parasympathetic system has a counterbalancing effect—it slows your heart rate, narrows the airways, and increases the flow of digestive juices.

THE BRAIN AND MAJOR NERVES OF THE HUMAN BODY

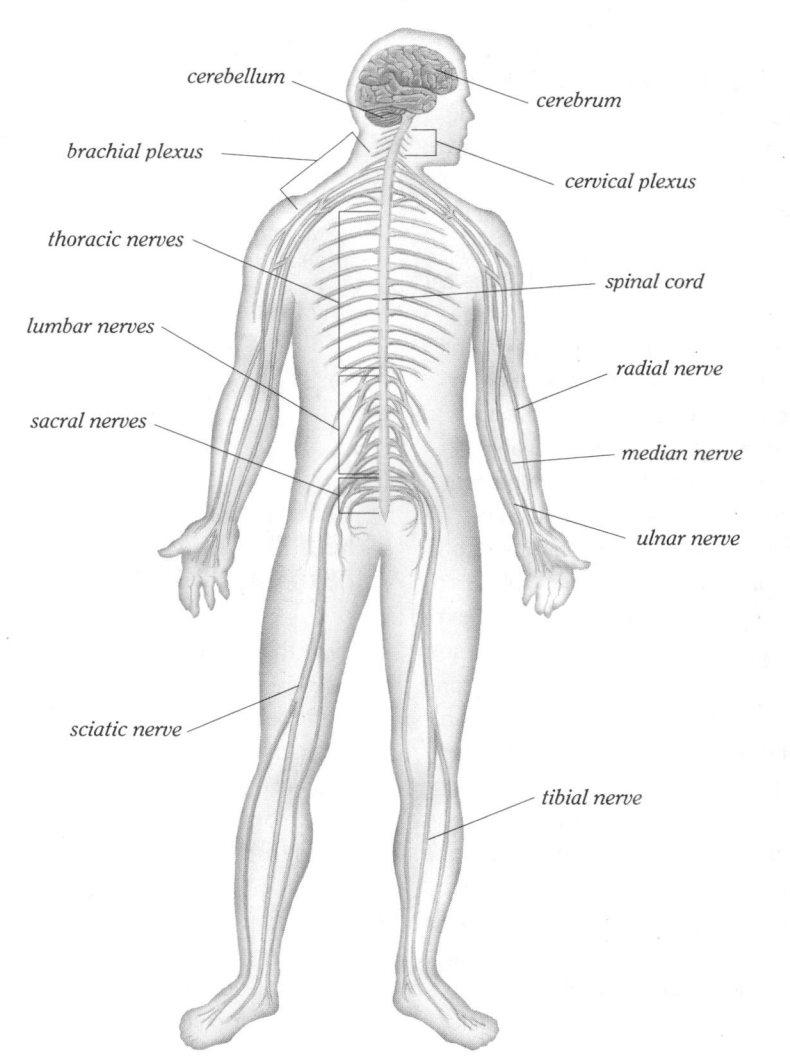

cerebellum
cerebrum
brachial plexus
cervical plexus
thoracic nerves
spinal cord
lumbar nerves
radial nerve
sacral nerves
median nerve
ulnar nerve
sciatic nerve
tibial nerve

The fundamental unit of the nervous system is the neuron, or nerve cell. Your brain, which weighs about three pounds, contains billions of individual neurons. Each neuron consists of a cell body with a central nucleus, a major projection termed an axon, and numerous smaller filaments called dendrites. Axons—some of which are very long, reaching a length of more than three feet—conduct electrical impulses away from the cell body, while the dendrites receive electrical signals from other neurons. Each neuron makes contact with an adjacent nerve cell at a point termed the synapse. When a neuron is stimulated, an electrical impulse travels down its axon to the synapse, where it triggers the release of chemical neurotransmitters. These substances then bind to receptor sites on a target cell, stimulating a response in that cell. Electrical and chemical impulses sprint from neuron to neuron in this fashion until the message reaches its destination and produces the desired effect.

Although your brain probably accounts for only about two percent of your total body weight, it commands 20 percent of your heart's output of blood. To maintain stable brain function, a so-called blood-brain barrier exists that controls the flow of molecules to your brain. This barrier consists of a highly impermeable layer of cells in the brain capillaries surrounded by a layer of astrocytes (supporting nerve cells). Relatively small molecules such as oxygen, water, and glucose easily penetrate this barrier, but many drugs and chemicals are unable to do so. Brain inflammation, however, can increase the permeability of many drugs that normally fail to penetrate the blood-brain barrier.

MAJOR CLASSES OF PSYCHIATRIC DRUGS

BENZODIAZEPINES
Alprazolam
Chlordiazepoxide
Clorazepate Dipotassium
Clonazepam
Diazepam
Estazolam
Flurazepam Hydrochloride
Lorazepam
Oxazepam
Prazepam
Quazepam
Temazepam
Triazolam

ANTIPSYCHOTICS
Chlorpromazine Hydrochloride
Clozapine
Fluphenazine
Haloperidol
Hydroxyzine Hydrochloride
Loxapine
Molindone
Olanzapine
Perphenazine
Prochlorperazine
Risperidone
Thioridazine Hydrochloride
Thiothixene
Trifluoperazine Hydrochloride

BARBITURATES
Amobarbital Sodium
Amobarbital/Secobarbital
Phenobarbital
Pentobarbital Sodium

ANTIDEPRESSANTS
Tricyclic Antidepressants
Amitriptyline Hydrochloride
Amoxapine
Clomipramine Hydrochloride
Desipramine Hydrochloride
Doxepin Hydrochloride
Imipramine
Nortriptyline Hydrochloride
Protriptyline Hydrochloride

MAO Inhibitors
Phenelzine Sulfate
Tranylcypromine Sulfate

SSRIs
Citalopram Hydrobromide
Fluoxetine Hydrochloride
Fluvoxamine Maleate
Paroxetine Hydrochloride
Sertraline Hydrochloride

ANTIMANIC DRUGS
Lithium

▼ DRUG THERAPY FOR COMMON NEUROLOGIC AND PSYCHIATRIC DISORDERS

Many of the disorders affecting the nervous system are highly complex. Biochemical, electrical, and structural changes in nervous tissue and problems affecting the blood vessels supplying the brain account for most neurologic disorders. Improvements in diagnosis and better understanding of brain function have led to significant advances in treatment in recent years, but for some neurologic disorders, drug therapy can still offer only partial relief of symptoms.

◆ Analgesics

When your tissues are damaged as a result of trauma, infection, or inflammation, they produce prostaglandins. These chemicals stimulate local nerve cells to generate a signal that is then transmitted to your brain, where it is interpreted as pain. The primary classes of drugs used to relieve pain are narcotics and non-narcotic analgesics (painkillers). Non-narcotic analgesics such as aspirin and other nonsteroidal anti-inflammatory drugs (see NSAIDs, page 26) block the production of prostaglandins at the site of injury so that no pain signals travel to the brain. The non-NSAID, non-narcotic painkiller, acetaminophen, decreases the production of prostaglandins in the brain but it does not alter prostaglandin production elsewhere in the body and so does not diminish inflammation. Narcotic analgesics, also called opioids, bind to receptors in the brain and apparently interfere with the transmission of pain signals within the brain and also in the spinal cord.

◆ Antimigraine Drugs
Migraine headaches are marked by severe, throbbing pain caused by an initial constriction of blood vessels surrounding the brain followed by the dilation of blood vessels in the scalp. Drugs used to prevent migraine, such as methysergide maleate, block the action of certain chemicals that provoke the initial blood vessel constriction leading to the migraine attack. Agents given to abort an acute attack, such as sumatriptan succinate, constrict the dilated blood vessels, thereby relieving the severe pain.

◆ Anticonvulsants
Epileptic seizures are characterized by episodes of uncontrolled electrical activity in the brain, leading to involuntary movements and altered consciousness. If you are epileptic, your physician may prescribe anticonvulsant drugs to prevent seizures or to halt one that is already underway. Anticonvulsants exert an inhibitory effect on brain cells and prevent the excessive electrical activity that provokes a seizure.

◆ Antiparkinsonism Drugs
Parkinson's disease, a degenerative neurologic disorder marked by shaking of the head and limbs, rigidity, and loss of facial expression, is caused by an imbalance between the neurotransmitters dopamine and acetylcholine in the brain. Antiparkinsonism drugs produce their effects by attempting to restore the normal balance between these two neurotransmitters. Anticholinergic agents decrease the effects of acetylcholine by blocking the brain receptors for this chemical and restoring the normal balance with dopamine. Dopamine-boosting agents, on the other hand, increase dopamine activity and restore the natural balance with acetylcholine.

◆ Antianxiety Drugs
Anxiety, a state of fear or apprehension about some ill-defined danger, results from a disruption of the normal balance of certain chemicals in the brain. The major classes of drugs used to treat this disorder are benzodiazepines and beta-blockers. Benzodiazepines appear to relieve anxiety by promoting the effect of gamma-aminobutyric acid (GABA), a brain chemical that normally inhibits brain activity in the portion of the brain that controls emotion. The beta-blockers, commonly used to treat high blood pressure (see page 22), are also used to ease physical symptoms of anxiety, such as trembling and palpitations, that are associated with increased activity of the sympathetic nervous system.

◆ Sedative and Hypnotic Drugs
Your physician may prescribe a sedative or hypnotic drug if you have persistent insomnia that fails to respond to simple remedies. Most sedatives work by decreasing communications between nerve cells, thereby reducing brain activity and allowing you to fall asleep more readily. Benzodiazepines (see Antianxiety Drugs, above) are the most commonly used sleeping drugs. Barbiturates were once widely used as sedatives, but they are now rarely prescribed for insomnia because of the risks of dependency and toxicity in overdose.

◆ Antidepressant Drugs
There are three major types of drugs used to treat significant depression: tricyclics, selective serotonin reuptake inhibitors (SSRIs), and monoamine oxidase (MAO) inhibitors. In depression, decreased neurotransmitter activity results in insufficient stimulation of brain cells. Tricyclic antidepressants boost neurotransmitter action by blocking their reabsorption and thereby prolonging the stimulatory effect of these chemicals on brain cells. The SSRIs exert their effect by slowing the uptake of the neurotransmitter serotonin by brain cells. The MAO inhibitor antidepressants increase the action of the excitatory neurotransmitters by blocking a brain enzyme (monoamine oxidase) that normally breaks down these chemicals.

◆ Antipsychotic Drugs
Psychotic disorders, including schizophrenia, manic depression, and paranoia, are marked by disturbances in thinking, inappropriate emotional reactions, and unusual behavior. In some forms of psychotic illness, brain cells release excessive amounts of the neurotransmitter dopamine. The resulting overstimulation of brain cells is thought to disturb normal thought processes and lead to abnormal behavior. Antipsychotic drugs bind to dopamine receptors on brain cells, thereby rendering the cells less sensitive to dopamine and decreasing the transmission of nerve impulses.

The Immune System and Infections

The immune system acts as the body's sentry, defending it against invading microorganisms and even protecting it from aberrant behavior by its own cells. Your body is constantly being exposed to millions of microbes, including viruses, bacteria, fungi, and protozoa. (Not all of these organisms are harmful, however: many benign bacteria reside on your skin's surface, and some intestinal bacteria are actually beneficial, helping to produce essential vitamins.)

Your body has several lines of defense against potentially damaging microorganisms, or pathogens. For example, skin presents a mechanical barrier to invasion, and acidic stomach secretions as well as enzymes in tears and saliva mount a chemical defense against infection. Infectious organisms that manage to breach these physical and chemical barriers and enter your body are then set upon.

In many cases, pathogens provoke an initial inflammatory response that prevents further spread of the infection. In this type of reaction, the foreign organism damages the local tissue, causing it to release prostaglandins and histamine. These chemicals attract special types of white blood cells termed neutrophils, which engulf and destroy the invading organisms.

If this rapid inflammatory response fails to halt the infection, specialized white blood cells called lymphocytes may be mobilized to eradicate the organisms. Two major classes of lymphocytes have been identified: B cells and T cells. The B cells produce antibodies that recognize and neutralize the infecting organism. The T cells, by contrast, attack and destroy the invading organisms directly by secreting power-ful chemicals called lymphokines. The T cells also attack cancerous cells, helping prevent tumor growth. After your immune system comes into contact with a specific invader, it produces so-called memory T and B cells, which recognize the invader and enable the immune system to mount a more rapid response when it is exposed again to the same foreign substance.

Lymphocytes circulate in the blood and are present in the bone marrow, spleen, thymus, and lymph nodes. They are also found in lymph, a thin, almost colorless fluid that circulates through the lymphatic vessels and is

ORGANS OF THE IMMUNE SYSTEM

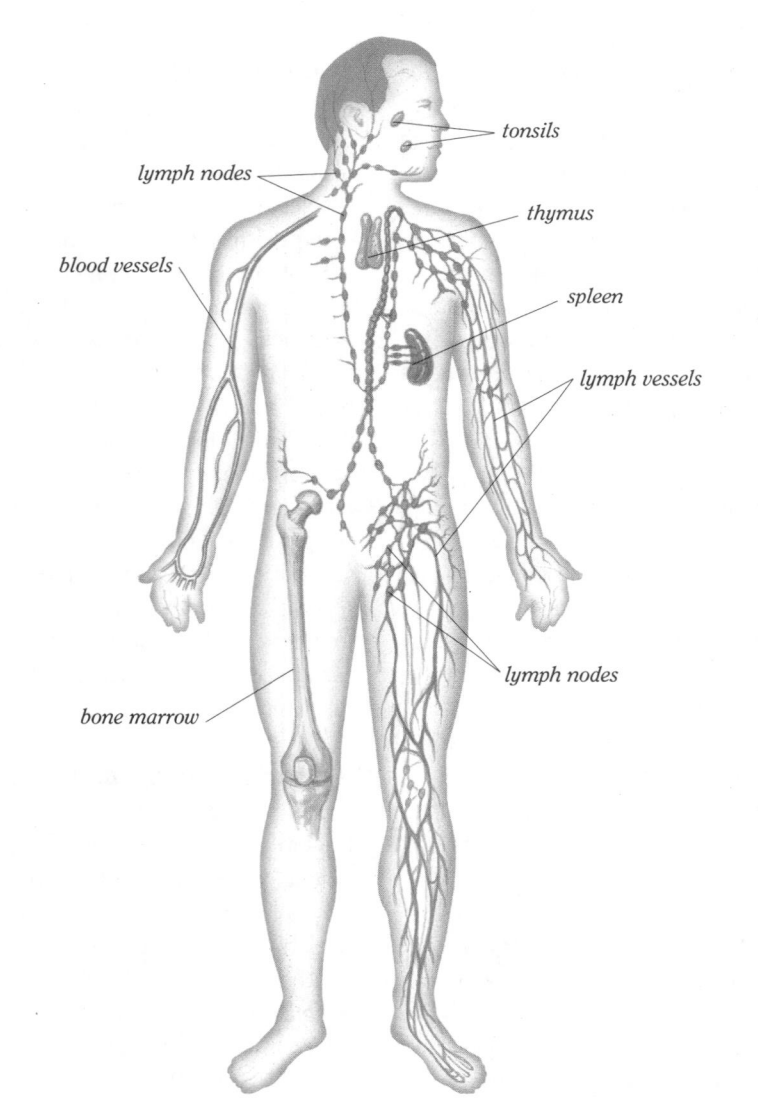

tonsils

lymph nodes

thymus

blood vessels

spleen

lymph vessels

lymph nodes

bone marrow

filtered by the lymph nodes, masses of lymph tissue enclosed by a fibrous capsule. The lymph nodes are located primarily in your neck, armpits, abdomen, and groin. All lymphocytes originate in the bone marrow as stem cells. Some stem cells migrate to the lymph nodes where they develop into B cells, while other stem cells travel to the thymus, where they replicate and mature into T cells.

This wonderful immune system, however, is not invincible, and infections do occur. It can also malfunction by mounting an attack on the body's own tissues, producing autoimmune diseases such as rheumatoid arthritis, or by overreacting to relatively harmless substances, such as pollen, particular foods, or insect venom. Allergic reactions are marked by the release of excessive amounts of chemicals such as histamine, which can produce rash, swelling, and narrowing of the airways. Common allergic reactions to certain drugs, such as penicillin, insulin, and barbiturates, include itchy rashes, hives, and a low fever. In such cases, the medication must be discontinued.

The immune system can be impaired by aging and by various medications, including corticosteroids. Infection with the human immunodeficiency virus (HIV) also subverts the normal immune response by invading and progressively destroying T cells.

▼ DRUG THERAPY FOR INFECTIONS AND IMMUNE-RELATED DISORDERS

◆ *Antibiotics*

Antibiotics, or drugs that combat disease-causing germs, are among the great success stories of modern medi-

MAJOR CLASSES OF ANTIBACTERIALS

CEPHALOSPORIN ANTIBIOTICS
Cefaclor
Cefadroxil
Cefamandole
Cefazolin
Cefepime
Cefixime
Cefotetan Disodium
Cefpodoxime Proxetil
Cefprozil
Cefuroxime
Cephalexin
Cephradine

AMINOGLYCOSIDES
Gentamicin
Tobramycin

SULFA DRUGS
Sulfasalazine
Sulfisoxazole Systemic

PENICILLIN ANTIBIOTICS
Amoxicillin
Ampicillin
Bacampicillin Hydrochloride
Carbenicillin Indanyl Sodium
Dicloxacillin Sodium
Oxacillin
Penicillin G
Penicillin V

MACROLIDES/AZALIDES
Azithromycin
Clarithromycin
Dirithromycin
Erythromycin Systemic

TETRACYCLINE ANTIBIOTICS
Doxycycline
Minocycline
Tetracycline Hydrochloride

cine. Since the discovery of penicillin in the 1930s, hundreds of antibiotics have been developed; in many cases they have been curing life-threatening infections quickly, efficiently, and relatively inexpensively.

The term antibiotics is commonly used to refer to drugs that kill or inhibit the growth and spread of infectious bacteria in particular, as opposed to other types of microorganisms. However, other types of anti-infective drugs are also available. Antivirals, for example, are active against viruses such as HIV, the cause of AIDS. Antifungals are used to treat athlete's foot, ringworm, and other fungal infections. And antiparasitics are effective against malaria, worms, head lice, and other types of parasites.

Antibacterials. Antibacterials are used to treat a wide variety of infections due to disease-causing bacteria, including bacterial pneumonias; some

infections of the eyes, ears, skin, blood, or bone; and certain sexually transmitted diseases. They are not effective against infections caused by viruses, including colds or flu.

Antibacterials are grouped into different classes according to their chemical structures and activity against particular types of bacteria. This helps doctors to select the right type of antibiotic for a given infection. If you know you are allergic to an antibiotic from one class, such as penicillin, it is likely that you will be allergic as well to related antibiotics, such as amoxicillin.

Unfortunately, many people continue to receive antibiotic prescriptions for colds, bronchitis, or upper respiratory infections caused by viruses, which are impervious to these drugs. Indiscriminate use of antibiotics has contributed to the emergence of drug-resistant bacteria that do not respond to most, or even any, antibiotics. The problem is compounded by patients who fail to complete a prescribed course of antibiotic therapy (often 10 days or longer), a dangerous practice that may allow the hardier bacteria, not killed off early in a course of antibiotic therapy, to flourish. It is important that antibiotics be taken only when necessary, and that the full course of therapy be completed.

Antiviral Drugs. While there is still no cure for the common cold, the emergence of AIDS has spurred the development of new drugs active against HIV, cytomegalovirus (CMV), herpes, and other viruses. Drug therapy for viruses has been especially difficult, because unlike other infectious organisms, viruses insinuate themselves into otherwise healthy cells and use the host cell's own genetic machinery to multiply. Most attempts to inhibit or kill the virus are also very likely to injure normal host cells.

A promising new group of AIDS drugs is the protease inhibitors, which block production of a key viral enzyme, protease, that HIV needs to replicate itself. Examples of protease inhibitors (also called protease drugs) are saquinavir mesylate, ritonavir, and indinavir sulfate.

◆ *Antihistamines and Anti-Allergy Medications*
A wide array of substances or factors (allergens) can trigger an allergic reaction. Pollens, dust, and molds, for example, are common triggers of seasonal allergies and hay fever (allergic rhinitis). Specific foods or drugs, plants such as poison ivy or poison oak, and in some cases even cold or exercise can also set off an allergic response in susceptible persons.

Allergies typically develop over time after repeated exposures to a specific allergen. The body protects itself from further invasion by releasing the inflammation-causing substance histamine into the nasal passages, the skin, or other tissues. The result is such familiar symptoms as sneezing, sniffling, red and watery eyes, wheezing, asthma, or itchy skin and hives. When severe, allergic reactions can be life-threatening (see Special Concerns, page 18).

Antihistamines, drugs that block the irritating effect of histamine on tissues, can be very effective for relief of allergy symptoms. They are often combined with a decongestant, which shrinks swollen membranes in the nasal passages. Some antihistamines cause drowsiness—an effect that may make these drugs useful for inducing sleep as well. Antihistamines are also employed sometimes to relieve motion sickness or vertigo (dizziness).

Other drugs are also used to treat allergies. Cromolyn sodium actually stops the release of histamine before it begins. If it is used prior to allergen exposure; it may prevent symptoms. Inhaled and ophthalmic corticosteroids (see pages 35 and 46) can also be effective against allergies.

◆ *Immunosuppressant Drugs*
Drugs that suppress the immune system (immunosuppressants) are essential to the success of organ transplants. When a foreign organ is introduced into the body, immune system cells try to destroy it, just as they would a foreign virus or bacteria. To help short-circuit this mechanism, virtually all transplant recipients must take multiple medications for the rest of their lives. The mainstays of post-

ANTIHISTAMINES

ANTIHISTAMINES
Azelastine
Brompheniramine Maleate
Cetirizine
Chlorpheniramine Maleate Oral
Clemastine Fumarate
Cyproheptadine Hydrochloride
Dimenhydrinate
Diphenhydramine Hydrochloride
Fexofenadine
Hydroxyzine
Levocabastine
Loratadine
Olopatadine
Promethazine Hydrochloride
Triprolidine Hydrochloride

transplant therapy are cyclosporine (introduced in 1983) and the newer, more potent drug tacrolimus. Both medications inhibit tissue-destroying T cells but have a minimal effect on B cells, which are needed to produce antibodies to fight infection.

Other drugs used by organ transplant recipients include corticosteroids (especially prednisone), azathioprine, and cyclophosphamide, which alter certain chemical reactions involved in the immune response. There are also newer drugs such as mycophenolate mofetil. Taken with cyclosporine or tacrolimus, these medications prevent rejection without destroying the body's ability to fight disease.

Corticosteroids and other drugs with immunosuppressant effects are also used to treat certain forms of cancer and rheumatoid arthritis, lupus, and other conditions associated with an overactive immune response.

COMMON DISORDERS AND THE DRUGS PRESCRIBED FOR THEM

As a rule, your doctor can choose from a variety of drugs to treat a particular medical condition. He or she will determine which drug or combination of drugs should be right for you, based on the duration and severity of your illness, other medications you may be taking, your age and general health, any accompanying medical problems, plus such additional factors as drug allergies or past experiences with particular medications. If you think that a drug is not working well or you cannot tolerate its side effects, consult with your doctor about trying another medication. Do not, however, discontinue the drug on your own, and never borrow prescription medicines from others.

The drugs covered in this book are grouped below according to the specific diseases, disorders, symptoms, and conditions for which they are typically used. The list is not exhaustive; it is meant to be a general resource to explore which drugs may be useful for a specific medical concern. Don't be alarmed if a drug you are taking is not listed under your condition. Only indications that have been approved by the Food and Drug Administration (FDA) are included here. However, it's important to note that once a drug has been FDA-approved for one indication, doctors are free to prescribe it for other purposes—a common and often effective practice known as "off-label use."

ABRASIONS AND CUTS
Bacitracin
Benzocaine
Iodine Topical
Lidocaine HCl Topical
Neomycin/Polymyxin B/
  Bacitracin Topical

ACID INDIGESTION AND UPSET STOMACH
Aluminum Salts
Bismuth Subsalicylate
Cimetidine
Famotidine
Magaldrate
Magnesium Oxide
Milk of Magnesia
Nizatidine
Omeprazole
Pantoprazole Sodium
Rabeprazole
Ranitidine
Simethicone
Sodium Bicarbonate

ACNE
Adapalene
Benzoyl Peroxide
Clindamycin
Doxycycline
Isotretinoin
Minocycline
Resorcinol
Sulfur Topical

Tazarotene
Tetracycline Hydrochloride
Tretinoin

AIDS (HIV INFECTION)
Abacavir Sulfate
Amprenavir
Cidofovir
Delavirdine
Didanosine (ddI)
Efavirenz
Foscarnet Sodium
Ganciclovir Sodium
Indinavir Sulfate
Interferon beta-1b
Lamivudine
Lamivudine/Zidovudine
Nelfinavir
Nevirapine
Rifabutin
Ritonavir
Saquinavir Mesylate
Stavudine
Zalcitabine (ddC)
Zidovudine

ALCOHOLISM
Disulfiram
Naltrexone

ALCOHOL WITHDRAWAL
Chlordiazepoxide
Clorazepate Dipotassium
Diazepam

Hydroxyzine Hydrochloride
Oxazepam

ALLERGIES AND ALLERGIC REACTIONS
Azelastine
Beclomethasone Inhalant
  and Nasal
Betamethasone Systemic
Brompheniramine
Budesonide
Cetirizine
Chlorpheniramine Maleate
  Oral
Clemastine Fumarate
Cortisone Oral
Cromolyn Sodium Oph.
Cyproheptadine HCl
Dexamethasone Inhalant
  and Nasal
Dexamethasone Ophthalmic
Dexamethasone Systemic
Diphenhydramine HCl
Epinephrine Hydrochloride
Fexofenadine Hydrochloride
Fexofenadine/
  Pseudoephedrine
Flunisolide
Hydrocortisone Systemic
Hydroxyzine Hydrochloride
Loratadine
Loratadine/Pseudoephedrine
Methylprednisolone
Mometasone Furoate Nasal

Olopatadine Hydrochloride
Oxymetazoline Nasal
Prednisolone Ophthalmic
Prednisolone Systemic
Prednisone
Promethazine Hydrochloride
Triamcinolone Inhalant and
  Nasal
Triamcinolone Systemic
Triprolidine Hydrochloride

ALTITUDE SICKNESS
Acetazolamide

ALZHEIMER'S DISEASE
Donepezil Hydrochloride
Rivastigmine Tartrate
Tacrine

AMOEBA INFECTIONS
Chloroquine
Metronidazole

AMYOTROPHIC LATERAL SCLEROSIS (ALS)
Riluzole

ANEMIA
Betamethasone Systemic
Cortisone Oral
Dexamethasone Systemic
Epoetin Alfa
Ferrous Salts
Fluoxymestrone

Folic Acid
Hydrocortisone Systemic
Leucovorin Calcium
Methylprednisolone
Prednisolone Systemic
Prednisone
Triamcinolone Systemic

ANGINA PECTORIS
Amlodipine
Amyl Nitrate
Atenolol
Diltiazem Hydrochloride
Isosorbide Dinitrate
Isosorbide Mononitrate
Metoprolol
Nadolol
Nicardipine HCl Oral
Nifedipine
Nitroglycerin
Propranolol Hydrochloride
Verapamil Hydrochloride

ANOREXIA
Megestrol Acetate

ANXIETY
Alprazolam
Amobarbital/Secobarbital
Amobarbital Sodium
Buspirone Hydrochloride
Chlordiazepoxide
Chlordiazepoxide/
  Amitriptyline
Clorazepate Dipotassium
Diazepam
Hydroxyzine Hydrochloride
Lorazepam
Maprotiline Hydrochloride
Meprobamate
Oxazepam
Pentobarbital Sodium
Perphenazine/Amitriptyline
Prazepam

ARTHRITIS
Acetaminophen/Aspirin/
  Caffeine

Aspirin
Aspirin/Caffeine
Auranofin
Azathioprine
Capsaicin
Celecoxib
Cortisone Oral
Dexamethasone Systemic
Diclofenac Systemic
Diclofenac/Misoprostol
Diflunisal
Etanercept
Etodolac
Fenoprofen Calcium
Flurbiprofen Oral
Gold Sodium Thiomalate
Hydrocortisone Systemic
Hydroxychloroquine Sulfate
Ibuprofen
Indomethacin
Ketoprofen
Leflunomide
Meclofenamate Sodium
Meloxicam
Methotrexate
Methylprednisolone
Nabumetone
Naproxen
Oxaprozin
Penicillamine
Piroxicam
Prednisolone Systemic
Prednisone
Rofecoxib
Salsalate
Sulindac
Tolmetin Sodium
Triamcinolone Systemic

ASTHMA
Albuterol
Aminophylline
Beclomethasone Inhalant
  and Nasal
Betamethasone Systemic
Bitolterol Mesylate
Budesonide

Cortisone Oral
Cromolyn Sodium Inhalant
  and Nasal
Dexamethasone Inhalant
  and Nasal
Dexamethasone Systemic
Ephedrine
Epinephrine Hydrochloride
Flunisolide
Isoetharine
Isoproterenol
Metaproterenol Sulfate
Methylprednisolone
Montelukast
Nedocromil Sodium Inhalant
Nifedipine
Pirbuterol Acetate
Prednisolone Systemic
Prednisone
Salmeterol Xinafoate
Terbutaline Sulfate
Theophylline
Triamcinolone Inhalant
Triamcinolone Systemic
Zafirlukast
Zileuton

ATHLETE'S FOOT
Butenafine Hydrochloride
Clotrimazole
Econazole Nitrate
Griseofulvin
Haloprogin
Ketoconazole Topical
Ketoconazole Oral
Miconazole
Terbinafine Hydrochloride
Tolnaftate
Undecylenic Acid

ATTENTION DEFICIT HYPERACTIVITY DISORDER (ADHD)
Amphetamine
Amphetamine/
  Dextroamphetamine
Dextroamphetamine Sulfate
Methamphetamine HCl

Methylphenidate HCl
Pemoline

BALDNESS
Minoxidil Topical

BED WETTING
Desmopressin Acetate
Imipramine Hydrochloride

BEE STING ALLERGIES
Epinephrine Hydrochloride

BEHAVIOR PROBLEMS IN CHILDREN
Haloperidol

BIPOLAR (MANIC DEPRESSIVE) DISORDER
Lithium

BLADDER INFECTIONS
(see Urinary Tract
  Infections)

BLEEDING, ABNORMAL UTERINE
Estradiol
Estrogens, Conjugated
Estrogens, Conjugated/Med-
  roxyprogesterone Acetate
Ethinyl Estradiol
Medroxyprogesterone
  Acetate
Norethindrone
Progesterone Systemic

BLOOD CLOTS AND DISORDERS
Aminocaproic Acid
Clopidogrel Bisulfate
Dalteparin Sodium
Dipyridamole
Enoxaparin Sodium Injection
Ticlopidine Hydrochloride
Warfarin

BREAST DISEASE, FIBROCYSTIC
Danazol

BREAST MILK SUPPRESSION
Bromocriptine Mesylate

BRONCHITIS
Acetylcysteine
Albuterol
Aminophylline
Amoxicillin
Ampicillin
Azithromycin
Bitolterol Mesylate
Cefepime
Cefixime
Cefpodoxime Proxetil
Cefprozil
Cefuroxime
Cephradine
Ciprofloxacin Systemic
Clarithromycin
Dicloxacillin Sodium
Dirithromycin
Doxycycline
Ephedrine
Epinephrine Hydrochloride
Erythromycin Systemic
Gatifloxacin
Ipratropium Bromide
Isoetharine
Isoproterenol
Levofloxacin
Lomefloxacin Hydrochloride
Loracarbef
Metaproterenol Sulfate
Minocycline
Moxifloxacin Hydrochloride
Ofloxacin Oral
Penicillin V
Pirbuterol Acetate
Sparfloxacin
Terbutaline Sulfate
Tetracycline Hydrochloride
Theophylline

Trimethoprim/
  Sulfamethoxazole

BURNS
Benzocaine
Lidocaine HCl Topical
Somatropin

BURSITIS AND JOINT INFLAMMATION
Betamethasone Systemic
Cortisone Oral
Dexamethasone Systemic
Hydrocortisone Systemic
Methylprednisolone
Prednisolone Systemic
Triamcinolone Systemic

CANCER
Alitretinoin
Altretamine
Anastrozole
Capecitabine
Carmustine
Chlorambucil
Chlorotrianisene
Cyclophosphamide
Dacarbazine
Diethylstilbestrol (DES)
Estradiol
Estramustine Phosphate
  Sodium
Estrogens, Conjugated
Ethinyl Estradiol
Etoposide
Exemestane
Fluorouracil (5-FU)
Fluoxymesterone
Flutamide
Goserelin Acetate
Hydroxyurea
Interferon alfa-2a
Interferon alfa-2b
Interferon beta-1b
Interferon gamma-1b
Letrozole
Leucovorin Calcium
Leuprolide Acetate

Levamisole Hydrochloride
Levothyroxine Sodium
Lomustine
Medroxyprogesterone
  Acetate
Megestrol Acetate
Melphalan
Methotrexate
Mitotane
Nilutamide
Octreotide Acetate
Paclitaxel Injection
Tamoxifen Citrate
Testolactone
Testosterone
Toremifene
Uracil Mustard

CANKER SORES
Amlexanox
Benzocaine
Lidocaine HCl Topical

CHICKENPOX
Acyclovir

CHLAMYDIA
Azithromycin
Erythromycin Systemic
Ofloxacin Oral
Sulfacetamide
Sulfisoxazole Systemic
Trovafloxacin

CHOLESTEROL, HIGH LEVELS OF
Atorvastatin
Cholestyramine
Colestipol Hydrochloride
Fluvastatin
Gemfibrozil
Lovastatin
Pravastatin Sodium
Simvastatin

COLDS AND COUGH
Acetaminophen
Brompheniramine

Chlorpheniramine Maleate
  Oral
Codeine
Cyproheptadine HCl
Dextromethorphan
Diphenhydramine HCl
Ephedrine
Guaifenesin
Phenylephrine HCl Oph.
Phenylephrine HCl Systemic
Phenylpropanolamine HCl
Phenylpropanolamine/
  Guaifenesin
Promethazine Hydrochloride
Pseudoephedrine
Pseudoephedrine/
  Guaifenesin
Triprolidine Hydrochloride

COLD SORES
Benzocaine
Lidocaine HCl Topical
Penciclovir

COLITIS
(see Inflammatory Bowel
  Disease)

CONGESTION, NASAL AND SINUS
Brompheniramine
Chlorpheniramine Maleate
  Oral
Clemastine Fumarate
Diphenhydramine HCl
Ephedrine
Loratadine
Mometasone Furoate Nasal
Oxymetazoline Nasal
Phenylephrine HCl Systemic
Phenylpropanolamine HCl
Promethazine Hydrochloride
Pseudoephedrine
Triprolidine Hydrochloride

CONGESTIVE HEART FAILURE
Captopril
Carvedilol
Digitoxin
Digoxin
Enalapril Maleate
Lisinopril
Nitroglycerin

CONJUNCTIVITIS (ITCHY EYES) DUE TO ALLERGIES
Brompheniramine
Cetirizine
Chlorpheniramine Maleate Oral
Clemastine Fumarate
Cortisone Oral
Cyproheptadine HCl
Dexamethasone Ophthalmic
Dexamethasone Systemic
Dimenhydrinate
Diphenhydramine HCl
Emedastine Difumarate
Hydrocortisone Ophthalmic
Hydrocortisone Systemic
Hydroxyzine Hydrochloride
Ketorolac Tromethamine Ophthalmic
Ketotifen Fumarate
Loratadine
Loteprednol Etabonate
Medrysone
Methylprednisolone
Mometasone Furoate Nasal
Nedocromil Sodium Oph.
Olopatadine
Prednisolone Ophthalmic
Prednisolone Systemic
Prednisone
Promethazine Hydrochloride
Triamcinolone Systemic
Triprolidine Hydrochloride

CONJUNCTIVITIS (PINK EYE) DUE TO INFECTION
Ciprofloxacin Ophthalmic
Erythromycin Ophthalmic
Gentamicin
Natamycin
Norfloxacin
Ofloxacin Ophthalmic
Sulfacetamide
Sulfisoxazole Ophthalmic

CONSTIPATION
(see also Laxatives)
Bisacodyl
Castor Oil
Docusate
Glycerin Rectal
Lactulose
Magnesium Citrate
Magnesium Oxide
Magnesium Sulfate
Psyllium
Senna
Sodium Phosphate/Sodium Biphosphate

CONTRACEPTION
Contraceptives, Oral (Combination Products)
Contraceptives, Oral (Progestin)
Levonorgestrel Implants
Medroxyprogesterone Acetate
Progesterone Intrauterine System

CONVULSIONS
(see Epilepsy and Seizures)

COUGHING
Brompheniramine Maleate
Chlorpheniramine Maleate Oral
Codeine
Dextromethorphan
Diphenhydramine HCl
Ephedrine
Guaifenesin
Hydromorphone HCl
Morphine
Promethazine Hydrochloride
Pseudoephedrine/ Guaifenesin
Triprolidine Hydrochloride

CRAB LICE
Lindane
Pyrethrins and Piperonyl Butoxide

CROHN'S DISEASE
(see Inflammatory Bowel Disease)

CUSHING'S DISEASE/SYNDROME
Dexamethasone Systemic

CYSTIC FIBROSIS
Acetylcysteine
Amiloride Hydrochloride
Dornase Alfa
Tobramycin

CYSTITIS
(see Urinary Tract Infections)

DANDRUFF
Coal Tar
Ketoconazole Topical

DEMENTIA
Ergoloid Mesylates
Tacrine

DEPRESSION
Amitriptyline Hydrochloride
Amoxapine
Bupropion Hydrochloride
Citalopram Hydrobromide
Desipramine Hydrochloride
Doxepin Hydrochloride
Fluoxetine Hydrochloride
Fluvoxamine Maleate
Imipramine
Maprotiline Hydrochloride
Mirtazapine
Nefazodone Hydrochloride
Nortriptyline Hydrochloride
Paroxetine Hydrochloride
Phenelzine Sulfate
Protriptyline Hydrochloride
Sertraline Hydrochloride
Tranylcypromine Sulfate
Trazodone
Venlafaxine

DIABETES
Acarbose
Acetohexamide
Chlorpropamide
Glimepiride
Glipizide
Glyburide
Insulin Glargine (rDNA origin)
Insulin Lispro (rDNA origin)
Insulin (NPH)
Insulin (regular)
Insulin (Ultralente)
Metformin
Miglitol
Pioglitazone Hydrochloride
Repaglinide
Rosiglitazone
Tolazamide
Tolbutamide

DIABETES INSIPIDUS
Desmopressin Acetate
Vasopressin

DIAPER RASH
Clotrimazole
Econazole Nitrate
Nystatin
Petrolatum
Triamcinolone Topical
Undecylenic Acid
Zinc Oxide

DIARRHEA
Attapulgite
Bismuth Subsalicylate
Charcoal, Activated

Diphenoxylate HCl/
  Atropine Sulfate
Kaolin with Pectin
Loperamide Hydrochloride
Loperamide/Simethicone
Vancomycin

DIPHTHERIA
Diphtheria and Tetanus Tox-
  oids and Pertussis Vaccine
Erythromycin Systemic
Penicillin G
Penicillin V

DIZZINESS (VERTIGO)
Dimenhydrinate
Diphenhydramine HCl
Meclizine
Promethazine Hydrochloride

DROWSINESS
Caffeine

DRUG ADDICTION
Levomethadyl Acetate HCl
Methadone Hydrochloride
Naltrexone

EAR INFECTIONS
Amoxicillin
Amoxicillin/Potassium
  Clavulanate
Ampicillin
Bacampicillin Hydrochloride
Cefepime
Cefixime
Cefpodoxime Proxetil
Cefprozil
Cefuroxime
Cephalexin
Cephradine
Chloramphenicol Otic
Clarithromycin
Colistin/Neomycin/
  Hydrocortisone Otic
Doxycycline
Erythromycin Systemic
Gentamicin

Loracarbef
Minocycline
Ofloxacin Otic
Penicillin G
Penicillin V
Sulfisoxazole Systemic
Tetracycline Hydrochloride
Trimethoprim/
  Sulfamethoxazole

ECZEMA
(see Skin Inflammations,
  Irritations, and Rashes)

EDEMA
(see Fluid Retention)

ENDOMETRIOSIS
Danazol
Goserelin Acetate
Leuprolide Acetate
Nafarelin Acetate
Norethindrone

EPILEPSY AND SEIZURES
Acetazolamide
Carbamazepine
Clonazepam
Clorazepate Dipotassium
Ethosuximide
Felbamate
Gabapentin
Lamotrigine
Levetiracetam
Magnesium Sulfate
Mephenytoin
Pentobarbital Sodium
Phenobarbital
Phenytoin
Primidone
Tiagabine Hydrochloride
Topiramate
Valproic Acid (Divalproex)

ERECTILE DYSFUNCTION
Alprostadil Injection
Papaverine Hydrochloride

Sildenafil Citrate
Yohimbine

EYE INFECTIONS AND INFLAMMATION
Atropine Sulfate Ophthalmic
Brompheniramine
Chloramphenicol Oph-
  thalmic
Chlorpheniramine Maleate
  Oral
Ciprofloxacin Ophthalmic
Clemastine Fumarate
Cortisone Oral
Cromolyn Sodium Oph.
Cyclosporine
Cyproheptadine HCl
Dexamethasone Ophthalmic
Dexamethasone Systemic
Diclofenac Ophthalmic
Dimenhydrinate
Diphenhydramine HCl
Erythromycin Ophthalmic
Fexofenadine
Fexofenadine/
  Pseudoephedrine
Foscarnet Sodium
Ganciclovir Sodium
Gentamicin
Hydrocortisone Systemic
Hydroxyzine Hydrochloride
Idoxuridine
Ketorolac Tomethamine
  Ophthalmic
Loratadine
Loratadine/
  Pseudoephedrine
Loteprednol Etabonate
Medrysone
Methylprednisolone
Mometasone Furoate Nasal
Natamycin
Neomycin/Polymyxin B/
  Bacitracin Ophthalmic
Neomycin/Polymyxin B/
  Hydrocortisone Oph.
Norfloxacin
Ofloxacin Ophthalmic

Olopatadine
Oxymetazoline Ophthalmic
Pilocarpine Ophthalmic
Prednisolone Ophthalmic
Prednisolone Systemic
Prednisone
Promethazine Hydrochloride
Scopolamine Ophthalmic
Sulfacetamide
Sulfisoxazole Ophthalmic
Triamcinolone Systemic
Triprolidine Hydrochloride
Zinc Sulfate Ophthalmic
  Solution

FATIGUE
Caffeine

FEVER
Acetaminophen
Aspirin
Aspirin/Caffeine
Ibuprofen
Naproxen
Salsalate

FEVER BLISTERS
Benzocaine
Lidocaine HCl Topical

FLU
Amantadine Hydrochloride
Influenza Virus Vaccine
Oseltamivir Phosphate
Rimantadine Hydrochloride
Zanamavir

FLUID RETENTION
Bumetanide
Chlorothiazide
Ethacrynate and Ethacrynic
  Acid
Furosemide
Hydrochlorothiazide
Hydrochlorothiazide/
  Triamterene
Indapamide

Metolazone
Spironolactone
Torsemide
Triamterene

FUNGAL INFECTIONS
Amphotericin B
Betamethasone/Clotrimazole
Butoconazole Nitrate
Clotrimazole
Econazole Nitrate
Fluconazole
Itraconazole
Ketoconazole Oral
Ketoconazole Topical
Miconazole
Nystatin
Terbinafine Hydrochloride
Terconazole
Tolnaftate

GALLSTONES
Ursodiol

GAS
Charcoal, Activated
Loperamide/Simethicone
Simethicone

GENITAL WARTS
Imiquimod
Interferon alfa-2b
Interferon alfa-n1
Interferon alfa-n3
Podofilox

GIARDIASIS
Quinacrine Hydrochloride

GINGIVITIS AND GUM DISEASE
Chlorhexidine Gluconate
Doxycycline
Minocycline
Penicillin G
Penicillin V
Tetracycline Hydrochloride

GLAUCOMA
Acetazolamide
Betaxolol Ophthalmic
Brimonidine Tartrate
Brinzolamide
Carteolol HCl Ophthalmic
Dipivefrin
Dorzolamide Hydrochloride
Epinephrine Hydrochloride
Glycerin Oral
Latanoprost
Levobunolol
Pilocarpine Ophthalmic
Timolol Maleate Ophthalmic

GOITER
Levothyroxine Sodium
Liothyronine Sodium

GONORRHEA
Amoxicillin
Cefepime
Cefixime
Cefotetan Disodium
Cefpodoxime Proxetil
Cefuroxime
Enoxacin
Erythromycin Systemic
Gatifloxacin
Norfloxacin
Ofloxacin Oral
Trovafloxacin

GOUT
Allopurinol
Betamethasone Systemic
Colchicine
Cortisone Oral
Dexamethasone Systemic
Hydrocortisone Systemic
Indomethacin
Methylprednisolone
Naproxen
Prednisolone Systemic
Prednisone
Probenecid
Sulfinpyrazone

Sulindac
Triamcinolone Systemic

GROWTH FAILURE
Somatrem
Somatropin
Testosterone

HAIR LOSS
Minoxidil Topical

HAY FEVER
(see Allergies)

HEADACHES— MIGRAINE, SINUS, TENSION, VASCULAR
(see Pain Relievers for
    relief of simple
    headaches)
Acetaminophen/Aspirin/
    Caffeine
Butalbital/Acetaminophen/
    Caffeine
Butalbital/Acetaminophen/
    Caffeine/Codeine
Butalbital/Aspirin/Caffeine
Butalbital/Aspirin/Caffeine/
    Codeine Phosphate
Dihydroergotamine Mesylate
Ergotamine/Belladonna/
    Phenobarbital
Methysergide Mesylate
Naratriptan Hydrochloride
Propranolol Hydrochloride
Rizatriptan Benzoate
Sumatriptan Succinate
Timolol Maleate Oral
Valproic Acid (Divalproex)
Zolmitriptan

HEAD LICE
Lindane
Permethrin
Pyrethrins and Piperonyl
    Butoxide

HEART ATTACK PREVENTION
Aspirin
Atenolol
Clopidogrel Bisulfate
Dipyridamole
Metoprolol
Propranolol Hydrochloride
Timolol Maleate Oral
Warfarin

HEARTBURN
Aluminum Salts
Cimetidine
Cisapride
Famotidine
Magaldrate
Magnesium Oxide
Metoclopramide HCl
Nizatadine
Omeprazole
Pantoprazole Sodium
Rabeprazole Sodium
Ranitidine

HEART FAILURE
(see Congestive Heart
    Failure)

HEART RHYTHM DISORDERS
Amiodarone
Digitoxin
Digoxin
Diltiazem Hydrochloride
Disopyramide
Flecainide Acetate
Mexiletine Hydrochloride
Phenylephrine HCl Systemic
Procainamide Hydrochloride
Propafenone
Propranolol Hydrochloride
Quinidine
Sotalol Hydrochloride
Tocainide Hydrochloride
Verapamil Hydrochloride

HEMORRHOIDS
Benzocaine
Hydrocortisone Topical

HEPATITIS
Hepatitis A Vaccine
Hepatitis B Vaccine
Interferon Alfa-2b
Interferon Beta-1b

HERPES, GENITAL
Acyclovir

HICCUPS, INTRACTABLE
Chlorpromazine HCl

HIGH BLOOD PRESSURE
Acebutolol Hydrochloride
Amiloride Hydrochloride
Amlodipine
Atenolol
Atenolol/Chlorthalidone
Benazepril Hydrochloride
Betaxolol Oral
Bisoprolol Fumarate
Bisoprolol/
  Hydrochlorothiazide
Candesartan Cilexetil
Captopril
Carteolol Hydrochloride Oral
Carvedilol
Chlorthalidone
Chlorothiazide
Clonidine Hydrochloride
Diltiazem Hydrochloride
Doxazosin Mesylate
Enalapril Maleate
Enalapril Maleate/Diltiazem
  Malate
Enalapril Maleate/Felodipine
Enalapril/
  Hydrochlorothiazide
Felodipine
Fosinopril Sodium
Furosemide
Guanabenz Acetate
Guanadrel Sulfate
Guanethidine Monosulfate

Guanfacine Hydrochloride
Hydralazine Hydrochloride
Hydrochlorothiazide
Hydrochlorothiazide/
  Triamterene
Indapamide
Irbesartan
Isradipine
Labetalol Hydrochloride
Lisinopril
Lisinopril/
  Hydrochlorothiazide
Losartan Potassium
Methyldopa and Methyl-
  dopate Hydrochloride
Metolazone
Metoprolol
Minoxidil Oral
Moexipril Hydrochloride
Moexipril Hydrochloride/
  Hydrochlorothiazide
Nadolol
Nicardipine HCl Oral
Nifedipine
Penbutolol Sulfate
Perindopril Erbumine
Pindolol
Prazosin
Propranolol Hydrochloride
Propranolol/
  Hydrochlorothiazide
Quinapril Hydrochloride
Quinapril Hydrochloride/
  Hydrochlorothiazide
Ramipril
Spironolactone
Spironolactone/
  Hydrochlorothiazide
Telmisartan
Terazosin
Timolol Maleate Oral
Torsemide
Trandolapril
Trandolapril/Verapamil HCl
Triamterene
Valsartan

Valsartan/
  Hydrochlorothiazide
Verapamil Hydrochloride

HIV INFECTION
(see AIDS)

HIVES
Brompheniramine
Cetirizine
Chlorpheniramine Maleate
  Oral
Clemastine Fumarate
Cyproheptadine HCl
Dimenhydrinate
Diphenhydramine HCl
Fexofenadine
Fexofenadine/
  Pseudoephedrine
Hydroxyzine Hydrochloride
Loratadine
Loratadine/
  Pseudoephedrine
Mometasone Furoate Nasal
Promethazine Hydrochloride
Triprolidine Hydrochloride

HYPERTHYROIDISM
Iodine, Strong
Methimazole
Propylthiouracil

HYPOGLYCEMIA
Diazoxide
Glucagon

HYPOTHYROIDISM
Levothyroxine Sodium
Liothyronine Sodium

IMPETIGO
Mupirocin

INDIGESTION
(see Acid Indigestion and
  Upset Stomach)

INFERTILITY
Bromocriptine Mesylate
Clomiphene Citrate
Progesterone Systemic

INFLAMMATORY BOWEL DISEASE
Aminosalicylate Sodium
Betamethasone Systemic
Budesonide
Cortisone Oral
Dexamethasone Systemic
Hydrocortisone Systemic
Hydrocortisone Topical
Mesalamine
Methylprednisolone
Olsalazine Sodium
Prednisolone Systemic
Prednisone
Sulfasalazine
Triamcinolone Systemic

INSECT BITES AND STINGS
Benzocaine
Calamine
Epinephrine Hydrochloride
Lidocaine HCl Topical

INSOMNIA
Chloral Hydrate
Diazepam
Diphenhydramine HCl
Estazolam
Ethchlorvynol
Flurazepam Hydrochloride
Lorazepam
Pentobarbital Sodium
Quazepam
Temazepam
Triazolam
Zaleplon
Zolpidem

IRREGULAR HEARTBEATS
(see Heart Rhythm
  Disorders)

IRRITABLE BOWEL SYNDROME
Alosetron HCl (women only)
Atropine Sulfate Oral
Atropine Sulfate/Scopo-
    lamine Hydrobromide/
    Hyoscyamine Sulfate/
    Phenobarbital
Dicyclomine Hydrochloride
Loperamide Hydrochloride
Phenobarbital
Psyllium

JOCK ITCH
Clotrimazole
Econazole Nitrate
Griseofulvin
Haloprogin
Ketoconazole Topical
Miconazole
Terbinafine Hydrochloride
Tolnaftate
Undecylenic Acid

KIDNEY STONES
Allopurinol

LEG CRAMPS
Pentoxifylline

LEGIONNAIRES' DISEASE
Dirithromycin
Erythromycin Systemic

LEUKEMIA
Betamethasone Systemic
Busulfan
Chlorambucil
Cortisone Oral
Cyclophosphamide
Dexamethasone Systemic
Hydrocortisone Systemic
Hydroxyurea
Interferon Alfa-2a
Interferon Alfa-2b
Interferon Alfa-n1
Mercaptopurine
Methotrexate

Methylprednisolone
Mitoxantrone Hydrochloride
Prednisolone Systemic
Prednisone
Thioguanine
Tretinoin
Triamcinolone Systemic
Uracil Mustard

LICE
Lindane
Permethrin
Pyrethrins and Piperonyl
    Butoxide

LOW BLOOD PRESSURE
Midodrine Hydrochloride

LISTERIOSIS
Erythromycin Systemic
Penicillin G

LOU GEHRIG'S DISEASE
(see Amyotrophic Lateral
    Sclerosis)

LUNG DISEASE
Albuterol
Aminophylline
Bitolterol Mesylate
Ephedrine
Epinephrine Hydrochloride
Ipratropium Bromide
Isoetharine
Isoproterenol
Metaproterenol Sulfate
Phenylephrine HCl Systemic
Pirbuterol Acetate
Terbutaline Sulfate
Theophylline

LUPUS
Betamethasone Systemic
Cortisone Oral
Cyclophosphamide
Dexamethasone
Fluticasone

Hydrocortisone Topical
Hydroxychloroquine Sulfate
Methylprednisolone
Mometasone Furoate Topical
Prednisolone Systemic
Triamcinolone Systemic

LYME DISEASE
Cefuroxime
Lyme Disease Vaccine
    (Recombinant OspA)

MALARIA
Chloroquine
Doxycycline
Hydroxychloroquine Sulfate
Mefloquine Hydrochloride
Primaquine
Quinacrine Hydrochloride
Quinidine
Sulfisoxazole Systemic

MANIC-DEPRESSIVE ILLNESS
Lithium

MEASLES
Measles, Mumps, Rubella
    Vaccine

MELANOMA
Hydroxyurea
Interferon Alfa-n1
Interferon Beta-1b
Melphalan

MENOPAUSE
Chlorotrianisene
Ergotamine/Belladonna/
    Phenobarbital
Estradiol
Estrogens, Conjugated
Estrogens, Conjugated/Med-
    roxyprogesterone Acetate
Estropipate
Ethinyl Estradiol

MENSTRUAL CRAMPS
Diclofenac Systemic
Ibuprofen
Ketoprofen
Meclofenamate Sodium
Mefenamic Acid
Naproxen

MENSTRUAL PERIODS, REGULATION OF
Bromocriptine Mesylate
Medroxyprogesterone
    Acetate
Norethindrone
Progesterone Systemic

MENTAL CAPACITY, DECLINE IN
Ergoloid Mesylates

MIGRAINES
(see Headaches)

MOTION SICKNESS
Dimenhydrinate
Diphenhydramine HCl
Meclizine
Promethazine Hydrochloride
Scopolamine Systemic

MOUNTAIN SICKNESS (HIGH ALTITUDE ILLNESS)
Acetazolamide

MULTIPLE SCLEROSIS
Baclofen
Betamethasone Systemic
Colchicine
Cortisone Oral
Dexamethasone Systemic
Glatiramer Acetate
Hydrocortisone Systemic
Interferon Beta-1a
Interferon Beta-1b
Methylprednisolone
Prednisolone Systemic
Prednisone
Triamcinolone Systemic

MUMPS
Measles, Mumps, Rubella Vaccine

MUSCLE SPASM
Carisoprodol
Chlorzoxazone
Cyclobenzaprine
Dantrolene Sodium
Methocarbamol
Orphenadrine Citrate
Tizanidine Hydrochloride

MYASTHENIA GRAVIS
Neostigmine

NAIL FUNGUS
Griseofulvin
Terbinafine Hydrochloride

NARCOLEPSY
Amphetamine
Amphetamine/
 Dextroamphetamine
Dextroamphetamine Sulfate
Ephedrine
Methylphenidate HCl

NASAL CONGESTION
(see Congestion, Nasal and Sinus)

NASAL POLYPS
Beclomethasone Inhalant and Nasal
Betamethasone Systemic
Budesonide
Cortisone Oral
Dexamethasone Inhalant and Nasal
Dexamethasone Systemic
Flunisolide
Hydrocortisone Systemic
Methylprednisolone
Prednisolone Systemic
Prednisone
Triamcinolone Systemic

NAUSEA AND VOMITING
(see also Motion Sickness)
Bismuth Subsalicylate
Chlorpromazine HCl
Dronabinol
Hydroxyzine Hydrochloride
Metoclopramide HCl
Ondansetron Hydrochloride
Perphenazine
Prochlorperazine
Promethazine Hydrochloride
Trimethobenzamide HCl

NEURALGIA/NERVE DYSFUNCTION
(see also Trigeminal Neuralgia)
Capsaicin
Nimodipine

OBESITY
Amphetamine
Benzphetamine
Dexfenfluramine
Dextroamphetamine Sulfate
Diethylpropion HCl
Orlistat
Phentermine
Phenylpropanolamine HCl
Sibutramine Hydrochloride Monohydrate

OBSESSIVE-COMPULSIVE DISORDERS
Clomipramine Hydrochloride
Fluoxetine Hydrochloride
Fluvoxamine Maleate
Paroxetine Hydrochloride

OSTEOARTHRITIS
(see Arthritis)

OSTEOPOROSIS
Alendronate Sodium
Calcitonin-Salmon
Estrogens, Conjugated

Estrogens, Conjugated/Medroxyprogesterone Acetate
Estradiol
Estropipate
Ethinyl Estradiol
Raloxifene Hydrochloride
Risedronate Sodium

PAGET'S DISEASE OF BONE
Alendronate Sodium
Calcitonin-Salmon
Etidronate Disodium
Risedronate Sodium
Tiludronate Disodium

PAIN RELIEVERS
Acetaminophen
Acetaminophen/Codeine Phosphate
Aspirin
Aspirin/Caffeine
Benzocaine
Butorphanol Tartrate
Clonidine Hydrochloride
Codeine
Diclofenac Systemic
Diflunisal
Etodolac
Fenoprofen Calcium
Fentanyl Transdermal
Fentanyl Transmucosal
Hydrocodone Bitartrate/ Acetaminophen
Hydrocodone Bitartrate/ Ibuprofen
Hydromorphone HCl
Ibuprofen
Ketoprofen
Ketorolac Tromethamine Systemic
Lidocaine HCl Topical
Meclofenamate Sodium
Mefenamic Acid
Meperidine Hydrochloride
Methadone Hydrochloride
Morphine
Nalbuphine Hydrochloride

Naproxen
Nifedipine
Oxycodone Hydrochloride
Oxycodone/Acetaminophen
Oxycodone/Aspirin
Pentazocine
Promethazine Hydrochloride
Propoxyphene
Propoxyphene/ Acetaminophen
Rofecoxib
Ropivacaine Hydrochloride Monohydrate
Salsalate
Simethicone
Sulindac
Tolmetin Sodium
Tramadol Hydrochloride

PANCREATIC ENZYME DEFICIENCY
Pancrelipase

PANIC ATTACKS
Alprazolam
Paroxetine Hydrochloride

PARASITIC INFECTIONS
(see also Malaria)
Albendazole
Atovaquone
Mebendazole
Pentamidine Isethionate
Piperazine Citrate
Praziquantel
Pyrantel Pamoate
Quinacrine Hydrochloride
Thiabendazole

PARKINSON'S DISEASE
Amantadine Hydrochloride
Benztropine Mesylate
Biperiden
Bromocriptine Mesylate
Diphenhydramine HCl
Entacapone
Levodopa
Levodopa/Carbidopa

Pergolide Mesylate
Pramipexole
Procyclidine
Ropinirole Hydrochloride
Selegiline Hydrochloride
Tolcapone
Trihexyphenidyl HCl

PELVIC INFECTIONS
Ampicillin Sodium/
  Sulbactam Sodium
Cefotetan Disodium
Clindamycin
Gatifloxacin
Metronidazole
Trovafloxacin

PERTUSSIS
(see Whooping Cough)

PIMPLES
(see Acne)

PINKEYE
(see Eye Infections,
  Conjunctivitis)

PINWORMS
Albendazole
Mebendazole
Piperazine Citrate
Pyrantel Pamoate

PNEUMONIA
Acetylcysteine
Amoxicillin
Amoxicillin/Potassium
  Clavulanate
Ampicillin
Atovaquone
Azithromycin
Bacampicillin Hydrochloride
Clindamycin
Carbenicillin Indanyl Sodium
Cefaclor
Cefamandole Nafate
Cefazolin
Cefepime

Cefotetan Disodium
Cefpodoxime Proxetil
Cefuroxime
Cephalexin
Cephradine
Ciprofloxacin Systemic
Clarithromycin
Clindamycin
Dicloxacillin Sodium
Doxycycline
Erythromycin Systemic
Flucytosine
Gatifloxacin
Gentamicin
Levofloxacin
Linezolid
Loracarbef
Metronidazole
Minocycline
Moxifloxacin
Ofloxacin Oral
Penicillin G
Pentamidine Isethionate
Pneumococcal Vaccine
Primaquine
Sparfloxacin
Tetracycline Hydrochloride
Tobramycin
Trimethoprim/
  Sulfamethoxazole
Trovafloxacin

POISONING
Charcoal, Activated
Ipecac Syrup

POLIO
Poliovirus Vaccine, Oral

PROSTATE ENLARGEMENT, BENIGN
Doxazosin Mesylate
Finasteride
Terazosin

PSORIASIS
Acitretin
Betamethasone Topical

Calcipotriene
Coal Tar
Fluticasone
Hydrocortisone Topical
Mometasone Furoate Topical
Resorcinol
Tazarotene

PSYCHOTIC DISORDERS
Chlorpromazine HCl
Clozapine
Fluphenazine
Haloperidol
Loxapine
Molindone
Olanzapine
Perphenazine
Prochlorperazine
Quetiapine Fumarate
Risperidone
Thioridazine Hydrochloride
Thiothixene
Trifluoperazine HCl

RASHES
(see Skin Irritations,
  Inflammation, and
  Rashes)

RHEUMATIC FEVER
Aspirin
Erythromycin Systemic
Penicillin G
Penicillin V
Salsalate

RHEUMATOID ARTHRITIS
(see Arthritis)

RINGWORM
Clotrimazole
Econazole Nitrate
Griseofulvin
Haloprogin
Ketoconazole Topical
Miconazole
Terfenadine Hydrochloride

Tolnaftate
Undecylenic Acid

ROCKY MOUNTAIN SPOTTED FEVER
Chloramphenicol Oral
Doxycycline
Minocycline
Tetracycline Hydrochloride

RUBELLA
Measles, Mumps, Rubella
  Vaccine

RUNNY NOSE AND POSTNASAL DRIP
Brompheniramine
Cetirizine
Chlorpheniramine Maleate
  Oral
Clemastine Fumarate
Cyproheptadine HCl
Dimenhydrinate
Diphenhydramine HCl
Hydroxyzine Hydrochloride
Ipratropium Bromide
Loratadine
Mometasone Furoate Nasal
Oxymetazoline Nasal
Promethazine Hydrochloride
Triprolidine Hydrochloride

SCABIES
Lindane
Permethrin
Sulfur Topical

SCHIZOPHRENIA
(see also Psychotic
  Disorders)
Clozapine
Molindone
Olanzapine
Quetiapine Fumarate

SEBORRHEA
(see Skin Irritations)

SEIZURES
(see Epilepsy and Seizures)

SHINGLES (HERPES ZOSTER)
Acyclovir
Famciclovir
Valacyclovir Hydrochloride

SICKLE CELL DISEASE
Hydroxyurea

SINUS CONGESTION
(see Congestion, Nasal and Sinus)

SINUS INFECTION
Amoxicillin
Amoxicillin/Potassium
  Clavulanate
Ampicillin
Bacampicillin Hydrochloride
Clarithromycin
Doxycycline
Erythromycin Systemic
Gatifloxacin
Levofloxacin
Loracarbef
Minocycline
Moxifloxacin
Oxacillin
Sparfloxacin
Tetracycline Hydrochloride

SKIN IRRITATIONS, INFLAMMATION, AND RASHES
Benzocaine
Betamethasone Systemic
Betamethasone Topical
Betamethasone/Clotrimazole
Calamine
Coal Tar
Cortisone Oral
Dexamethasone Systemic
Dexamethasone Topical
Fluticasone

Hydrocortisone Systemic
Hydrocortisone Topical
Lidocaine HCl Topical
Masoprocol
Methylprednisolone
Mometasone Furoate Topical
Prednisolone Systemic
Prednisone
Resorcinol
Sulfur Topical
Triamcinolone Systemic
Triamcinolone Topical

SLEEP PROBLEMS
(see Insomnia, Narcolepsy)

SMOKING CESSATION
Nicotine

SNEEZING
Azelastine
Brompheniramine
Chlorpheniramine Maleate
  Oral
Clemastine Fumarate
Cyproheptadine HCl
Diphenhydramine HCl
Fexofenadine
Fexofenadine/
  Pseudoephedrine
Hydroxyzine Hydrochloride
Loratadine
Loratadine/
  Pseudoephedrine
Mometasone Furoate Nasal
Promethazine Hydrochloride
Triprolidine Hydrochloride

SPASTIC COLON
(see Irritable Bowel Disease)

STINGS, INSECT
Epinephrine Hydrochloride

STREP THROAT
Azithromycin

Clarithromycin
Dirithromycin
Doxycycline
Erythromycin Systemic

SUNBURN
Betamethasone Topical
Fluticasone
Hydrocortisone Topical
Triamcinolone Topical
Zinc Oxide

SYPHILIS
Doxycycline
Erythromycin Systemic
Minocycline
Penicillin G
Tetracycline Hydrochloride

TETANUS
Amobarbital Sodium
Chlorpromazine HCl
Diphtheria and Tetanus Tox-
  oids and Pertussis Vaccine
Penicillin G
Pentobarbital Sodium
Phenobarbital

THRUSH
Clotrimazole
Fluconazole
Ketoconazole Oral
Miconazole
Nystatin

THYROID HORMONE DEFICIENCY
Levothyroxine Sodium

THYROID DISEASE
(see Hyperthyroidism, Hypothyroidism)

TONSILLITIS
Cefaclor
Cefadroxil
Cefepime
Cefixime

Cefpodoxime Proxetil
Cefprozil
Cefuroxime
Cephradine

TOOTHACHE
Benzocaine

TOURETTE'S SYNDROME
Haloperidol

TOXOPLASMOSIS
Sulfisoxazole Systemic

TRANSPLANT REJECTION
Azathioprine
Cyclosporine
Muromonab-CD3
Mycophenolate Mofetil
Tacrolimus (FK506)

TRAVELER'S DIARRHEA
Loperamide Hydrochloride
Trimethoprim/
  Sulfamethoxazole

TREMORS
Propranolol Hydrochloride

TRIGEMINAL NEURALGIA (TIC DOULOUREUX)
Carbamazepine

TUBERCULOSIS
Acetylcysteine
Aminosalicylate Sodium
Betamethasone Systemic
Cortisone Oral
Cycloserine
Dexamethasone Systemic
Hydrocortisone Systemic
Isoniazid
Methylprednisolone
Prednisolone Systemic
Prednisone
Pyrazinamide
Rifabutin
Rifampin

Rifapentine
Triamcinolone Systemic

TYPHOID FEVER
Chloramphenicol Oral
Ciprofloxacin Systemic

TYPHUS FEVER
Chloramphenicol Oral
Doxycycline
Minocycline
Tetracycline Hydrochloride

ULCERS
Aluminum Salts
Atropine Sulfate Oral
Cimetidine
Clarithromycin
Famotidine
Glycopyrrolate
Lansoprazole
Magaldrate
Magnesium Oxide
Milk of Magnesia
Misoprostol
Nizatidine
Omeprazole
Pantoprazole Sodium
Propantheline Bromide
Rabeprazole Sodium
Ranitidine
Ranitidine Bismuth Citrate
Sodium Bicarbonate
Sucralfate

URINARY TRACT INFECTIONS
Amoxicillin
Amoxicillin/Potassium
   Clavulanate
Ampicillin
Bacampicillin Hydrochloride
Carbenicillin Indanyl Sodium
Cefaclor
Cefadroxil
Cefamandole Nafate
Cefazolin
Cefepime

Cefixime
Cefotetan Disodium
Cefpodoxime Proxetil
Cefuroxime
Cephalexin
Cephradine
Ciprofloxacin Systemic
Doxycycline
Enoxacin
Flavoxate
Flucytosine
Fosfomycin Tromethamine
Gatifloxacin
Gentamicin
Levofloxacin
Lomefloxacin Hydrochloride
Loracarbef
Methenamine and
   Methenamine Salts
Minocycline
Nalidixic Acid
Nitrofurantoin
Norfloxacin
Ofloxacin Oral
Pentosan Polysulfate Sodium
Sulfisoxazole Systemic
Tetracycline Hydrochloride
Tobramycin
Trimethoprim/
   Sulfamethoxazole

URINARY TRACT PAIN/DISORDERS
Bethanechol Chloride
Flavoxate
Methenamine
Oxybutynin Chloride
Pentosan Polysulfate Sodium
Phenazopyridine HCl

VAGINAL IRRITATION OR INFECTION
(see also Yeast Infections)
Chlorotrianisene
Clindamycin
Estradiol
Estrogens, Conjugated
Estrogens, Conjugated/Med-

roxyprogesterone Acetate
Estropipate
Ethinyl Estradiol
Medroxyprogesterone
   Acetate
Metronidazole

VERTIGO
(see Dizziness)

VITAMIN AND MINERAL DEFICIENCY/DIETARY SUPPLEMENTS
Beta Carotene
Biotin
Calcitriol
Calcium
Folacin (Folic Acid, Folate)
Potassium Chloride
Vitamin A
Vitamin B1
Vitamin B2
Vitamin B3
Vitamin B6
Vitamin B12
Vitamin C
Vitamin D
Vitamin E
Vitamin K1
Zinc Sulfate Systemic

VOMITING
(see also Nausea)
Ipecac Syrup (to induce)
Metoclopramide HCl
Ondansetron Hydrochloride
Prochlorperazine
Promethazine Hydrochloride
Trimethobenzamide HCl

WARTS
Resorcinol

WASTING (IN AIDS)
Dronabinol
Megestrol Acetate
Somatropin
Testosterone

WEIGHT LOSS
(see Obesity)

WHEEZING
(see Asthma)

WHOOPING COUGH (PERTUSSIS)
Diphtheria and Tetanus Tox-
   oids and Pertussis Vaccine
Erythromycin Systemic

WORMS
(see Parasitic Infections)

WOUNDS AND CUTS
Bacitracin
Benzocaine
Iodine Topical
Lidocaine HCl Topical
Neomycin/Polymyxin B/
   Bacitracin Topical

WRINKLES
Tretinoin

YEAST INFECTIONS, VAGINAL
Butoconazole Nitrate
Clotrimazole
Econazole Nitrate
Fluconazole
Miconazole
Nystatin
Terconazole
Tioconazole

COLOR PILL LOCATOR

Nicotine 2 mg Nicorette HOECHST MARION ROUSSEL	**Cyclosporine** 100 mg Sandimmune SANDOZ	**Cyclosporine** 25 mg Sandimmune SANDOZ	**Thioridazine Hydrochloride** 25 mg Generic CREIGHTON
Thiothixene 5 mg Generic MYLAN	**Olsalazine Sodium** 250 mg Dipentum PHARMACIA	**Verapamil Hydrochloride** 120 mg Isoptin SR KNOLL	**Zalcitabine** 0.375 mg HIVID ROCHE
Cimetidine 300mg Tagamet SMITHKLINE BEECHAM	**Levodopa/Carbidopa** 200/50 mg Sinemet DUPONT	**Lamotrigine** 100 mg Lamictal GLAXO WELLCOME	**Pancrelipase** 30,000/8,000/30,000 units Viokase A.H. ROBINS
Famotidine 20 mg Pepcid MERCK	**Cefprozil** 250 mg Cefzil BRISTOL-MYERS SQUIBB	**Ofloxacin** 400 mg Floxin ORTHO	**Ofloxacin Oral** 200 mg Floxin ORTHO
Phenolphthalein 90 mg Ex-Lax SANDOZ	**Nizatidine** 75 mg Axid AR WHITEHALL-ROBINS	**Primidone** 250 mg Mysoline WYETH-AYERST	**Dexamethasone** 0.5 mg Generic ROXANE

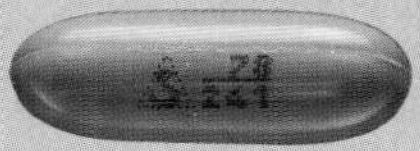

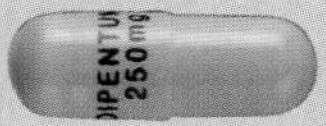

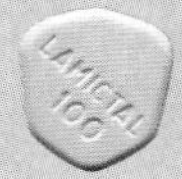

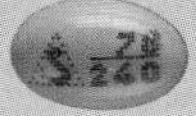

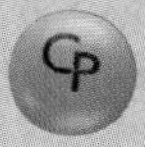

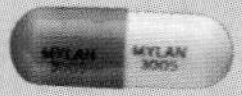

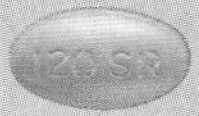

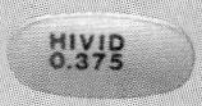

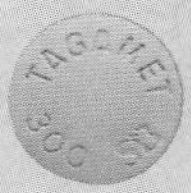

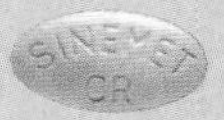

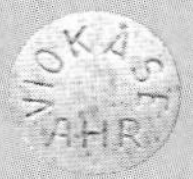

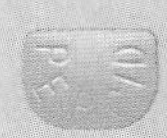

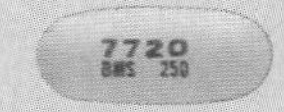

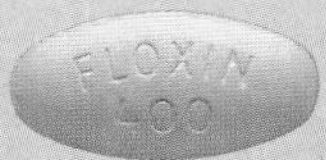

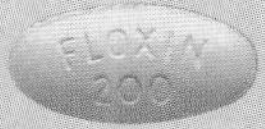

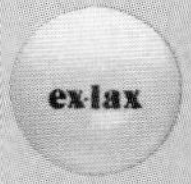

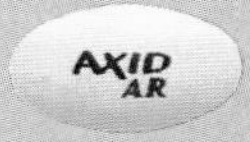

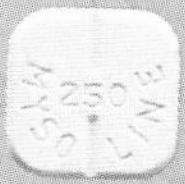

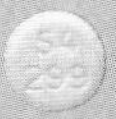

COLOR PILL LOCATOR

▼

Moexipril HCl/HCTZ 7.5/12.5 mg Uniretic SCHWARZ PHARMA	**Naltrexone** 50 mg Revia DUPONT	**Pantoprazole Sodium** 40 mg Protonix WYETH	**Simvastatin** 5 mg Zocor MERCK
Verapamil Hydrochloride 240 mg Isoptin SR KNOLL	**Mebendazole** 100 mg Generic COPLEY	**Dronabinol** 2.5 mg Marinol ROXANE	**Fluoxymesterone** 5 mg Halotestin UPJOHN
Clozapine 25 mg Clozaril NOVARTIS	**Levothyroxine Sodium** 0.1 mg Levoxyl DANIELS	**Amoxicillin** 500 mg Generic BIOCRAFT	**Nimodipine** 30 mg Nimotop BAYER
Doxepin Hydrochloride 50 mg Generic MYLAN	**Amiloride Hydrochloride** 5 mg Midamor MERCK	**Pergolide Mesylate** 0.05 mg Permax ATHENA	**Thioguanine** 40 mg Generic GLAXO WELLCOME
Nefazodone Hydrochloride 200 mg Serzone BRISTOL-MYERS SQUIBB	**Phenytoin** 50 mg Dilantin PARKE-DAVIS	**Chlorthalidone** 25 mg Generic MYLAN	**Folic Acid** 1 mg Generic WEST-WARD

COLOR PILL LOCATOR

Methylphenidate
5 mg
Generic
MD PHARM

Aspirin
81 mg
Bayer Adult Low Strength
BAYER

Simethicone
150 mg
Maalox Anti-Gas Extra Strength
NOVARTIS

Propranolol Hydrochloride
80 mg
Generic
WATSON

Chlorpheniramine Maleate
8 mg
Chlor-Trimeton Allergy 8 Hour
SCHERING-PLOUGH

Clarithromycin
250 mg
Biaxin
ABBOTT

Penicillamine
125 mg
Cuprimine
MERCK

Clarithromycin
500 mg
Biaxin
ABBOTT

Salsalate
750 mg
Generic
SIDMAK

Estropipate
0.75 mg
Generic
WATSON

Methotrexate
2.5 mg
Generic
MYLAN

Desipramine Hydrochloride
25 mg
Generic
SIDMAK

Phenylpropanolamine
75 mg
Dexatrim Maximum Strength
THOMPSON MEDICAL

Probenecid
500 mg
Generic
SCHEIN

Salsalate
500 mg
Generic
SIDMAK

Aspirin
81 mg
Generic
LNK

Tiagabine Hydrochloride
4 mg
Gabitril
ABBOTT

Acetaminophen
500 mg
Tylenol Extra Strength
MCNEIL

Azathioprine
50 mg
Generic
ROXANE

Nadolol
40 mg
Generic
MYLAN

Fluvoxamine Maleate 50 mg Luvox SOLVAY	**Chlorpheniramine Maleate** 4 mg Chlor-Trimeton Allergy 4 Hour SCHERING-PLOUGH	**Haloperidol** 1 mg Generic GENEVA	**Colestipol Hydrochloride** 1 gram Colestid PHARMACIA & UPJOHN
Vitamin K1 5 mg Mephyton MERCK	**Mirtazapine** 15 mg Remeron ORGANON	**Felbamate** 400 mg Felbatol WALLACE	**Cyclobenzaprine** 10 mg Generic MYLAN
Levodopa/Carbidopa 100/25 mg Generic LEMMON	**Procarbazine Hydrochloride** 50 mg Matulane SIGMA-TAU	**Chlorpheniramine Maleate** 4 mg Generic ADVANCE	**Clofibrate** 500 mg Generic ROSEMONT
Carbenicillin Indanyl Sodium 382 mg Geocillin ROERIG	**Nifedipine** 10 mg Generic PUREPAC	**Estrogen, Conjugated** 1.25 mg Premarin WYETH-AYERST	**Prochlorperazine** 5 mg Compazine SMITHKLINE BEECHAM
Ibuprofen 200 mg Nuprin BRISTOL-MYERS SQUIBB	**Penbutolol Sulfate** 20 mg Levatol SCHWARZ PHARMA	**Phentermine** 30 mg Generic EON	**Rabeprazole Sodium** 20 mg Aciphex EISAI INC./JANSSEN PHARMACEUTICA

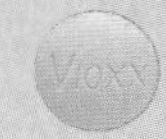

COLOR PILL LOCATOR

Rofecoxib
25 mg
Vioxx
MERCK

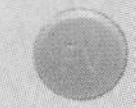

Letrozole
2.5 mg
Femara
NOVARTIS

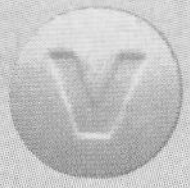

Caffeine
200 mg
Vivarin
SMITHKLINE BEECHAM

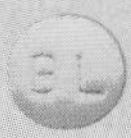

Imipramine
10 mg
Generic
BIOCRAFT

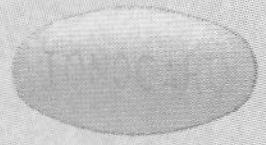

Tocainide Hydrochloride
400 mg
Tonocard
ASTRA MERCK

Ondansetron Hydrochloride
8 mg
Zofran
GLAXO WELLCOME

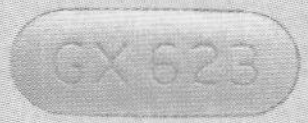

Abacavir Sulfate
300 mg
Ziagen
GLAXO WELLCOME

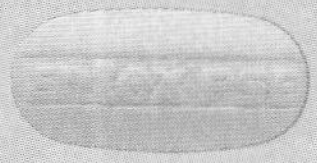

Pseudoephedrine/Guaifenesin
120/600 mg
Entex PSE
WELPHARM

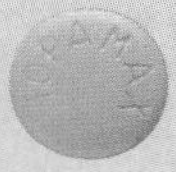

Topiramate
100 mg
Topamax
MCNEIL

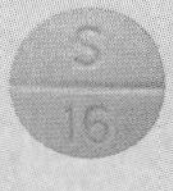

Sulindac
150 mg
Generic
MYLAN

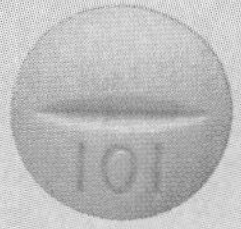

Sulfasalazine
500 mg
Azulfidine
PHARMACIA

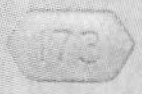

Enalapril Maleate/HCTZ
5/12.5 mg
Generic
MERCK

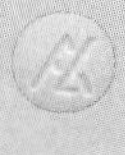

Levothyroxine Sodium
0.3 mg
Levothroid
FOREST

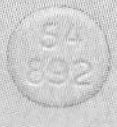

Dexamethasone
4 mg
Generic
ROXANE

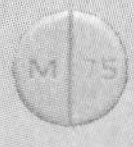

Chlorthalidone
50 mg
Generic
MYLAN

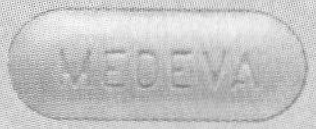

Guaifenesin
600 mg
Humibid L.A.
MEDEVA

Calcium
500 mg
Os-Cal 500
SMITHKLINE BEECHAM

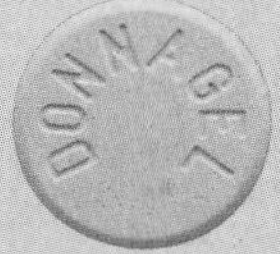

Attapulgite
600 mg
Donnagel
WYETH-AYERST

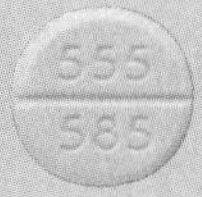

Chlorzoxazone
500 mg
Generic
BARR

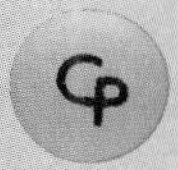

Thioridazine Hydrochloride
100 mg
Generic
CREIGHTON

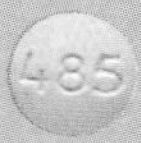

COLOR PILL LOCATOR

Leucovorin Calcium
25 mg
Generic
BARR

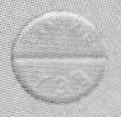

Digoxin
0.125 mg
Lanoxin
GLAXO WELLCOME

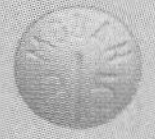

Molindone
25 mg
Moban
GATE

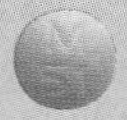

Amitriptyline Hydrochloride
25 mg
Generic
MYLAN

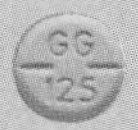

Haloperidol
5 mg
Generic
GENEVA

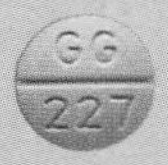

Isosorbide Dinitrate
20 mg
Generic
GENEVA

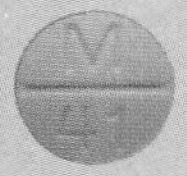

Spironolactone/HCTZ
25/25 mg
Generic
MYLAN

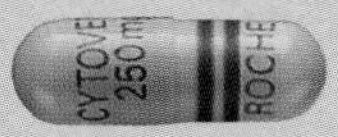

Ganciclovir
250 mg
Cytovene
ROCHE

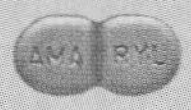

Glimepiride
2 mg
Amaryl
HOECHST MARION ROUSSEL

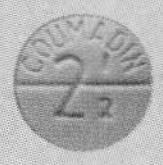

Warfarin
2.5 mg
Coumadin
DUPONT

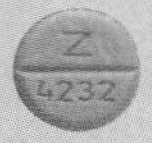

Bumetanide
0.5 mg
Generic
ZENITH

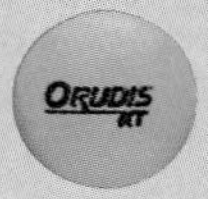

Ketoprofen
12.5 mg
Orudis KT
WHITEHALL-ROBINS

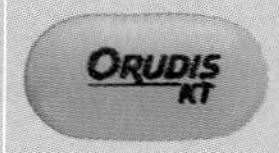

Ketoprofen
12.5 mg
Orudis KT Caplets
WHITEHALL-ROBINS

Ferrous Gluconate
320 mg
Fergon
BAYER

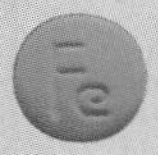

Ferrous Gluconate
300 mg
Generic
UPSHER-SMITH

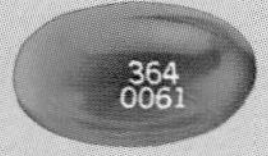

Chloral Hydrate
500 mg
Generic
SCHEIN

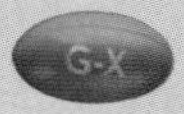

Simethicone
125 mg
Gas-X Extra Strength
NOVARTIS

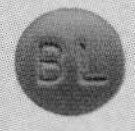

Imipramine
50 mg
Generic
BIOCRAFT

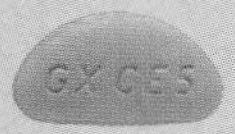

Naratriptan Hydrochloride
2.5 mg
Amerge
GLAXO WELLCOME

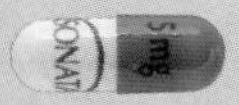

Zaleplon
5 mg
Sonata
WYETH

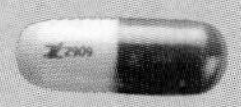

Hydroxyzine Pamoate
50 mg
Generic
ZENITH

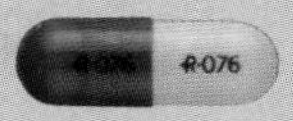

Temazepam
15 mg
Generic
PUREPAC

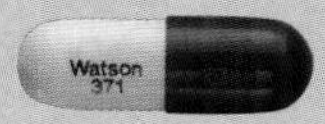

Loxapine
25 mg
Generic
WATSON

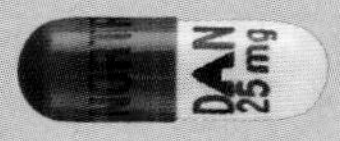

Nortriptyline Hydrochloride
25 mg
Generic
SCHEIN/DANBURY

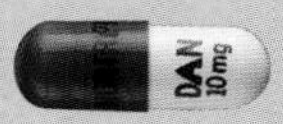

Nortriptyline Hydrochloride
10 mg
Generic
SCHEIN/DANBURY

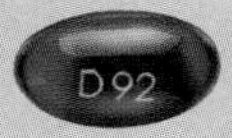

Vitamin D
50,000 IU
Drisdol
SANOFI WINTHROP

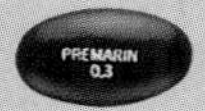

Estrogen, Conjugated
0.3 mg
Premarin
WYETH-AYERST

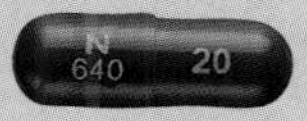

Piroxicam
20 mg
Generic
NOVOPHARM

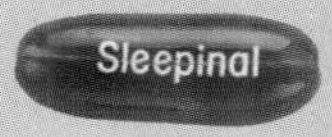

Diphenhydramine HCl
50 mg
Sleepinal Softgels Max. Strength
THOMPSON MEDICAL

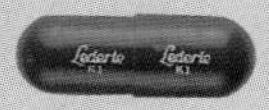

Ketoprofen
25 mg
Generic
LEDERLE

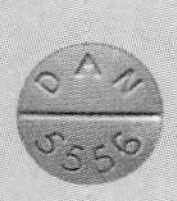

Propranolol Hydrochloride
40 mg
Generic
SCHEIN/DANBURY

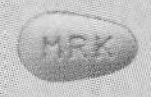

Losartan Potassium
25 mg
Cozaar
MERCK

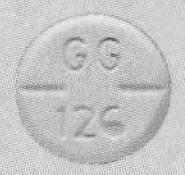

Haloperidol
10 mg
Generic
GENEVA

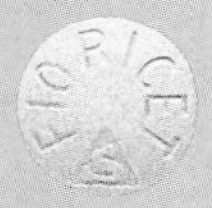

Butalbital/APAP/Caffeine
50/325/40 mg
Fioricet
NOVARTIS

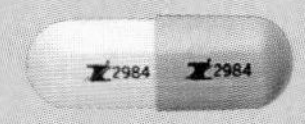

Doxycycline
500 mg
Generic
ZENITH

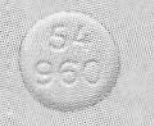

Dexamethasone
0.75 mg
Generic
ROXANE

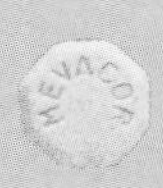

Lovastatin
20 mg
Mevacor
MERCK

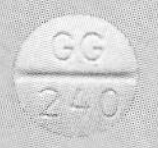

Glyburide
5 mg
Generic
GENEVA

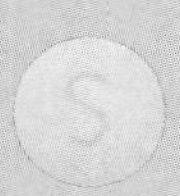

Diphenhydramine HCl
25 mg
Sominex
SMITHKLINE BEECHAM

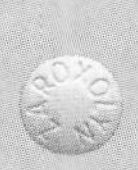

Metolazone
5 mg
Zaroxolyn
FISONS

COLOR PILL LOCATOR

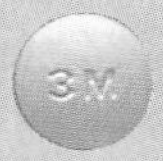

Flecainide Acetate 100 mg Tambocor 3M	**Levothyroxine Sodium** 0.15 mg Levoxyl DANIELS	**Naproxen** 220 mg Aleve BAYER	**Levodopa/Carbidopa** 250/25 mg Generic LEMMON
Levodopa/Carbidopa 100/10 mg Generic LEMMON	**Nelfinavir** 250 mg Viracept AGOURON	**Chlorpropamide** 100 mg Generic SIDMAK	**Dicyclomine Hydrochloride** 20 mg Generic UDL
Propranolol Hydrochloride 20 mg Generic SCHEIN/DANBURY	**Procainamide Hydrochloride** 500 mg Procanbid PARKE-DAVIS	**Isosorbide Dinitrate** 40 mg Sorbitrate ZENECA	**Doxycycline** 100 mg Generic SCHEIN/DANBURY
Acyclovir 200 mg Zovirax GLAXO WELLCOME	**Flurazepam Hydrochloride** 15 mg Generic MYLAN	**Maprotiline Hydrochloride** 50 mg Generic MYLAN	**Finasteride** 5 mg Proscar MERCK
Phenolphthalein 135 mg Ex-Lax Maximum Relief SANDOZ	**Pseudoephedrine** 240 mg Efidac 24 Once Daily NOVARTIS	**Sildenafil Citrate** 50 mg Viagra PFIZER	**Cefuroxime** 500 mg Ceftin GLAXO WELLCOME

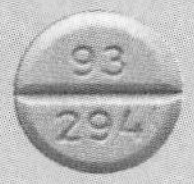

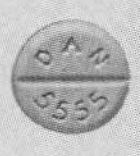

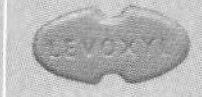

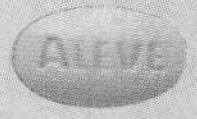

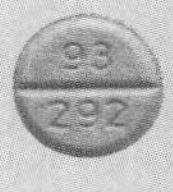

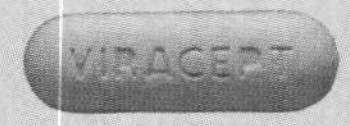

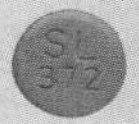

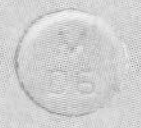

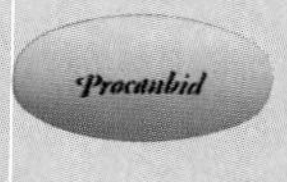

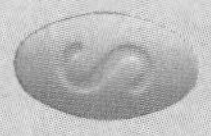

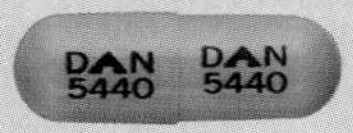

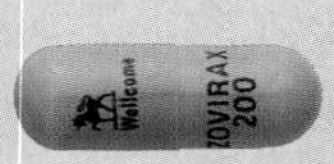

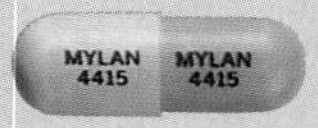

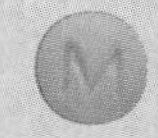

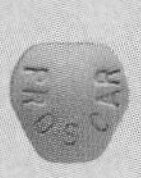

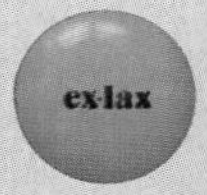

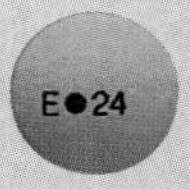

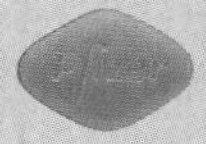

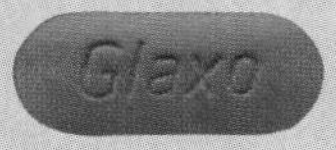

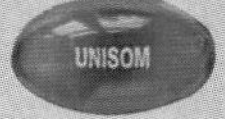

COLOR PILL LOCATOR

Diphenhydramine HCl 50 mg Unisom SleepGels PFIZER	**Prazosin** 5 mg Generic LEDERLE	**Valacyclovir Hydrochloride** 500 mg Valtrex GLAXO WELLCOME	**Orlistat** 120 mg Xenical ROCHE
Enoxacin 400 mg Generic RHONE-POULENC RORER	**Sertraline Hydrochloride** 50 mg Zoloft ROERIG	**Flurbiprofen** 100 mg Ansaid UPJOHN	**Morphine** 15 mg M S Contin PURDUE FREDERICK
Nadolol 20 mg Corgard BRISTOL-MYERS SQUIBB	**Salsalate** 500 mg Salsitab UPSHER-SMITH	**Acetaminophen** 160 mg Tempra Quicklets Junior Strength BRISTOL-MYERS SQUIBB	**Acetaminophen** 80 mg Tylenol Children's MCNEIL
Acetaminophen 160 mg Tylenol Junior Strength MCNEIL	**Diphenhydramine HCl** 12.5 mg Benadryl Allergy Chewables PARKE-DAVIS	**Warfarin** 2 mg Coumadin DUPONT	**Sucralfate** 1 g Carafate HOECHST MARION ROUSSEL
Omeprazole 20 mg Prilosec ASTRA MERCK	**Morphine** 30 mg M S Contin PURDUE FREDERICK	**Trifluoperazine Hydrochloride** 1 mg Generic GENEVA	**Trifluoperazine Hydrochloride** 2 mg Generic GENEVA

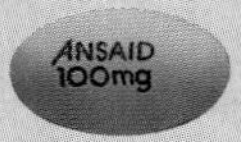

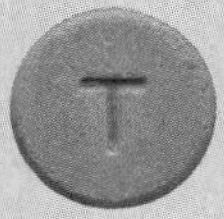

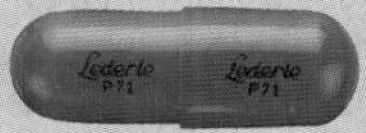

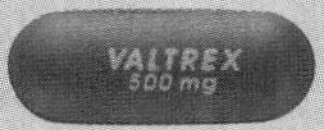

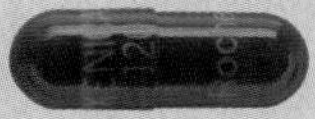

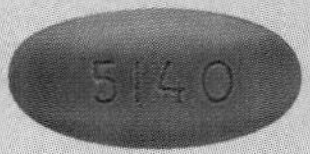

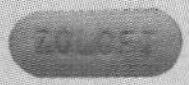

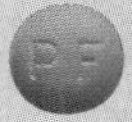

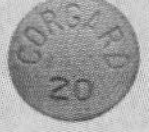

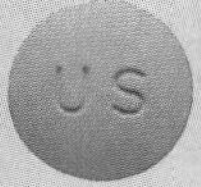

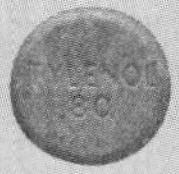

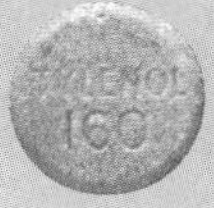

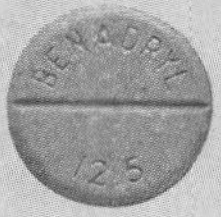

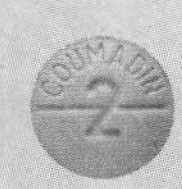

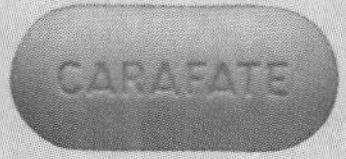

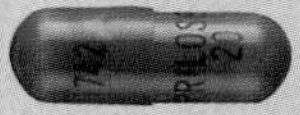

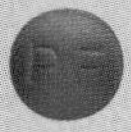

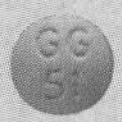

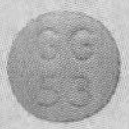

Trifluoperazine Hydrochloride 5 mg Generic GENEVA	**Trifluoperazine Hydrochloride** 10 mg Generic GENEVA	**Metolazone** 2.5 mg Zaroxolyn FISONS	**Digitoxin** 0.1 mg Generic LILLY
Fludrocortisone 0.1 mg Florinef Acetate APOTHECON	**Haloperidol** 2 mg Generic GENEVA	**Glyburide** 2.5 mg Generic GENEVA	**Isosorbide Dinitrate** 5 mg Generic GENEVA
Guanfacine Hydrochloride 1 mg Generic WATSON	**Primaquine Phosphate** 26.3 mg Generic SANOFI WINTHROP	**Ranitidine** 75 mg Zantac 75 GLAXO WELLCOME	**Famotidine** 10 mg Pepcid AC MERCK
Oxycodone Hydrochloride 20 mg Oxycontin PURDUE	**Methylprednisolone** 2 mg Medrol UPJOHN	**Benazepril Hydrochloride** 20 mg Lotensin NOVARTIS	**Isradipine** 5 mg DynaCirc NOVARTIS
Phenylpropanolamine HCl 75 mg Acutrim Late Day Strength NOVARTIS	**Phenylpropanolamine HCl** 75 mg Acutrim Maximum Strength NOVARTIS	**Hydrochlorothiazide** 25 mg Generic GOLDLINE	**Guanabenz Acetate** 4 mg Generic COPLEY

COLOR PILL LOCATOR

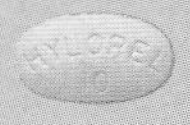 **Guanadrel Sulfate** 10 mg Hylorel FISONS	**Felodipine** 5 mg Plendil ASTRA MERCK	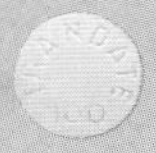 **Labetalol Hydrochloride** 100 mg Trandate GLAXO WELLCOME	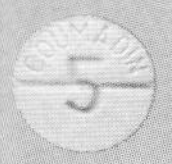 **Warfarin** 5 mg Coumadin DUPONT
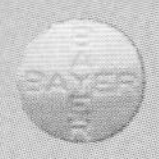 **Aspirin** 81 mg Bayer Children's BAYER	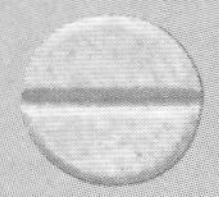 **Ibuprofen** 50 mg Motrin Children's MCNEIL	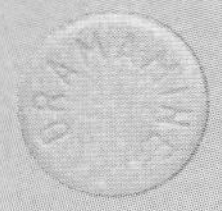 **Dimenhydrinate** 50 mg Dramamine Chewable UPJOHN	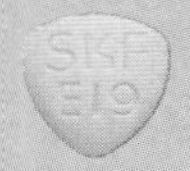 **Dextroamphetamine Sulfate** 5 mg Generic SMITHKLINE BEECHAM
Methyldopa 500 mg Generic LEDERLE	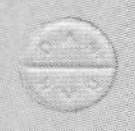 **Prednisolone** 5 mg Generic SCHEIN	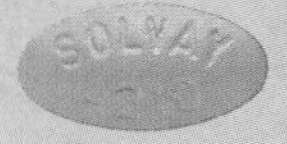 **Fluvoxamine Maleate** 100 mg Luvox SOLVAY	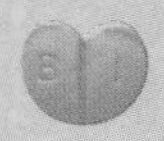 **Bisoprolol Fumarate** 5 mg Zebeta LEDERLE
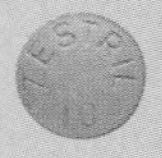 **Lisinopril** 10 mg Zestril ZENECA	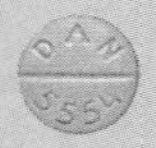 **Propranolol Hydrochloride** 10 mg Generic SCHEIN/DANBURY	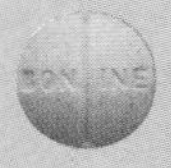 **Meclizine** 25 mg Bonine PFIZER	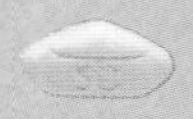 **Rosiglitazone Maleate** 2 mg Avandia SMITHKLINE BEECHAM
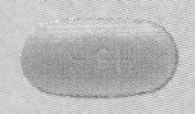 **Valsartan/HCTZ** 80/12.5 mg Diovan HCT NOVARTIS	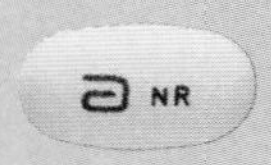 **Valproic Acid** 250 mg Depakote ABBOTT	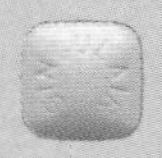 **Montelukast Sodium** 10 mg Singulair MERCK	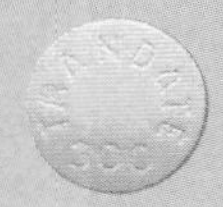 **Labetalol Hydrochloride** 300 mg Trandate GLAXO WELLCOME

Ibuprofen 100 mg Advil Junior Strength WHITEHALL-ROBINS	**Medroxyprogesterone** 10 mg Cycrin ESI	**Rimantadine Hydrochloride** 100 mg Flumadine FOREST	**Nefazodone Hydrochloride** 150 mg Serzone BRISTOL-MYERS SQUIBB
Quazepam 7.5 mg Doral WALLACE	**Trandolapril** 1 mg Mavic KNOLL	**Prednisone** 20 mg Generic SCHEIN	**Venlafaxine** 37.5 mg Effexor WYETH-AYERST
Levothyroxine Sodium 0.025 mg Levoxyl DANIELS	**Ranitidine** 150 mg Zantac GLAXO WELLCOME	**Pemoline** 37.5 mg Cylert ABBOTT	**Norfloxacin** 400 mg Noroxin MERCK
Lithium 300 mg Generic ROXANE	**Ursodiol** 300 mg Actigall SUMMIT	**Prazosin** 1 mg Generic LEDERLE	**Propoxyphene** 65 mg Darvon LILLY
Fluconazole 100 mg Diflucan ROERIG	**Fluconazole** 200 mg Diflucan ROERIG	**Levothyroxine Sodium** 0.2 mg Levoxyl DANIELS	**Zolpidem** 5 mg Ambien SEARLE

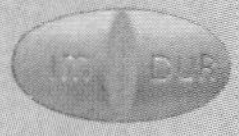

COLOR PILL LOCATOR

Isosorbide Mononitrate 30 mg IMDUR KEY	**Levofloxacin** 250 mg Levaquin MCNEIL	**Valproic Acid** 500 mg Depakote ABBOTT	**Erythromycin** 250 mg Ery-Tab ABBOTT
Amiodarone 200 mg Cordarone WYETH-AYERST	**Acetaminophen** 80 mg Panadol Children's SMITHKLINE BEECHAM	**Carbamazepine** 200 mg Tegretol BASEL	**Paroxetine Hydrochloride** 20 mg Paxil SMITHKLINE BEECHAM
Bismuth Subsalicylate 262 mg Pepto-Bismol Caplets PROCTER & GAMBLE	**Levodopa** 100 mg Larodopa ROCHE	**Verapamil Hydrochloride** 180 mg Isoptin SR KNOLL	**Midodrine Hydrochloride** 5 mg Proamatine ROBERTS
Hydralazine Hydrochloride 10 mg Generic PAR	**Metoprolol** 50 mg Generic MYLAN	**Acetaminophen** 80 mg Tylenol Children's MCNEIL	**Oxazepam** 10 mg Generic PUREPAC
Pentoxifylline 400 mg Trental HOECHST MARION ROUSSEL	**Estrogen/Medroxyprogesterone** 0.625/2.5 mg Prempro AYERST LAB	**Bismuth Subsalicylate** 262 mg Pepto-Bismol PROCTER & GAMBLE	**Diphenhydramine HCl** 25 mg Benadryl Allergy PARKE-DAVIS

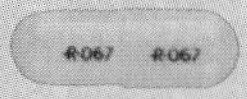

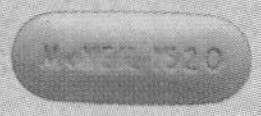

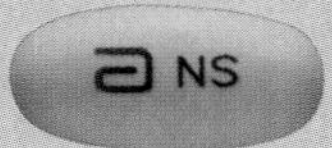

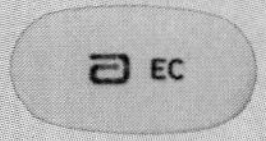

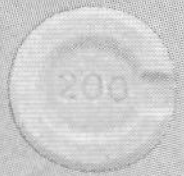

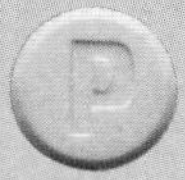

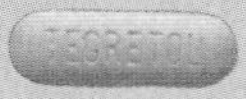

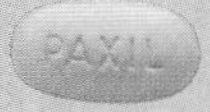

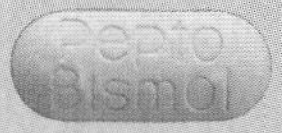

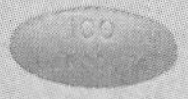

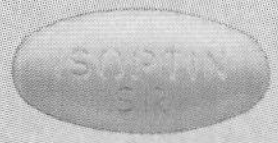

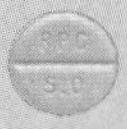

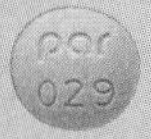

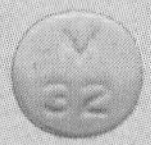

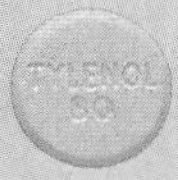

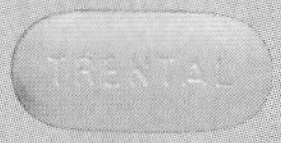

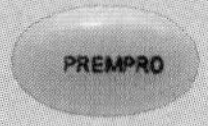

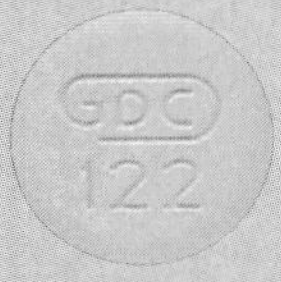

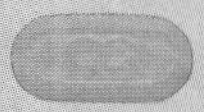

COLOR PILL LOCATOR

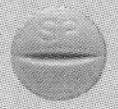

Moexipril Hydrochloride 7.5 mg Univasc SCHWARZ PHARMA	**Pravastatin** 10 mg Pravachol BRISTOL-MYERS SQUIBB	**Repaglinide** 2 mg Prandin NOVO NORDISK	**Quetiapine Fumarate** 25 mg Seroquel ZENECA
Diphenhydramine HCl 50 mg Generic BARR	**Ethinyl Estradiol** 0.05 mg Estinyl SCHERING-PLOUGH	**Lisinopril** 20 mg Zestril ZENECA	**Erythromycin** 250 mg Erythrocin ABBOTT
Amitriptyline Hydrochloride 10 mg Generic SIDMAK	**Bisacodyl** 5 mg Correctol SCHERING-PLOUGH	**Chloroquine** 500 mg Aralen Phosphate SANOFI WINTHROP	**Vitamin B12 (Cyanocobalamin)** 1,000 mcg Generic GOLDLINE
Diphenhydramine HCl 25 mg Generic PUREPAC	**Mexiletine Hydrochloride** 200 mg Mexitil BOEHRINGER INGELHEIM	**Aspirin** 227 mg Aspergum SCHERING-PLOUGH	**Simethicone** 125 mg Phazyme Maximum Strength BLOCK
Simethicone 95 mg Phazyme BLOCK	**Citalopram Hydrobromide** 20 mg Celexa FOREST PHARMACEUTICALS	**Pseudoephedrine** 30 mg Sudafed GLAXO WELLCOME	**Hydralazine Hydrochloride** 25 mg Generic LEDERLE

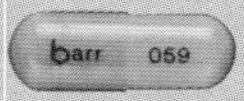

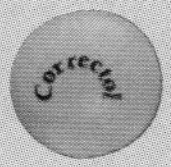

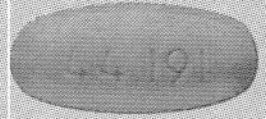

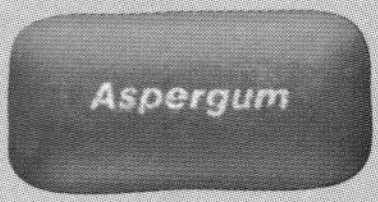

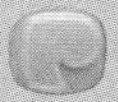

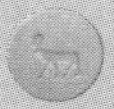

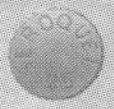

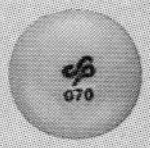

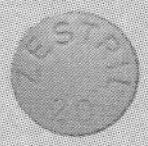

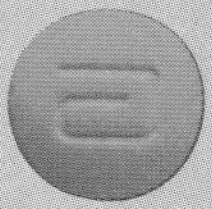

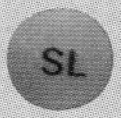

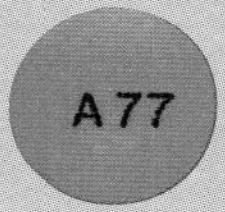

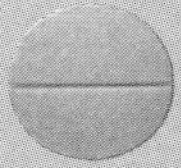

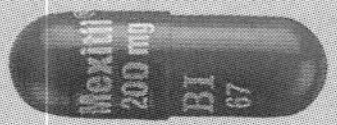

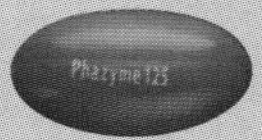

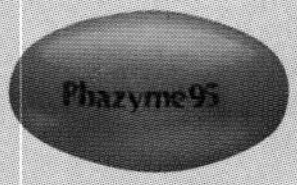

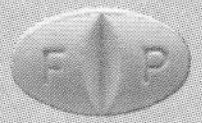

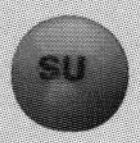

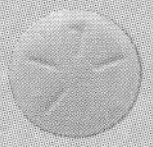

COLOR PILL LOCATOR

Clopidogrel Bisulfate
75 mg
Plavix
SANOFI

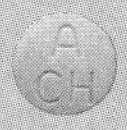

Candesartan Cilexetil
16 mg
Atacand
ASTRO PHARMACEUTICALS

Activated Charcoal
200 mg
Charcoal Plus
KRAMER LABORATORIES

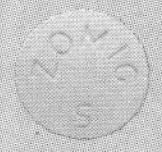

Zolmitriptan
5 mg
Zomig
ZENETH

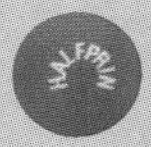

Aspirin
162 mg
Halfprin
KRAMER

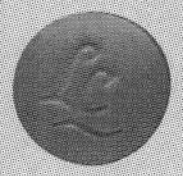

Hydralazine Hydrochloride
50 mg
Generic
LEDERLE

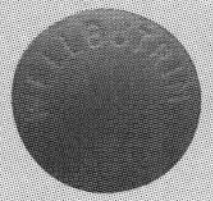

Bupropion Hydrochloride
100 mg
Wellbutrin
GLAXO WELLCOME

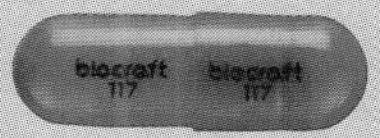

Cephalexin
500 mg
Generic
BIOCRAFT

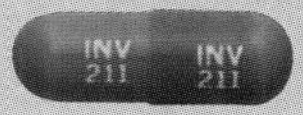

Amantadine Hydrochloride
100 mg
Generic
INVAMED

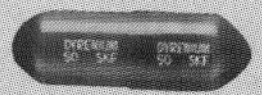

Triamterene
50 mg
Dyrenium
SMITHKLINE BEECHAM

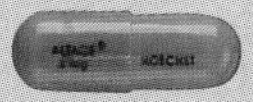

Ramipril
5 mg
Altace
HOECHST MARION ROUSSEL

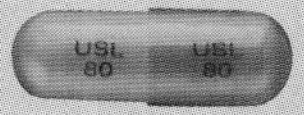

Zinc Sulfate
220 mg
Generic
UPSHER-SMITH

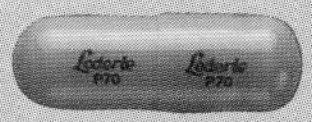

Prazosin
2 mg
Generic
LEDERLE

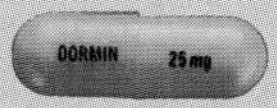

Diphenhydramine HCl
25 mg
Dormin
RANDOB LABS

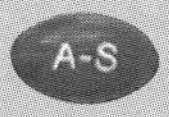

Simethicone
125 mg
Alka-Seltzer Liquid Gelcaps
BAYER

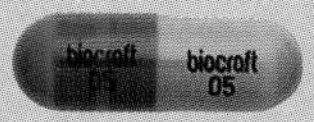

Ampicillin
250 mg
Generic
BIOCRAFT

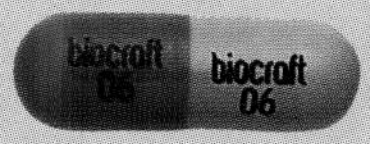

Ampicillin
500 mg
Generic
BIOCRAFT

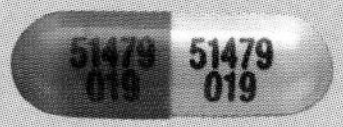

Cycloserine
250 mg
Seromycin
DURA

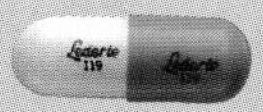

Indomethacin
25 mg
Generic
LEDERLE

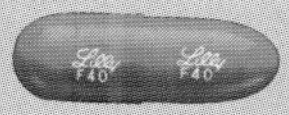

Secobarbital Sodium
100 mg
Seconal Sodium
LILLY

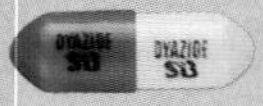

HCTZ/Triamterene 25/37.5 mg Dyazide SMITHKLINE BEECHAM	**Cefadroxil** 500 mg Duricef BRISTOL-MYERS SQUIBB	**Ethchlorvynol** 500 mg Placidyl ABBOTT	**Ethchlorvynol** 200 mg Placidyl ABBOTT
Docusate 240 mg Surfak UPJOHN	**Vitamin A (Retinol)** 25,000 IU Aquasol A ASTRA	**Docusate** 100 mg Generic SCHERER	**Amitriptyline Hydrochloride** 50 mg Generic SIDMAK
Tranylcypromine Sulfate 10 mg Parnate SMITHKLINE BEECHAM	**Imipramine** 25 mg Generic BIOCRAFT	**Rifabutin** 150 mg Mycobutin PHARMACIA	**Nystatin** 500,000 units Generic LEMMON
Perphenazine /Amitriptyline 4/10 mg Generic GENEVA	**Stavudine** 20 mg Zerit BRISTOL-MYERS SQUIBB	**Nifedipine** 60 mg Adalat CC BAYER	**Quinapril Hydrochloride** 20 mg Accupril PARKE-DAVIS
Quinapril Hydrochloride 10 mg Accupril PARKE-DAVIS	**Quinapril Hydrochloride** 5 mg Accupril PARKE-DAVIS	**Acetazolamide** 500 mg Diamox STORZ	**Propoxyphene/Acetaminophen** 65/650 mg Generic MYLAN

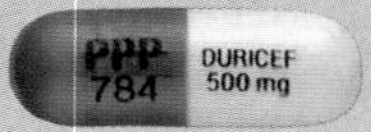

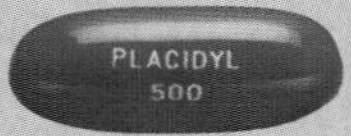

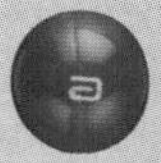

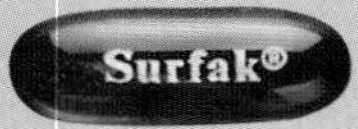

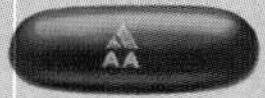

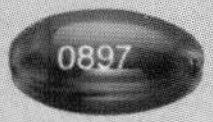

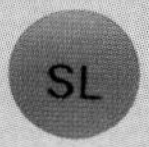

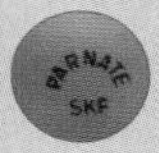

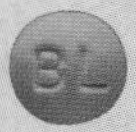

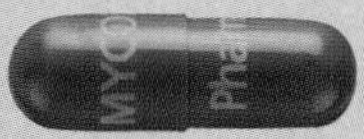

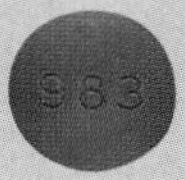

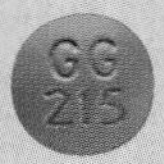

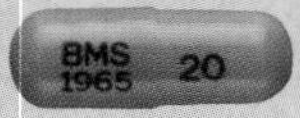

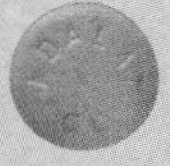

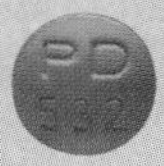

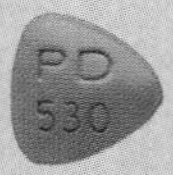

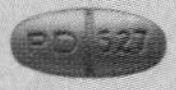

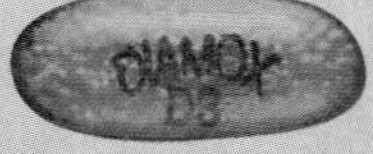

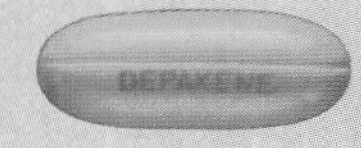

COLOR PILL LOCATOR

Valproic Acid
250 mg
Depakene
ABBOTT

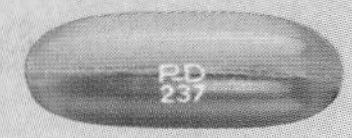

Ethosuximide
250 mg
Zarontin
PARKE-DAVIS

Phenylpropanolamine HCl
75 mg
Permathene-12
CCA INDUSTRIES

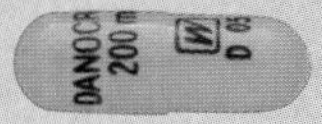

Danazol
200 mg
Danocrine
SANOFI WINTHROP

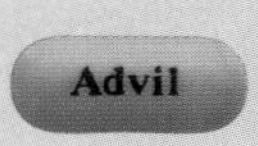

Ibuprofen
200 mg
Advil
WHITEHALL

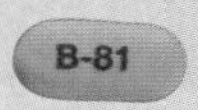

Aspirin
81 mg
Bufferin Low Dose
BRISTOL-MYERS SQUIBB

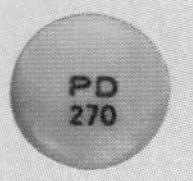

Phenelzine Sulfate
15 mg
Nardil
PARKE-DAVIS

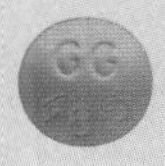

Fluphenazine
5 mg
Generic
GENEVA

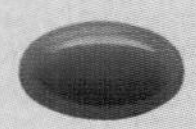

Beta-Carotene
25,000 IU
Generic
MAJOR PHARMACEUTICALS

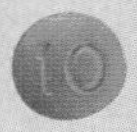

Chlorpromazine Hydrochloride
10 mg
Generic
GENEVA

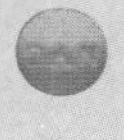

Hydroxyzine Hydrochloride
10 mg
Generic
SCHEIN/DANBURY

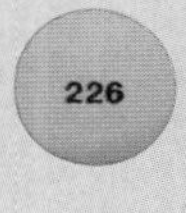

Aspirin
325 mg
Generic
TIME-CAP

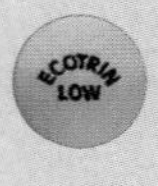

Aspirin (Enteric Coated)
81 mg
Ecotrin
SMITHKLINE BEECHAM

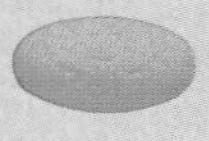

Cefpodoxime Proxetil
100 mg
Vantin
UPJOHN

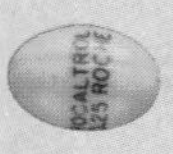

Calcitriol
0.25 mcg
Rocaltrol
ROCHE

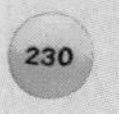

Bisacodyl
5 mg
Generic
PADDOCK

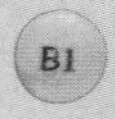

Bisacodyl
5 mg
Dulcolax
BOEHRINGER INGELHEIM

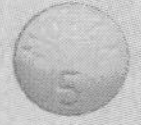

Molindone
5 mg
Moban
GATE

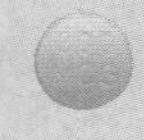

Cerivastatin
0.3 mg
Baycol
BAYER

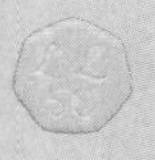

Amoxapine
50 mg
Asendin
LEDERLE

Fluphenazine
1 mg
Generic
GENEVA

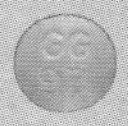

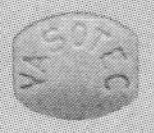

Enalapril Maleate
10 mg
Vasotec
MERCK

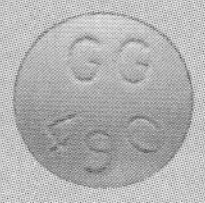

Fluphenazine
10 mg
Generic
GENEVA

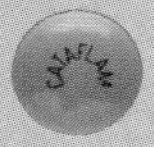

Diclofenac
50 mg
Cataflam
GEIGY

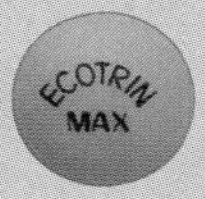

Aspirin (Enteric Coated)
500 mg
Ecotrin Maximum Strength
SMITHKLINE BEECHAM

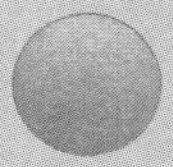

Vitamin B 2 (Riboflavin)
100 mg
Riboflavin
REXALL

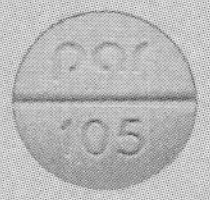

Allopurinol
300 mg
Generic
PAR

Diflunisal
500 mg
Generic
ENDO

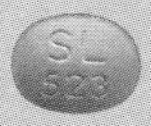

Protriptyline Hydrochloride
5 mg
Generic
SIDMAK

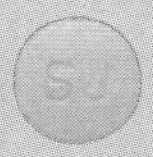

Aspirin
81 mg
St. Joseph Adult Chewable
SCHERING-PLOUGH

Fluphenazine
2.5 mg
Generic
GENEVA

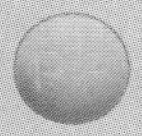

Morphine
60 mg
M S Contin
PURDUE FREDERICK

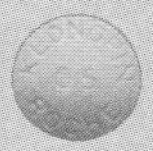

Clonazepam
0.5 mg
Klonopin
ROCHE

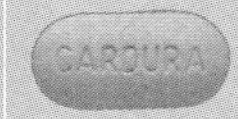

Doxazosin Mesylate
4 mg
Cardura
ROERIG

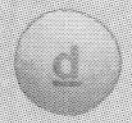

Phenylpropanolamine HCl
75 mg
Dexatrim Extended Duration
THOMPSON MEDICAL

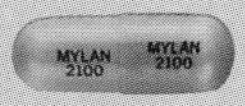

Loperamide Hydrochloride
2 mg
Generic
MYLAN

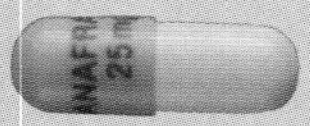

Clomipramine Hydrochloride
25 mg
Anafranil
NOVARTIS

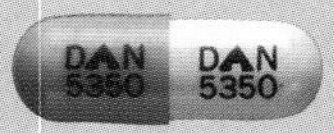

Procainamide Hydrochloride
375 mg
Generic
SCHEIN/DANBURY

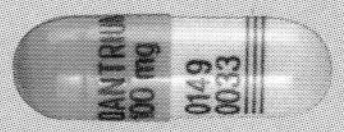

Dantrolene Sodium
100 mg
Dantrium
P&GP

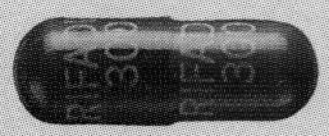

Rifampin
300 mg
Rifadin
HOECHST MARION ROUSSEL

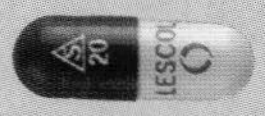

COLOR PILL LOCATOR

Fluvastatin 20 mg Lescol NOVARTIS	**Mexiletine Hydrochloride** 150 mg Mexitil BOEHRINGER INGELHEIM	**Cephalexin** 250 mg Generic BIOCRAFT	**Ibuprofen** 200 mg Advil Gel Caplets WHITEHALL
Phenoxybenzamine HCl 10 mg Dibenzyline SMITHKLINE BEECHAM	**Stavudine** 15 mg Zerit BRISTOL-MYERS SQUIBB	**Procainamide Hydrochloride** 500 mg Generic ZENITH	**Tetracycline Hydrochloride** 250 mg Generic ZENITH
Fenoprofen Calcium 300 mg Nalfon DISTA	**Nizatidine** 150 mg Axid LILLY	**Mefenamic Acid** 250 mg Ponstel PARKE-DAVIS	**Clomipramine Hydrochloride** 50 mg Anafranil NOVARTIS
Simethicone 62.5 mg Mylanta Gas Maximum Strength JOHNSON & JOHNSON/MERCK	**Tacrine** 10 mg Cognex PARKE-DAVIS	**Piroxicam** 10 mg Generic MYLAN	**Chlordiazepoxide** 10 mg Generic BARR
Fluoxetine Hydrochloride 20 mg Prozac DISTA	**Dicloxacillin Sodium** 250 mg Generic BIOCRAFT	**Dicloxacillin Sodium** 500 mg Generic BIOCRAFT	**Cephradine** 250 mg Generic BIOCRAFT

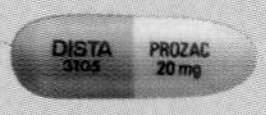

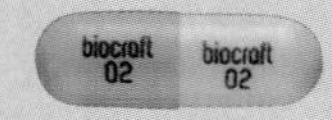

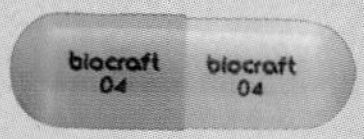

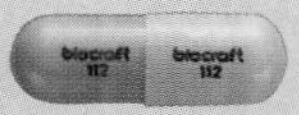

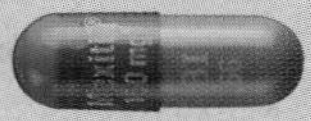

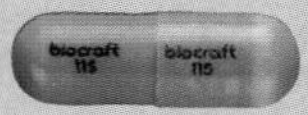

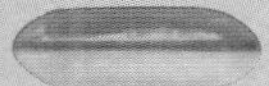

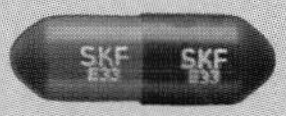

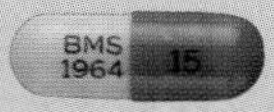

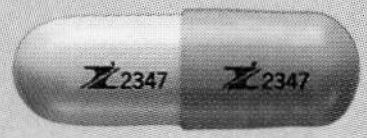

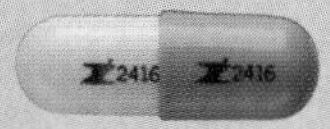

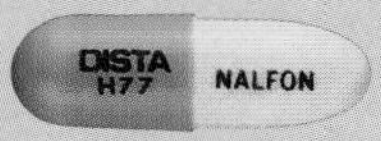

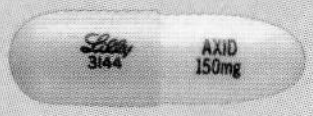

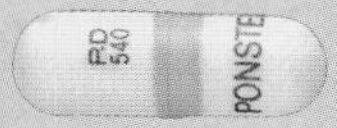

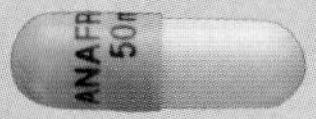

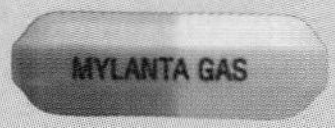

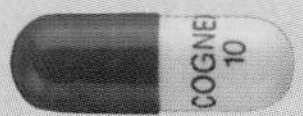

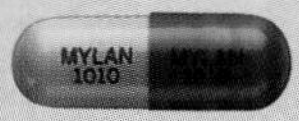

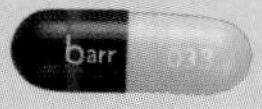

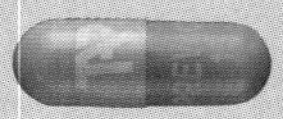

COLOR PILL LOCATOR

Lansoprazole
15 mg
Prevacid
TAP

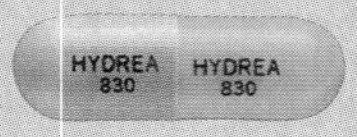

Hydroxyurea
500 mg
Hydrea
BRISTOL-MYERS SQUIBB

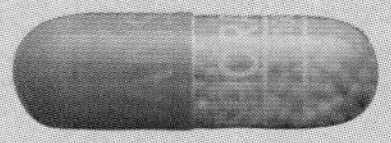

Itraconazole
100 mg
Sporanox
JANSSEN

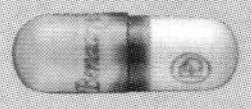

Diphenhydramine HCl
25 mg
Benadryl Allergy
PARKE-DAVIS

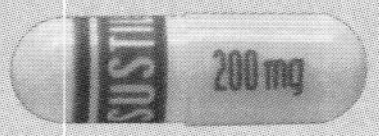

Efavirenz
200 mg
Sustiva
DUPONT

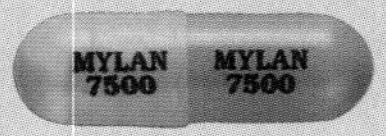

Cefaclor
500 mg
Generic
MYLAN

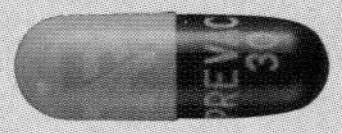

Lansoprazole
30 mg
Prevacid
TAP

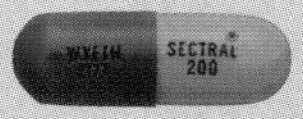

Acebutolol Hydrochloride
200 mg
Sectral
WYETH-AYERST

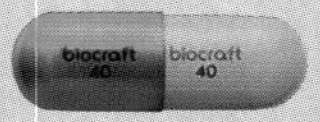

Disopyramide
100 mg
Generic
BIOCRAFT

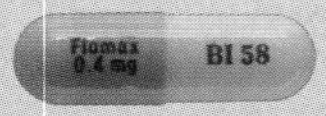

Tamsulosin Hydrochloride
0.4 mg
Flomax
YAMANOUCHI

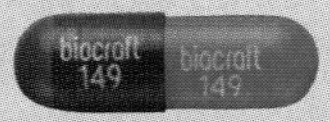

Clindamycin
150 mg
Generic
BIOCRAFT

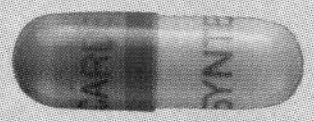

Nicardipine Hydrochloride
30 mg
Cardene
SYNTEX

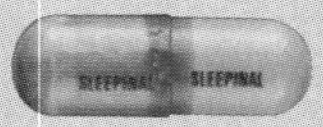

Diphenhydramine HCl
50 mg
Sleepinal Maximum Strength
THOMPSON MEDICAL

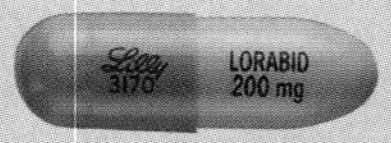

Loracarbef
200 mg
Lorabid
LILLY

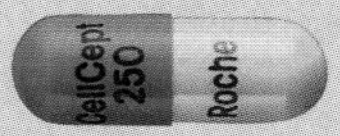

Mycophenolate Mofetil
250 mg
CellCept
ROCHE

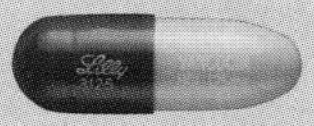

Vancomycin
125 mg
Vancocin
LILLY

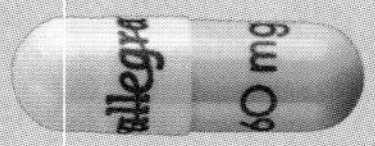

Fexofenadine
60 mg
Allegra
HOECHST MARION ROUSSEL

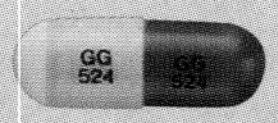

Meclofenamate Sodium
50 mg
Generic
GENEVA

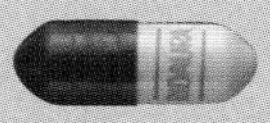

Auranofin
3 mg
Ridaura
SMITHKLINE BEECHAM

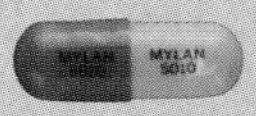

Thiothixene
10 mg
Generic
MYLAN

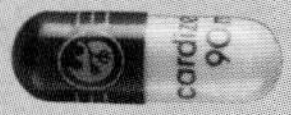

COLOR PILL LOCATOR

Diltiazem Hydrochloride
90 mg
Cardizem SR
HOECHST MARION ROUSSEL

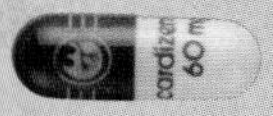

Diltiazem Hydrochloride
60 mg
Cardizem SR
HOECHST MARION ROUSSEL

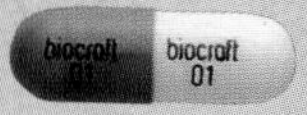

Amoxicillin
250 mg
Generic
BIOCRAFT

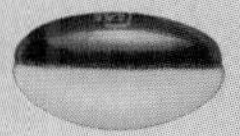

Docusate
100 mg
Colace
ROBERTS

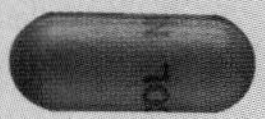

Mesalamine
400 mg
Asacol
P&GP

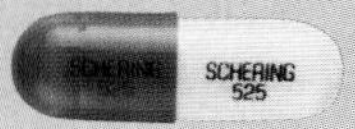

Flutamide
125 mg
Eulexin
SCHERING-PLOUGH

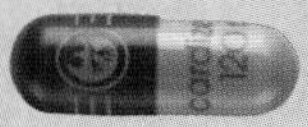

Diltiazem Hydrochloride
120 mg
Cardizem SR
HOECHST MARION ROUSSEL

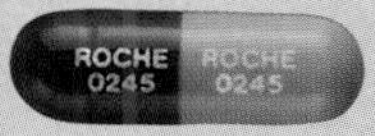

Saquinavir
200 mg
Invirase
ROCHE

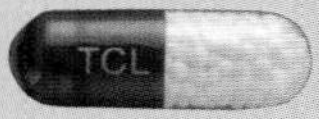

Papaverine Hydrochloride
150 mg
Generic
TIME-CAP

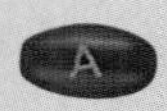

Phenolphthalein
60 mg
Alophen
PARKE-DAVIS

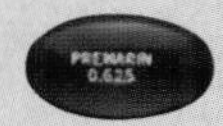

Estrogen, Conjugated
0.625 mg
Premarin
WYETH-AYERST

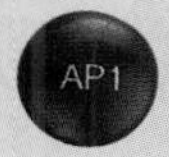

Phenazopyridine HCl
100 mg
Generic
ABLE

Ferrous Sulfate
324 mg
Generic
CHASE

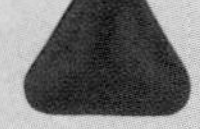

Ferrous Sulfate
200 mg
Feosol
SMITHKLINE BEECHAM

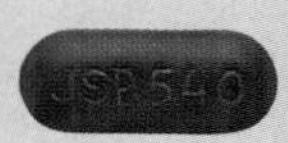

Methenamine
500 mg
Generic
JEROME STEVENS

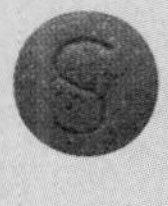

Senna
8.6 mg
Senokot
PURDUE FREDERICK

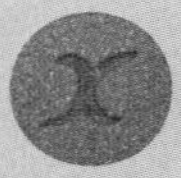

Senna
17 mg
SenokotXTRA
PURDUE FREDERICK

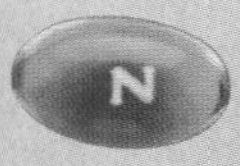

Diphenhydramine HCl
50 mg
Nytol Quickgels Max. Strength
BLOCK

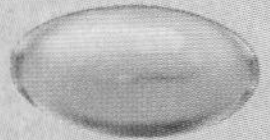

Vitamin E
400 IU
Generic
GOLD CAPS

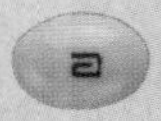

Terazosin
1 mg
Hytrin
ABBOTT

85

Simvastatin 10 mg Zocor MERCK	**Zidovudine** 100 mg Retrovir GLAXO WELLCOME	**Phenytoin** 100 mg Dilantin PARKE-DAVIS	**Doxepin Hydrochloride** 25 mg Generic GENEVA
Thiothixene 1 mg Generic MYLAN	**Etodolac** 200 mg Lodine WYETH-AYERST	**Nitrofurantoin** 50 mg Generic ZENITH	**Minocycline** 50 mg Dynacin MEDICIS
Theophylline 50 mg Slo-Bid RHONE-POULENC RORER	**Theophylline** 100 mg Slo-Bid RHONE-POULENC RORER	**Acetaminophen** 325 mg Tylenol Hospital MCNEIL	**Aspirin** 500 mg Bayer Extra Strength BAYER
Pseudoephedrine 120 mg Sudafed 12 Hour GLAXO WELLCOME	**Ticlopidine Hydrochloride** 250 mg Ticlid ROCHE	**Altretamine** 50 mg Hexalen US BIOSCIENCE	**Indinavir Sulfate** 200 mg Crixivan MERCK
Gabapentin 100 mg Neurontin PARKE-DAVIS	**Ibuprofen** 200 mg Motrin IB PHARMACIA & UPJOHN	**Thiothixene** 5 mg Generic GENEVA	**Flucytosine** 500 mg Ancobon ROCHE

COLOR PILL LOCATOR

Ritonavir 100 mg Norvir ABBOTT	**Loxapine** 5 mg Generic WATSON	**Pentosan Polysulfate Sodium** 100 mg Elmiron BAKER NORTON	**Lomustine** 10 mg CeeNU BRISTOL-MYERS SQUIBB
Celecoxib 100 mg Celecoxib PFIZER	**Tacrolimus** 1 mg Prograf FUJISAWA	**Sibutramine HCl Monohydrate** 10 mg Meridia KNOLL	**Trimethobenzamide HCl** 100 mg Tigan ROBERTS LABS
Ibuprofen 100 mg Motrin Junior Strength MCNEIL	**Ethacrynic Acid** 25 mg Edecrin MERCK	**Riluzole** 50 mg Rilutek RHONE-POLENC RORER	**Sotalol Hydrochloride** 80 mg Betapace BERLEX
Clemastine Fumarate 1.34 mg Tavist-1 12 Hour NOVARTIS	**Torsemide** 5 mg Demadex BOEHRINGER MANNHEIM	**Fosinopril** 20 mg Monopril BRISTOL-MYERS SQUIBB	**Risperidone** 1 mg Risperdal JANSSEN
Tramadol 50 mg Ultram MCNEIL	**Diphenhydramine HCl** 25 mg Nytol Quick Caps BLOCK	**Hydroxychloroquine Sulfate** 200 mg Generic APOTHECON	**Terbutaline Sulfate** 2.5 mg Brethine GEIGY

Aspirin 325 mg Bayer BAYER	**Caffeine** 200 mg Nodoz BRISTOL-MYERS SQUIBB	**Carteolol** 5 mg Cartrol ABBOTT	**Acetohexamide** 250 mg Generic SCHEIN
Captopril 100 mg Capoten BRISTOL-MYERS SQUIBB	**Theophylline** 300 mg Theo-Dur KEY	**Theophylline** 200 mg Theo-Dur KEY	**Atorvastatin** 20 mg Lipitor PARKE-DAVIS
Meclizine 25 mg Generic PAR	**Torsemide** 10 mg Demadex BOEHRINGER MANNHEIM	**Alprazolam** 0.25 mg Generic GENEVA	**Benztropine Mesylate** 1 mg Generic PAR
Cetirizine 10 mg Zyrtec PFIZER	**Cimetidine** 200 mg Tagamet HB SMITHKLINE BEECHAM	**Lamivudine** 150 mg Epivir GLAXO WELLCOME	**Etidronate Disodium** 200 mg Didronel PROCTER & GAMBLE
Nefazodone Hydrochloride 100 mg Serzone BRISTOL-MYERS SQUIBB	**Amlodipine** 5 mg Norvasc PFIZER	**Buspirone Hydrochloride** 5 mg BuSpar MEAD JOHNSON	**Estazolam** 1 mg ProSom ABBOTT

COLOR PILL LOCATOR

▼

Telmisartan 40 mg Micardis BOEHRINGER-INGELHEIM	**Irbesartan** 150 mg Avapro BRISTOL-MYERS SQUIBB	**Misoprostol** 0.2 mg Cytotec SEARLE	**Levothyroxine Sodium** 0.05 mg Levoxyl DANIELS
Pindolol 10 mg Visken NOVARTIS	**Fosinopril** 10 mg Monopril BRISTOL-MYERS SQUIBB	**Enalapril Maleate** 5 mg Vasotec MERCK	**Famotidine** 10 mg Mylanta AR MERCK
Lisinopril 5 mg Prinivil MERCK	**Medroxyprogesterone** 2.5 mg Cycrin ESI	**Trimethoprim** 100 mg Generic SCHEIN	**Triamcinolone** 4 mg Generic SCHEIN
Triazolam 0.125 mg Generic GENEVA	**Methylprednisolone** 4 mg Medrol UPJOHN	**Norethindrone** 5 mg Aygestin LEDERLE	**Ergoloid Mesylates** 1 mg Generic ZENITH-GOLDLINE
Selegiline Hydrochloride 5 mg Eldepryl SOMERSET	**Lamotrigine** 25 mg Lamictal GLAXO WELLCOME	**Lorazepam** 0.5 mg Generic SCHEIN/DANBURY	**Nitroglycerin** 0.4 mg Nitrostat PARKE-DAVIS

COLOR PILL LOCATOR

Atenolol 25 mg Generic LEDERLE	**Thyroid** 15 mg Armour Thyroid FOREST	**Estradiol** 0.5 mg Generic APOTHECON	**Diphenoxylate HCl/Atropine Sulfate** 2.5/0.025 mg Lonox GENEVA
Prednisone 1 mg Generic ROXANE	**Ropinirole Hydrochloride** 0.25 mg Requip SMITHKLINE BEECHAM	**Thyroid** 30 mg Armour Thyroid FOREST	**Methimazole** 5 mg Tapazole LILLY
Hydromorphone Hydrochloride 2 mg Generic ROXANE	**Desipramine Hydrochloride** 10 mg Generic GENEVA	**Captopril** 12.5 mg Generic APOTHECON	**Furosemide** 20 mg Generic ROXANE
Propantheline Bromide 15 mg Generic ROXANE	**Carvedilol** 3.125 mg Coreg SMITHKLINE BEECHAM	**Dipyridamole** 25 mg Generic BARR	**Raloxifene Hydrochloride** 60 mg Evista ELI LILLY
Phenylpropanolamine HCl 75 mg Acutrim 16-Hr Steady Control NOVARTIS	**Diethylstilbestrol** 1 mg Generic LILLY	**Dexamethasone** 2 mg Generic ROXANE	**Clonidine Hydrochloride** 0.1 mg Generic MYLAN

COLOR PILL LOCATOR

Topiramate 25 mg Topamax MCNEIL	**Sumatriptan Succinate** 25 mg Imitrex GLAXO WELLCOME	**Loratadine** 10 mg Claritin SCHERING-PLOUGH	**Benztropine Mesylate** 0.5 mg Generic PAR
Colchicine 0.5 mg Generic WEST-WARD	**Timolol Maleate** 5 mg Generic GENEVA	**Pseudoephedrine** 30 mg Generic ROXANE	**Clonidine Hydrochloride** 0.2 mg Generic MYLAN
Chlorambucil 2 mg Leukeran GLAXO WELLCOME	**Furosemide** 40 mg Generic ROXANE	**Tolterodine Tartrate** 1 mg Detrol PHARMACIA & UPJOHN	**Pramipexole Dihydrocholoride** 0.125 mg Mirapex PHARMACIA & UPJOHN
Pilocarpine 5 mg Salagen BOEHRINGER-INGELHEIM	**Anastrozole** 1 mg Arimidex ZENECA	**Prednisone** 5 mg Generic SCHEIN	**Methadone Hydrochloride** 5 mg Generic ROXANE
Meperidine Hydrochloride 50 mg Generic WYETH-AYERST	**Codeine** 15 mg Generic ROXANE	**Codeine** 30 mg Generic ROXANE	**Dipyridamole** 50 mg Generic BARR

COLOR PILL LOCATOR

Oxycodone Hydrochloride 10 mg Oxycontin PURDUE	**Digoxin** 0.25 mg Lanoxin GLAXO WELLCOME	**Ketoprofen** 12.5 mg Actron BAYER	**Indapamide** 2.5 mg Generic RHONE-POULENC RORER
Levamisole Hydrochloride 50 mg Ergamisol JANSSEN	**Cortisone Acetate** 5 mg Generic UPJOHN	**Cortisone** 5 mg Generic UPJOHN	**Phenobarbital** 30 mg Generic ROXANE
Diethylstilbestrol 5 mg Generic LILLY	**Donepezil** 5 mg Aricept EISAI	**Pemoline** 18.75 mg Cylert ABBOTT	**Acarbose** 50 mg Precose BAYER
Cyproheptadine Hydrochloride 4 mg Generic SIDMAK	**Melphalan** 2 mg Alkeran GLAXO WELLCOME	**Metaproterenol Sulfate** 10 mg Generic PAR	**Atenolol** 50 mg Generic GENEVA
Benztropine Mesylate 2 mg Generic PAR	**Busulfan** 2 mg Myleran GLAXO WELLCOME	**Procyclidine** 5 mg Kemadrin GLAXO WELLCOME	**Morphine** 100 mg M S Contin PURDUE FREDERICK

Metoclopramide Hydrochloride 10 mg Generic SCHEIN	**Liothyronine Sodium** 25 mcg Cytomel SMITHKLINE BEECHAM	**Diltiazem Hydrochloride** 30 mg Generic MYLAN	**Isosorbide Dinitrate** 10 mg Generic GENEVA
Bromocriptine Mesylate 2.5 mg Parlodel NOVARTIS	**Aspirin** 81 mg Ascriptin Adult Low Strength NOVARTIS	**Albuterol** 2 mg Generic BIOCRAFT	**Perphenazine** 4 mg Generic GENEVA
Methylphenidate 10 mg Generic MD PHARM	**Minoxidil** 2.5 mg Generic SCHEIN/DANBURY	**Captopril** 25 mg Generic APOTHECON	**Zafirlukast** 20 mg Accolate ZENECA
Tamoxifen Citrate 10 mg Nolvadex ZENECA	**Sodium Bicarbonate** 324 mg Generic CONCORD	**Leucovorin Calcium** 5 mg Wellcovorin GLAXO WELLCOME	**Propylthiouracil** 50 mg Generic LEDERLE
Oxybutynin Chloride 5 mg Generic SIDMAK	**Prednisone** 10 mg Generic SCHEIN	**Diazepam** 2 mg Generic PUREPAC	**Atropine Sulfate** 0.4 mg Generic LILLY

Hydrocortisone 5 mg Cortef Upjohn	**Vitamin B3** 50 mg Generic Nutro	**Terbutaline Sulfate** 5 mg Brethine Geigy	**Megestrol Acetate** 20 mg Generic PAR
Codeine 60 mg Generic Roxane	**Glipizide** 5 mg Generic Mylan	**Cyclophosphamide** 25 mg Cytoxan Bristol-Myers Squibb	**Propranolol/HCTZ** 40/25 mg Generic Purepac
Perphenazine 8 mg Generic Geneva	**Verapamil Hydrochloride** 80 mg Generic Geneva	**Thioridazine Hydrochloride** 50 mg Generic Creighton	**Biperiden** 2 mg Akineton Knoll
Promethazine Hydrochloride 25 mg Phenergan Wyeth-Ayerst	**Cortisone** 25 mg Generic Rugby	**Dimenhydrinate** 50 mg Dramamine Upjohn	**Clomiphene Citrate** 50 mg Generic Lemmon
Baclofen 10 mg Generic Zenith	**Atenolol** 100 mg Generic Mylan	**Biotin** 300 mcg Generic Tishcon	**Olanzapine** 5 mg Zyprexa Lilly

COLOR PILL LOCATOR

Cisapride 10 mg Propulsid JANSSEN	**Warfarin** 10 mg Coumadin DUPONT	**Prednisone** 50 mg Generic ROXANE	**Testolactone** 50 mg Teslac BRISTOL-MYERS SQUIBB
Tolazamide 100 mg Generic ZENITH	**Ibuprofen** 200 mg Motrin IB PHARMACIA & UPJOHN	**Vitamin B1** 50 mg Generic NUTRO	**Aminophylline** 100 mg Generic WEST-WARD
Propafenone 150 mg Rythmol KNOLL	**Diltiazem Hydrochloride** 60 mg Generic MYLAN	**Trihexyphenidyl Hydrochloride** 5 mg Generic LEDERLE	**Ketoconazole** 200 mg Nizoral JANSSEN
Metronidazole 250 mg Generic SCHEIN/DANBURY	**Atenolol/Chlorthalidone** 50/25 mg Tenoretic ZENECA	**Betaxolol** 10 mg Generic AMIDE PHARMACEUTICAL	**Bisoprolol/HCTZ** 10 mg Ziac LEDERLE
Cilostazol 100 mg Pletal PHARMACIA & UPJOHN	**Glycopyrrolate** 1 mg Robinul A.H. ROBINS	**Ketorolac Tromethamine** 10 mg Tromethamine SYNTEX	**Lisinopril/HCTZ** 20/12.5 mg Zestoretic ZENECA

Leflunomide
10 mg
Arava
HOECHST MARION ROUSSEL

Spironolactone
25 mg
Generic
MYLAN

Pioglitazone Hydrochloride
15 mg
Actos
TAKEDA PHARM

Trazodone
50 mg
Generic
PUREPAC

Sulfinpyrazone
100 mg
Anturane
NOVARTIS

Naproxen
250 mg
Generic
MYLAN

Penicillin V
250 mg
Generic
BIOCRAFT

Acetaminophen
325 mg
Tylenol Regular Strength
MCNEIL

Labetalol Hydrochloride
200 mg
Trandate
GLAXO WELLCOME

Disulfiram
250 mg
Generic
SIDMAK

Chlordiazepoxide/Amitriptyline
10\25 mg
Generic
MYLAN

Chlorothiazide
250 mg
Generic
WEST POINT

Aspirin
325 mg
Bayer
BAYER

Alendronate Sodium
10 mg
Fosamax
MERCK

Mercaptopurine
50 mg
Purinethol
GLAXO WELLCOME

Allopurinol
100 mg
Generic
SCHEIN/DANBURY

Vitamin C
250 mg
Generic
NUTRO

Carbamazepine
100 mg
Tegretol
BASEL

Ciprofloxacin
250 mg
Cipro
BAYER

Magnesium Oxide
400 mg
Generic
BLAINE

COLOR PILL LOCATOR

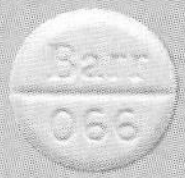 **Isoniazid** 100 mg Generic **BARR**	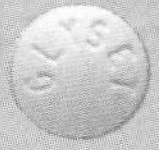 **Miglitol** 100 mg Glyset **UPJOHN**	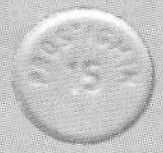 **Neostigmine** 15 mg Prostigmin **ICN PHARMACEUTICALS**	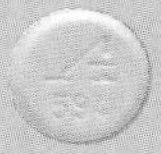 **Tizanidine Hydrochloride** 4 mg Zanaflex **SANDOZ PHARMA**
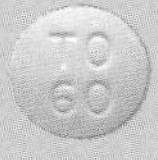 **Toremifene Citrate** 60 mg Fareston **ROBERTS PHARMACEUTICAL**	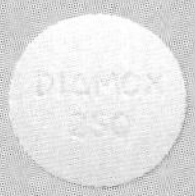 **Acetazolamide** 250 mg Diamox **STORZ**	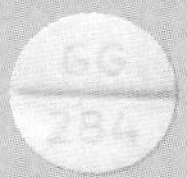 **Isoxsuprine Hydrochloride** 20 mg Generic **GENEVA**	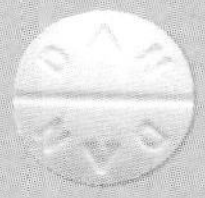 **Quinidine** 300 mg Generic **SCHEIN**
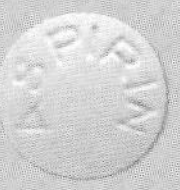 **Aspirin** 325 mg Generic **LNK**	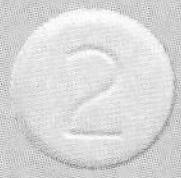 **Acetaminophen/Codeine** 300/15 mg Generic **GOLDLINE**	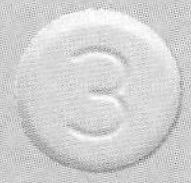 **Acetaminophen/Codeine** 300/30 mg Generic **GOLDLINE**	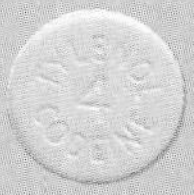 **Acetaminophen/Codeine** 300/60 mg Tylenol With Codeine **MCNEIL**
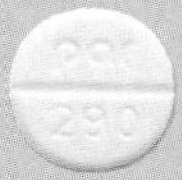 **Megestrol Acetate** 40 mg Generic **PAR**	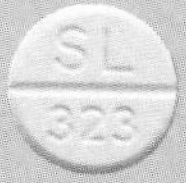 **Bethanechol Chloride** 5 mg Generic **SIDMAK**	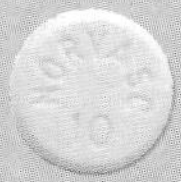 **Amlodipine** 10 mg Norvasc **PFIZER**	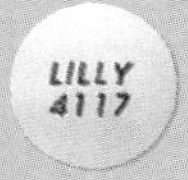 **Olanzapine** 10 mg Zyprexa **LILLY**
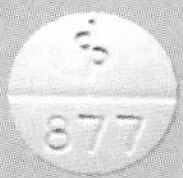 **Yohimbine** 5.4 mg Generic **MIKART**	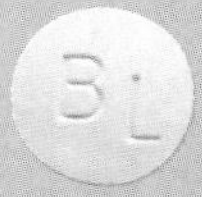 **Penicillin V** 500 mg Generic **BIOCRAFT**	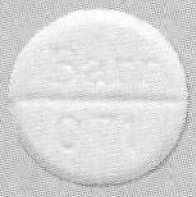 **Isoniazid** 300 mg Generic **BARR**	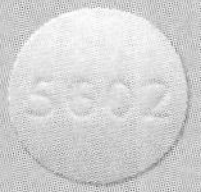 **Verapamil Hydrochloride** 120 mg Generic **SCHEIN/DANBURY**

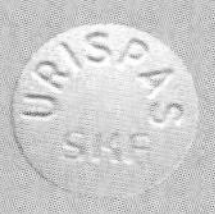

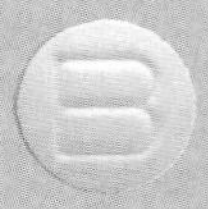

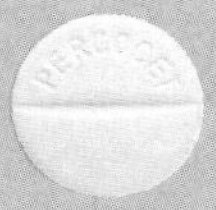

COLOR PILL LOCATOR

Flavoxate	**Aspirin**	**Vitamin C**	**Oxycodone/Acetaminophen**
100 mg	325 mg	500 mg	5/325 mg
Urispas	Bufferin	Generic	Percocet
SMITHKLINE BEECHAM	BRISTOL-MYERS SQUIBB	NUTRO	DUPONT
Albendazole	**Amoxicillin/Potassium Clavulanate**	**Diclofenac/Misoprostol**	**Mefloquine Hydrochloride**
200 mg	500/125 mg	50 mg/200 mcg	250 mg
Albenza	Augmentin	Arthrotec 50	Lariam
SMITHKLINE BEECHAM	SMITHKLINE BEECHAM	SEARLE	HOFFMANN-LAROCHE
Milk of Magnesia	**Vitamin B 6 (Pyridoxine)**	**Sparfloxacin**	**Terbinafine Hydrochloride**
311 mg	50 mg	200 mg	250 mg
Phillips' Chewable	Generic	Zagam	Lamisil
BAYER	UDL	RHONE-POULENC RORER	SANDOZ PHARMA
Famciclovir	**Azithromycin**	**Griseofulvin**	**Tolmetin Sodium**
500 mg	600 mg	125 mg	600 mg
Famvir	Zithromax	Gris-PEG	Generic
SMITHKLINE BEECHAM	PFIZER	WYETH-AYERST	PUREPAC
Dirithromycin	**Trimethoprim/Sulfamethoxazole**	**Methocarbamol**	**Nevirapine**
250 mg	160/800 mg	750 mg	200 mg
Dynabac	Generic	Generic	Viramune
BOCK	SCHEIN/DANBURY	GENEVA	BOEHRINGER INGELHEIM

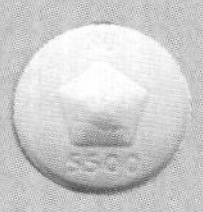

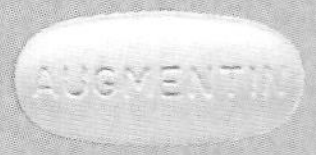

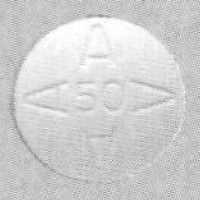

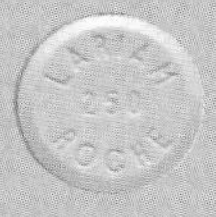

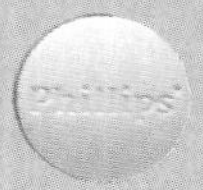

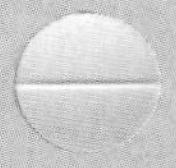

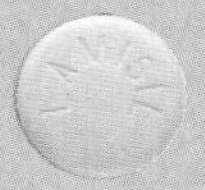

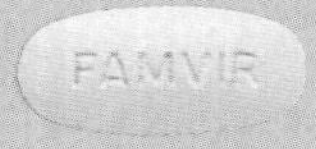

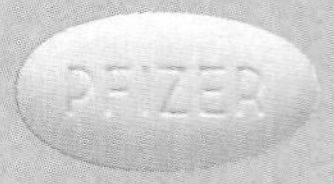

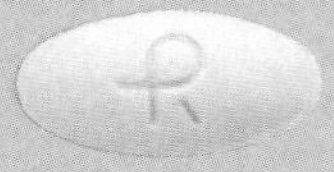

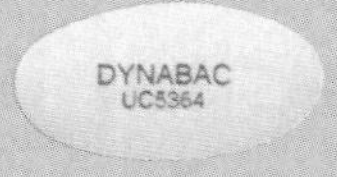

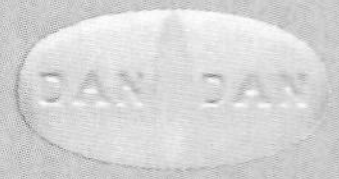

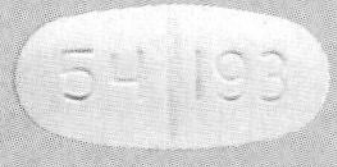

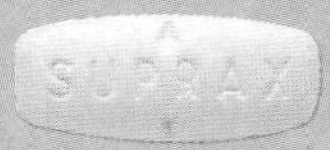

Cefixime
400 mg
Suprax
LEDERLE

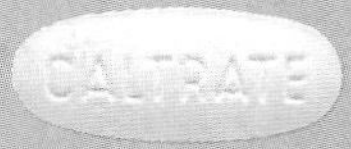

Calcium
600 mg
Caltrate 600
LEDERLE

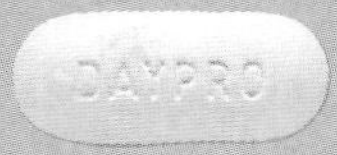

Oxaprozin
600 mg
DayPro
SEARLE

Acetaminophen
650 mg
Tylenol Extended Relief
MCNEIL

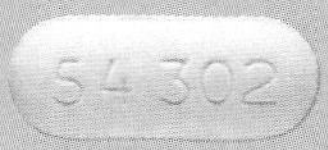

Calcium Carbonate
1.25 g
Generic
ROXANE

Theophylline
450 mg
Theo-Dur
KEY

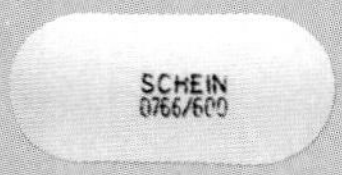

Ibuprofen
600 mg
Generic
SCHEIN

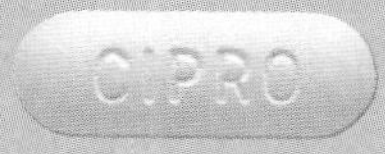

Ciprofloxacin
750 mg
Cipro
BAYER

Praziquantel
600 mg
Biltricide
BAYER

Potassium Chloride
1,500 mg
K-Dur 20
KEY

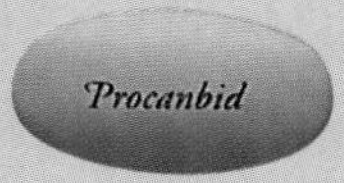

Procainamide Hydrochloride
1,000 mg
Procanbid
PARKE-DAVIS

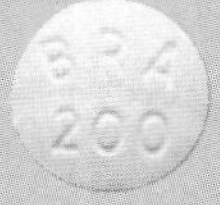

Calcium Acetate
667 mg
Phoslo
BRAINTREE

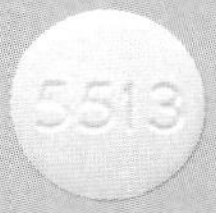

Carisoprodol
350 mg
Generic
SCHEIN/DANBURY

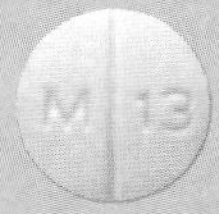

Tolbutamide
500 mg
Generic
MYLAN

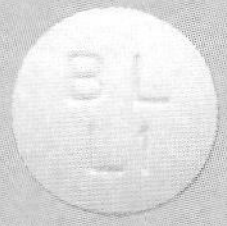

Mitotane
500 mg
Lysodren
BRISTOL-MYERS SQUIBB

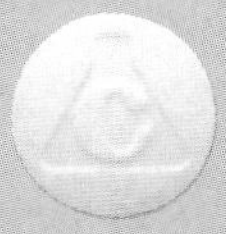

Quinidine
324 mg
Quinaglute
BERLEX

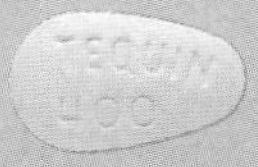

Gatifloxacin
400 mg
Tequin
BRISTOL-MYERS SQUIBB

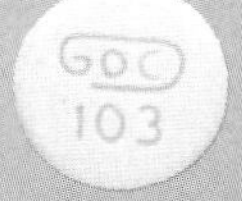

Simethicone
80 mg
Generic
GOLDLINE

Metformin
850 mg
Glucophage
BRISTOL-MYERS SQUIBB

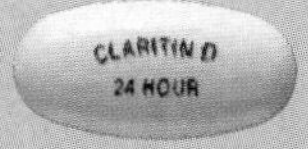

Loratadine/Pseudoephedrine
10/240 mg
Claritin-D 24 hr.
SCHERING CORP

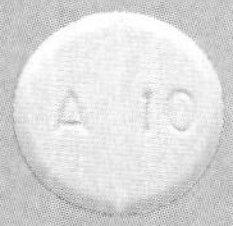

COLOR PILL LOCATOR

Aminocaproic Acid
500 mg
Amicar
IMMUNEX

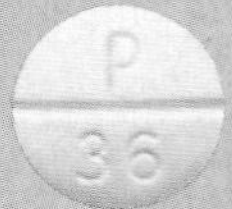

Pyrazinamide
500 mg
Generic
LEDERLE

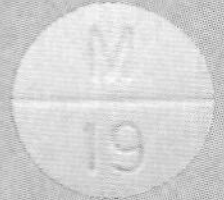

Methyldopa
250 mg
Generic
LEDERLE

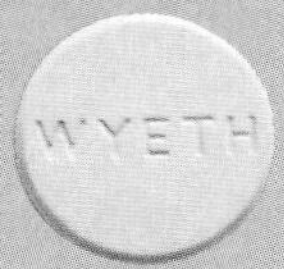

Aluminum Hydroxide
600 mg
Amphojel
WYETH-AYERST

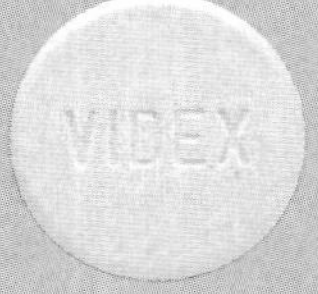

Didanosine
100 mg
Videx
BRISTOL-MYERS SQUIBB

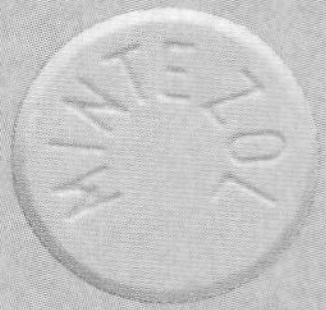

Thiabendazole
500 mg
Mintezol
MERCK

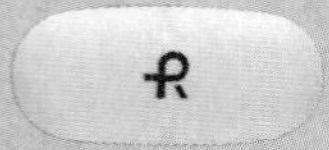

Gemfibrozil
600 mg
Generic
LEMMON

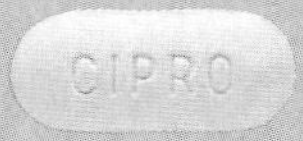

Ciprofloxacin
500 mg
Cipro
BAYER

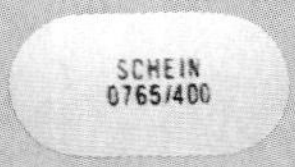

Ibuprofen
400 mg
Generic
SCHEIN

Diphenhydramine HCl
50 mg
Compoz Maximum Strength
MEDTECH

Diltiazem Hydrochloride
90 mg
Generic
MYLAN

Lomefloxacin Hydrochloride
400 mg
Maxaquin
SEARLE

Potassium Chloride
750 mg
K-Dur 10
KEY

Acetaminophen/Aspirin/Caffeine
250/250/65 mg
Excedrin
BRISTOL-MYERS SQUIBB

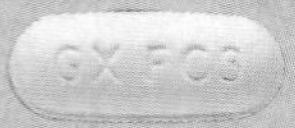

Lamivudine/Zidovudine
150/300 mg
Combivir
GLAXO WELLCOME

Diethylpropion Hydrochloride
75 mg
Tenuate Dospan
HOECHST MARION ROUSSEL

Fexofenadine/Pseudoephedrine
60/120 mg
Allegra-D
HOECHST MARION ROUSSEL

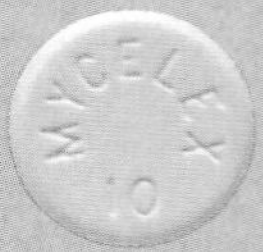

Clotrimazole
10 mg
Mycelex Troche
BAYER

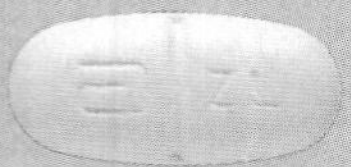

Zileuton
600 mg
Zyflo
ABBOTT

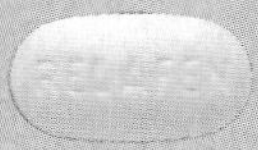

Nabumetone
500 mg
Relafen
SMITHKLINE BEECHAM

ABACAVIR SULFATE

Available in: Tablets, oral solution
Available OTC? No   **As Generic?** No
Drug Class: Antiviral/reverse transcriptase inhibitor

▼ USAGE INFORMATION

WHY IT'S PRESCRIBED
To treat human immunodeficiency virus (HIV) infection in combination with other drugs. While not a cure for HIV, such drugs may suppress the replication of the virus and delay the progression of the disease.

HOW IT WORKS
Abacavir prevents HIV from reproducing in two ways. A metabolite of the drug inhibits the activity of an enzyme needed for the replication of DNA in viral cells. The metabolite is also incorporated into viral DNA and terminates the formation of the complete DNA.

▼ DOSAGE GUIDELINES

RANGE AND FREQUENCY
Adults: To start, 300 mg 2 times a day. The drug must be taken in combination with other drugs for HIV, to delay the development of resistant strains of the virus. Children 3 months to 16 years: 8 mg per 2.2 lbs (1 kg) of body weight 2 times a day in combination with other drugs for HIV. Children should take no more than 300 mg twice a day.

ONSET OF EFFECT
Unknown. With most antiretroviral drugs, an early response can be seen within the first few days of therapy, but the maximum effect may take 12 to 16 weeks.

DURATION OF ACTION
Unknown.

DIETARY ADVICE
Abacavir can be taken with or without food.

STORAGE
Store at room temperature in a tightly sealed container away from heat, moisture, and direct light. The oral solution may be refrigerated, but should not be allowed to freeze.

MISSED DOSE
Take it as soon as you remember. If it is near the time for the next dose, skip the missed dose and resume your regular dosage schedule. Do not double the next dose. It is especially important to take abacavir on schedule, to assure constant, proper blood levels of the drug.

STOPPING THE DRUG
The decision to stop taking the drug should be made in consultation with your physician.

PROLONGED USE
See your doctor regularly for tests and examinations.

▼ PRECAUTIONS

Over 60: It is not known whether abacavir causes different or more severe side effects in older patients.

Driving and Hazardous Work: Avoid such activities until you determine how the medicine affects you.

Alcohol: Alcohol may raise blood levels of the drug.

Pregnancy: Abacavir has been shown to cause birth defects in animals. Human studies have not been done. This medication should be given during pregnancy only if potential benefits outweigh the risks to the unborn child.

Breast Feeding: Women with HIV should not breast feed, to avoid transmitting the virus to an uninfected child.

Infants and Children: Your pediatrician will determine the appropriate dosage based on your child's weight. Call your doctor immediately if you notice rash or any other side effects while your child is taking abacavir. The drug has not been tested in infants less than 3 months of age.

Special Concerns: See Serious Side Effects. If you must stop taking this drug because of this serious reaction, never take abacavir again. If you take this drug again after you have had this reaction, within hours you may experience life-threatening symptoms that may include lowering of blood pressure or death. Use of abacavir does not eliminate the risk of passing the AIDS virus to other persons. You should take appropriate preventive measures.

OVERDOSE
Symptoms: No cases of overdose have been reported.

What to Do: If you suspect an overdose or if someone takes a much larger dose than prescribed, call your doctor, emergency medical services (EMS), or the nearest poison control center immediately.

▼ INTERACTIONS

DRUG INTERACTIONS
Currently, there are no clinically significant drug interactions. Further studies are being conducted.

FOOD INTERACTIONS
No known food interactions.

DISEASE INTERACTIONS
Currently, there are no clinically significant disease interactions. Further studies are being conducted.

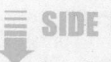

SIDE EFFECTS

SERIOUS
Uncommon (in approximately 5% of patients) and possibly fatal hypersensitivity reactions have been reported. Symptoms may include fever, skin rash, fatigue, nausea, vomiting, diarrhea, abdominal pain, weakness, lethargy, muscle and joint pain, swelling, shortness of breath, numbness, tingling, or prickling sensations, conjunctivitis, and mouth sores. Stop taking the drug and call your doctor immediately. Rarely, abacavir can also cause lactic acidosis (which is often fatal) and a greatly enlarged liver.

COMMON
Nausea, vomiting, weakness, fatigue, headache, loss of appetite, and diarrhea.

LESS COMMON
Insomnia and other sleep disorders.

ACARBOSE

Available in: Tablets
Available OTC? No   **As Generic?** No
Drug Class: Antidiabetic agent

▼ USAGE INFORMATION

WHY IT'S PRESCRIBED
As an adjunct (supplemental) therapy in patients with diabetes who do not require insulin injections yet are unable to control their blood glucose levels with diet alone or with other medications.

HOW IT WORKS
Acarbose inhibits the activity of enzymes required to break carbohydrates down into simple sugars within the intestine. This effect delays the digestion of carbohydrates and thus reduces the rise in blood sugar that typically occurs after meals.

▼ DOSAGE GUIDELINES

RANGE AND FREQUENCY
Initially, 25 mg, 1 to 3 times a day. The dose may be increased (at 4- to 8-week intervals) to a maximum of 100 mg, 3 times daily.

ONSET OF EFFECT
Within 1 hour.

DURATION OF ACTION
Up to 2 hours.

DIETARY ADVICE
This medicine should be taken with the first bite of breakfast, lunch, and dinner. Follow your doctor's advice regarding diet, weight loss, and exercise.

STORAGE
Keep in a tightly sealed container away from heat and direct light.

MISSED DOSE
If you have finished a meal without taking the medication, skip the missed dose and resume your regular dosing schedule with the next meal. Do not double the next dose.

STOPPING THE DRUG
Take it as prescribed for the full treatment period.

PROLONGED USE
Since non-insulin-dependent (type 2) diabetes is a chronic condition, use of acarbose will be ongoing. Blood glucose levels should be checked regularly during treatment so that the dosage may be adjusted if necessary.

▼ PRECAUTIONS

Over 60: No special precautions required.

Driving and Hazardous Work: Acarbose should not impair your ability to perform such tasks safely.

Alcohol: Drink only in moderation when taking acarbose.

Pregnancy: Consult your doctor for advice. Insulin is usually the treatment of choice for pregnant diabetic patients.

Breast Feeding: Trace amounts of acarbose can be found in breast milk; however, adverse effects in infants have not been documented. Consult your doctor for advice.

Infants and Children: Safety and effectiveness have not been established for patients under 18 years of age. Consult your doctor for specific advice.

Special Concerns: You should not take acarbose if you've had an allergic reaction to it previously or if you are taking, or took within the past 14 days, a monoamine oxidase (MAO) inhibitor (a class of antidepressant drugs).

OVERDOSE
Symptoms: Increased gas, diarrhea, and stomach pain.

What to Do: These symptoms usually subside on their own within a short period of time. If not, consult your doctor for advice. Symptoms of hypoglycemia should not occur when taking acarbose alone, but may occur if a patient is also taking sulfonylurea or insulin for diabetes.

▼ INTERACTIONS

DRUG INTERACTIONS
Do not take acarbose if you are taking, or took within the past 14 days, an MAO inhibitor. Consult your doctor for specific advice if you are taking any of the following drugs that may interact with acarbose: digestive enzyme preparations containing amylase or pancreatin, intestinal absorbents (such as charcoal), insulin, or sulfonylureas (oral antidiabetic agents).

FOOD INTERACTIONS
Avoid foods that contain large amounts of sugar (for example, cake, cookies, candy, acidic fruits). Closely follow the diet your doctor has prescribed.

DISEASE INTERACTIONS
This drug should not be taken by patients with a history of diabetic ketoacidosis, intestinal disorders (including malabsorption or obstruction), inflammatory bowel disease (for example, Crohn's disease or ulcerative colitis), liver or kidney disease, or gastric ulcers.

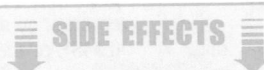

SIDE EFFECTS

SERIOUS
There are no serious side effects associated with acarbose.

COMMON
Feelings of bloating, gas, abdominal discomfort, diarrhea. These symptoms tend to decrease over time.

LESS COMMON
Rise in liver enzymes, causing yellowish tinge to eyes or skin (jaundice), when maximal dose is exceeded. When used in combination with sulfonylureas, may cause symptoms of low blood sugar, which include sweating, tremor, anxiety, hunger, confusion, seizures, rapid heartbeat, vision changes, dizziness, headache, loss of consciousness. Hypoglycemia must be treated by ingestion of glucose (dextrose). Sucrose (table sugar) and foods or drinks containing sugars or starches are ineffective because acarbose prevents their breakdown and absorption.

ACEBUTOLOL HYDROCHLORIDE

Available in: Capsules
Available OTC? No   **As Generic?** Yes
Drug Class: Beta-blocker

▼ USAGE INFORMATION

WHY IT'S PRESCRIBED
To treat mild to moderate high blood pressure; also used to prevent or control heartbeat irregularities (cardiac arrhythmias).

HOW IT WORKS
Acebutolol slows the rate and force of contraction of the heart by blocking certain nerve impulses, thus reducing blood pressure. By modifying nerve impulses to the heart, the drug also helps to stabilize heart rhythm.

▼ DOSAGE GUIDELINES

RANGE AND FREQUENCY
Adults: Initially, 400 mg a day, either as a single dose in the morning or as two 200 mg doses taken in the morning and evening (12 hours apart). Maximum daily dose is 1,200 mg; for those over 65, daily dose should not exceed 800 mg.

ONSET OF EFFECT
1 to 1 ½ hours.

DURATION OF ACTION
Up to 24 hours.

DIETARY ADVICE
Follow your doctor's dietary recommendations to improve control over high blood pressure and heart disease.

STORAGE
Store away from heat, moisture, and direct light.

MISSED DOSE
Take it as soon as you remember. If it is within 4 hours of the next scheduled dose, skip the missed dose and resume your regular dosage schedule. Do not double the next dose.

STOPPING THE DRUG
Suddenly stopping acebutolol may cause blood pressure to rise (rebound) to high or even dangerous levels, possibly triggering angina or a heart attack in patients with advanced heart disease. Slow reduction of the dose over a period of 2 to 3 weeks is advised, under careful supervision by your doctor.

PROLONGED USE
Regular visits to your doctor are needed to evaluate the drug's ongoing, long-term effectiveness.

▼ PRECAUTIONS

Over 60: Many elderly patients are more sensitive to the drug than younger persons. Smaller doses and frequent blood pressure checks may be advised.

Driving and Hazardous Work: Use caution until you determine how the medication affects you.

Alcohol: Drink in careful moderation, if at all. Alcohol may interact with the drug and cause a dangerous drop in blood pressure.

Pregnancy: Discuss with your doctor the relative risks and benefits of using this drug while pregnant.

Breast Feeding: Trace amounts of this drug can be found in breast milk, though adverse effects in infants have not been documented. Consult your doctor for advice.

Infants and Children: Not recommended.

Special Concerns: Use of the drug should be considered but one element of a comprehensive therapeutic program that includes weight control, smoking cessation, regular exercise, and a healthy low-salt, low-fat diet.

OVERDOSE
Symptoms: Unusually slow or rapid heartbeat, severe dizziness or fainting, poor circulation in the hands (bluish skin), breathing difficulty, seizures.

What to Do: Contact your doctor immediately.

▼ INTERACTIONS

DRUG INTERACTIONS
Consult your doctor for specific advice if you are taking amphetamines, oral antidiabetic agents, asthma medication (such as aminophylline or theophylline), calcium channel blockers, clonidine, guanabenz, halothane, allergy shots, insulin, MAO inhibitors, reserpine, or other beta-blockers.

FOOD INTERACTIONS
None reported.

DISEASE INTERACTIONS
Acebutolol should be used with caution in people with diabetes, especially insulin-dependent diabetes, since the drug may mask symptoms of hypoglycemia. Consult your doctor for specific advice if you have a history of allergies or asthma, heart or blood vessel disease (including congestive heart failure and peripheral vascular disease), hyperthyroidism, irregular (slow) heartbeat, myasthenia gravis, psoriasis, respiratory problems such as bronchitis or emphysema, kidney or liver disease, or mental depression.

≋ SIDE EFFECTS ≋

SERIOUS
Severe shortness of breath and rapid heartbeat (symptoms of congestive heart failure), worsening of asthma, severe allergic reaction (skin rash, itching, wheezing, swelling of lips, tongue, and throat). If any of these symptoms develop, seek medical attention immediately.

COMMON
Cough, diarrhea, decreased sexual ability, depression, drowsiness, dizziness, fatigue, frequent urination, gas, indigestion, nausea, trouble sleeping, cold hands and feet, numbness or tingling in fingers or toes.

LESS COMMON
Fever, sore throat, abdominal pain, headache, anxiety, joint or back pain, dry or burning eyes, unusual bleeding or bruising, dark urine, nightmares or unusually vivid dreams.

ACETAMINOPHEN

Available in: Capsules, caplets, tablets, powder, liquid, suppositories
Available OTC? Yes   **As Generic?** Yes
Drug Class: Analgesic; antipyretic (fever reducer)

▼ USAGE INFORMATION

WHY IT'S PRESCRIBED
To treat mild to moderate pain and fever, including simple headaches, muscle aches, and mild forms of arthritis. Acetaminophen is useful for patients who cannot take aspirin, such as those taking anticoagulants or suffering from gastrointestinal ulcers or bleeding disorders.

HOW IT WORKS
Acetaminophen appears to interfere with the action of prostaglandins, substances in the body that cause inflammation and make nerves more sensitive to pain impulses. It also relieves fever, probably by acting on the heat-regulating center of the brain.

▼ DOSAGE GUIDELINES

RANGE AND FREQUENCY
For adults and teenagers: 325 to 650 mg every 4 to 6 hours, or 1 g, 3 to 4 times a day, as needed. Extended-release caplets: Take 2 every 8 hours. Maximum dosage with short-term therapy should not exceed 4 g a day; with long-term therapy it should not exceed 2.6 g a day unless otherwise prescribed by your doctor. For children 12 years and under: Consult a pediatrician for proper dose. Liquid form may be recommended for young children.

ONSET OF EFFECT
Within 15 to 30 minutes.

DURATION OF ACTION
3 to 4 hours; 8 hours for extended-release form.

DIETARY ADVICE
Take it with water 30 minutes before or 2 hours after meals. It may be taken with milk to minimize stomach upset. If you are on a salt-restricted diet, be sure to account for the sodium present in the powder form of acetaminophen.

STORAGE
Store in a tightly sealed container away from heat and direct light. Refrigerate liquid forms (to make them more palatable) and rectal suppositories. Do not allow the medication to freeze.

SIDE EFFECTS

SERIOUS
Allergic reaction causing rash, itching, hives, swelling, or breathing difficulty; yellow-tinged skin and eyes (indicating liver damage). Seek medical assistance immediately.

COMMON
No common side effects have been reported.

LESS COMMON
Sore throat and fever (not present before treatment and not caused by the condition being treated), extreme fatigue or weakness, unexplained bleeding or bruising, blood in urine, painful, decreased, or frequent urination.

MISSED DOSE
Take it as soon as you remember. If it is near the time for the next dose, skip the missed dose and resume your regular dosage schedule. Do not double the next dose.

STOPPING THE DRUG
Unless directed otherwise by your doctor, limit use to 5 days for children under age 12 and 10 days for adults.

PROLONGED USE
Prolonged use may lead to liver problems, kidney problems, or anemia in some patients. Talk to your doctor about the need for periodic physical examinations and laboratory tests.

▼ PRECAUTIONS

Over 60: Adverse reactions may be more likely and more severe in older patients; lower doses may be warranted.

Driving and Hazardous Work: No problems are expected.

Alcohol: Avoid alcohol; combining the two can cause serious liver problems. Patients with a history of alcohol abuse should not use acetaminophen except under close supervision by a doctor.

Pregnancy: No problems have been reported. Consult your doctor if you are or plan to become pregnant.

Breast Feeding: No problems have been reported.

Infants and Children: No problems are expected; however, some formulations are sweetened with aspartame, which should not be consumed by children with phenylketonuria.

OVERDOSE
Symptoms: Nausea, vomiting, appetite loss, abdominal pain, excessive sweating, confusion, drowsiness or exhaustion, stomach tenderness, heartbeat irregularities, yellowing of the skin and eyes.

What to Do: If you suspect an overdose, seek medical aid immediately, even if no symptoms are present. Steps must be taken promptly to avoid potentially fatal liver damage.

▼ INTERACTIONS

DRUG INTERACTIONS
Consult your doctor for specific advice if you are taking anticoagulants (such as warfarin), aspirin, an NSAID, barbiturates, carbamazepine, hydantoins, rifampin, sulfinpyrazone, isoniazid, nicotine, or zidovudine.

FOOD INTERACTIONS
No known food interactions.

DISEASE INTERACTIONS
Consult your doctor if you have liver or kidney disease, diabetes mellitus, phenylketonuria, or a history of alcohol abuse.

ACETAMINOPHEN WITH CODEINE PHOSPHATE

Available in: Capsules, tablets, oral solution, oral suspension
Available OTC? No   **As Generic?** Yes
Drug Class: Opioid (narcotic) analgesic/antipyretic

▼ USAGE INFORMATION

WHY IT'S PRESCRIBED
To relieve mild to severe pain when nonprescription pain relievers prove inadequate. A narcotic analgesic such as codeine, in combination with acetaminophen, may provide better pain relief than either medicine used alone. Used together, pain relief may be achieved at lower doses of the two medications.

HOW IT WORKS
Acetaminophen appears to interfere with the action of prostaglandins, naturally occurring substances in the body that cause inflammation and make nerves more sensitive to pain impulses. It also relieves fever, probably by acting on the heat-regulating center of the brain. Unlike aspirin, however, acetaminophen does not reduce inflammation. Codeine, a narcotic analgesic, is believed to relieve pain by acting on specific areas in the spinal cord and brain that process pain signals from nerves throughout the body.

▼ DOSAGE GUIDELINES

RANGE AND FREQUENCY
Adults— Capsules or tablets: 1 or 2 capsules containing 15 or 30 mg of codeine with acetaminophen or 1 capsule containing 60 mg of codeine with acetaminophen, every 4 hours as needed. Oral solution or suspension: 1 tablespoon every 4 hours as needed. Children— Oral solution or suspension: Ages 3 to 6: 1 teaspoon 3 or 4 times a day as needed. Ages 7 to 12: 2 teaspoons 3 or 4 times a day as needed.

ONSET OF EFFECT
Acetaminophen: Rapid. Codeine: Within 2 hours.

DURATION OF ACTION
Up to 4 hours.

DIETARY ADVICE
Take this drug with meals or milk to avoid stomach upset, unless doctor directs you to do otherwise.

STORAGE
Store in a tightly sealed container away from heat, moisture, and direct light. Keep liquid forms from freezing.

MISSED DOSE
If you are taking acetaminophen with codeine on a fixed schedule, take it as soon as you remember. If it is near the time for the next dose, skip the missed dose and resume your regular dosage schedule. Do not double the next dose.

STOPPING THE DRUG
You should take the drug as prescribed for the full treatment period, but you may stop taking it if you are feeling better before the scheduled end of therapy. This drug should never be stopped abruptly after long-term regular use.

PROLONGED USE
Narcotic drugs, such as codeine, may cause physical dependence. Taking too much acetaminophen may cause liver damage. Therapy with acetaminophen and codeine should not continue for more than 2 weeks and may actually cease to be effective before then.

▼ PRECAUTIONS

Over 60: Adverse reactions may be more likely and more severe in older patients.

Driving and Hazardous Work: This drug can cause dizziness or drowsiness; proceed with caution.

Alcohol: Avoid alcohol. The combination of alcohol and this drug may increase the depressant effects of the medicine. Drinking alcohol-containing beverages while taking acetaminophen greatly increases the risk of liver damage.

Pregnancy: Use of this drug during pregnancy can cause fetal addiction and may cause breathing problems in the newborn infant if taken during or just before delivery. Consult your doctor for specific guidelines and advice and discuss the relative risks and benefits of using this drug while pregnant.

Breast Feeding: Acetaminophen with codeine passes into breast milk; avoid or discontinue nursing while taking this drug.

Infants and Children: This medicine should not be given to infants. The drug may be used by children over the age of 3, but only with extreme caution and under the careful supervision of your doctor. Children are generally prescribed the oral solution or suspension instead of the capsule or tablet.

Special Concerns: Taking a narcotic, such as codeine, for an extended period of time can lead to physical dependence. When discontinuing the drug after using it for an extended period, it is important to decrease the dosage gradually under the supervision of your doctor to reduce the risk of suffering from withdrawal symptoms. Call your doctor if you notice these symptoms after discon-

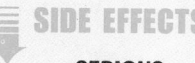

SIDE EFFECTS

SERIOUS
See Overdose and Special Concerns.

COMMON
Dizziness, lightheadedness, nausea or vomiting, drowsiness, constipation, unusual fatigue.

LESS COMMON
Stomach pain, allergic reaction, false sense of well-being (euphoria), depression, loss of appetite, blurring or change in vision, nightmares or unusual dreams, dry mouth, general feeling of illness, headache, nervousness, insomnia.

(continued)

tinuing the drug: shivering or trembling; insomnia; gooseflesh; nausea or vomiting; body aches; loss of appetite; stomach cramps; weakness; diarrhea; restlessness, nervousness, or irritability; rapid heartbeat; runny nose, sneezing, or fever; increased yawning; or increased sweating. Overuse of acetaminophen with codeine may also lead to anemia, liver problems, or central nervous system disorders. Contact your doctor as soon as possible if you experience any of the following symptoms during or after the use of this drug: bloody, dark, or cloudy urine; severe pain in the lower back or side; frequent urge to urinate; painful or difficult urination; sudden decrease in urine output; pale or black, tarry stools; yellow discoloration of the eyes or skin (jaundice); hallucinations; unusual bleeding or bruising; skin rash, hives, or itching; pinpoint red spots on skin; sore throat and fever; unusual excitability; trembling or uncontrolled muscle movements; redness, flushing, or swelling of the face.

OVERDOSE

Symptoms: Severe dizziness or drowsiness; cold, clammy skin; difficult or slow breathing or shortness of breath; severe confusion; seizures; stomach cramps or pain; diarrhea; low blood pressure; increased sweating; constricted pupils; nausea or vomiting; irregular heartbeat; severe weakness.

What to Do: Call your doctor, emergency medical services (EMS), or the nearest poison control center immediately.

▼ INTERACTIONS

DRUG INTERACTIONS

Some drugs may interact with acetaminophen and codeine. Consult your doctor for specific advice if you are taking any prescription or over-the-counter drugs, especially if they contain acetaminophen; central nervous system depressants, such as antihistamines or medicine for hay fever, allergies, or colds; barbiturates; seizure medicine; muscle relaxants; anesthetics; or tranquilizers, sedatives, or sleep medications.

FOOD INTERACTIONS

No significant food interactions have been reported.

DISEASE INTERACTIONS

Consult your doctor if you have a head injury or brain disease, an underactive thyroid, an enlarged prostate, seizures, kidney or liver disease, gallbladder problems, a blood disorder, or a history of alcohol or drug abuse. These conditions may increase the likelihood of side effects from acetaminophen and codeine.

ACETAMINOPHEN/ASPIRIN/CAFFEINE

BRAND NAMES

Buffets II, Duradyne, Excedrin Extra-Strength, Excedrin Migraine, Gelpirin, Goody's Extra Strength Tablets, Goody's Headache Powders, Supac, Vanquish Caplets

Available in: Tablets, caplets, oral powder
Available OTC? Yes   **As Generic?** No
Drug Class: Analgesic

▼ USAGE INFORMATION

WHY IT'S PRESCRIBED
For the temporary relief of mild to moderate pain associated with arthritis or migraines.

HOW IT WORKS
Acetaminophen and aspirin both appear to interfere with the production of prostaglandins, naturally occurring substances in the body that cause inflammation and make nerves more sensitive to pain impulses. Caffeine is believed to enhance the effectiveness of pain relievers.

▼ DOSAGE GUIDELINES

RANGE AND FREQUENCY
Because the amount of each of the components varies with different brands, consult your doctor for the appropriate dose. The following are general guidelines. Adults and teenagers— Tablets and caplets: 1 to 2 pills every 3 to 6 hours, as needed and depending on the strength of the product. Do not take more than 8 pills in a 24-hour period. Oral powder: 1 packet followed immediately by a full glass of water every 6 hours. Children— Generally not recommended for children.

ONSET OF EFFECT
Unknown.

DURATION OF ACTION
Unknown.

DIETARY ADVICE
Should be taken with food or a full glass of water to minimize stomach upset.

STORAGE
Store in a tightly sealed container away from heat, moisture, and direct light.

MISSED DOSE
Skip the missed dose and then resume your regular dosage schedule. Do not double the next dose.

STOPPING THE DRUG
You may stop taking the drug whenever you choose.

PROLONGED USE
This combination is indicated for short-term use only. Side effects are more likely with prolonged use.

▼ PRECAUTIONS

Over 60: Adverse reactions may be more likely and more severe.

Driving and Hazardous Work: May cause drowsiness or vision difficulties.

Alcohol: Do not consume more than 2 alcohol-containing beverages a day.

Pregnancy: Discuss with your doctor the relative risks and benefits of using this drug while pregnant. This drug should not be used during the last 3 months of pregnancy.

Breast Feeding: This drug may pass into breast milk; consult your doctor for specific advice.

Infants and Children: Consult your pediatrician. This drug is not recommended for children under age 16, since the aspirin component may cause a rare but life-threatening condition known as Reye's syndrome.

Special Concerns: Be sure your doctor knows you are taking this medication; it can interfere with the results of some blood and urine tests. Patients allergic to aspirin should not take this drug.

OVERDOSE
Symptoms: Nausea and vomiting, disorientation, seizures, rapid breathing, ringing or buzzing in the ears, fever, appetite loss, abdominal pain, excessive sweating, drowsiness or exhaustion, stomach tenderness, heartbeat irregularities, yellow discoloration of the skin and eyes, agitation, anxiety, restlessness, delirium.

What to Do: Call your doctor, emergency medical services (EMS), or the nearest poison control center immediately.

▼ INTERACTIONS

DRUG INTERACTIONS
Consult your doctor before taking this drug if you are currently taking any of the following: blood pressure medication, gout or arthritis drugs, anticoagulants such as warfarin, antidiabetic agents, steroids, seizure medication, NSAIDs, barbiturates, nicotine, zidovudine (AZT), isoniazid, any central nervous system stimulant, a MAO inhibitor, amantadine, over-the-counter cold and allergy medications, or asthma medicine.

FOOD INTERACTIONS
Do not drink large amounts of caffeine-containing beverages like coffee, tea, cola, cocoa, or chocolate milk.

DISEASE INTERACTIONS
Consult your doctor if you have liver or kidney disease, diabetes, phenylketonuria, a history of alcohol abuse, asthma, a bleeding disorder, congestive heart failure, gout, high blood pressure, thyroid disease, peptic ulcer, anxiety or panic attacks, agoraphobia, or insomnia.

 SIDE EFFECTS

SERIOUS
Difficulty swallowing; dizziness, lightheadedness, or fainting; flushing, redness, or change in color of skin; difficulty breathing, shortness of breath, tightness in the chest, or wheezing; sudden decrease in urine output; swelling of face, eyelids, or lips; black or tarry stools; unusual bleeding or bruising; yellow discoloration of the skin and eyes (indicating liver damage). Call your doctor immediately.

COMMON
Indigestion, nausea and vomiting, stomach pain.

LESS COMMON
Sleeping difficulty, nervousness, irritability.

ACETAZOLAMIDE

Available in: Tablets, extended-release capsules, injection
Available OTC? No **As Generic?** Yes
Drug Class: Carbonic anhydrase inhibitor; anticonvulsant

▼ USAGE INFORMATION

WHY IT'S PRESCRIBED
To treat glaucoma, seizures, familial periodic paralysis; to prevent or treat mountain (altitude) sickness; to prevent one type of kidney stones.

HOW IT WORKS
For glaucoma: Blocks the enzyme carbonic anhydrase, thus decreasing the normal secretion of fluid inside the eyeball. For seizures: Appears to reduce the firing of neurons in the brain. For paralysis: Stabilizes muscle membranes. For mountain sickness: Stimulates greater oxygen intake, improves blood flow to the brain, and improves release of oxygen from red blood cells. For kidney stones: Increases alkalinity of urine, which reduces stone formation.

▼ DOSAGE GUIDELINES

RANGE AND FREQUENCY
Tablets— For glaucoma: Adults: 250 mg, 1 to 4 times a day. Children: 4.5 to 6.8 mg per lb of body weight per day in divided doses. For seizures: 4.5 mg per lb daily in divided doses. For altitude sickness: 250 mg, 2 to 4 times a day. Extended-release capsules— For glaucoma: 500 mg twice a day (morning and evening). For altitude sickness: 500 mg, 1 to 2 times a day. Injection— For glaucoma: Adults: 500 mg once a day. Children: 2.3 to 4.5 mg per lb every 6 hours.

ONSET OF EFFECT
Tablets: Within 60 to 90 minutes. Extended-release capsules: 2 hours. Injection: 2 minutes.

DURATION OF ACTION
Tablets: 8 to 12 hours. Extended-release capsules: 18 to 24 hours. Injection: 4 to 5 hours.

DIETARY ADVICE
Take oral acetazolamide with food or milk to avoid stomach upset. Tablets can be crushed and mixed with sweet foods to cover taste. (Do not crush extended-release capsules.) Eat foods high in potassium.

STORAGE
Store in a tightly sealed container away from heat, moisture, and direct light.

MISSED DOSE
Take it as soon as you remember. If it is near the time for the next dose, skip the missed dose and resume your regular dosage schedule. Do not double the next dose.

STOPPING THE DRUG
The decision to stop taking the drug should be made by your doctor. Do not stop taking the drug abruptly.

PROLONGED USE
Prolonged use of this drug may require increased potassium intake.

▼ PRECAUTIONS

Over 60: Adverse reactions may be more likely and more severe in older patients.

Driving and Hazardous Work: Avoid such activities until you determine how the medicine affects you.

Alcohol: Alcohol may interfere with seizure control.

Pregnancy: Adequate studies have not been done; discuss the relative risks and benefits with your doctor.

Breast Feeding: It may be necessary to switch medications or discontinue breast feeding.

Infants and Children: No problems are expected.

Special Concerns: May increase urine output, especially at first, as your body adapts to the drug. To keep this condition from disrupting sleep, take a single dose after breakfast if possible; if you take multiple daily doses, take the last one before 6 pm, unless your doctor instructs otherwise.

OVERDOSE
Symptoms: Drowsiness, numbness, nausea, thirst, vomiting, seizures, coma.

What to Do: Call your doctor, emergency medical services (EMS), or the nearest poison control center immediately.

▼ INTERACTIONS

DRUG INTERACTIONS
Do not take acetazolamide with high doses of aspirin or amphetamines, as this may be toxic. Do not take it if you are allergic to sulfa-type drugs. Consult your doctor if you are taking mecamylamine, quinidine, lithium, methenamine, or oral hypoglycemia agents.

FOOD INTERACTIONS
Avoid black licorice. Include high-potassium foods, such as bananas and citrus fruits, in your diet.

DISEASE INTERACTIONS
Do not take acetazolamide if you have serious liver or kidney disease, Addison's disease, low blood levels of potassium or sodium, or diabetes mellitus. Consult your doctor if you have gout or a lung disease, such as emphysema, or a history of kidney stones.

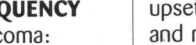

SIDE EFFECTS

SERIOUS
Breathing difficulty, seizures, serious allergic reaction (hives, itching, swelling of eyes, lips, and throat).

COMMON
Unusual fatigue; diarrhea; increase in volume and frequency of urination; loss of appetite and weight; metallic taste in mouth; numbness, tingling, or prickling sensations in hands, feet, fingers, toes, lips, and elsewhere.

LESS COMMON
Worsening nearsightedness, dark or bloody urine, painful urination, depression, lower back or flank pain, sudden decrease in urine output, unusual bruising or bleeding, bloody, black, pale, or tarry stools, confusion, clumsiness.

ACETOHEXAMIDE

Available in: Tablets
Available OTC? No   **As Generic?** Yes
Drug Class: Antidiabetic agent/sulfonylurea

▼ USAGE INFORMATION

WHY IT'S PRESCRIBED
Used as an adjunct (supplemental) therapy to dietary modification to help control sugar levels in patients with non-insulin-dependent (type 2) diabetes mellitus.

HOW IT WORKS
It stimulates the pancreas to produce more insulin. Increased insulin levels reduce blood glucose levels and promote the transport of glucose into muscle cells and other tissues, where it is burned for energy.

▼ DOSAGE GUIDELINES

RANGE AND FREQUENCY
Starting at 250 mg once a day, increased as needed to a maximum of 1.5 g per day. In patients receiving less than 1 g per day, sugar levels can usually be controlled with a once-a-day dose; for those receiving between 1 and 1.5 g, the drug is given in two daily doses, morning and evening.

ONSET OF EFFECT
Within 1 hour.

DURATION OF ACTION
12 to 24 hours.

DIETARY ADVICE
Take it with food or liquid to minimize stomach upset.

STORAGE
Store in a tightly sealed container away from heat, moisture, and direct light.

MISSED DOSE
If you miss a dose, take it as soon as you remember unless it is almost time for the next dose. In that case, skip the missed dose and return to your regular schedule. Do not double the next dose.

STOPPING THE DRUG
Do not stop taking acetohexamide without consulting your doctor.

PROLONGED USE
The dosage may need to be adjusted with prolonged use. Over time, many patients become resistant to the effects of the medication and may require treatment with insulin instead.

▼ PRECAUTIONS

Over 60: A smaller dosage is usually warranted for older patients.

Driving and Hazardous Work: No problems are expected.

Alcohol: Drink in moderation only. Small amounts of alcohol at mealtimes usually cause no problems with blood sugar; however, alcohol may cause unpleasant flushing in the face, arms, and neck, up to 12 hours after ingestion.

Pregnancy: Acetohexamide is not usually given during pregnancy. Insulin is generally the treatment of choice for pregnant diabetic patients.

Breast Feeding: Acetohexamide may pass into breast milk; caution is advised. Consult your doctor if you are considering breast feeding.

Infants and Children: Safety and effectiveness have not been established for young patients.

Special Concerns: Follow carefully your doctor's advice about diet, exercise, and weight control. These aspects of treatment are just as essential to the proper control of diabetes as taking the medication. Be sure to carry at all times some form of medical identification that indicates you have diabetes and that lists all of the drugs you are taking.

OVERDOSE

Symptoms: Excessive hunger, nausea, anxiety, cold sweats, drowsiness, rapid heartbeat, weakness, changes in mental state, loss of consciousness (indications of hypoglycemia). Overdose is most likely to occur after you have delayed or missed a meal, have exercised more than usual, or have consumed more than a small amount of alcohol.

What to Do: Call your doctor, emergency medical services (EMS), or local hospital immediately.

▼ INTERACTIONS

DRUG INTERACTIONS
The effects of acetohexamide can be altered by anticoagulants, antidepressants, aspirin, over-the-counter cold preparations containing aspirin, some diuretics, glucagon, beta-blockers, steroids, phenylbutazone, probenecid, rifampin, nonprescription drugs for colds, hay fever, and appetite control, and sulfa-containing antibiotics.

FOOD INTERACTIONS
A special diet is essential for proper control of blood glucose levels. Avoid foods high in sugar.

DISEASE INTERACTIONS
Liver disease, overactive or underactive thyroid, and kidney disease can affect the activity of the drug.

 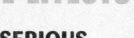 **SIDE EFFECTS**

SERIOUS
Hypoglycemia (blood sugar levels that are too low), resulting in shakiness, headache, cold sweats, anxiety, and changes in mental state. Stop taking the drug and seek medical help immediately. Severe diarrhea, bleeding, bruising, chills, fever, stomach pain, or heartburn may also occur; stop taking the drug and notify your doctor. Other serious but less-common side effects include bone marrow suppression, hemolytic anemia, and elevation of liver-associated enzymes; these problems can be detected by your doctor.

COMMON
Increased skin sensitivity to sunlight.

LESS COMMON
Fatigue, itchy skin, sore throat, ringing in ears, weakness.

ACETYLCYSTEINE

Available in: Inhalant solution
Available OTC? No   **As Generic?** Yes
Drug Class: Decongestant/cough drug

▼ USAGE INFORMATION

WHY IT'S PRESCRIBED
To relieve congestion and make breathing easier in lung conditions associated with the production of large amounts of thick mucus, such as bronchiectasis (irreversible destruction of the bronchial walls), bronchitis, pneumonia, and cystic fibrosis. It may also be used in patients who have undergone tracheostomy (surgical opening in the neck to establish an airway when the throat is obstructed), or who have a collapsed lobe of the lung due to a plug of mucus blocking an airway.

HOW IT WORKS
Acetylcysteine liquefies and thins mucus so that it may be coughed up (or removed with suction if necessary).

▼ DOSAGE GUIDELINES

RANGE AND FREQUENCY
3 to 5 ml of 20% solution, or 6 to 10 ml of 10% solution by nebulizer every 2 to 6 hours. (The medicine may be inhaled through a face mask, mouthpiece, or via tracheostomy.) Or, 1 to 2 ml of 10% or 20% solution placed directly into the trachea via catheter every hour. The dosage differs from patient to patient; follow your doctor's directions carefully.

ONSET OF EFFECT
Within 1 minute.

DURATION OF ACTION
Up to several hours.

DIETARY ADVICE
This drug should not be taken with meals. Be sure to drink plenty of fluids.

STORAGE
Before opening, store container away from heat and direct light. After opening, store it in the refrigerator, but do not allow it to freeze. Discard the container 96 hours after opening.

MISSED DOSE
Take it as soon as you remember. Take the rest of the day's doses at evenly spaced intervals.

STOPPING THE DRUG
The decision to stop taking the drug should be made by your doctor.

PROLONGED USE
No special problems are expected.

▼ PRECAUTIONS

Over 60: No special problems are expected.

Driving and Hazardous Work: Be cautious if acetylcysteine makes you drowsy.

Alcohol: Alcohol intake should be limited.

Pregnancy: The effects of acetylcysteine on the human fetus have not been documented; consult your doctor or OB/GYN for specific advice if you are pregnant or plan to become pregnant.

Breast Feeding: It is not known whether acetylcysteine passes into breast milk; problems have not been documented. Consult your doctor for specific advice before deciding to nurse while using this drug.

Infants and Children: No special problems are expected.

Special Concerns: Be sure to tell your doctor if you have ever had any unusual or allergic reaction to acetylcysteine, or if you are allergic to any other substances, including foods, preservatives, latex, or dyes. If you use a nebulizer to administer the medication, it should be cleaned immediately after use, since residues of the medicine can be sticky and may clog the apparatus. Nebulized solution may be inhaled directly from the nebulizer, or the nebulizer may be fitted with a plastic face mask or mouthpiece. When acetylcysteine is used by patients with asthma or other types of hypersensitivity of the airways, a bronchodilator should be administered first to prevent bronchospasm.

OVERDOSE
Symptoms: Unusual breathing difficulties.

What to Do: Call your doctor, emergency medical services (EMS), or local hospital immediately.

▼ INTERACTIONS

DRUG INTERACTIONS
Simultaneous use of acetylcysteine with tetracycline, erythromycin, lactobionate, amphotericin B, ampicillin, chymotrypsin, or hydrogen peroxide in the same solution should be avoided. Such medications should be taken at another time.

FOOD INTERACTIONS
No known food interactions.

DISEASE INTERACTIONS
Acetylcysteine can aggravate asthma or other respiratory diseases.

≣ SIDE EFFECTS ≣

SERIOUS
Wheezing, tightness in the chest, and breathing difficulty (especially among patients with asthma); spitting up of blood. Contact your doctor immediately if any such symptoms arise.

COMMON
Acetylcysteine does not commonly cause side effects.

LESS COMMON
Clammy skin, fever, increased mucus production in the lungs, pain or irritation around the mouth or throat, nausea and vomiting, runny nose, drowsiness. Such symptoms are likely to diminish as your body adjusts to the medication.

ACITRETIN

Available in: Capsules
Available OTC? No   **As Generic?** No
Drug Class: Retinoid

▼ USAGE INFORMATION

WHY IT'S PRESCRIBED
To treat severe psoriasis. Acitretin is used only when other medications to treat psoriasis prove ineffective.

HOW IT WORKS
The exact mechanism of action of acitretin is unknown. It appears to establish a more normal pattern of growth and shedding of skin cells.

▼ DOSAGE GUIDELINES

RANGE AND FREQUENCY
To start, 25 mg once a day. A maintenance dose, given after the initial response to therapy, is 25 to 50 mg once a day. If the response to the drug is unsatisfactory after 4 weeks and there are minimal side effects, the dose may be increased by your doctor, depending on your condition and body weight.

ONSET OF EFFECT
It may take 2 or 3 months to attain the full therapeutic benefit of acitretin.

DURATION OF ACTION
Unknown.

DIETARY ADVICE
Acitretin is best taken with the main meal of the day.

STORAGE
Store in a tightly sealed container away from heat, moisture, and direct light.

MISSED DOSE
Take it as soon as you remember. If it is near the time for the next dose, skip the missed dose and resume your regular dosage schedule. Do not double the next dose.

STOPPING THE DRUG
You should take it as prescribed for the full treatment period, but you may stop taking the drug before the scheduled end of therapy if the symptoms have sufficiently resolved. Consult your doctor.

PROLONGED USE
Acitretin is generally prescribed for 1-month periods. See your doctor regularly for tests and examinations to assess the effectiveness and safety of the drug.

▼ PRECAUTIONS

Over 60: Adverse reactions may be more likely and more severe in older patients.

Driving and Hazardous Work: Do not drive or engage in hazardous work until you determine how the medicine affects you.

Alcohol: Avoid alcohol during and for two months after completing therapy.

Pregnancy: Acitretin can cause serious birth defects. Before your doctor will prescribe it, you must sign a waiver agreeing to use contraceptive measures for one month prior to therapy and three years afterward. You must receive a negative result on a pregnancy test within one week of beginning treatment.

Breast Feeding: Acitretin may pass into breast milk and cause serious harm. Do not nurse while taking this drug.

Infants and Children: No studies have been done with children, although it is believed that acitretin could adversely affect growth.

Special Concerns: You may experience increased sensitivity to contact lenses while taking acitretin. If it causes increased sensitivity to sunlight, wear protective clothing, use a sun block, and try to avoid exposure to sunlight. Do not donate blood while you take acitretin and for three years afterward. Many patients will experience a relapse and require further treatment after they stop taking acitretin.

OVERDOSE
Symptoms: No cases of overdose have been reported.

What to Do: An overdose of acitretin is unlikely to be life-threatening. However, if someone takes a much larger dose than prescribed, call your doctor, emergency medical services (EMS), or the nearest poison control center immediately.

▼ INTERACTIONS

DRUG INTERACTIONS
Other drugs may interact with acitretin. Consult your doctor if you are taking vitamin A, any other retinoid, or methotrexate. Also tell your doctor if you are taking any other prescription or over-the-counter drug.

FOOD INTERACTIONS
No known food interactions.

DISEASE INTERACTIONS
Consult your doctor for advice if you have diabetes mellitus, liver disease, or any other medical condition.

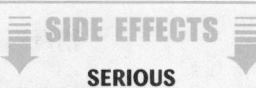

SIDE EFFECTS

SERIOUS
Severe headache, liver damage, eye lesions, joint pain, abnormal spinal bone growth, rigidity, violent shivering associated with chills and fever. Call your doctor as soon as possible.

COMMON
Dry mouth, dryness and cracking of the lips, runny nose, nosebleeds, skin peeling, hair loss, dry skin, nail problems, itching, rash, increased sensitivity to touch, numbness or tingling, inflammation of fingers or toes, sticky skin, dry eyes, irritation of eyes, loss of eyebrows and eyelashes.

LESS COMMON
Bleeding gums, increased saliva, thirst, inflammation of the mouth, abnormal skin odor, blisters, cold and clammy skin, increased sweating, skin infection, ulcerations, sunburn, abnormal or blurred vision, reduced night vision, joint pain, back pain, muscle pain, mild headache, abdominal pain, diarrhea, nausea, odd taste in mouth, ringing in ears, depression, insomnia.

ACYCLOVIR

Available in: Capsules, tablets, liquid, ointment, injection
Available OTC? No   **As Generic?** Yes
Drug Class: Antiviral

▼ USAGE INFORMATION

WHY IT'S PRESCRIBED
To treat herpes virus infections such as genital herpes, shingles, herpes simplex, and chicken pox.

HOW IT WORKS
Acyclovir interferes with the activity of enzymes needed for the replication of viral DNA in cells. This prevents the virus from multiplying.

▼ DOSAGE GUIDELINES

RANGE AND FREQUENCY
Oral forms— For genital herpes: Up to 1,200 mg a day in evenly distributed doses, every 4 or 8 hours. For shingles: Up to 4,000 mg a day in evenly distributed doses every 4 hours. For chicken pox: Up to 800 mg, 4 times a day, not to exceed 3,200 mg a day. Topical form— To relieve herpes symptoms: Apply a small amount to lesions every 3 hours (6 times a day) for 7 days. Use a glove or finger cot when applying medication.

ONSET OF EFFECT
2 hours or more.

DURATION OF ACTION
Up to 5 hours following the final dose.

DIETARY ADVICE
Capsule, tablet, and liquid forms should all be taken with food and with a full (8 oz) glass of water.

STORAGE
Store in a dry place at room temperature, away from direct sunlight. Refrigerate any liquid form of acyclovir, but do not allow it to freeze.

MISSED DOSE
If you miss a tablet, capsule, or liquid dose, take it as soon as you remember, up to 2 hours late. If more than 2 hours, wait for the next scheduled dose. Do not double the next dose. For ointment, apply dose as soon as you remember, then return to your regular dosing schedule.

STOPPING THE DRUG
Take the drug as prescribed for the full treatment period,
even if you begin to feel better before the scheduled end of therapy, but do not take it for longer than the recommended period.

PROLONGED USE
Women with genital herpes are at increased risk of developing cervical cancer; annual Pap smears are recommended for these patients.

▼ PRECAUTIONS

Over 60: Adverse reactions and side effects may be more common in older persons. Such effects can be minimized by drinking at least 2 to 3 quarts of liquid per day.

Driving and Hazardous Work: The use of acyclovir should not impair your ability to perform such tasks safely.

Alcohol: Alcohol may accentuate the side effects of lightheadedness and dizziness.

Pregnancy: Acyclovir has been used by pregnant women and no birth defects or other related problems have been reported; however, studies in humans have been limited and inconclusive. Consult your doctor about using acyclovir if you are pregnant or plan to become pregnant.

Breast Feeding: Acyclovir may pass into breast milk. Breast feeding should be avoided while taking any oral form of the drug. No problems are expected with the topical form.

Infants and Children: Acyclovir should not be used for children under 2 years of age.
Its use for children under age 12 should be carefully supervised by a physician.

Special Concerns: Be sure to tell your doctor if you have ever had any unusual or allergic reaction to acyclovir. It is important to remember that the use of acyclovir is not a cure and will not help prevent you from spreading herpes infections to others.

OVERDOSE
Symptoms: No specific ones have been reported.

What to Do: An overdose of acyclovir is unlikely to be life-threatening. However, if someone takes a much larger dose than prescribed, call your doctor, emergency medical services (EMS), or the nearest poison control center right away for advice. Prolonged overdose may lead to kidney damage.

▼ INTERACTIONS

DRUG INTERACTIONS
Consult your doctor for specific advice if you are taking cyclosporine, probenecid, meperidine, or zidovudine.

FOOD INTERACTIONS
No significant food interactions have been reported.

DISEASE INTERACTIONS
Use of acyclovir may cause complications in patients with liver or kidney disease, since these organs work together to remove the medication from the body.

 SIDE EFFECTS

SERIOUS
No serious side effects have been reported.

COMMON
Rash, nausea and vomiting. Ointment can cause pain, burning, or itching at the site where it is applied. Should such adverse symptoms persist, notify your doctor. Injection can cause inflammation of the vein (phlebitis); call your doctor if this occurs.

LESS COMMON
Diarrhea, stomach pain, lightheadedness, dizziness, confusion, tremor. In rare cases kidney function may be altered when the drug is given by injection, causing such symptoms as decreased urine output.

ADAPALENE

Available in: Topical gel
Available OTC? No   **As Generic?** No
Drug Class: Acne drug

▼ USAGE INFORMATION

WHY IT'S PRESCRIBED
To treat acne.

HOW IT WORKS
Its exact mechanism of action is unclear, but adapalene appears to bind with specific receptors in skin cells in a way that encourages the formation of normal skin cells and discourages the formation of acne lesions.

▼ DOSAGE GUIDELINES

RANGE AND FREQUENCY
After washing affected areas, apply a thin film of adapalene once a day to affected skin areas before bedtime.

ONSET OF EFFECT
Becomes noticeable after 8 to 12 weeks. During the first few weeks of therapy, acne may actually get worse before it begins to get better. This is because the drug is affecting previously unseen lesions, and it should not be considered a reason to stop using the medication.

DURATION OF ACTION
Unknown.

DIETARY ADVICE
Adapalene can be used without regard to diet.

STORAGE
Store in a tightly sealed container away from heat and direct light.

MISSED DOSE
Apply it as soon as you remember. If it is near the time for the next dose, skip the missed dose and resume your regular dosage schedule. Do not double the next dose.

STOPPING THE DRUG
The decision to stop using the drug should be made by your doctor.

PROLONGED USE
No problems are expected with prolonged use.

▼ PRECAUTIONS

Over 60: No special precautions are required.

Driving and Hazardous Work: No special precautions are required.

Alcohol: No special precautions are required.

≡ SIDE EFFECTS ≡

SERIOUS
No serious side effects have been reported.

COMMON
Redness, dryness, and scaling of skin; itching or burning immediately after application.

LESS COMMON
Skin irritation, sunburn, flareups of acne. These usually occur during the first month of treatment and then decrease in severity and frequency.

Pregnancy: In some tests, large doses of adapalene caused minor birth defects (an excess number of ribs) in animals, and theoretically could cause major birth defects. Human tests have not been done. Generally, adapalene should not be used during pregnancy. Consult your doctor for specific advice.

Breast Feeding: Adapalene may pass into breast milk; caution is advised. Consult your doctor for specific advice.

Infants and Children: The safety and effectiveness of adapalene in children under the age of 12 have not been established.

Special Concerns: Anyone with a history of allergy to adapalene or any ingredients in the gel should not use this medication. Acne may appear to worsen temporarily during the first weeks of adapalene therapy; cosmetic improvement should become apparent after 8 to 12 weeks. The medicine should be kept away from the eyes, lips, nostrils, and mucous membranes. It should not be applied to cuts, abrasions, scaly or flaky skin, or patches of sunburned skin. The extremes of winter weather, including high winds and cold temperatures, can cause extra skin irritation and dryness. In sunny conditions, protect the treated area with sunscreen products (with a minimum sun protection factor, or SPF, of 15) and adequate clothing; keep exposure to sunlight to a minimum. If you get a sunburn, adapalene therapy should be stopped or delayed until the sunburned areas return to normal. Use of skin products containing alcohol, astringents, spices, or lime should be avoided.

OVERDOSE
Symptoms: Excessive application of adapalene may lead to redness, pain, and peeling of the skin.

What to Do: Discontinue the drug and consult your doctor. If accidentally ingested, seek emergency medical aid right away.

▼ INTERACTIONS

DRUG INTERACTIONS
Some drugs may interact with adapalene. Consult your doctor for specific advice if you are taking other products that can irritate the skin, such as medicated or abrasive soaps and cleansers and products containing sulfur, resorcinol, or salicylic acid. They generally should not be used during adapalene therapy unless otherwise recommended by your doctor.

FOOD INTERACTIONS
No food interactions have been documented.

DISEASE INTERACTIONS
Caution is advised when using adapalene. Consult your doctor if you have any other skin condition.

ALBENDAZOLE

Albenza

Available in: Tablets
Available OTC? No **As Generic?** No
Drug Class: Anthelmintic

▼ USAGE INFORMATION

WHY IT'S PRESCRIBED
To treat hydatid disease and neurocysticercosis. Hydatid disease is a parasitic infection, usually of the liver, caused by echinococcus (dog tapeworm) larvae. Humans can become infected through ingestion of tapeworm eggs in dog feces. Neurocysticercosis is a parasitic infection of the nervous system, caused by taenia solium (pork tapeworm) larvae. It can be contracted by ingesting egg-containing feces from an infected person, owing to food mishandling. Albendazole may be used to treat a variety of other roundworm infections and may be useful in treating a type of intestinal protozoan common in AIDS patients, but it is not licensed for such uses in the United States.

HOW IT WORKS
Albendazole interferes with various energy-producing processes of helminths (worms), including impairing the uptake of glucose (sugar) for energy.

▼ DOSAGE GUIDELINES

RANGE AND FREQUENCY
For hydatid disease— Patients weighing more than 132 lbs (60 kg): 1 cycle consisting of 400 mg twice a day for 28 days followed by a 14-day albendazole-free period; repeat for at least 3 cycles. Patients weighing less than 132 lbs (60 kg): 1 cycle consisting of 7.5 mg per 2.2 lbs (1 kg) of body weight twice a day for 28 days followed by a 14-day albendazole-free period; repeat for at least 3 cycles. For neurocysticercosis— Patients weighing more than 132 lbs (60 kg): 400 mg twice a day for 8 to 30 days. Patients weighing less than 132 lbs (60 kg): 7.5 mg per 2.2 lbs twice a day for 8 to 30 days. Corticosteroids are often administered concurrently for therapy of neurocysticercosis to control the inflammation caused by dying larvae.

ONSET OF EFFECT
Unknown.

DURATION OF ACTION
Unknown.

DIETARY ADVICE
Take it with meals high in fat content to help the body better absorb the drug.

STORAGE
Store in a tightly sealed container away from heat, moisture, and direct light.

MISSED DOSE
Take it as soon as you remember. If it is near the time for the next dose, skip the missed dose and resume your regular dosage schedule. Do not double the next dose.

STOPPING THE DRUG
Take it as prescribed for the full treatment period even if you begin to feel better before the scheduled end of therapy. The decision to stop taking the drug should be made by your doctor.

PROLONGED USE
See your doctor regularly for tests and examinations every 2 weeks if you must take this medicine for a prolonged period of time.

▼ PRECAUTIONS

Over 60: No studies have been done specifically on older patients; adverse reactions may be more likely or more severe.

Driving and Hazardous Work: Do not drive or engage in hazardous work until you determine how the medicine affects you.

Alcohol: No special precautions are necessary.

Pregnancy: Pregnant women should not use albendazole except when no other alternative is available. Discuss with your doctor the relative risks and benefits of using this drug while pregnant.

Breast Feeding: Albendazole may pass into breast milk; caution is advised. Consult your doctor for specific advice.

Infants and Children: No special problems are expected.

OVERDOSE
Symptoms: No cases of overdose have been reported.

What to Do: If someone takes a much larger dose than prescribed, call your doctor, emergency medical services (EMS), or the nearest poison control right away.

▼ INTERACTIONS

DRUG INTERACTIONS
Other drugs may interact with albendazole. Consult your doctor for specific advice if you are taking dexamethasone, praziquantel, cimetidine, theophylline, or any other prescription or over-the-counter medication.

FOOD INTERACTIONS
No known food interactions.

DISEASE INTERACTIONS
Dosage may need to be adjusted in patients with cirrhosis. Consult your doctor for specific advice if you have any other medical condition.

SIDE EFFECTS

SERIOUS
Neutropenia (low white blood cell count), thrombocytopenia (low platelet count), and hepatitis can occur during prolonged therapy, but are reversible by discontinuing the drug. If fever, sore throat, abdominal pain, loss of appetite, unusual fatigue, skin rash, or itching occur, call your doctor immediately.

COMMON
No common side effects are associated with albendazole.

LESS COMMON
Nausea, vomiting, dizziness, stomach upset, diarrhea, headache. Alopecia (thinning or loss of hair), a rare side effect, can occur, but is reversible by stopping the drug.

ALBUTEROL

BRAND NAMES
Airet, Proventil, Ventolin, Volmax

Available in: Inhaler, solution, capsules, tablets, syrup
Available OTC? No   **As Generic?** Yes
Drug Class: Bronchodilator/sympathomimetic

▼ USAGE INFORMATION

WHY IT'S PRESCRIBED
To dilate air passages in the lungs that have become narrowed as a result of disease or inflammation. It is used in the treatment of asthma and chronic obstructive pulmonary disease (COPD).

HOW IT WORKS
Albuterol widens constricted airways by relaxing the smooth muscles that surround the bronchial passages.

▼ DOSAGE GUIDELINES

RANGE AND FREQUENCY
Use it when needed to relieve breathing difficulty. For bronchospasm: 1 to 2 puffs of aerosol inhaler every 4 to 6 hours; or 2.5 mg of solution delivered via nebulizer 3 to 4 times a day; or 200 micrograms (mcg) of capsules for inhalation using Rotahaler every 4 to 6 hours; or 2 to 4 mg of tablets 3 or 4 times a day, not to exceed 32 mg per day. Children may require a smaller dose, and the syrup form of the drug may be preferable to young patients. For prevention of exercise-induced asthma: 1 or 2 inhalations (at least 1 full minute apart), 15 minutes prior to exercise.

ONSET OF EFFECT
Inhalant: Within 5 minutes. Oral forms: 15 to 30 minutes.

DURATION OF ACTION
Inhalant: 3 to 6 hours. Oral forms: 8 hours.

DIETARY ADVICE
Can be taken on an empty stomach or with food or milk.

STORAGE
Contents of aerosol canisters are under pressure; do not puncture. Store canister away from heat, open flame, and direct light.

MISSED DOSE
Skip the missed dose and resume your regular dosage schedule. Do not double the next dose.

STOPPING THE DRUG
It may not be necessary to finish the recommended course of therapy. Consult your doctor.

PROLONGED USE
Therapy may require months or years. Excessive use may result in temporary loss of effectiveness.

▼ PRECAUTIONS

Over 60: Adverse reactions may be more likely and more severe in older patients.

Driving and Hazardous Work: Dizziness may occur as a side effect and interfere with your ability to perform such tasks safely. Do not drive or engage in hazardous work until you determine how the medicine affects you.

Alcohol: No special precautions are necessary.

Pregnancy: Consult your doctor for advice.

Breast Feeding: Albuterol may pass into breast milk; caution is advised. Consult your doctor for advice.

Infants and Children: Not recommended for use by children under the age of 2.

Special Concerns: The inhaler should be primed prior to the first use and in cases when it has not been used for more than two weeks. Prime it by releasing four test sprays in the air away from the face. You should wash your rotahaler (once every two weeks) and inhaler (once a week) to prevent medication build-up and blockage. Wash the two halves of the rotahaler or the mouthpiece of the inhaler (with the canister removed) with warm water and shake to remove excess water. Both the rotahaler and the inhaler should be air-dried thoroughly.

OVERDOSE
Symptoms: Confusion, delirium, severe anxiety, seizures, nervousness, headache, nausea, dry mouth, dizziness, insomnia, chest pain, muscle tremors, profound weakness, rapid and irregular pulse.

What to Do: Call your doctor, emergency medical services (EMS), or your local hospital immediately.

▼ INTERACTIONS

DRUG INTERACTIONS
Albuterol should not be used within 14 days of using an MAO inhibitor or tricyclic antidepressants. Consult your doctor if you are taking beta-blockers, loop or thiazide diuretics, high blood pressure medication, digitalis drugs, epinephrine, ergot, finasteride, furazolidone, guanadrel, guanethidine, maprotiline, methyldopa, any nitrate, a phenothiazine, pseudoephedrine-containing products, rauwolfia alkaloids, terazosin, theophylline or other asthma medications, or thyroid hormone.

FOOD INTERACTIONS
No known food interactions.

DISEASE INTERACTIONS
Consult your doctor if you have an overactive thyroid, diabetes mellitus, a history of seizures, heart problems, high blood pressure, or blood vessel disease.

≡ SIDE EFFECTS ≡

SERIOUS
Inhaled form: May become ineffective if used too often, resulting in more-severe breathing difficulty that does not improve. Signs include persistent wheezing, coughing, or shortness of breath; confusion; bluish color to lips or fingernails; inability to speak. Ingested form: Chest pain or heaviness; heart palpitations; lightheadedness; fainting; severe weakness; severe headache.

COMMON
Nervousness, tremor, dizziness, headache, insomnia.

LESS COMMON
Dryness and irritation of the nose, mouth, and throat; heartburn; nausea; muscle cramps.

ALCLOMETASONE

Available in: Cream, ointment
Available OTC? No   **As Generic?** No
Drug Class: Topical corticosteroid

BRAND NAME

Aclovate

▼ USAGE INFORMATION

WHY IT'S PRESCRIBED
To relieve swelling, itching, redness, and other kinds of discomfort associated with certain skin conditions.

HOW IT WORKS
Alclometasone appears to interfere with the formation of natural substances within the body that are directly responsible for the process of inflammation, which produces swelling, redness, and itching.

▼ DOSAGE GUIDELINES

RANGE AND FREQUENCY
Apply sparingly (as a thin film), 2 or 3 times a day, only to the specific areas of skin where it is needed. Prior to application, wash or soak the affected area and allow it to dry; this may improve the absorption of the medication.

ONSET OF EFFECT
Rapid, but may take 24 to 48 hours to see the effect.

DURATION OF ACTION
Unknown.

DIETARY ADVICE
No special precautions.

STORAGE
Store in a tightly sealed container away from heat and direct light.

MISSED DOSE
Apply it as soon as you remember. If it is close to the next application, skip the missed dose and resume your regular dosage schedule as prescribed.

STOPPING THE DRUG
Take it as prescribed for the full treatment period, even if you begin to feel better before the scheduled end of therapy. For some conditions, you may be directed to taper off the medication if symptoms and rash abate.

PROLONGED USE
See your doctor regularly for tests and examinations if you must use this drug for a prolonged period; use of this drug for more than 14 days is generally not recommended unless your doctor advises otherwise. Avoid prolonged use, particularly near the eyes, on the face in general, on genital or rectal areas, or in the folds of the skin.

▼ PRECAUTIONS

Over 60: Side effects may be more likely and more severe in elderly patients; therapy with topical corticosteroids should therefore be brief and infrequent.

Driving and Hazardous Work: Use of alclometasone should not impair your ability to perform such tasks safely.

Alcohol: No special precautions are necessary.

Pregnancy: Should not be used for prolonged periods by pregnant women or by women trying to become pregnant.

Breast Feeding: Although problems have not been documented, caution is advised. Do not apply to breasts prior to nursing.

Infants and Children: Should not be used for more than 2 weeks on children and adolescents, unless otherwise directed by your doctor. Do not use tight-fitting diapers or plastic pants on children when treating skin irritation in the diaper area.

Special Concerns: Do not use alclometasone longer or more frequently than recommended by your doctor. Do not use it for other skin problems without a doctor's approval. Do not bandage or otherwise wrap the skin unless directed by your doctor. Wash the skin gently and allow it to dry and cool before applying. Be careful not to get the medicine in your eyes; if you do, flush your eyes with water. Wash hands after applying it with your fingers. Do not apply it to the face, mucous membranes, armpits, groin, or under breasts unless your doctor so directs. When treating a hairy site, part the hair and apply directly to the lesion.

OVERDOSE
Symptoms: No cases of overdose have been reported.

What to Do: An overdose is unlikely. However, in the event of accidental ingestion, call your doctor, emergency medical services (EMS), or the nearest poison control center immediately.

▼ INTERACTIONS

DRUG INTERACTIONS
Do not mix topical alclometasone with other products, especially alcohol-containing preparations (which include colognes, aftershave, and many moisturizer lotions), since this may cause dryness and irritation, or increase the risk of an allergic reaction. Consult your doctor if you are taking antifungal agents or antibiotics.

FOOD INTERACTIONS
No known food interactions.

DISEASE INTERACTIONS
Consult your doctor if you have cataracts; diabetes mellitus; glaucoma; infection, sores, or ulcerations of the skin; infection elsewhere in your body; or tuberculosis.

⚟ SIDE EFFECTS ⚟

SERIOUS
Failure of skin to heal; severe burning and continued itching of skin. Seek medical assistance immediately.

COMMON
Burning, itching, irritation, redness, dryness, acne, stinging and cracking of skin.

LESS COMMON
Prolonged use, especially in covered areas, may produce blistering and pus near hair follicles, unusual bleeding or easy bruising, darkening or prominence of small surface veins, or increased susceptibility to infection.

ALENDRONATE SODIUM

Available in: Tablets
Available OTC? No   **As Generic?** No
Drug Class: Bisphosphonate inhibitor of bone resorption

▼ USAGE INFORMATION

WHY IT'S PRESCRIBED
To prevent and treat osteoporosis in postmenopausal women. Alendronate also treats glucocorticoid-induced osteoporosis in those receiving corticosteroids in a daily dosage equivalent to 7.5 mg or greater of prednisone and who have low bone mineral density. Also used to treat Paget's disease, a disorder characterized by rapid breakdown and reformation of bone, which can lead to bone fragility and malformation.

HOW IT WORKS
Healthy bones are continuously remodeled (broken down and then reformed); the minerals and other components of bones are reabsorbed by one set of cells (osteoclasts) and replaced by another set of cells to form new bone. Alendronate suppresses the activity of osteoclasts; consequently, the breakdown of bone tissue occurs more slowly than the laying down of new bone. This action preserves bone density and strength.

▼ DOSAGE GUIDELINES

RANGE AND FREQUENCY
For prevention of osteoporosis: 5 mg once a day. For treatment of osteoporosis: 10 mg once a day. For glucocorticoid-induced osteoporosis in men and women: 5 mg once a day; postmenopausal women not receiving estrogen should take 10 mg once a day. For Paget's disease: 40 mg once a day. The dose is taken in the morning. Swallow tablets whole; do not suck or chew them. Do not lie down for 30 minutes following your dosage. The tablet must be taken with an 8 oz glass of water at least 30 minutes before any food or other medication.

ONSET OF EFFECT
Within 2 hours.

DURATION OF ACTION
24 hours.

DIETARY ADVICE
Take alendronate at least 30 minutes before your first food or beverage of the day, with a full glass of water. Some patients may be advised to take calcium or vitamin C supplements to aid in the formation of new bone tissue.

STORAGE
Store in a tightly sealed container away from heat, moisture, and direct light.

MISSED DOSE
Take it as soon as you remember. If it is near the time for the next dose, skip the missed dose and resume your regular dosage schedule. Do not double the next dose.

STOPPING THE DRUG
The decision to stop taking the drug should be made by your doctor. In most cases, patients with Paget's disease are treated for 6 months; the drug is then stopped. Retreatment may be necessary if such patients show signs of relapse after a subsequent 6-month observation period.

PROLONGED USE
No special precautions.

▼ PRECAUTIONS

Over 60: No special problems are expected.

Driving and Hazardous Work: No special warnings.

Alcohol: Alcohol should be restricted in high-risk women because it is a risk factor for osteoporosis.

Pregnancy: Alendronate is normally not used in premenopausal women.

Breast Feeding: Alendronate may pass into breast milk; caution is advised. Consult your doctor for advice.

Infants and Children: Use not recommended for infants and children.

Special Concerns: Patients taking alendronate are encouraged to engage in regular weight-bearing exercise and should avoid cigarettes and limit alcohol, which inhibit healthy bone production.

OVERDOSE
Symptoms: Severe heartburn, stomach cramps, or throat irritation might occur if an overdose disturbs the body's electrolyte (mineral) balance.

What to Do: Few overdoses have been reported. However, if someone takes a much larger dose than prescribed, call a doctor or the nearest poison control center.

▼ INTERACTIONS

DRUG INTERACTIONS
Consult your doctor for specific advice if you are taking antacids, calcium supplements, aspirin or other nonsteroidal anti-inflammatory drugs (NSAIDs), or hormone replacement therapy. Wait at least 30 minutes after taking alendronate before taking any other drugs.

FOOD INTERACTIONS
Any food eaten within 30 minutes of taking alendronate decreases its effect. Mineral water, coffee, tea, and fruit juice can interfere with the absorption of alendronate.

DISEASE INTERACTIONS
Kidney impairment or a gastrointestinal disease may increase the risk of side effects. Low blood calcium levels and vitamin D deficiency must be treated before using alendronate.

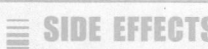
SIDE EFFECTS

SERIOUS
No serious side effects have been reported.

COMMON
Abdominal pain or bloating (persistent abdominal pain should be reported to your doctor), indigestion, heartburn, nausea.

LESS COMMON
Headache, constipation, diarrhea, gas, swallowing difficulty, throat irritation, abdominal swelling or tightness, muscle or bone pain, changes in taste perception.

ALITRETINOIN

Available in: Topical gel
Available OTC? No   **As Generic?** No
Drug Class: Retinoid

BRAND NAME
Panretin

▼ USAGE INFORMATION

WHY IT'S PRESCRIBED
To treat skin lesions topically in patients with AIDS-related Kaposi's sarcoma (a type of skin cancer that commonly affects immunocompromised patients). Not for use when systemic anti-Kaposi's sarcoma therapy is required.

HOW IT WORKS
Alitretinoin, a vitamin A-related retinoid found naturally in the body, inhibits the growth of Kaposi's sarcoma cells.

▼ DOSAGE GUIDELINES

RANGE AND FREQUENCY
To start, apply a generous layer of gel to the skin lesions twice a day. Frequency of application may be gradually increased by your doctor to 3 to 4 times a day.

ONSET OF EFFECT
A response to the gel may be seen as soon as 2 weeks after the initiation of therapy. However, some patients require up to 14 weeks of therapy before a response is noted.

DURATION OF ACTION
Unknown.

DIETARY ADVICE
No special restrictions.

STORAGE
Store in a tightly sealed container away from heat, moisture, and direct light.

MISSED DOSE
If you fail to apply the medication on one day, return to your regular schedule the next day; do not apply an extra amount in an attempt to compensate for the missed dose.

STOPPING THE DRUG
Use of alitretinoin should be continued as long as its benefit persists. Consult your doctor before discontinuing treatment.

PROLONGED USE
Long-term therapy with this medication is often required.

▼ PRECAUTIONS

Over 60: Information is inadequate, but no special problems are expected.

Driving and Hazardous Work: The use of alitretinoin should not impair your ability to perform such tasks safely.

Alcohol: No special precautions are necessary.

Pregnancy: Alitretinoin should not be used if you are pregnant or plan to become pregnant. Adequate birth-control methods should be practiced when alitretinoin is used in women of child-bearing age.

Breast Feeding: Alitretinoin may pass into breast milk. However, women infected with HIV should not breast-feed, so as to avoid transmitting the virus to an uninfected child.

Infants and Children: Not recommended for use by children.

Special Concerns: Avoid applying the gel to unaffected skin, as skin irritation may result. Allow the gel to dry for 3 to 5 minutes before covering with clothing. Do not apply near mucous membranes, such as the nose, eyes, and mouth. Patients with cutaneous T-cell lymphoma are less tolerant to the drug.

OVERDOSE
Symptoms: Excessive use of alitretinoin may lead to skin redness, peeling, or discomfort.

What to Do: An overdose is unlikely to occur. If someone accidentally ingests alitretinoin, call your doctor.

▼ INTERACTIONS

DRUG INTERACTIONS
If you are using alitretinoin, do not use any products containing DEET, a common ingredient in some insect repellents.

FOOD INTERACTIONS
No known food interactions.

DISEASE INTERACTIONS
Consult your doctor if you have any other skin condition before using alitretinoin.

  SIDE EFFECTS

SERIOUS
No serious side effects are associated with alitretinoin.

COMMON
Redness, rash, itching, numbness and tingling, skin cracking, scabbing, swelling, burning sensation, and pain at application site.

LESS COMMON
No less common side effects are associated with alitretinoin.

ALLOPURINOL

Available in: Tablets
Available OTC? No   **As Generic?** Yes
Drug Class: Antigout drug

▼ USAGE INFORMATION

WHY IT'S PRESCRIBED
To treat chronic gout or excessive uric acid buildup caused by kidney disorders, cancer, or the use of chemotherapy drugs for cancer. Also prescribed to prevent recurrence of uric acid kidney stones. Allopurinol should not be used for treating acute gout attacks in progress.

HOW IT WORKS
Allopurinol blocks the enzyme xanthine oxidase, which is required for the production of uric acid, thus reducing blood levels of uric acid.

▼ DOSAGE GUIDELINES

RANGE AND FREQUENCY
Adults: Initially 100 mg per day, increased by 100 mg per week to a maximum of 800 mg per day. 100 mg doses are administered once a day; doses of 300 mg or more are taken in 2 or 3 evenly divided portions throughout the day.

Children ages 6 to 10: 300 mg per day for certain types of cancer. Children age 6 and under: 50 mg per day in 3 evenly divided portions.

ONSET OF EFFECT
Reduces uric acid levels in 2 to 3 days; may take 6 months for full effect to occur.

DURATION OF ACTION
1 to 2 weeks.

DIETARY ADVICE
Take it with food or milk to avoid stomach irritation. Drink 10 to 12 glasses (8 oz each) of water a day.

STORAGE
Store in a tightly sealed container away from heat and direct light.

MISSED DOSE
Take it as soon as you remember. However, if it is near the time for the next dose, skip the missed dose and resume your regular dosage schedule. Do not double the next dose.

STOPPING THE DRUG
Take allopurinol as prescribed for the full treatment period, even if you begin to feel better before the scheduled end of therapy.

PROLONGED USE
Consult your doctor about the need for tests of liver function, kidney function, blood counts, and blood and urine levels of uric acid.

▼ PRECAUTIONS

Over 60: Adverse reactions may be more likely and more severe in older patients.

Driving and Hazardous Work: Allopurinol may cause drowsiness. If possible, avoid driving and hazardous work.

Alcohol: No special precautions are necessary.

Pregnancy: Caution is advised; consult your doctor about whether the benefits outweigh potential risks to the unborn child.

Breast Feeding: Allopurinol passes into breast milk; avoid the drug or discontinue use while nursing.

Infants and Children: Follow your doctor's instructions carefully for children.

OVERDOSE
Symptoms: No specific symptoms have been reported.

What to Do: An overdose of allopurinol is unlikely to be life-threatening. However, if someone takes a much larger dose than prescribed, contact your doctor, poison control center, or local emergency room for instructions.

▼ INTERACTIONS

DRUG INTERACTIONS
Consult your doctor for specific advice if you are taking an antibiotic (such as amoxicillin, ampicillin, or bacampicillin), an anticoagulant (warfarin, dicumarol), an anticancer (chemotherapy) drug, chlorpropamide, a diuretic, or theophylline.

FOOD INTERACTIONS
None are likely, but a low-purine diet is recommended to reduce the risk of gout attacks. Foods high in purines include anchovies, sardines, legumes, poultry, sweetbreads, liver, kidneys, and other organ meats.

DISEASE INTERACTIONS
Caution is advised when taking allopurinol. Consult your doctor if you have high blood pressure, diabetes mellitus, kidney disease, or impaired iron metabolism.

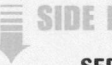
SIDE EFFECTS

SERIOUS
Anemia or other blood or bone marrow disorders that may produce fatigue, bleeding, or bruising; yellowish tinge to eyes or skin (signifying hepatitis or liver damage); severe skin reactions (marked by rashes, skin ulcers, hives, intense itching); chest tightness; weakness. Call your doctor right away if such symptoms arise.

COMMON
Mild rash, drowsiness, nausea, diarrhea. The frequency of gout attacks may increase during the first weeks of use.

LESS COMMON
Headache, abdominal pain, boils on face, chills or fever, vomiting, hair loss.

ALOSETRON HYDROCHLORIDE

Available in: Tablets
Available OTC? No   **As Generic?** No
Drug Class: Selective 5-HT3 (serotonin) receptor antagonist

BRAND NAME
Lotronex

▼ USAGE INFORMATION

WHY IT'S PRESCRIBED
To treat irritable bowel syndrome (IBS) in women whose primary symptom is diarrhea. (Alosetron has not been shown to be effective in men.) NOTE: Due to reports of rare but serious side effects, the drug's manufacturer has voluntarily removed it from the market. If you currently use alosetron, consult your doctor about alternative medications as soon as possible.

HOW IT WORKS
By blocking the action of serotonin, alosetron inhibits the excitation of nerves along the gastrointestinal tract that may be hypersensitive in IBS sufferers. It also slows the movement of food through the bowel and may ease the pain and discomfort of IBS.

▼ DOSAGE GUIDELINES

RANGE AND FREQUENCY
1 mg twice a day.

ONSET OF EFFECT
1 to 4 weeks.

DURATION OF ACTION
Alosetron is effective as long as you continue to take it.

DIETARY ADVICE
Alosetron may be taken with or without food.

STORAGE
Store in a tightly sealed container away from heat, moisture, and direct light.

MISSED DOSE
Take it as soon as you remember. However, if it is near the time for the next dose, skip the missed dose and resume your regular dosage schedule. Do not double the next dose.

STOPPING THE DRUG
The decision to stop taking the drug should be made in consultation with your physician. Because alosetron does not cure IBS or work for everyone, quit using it if your symptoms do not improve within 4 weeks.

PROLONGED USE
The safety and efficacy of alosetron for treatment beyond 12 months have not been established.

▼ PRECAUTIONS

Over 60: No special problems are expected.

Driving and Hazardous Work: No special warnings.

Alcohol: Avoid alcohol while taking this medication, as it may aggravate your condition.

Pregnancy: In animal tests, alosetron has not caused problems. Human tests have not been done. Before you take alosetron, tell your doctor if you are pregnant or plan to become pregnant.

Breast Feeding: Alosetron may pass into breast milk; caution is advised. Consult your doctor for advice on whether to discontinue nursing or discontinue the drug.

Infants and Children: The safety and effectiveness of this drug have not been established for children under the age of 18.

Special Concerns: When you stop taking alosetron, IBS symptoms are likely to return within 1 week.

OVERDOSE
Symptoms: No cases of overdose have been reported. However, symptoms may include difficulty breathing, subdued behavior, coordination difficulties, tremor, and seizures.

What to Do: If you suspect an overdose or if someone takes a much larger dose than prescribed, call your doctor, emergency medical services (EMS), or the nearest poison control center immediately.

▼ INTERACTIONS

DRUG INTERACTIONS
No known drug interactions.

FOOD INTERACTIONS
No known food interactions.

DISEASE INTERACTIONS
Do not start taking alosetron when you are constipated or if you are constipated most of the time. Do not take alosetron if you have a history of ischemic colitis or other intestinal disorders, such as Crohn's disease, ulcerative colitis, or active diverticulitis.

≡ SIDE EFFECTS ≡

SERIOUS
If you have severe or worsening constipation while taking alosetron, stop using it immediately and call your doctor. Rarely, acute ischemic colitis (insufficient flow of blood to the colon) has been reported in some patients taking alosetron. The exact relationship between this drug and acute colitis has not been determined. However, if you experience rectal bleeding or bloody diarrhea, low-grade fever, and abdominal distention and tenderness, discontinue alosetron and contact your doctor immediately.

COMMON
Constipation.

LESS COMMON
High blood pressure, runny nose, nausea, abdominal discomfort and pain, gas, increased susceptibility to viral gastrointestinal infections, heartburn, abdominal swelling, hemorrhoids, sleep problems, depression.

ALPRAZOLAM

BRAND NAME

Xanax

Available in: Tablets, oral solution
Available OTC? No   **As Generic?** Yes
Drug Class: Benzodiazepine tranquilizer; antianxiety agent

▼ USAGE INFORMATION

WHY IT'S PRESCRIBED
To treat anxiety and panic disorder.

HOW IT WORKS
In general, alprazolam produces mild sedation by depressing activity in the central nervous system. In particular, alprazolam appears to enhance the effect of gamma-aminobutyric acid (GABA), a natural chemical that inhibits the firing of neurons and dampens the transmission of nerve signals, thus decreasing nervous excitation.

▼ DOSAGE GUIDELINES

RANGE AND FREQUENCY
Adults: Initial dose is 1.5 mg a day, taken in 3 divided doses; may be gradually increased to a maximum dose of 4 mg a day. Older adults: Initial dose is 0.5 to 0.75 mg per day, taken in 2 or 3 divided doses; may be gradu-

ally increased to a maximum dose of 2 mg a day. Children: Not usually prescribed.

ONSET OF EFFECT
2 hours.

DURATION OF ACTION
Up to 6 hours.

DIETARY ADVICE
Alprazolam can be taken on an empty stomach or with food or milk.

STORAGE
Store in a tightly sealed container away from heat and direct light.

MISSED DOSE
If you miss a dose, take it if you remember within 1 hour. Otherwise, skip the missed dose and take the next one at the regular time. Do not double the next dose.

STOPPING THE DRUG
Never stop taking the drug abruptly, as this can cause withdrawal symptoms

(seizures, sleep disruption, nervousness, irritability, diarrhea, abdominal cramps, muscle aches, memory impairment). Dosage should be reduced gradually as directed by your doctor.

PROLONGED USE
Short-term therapy (8 weeks or less) is typical; do not take it for a longer period unless so advised by your doctor.

▼ PRECAUTIONS

Over 60: Use with caution; side effects such as drowsiness and dizziness may be more pronounced in older patients.

Driving and Hazardous Work: Alprazolam can impair mental alertness and physical coordination. Adjust your activities accordingly.

Alcohol: Alcohol intake should be extremely moderate or stopped altogether while taking alprazolam.

Pregnancy: Use of this drug during pregnancy should be avoided if possible. Be sure to tell your doctor if you are pregnant or plan to become pregnant.

Breast Feeding: Alprazolam passes into breast milk; do not take it while nursing.

Infants and Children: Safety and effectiveness have not been established for children under age 18.

Special Concerns: Use of this drug can lead to psychological or physical dependence. Short-term therapy (8 weeks

or less) is typical; patients should not take the drug for a longer period unless so advised by their doctor. Never take more than the prescribed daily dose.

OVERDOSE
Symptoms: Extreme drowsiness, confusion, slurred speech, slow reflexes, poor coordination, staggering gait, tremor, slowed breathing, loss of consciousness.

What to Do: Call your doctor, emergency medical services (EMS), or the nearest poison control center immediately.

▼ INTERACTIONS

DRUG INTERACTIONS
Other drugs may interact with alprazolam. Consult your doctor for specific advice if you are taking any drugs that depress the central nervous system; these include antihistamines, antidepressants (including nefazodone) or other psychiatric medications, barbiturates, sedatives, cough medicines, decongestants, and painkillers. Be sure your doctor knows about any over-the-counter medication you may take.

FOOD INTERACTIONS
None reported.

DISEASE INTERACTIONS
Consult your doctor if you have a history of alcohol or drug abuse, stroke or other brain disease, any chronic lung disease, hyperactivity, depression or other mental illness, myasthenia gravis, sleep apnea, epilepsy, porphyria, kidney disease, or liver disease.

SIDE EFFECTS

SERIOUS
Difficulty concentrating, outbursts of anger, other behavior problems, depression, hallucinations, low blood pressure (causing faintness or confusion), memory impairment, muscle weakness, skin rash or itching, sore throat, fever and chills, sores or ulcers in throat or mouth, unusual bruising or bleeding, extreme fatigue, yellowish tinge to eyes or skin. Call your doctor immediately.

COMMON
Drowsiness, loss of coordination, unsteady gait, dizziness, lightheadedness, slurred speech.

LESS COMMON
Change in sexual desire or ability, constipation, false sense of well-being, nausea and vomiting, urinary problems, unusual fatigue.

ALPROSTADIL INJECTION

Available in: Injection
Available OTC? No **As Generic?** Yes
Drug Class: Vasodilator

▼ USAGE INFORMATION

WHY IT'S PRESCRIBED
To treat erectile dysfunction (impotence) in men; also, to help maintain adequate blood flow in infants during heart surgery.

HOW IT WORKS
Alprostadil causes dilation of blood vessels, thereby increasing blood flow to the tissues supplied by the vessels affected by the drug. When injected into the penis, alprostadil causes the penile arteries to dilate, thus promoting erection.

▼ DOSAGE GUIDELINES

RANGE AND FREQUENCY
For adult men: Injection of 0.001 to 0.04 mg, self-administered at the base of the penis as needed. It should not be administered more than once a day. For infants: Injection of 0.005 to 0.01 mg before surgery.

ONSET OF EFFECT
5 to 10 minutes.

DURATION OF ACTION
30 minutes to 3 hours.

DIETARY ADVICE
Diet is not significant in alprostadil therapy.

STORAGE
Keep the liquid form of alprostadil refrigerated, but do not allow it to freeze.

MISSED DOSE
Not applicable; the drug is taken only when the patient chooses.

STOPPING THE DRUG
Consult your doctor if you wish to discontinue therapy or if you feel alprostadil is losing its effectiveness.

PROLONGED USE
Alprostadil should not be used more frequently than a physician recommends, which is generally not more than 3 times a week, with at least 24 hours between each dose. Patients who self-administer alprostadil should visit their doctor every 3 months for evaluation; dosage adjustments or the decision to stop using the drug will be made

at these times. Never increase the dosage without consulting your doctor.

▼ PRECAUTIONS

Over 60: Information about use specifically in older persons is not available, though elderly patients are more likely to suffer from circulatory problems and thus may be less responsive to the drug than their younger counterparts. Your doctor may need to adjust the dosage.

Driving and Hazardous Work: No special precautions are necessary.

Alcohol: No special precautions are necessary.

Pregnancy: Not applicable; the drug is used only in men and infants. No problems have been reported in women who became pregnant by partners using alprostadil.

Breast Feeding: Not applicable; the drug is used only by men or in infants.

Infants and Children: Prostin VR Pediatric should be used for infants only in a hospital setting.

Special Concerns: Your doctor should instruct you on how to administer the injection of alprostadil before you attempt to do it yourself. Only men who have been diagnosed with and are being medically treated for erectile dysfunction should use this drug as a sexual aid.

OVERDOSE
Symptoms: Painful erection

or an erection that persists for more than 4 hours.

What to Do: Call your doctor, emergency medical services (EMS), or your local hospital right away. Prolonged erection may result in permanent damage to the tissues of the penis and the inability to achieve subsequent erections.

▼ INTERACTIONS

DRUG INTERACTIONS
None reported in infants. Adults should notify their doctor if they are taking any other drugs.

FOOD INTERACTIONS
No significant interactions have been reported.

DISEASE INTERACTIONS
An adult who has a blood coagulation defect, liver disease, sickle cell disease, or a history of priapism (erections lasting more than 4 hours) should inform his physician before using alprostadil.

≡ SIDE EFFECTS ≡

SERIOUS
Painful or prolonged erection (lasting more than 4 hours), usually as a result of excessive dosage. If erection does not resolve on its own in a reasonable amount of time, seek medical help promptly. If erection does resolve on its own, subsequent doses should be reduced; consult your doctor for specific guidelines.

COMMON
Pain, itching, or burning at site of injection.

LESS COMMON
Bruising or bleeding at site of injection.

ALTRETAMINE

Available in: Capsules
Available OTC? No   **As Generic?** No
Drug Class: Antineoplastic (anticancer) agent

▼ USAGE INFORMATION

WHY IT'S PRESCRIBED
To treat persistent or recurrent ovarian cancer. This drug is generally used following first-line treatment with other chemotherapy agents.

HOW IT WORKS
The exact mechanism of action of altretamine is not known, but the drug appears to interfere with the synthesis of genetic material within cells, thereby inhibiting the growth of cancer cells.

▼ DOSAGE GUIDELINES

RANGE AND FREQUENCY
260 mg per square meter of body size, in 4 equally divided doses per day (at mealtimes and at bedtime), generally given 14 or 21 consecutive days out of a 28-day cycle. The actual dose will depend on how much toxicity has occurred in previous cycles of chemotherapy.

ONSET OF EFFECT
Peak blood levels are achieved within 3 hours.

DURATION OF ACTION
Up to 10 hours.

DIETARY ADVICE
Take it after meals to minimize nausea and vomiting. Maintain adequate intake of food and fluids.

STORAGE
Store in a tightly sealed container away from heat and direct light.

MISSED DOSE
Take it as soon as you remember, unless it is almost time for the next dose. In that case, skip the missed dose and take the next one. If you miss more than one dose, call your doctor.

STOPPING THE DRUG
The decision to stop taking the drug should be made in consultation with your doctor.

PROLONGED USE
Prolonged use can increase the incidence of nausea and vomiting, which can be treated by antiemetic drugs. Blood tests should be taken every 2 to 4 weeks and prior to the beginning of each new course of therapy with altretamine. Neurological exams should be performed regularly as well to determine whether altretamine is causing any nerve damage.

▼ PRECAUTIONS

Over 60: No special problems are expected.

Driving and Hazardous Work: This drug may produce side effects such as dizziness or nausea; avoid any potentially dangerous activities until you determine how the medication affects you.

Alcohol: Alcohol intake should be limited; drink only in moderation while taking this drug.

Pregnancy: Altretamine should not be used during pregnancy because it may cause birth defects. When using this drug, a reliable method of birth control is recommended.

Breast Feeding: Breast feeding is not recommended; altretamine passes into breast milk and may harm the nursing child.

Infants and Children: No specific information on use in children is available.

Special Concerns: This drug may affect your ability to resist infections. If possible, avoid others who are sick with any sort of infection. Be careful when using a toothbrush, dental floss, or a toothpick, and check with your doctor before having any dental work done. Avoid touching your eyes, nose, or mouth, unless your hands are very clean. Be careful not to cut yourself with objects such as razors or nail clippers, and avoid contact sports or any other activities that could result in injuries.

OVERDOSE
Symptoms: The symptoms of an overdose have not been well-defined, but an overdose may be life-threatening.

What to Do: If someone takes a much larger dose than prescribed, call emergency medical services (EMS) immediately to receive evaluation and treatment in the closest emergency facility.

▼ INTERACTIONS

DRUG INTERACTIONS
Consult your doctor if you are taking amphotericin B (by injection), antithyroid drugs, azathioprine, chlorambucil, colchicine, flucytosine, ganciclovir, interferon, plicamycin, zidovudine, or an MAO inhibitor (a class of antidepressants). Do not get vaccinated against bacteria or viruses while you are taking altretamine.

FOOD INTERACTIONS
None expected.

DISEASE INTERACTIONS
Caution is advised when taking altretamine. Consult your doctor if you have any of the following conditions: bone marrow depression, chicken pox, shingles, any infection, or reduced kidney function.

≡ SIDE EFFECTS ≡

SERIOUS
Anemia or other blood problems that cause fatigue, bleeding, bruising, fever, and chills; anxiety, confusion, dizziness, weakness, and loss of balance or coordination; numbness or tingling in the arms and legs. Call your doctor right away.

COMMON
Dizziness, drowsiness, mood changes, nausea, vomiting.

LESS COMMON
Diarrhea, loss of appetite, abdominal cramps, skin rash, temporary hair loss.

ALUMINUM SALTS

BRAND NAMES

AlternaGEL Liquid, Alu-Cap, Alu-Tab, Amphojel, Basaljel, Dialume, Phosphaljel, Rolaids

Available in: Tablets, capsules, oral suspension, gel
Available OTC? Yes   **As Generic?** Yes
Drug Class: Antacid

▼ USAGE INFORMATION

WHY IT'S PRESCRIBED
To treat heartburn, acid indigestion, sour stomach, peptic ulcers, gastritis, esophagitis, and gastroesophageal reflux. May also be used to treat or prevent excess phosphate in the blood or to prevent urinary phosphate stones.

HOW IT WORKS
Aluminum salts neutralize stomach acid and reduce the action of pepsin, a digestive enzyme. This provides symptomatic relief from excess stomach acid.

▼ DOSAGE GUIDELINES

RANGE AND FREQUENCY
1 to 2 tablets or capsules or 5 to 30 ml suspension or gel as often as every 2 hours, up to 12 times per day. Take the dose between meals unless your doctor directs otherwise. When used as sole treatment

of peptic ulcer or esophagitis, take it 1 and 3 hours after meals and at bedtime. Tablets should be chewed.

ONSET OF EFFECT
Within minutes.

DURATION OF ACTION
20 minutes to 3 hours.

DIETARY ADVICE
Avoid a low-phosphate diet during prolonged use, unless your doctor directs otherwise. Some recommended high-phosphate foods include red meat, poultry, fish, eggs, dark green leafy vegetables, dairy products, and nuts.

STORAGE
Store in a tightly sealed container away from heat, moisture, and direct light. Keep liquid forms refrigerated.

MISSED DOSE
Take it as soon as you remember. Do not double the next dose.

STOPPING THE DRUG
Take as directed.

PROLONGED USE
Do not take it for more than 2 weeks unless your doctor recommends otherwise.

▼ PRECAUTIONS

Over 60: Constipation or intestinal trouble is more common in older persons. Older patients who have or who are at high risk for osteoporosis or other bone disorders should avoid frequent use of this medicine.

Driving and Hazardous Work: No special precautions are necessary.

Alcohol: Alcohol decreases the effect of antacids.

Pregnancy: Consult your doctor before taking aluminum salts while pregnant.

Breast Feeding: Aluminum-containing antacids pass into breast milk. It is unknown whether this poses any risk to nursing infants. Consult your doctor for advice.

Infants and Children: Antacids should not be dispensed to children under age 6 unless otherwise instructed by a physician.

Special Concerns: Use over-the-counter antacids only occasionally unless otherwise directed by your doctor. Persistent heartburn not readily relieved by antacids may be signaling a heart attack or another serious disorder. In such cases, seek medical help promptly.

OVERDOSE
Symptoms: Shallow breathing, dry mouth, constipation or diarrhea, confusion, headache, weakness or fatigue, bone pain, stupor.

What to Do: Seek medical assistance immediately.

▼ INTERACTIONS

DRUG INTERACTIONS
Other medications may lose their effectiveness when taken within 1 hour of antacids. Consult your doctor for specific advice if you are taking amphetamines, bisacodyl, citrates, chenodiol, digoxin, enteric-coated medications, iron salts, isoniazid, ketoconazole, mecamylamine, methenamine, penicillamine, phosphates, nitrofurantoin, quinidine, salicylates, or tetracyclines.

FOOD INTERACTIONS
Taking an aluminum salt with food can decrease its activity. Wait at least 60 minutes after eating before taking it.

DISEASE INTERACTIONS
Do not take aluminum salts if you have any symptoms of appendicitis or an inflamed bowel (abdominal pain, cramps, soreness, bloating, nausea, vomiting). Aluminum salts are not recommended for Alzheimer's patients. Consult your doctor if you have chronic constipation, colitis, ileostomy, colostomy, intestinal or stomach blockage, bone fractures, diarrhea, kidney disease, hypophosphatemia, heart disease, liver disease, edema, stomach bleeding, intestinal bleeding.

≡ SIDE EFFECTS ≡

SERIOUS
Severe and continuing constipation, dizziness, lightheadedness, and heartbeat irregularities. Bone loss may occur, especially with prolonged use in dialysis patients. Hypophosphatemia (too little phosphate in the blood) may occur with prolonged use and a low-phosphate diet; symptoms include bone pain, fractures, muscle weakness, loss of appetite, mood changes, a general feeling of discomfort, swelling of the wrists and ankles, unusual weight loss, and anemia (decreased number of red blood cells; symptoms include weakness and fatigue).

COMMON
Chalky taste.

LESS COMMON
Mild constipation, stomach cramps, speckling or whitish coloration of stools, increased thirst, nausea and vomiting.

AMANTADINE HYDROCHLORIDE

Available in: Tablets, syrup
Available OTC? No **As Generic?** Yes
Drug Class: Antiviral/antiparkinsonism agent

▼ USAGE INFORMATION

WHY IT'S PRESCRIBED
To prevent or treat type A influenza; to treat Parkinson's disease. It may also be used to minimize stiffness and shaking caused by certain other drugs prescribed for treating nervous, mental, or emotional disorders.

HOW IT WORKS
The exact mechanism of action is unknown, though amantadine appears to prevent the influenza A virus from penetrating and entering healthy cells. In Parkinsonism, it increases the release and activity of dopamine, which plays a key role in the control of muscle movement. The increased availability of dopamine in the brain helps compensate for the reduction in the natural supply caused by the disease, and so eases symptoms of Parkinsonism.

▼ DOSAGE GUIDELINES

RANGE AND FREQUENCY
For treatment or prevention of influenza— Adults: 100 to 200 mg a day in 1 or 2 doses for 5 days. Children: Up to 150 mg once a day. For Parkinsonism— Adults: 100 mg, 2 times a day. In some cases the maximum dose may be increased to 400 mg a day. Older patients and those with a history of seizure disorders are usually given reduced doses, generally 100 mg a day.

ONSET OF EFFECT
For influenza A: 2 hours. For Parkinsonism: 48 hours.

DURATION OF ACTION
Up to 12 hours.

DIETARY ADVICE
Take it with or after meals.

STORAGE
Store in a tightly sealed container away from heat and direct light.

MISSED DOSE
If you miss a dose, take it as soon as you remember unless it is almost time for your next dose. In that case, skip the missed dose and return to your regular schedule. Do not double the next dose.

STOPPING THE DRUG
Influenza: For prevention, take amantadine for the full treatment period as recommended by your doctor; for treatment, do not stop taking amantadine without consulting your doctor. Parkinsonism: Doses must be decreased gradually according to your doctor's instructions.

PROLONGED USE
Prolonged use requires periodic checks by your doctor.

▼ PRECAUTIONS

Over 60: Older persons are generally more sensitive to amantadine and more likely to experience adverse side effects. Smaller doses may be warranted.

Driving and Hazardous Work: Amantadine can cause drowsiness, dizziness, blurred vision, or confusion. Avoid driving and hazardous work until you determine how the medicine affects you.

Alcohol: Avoid alcohol since it may increase side effects such as dizziness and blurred vision.

Pregnancy: In some animal studies, amantadine has been shown to cause birth defects, though human studies have not been done. Accordingly, the drug should be avoided during the first 3 months of pregnancy. Notify your doctor if you are pregnant or plan to become pregnant.

Breast Feeding: Amantadine passes into breast milk and should not be taken while breast feeding.

Infants and Children: Safety for children under the age of 1 has not been established.

Special Concerns: Individuals with kidney disease must take reduced dosages and be closely monitored.

OVERDOSE
Symptoms: Hyperactivity, disorientation, confusion, visual hallucinations, seizures, drop in blood pressure, palpitations or heart rhythm disturbances.

What to Do: Call your doctor, emergency medical services (EMS), or the nearest poison control center immediately.

▼ INTERACTIONS

DRUG INTERACTIONS
The effects of amantadine can be altered by amphetamines, diet pills, asthma and cold medicines, methylphenidate, nabilone, and pemoline. Anticholinergic drugs can increase the side effects of amantadine.

FOOD INTERACTIONS
None are expected.

DISEASE INTERACTIONS
Caution is advised when taking this medication. Consult your doctor if you have eczema, epilepsy, heart disease, circulation problems, kidney disease, or an emotional disorder.

≡ SIDE EFFECTS ≡

SERIOUS
Skin rash, confusion, seizures, hallucinations, swollen feet or arms, difficulty breathing. Call your doctor at once.

COMMON
Dizziness, irritability, distractibility, difficulty sleeping. Consult your doctor if such symptoms persist.

LESS COMMON
Mild skin rash, weakness, depression, fatigue, anxiety, headache, lightheadedness, loss of appetite, nausea, constipation, dry mouth. Consult your doctor if such symptoms persist.

AMILORIDE HYDROCHLORIDE

Available in: Capsules, tablets
Available OTC? No   **As Generic?** Yes
Drug Class: Potassium-sparing diuretic

▼ USAGE INFORMATION

WHY IT'S PRESCRIBED
As adjunctive (supplementary) treatment with other diuretics to increase excretion of sodium and water in the urine, while conserving potassium.

HOW IT WORKS
Amiloride promotes loss of sodium and water from the body by altering kidney enzymes that control urine production. Unlike other types of diuretics, amiloride belongs to a class that promotes excretion of excess water but does not deplete normal levels of potassium. In conjunction with thiazide or loop diuretics, amiloride reduces the overall fluid volume in the body and helps to control symptoms of heart disease, kidney disease, and liver disease.

▼ DOSAGE GUIDELINES

RANGE AND FREQUENCY
In most cases, 5 mg a day, increased to 10 mg a day if necessary. Maximum dose is 20 mg a day. The drug is usually taken in one daily dose, preferably in the morning.

ONSET OF EFFECT
2 to 4 hours.

DURATION OF ACTION
Up to 24 hours.

DIETARY ADVICE
Amiloride can be taken with liquid or food to lessen stomach irritation. Avoid large quantities of high-potassium foods (see Food Interactions).

STORAGE
Store in a tightly sealed container away from heat and direct light.

MISSED DOSE
Take it as soon as you remember. If it is near the time for the next dose, skip the missed dose and resume your regular dosage schedule. Do not double the next dose.

STOPPING THE DRUG
The decision to stop taking the drug should be made by your doctor.

PROLONGED USE
No apparent problems.

▼ PRECAUTIONS

Over 60: No special precautions are warranted.

Driving and Hazardous Work: No special warnings.

Alcohol: No special warnings.

Pregnancy: Animal studies have not shown birth defects. Adequate human studies have not been done. Consult your doctor about taking amiloride during pregnancy.

Breast Feeding: It is not known whether amiloride passes into breast milk. Consult your doctor about its use while nursing.

Infants and Children: A small dose (0.625 mg per day) may be used in young children.

OVERDOSE
Symptoms: Rapid, irregular heartbeat, shortness of breath, nervousness, confusion, weakness, stupor.

What to Do: Call your doctor, emergency medical services (EMS), or the nearest poison control center immediately.

▼ INTERACTIONS

DRUG INTERACTIONS
Tell your doctor if you are taking other drugs, especially ACE inhibitors, nonsteroidal anti-inflammatory drugs (NSAIDs), digoxin, lithium, potassium supplements, or another diuretic.

FOOD INTERACTIONS
Avoid consuming large servings of high-potassium foods, which include bananas, citrus fruits and juices, melons, prunes, (and most fruits in general), avocados, potatoes, nuts, baked beans, brussels sprouts, and skim milk.

DISEASE INTERACTIONS
Caution is advised when taking amiloride. Consult your doctor if you have any of the following: diabetes mellitus, gout, kidney stones, liver disease, or kidney disease.

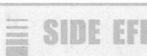 **SIDE EFFECTS**

SERIOUS
Heartbeat irregularities, lightheadedness (caused by high blood potassium levels). Notify your doctor at once.

COMMON
There are no common side effects associated with the use of amiloride.

LESS COMMON
Headache, nausea, loss of appetite, weight loss, diarrhea, vomiting, weakness, dizziness, drowsiness, abdominal pain, constipation, impotence, increased skin sensitivity to sunlight, nervousness, irregular heartbeat, shortness of breath, tingling in hands, feet, or lips.

AMINOCAPROIC ACID

Available in: Tablets, syrup, injection
Available OTC? No   **As Generic?** Yes
Drug Class: Antifibrolytic (bleeding prevention) agent

▼ USAGE INFORMATION

WHY IT'S PRESCRIBED
To treat serious bleeding that occurs after surgery or dental work or to prevent potentially life-threatening bleeding during surgery in patients with hemophilia, low blood platelet counts, or similar problems.

HOW IT WORKS
Aminocaproic acid inhibits certain biochemical reactions that involve enzymes, including the activation of plasminogen, a natural enzyme that dissolves blood clots. As a result, blood becomes more prone to clotting, which helps to stanch episodes of uncontrolled bleeding.

▼ DOSAGE GUIDELINES

RANGE AND FREQUENCY
Adults: Initial dose is 5 g, then 1 or 1.25 g per hour, 3 or 4 times a day after the initial dose. The maximum daily dose is 30 g per day. It may be taken by mouth or intravenously. Children: Initial dose is 45.5 mg per lb of body weight, followed by 15.1 mg per lb, 3 or 4 times a day, for 2 to 8 days.

ONSET OF EFFECT
Within 1 hour.

DURATION OF ACTION
3 to 4 hours.

DIETARY ADVICE
Tablet or syrup forms may be taken with food to prevent stomach irritation.

STORAGE
Store in a tightly sealed container away from heat and direct light.

MISSED DOSE
Take the missed dose as soon as you remember, unless it is almost time for the next dose. In that case, double the next dose. Then resume your regular dosage schedule.

≡ SIDE EFFECTS ≡

SERIOUS
Shortness of breath; weakness or numbness of arm or leg; slurred speech; severe and sudden headache; sharp pain in the chest, upper arm, or legs; vision changes. Although rare, such symptoms may be signaling a stroke or heart attack. Other rare but serious side effects include bleeding problems, seizures, and hallucinations. Discontinue the medication and seek emergency medical treatment immediately.

COMMON
Nausea, diarrhea, severe menstrual cramps, muscle cramps and aches, vomiting. Notify your doctor if such symptoms persist.

LESS COMMON
Dizziness; headache; muscle weakness and fatigue; ringing in the ears; skin rash; abdominal pain; rapid weight gain; swelling in the feet, face, and legs; nasal congestion; delirium; confusion.

STOPPING THE DRUG
Do not stop taking aminocaproic acid without your doctor's consent, unless a serious problem occurs, at which time discontinue the drug immediately. Gradual reduction of the dosage may be necessary if you have taken the drug for a long time. Consult your doctor for specific guidelines. Never take more than 30 g per day.

PROLONGED USE
Ask your doctor about the need for medical examinations or laboratory studies with prolonged use.

▼ PRECAUTIONS

Over 60: No special problems are expected.

Driving and Hazardous Work: Do not drive or engage in hazardous work until you determine how the drug affects you.

Alcohol: Avoid alcohol because it decreases the therapeutic effect of the drug.

Pregnancy: It is not known whether aminocaproic acid causes fetal harm. It should be used during pregnancy only if clearly necessary, after a detailed discussion with your doctor.

Breast Feeding: Aminocaproic acid passes into breast milk, although it has not been reported to cause health problems in nursing infants. Consult your doctor or pediatrician for advice.

Infants and Children: Safety and effectiveness in young patients have not been established; this drug should be used in children only under a doctor's careful supervision.

OVERDOSE
Symptoms: Few cases of overdose have been reported. However, symptoms following high doses of injectable aminocaproic acid may include dizziness, confusion, slow heartbeat, fainting, sluggishness, fatigue, confusion, seizures, increased urination, gastrointestinal bleeding.

What to Do: Discontinue the medication and call your doctor, emergency medical services (EMS), or local hospital immediately.

▼ INTERACTIONS

DRUG INTERACTIONS
Oral contraceptives and estrogens boost the the clotpromoting effect of aminocaproic acid, which may therefore increase the risk of potentially dangerous blood clot formation. Thrombolytic (blood-clot-dissolving) agents such as streptokinase decrease the effect of aminocaproic acid.

FOOD INTERACTIONS
No significant food interactions have been reported.

DISEASE INTERACTIONS
Patients with a history of disseminated intravascular coagulation (also known as DIC, a rare disorder marked by excessive blood coagulation) should not take aminocaproic acid. If you are pregnant or have heart disease, kidney disease, or liver disease, you may be at increased risk for side effects.

AMINOPHYLLINE

BRAND NAMES

Aminophyllin, Phyllocontin, Truphylline

Available in: Tablets, liquid, injection, suppositories
Available OTC? No   **As Generic?** Yes
Drug Class: Bronchodilator/xanthine

▼ USAGE INFORMATION

WHY IT'S PRESCRIBED
To widen the airways (bronchodilation) and so prevent the wheezing and constriction of the airways associated with asthma and other breathing disorders, such as chronic bronchitis, emphysema, and chronic obstructive pulmonary disease (COPD).

HOW IT WORKS
An asthma attack occurs when the smooth muscles in the bronchial passages of the lungs go into a spasm (bronchospasm). Aminophylline relaxes these muscles, thus helping to widen the constricted airways and restore normal breathing.

▼ DOSAGE GUIDELINES

RANGE AND FREQUENCY
Adults: 6 to 8 mg per day per 2.2 lbs (1 kg) of body weight. Children: 18 mg per day per 2.2 lbs of body weight. The dosage must be adjusted for each person. Higher doses are warranted during an acute asthma attack and taken as needed. Maintenance dose is taken every 6 to 8 hours.

ONSET OF EFFECT
15 to 60 minutes.

DURATION OF ACTION
Several hours, depending on dosage and form.

DIETARY ADVICE
Best taken 1 hour before or 2 hours after eating. Can be taken with meals to lessen any stomach upset.

STORAGE
Keep in a tightly sealed container away from heat, moisture, and direct light.

MISSED DOSE
If you miss a dose, take it as soon as you remember up to 2 hours late. If more than 2 hours, wait for the next scheduled dose. Do not double the next dose.

STOPPING THE DRUG
Take it as long as your doctor advises. See your doctor for regular checkups.

PROLONGED USE
If used properly, aminophylline can be taken safely for a lifetime; no specific problems are expected.

▼ PRECAUTIONS

Over 60: Adverse reactions may be more likely and more severe in older patients.

Driving and Hazardous Work: Do not engage in such activities until you determine how the drug affects you. If you experience side effects such as dizziness and lightheadedness, proceed with caution.

Alcohol: No special precautions are necessary.

Pregnancy: It is unclear whether aminophylline causes fetal harm; discuss the risks with your doctor. Generally, this drug should be used only if necessary and if a substitute cannot be prescribed.

Breast Feeding: Aminophylline passes into breast milk and may be toxic to nursing infants; avoid the drug or discontinue breast feeding.

Infants and Children: Be alert for side effects such as agitation, irritability, fever, lethargy, rapid heartbeat and breathing, or seizures. The liquid form of aminophylline is often recommended for children to make it easier to use and ensure a more accurate dosage.

Special Concerns: Aminophylline should not be used by patients who have had prior allergic reactions to it or its components (including ethylenediamide).

OVERDOSE

Symptoms: Acute restlessness, irritability, confusion, breathing difficulties, heart rhythm irregularities, delirium, seizures.

What to Do: Stop taking the drug and contact your doctor, emergency medical services (EMS), or the nearest poison control center immediately.

▼ INTERACTIONS

DRUG INTERACTIONS
Consult your doctor for specific advice if you are taking allopurinol, cimetidine, ciprofloxacin, erythromycin, troleandomycin, lithium, oral contraceptives, phenytoin, propranolol, or rifampin.

FOOD INTERACTIONS
Avoid excessive use of caffeine-containing beverages. High-carbohydrate and high-fat meals can decrease the effect of aminophylline.

DISEASE INTERACTIONS
You should not take aminophylline if you have active peptic ulcer disease or an underlying disorder that causes seizures (unless you are also taking appropriate anticonvulsant medication). The suppository form should not be used by people with inflammation or infection of the rectum or lower colon. Use caution when taking aminophylline if you have heart disease, liver disease, or an underactive thyroid (hypothyroidism). Consult your doctor in such cases.

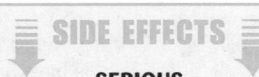

SIDE EFFECTS

SERIOUS
Although very rare, aminophylline may lead to heartbeat irregularities, seizures, or extreme breathing difficulty. Seek emergency medical assistance immediately.

COMMON
Headache, irritability, nervousness, nausea, vomiting, rapid breathing or heartbeat, restlessness, insomnia, stomach pain, increased urine output.

LESS COMMON
Hives or skin rash, diarrhea, dizziness, lightheadedness, loss of appetite, fatigue.

AMINOSALICYLATE SODIUM

BRAND NAMES

Sodium P.A.S., Tubasal

Available in: Tablets
Available OTC? No   **As Generic?** No
Drug Class: Anti-infective/antitubercular agent

▼ USAGE INFORMATION

WHY IT'S PRESCRIBED
To treat active tuberculosis; must be used in conjunction with other antitubercular agents, such as isoniazid, streptomycin, and rifampin.

HOW IT WORKS
Aminosalicylate kills tuberculosis bacteria by preventing them from utilizing folic acid, a vitamin necessary for cell growth and reproduction.

▼ DOSAGE GUIDELINES

RANGE AND FREQUENCY
Adults and teenagers: 4 to 6 grams every 12 hours; usually not more than 68 to 91 mg per lb of body weight a day. Children age 12 and under: 23 to 34 mg per lb of body weight every 12 hours. Aminosalicylate is taken in conjunction with other antitubercular agents.

ONSET OF EFFECT
Unknown.

DURATION OF ACTION
Unknown.

DIETARY ADVICE
Take it with or after meals or with an antacid to minimize stomach irritation.

STORAGE
Store in a tightly sealed container away from heat, moisture, and direct light.

MISSED DOSE
Take it as soon as you remember. This will help keep a constant level of medication in your system. If it is near the time for the next dose, skip the missed dose and resume your regular dosage schedule. Do not double the next dose.

STOPPING THE DRUG
Take it as prescribed for the full treatment period, even if you begin to feel better before the scheduled end of therapy. Treatment may continue for months or years. The decision to stop taking the drug should be made by your doctor.

PROLONGED USE
Prolonged use with high doses may cause swelling in the front of the neck, menstrual changes in women, decreased sexual ability in men, unusual weight gain, and dry, puffy skin. Consult your doctor about the need for periodic medical examinations and laboratory tests if you take this medication for a prolonged period.

▼ PRECAUTIONS

Over 60: Adverse reactions may be more likely and more severe in older patients.

Driving and Hazardous Work: Do not drive or engage in hazardous work until you determine how the medicine affects you.

Alcohol: No special precautions are necessary.

Pregnancy: Adequate studies of aminosalicylate use during pregnancy have not been done. Consult your doctor for specific advice if you are pregnant or plan to become pregnant.

Breast Feeding: Aminosalicylate passes into breast milk, but no problems have been documented.

Infants and Children: No special warnings; children may tolerate the drug better than adults.

Special Concerns: Do not take tablets that are brown or purple in color.

OVERDOSE
Symptoms: An overdose with aminosalicylate is unlikely.

What to Do: Emergency instructions not applicable.

▼ INTERACTIONS

DRUG INTERACTIONS
Do not take rifampin within 6 hours of taking aminosalicylate. Other drugs may interact with aminosalicylate. Consult your doctor if you are taking aminobenzoates or other over-the-counter or prescription medications.

FOOD INTERACTIONS
None are anticipated, although aminosalicylate can interfere with the absorption of vitamin B12 and other nutrients; vitamin supplementation may be necessary.

DISEASE INTERACTIONS
Caution is advised when taking aminosalicylate. Consult your doctor if you have any of the following: gastric ulcers, epilepsy, heart disease, cancer, an overactive thyroid, or adrenal insufficiency. Use of aminosalicylate may cause complications in patients with liver or kidney disease, since these organs work together to remove the medication from the body.

  SIDE EFFECTS

SERIOUS
Joint pain, fever, unusual fatigue, skin rash or itching, lower back pain, yellow discoloration of the eyes or skin, severe abdominal pain, sore throat, pale skin, headache, pain or burning while urinating. Call your doctor immediately.

COMMON
Abdominal discomfort, nausea and vomiting, diarrhea, loss of weight and appetite.

LESS COMMON
Peptic ulcer disease, intestinal bleeding, lowered white and red blood cell counts.

AMIODARONE

Available in: Tablets
Available OTC? No   **As Generic?** Yes
Drug Class: Antiarrhythmic

▼ USAGE INFORMATION

WHY IT'S PRESCRIBED
To prevent and treat heartbeat irregularities, including atrial fibrillation and ventricular tachycardia. The relative risks of using this drug must be weighed carefully against its benefits, since amiodarone can be toxic, especially when taken at high doses or for long periods of time.

HOW IT WORKS
Amiodarone slows and helps regulate nerve impulses in the heart, and acts directly on the tissue of the heart, making heart muscle less responsive to abnormal stimuli.

▼ DOSAGE GUIDELINES

RANGE AND FREQUENCY
Adults: 800 to 2,400 mg per day in 3 or 4 equally divided doses at first; then 600 to 800 mg per day for one month; then 200 to 400 mg per day. Children: Dosage schedule varies according to the severity of the arrhythmia and often according to individual physician preferences.

ONSET OF EFFECT
2 or 3 days to 2 to 3 weeks.

DURATION OF ACTION
10 days to several months depending on total amount of time the drug has been prescribed and total quantity consumed.

DIETARY ADVICE
Amiodarone be taken with liquid or food to minimize the risk of stomach upset.

STORAGE
Store in a tightly sealed container away from heat, moisture, and direct light.

SIDE EFFECTS

SERIOUS
Cough, shortness of breath, increased palpitations, loss of voice (rare). Seek medical assistance immediately. Nausea, vomiting, and yellow-tinged skin or eyes (jaundice) may occur as an indication of serious liver problems; notify your doctor right away if such symptoms arise.

COMMON
Stomach upset; nausea; vomiting; constipation; loss of appetite; low-grade fever; heightened skin sensitivity to sun, resulting in greater predisposition to sunburn; numbness or tingling in the fingers or toes; trembling or shaking; unsteadiness when walking; headache.

LESS COMMON
Bitter or metallic taste in the mouth, blue-gray discoloration of skin, vision disturbances, dry eyes, dry, puffy skin, coldness or chills, dizziness, nervousness or restlessness, diminished sex drive in males, scrotal pain and swelling, slow heartbeat, unusual or profuse sweating, insomnia, fatigue, unexpected gain or loss of weight.

MISSED DOSE
Skip the missed dose and return to your regular schedule. Do not double next dose.

STOPPING THE DRUG
The decision to stop taking the drug should be made by your doctor. Be sure to report any unusual symptoms after you discontinue the medication.

PROLONGED USE
Dosage is typically reduced (to 100 to 200 mg daily) with prolonged use.

▼ PRECAUTIONS

Over 60: Side effects may be more likely and more severe. Thyroid problems (both hypo- and hyperthyroidism) as well as walking difficulty, and numbness, tingling, trembling, or weakness in the hands and feet are likely to develop.

Driving and Hazardous Work: Proceed with caution until you determine how the drug affects you.

Alcohol: Drink only in strict moderation if at all.

Pregnancy: Studies have indicated that amiodarone may cause thyroid and heart problems in unborn children. Nonetheless, the drug may be needed if a history of serious cardiac arrhythmia is a threat to the mother's life. Discuss the relative risks and benefits with your doctor.

Breast Feeding: Amiodarone passes into breast milk; consult your doctor for advice.

Infants and Children: Amiodarone can be used in children who have symptomatic or life-threatening arrhythmias. Discuss relative risks and benefits with your doctor.

Special Concerns: To screen for early signs of side effects, most patients should have regular blood tests for liver, thyroid, and pulmonary function, and have eye exams at least annually. Before dental work, emergency treatment, or surgery requiring general anesthesia, be sure to tell the attending doctor or dentist that you are taking amiodarone.

OVERDOSE
Symptoms: Seizures, irregular or very slow heartbeat, loss of consciousness.

What to Do: Call your doctor, emergency medical services (EMS), or the nearest poison control center immediately.

▼ INTERACTIONS

DRUG INTERACTIONS
Consult your doctor for specific advice if you are taking anticoagulants, other heart medications, theophylline, or phenytoin. The blood-thinning effect of warfarin may be drastically enhanced within days of starting amiodarone. Usually the dose of warfarin is reduced once amiodarone is prescribed; prothrombin time is monitored carefully.

FOOD INTERACTIONS
None are expected.

DISEASE INTERACTIONS
Consult your doctor if you have liver or kidney disease, or a thyroid disorder.

AMITRIPTYLINE HYDROCHLORIDE

Available in: Tablets
Available OTC? No **As Generic?** Yes
Drug Class: Tricyclic antidepressant; antimanic agent

BRAND NAMES

Amitid, Amitril, Elavil, Emitrip, Endep, Enovil, Vanatrip

▼ USAGE INFORMATION

WHY IT'S PRESCRIBED
To relieve symptoms of major depression and chronic pain.

HOW IT WORKS
Amitriptyline affects levels of specific brain chemicals (serotonin, norepinephrine, and acetylcholine) that are thought to be linked to mood, emotions, and mental state.

▼ DOSAGE GUIDELINES

RANGE AND FREQUENCY
Adults: To start, 25 mg, 2 to 4 times a day; may be increased to 150 mg a day. Teenagers: 10 mg, 3 times a day, and 20 mg at bedtime. Children ages 6 to 12: 10 to 30 mg a day. Older adults: To start, 25 mg a day at bedtime; may be increased to 100 mg a day.

ONSET OF EFFECT
1 to 6 weeks.

DURATION OF ACTION
Unknown.

DIETARY ADVICE
To lessen stomach upset, take with food, unless your doctor instructs otherwise. Increase intake of fiber and fluids.

STORAGE
Store in a tightly sealed container away from heat, moisture, and direct light.

MISSED DOSE
If you take a one-time daily bedtime dose, do not take the missed dose in the morning; it may cause drowsiness. Call your doctor. If you take more than 1 dose a day, take it as soon as you remember. If it is near the time for the next dose, skip the missed dose and resume your regular dosage schedule. Do not double the next dose.

STOPPING THE DRUG
Take it as prescribed for the full treatment period, even if you feel better before the scheduled end of therapy. The decision to stop taking the drug should be made in consultation with your doctor. The dosage should be gradually tapered over 5 to 7 days when stopping.

PROLONGED USE
The usual course of therapy lasts 6 months to 1 year; some patients may benefit from additional therapy.

▼ PRECAUTIONS

Over 60: Adverse reactions are more likely and more severe in older patients. Amitriptyline is generally not recommended, as there are safer alternatives for older patients. A lower dose may be warranted.

Driving and Hazardous Work: Exercise caution until you determine how the medicine affects you. Drowsiness or lightheadedness can occur.

Alcohol: Avoid alcohol.

Pregnancy: Adequate human studies have not been done in pregnant women. Consult your doctor for advice.

Breast Feeding: Amitriptyline passes into breast milk; do not use it while nursing.

Infants and Children: Not prescribed for children under the age of 6.

Special Concerns: This is a potentially dangerous drug, especially if taken in excess. Tricyclic antidepressants should not be within easy reach of suicidal patients. If dry mouth occurs, use sugarless gum or candy.

OVERDOSE
Symptoms: Breathing difficulty, fever, severe fatigue, impaired concentration, mental confusion, hallucinations, dilated pupils, irregular heartbeat or palpitations, and seizures.

What to Do: Call your doctor, emergency medical services (EMS), or the nearest poison control center immediately.

▼ INTERACTIONS

DRUG INTERACTIONS
Consult your doctor for specific advice if you are taking antithyroid agents, cimetidine, cisapride, clonidine, guanadrel, guanethidine, metrizamide, appetite suppressants, isoproterenol, ephedrine, epinephrine, amphetamines, phenylephrine, antipsychotic drugs, pimozide, methyldopa, metyrosine, metoclopramide, pemoline, promethazine, trimeprazine, rauwolfia alkaloids, MAO inhibitors, or any drugs that depress the central nervous system.

FOOD INTERACTIONS
No known food interactions.

DISEASE INTERACTIONS
Consult your doctor if you have any of the following: a history of alcohol abuse, difficulty urinating, asthma, bipolar disorder, high blood pressure, stomach or intestinal problems, glaucoma, overactive thyroid, enlarged prostate, schizophrenia, seizures, a blood disorder, or kidney, heart, or liver disease.

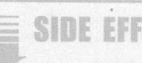

SIDE EFFECTS

SERIOUS
Confusion, heartbeat irregularities, hallucinations, seizures, extreme fatigue or drowsiness, blurred or altered vision, breathing difficulty, constipation, impaired concentration, difficult urination, fever, extreme and persistent restlessness, loss of coordination and balance, difficulty swallowing or speaking, dilated pupils, eye pain, fainting. Also trembling, shaking, weakness, and stiffness in the extremities; shuffling gait. Call your doctor immediately.

COMMON
Drowsiness, dizziness, or lightheadedness, headache, dry mouth or unpleasant taste, fatigue, heightened sensitivity to light, unusual weight gain, increased appetite, nausea.

LESS COMMON
Heartburn, insomnia or restlessness, diarrhea, increased sweating, vomiting.

AMLEXANOX

BRAND NAME

Aphthasol

Available in: Adhesive oral paste
Available OTC? No   **As Generic?** No
Drug Class: Antiaphthous ulcer drug

▼ USAGE INFORMATION

WHY IT'S PRESCRIBED
To help heal aphthous ulcers (canker sores) of the mouth. Amlexanox works best if it is taken as soon as such ulcers are diagnosed.

HOW IT WORKS
The exact way in which amlexanox works is unknown. Studies have suggested that it inhibits the formation and release of substances in the body associated with allergic reactions and inflammation.

▼ DOSAGE GUIDELINES

RANGE AND FREQUENCY
Apply ¼ inch of paste on each lesion (mouth ulcer), 4 times a day.

ONSET OF EFFECT
Unknown.

DURATION OF ACTION
Unknown.

DIETARY ADVICE
The paste is best applied after each meal and at bedtime.

STORAGE
Store in a tightly sealed container away from heat and direct light.

MISSED DOSE
Apply it as soon as you remember. If it is near the time for the next dose, skip the missed dose and resume your regular dosage schedule. Do not double the next dose.

STOPPING THE DRUG
Use this drug as prescribed for the full treatment period, even if you begin to feel better before the scheduled end of therapy.

PROLONGED USE
You should see your doctor regularly for tests and examinations if you take this medicine for a prolonged period. If ulcers have not healed significantly or pain has not been reduced after 10 days, consult your doctor.

▼ PRECAUTIONS

Over 60: It is unknown whether amlexanox causes side effects in older patients different from or more severe than those in younger patients.

Driving and Hazardous Work: The use of amlexanox should not impair your ability to perform such tasks safely.

Alcohol: No special precautions are necessary.

Pregnancy: In animal studies, amlexanox has not caused birth defects or other problems. Human studies have not been done. Before you take amlexanox, tell your doctor if you are pregnant or plan to become pregnant.

Breast Feeding: Amlexanox may pass into breast milk; caution is advised. Consult your doctor for advice.

Infants and Children: The safety and effectiveness of amlexanox in children have not been established.

Special Concerns: Wash your hands immediately after applying amlexanox. Flush your eyes with water promptly if they come in contact with the paste. If a rash or inflammation of the mucous membranes develops, discontinue use of amlexanox and contact your doctor.

OVERDOSE
Symptoms: None have been reported.

What to Do: An overdose of amlexanox is very unlikely to occur. Emergency instructions are not applicable.

▼ INTERACTIONS

DRUG INTERACTIONS
Consult your doctor for specific advice if you are taking any other prescription or over-the-counter drug.

FOOD INTERACTIONS
No known food interactions.

DISEASE INTERACTIONS
Caution is advised when tak-

ing amlexanox. Consult your doctor for specific advice if you have any other medical condition, especially a weakened immune system, which is prevalent in people receiving immunosuppressant drugs or chemotherapy, as well as those with acquired immuno-deficiency syndrome (AIDS). The safety and effectiveness of amlexanox in persons with a weakened immune system have not been established. In addition, amlexanox should not be used by anyone who has had a previous allergic reaction to the medication or any other ingredient in the formulation.

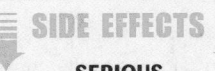
SIDE EFFECTS

SERIOUS
No serious side effects are associated with amlexanox.

COMMON
Transient pain, stinging, or burning at site of application.

LESS COMMON
Nausea, diarrhea, inflammation of the mucous membranes.

AMLODIPINE

Available in: Tablets, capsules
Available OTC? No   **As Generic?** No
Drug Class: Calcium channel blocker

▼ USAGE INFORMATION

WHY IT'S PRESCRIBED
To relieve angina (chest pain associated with heart disease) and to treat hypertension.

HOW IT WORKS
Amlodipine interferes with the movement of calcium into heart muscle cells and the smooth muscle cells in the walls of the arteries. This action relaxes blood vessels (causing them to widen), which lowers blood pressure, increases the blood supply to the heart, and decreases the heart's overall workload.

▼ DOSAGE GUIDELINES

RANGE AND FREQUENCY
2.5 to 10 mg per day in one daily dose (usually in the morning, with breakfast).

ONSET OF EFFECT
1 to 2 hours.

DURATION OF ACTION
24 hours.

DIETARY ADVICE
It can be taken with or after meals to minimize stomach irritation. Be sure to follow a low-sodium, low-fat diet if your doctor so advises.

STORAGE
Store in a tightly sealed container away from heat and direct light.

MISSED DOSE
If you miss a dose, take it as soon as you remember, unless the next dose is less than 4 hours away. In that case, skip the missed dose and go back to your regular schedule. Do not double the next dose.

STOPPING THE DRUG
Take as prescribed for the full treatment period. Do not stop taking this drug suddenly, as this may cause potentially serious health problems. If therapy is to be discontinued, dosage should be reduced gradually, according to doctor's instructions.

PROLONGED USE
In some cases amlodipine therapy may be required for years or even a lifetime. Consult your doctor about the need for medical or laboratory tests of heart activity, blood pressure, kidney function, and liver function.

▼ PRECAUTIONS

Over 60: Adverse reactions may be more likely and more severe in older patients. Smaller doses (2.5 mg per day) are generally prescribed.

Driving and Hazardous Work: Avoid driving or engaging in hazardous work until you determine how this medication affects you. Be cautious if it causes dizziness.

Alcohol: Alcohol should be used with caution because it may increase the effect of the drug and cause an excessive drop in blood pressure.

Pregnancy: Amlodipine should not be taken during the first 3 months of pregnancy and should be used in the last 6 months only if your doctor so advises.

Breast Feeding: Amlodipine should not be taken by nursing mothers.

Infants and Children: Amlodipine is not usually prescribed for patients under the age of 12.

Special Concerns: Amlodipine should not be taken by anyone who has had a prior adverse reaction to it. When taking amlodipine, avoid sudden changes in position, especially standing up quickly after sitting or lying down; such movements may cause dizziness.

OVERDOSE

Symptoms: Severe drop in blood pressure resulting in weakness, dizziness, drowsiness, confusion, or slurred speech.

What to Do: Call your doctor, emergency medical services (EMS), or your local hospital immediately.

▼ INTERACTIONS

DRUG INTERACTIONS
Other heart drugs taken with amlodipine can cause heart rate and rhythm problems. In general, consult your doctor if you are taking any other prescription or nonprescription medications.

FOOD INTERACTIONS
Avoid excessive intake of foods high in sodium.

DISEASE INTERACTIONS
Consult your doctor if you have kidney disease, liver disease, high blood pressure, or any heart disease other than coronary artery disease.

 SIDE EFFECTS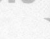

SERIOUS
Increased angina attacks, dizziness upon arising from a sitting or lying position, shortness of breath, weakness, very slow heartbeat. Call your doctor immediately.

COMMON
Headache; flushing in the face and body; water retention causing decreased urination, swelling of the feet and ankles, weight gain.

LESS COMMON
Fatigue, dizziness, drowsiness, palpitations, nausea, abdominal pain.

AMOBARBITAL/SECOBARBITAL

BRAND NAME

Tuinal

Available in: Capsules
Available OTC? No   **As Generic?** No
Drug Class: Barbiturate; central nervous system depressant

▼ USAGE INFORMATION

WHY IT'S PRESCRIBED
Amobarbital/secobarbital was previously used for the short-term treatment of insomnia. It is now prescribed only rarely by doctors, usually for the purpose of sedation.

HOW IT WORKS
This medication is actually two barbiturates, amobarbital and secobarbital, in combination. These drugs act on the central nervous system as a powerful sedative.

▼ DOSAGE GUIDELINES

RANGE AND FREQUENCY
100 or 200 mg at bedtime.

ONSET OF EFFECT
Within 15 minutes.

DURATION OF ACTION
From 3 to 8 hours.

DIETARY ADVICE
The capsules may be crushed and taken with food or liquids.

STORAGE
Store in a tightly sealed container away from heat, moisture, and direct light.

MISSED DOSE
Amobarbital/secobarbital is prescribed for once-daily use at bedtime only. If you are unable to take this medication on a particular night, resume only your regularly scheduled dose the following night. Do not double the next dose.

STOPPING THE DRUG
Never stop taking the drug abruptly, as this can cause withdrawal symptoms (seizures, sleep disruption, nervousness, irritability, diarrhea, abdominal cramps, muscle aches, memory impairment). Dosage should be reduced gradually, as directed by your doctor.

PROLONGED USE
Barbiturates are habit-forming. Prolonged use of amobarbital/secobarbital increases the risk of dependency. Amobarbital/secobarbital should not be prescribed for long-term therapy because safer and more effective drugs are available.

▼ PRECAUTIONS

Over 60: Adverse reactions may be more likely and more severe in older patients.

Driving and Hazardous Work: The use of amobarbital/secobarbital may impair your ability to perform such tasks safely.

Alcohol: Avoid alcohol completely; the combination of alcohol and barbiturates is potentially lethal.

Pregnancy: Discuss with your doctor the relative risks and benefits of using this drug while pregnant.

Breast Feeding: Do not use this drug while nursing.

Infants and Children: Not recommended for children.

Special Concerns: Amobarbital/secobarbital is a potentially dangerous drug. Barbiturates should not be used for the treatment of anxiety or stress.

OVERDOSE
Symptoms: Lethargy, excessive sleepiness, slurred speech, severe clumsiness, difficulty walking, confusion, extremely slow, noisy breathing, loss of consciousness. Some patients may become agitated and unusually excited (paradoxical excitation). Pupils may become very tiny, although with severe overdose the pupils may become very dilated.

What to Do: Contact emergency medical services (EMS) immediately.

▼ INTERACTIONS

DRUG INTERACTIONS
The risk of an undesirable interaction is increased when amobarbital/secobarbital is used with any or all of the following drugs: alcohol-containing medicines, antihistamines, allergy medications, sedatives, antiseizure medications, pain medications (especially prescription pain relievers and narcotics), muscle relaxants, and antidepressants. Use of amobarbital/secobarbital may cause the following to be less effective: blood thinners, birth control pills, and medications similar to cortisone.

FOOD INTERACTIONS
No known food interactions.

DISEASE INTERACTIONS
Patients with kidney or liver disease should avoid amobarbital/secobarbital. The drug may make the following conditions worse: asthma, emphysema, and other respiratory diseases; mental depression; porphyria; and diabetes mellitus.

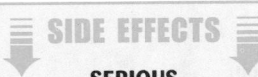
SIDE EFFECTS

SERIOUS
Extreme confusion, severe drowsiness, shortness of breath, wheezing or difficulty breathing, fever, bleeding, rash, hives, hallucinations. Stop taking the drug and call your doctor immediately if you experience any of these side effects.

COMMON
Clumsiness or unsteadiness, dizziness or lightheadedness, drowsiness, hangover-like feelings.

LESS COMMON
Nausea, vomiting, constipation, headache, irritability, sleep disturbances, including nightmares and difficulty falling asleep.

AMOXAPINE

Available in: Tablets
Available OTC? No   **As Generic?** Yes
Drug Class: Tricyclic antidepressant

▼ USAGE INFORMATION

WHY IT'S PRESCRIBED
To relieve symptoms of major depression.

HOW IT WORKS
Amoxapine affects levels of norepinephrine, a brain chemical that is thought to be linked to mood, emotions, and mental state.

▼ DOSAGE GUIDELINES

RANGE AND FREQUENCY
Adults: To start, 50 mg, 2 to 3 times a day. Older adults: To start, 25 mg, 2 to 3 times a day. Dosages may be gradually increased, as determined by your doctor.

ONSET OF EFFECT
1 to 6 weeks.

DURATION OF ACTION
Unknown.

DIETARY ADVICE
To lessen stomach upset, take with food, unless your doctor instructs otherwise. Increase intake of fiber and fluids.

STORAGE
Store in a tightly sealed container away from heat, moisture, and direct light.

MISSED DOSE
If you take a one-time daily bedtime dose, do not take a missed dose in the morning because it may cause drowsiness. Call your doctor. If you take more than 1 dose a day, take it as soon as you remember. If it is near the time for the next dose, skip the missed dose and resume your regular dosage schedule. Do not double the next dose.

STOPPING THE DRUG
Take it as prescribed for the full treatment period, even if you feel better before the scheduled end of therapy. The decision to stop taking the drug should be made in consultation with your doctor. The dosage should be gradually tapered over several days when stopping.

PROLONGED USE
The usual course of therapy lasts 6 months to 1 year; some patients may benefit from additional therapy. There is increased risk of movement disorders with prolonged use.

▼ PRECAUTIONS

Over 60: Adverse reactions may be more likely and more severe in older patients. A lower dose may be warranted.

Driving and Hazardous Work: Use caution when driving or engaging in hazardous work until you determine how the medication affects you. Drowsiness and lightheadedness can occur.

Alcohol: Avoid alcohol.

Pregnancy: Adequate human studies have not been done. Consult your doctor.

Breast Feeding: Amoxapine passes into breast milk; do not use it while nursing.

Infants and Children: Not prescribed for children under the age of 6.

Special Concerns: This is a potentially dangerous drug, especially if taken in excess. Tricyclic antidepressants

should not be within easy reach of suicidal patients. If dry mouth occurs, use sugarless gum or candy for relief.

OVERDOSE
Symptoms: Difficulty breathing, severe fatigue, seizures, confusion, hallucinations, dilated pupils, irregular heartbeat, heart palpitations, fever, difficulty concentrating.

What to Do: Call your doctor, emergency medical services (EMS), or the nearest poison control center immediately.

▼ INTERACTIONS

DRUG INTERACTIONS
Consult your doctor for specific advice if you are taking antithyroid agents, cimetidine, cisapride, clonidine, guanadrel, guanethidine, metrizamide, appetite suppressants, isoproterenol, ephedrine, epinephrine, amphetamines, phenylephrine, antipsychotic drugs, pimozide, methyldopa, metyrosine, metoclopramide, pemoline, promethazine, trimeprazine, rauwolfia alkaloids, MAO inhibitors, or central nervous system depressants.

FOOD INTERACTIONS
No known food interactions.

DISEASE INTERACTIONS
Consult your doctor if you have any of the following: a history of alcohol abuse, difficulty urinating, asthma, bipolar disorder, high blood pressure, stomach or intestinal problems, glaucoma, overactive thyroid, enlarged prostate, schizophrenia, seizures, a blood disorder, or kidney, heart, or liver disease.

SIDE EFFECTS

SERIOUS
Confusion; sexual dysfunction; heartbeat irregularities; hallucinations; seizures; extreme fatigue or drowsiness; blurred or altered vision; breathing difficulty; constipation; staring and absence of facial expression; impaired concentration; difficult urination; fever; extreme and persistent restlessness; loss of coordination and balance; difficulty swallowing or speaking; dilated pupils; eye pain; fainting; trembling, shaking, weakness, and stiffness in the extremities; shuffling gait; persistent, uncontrolled chewing, lip-smacking, or tongue movements; uncontrolled movements, including tics, twitching, twisting movements, and muscle spasms in the face, arms hands, and legs. Call your doctor immediately.

COMMON
Drowsiness or dizziness, headache, dry mouth or unpleasant taste, fatigue, heightened sensitivity to light, nausea, weight gain, increased appetite.

LESS COMMON
Heartburn, insomnia, diarrhea, sweating, vomiting.

AMOXICILLIN

Available in: Capsules, oral suspension, chewable tablets, liquid drops
Available OTC? No   **As Generic?** Yes
Drug Class: Penicillin antibiotic

▼ USAGE INFORMATION

WHY IT'S PRESCRIBED
To treat bacterial infections of the ear, nose, and throat, genitourinary tract, skin and soft tissues, and the lower respiratory tract. It is used, often with other drugs, to treat uncomplicated gonorrhea. It is also prescribed preventively before surgery or dental work to patients at risk for endocarditis (infection of the interior lining of the heart). It is also used to treat some stages of Lyme disease and, along with other drugs, to treat H. pylori infection (the cause of stomach ulcers).

HOW IT WORKS
Amoxicillin blocks the formation of bacterial cell walls, rendering bacteria unable to multiply and spread.

▼ DOSAGE GUIDELINES

RANGE AND FREQUENCY
For infections— Adults: 250 to 500 mg every 8 hours (3 doses per day). Children: 3 to 6 mg per lb of body weight every 8 hours (3 doses per day). To treat gonorrhea— 3 g in a single oral dose.

ONSET OF EFFECT
Rapid; within 2 hours.

DURATION OF ACTION
8 hours.

DIETARY ADVICE
Best taken on an empty stomach, but may be taken with food to minimize stomach irritation or diarrhea.

STORAGE
Store in a tightly sealed container away from heat and direct light. Keep any liquid form refrigerated, but do not allow it to freeze, and discard after 14 days.

MISSED DOSE
Take it as soon as you remember. If it is near the time for the next dose, skip the missed dose and resume your regular dosage schedule. Do not double the next dose.

STOPPING THE DRUG
Take as prescribed for the full treatment period, even if you begin to feel better before the scheduled end of therapy. Stopping the drug prematurely may slow your recovery or lead to a rebound infection, also known as superinfection, in which the heartier strains of bacteria survive and multiply, leading to a more serious and drug-resistant infection.

PROLONGED USE
Prolonged use of any antibiotic increases the risk of superinfection; caution is advised.

▼ PRECAUTIONS

Over 60: No special problems are expected.

Driving and Hazardous Work: The use of amoxicillin should not impair your ability to perform such tasks safely.

Alcohol: No special precautions are necessary.

Pregnancy: Adequate studies of the use of this drug during pregnancy have not been done; however, no problems have been reported.

Breast Feeding: Amoxicillin passes into breast milk and may cause diarrhea, fungal infections, and allergic reactions in nursing infants; avoid use while nursing.

Infants and Children: No special problems are expected.

Special Concerns: Amoxicillin can cause false results on some urine sugar tests for diabetics. Those who are prone to asthma, hay fever, hives, or allergies may be more likely to have an allergic reaction to a penicillin antibiotic. Oral contraceptives may not be effective while you are taking amoxicillin; use other methods of contraception to avoid unplanned pregnancy.

OVERDOSE
Symptoms: Severe nausea, vomiting, diarrhea, muscle spasticity, seizures.

What to Do: Call your doctor, emergency medical services (EMS), or the nearest poison control center immediately.

▼ INTERACTIONS

DRUG INTERACTIONS
Consult your doctor for specific advice if you are taking: aminoglycosides, ACE inhibitors, diuretics, potassium supplements or potassium-containing medications, anticoagulants or other anticlotting drugs, nonsteroidal anti-inflammatory drugs (NSAIDS), sulfinpyrazone, cholestyramine, colestipol, oral contraceptives, methotrexate, probenecid, allopurinol, or rifampin.

FOOD INTERACTIONS
No known food interactions.

DISEASE INTERACTIONS
Consult your doctor if you have a history of allergies, asthma, congestive heart failure, gastrointestinal disorders (especially colitis associated with the use of antibiotics), or impaired kidney function.

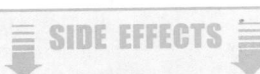

SIDE EFFECTS

SERIOUS
Irregular, rapid, or labored breathing; lightheadedness or sudden fainting; joint pain; fever; severe abdominal pain and cramping with watery or bloody stools; severe allergic reaction (marked by sudden swelling of the lips, tongue, face, or throat; breathing difficulty; skin rash, itching, or hives); unusual bleeding or bruising; yellowish tinge to eyes or skin. Call your doctor immediately.

COMMON
Rash, mild diarrhea, nausea, vomiting, headache, vaginal discharge and itching, pain or white patches in the mouth or on the tongue.

LESS COMMON
Diminished urine output, chills, weakness, fatigue.

AMOXICILLIN/POTASSIUM CLAVULANATE

BRAND NAME

Augmentin

Available in: Tablets, chewable tablets, oral suspension
Available OTC? No   **As Generic?** No
Drug Class: Penicillin antibiotic combination

▼ USAGE INFORMATION

WHY IT'S PRESCRIBED
To treat a variety of bacterial infections, including those of the sinuses and middle ear, skin and soft tissues, genitourinary tract, and the respiratory tract. The medication is effective only against infections caused by bacteria, not against those caused by viruses, fungi, or other microorganisms.

HOW IT WORKS
Amoxicillin blocks the formation of bacterial cell walls, rendering bacteria unable to multiply and spread. Clavulanate enhances the effectiveness of amoxicillin by inhibiting the activity of a specific enzyme (beta-lactamase) produced by certain drug-resistant strains of bacteria.

▼ DOSAGE GUIDELINES

RANGE AND FREQUENCY
Tablets— Adults and children more than 88 lbs: 250 to 500 mg of amoxicillin with 125 mg of clavulanate every 8 hours. Children up to 88 lbs: 6.7 to 13.3 mg of amoxicillin with 1.7 to 3.3 mg of clavulanate per 2.2 lbs (1 kg) of body weight every 8 hours. Chewable tablets and oral suspension— Adults and children more than 88 lbs: 250 to 500 mg of amoxicillin with 62.5 to 125 mg of clavulanate every 8 hours. Children up to 88 lbs: 6.7 to 13.3 mg of amoxicillin with 1.7 to 3.3 mg of clavulanate per 2.2 lbs (1 kg) of body weight every 8 hours. Newer dosage for adults: 875 mg of amoxicillin with 125 mg of clavulanate twice a day.

ONSET OF EFFECT
1 to 2 hours.

DURATION OF ACTION
6 to 8 hours.

DIETARY ADVICE
Best taken on an empty stomach, but may be taken with food to minimize stomach irritation or diarrhea.

STORAGE
Store in a tightly sealed container away from heat and direct light. Keep the liquid form refrigerated, but do not allow it to freeze.

MISSED DOSE
Take it as soon as you remember unless it is almost time for the next dose. In that case, skip the missed dose and take the next one. Do not double the next dose.

STOPPING THE DRUG
Take this medication as prescribed for the full treatment period, even if you begin to feel better before the scheduled end of therapy.

PROLONGED USE
Prolonged use can make you more susceptible to bacterial or fungal infections (such as yeast infections).

▼ PRECAUTIONS

Over 60: No special problems are expected.

Driving and Hazardous Work: Do not drive or engage in hazardous work until you determine how the medicine affects you.

Alcohol: No special warnings.

Pregnancy: Limited studies have found no evidence of birth defects. Consult your doctor if you are pregnant or plan to become pregnant.

Breast Feeding: Amoxicillin/clavulanate may pass into breast milk and cause problems in the nursing infant; avoid use while breast feeding.

Infants and Children: No special problems are expected.

Special Concerns: Those who are prone to asthma, hay fever, hives, or allergies may be more likely to have an allergic reaction to a penicillin antibiotic. If severe diarrhea occurs as a side effect of this drug, do not take antidiarrheal medications; call your doctor for advice instead. This drug can cause false results on some urine sugar tests for patients who have diabetes.

OVERDOSE
Symptoms: Severe diarrhea, nausea, unusual excitability, seizures, or vomiting.

What to Do: Call your doctor, emergency medical services (EMS), or the nearest poison control center immediately.

▼ INTERACTIONS

DRUG INTERACTIONS
Consult your doctor for advice if you are taking erythromycins, disulfiram, anticoagulants, tetracyclines, oral contraceptives, or gout drugs.

FOOD INTERACTIONS
None expected.

DISEASE INTERACTIONS
Consult your doctor if you have a history of allergies, asthma, congestive heart failure, gastrointestinal disorders (especially colitis associated with the use of antibiotics), or impaired kidney function.

≋ SIDE EFFECTS ≋

SERIOUS
Irregular, rapid, or labored breathing; lightheadedness or sudden fainting; seizures; joint pain; fever; severe abdominal pain and cramping with watery or bloody stools; severe allergic reaction (marked by sudden swelling of the lips, tongue, face, or throat; breathing difficulty; skin rash, itching, or hives); unusual bleeding or bruising; yellowish tinge to eyes or skin. Call your doctor immediately.

COMMON
Rash, mild diarrhea, nausea, vomiting, headache, vaginal discharge and itching, pain or white patches in the mouth or on the tongue.

LESS COMMON
Weakness, fatigue.

AMPHETAMINE

Available in: Tablets
Available OTC? No   **As Generic?** Yes
Drug Class: Central nervous system stimulant/amphetamine

▼ USAGE INFORMATION

WHY IT'S PRESCRIBED
To treat narcolepsy and attention-deficit hyperactivity disorder (ADHD) in children and adults.

HOW IT WORKS
Amphetamine activates nerve cells in the brain and spinal cord to increase motor activity, boost alertness, and lessen drowsiness and fatigue.

▼ DOSAGE GUIDELINES

RANGE AND FREQUENCY
For narcolepsy— Adults: 5 to 60 mg a day, 1 to 3 times a day; not to exceed 60 mg a day. Teenagers: 5 mg twice a day. Children ages 6 to 12: 2.5 mg twice a day.
For ADHD— Adults and children age 6 and older: 5 to 40 mg a day, 1 to 3 times a day; not to exceed 40 mg a day. Children ages 3 to 6: 2.5 mg once a day.

ONSET OF EFFECT
Variable.

DURATION OF ACTION
Variable.

DIETARY ADVICE
Swallow with liquid. May be taken with or without food. Avoid caffeine-containing beverages like tea, coffee, and some carbonated colas. Avoid acidic foods rich in vitamin C, such as fruit juices and other citrus products. Avoid vitamin C tablets.

STORAGE
Store in a tightly sealed container away from heat, moisture, and direct light.

MISSED DOSE
If dosage is once daily, take your missed dose as soon as you remember, unless your bedtime is within the next 6 hours. If so, do not take the missed dose. Take your next dose at the proper time and resume your regular schedule. Do not double the next dose. If dosage is more than once daily, take your missed dose as soon as you remember, unless the time for your next scheduled dose is within the next 2 hours. If so, do not take the missed dose. Take your next dose at the proper time and resume your regular schedule. Do not double the next dose.

STOPPING THE DRUG
Take amphetamine as prescribed for the full treatment period, even if you begin to feel better before the scheduled end of therapy. The decision to stop taking the drug should be made by your doctor. The doctor may decrease your dosage gradually to reduce the possibility of withdrawal symptoms.

PROLONGED USE
Amphetamines may be habit-forming, and prolonged use may increase the risk of dependency.

▼ PRECAUTIONS

Over 60: Adverse reactions may be more likely and more severe in older patients.

Driving and Hazardous Work: Do not drive or engage in hazardous work until you determine how the medicine affects you.

Alcohol: Avoid alcohol.

Pregnancy: Amphetamine taken during pregnancy may cause premature delivery, low birth weight, and birth defects. Discuss with your doctor the relative risks and benefits of using this drug while pregnant.

Breast Feeding: Amphetamine passes into breast milk; avoid or discontinue use while nursing. Consult your doctor for specific advice.

Infants and Children: Long-term amphetamine use by children can affect behavior and growth. Discuss the use of the drug and its relative risks and benefits with your doctor.

OVERDOSE
Symptoms: Extreme degrees of restlessness, agitation, bizarre behavior; panic; rapid breathing; confusion; high fever; hallucinations; seizures; coma.

What to Do: Call your doctor, emergency medical services (EMS), or the nearest poison control center immediately.

▼ INTERACTIONS

DRUG INTERACTIONS
The following drugs may interact with amphetamine. Consult your doctor for specific advice if you are taking tricyclic antidepressants, caffeine, beta-blockers, digitalis drugs, central nervous system stimulants, meperidine, MAO inhibitors, sympathomimetic agents, or thyroid hormones.

FOOD INTERACTIONS
Citrus juices and caffeinated beverages and foods may interact with amphetamine.

DISEASE INTERACTIONS
Caution is advised when taking amphetamine. Consult your doctor if you have any of the following: advanced blood vessel disease, heart disease, hyperthyroidism, high blood pressure, severe anxiety, Tourette's syndrome, glaucoma, or a history of drug abuse.

≡ SIDE EFFECTS ≡

SERIOUS
Irregular heartbeat, chest pain, increased blood pressure, skin rash, uncontrollable movements of arms and legs, mental changes, unusual weakness, very high fever. Call your doctor immediately.

COMMON
Mood changes, insomnia, drowsiness, restlessness.

LESS COMMON
Blurred vision, constipation, diarrhea, loss of appetite, headache, increased sweating, stomach cramps or pain, nausea or vomiting, changes in sexual desire or decreased sexual ability.

AMPHETAMINE/DEXTROAMPHETAMINE

Available in: Tablets
Available OTC? No   **As Generic?** No
Drug Class: Central nervous system stimulant/amphetamine

▼ USAGE INFORMATION

WHY IT'S PRESCRIBED
To treat narcolepsy and attention-deficit hyperactivity disorder (ADHD) in children and adults.

HOW IT WORKS
Amphetamine and dextroamphetamine activate nerve cells in the brain and spinal cord to increase motor activity and alertness and lessen drowsiness and fatigue. In hyperactivity disorders and narcolepsy, amphetamines improve mental focus and the ability to stay awake or concentrate.

▼ DOSAGE GUIDELINES

RANGE AND FREQUENCY
For narcolepsy– Adults: 5 to 60 mg a day, 1 to 3 times a day; not to exceed 60 mg a day. Teenagers: To start, 10 mg a day. Children ages 6 to 12: To start, 5 mg a day. To treat ADHD– Children age 6 and older: To start, 5 mg, 1 or 2 times a day. Children ages 3 to 6: To start, 2.5 mg a day.

ONSET OF EFFECT
Within 30 to 45 minutes.

DURATION OF ACTION
Adults: 8 to 12 hours. Children: 6 to 10 hours.

DIETARY ADVICE
Take it with liquid 30 to 45 minutes before meals. Avoid caffeinated beverages, acidic foods rich in vitamin C, and vitamin C tablets.

STORAGE
Store in a tightly sealed container away from heat, moisture, and direct light.

MISSED DOSE
If dosage is once daily, take your missed dose as soon as you remember, unless your bedtime is within the next 6 hours. If so, do not take the missed dose. Take your next dose at the proper time and resume your regular schedule. Do not double the next dose. If dosage is more than once daily, take your missed dose as soon as you remember, unless the time for your next scheduled dose is within the next 2 hours. If so, do not take the missed dose. Take your next dose at the proper time and resume your regular schedule. Do not double the next dose.

STOPPING THE DRUG
Take it as prescribed for the full treatment period, even if you begin to feel better before the scheduled end of therapy. The decision to stop taking the drug should be made by your doctor. The doctor may taper your dosage gradually to reduce the risk of withdrawal symptoms.

PROLONGED USE
Prolonged use may increase the risk of drug dependency.

▼ PRECAUTIONS

Over 60: Adverse reactions may be more likely and more severe in older patients.

Driving and Hazardous Work: Do not drive or engage in hazardous work until you determine how the medicine affects you.

Alcohol: Avoid alcohol.

Pregnancy: Amphetamines taken during pregnancy may cause premature delivery, low birth weight, and birth defects. Discuss with your doctor the relative risks and benefits of using this drug while pregnant.

Breast Feeding: Amphetamine passes into breast milk; avoid or discontinue use while nursing.

Infants and Children: Not recommended for use by children under age 3.

Special Concerns: Take only as directed and do not increase the dose on your own. Fatigue, excessive drowsiness, or depression while taking stimulants may mean an emergency situation is developing. Difficulty sleeping may be improved by taking the last scheduled dose several hours before bedtime.

OVERDOSE
Symptoms: Extreme restlessness, agitation, or bizarre behavior; panic; rapid breathing; confusion; high fever; hallucinations; seizures; coma.

What to Do: Call your doctor, emergency medical services (EMS), or the nearest poison control center immediately.

▼ INTERACTIONS

DRUG INTERACTIONS
Consult your doctor for specific advice if you are taking tricyclic antidepressants, caffeine, beta-blockers, digitalis drugs, central nervous system stimulants, meperidine, MAO inhibitors, sympathomimetic agents (such as ephedrine, phenylephrine, and diethylpropion), or thyroid hormones.

FOOD INTERACTIONS
Citrus juices and caffeine may interact with this drug.

DISEASE INTERACTIONS
Consult your doctor if you have any of the following: advanced blood vessel disease, heart disease, hyperthyroidism, high blood pressure, severe anxiety, Tourette's syndrome, glaucoma, or a history of drug abuse.

SIDE EFFECTS

SERIOUS
Irregular heartbeat, chest pain, increased blood pressure, skin rash, uncontrollable movements of arms and legs, mental changes, unusual weakness, very high fever. Call your doctor immediately.

COMMON
Mood changes, insomnia, drowsiness, restlessness.

LESS COMMON
Blurred vision, constipation, diarrhea, loss of appetite, headache, increased sweating, stomach cramps or pain, nausea or vomiting, changes in sexual desire or decreased sexual ability.

AMPHOTERICIN B

BRAND NAMES

Abelcet, AmBisome, Amphocin, Fungizone, Fungizone Intravenous

Available in: Cream, lotion, ointment, injection
Available OTC? No   **As Generic?** Yes
Drug Class: Antifungal

▼ USAGE INFORMATION

WHY IT'S PRESCRIBED
To treat serious and potentially life-threatening fungal infections.

HOW IT WORKS
Amphotericin B prevents fungal organisms from producing vital substances required for growth and function. This drug is effective only for infections caused by fungal organisms. It will not work for bacterial or viral infections.

▼ DOSAGE GUIDELINES

RANGE AND FREQUENCY
Topical forms: Apply a liberal amount to the affected area 2 to 4 times a day, according to doctor's instructions. It should be applied externally only. Injection: Dose is determined by your doctor based on many factors.

ONSET OF EFFECT
Topical: Not applicable. Injection: Immediate.

DURATION OF ACTION
Injection and topical: Unknown.

DIETARY ADVICE
Increase fluid intake to 2 to 3 quarts a day.

STORAGE
Can be stored at room temperature for 24 hours or in the refrigerator for 7 days in a tightly sealed container away from heat, moisture, and direct light. Keep it from freezing.

MISSED DOSE
Tell your doctor if you miss an injected dose. If you miss a topical dose, apply it as soon as you remember, then resume your regular dosage schedule.

STOPPING THE DRUG
Take it as prescribed for the full treatment period, even if you begin to feel better before the scheduled end of therapy. The decision to stop taking the drug should be made by your doctor.

PROLONGED USE
Topical forms are generally prescribed for short-term therapy (1 to 4 weeks). Consult your doctor if your condition does not improve, or worsens, within 1 to 2 weeks. The injection may be prescribed for up to 12 months. Your doctor will determine the proper length of therapy.

▼ PRECAUTIONS

Over 60: Adverse reactions may be more likely and more severe in older patients.

Driving and Hazardous Work: Avoid such activities until you determine how the medicine affects you.

Alcohol: Avoid alcohol.

Pregnancy: Adequate studies of the use of amphotericin B use during pregnancy have not been done. Consult your doctor for specific advice if you are pregnant or plan to become pregnant.

Breast Feeding: Amphotericin B may pass into breast milk; caution is advised. Consult your doctor for advice.

Infants and Children: No special problems are expected.

Special Concerns: Use gloves when applying the topical form of amphotericin B, as it can stain or discolor skin and clothing. The stain may be removed by hand washing with warm water and soap. Do not use an airtight dressing to cover the topical form, since this may increase the risk of infection.

OVERDOSE
Symptoms: Heartbeat irregularities; breathing difficulty.

What to Do: Treatment should be discontinued. Call your doctor, emergency medical services (EMS), or the nearest poison control center immediately.

▼ INTERACTIONS

DRUG INTERACTIONS
Consult your doctor for specific advice if you are taking corticosteroids, corticotropin, digitalis drugs, potassium-sparing diuretics, bone marrow depressants, nephrotoxic medications, or other topical prescription or over-the-counter medications. Also consult your doctor if you are undergoing radiation therapy.

FOOD INTERACTIONS
No known food interactions.

DISEASE INTERACTIONS
Caution is advised when taking amphotericin B. Consult your doctor if you have any other medical problem, especially kidney disease.

 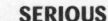 SIDE EFFECTS

SERIOUS
Topical: Redness, burning, itching, or irritation not present prior to therapy. Injection into a vein: Headache, fever, muscle pain or cramps, fatigue, chills, heartbeat irregularities, seizures, increased or decreased urine output, nausea, vomiting, pain at site of injection, change in or blurred vision, skin rash or itching, breathing difficulties, tightness in chest, unusual bleeding or bruising, sore throat. Injection into the spinal column: Urination difficulties, change in or blurred vision, numbness, tingling, fatigue, or weakness.

COMMON
Topical: None reported. Injection: Mild headache, diarrhea, indigestion, stomach pain, loss of appetite, mild nausea or vomiting.

LESS COMMON
Topical (cream only): Dry skin. Injection into the spinal column: Severe nausea or vomiting, dizziness or lightheadedness, headache, pain in the back, leg, or neck.

AMPICILLIN

Available in: Capsules, oral suspension, injection (available only in hospitals)
Available OTC? No **As Generic?** Yes
Drug Class: Penicillin antibiotic

▼ USAGE INFORMATION

WHY IT'S PRESCRIBED
Oral ampicillin is used to treat infections of the skin, urinary tract, and respiratory tract (sinuses, tonsils, and lung) caused by certain bacteria known to be susceptible to this antibiotic. Injectable ampicillin is used to treat more serious infections in hospitalized patients.

HOW IT WORKS
Ampicillin blocks the formation of bacterial cell walls, rendering bacteria unable to multiply and spread.

▼ DOSAGE GUIDELINES

RANGE AND FREQUENCY
Adults or children weighing more than 44 lbs (20 kg): 250 to 500 mg, 4 times a day. The dosage for smaller children must be adjusted according to weight.

ONSET OF EFFECT
Within 2 hours of oral dose.

DURATION OF ACTION
6 to 8 hours with oral dose.

DIETARY ADVICE
Should be taken on an empty stomach with plenty of water.

STORAGE
Store in a tightly sealed container away from heat and direct light. Keep the suspension refrigerated, but do not allow it to freeze.

MISSED DOSE
Take it as soon as you remember. If it is within 60 to 90 minutes of the next dose, skip the missed dose and resume your regular dosage schedule. Do not double the next dose.

STOPPING THE DRUG
Take it as prescribed for the full treatment period, even if you begin to feel better before the scheduled end of therapy. Stopping the drug prematurely may slow your recovery or lead to a rebound infection, also known as superinfection, in which the heartier strains of bacteria survive and multiply, leading to a more serious and drug-resistant infection.

PROLONGED USE
Therapy with ampicillin is usually completed within 7 to 10 days. Prolonged use may promote infection by bacteria resistant to the medication's effects (superinfection).

▼ PRECAUTIONS

Over 60: No special problems are expected.

Driving and Hazardous Work: No problems are expected.

Alcohol: No interactions are expected, but alcohol may dampen the immune system's response against infection and may increase the risk of stomach upset when taking this drug.

Pregnancy: Ampicillin may be used during pregnancy under certain conditions. Consult your doctor for guidelines.

Breast Feeding: Ampicillin may pass into breast milk and cause problems in the nursing infant; avoid use while nursing.

Infants and Children: No special problems are expected.

Special Concerns: If severe diarrhea occurs as a side effect of this drug, do not take antidiarrheal medications; call your doctor. Oral contraceptives may not be effective while you are taking ampicillin; consider other methods of birth control. Those who are prone to asthma, hay fever, hives, or allergies may be more likely to have an allergic reaction to a penicillin antibiotic.

OVERDOSE
Symptoms: Severe nausea, vomiting, diarrhea, muscle spasticity, seizures.

What to Do: Call your doctor, emergency medical services (EMS), or the nearest poison control center immediately.

▼ INTERACTIONS

DRUG INTERACTIONS
Consult your doctor for specific advice if you are taking aminoglycosides, ACE inhibitors, diuretics, potassium supplements or potassium-containing medications, anticoagulants or other anticlotting drugs, nonsteroidal anti-inflammatory drugs, sulfinpyrazone, cholestyramine, colestipol, oral contraceptives, methotrexate, probenecid, allopurinol, or rifampin.

FOOD INTERACTIONS
Acidic fruits or juices can interfere with this drug's therapeutic effect.

DISEASE INTERACTIONS
Consult your doctor if you have a history of allergies, asthma, congestive heart failure, gastrointestinal disorders (especially colitis associated with the use of antibiotics), infectious mononucleosis, or impaired kidney function.

SIDE EFFECTS

SERIOUS
Irregular, rapid, or labored breathing; lightheadedness or sudden fainting; joint pain; fever; severe abdominal pain and cramping with watery or bloody stools; severe allergic reaction (marked by sudden swelling of the lips, tongue, face, or throat; breathing difficulty; skin rash, itching, or hives); unusual bleeding or bruising; yellowish tinge to eyes or skin. Call your doctor immediately.

COMMON
Mild rash, mild diarrhea, nausea, vomiting, headache, vaginal discharge and itching, pain or white patches in the mouth or on the tongue.

LESS COMMON
Diminished urine output, chills, weakness, fatigue, seizures.

AMPICILLIN SODIUM/SULBACTAM SODIUM

Available in: Injection (available primarily in hospitals and nursing facilities)
Available OTC? No   **As Generic?** No
Drug Class: Penicillin antibiotic

▼ USAGE INFORMATION

WHY IT'S PRESCRIBED
Ampicillin sodium/sulbactam sodium is used to treat moderately severe bacterial infections requiring hospitalization. These infections are frequently caused by bacteria that are likely to be resistant to penicillin and not treatable with oral antibiotics alone.

HOW IT WORKS
Ampicillin blocks the formation of bacterial cell walls, rendering bacteria unable to multiply and spread; sulbactam is added to protect ampicillin from the effects of a destructive enzyme (betalactamase) produced by certain drug-resistant strains of bacteria.

▼ DOSAGE GUIDELINES

RANGE AND FREQUENCY
Adults: 1.5 to 3 g injected into a muscle or vein every 6 hours. Children age 1 and older: 300 mg per 2.2 lbs (1 kg) of body weight per day into a vein in divided doses every 6 hours.

ONSET OF EFFECT
Immediate with intravenous injection; unknown for intramuscular injection.

DURATION OF ACTION
Unknown.

DIETARY ADVICE
No special restrictions.

STORAGE
Not applicable.

MISSED DOSE
Not applicable; the dosage schedule is determined by a doctor or other health care professional.

STOPPING THE DRUG
The decision to stop treatment with this drug will be made by your doctor.

PROLONGED USE
Therapy with ampicillin sodium/sulbactam sodium is usually completed within 7 to 14 days. Infections in hospitalized patients may be more serious and can respond unpredictably to treatment. But treatment may also result in rapid improvement, and your doctor may stop intravenous or intramuscular ampicillin sodium/sulbactam sodium earlier than 7 to 14 days and begin oral therapy with another appropriate antibiotic in preparation for your discharge.

▼ PRECAUTIONS

Over 60: Adverse reactions may be more likely and more severe in older patients.

Driving and Hazardous Work: Not applicable; therapy with this drug generally requires hospitalization.

Alcohol: Avoid alcohol.

Pregnancy: Adequate studies of the use of penicillin antibiotics during pregnancy have not been done. Consult your doctor concerning the use of ampicillin sodium/sulbactam sodium if you are pregnant.

Breast Feeding: Avoid or discontinue the use of ampicillin sodium/sulbactam sodium while nursing.

Infants and Children: This drug is not recommended for infants and children under age 1.

Special Concerns: Anyone who has had a prior allergic reaction to penicillin or any penicillin antibiotic should not take this drug. Those who are prone to asthma, hay fever, hives, or allergies are at increased risk of having an allergic reaction to it.

OVERDOSE
Symptoms: Seizures may occur with very high doses; overdose is nonetheless unlikely.

What to Do: Call your doctor or emergency medical services (EMS) immediately if you suspect an overdose.

▼ INTERACTIONS

DRUG INTERACTIONS
Consult your doctor for specific advice if you are taking aminoglycosides, ACE inhibitors, diuretics, potassium supplements or potassium-containing medications, anticoagulants or other anticlotting drugs, nonsteroidal anti-inflammatory drugs, sulfinpyrazone, cholestyramine, colestipol, oral contraceptives, methotrexate, probenecid, allopurinol, or rifampin.

FOOD INTERACTIONS
No known food interactions.

DISEASE INTERACTIONS
Consult your doctor if you have a history of allergies, asthma, bleeding disorders (such as hemophilia), congestive heart failure, gastrointestinal disorders (especially colitis associated with the use of antibiotics), infectious mononucleosis, or impaired kidney function.

≡ SIDE EFFECTS ≡

SERIOUS
Irregular, rapid, or labored breathing; lightheadedness or sudden fainting; joint pain; fever; severe abdominal pain and cramping with watery or bloody stools; severe allergic reaction (marked by sudden swelling of the lips, tongue, face, or throat; breathing difficulty; skin rash, itching, or hives); unusual bleeding or bruising; yellowish tinge to eyes or skin. Call your doctor immediately.

COMMON
Mild rash, mild diarrhea, nausea, vomiting, headache, vaginal discharge and itching, pain or white patches in the mouth or on the tongue, pain at the site of injection.

LESS COMMON
Diminished urine output, chills, weakness, fatigue.

AMPRENAVIR

Available in: Capsules, oral solution
Available OTC? No   **As Generic?** No
Drug Class: Antiviral/protease inhibitor

▼ USAGE INFORMATION

WHY IT'S PRESCRIBED
To treat advanced HIV (human immunodeficiency virus) infection and AIDS (acquired immunodeficiency syndrome), usually in combination with other drugs. While not a cure for HIV infection, this drug may suppress the replication of the virus and delay the progression of the disease.

HOW IT WORKS
Amprenavir blocks the activity of a viral protease, an enzyme that is needed by HIV to reproduce. Blocking the protease causes HIV to make copies that cannot infect new cells.

▼ DOSAGE GUIDELINES

RANGE AND FREQUENCY
Capsules— Adults and children age 13 to 16: 1200 mg (8 capsules) 2 times a day, in combination with other antiretroviral drugs. Oral solution— Recommended for children age 4 and older: Consult pediatrician for proper dosage. The capsules and the oral solution are not interchangeable. Do not change forms without consulting your doctor.

ONSET OF EFFECT
Unknown. With most antiretroviral drugs, an early response can be seen within the first few days of therapy, but the maximum effect may take 12 to 16 weeks.

DURATION OF ACTION
Unknown.

DIETARY ADVICE
Amprenavir can be taken with or without food. However, taking it with a meal high in fat could reduce the absorption of the drug from the intestine.

STORAGE
Keep away from heat, moisture, and direct light. Do not refrigerate.

MISSED DOSE
If you miss a dose, take it as soon as you remember up to 4 hours late. Otherwise, wait for the next scheduled dose. Do not double the next dose.

STOPPING THE DRUG
The decision to stop taking the drug should be made in consultation with your physician.

PROLONGED USE
See your doctor regularly for tests and examinations.

≡ SIDE EFFECTS ≡

SERIOUS
Severe rash or moderate rash with other symptoms. Call your doctor immediately. Diabetes has developed in patients taking drugs of this class, although a cause-and-effect relationship has not been established. Call your doctor if you develop increased thirst or excessive urination.

COMMON
Nausea, vomiting, abdominal pain, rash, diarrhea.

LESS COMMON
Taste disorders; numbness, tingling, or prickling; depression.

▼ PRECAUTIONS

Over 60: It is not known whether amprenavir causes different or more severe side effects in older patients.

Driving and Hazardous Work: Do not drive or engage in hazardous work until you determine how the medicine affects you.

Alcohol: Avoid alcohol if liver function is impaired.

Pregnancy: Amprenavir has been shown to cause birth defects in animal studies. Adequate studies of use during pregnancy have not been done; consult your doctor for specific advice. There is no evidence that the drug will reduce the risk of transmitting the virus from the mother to the fetus.

Breast Feeding: It is unknown whether amprenavir passes into breast milk; however, to avoid transmitting the virus to an uninfected child, women infected with HIV should not breast feed.

Infants and Children: The safety and effectiveness of amprenavir have not been established for children under 4 years of age.

Special Concerns: Do not switch between the capsules and solution without consulting your doctor; the body absorbs them at different rates. Taking amprenavir does not eliminate the risk of passing the AIDS virus to other persons. Take appropriate preventive measures.

OVERDOSE
Symptoms: No cases of overdose have been reported.

What to Do: If you suspect an overdose, call your doctor, emergency medical services (EMS), or the nearest poison control center immediately.

▼ INTERACTIONS

DRUG INTERACTIONS
Amprenavir should not be used at the same time as astemizole, bepridil, cisapride, dihydroergotamine, ergotamine, midazolam, triazolam, rifampin, oral contraceptives, and vitamin E supplements. Use extreme caution if you are taking amiodarone, systemic lidocaine, tricyclic antidepressants, quinidine, warfarin, sildenafil, phenobarbital, phenytoin, carbamazepine, and statin (cholesterol-lowering) drugs. Patients taking antacids or didanosine should take them at least one hour before or after amprenavir. Rifabutin dosage may have to be adjusted by your doctor. Consult your doctor if you are taking any other prescription or over-the-counter medications.

FOOD INTERACTIONS
Meals high in fat could reduce the absorption of amprenavir.

DISEASE INTERACTIONS
Consult your doctor for advice if you have any other medical condition, especially hemophilia. Use of amprenavir can cause complications in patients with diseases of the liver, which works to remove the drug from the body.

AMYL NITRITE

Available in: Glass capsule
Available OTC? No   **As Generic?** Yes
Drug Class: Nitrate

▼ USAGE INFORMATION

WHY IT'S PRESCRIBED
To prevent or relieve attacks of angina (chest pain associated with heart disease).

HOW IT WORKS
Amyl nitrite relaxes the smooth muscle of the blood vessels and increases the supply of blood and oxygen to the heart. It also reduces the heart's workload and demand for oxygen.

▼ DOSAGE GUIDELINES

RANGE AND FREQUENCY
No fixed schedule; take as needed. When angina attack occurs, break the protective cloth-covered glass capsule between your fingers and inhale 1 to 6 times while seated. If inhaling 2 capsules in 10 minutes does not bring relief, seek medical assistance immediately. When inhaling 2 capsules, wait 3 to 5 minutes between capsules.

ONSET OF EFFECT
30 seconds to 5 minutes.

DURATION OF ACTION
3 to 5 minutes.

DIETARY ADVICE
Amyl nitrite can be taken without regard to diet.

STORAGE
Store away from direct light and heat. Heat may cause the medicine to break down. Do not store it in the kitchen, because amyl nitrite is flammable. Keep refrigerated, but do not allow it to freeze.

MISSED DOSE
Not applicable.

STOPPING THE DRUG
Consult your doctor before stopping use.

PROLONGED USE
Prolonged, too-frequent use can lead to tolerance of the drug, reducing its effectiveness. Notify your doctor if you experience an increase in angina attacks.

▼ PRECAUTIONS

Over 60: Adverse reactions and side effects may be more common and severe in older persons.

Driving and Hazardous Work: The use of amyl nitrite may impair your ability to perform such tasks safely.

Alcohol: Alcohol can increase the lightheadedness caused by amyl nitrite and may cause a serious drop in blood pressure. Consult your doctor for specific advice.

Pregnancy: Use is not recommended during pregnancy because of the danger to the unborn baby.

Breast Feeding: Amyl nitrite may pass into breast milk; caution is advised. Consult your doctor for advice.

Infants and Children: Safety and effectiveness have not been determined. Consult your pediatrician.

Special Concerns: Before use, extinguish all tobacco products and stay away from open flames, since amyl nitrite is highly flammable. Since dizziness is common after taking amyl nitrite, it is advisable to sit or lie down rather than remain standing while taking the medication. For relief of headache (very common following use of amyl nitrate), take acetaminophen.

OVERDOSE

Symptoms: Blue lips, palms of hands, or fingernails; extreme dizziness, extreme headache, or feeling of intense pressure in the head; fainting; shortness of breath; unusual weakness; weak and rapid heartbeat.

What to Do: Call your doctor, emergency medical services (EMS), or the nearest poison control center immediately.

▼ INTERACTIONS

DRUG INTERACTIONS
Consult your doctor for specific advice if you are taking drugs for high blood pressure, norepinephrine, or sympathomimetic drugs (such as ephedrine, phenylephrine, or epinephrine).

FOOD INTERACTIONS
No known food interactions.

DISEASE INTERACTIONS
Caution is advised when taking amyl nitrite. Consult your doctor if you have any of the following: severe anemia, recent head trauma, recent heart attack or brain hemorrhage, glaucoma, hyperthyroidism, or prior allergic reaction to nitrates.

 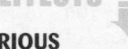 SIDE EFFECTS

SERIOUS
Shortness of breath; extreme dizziness or fainting; bluish appearance of lips, fingernails, and palms of hands; irregular heartbeat.

COMMON
Dizziness or lightheadedness, especially upon arising from a seated or lying position; rapid heartbeat and pulse; headache; restlessness; flushing in the face and neck. Such side effects tend to occur less frequently as your body adjusts to the medication. Contact your doctor if such symptoms do not subside quickly or if they interfere with your daily activities.

LESS COMMON
Unusual tiredness or weakness, skin rash.

ANASTROZOLE

BRAND NAME

Arimidex

Available in: Tablets
Available OTC? No   **As Generic?** No
Drug Class: Antiestrogen; antineoplastic (anticancer) agent

USAGE INFORMATION

WHY IT'S PRESCRIBED
Anastrozole is given for breast cancer chemotherapy. It is usually prescribed for postmenopausal women with breast cancer who have already undergone treatment with other antiestrogen medications such as tamoxifen.

HOW IT WORKS
The growth of some breast tumors is stimulated by estradiol, a hormone that is produced by adult females. Anastrozole is not directly toxic to cancer cells but rather reduces blood levels of estradiol in the body and thus inhibits the growth of such tumors.

DOSAGE GUIDELINES

RANGE AND FREQUENCY
1 mg or 10 mg tablet, taken once daily.

ONSET OF EFFECT
Unknown.

DURATION OF ACTION
Unknown.

DIETARY ADVICE
Maintain adequate food and fluid intake. Calorie, protein, and vitamin needs increase in patients with cancer. Good nutrition is essential to cope with the demands of chemotherapy.

STORAGE
Store safely and securely away from heat and light.

MISSED DOSE
Anastrozole is prescribed for once-daily use only. If you are unable to take this medication on a particular day, skip the missed dose and resume your regularly scheduled dose the following day. Do not double the next dose.

STOPPING THE DRUG
This medication is used to treat a chronic condition. You may need to remain on this medication for an extended period, and you should take the drug exactly as prescribed throughout the course of treatment. The decision to stop the drug must be made in consultation with your doctor. Do not stop taking anastrozole on your own, even if you are feeling better. Contact

your doctor if you have any questions about the way you feel while taking anastrozole, or if you think that you are experiencing a side effect that would require discontinuation of the drug.

PROLONGED USE
There is no standard duration of therapy with anastrozole, although you can expect to remain on it for several weeks in order to determine if it is effective. Your doctor will determine whether your response to the drug is satisfactory or not, and will recommend the continuation or discontinuation of therapy.

PRECAUTIONS

Over 60: Adverse reactions may be more likely and more severe in older patients.

Driving and Hazardous Work: The use of anastrozole may impair your ability to drive or operate machinery safely or perform hazardous work.

Alcohol: Avoid alcohol while taking this drug.

Pregnancy: Anastrozole must not be used in pregnant women. Although anastrozole is not generally prescribed for premeno-pausal women, it is important that patients be sure they are not pregnant before starting treatment with this drug.

Breast Feeding: Use of this drug is not recommended while breast feeding; the benefits must clearly outweigh potential risks. Consult your doctor for advice.

Infants and Children: Use of anastrozole is not approved for infants and children.

Special Concerns: Patients with cancer are very often weakened by their illness, by poor nutrition, and by the effects of chemotherapy, radiation, and surgery. Such patients are more likely to experience undesirable side effects of a medication. In addition, these side effects may be more pronounced. Follow all medication directions carefully.

OVERDOSE
Symptoms: No cases of overdose with anastrozole have been reported.

What to Do: An overdose is unlikely; however, if you have any reason to suspect that one has occurred, call emergency medical services (EMS) to receive evaluation and treatment in the closest emergency facility.

INTERACTIONS

DRUG INTERACTIONS
No significant interactions.

FOOD INTERACTIONS
No significant interactions.

DISEASE INTERACTIONS
No significant interactions.

SIDE EFFECTS

SERIOUS
No serious side effects have been reported.

COMMON
Headache, diarrhea, nausea, hot flashes, back pain, weakness, and a feeling of reduced energy (asthenia).

LESS COMMON
Dizziness; chest pain; tingling or numbness in the extremities (paresthesia); weight gain; abdominal pain; vaginal itching, dryness, and occasionally bleeding; swelling of the fingers and of skin around the eyes; rash; formation of blood clots.

ASPIRIN

Available in: Tablets, capsules
Available OTC? Yes **As Generic?** Yes
Drug Class: Nonsteroidal anti-inflammatory drug (NSAID); analgesic; anticoagulant

▼ USAGE INFORMATION

WHY IT'S PRESCRIBED
For mild to moderate every-day pain and inflammation; to reduce fever; to prevent the formation of blood clots, a primary cause of heart attack, stroke, and other circulatory problems; to ease the inflammation, joint pain, and stiffness associated with arthritis.

HOW IT WORKS
Nonsteroidal anti-inflammatory drugs (NSAIDs) such as aspirin inhibit the release of chemicals in the body called prostaglandins, which play a role in inflammation, though it is unknown exactly how they exert their pain-relieving, fever-reducing, and anti-inflammatory effects.

▼ DOSAGE GUIDELINES

RANGE AND FREQUENCY
For pain or fever: 325 to 650 mg every 4 hours as needed. For prevention of blood clots: 80 to 100 mg daily or every other day. For arthritis: 3,600 to 5,400 mg daily in divided doses.

ONSET OF EFFECT
30 minutes.

DURATION OF ACTION
For pain relief, up to 4 hours.

DIETARY ADVICE
Swallow aspirin with food or a full glass of water to lessen stomach irritation.

STORAGE
Store in a tightly sealed container away from heat and direct light.

MISSED DOSE
For pain and fever, take a missed dose as soon as you remember, then wait 4 hours for your next dose. For arthritis, take the aspirin as soon as you remember up to 2 hours late, then return to your regular schedule.

STOPPING THE DRUG
For pain and fever, stop when relief is achieved. For arthritis and blood clotting, consult your doctor about stopping.

PROLONGED USE
Talk to your doctor about the need for medical examinations or laboratory tests if you must take aspirin regularly for a prolonged period.

▼ PRECAUTIONS

Over 60: Gastrointestinal bleeding and irritation are more likely to occur in older persons.

Driving and Hazardous Work: The use of aspirin should not impair your ability to perform such tasks safely.

Alcohol: Alcohol intake should be limited because it increases the risk of stomach irritation and bleeding.

Pregnancy: Do not use aspirin during the last 3 months of pregnancy unless prescribed by your doctor.

Breast Feeding: Aspirin passes into breast milk. Avoid it or do not nurse.

Infants and Children: Do not give aspirin to children under age 16 unless your doctor instructs otherwise, since it may cause a very rare but life-threatening condition known as Reye's syndrome.

OVERDOSE
Symptoms: Nausea, disorientation, seizures, vomiting, rapid breathing, fever.

What to Do: Call your doctor, emergency medical services (EMS), or the nearest poison control center immediately.

▼ INTERACTIONS

DRUG INTERACTIONS
Consult your doctor before taking aspirin if you currently take a blood pressure medication, a medication for gout, an arthritis drug, an anticoagulant such as warfarin, a diabetes medication, a steroid, or an antiseizure medication.

FOOD INTERACTIONS
No known adverse food interactions. Taking aspirin with caffeine-containing foods or beverages may actually enhance the medicine's pain-relieving effects.

DISEASE INTERACTIONS
Consult your doctor about taking aspirin if you have asthma, a bleeding disorder, congestive heart failure, diabetes mellitus, gout, hemophilia, high blood pressure, kidney disease, liver disease, thyroid disease, or a peptic ulcer.

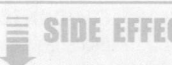
SIDE EFFECTS

SERIOUS
Vomiting, agitation, extreme fatigue, confusion; allergic reaction causing troubled breathing, redness of face, itching, swelling of face, lips, or eyelids. These are symptoms of Reye's syndrome, a rare but serious disorder that is most likely to affect patients under the age of 16. Seek emergency medical attention immediately.

COMMON
Stomach upset, rash, nausea, ringing in the ears.

LESS COMMON
Insomnia.

ASPIRIN/CAFFEINE

Available in: Tablets
Available OTC? Yes **As Generic?** No
Drug Class: Nonsteroidal anti-inflammatory drug (NSAID); analgesic; antirheumatic

▼ USAGE INFORMATION

WHY IT'S PRESCRIBED
For mild to moderate every-day pain and inflammation; to reduce fever; to ease the inflammation, joint pain, and stiffness associated with arthritis.

HOW IT WORKS
Aspirin appears to interfere with the production of prostaglandins, naturally occurring substances in the body that cause inflammation and make nerves more sensitive to pain impulses. Caffeine may enhance the effectiveness of pain relievers.

▼ DOSAGE GUIDELINES

RANGE AND FREQUENCY
Adults— For pain or fever: 325 to 650 mg every 4 hours as needed. For arthritis: 3,600 to 5,400 mg daily in divided doses. Children 9 years of age and older— For pain or fever: 325 to 400 mg every 4 hours as needed. For arthritis: 80 to 100 mg per 2.2 lbs (1 kg) of body weight a day in divided doses.

ONSET OF EFFECT
For pain, inflammation, or fever: within 30 minutes. For arthritis: May take 2 to 3 weeks to achieve maximum effect.

DURATION OF ACTION
For pain relief, up to 4 hours.

DIETARY ADVICE
Take with food or a full glass of water to lessen stomach irritation.

STORAGE
Store in a tightly sealed container away from heat, moisture, and direct light.

MISSED DOSE
For pain and fever, take a missed dose as soon as you remember, then wait 4 hours for your next dose. For arthritis, take as soon as you remember up to 2 hours late, then return to your regular schedule.

STOPPING THE DRUG
For pain and fever, stop when relief is achieved. For arthritis, consult your doctor about stopping.

PROLONGED USE
Talk to your doctor about the need for medical examinations or laboratory tests if you must take this medication regularly for a prolonged period.

▼ PRECAUTIONS

Over 60: Gastrointestinal bleeding and irritation are more likely to occur in older persons.

Driving and Hazardous Work: No special precautions are necessary.

Alcohol: Alcohol intake should be limited because it increases the risk of stomach irritation and bleeding.

Pregnancy: Do not use this drug during the last 3 months of pregnancy unless prescribed by your doctor.

Breast Feeding: Aspirin passes into breast milk. Avoid it or do not nurse.

Infants and Children: Do not give aspirin-containing products to children under age 16 unless your doctor instructs otherwise, since it may cause a very rare but life-threatening condition known as Reye's syndrome.

OVERDOSE
Symptoms: Nausea, disorientation, seizures, vomiting, rapid breathing, fever.

What to Do: Call your doctor, emergency medical services (EMS), or the nearest poison control center immediately.

▼ INTERACTIONS

DRUG INTERACTIONS
Consult your doctor before taking this drug if you currently take a blood pressure medication, a medication for gout, an arthritis drug, an anticoagulant such as warfarin, a diabetes medication, a steroid, or an antiseizure medication.

FOOD INTERACTIONS
No known interactions.

DISEASE INTERACTIONS
Consult your doctor about taking this drug if you have asthma, a bleeding disorder, congestive heart failure, diabetes mellitus, gout, hemophilia, high blood pressure, kidney disease, liver disease, thyroid disease, or a peptic ulcer.

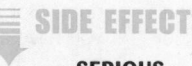
SIDE EFFECTS

SERIOUS
Vomiting, agitation, extreme fatigue, confusion; allergic reaction causing troubled breathing, redness of face, itching, swelling of face, lips, or eyelids. These are symptoms of Reye's syndrome, a rare but serious disorder that is most likely to affect patients under the age of 16. Seek emergency medical attention immediately.

COMMON
Stomach upset, rash, nausea, ringing in the ears.

LESS COMMON
Insomnia.

ATENOLOL

Available in: Tablets (Injection is for hospital use only.)
Available OTC? No **As Generic?** Yes
Drug Class: Beta-blocker

▼ USAGE INFORMATION

WHY IT'S PRESCRIBED
To treat mild to moderate high blood pressure and to treat angina; also used to prevent or control heartbeat irregularities (cardiac arrhythmias). The injectable form is used in hospitals to treat heart attack.

HOW IT WORKS
Atenolol slows the rate and force of contraction of the heart by blocking certain nerve impulses, thus reducing blood pressure. By modifying nerve impulses to the heart, the drug also helps to stabilize heart rhythm.

▼ DOSAGE GUIDELINES

RANGE AND FREQUENCY
50 to 100 mg, once a day. Smaller doses may be recommended for elderly patients or for those with impaired kidney function.

ONSET OF EFFECT
Oral: 1 to 2 hours; the full therapeutic effect may take 1 to 2 weeks. Injectable: Within 10 minutes.

DURATION OF ACTION
Up to 24 hours.

DIETARY ADVICE
Take atenolol on an empty stomach. Avoid alcohol and caffeine.

STORAGE
Store in a tightly sealed container away from heat and direct light.

MISSED DOSE
Take it as soon as you remember. If it is within 4 hours of the next scheduled dose, skip the missed dose and resume your regular schedule. Do not double the next dose.

STOPPING THE DRUG
Suddenly stopping atenolol may cause serious health problems. Slow reduction of

the dose over a period of 2 to 3 weeks is advised, under doctor's careful supervision.

PROLONGED USE
Therapy with atenolol may be lifelong; prolonged use may be associated with an increased risk of side effects.

▼ PRECAUTIONS

Over 60: Adverse reactions may be more likely and more severe in older patients; a reduction in dosage may be warranted.

Driving and Hazardous Work: In rare cases atenolol may impair your ability to drive or operate machinery safely or perform hazardous work. Use caution, especially soon after beginning therapy.

Alcohol: Drink in careful moderation if at all. Alcohol may interact with the drug and cause a dangerous drop in blood pressure.

Pregnancy: Discuss with your doctor the relative risks and benefits of using this drug while pregnant.

Breast Feeding: Avoid or discontinue the use of atenolol while nursing.

Infants and Children: Proper dose will be determined by pediatrician.

Special Concerns: Use of the drug should be considered but one element of a comprehensive therapeutic program that includes weight control, smoking cessation, regular exercise, and a healthy low-salt, low-fat diet.

OVERDOSE
Symptoms: Slow heartbeat; severe dizziness, lightheadedness or fainting; rapid or irregular heartbeat; difficulty breathing; extreme weakness; seizures; confusion; coma.

What to Do: Call your doctor, emergency medical services (EMS), or the nearest poison control center immediately.

▼ INTERACTIONS

DRUG INTERACTIONS
Consult your doctor if you are taking amphetamines, oral antidiabetic agents, asthma medication (such as aminophylline or theophylline), calcium channel blockers, clonidine, guanabenz, halothane, allergy shots, insulin, MAO inhibitors, reserpine, or other beta-blockers.

FOOD INTERACTIONS
None known.

DISEASE INTERACTIONS
Atenolol should be used with caution in people with diabetes, especially insulin-dependent diabetes, since the drug may mask symptoms of hypoglycemia. Consult your doctor for specific advice if you have allergies or asthma; heart or blood vessel disease (including congestive heart failure and peripheral vascular disease); irregular (slow) heartbeat; hyperthyroidism; myasthenia gravis; psoriasis; respiratory problems, such as bronchitis or emphysema; kidney or liver disease; or a history of mental depression.

SIDE EFFECTS

SERIOUS
Depression, shortness of breath, wheezing, slow heartbeat (especially less than 50 beats per minute), chest pain or tightness, swelling of the ankles, feet, and lower legs. If you experience such symptoms, stop taking atenolol and call your doctor immediately.

COMMON
Decreased sexual ability; decreased ability to engage in usual physical activities or exercise; dizziness or lightheadedness, especially when rising suddenly from a sitting or lying position; drowsiness, fatigue, or weakness; insomnia.

LESS COMMON
Anxiety, irritability; constipation; diarrhea; dry eyes; itching; nausea or vomiting; nightmares or intensely vivid dreams; numbness, tingling, or other unusual sensations in the fingers and toes; abdominal pain; nasal congestion.

ATENOLOL/CHLORTHALIDONE

Available in: Tablets
Available OTC? No **As Generic?** Yes
Drug Class: Beta-blocker/diuretic

▼ USAGE INFORMATION

WHY IT'S PRESCRIBED
To treat high blood pressure with or without concurrent angina.

HOW IT WORKS
Atenolol slows the rate and force of contraction of the heart by blocking certain nerve impulses, thus reducing blood pressure. Chlorthalidone (a diuretic) increases the elimination of urine from the body. By reducing the overall fluid volume and excess sodium in the body, diuretics reduce blood volume and so reduce pressure within the blood vessels.

▼ DOSAGE GUIDELINES

RANGE AND FREQUENCY
Initial dose is 1 tablet a day (each tablet contains 50 mg atenolol and 25 mg chlorthalidone). The dose can be increased to 2 tablets a day.

ONSET OF EFFECT
Within 1 hour.

DURATION OF ACTION
24 hours.

DIETARY ADVICE
This drug can be taken with or without food, as instructed by your doctor.

STORAGE
Store in a tightly sealed container away from heat and direct light.

MISSED DOSE
If you miss a dose, take it as soon as you remember unless the next dose is less than 8 hours away. In that case, skip the missed dose and go back to your regular schedule. Do not double the next dose.

STOPPING THE DRUG
Suddenly stopping this drug may cause blood pressure to rise dangerously high, possibly triggering angina or heart attack in patients with advanced heart disease. Slow reduction of the dose over a period of 2 to 3 weeks is advised, under careful supervision by your doctor.

PROLONGED USE
No special problems are expected, although prolonged use may increase the chance of side effects. Regular visits to your doctor are needed to evaluate the drug's ongoing, long-term effectiveness.

▼ PRECAUTIONS

Over 60: Older persons with reduced kidney function may require a lower dosage.

Driving and Hazardous Work: Be cautious about any activity that requires acuity since this medication may cause drowsiness and impaired alertness.

Alcohol: Drink in careful moderation if at all. Alcohol may interact with the drug and cause a dangerous drop in blood pressure.

Pregnancy: This drug may harm the developing child. Inform your doctor if you are pregnant or plan to become pregnant.

Breast Feeding: This drug passes into breast milk; avoid breast feeding while taking it.

Infants and Children: Not usually prescribed for infants or children.

Special Concerns: Use of the drug should be considered but one element of a comprehensive therapeutic program that includes weight control, smoking cessation, regular exercise, and a healthy low-salt, low-fat diet.

OVERDOSE
Symptoms: Breathing difficulties, slow heartbeat, sluggishness, extremely low blood pressure.

What to Do: Call your doctor, emergency medical services (EMS), or the nearest poison control center immediately.

▼ INTERACTIONS

DRUG INTERACTIONS
Consult your doctor for specific advice if you are taking amphetamines, oral antidiabetic agents, asthma medication (such as aminophylline or theophylline), calcium channel blockers, clonidine, guanabenz, halothane, allergy shots, insulin, MAO inhibitors, reserpine, or other beta-blockers.

FOOD INTERACTIONS
None expected.

DISEASE INTERACTIONS
Atenolol/chlorthalidone should be used with caution in people with diabetes, especially insulin-dependent diabetes, since atenolol can mask the symptoms of hypoglycemia. Consult your doctor if you have allergies or asthma; heart or blood vessel disease (including congestive heart failure and peripheral vascular disease); irregular (slow) heartbeat; hyperthyroidism; myasthenia gravis; psoriasis; respiratory problems, such as bronchitis or emphysema; kidney or liver disease; or a history of mental depression.

SIDE EFFECTS

SERIOUS
Mental depression; shortness of breath, wheezing; slow heartbeat (especially less than 50 beats per minute); chest pain or tightness; swelling of the ankles, feet, and lower legs. If you experience such symptoms, stop taking this drug and call your doctor immediately.

COMMON
Decreased sexual ability; decreased ability to engage in usual physical activities or exercise; dizziness or lightheadedness, especially when rising suddenly from a sitting or lying position; drowsiness, fatigue, or weakness; insomnia.

LESS COMMON
Anxiety, irritability; constipation; diarrhea; dry eyes; itching; nausea or vomiting; nightmares or intensely vivid dreams; numbness, tingling, or other unusual sensations in the fingers and toes; abdominal pain; visual disturbances.

ATORVASTATIN

Available in: Tablets
Available OTC? No   **As Generic?** No
Drug Class: Antilipidemic (cholesterol-lowering agent)

▼ USAGE INFORMATION

WHY IT'S PRESCRIBED
To treat high cholesterol. Usually prescribed after the first lines of treatment—including diet changes, weight loss, and exercise—fail to reduce to acceptable levels the amounts of total and low-density lipoprotein (LDL) cholesterol in the blood.

HOW IT WORKS
Atorvastatin blocks the action of an enzyme required for the manufacture of cholesterol, thereby interfering with its formation. By lowering the amount of cholesterol in the liver cells, atorvastatin increases the formation of receptors for LDL, and thereby reduces blood levels of total and LDL cholesterol. In addition to lowering LDL cholesterol, atorvastatin also modestly reduces triglyceride levels and raises HDL (the so-called "good") cholesterol.

▼ DOSAGE GUIDELINES

RANGE AND FREQUENCY
Initial dose is 10 mg a day, taken once daily. It may be increased by your doctor as needed up to a maximum dose of 80 mg per day. Unlike other "-statin" cholesterol-lowering drugs, atorvastatin does not have to be taken in the evening to be maximally effective.

ONSET OF EFFECT
2 to 4 weeks.

DURATION OF ACTION
The effect persists for the duration of therapy.

DIETARY ADVICE
Cholesterol-lowering drugs are only one part of a total program that should include regular exercise and a healthy low-fat, low-cholesterol, and high-fiber diet.

STORAGE
Store in a tightly sealed container in a dry place away from heat and direct light.

MISSED DOSE
Take it as soon as you remember. Take your next scheduled dose at the proper time and resume your regular dosage schedule. Do not double your next dose.

STOPPING THE DRUG
The decision to stop taking the drug should be made in consultation with your doctor. Once the medication is discontinued, blood cholesterol is likely to return to original elevated levels.

PROLONGED USE
Side effects are more likely with prolonged use. As you continue with atorvastatin, your doctor will periodically order blood tests to evaluate liver function.

▼ PRECAUTIONS

Over 60: No special problems are expected in older patients.

Driving and Hazardous Work: The use of atorvastatin should not impair your ability to perform such tasks safely.

Alcohol: No special precautions are necessary.

Pregnancy: Should not be used during pregnancy or by women who plan to become pregnant in the near future.

Breast Feeding: This drug is not recommended for women who are nursing.

Infants and Children: Safety and effectiveness are not known; this drug is rarely used in children. Consult your pediatrician.

Special Concerns: Important elements of treatment for high cholesterol include proper diet, weight loss, regular moderate exercise, and avoidance of certain medications that may increase cho-

lesterol levels. Because atorvastatin has potential side effects, it is important that you maintain a recommended healthy diet and cooperate with other treatments your doctor may suggest.

OVERDOSE
Symptoms: An overdose of atorvastatin is unlikely.

What to Do: Emergency instructions not applicable.

▼ INTERACTIONS

DRUG INTERACTIONS
Consult your doctor if you are taking cyclosporine, gemfibrozil, niacin, antibiotics, especially erythromycin, or medications for fungus infections. All of these drugs may increase the risk of myositis (muscle inflammation) when taken with atorvastatin and may lead to kidney failure.

FOOD INTERACTIONS
No known food interactions.

DISEASE INTERACTIONS
Consult your doctor if you have any of the following problems: liver, kidney, or muscle disease, or a medical history involving organ transplant or recent surgery.

  SIDE EFFECTS

SERIOUS
Fever, chest pain, unusual or unexplained muscle aches and tenderness. Call your doctor right away.

COMMON
Side effects occur in only 1% to 2% of patients. These include constipation or diarrhea, dizziness or lightheadedness, bloating or gas, heartburn, nausea, allergic reaction, stomach pain, rise in liver enzymes.

LESS COMMON
Sleeping difficulty, skin rash.

ATOVAQUONE

Available in: Oral suspension, tablets
Available OTC? No **As Generic?** No
Drug Class: Anti-infective/antiprotozoal

▼ USAGE INFORMATION

WHY IT'S PRESCRIBED
To treat mild to moderately severe Pneumocystis carinii pneumonia (PCP) in patients who cannot take the antibiotic trimethoprim/sulfamethoxazole (the standard therapy for PCP). This serious type of pneumonia is prevalent among patients with AIDS.

HOW IT WORKS
Atovaquone prevents infecting cells from manufacturing DNA and other substances necessary for growth and reproduction.

▼ DOSAGE GUIDELINES

RANGE AND FREQUENCY
Adults and teenagers– Oral suspension: 750 mg twice a day, with meals, for 21 days. Tablets: 750 mg, 3 times a day, with meals, for 21 days.

ONSET OF EFFECT
Unknown.

DURATION OF ACTION
Unknown.

DIETARY ADVICE
Take it with meals high in fat content to help the body absorb the medication.

STORAGE
Store in a tightly sealed container away from heat, moisture, and direct light. Do not allow to freeze. Keep away from extreme temperatures.

MISSED DOSE
Take it as soon as you remember. This will help keep a constant level of medication in your system. However, if it is near the time for the next dose, skip the missed dose and resume your regular dosage schedule. Do not double the next dose.

STOPPING THE DRUG
Take it as prescribed for the full treatment period, even if you begin to feel better before the scheduled end of therapy. The decision to stop taking the drug should be made in consultation with your doctor. Stopping the drug prematurely may slow your recovery or lead to a rebound infection.

PROLONGED USE
Therapy with atovaquone requires 21 days. Prolonged use of atovaquone beyond this period may be associated with an increased chance of side effects.

▼ PRECAUTIONS

Over 60: No studies have been done specifically on older patients; adverse reactions may be more likely or more severe.

Driving and Hazardous Work: Do not drive or engage in hazardous work until you determine how the medicine affects you.

Alcohol: No special precautions are necessary.

Pregnancy: Adequate human studies on the use of this drug in pregnant women have not been done. Before taking atovaquone, tell your doctor if you are pregnant or plan to become pregnant. Discuss with your doctor the relative risks and benefits of using this drug while pregnant.

Breast Feeding: Atovaquone may pass into breast milk; caution is advised. Consult your doctor for advice.

Infants and Children: Adequate studies of the use of atovaquone in children have not been done. Consult your pediatrician for advice.

Special Concerns: A regular teaspoon may not hold the correct amount of medication. Use a specially marked measuring spoon or other device to dispense each dose.

OVERDOSE
Symptoms: No cases of overdose have been reported.

What to Do: If someone takes a much larger dose than prescribed, call your doctor, emergency medical services (EMS), or the nearest poison control center as soon as possible.

▼ INTERACTIONS

DRUG INTERACTIONS
Other drugs may interact with atovaquone. Consult your doctor for specific advice if you are taking rifampin, rifabutin, sulfamethoxazole and trimethoprim combination, or zidovudine.

FOOD INTERACTIONS
No known food interactions.

DISEASE INTERACTIONS
Atovaquone may not work properly in patients with a stomach or an intestinal condition (such as colitis) that limits drug absorption. Consult your doctor for more information.

 SIDE EFFECTS

SERIOUS
Skin rash, fever. Call your doctor immediately.

COMMON
Insomnia, diarrhea, cough, headache, nausea or vomiting.

LESS COMMON
Lack of energy, fatigue, itching, stomach upset or abdominal pain, constipation, dizziness.

ATROPINE SULFATE OPHTHALMIC

Available in: Ophthalmic solution, ointment
Available OTC? No   **As Generic?** Yes
Drug Class: Eye muscle relaxant, pupil enlarger

▼ USAGE INFORMATION

WHY IT'S PRESCRIBED
Used for eye examinations, before and after eye surgery, and to treat certain types of eye conditions, including uveitis (inflammation of the uvea, or the central portion of the eye) and posterior synechiae (a potentially blinding eye disorder). May also be used to help determine the proper prescription for eyeglasses in young children.

HOW IT WORKS
Atropine sulfate relaxes the ciliary muscle, which controls the shape of the eye's lens as it focuses, and another eye muscle called the sphincter, which controls the narrowing and widening of the pupil. Relaxation of these muscles prevents the lens from focusing and widens the pupil. This allows the doctor to view the interior structures of the eye during an ophthalmologic procedure. And, by immobilizing the tiny structures within the eye, the drug prevents scarring of eye tissue and may also alleviate pain somewhat.

▼ DOSAGE GUIDELINES

RANGE AND FREQUENCY
For eye examination— Adults: Dose to be determined by your doctor. Children: Ophthalmic solution: 1 drop in the eye twice a day for 2 days before the examination. Ointment: A thin strip of ointment applied to the eye 3 times a day for up to 3 days before the examination. For uveitis— Adults: 1 drop in the eye or a thin strip of ointment applied to the eye 1 to 4 times a day. Children: 1 drop in the eye or a thin strip of ointment applied to the eye up to 3 times a day.

ONSET OF EFFECT
Unknown.

DURATION OF ACTION
From 6 to 12 days. The drug's effect on the lens's ability to focus may last longer than its effect on the size of the pupil.

DIETARY ADVICE
No special restrictions.

STORAGE
Store in a tightly sealed container away from heat, moisture, and direct light.

MISSED DOSE
If you miss a dose, apply the missed dose as soon as possible unless it is almost time for the next dose. In that case, skip the missed dose and go back to your regular schedule. Do not double the next dose.

STOPPING THE DRUG
The decision to stop using the drug should be made by your doctor.

PROLONGED USE
Call your doctor if symptoms persist more than 14 days.

▼ PRECAUTIONS

Over 60: Sleepiness and agitation are more likely.

Driving and Hazardous Work: Avoid such activities until temporary blurring of vision goes away.

Alcohol: No special warnings.

Pregnancy: Adequate human studies have not been done. Tell your doctor if you are pregnant or are planning a pregnancy.

Breast Feeding: Small amounts of this drug may pass into breast milk; extreme caution is advised. Infants exposed to atropine may exhibit a rapid pulse, fever, or dry skin.

Infants and Children: Infants, young children, and children with blond hair or blue eyes may be more sensitive to the effects of this drug and may have an increased risk of side effects. Use with extreme caution in these groups.

Special Concerns: Before administering the drug, wash your hands. Tilt your head back. Gently apply pressure to the inside corner of the eyelid and pull downward on the lower eyelid to make a space. Drop the medicine or put about ⅓ inch of ointment into this space and close your eye. Apply pressure for 1 or 2 minutes while the eye is closed. Wash your hands again. Make sure the tip of the applicator does not touch any other surface.

OVERDOSE
Symptoms: Impaired vision, extreme sensitivity to light, confusion, clumsiness, dizziness, hallucinations, irregular heartbeat, extreme drowsiness or weakness, unuusal dry skin or mouth.

What to Do: Call your doctor, emergency medical services (EMS), or the nearest poison control center immediately.

▼ INTERACTIONS

DRUG INTERACTIONS
Consult your doctor if you use tranquilizers, drugs for glaucoma or myasthenia gravis, or any other eye drops or medications.

FOOD INTERACTIONS
None expected.

DISEASE INTERACTIONS
Do not use if you have glaucoma, especially closed-angle glaucoma, without consulting your doctor. The drug may increase abdominal pain in gastrointestinal disorders.

▼ SIDE EFFECTS

SERIOUS
Hallucinations, confusion, extreme sleepiness, heart palpitations. Call your doctor immediately.

COMMON
Blurred vision, increased sensitivity of eyes to light.

LESS COMMON
Eye crusting or drainage, itching and redness of the eye, swelling within the eye, eye pain, dry eyes, dry skin, dry mouth, irritability, agitation, flushing, fever.

ATROPINE SULFATE ORAL

Available in: Tablets
Available OTC? No   **As Generic?** Yes
Drug Class: Anticholinergic; antispasmodic

▼ USAGE INFORMATION

WHY IT'S PRESCRIBED
To relieve painful cramps and spasms due to irritable bowel syndrome. It is also used rarely to treat stomach ulcers in conjunction with other drugs such as cimetidine, and as an antidote to poisoning with certain pesticides.

HOW IT WORKS
Nerve impulses are transmitted to muscles and glands throughout the body by the action of specialized, naturally occurring chemicals known as "neurotransmitters." Atropine blocks the ability of the neurotransmitter acetylcholine to stimulate certain muscles and glands. This produces effects ranging from drying of secretions (saliva, perspiration) to changing the size of the pupils and relief of intestinal muscle spasms.

▼ DOSAGE GUIDELINES

RANGE AND FREQUENCY
Adults and teenagers: 300 to 1,200 micrograms (mcg)

every 4 to 6 hours. Children: 4.5 mcg per lb of body weight every 4 to 6 hours, not exceeding 400 mcg per dose.

ONSET OF EFFECT
Within 30 to 60 minutes.

DURATION OF ACTION
From 4 to 6 hours.

DIETARY ADVICE
Take it 30 to 60 minutes before meals and at bedtime.

STORAGE
Store in a tightly sealed container away from heat, moisture, and direct light.

MISSED DOSE
Take it as soon as you remember. However, if it is near the time for the next dose, skip the missed dose and resume your regular dosage schedule. Do not double the next dose.

STOPPING THE DRUG
Take it as prescribed for the full treatment period, even if you feel better before the scheduled end of therapy.

PROLONGED USE
Therapy with this medication may require a period of several days to weeks. Prolonged use may increase the risk of an undesirable side effect.

▼ PRECAUTIONS

Over 60: Common side effects may be more likely and more severe in older patients, who may also develop confusion and drowsiness.

Driving and Hazardous Work: The use of atropine may impair your ability to perform such tasks safely.

Alcohol: Consume alcohol only in moderation.

Pregnancy: Although studies have been limited, atropine crosses the placenta and is not recommended during pregnancy. Before taking atropine, tell your doctor if you are pregnant or plan to become pregnant.

Breast Feeding: Atropine passes into breast milk and should not be used while breast feeding. This medication may also inhibit milk formation.

Infants and Children: Not recommended for use by children unless under close medical supervision. Infants and very young children are very susceptible to the effects of atropine.

Special Concerns: Atropine must be used with care; it is potentially a very dangerous drug. Use caution when exercising, especially when physical activity is sustained or

carried out in hot weather. By inhibiting perspiration, atropine may impair your ability to cool down; heat stroke may result.

OVERDOSE
Symptoms: Blurred or altered vision; dilated pupils; eye pain; hot, dry, or flushed skin; high fever; heartbeat irregularities; seizures; unusual agitation; bizarre behavior; hallucinations; fainting; coma.

What to Do: Call your doctor, emergency medical services (EMS), or the nearest poison control center immediately.

▼ INTERACTIONS

DRUG INTERACTIONS
Consult your doctor for specific advice if you are taking antacids or diarrhea medication; decongestants, antihistamines, and other medications for allergies or colds; ketoconazole; medicines that cause drowsiness, such as barbiturates, sedatives, and cough medicines; psychiatric medications, including antidepressants; alcohol-containing medicines; or painkillers.

FOOD INTERACTIONS
No known food interactions.

DISEASE INTERACTIONS
Consult your doctor if you have heart disease or a history of heart rhythm irregularities, pacemaker usage, or fainting; esophagitis or hiatal hernia; glaucoma; a history of intestinal obstruction, intestinal inflammation (colitis), or other gastrointestinal problems; myasthenia gravis; prostate enlargement or other urinary problems.

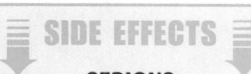
SIDE EFFECTS

SERIOUS
Blurring or changes in vision; large, dilated pupils; eye pain; hot, dry, or flushed skin; high fever; heartbeat irregularities; seizures; fainting; coma; unusual agitation; bizarre behavior; hallucinations. Call your doctor immediately.

COMMON
Dry mouth, nose, throat, or skin; constipation; decreased sweating.

LESS COMMON
Difficult urination, decreased breast milk production, difficulty swallowing, headache, memory loss, increased sensitivity of eyes to light, nausea or vomiting, unusual fatigue.

ATROPINE SULFATE/SCOPOLAMINE HYDROBROMIDE/ HYOSCYAMINE SULFATE/PHENOBARBITAL

Available in: Tablets, elixir, capsules, extended-release tablets
Available OTC? No **As Generic?** Yes
Drug Class: Anticholinergic; antispasmodic

▼ USAGE INFORMATION

WHY IT'S PRESCRIBED
To relieve symptoms of irritable bowel syndrome, peptic and duodenal ulcers, and gastrointestinal cramps.

HOW IT WORKS
Acetylcholine is a naturally occurring chemical in the body that is involved in the activity of nerves, muscles, glands, and other physiological processes. This drug interferes with the action of acetylcholine, leading to a variety of effects including the drying of secretions (saliva, perspiration), relief of muscle spasms in the intestines, and changing the size of the pupils.

▼ DOSAGE GUIDELINES

RANGE AND FREQUENCY
Capsules or tablets— Adults and teenagers: 1 or 2 capsules, 2 to 4 times a day. Children ages 2 to 12: ½ to 1 chewable tablet, 3 or 4 times a day. Elixir— Adults: 5 to 10 ml, 3 to 4 times a day. Children: 0.5 to 7.5 ml every 4 to 6 hours. Extended-release tablets— Adults and teenagers: 1 tablet every 8 to 12 hours. Children: Not recommended for children under age 13.

ONSET OF EFFECT
Unknown.

DURATION OF ACTION
Unknown.

DIETARY ADVICE
Take this medication 30 to 60 minutes before meals unless your doctor orders otherwise.

STORAGE
Store in a tightly sealed container away from heat, moisture, and direct light. Keep the liquid form refrigerated, but do not allow it to freeze.

MISSED DOSE
Take it as soon as you remember. If it is near the time for the next dose, skip the missed dose and resume your regular dosage schedule. Do not double the next dose.

STOPPING THE DRUG
The decision to stop taking the drug should be made in consultation with your doctor.

PROLONGED USE
No special problems are expected.

▼ PRECAUTIONS

Over 60: Adverse reactions may be more likely and more severe in older patients.

Driving and Hazardous Work: Do not drive or engage in hazardous work until you determine how the medicine affects you.

Alcohol: Avoid alcohol when using this medication.

Pregnancy: Tell your doctor if you are pregnant or plan to become pregnant before taking this medicine.

Breast Feeding: This drug may pass into breast milk; caution is advised. Consult your doctor for advice.

Infants and Children: The drug should not be prescribed for children under age 2. Adverse reactions may be more likely and more severe in infants and young children, especially those suffering from brain damage or spastic paralysis.

OVERDOSE
Symptoms: Nausea, vomiting, headache, blurred vision, dilated pupils, weak pulse, fever, hallucinations, seizures, unconsciousness, confusion, dry skin and mouth.

What to Do: Call your doctor, emergency medical services (EMS), or the nearest poison control center immediately.

▼ INTERACTIONS

DRUG INTERACTIONS
Other drugs may interact with this medication. Consult your doctor for specific advice if you are taking an anticholinergic (such as belladonna), an adrenocorticoid, an antacid, an anti-diarrheal medicine containing kaolin or attapulgite, ketoconazole, an anticoagulant (blood thinner), central nervous system depressants (such as antihistamines, cold medicines, sleep aids, or tranquilizers), an MAO inhibitor, haloperidol, or potassium chloride.

FOOD INTERACTIONS
No known food interactions.

DISEASE INTERACTIONS
Caution is advised when taking this drug. Consult your doctor if you have any of the following: a nerve disorder, asthma or other lung problems, an enlarged prostate, severe and continuing dry mouth, liver disease, kidney disease, Down syndrome, intestinal blockage or other intestinal problems, an overactive thyroid gland, heart disease, high blood pressure, glaucoma, or ulcerative colitis.

≡ SIDE EFFECTS ≡

SERIOUS
Yellow-tinged eyes or skin, skin rash or hives, eye pain, unusual bruising or bleeding, sore throat and fever. Call your doctor immediately.

COMMON
Constipation; dry mouth, nose, skin, or throat; decreased sweating; dizziness; drowsiness.

LESS COMMON
Loss of memory, difficult urination, blurred vision, nausea or vomiting, bloated feeling, unusual weakness or tiredness, difficulty swallowing, decreased flow of breast milk.

ATTAPULGITE

Available in: Oral suspension, tablets, chewable tablets
Available OTC? Yes   **As Generic?** Yes
Drug Class: Antidiarrheal

▼ USAGE INFORMATION

WHY IT'S PRESCRIBED
To treat diarrhea.

HOW IT WORKS
Attapulgite is believed to bind to and remove large volumes of bacteria and toxins from the digestive tract. It may also reduce the fluidity of the stool associated with diarrhea. There is some debate regarding attapulgite's effectiveness.

▼ DOSAGE GUIDELINES

RANGE AND FREQUENCY
Adults and teenagers—Suspension and tablets: 1,200 to 1,500 mg taken after each loose bowel movement; take no more than 9,000 mg in 24 hours. Chewable tablets: 1,200 mg after each loose bowel movement; take no more than 8,400 mg in 24 hours. Children ages 6 to 12—Suspension and chewable tablets: 600 mg after each loose bowel movement; take no more than 4,200 mg in 24 hours. Tablets: 750 mg after each loose bowel movement; take no more than 4,500 mg in 24 hours. Children ages 3 to 6— Suspension and chewable tablets: 300 mg after each loose bowel movement; take no more than 2,100 mg in 24 hours. Tablets: Should not be taken by children in this age group.

ONSET OF EFFECT
Unknown.

DURATION OF ACTION
Unknown.

DIETARY ADVICE
A mild diet is recommended when recovering from diarrhea. Bananas, rice, applesauce, and plain toast are good choices. Be sure to get plenty of fluids.

STORAGE
Store in a tightly sealed container away from heat, moisture, and direct light.

MISSED DOSE
Take it as soon as you remember. However, if it is near the time for the next dose, skip the missed dose and resume your regular dosage schedule. Do not double the next dose.

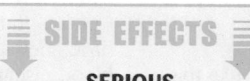

SIDE EFFECTS

SERIOUS
No serious side effects are associated with attapulgite. However, loss of body water due to diarrhea can cause dry mouth, increased thirst, dizziness, lightheadedness, decreased urination, and wrinkling of skin. Call your doctor immediately.

COMMON
Constipation.

LESS COMMON
There are no less-common side effects associated with the use of attapulgite.

STOPPING THE DRUG
You may stop taking the drug if you feel better before the scheduled end of therapy.

PROLONGED USE
If diarrhea has not improved or has gotten worse in 2 days, or if you develop a fever, call your doctor.

▼ PRECAUTIONS

Over 60: Older persons are more likely to experience excessive loss of body fluid and therefore are advised to increase their fluid intake accordingly.

Driving and Hazardous Work: The use of attapulgite should not impair your ability to perform such tasks safely.

Alcohol: Avoid alcohol.

Pregnancy: Attapulgite is not absorbed by the body and is not expected to cause problems during pregnancy.

Breast Feeding: Attapulgite is not absorbed by the body and is not expected to cause problems while nursing.

Infants and Children: Should not be given to children under the age of 3 without consulting your doctor. Be sure your child drinks a sufficient amount of fluids.

Special Concerns: In addition to taking attapulgite, it is important to replace the body fluids lost because of diarrhea. During the first day you should drink ample amounts of clear liquids, like decaffeinated colas, ginger ale, and decaffeinated tea, and eat gelatin. On the following day you should continue your fluid intake and eat bland foods, such as applesauce, cooked cereals, and bread. Do not take attapulgite if your diarrhea is accompanied by blood or mucus in the stools.

OVERDOSE
Symptoms: No cases of overdose have been reported.

What to Do: An overdose is unlikely to be life-threatening. However, if someone takes a much larger dose than prescribed, seek medical assistance immediately.

▼ INTERACTIONS

DRUG INTERACTIONS
Other drugs may interact with attapulgite. If you are taking any other medication, do not take it within 2 to 3 hours before or after taking attapulgite.

FOOD INTERACTIONS
Eating fried or spicy foods, bran, fruits, vegetables, or drinking caffeinated or alcoholic beverages can make diarrhea worse.

DISEASE INTERACTIONS
Consult your doctor if you have dysentery or any other medical condition.

AURANOFIN

Available in: Capsules
Available OTC? No   **As Generic?** No
Drug Class: Antirheumatic

BRAND NAME

Ridaura

▼ USAGE INFORMATION

WHY IT'S PRESCRIBED
To treat rheumatoid arthritis. Because of the risk of highly unpleasant side effects, auranofin is generally prescribed for patients who have not responded adequately to other more conservative arthritis treatments, such as nonsteroidal anti-inflammatory drugs, corticosteroids, and aspirin. (Auranofin is not appropriate for the treatment of osteoarthritis, which is much more common.)

HOW IT WORKS
Auranofin contains gold. It is not precisely known how gold compounds work, but evidently they reduce some of the painful joint inflammation associated with arthritis. Auranofin can halt the progress of severe rheumatoid arthritis, preventing further joint damage, and, in some cases, it may bring about a remission.

▼ DOSAGE GUIDELINES

RANGE AND FREQUENCY
Adults: 6 mg once a day, or 3 mg twice a day. After 6 months of therapy, your doctor may increase the dose to 3 mg, 3 times a day. Children: Consult your pediatrician for proper dosage.

ONSET OF EFFECT
Within 3 to 4 months.

DURATION OF ACTION
Unknown.

DIETARY ADVICE
Maintain your usual food and fluid intake.

STORAGE
Store in a tightly sealed container away from heat and direct light.

MISSED DOSE
Take the missed dose as soon as you remember. If you are within 2 hours of your next scheduled dose, skip the missed dose. Take your next scheduled dose at the proper time, then resume your regular dosage schedule. Do not double the next dose.

STOPPING THE DRUG
This medication should be taken as prescribed for the full treatment period. Do not stop taking it on your own if you are feeling better before the scheduled end of drug therapy unless you are experiencing a serious side effect.

PROLONGED USE
Several months of therapy may be necessary to determine whether this medication is helping you. Prolonged use of auranofin may increase the risk of side effects.

▼ PRECAUTIONS

Over 60: Adverse reactions may be more likely and more severe in older patients.

Driving and Hazardous Work: The use of auranofin may impair your ability to perform such tasks safely.

Alcohol: Avoid alcohol while taking this drug.

Pregnancy: Do not use this drug during pregnancy.

Breast Feeding: Auranofin passes into breast milk; discontinue use while nursing.

Infants and Children: Not recommended.

Special Concerns: Gold compounds may have many adverse effects resulting from gold toxicity. Your doctor will order periodic blood tests to determine if you are having any undesirable reactions to auranofin, such as anemia or low white blood cell count. Always contact your doctor if you have any concerns about the way you feel while taking auranofin. Auranofin may cause heightened sensitivity to sunlight. Avoid direct sunlight during peak hours, and wear protective clothing. Use sunscreens if possible.

OVERDOSE
Symptoms: No cases of overdose have been reported.

What to Do: If you are concerned about the possibility of an overdose, contact your doctor, emergency medical services (EMS), or the nearest poison control right away.

▼ INTERACTIONS

DRUG INTERACTIONS
Consult your doctor for specific advice if you are taking penicillamine.

FOOD INTERACTIONS
No known food interactions.

DISEASE INTERACTIONS
Consult your doctor if you have anemia or any other blood disease, skin disease, colitis or any other intestinal disease, ulcers or heartburn, kidney disease, or systemic lupus erythematosus (SLE).

SIDE EFFECTS

SERIOUS
Severe abdominal pain, widespread rash, neurological disturbances causing confusion or seizures.

COMMON
Itching, hives, sores or spots in mouth or throat, poor appetite, diarrhea, nausea, vomiting, rashes, fever, stomach pains, indigestion, heartburn, constipation.

LESS COMMON
Coughing, hoarseness, breathing difficulty, or wheezing; dark urine or reduced urine output; impaired vision; difficulty swallowing; sore throat; fever and chills; hair loss; hallucinations; painful urination; low back pain or flank pain; red, painful, itching eyes; unusual bleeding or bruising; red, thickened, or scaly patches on skin; swelling of face, legs, or feet; swollen or painful glands; excessive fatigue or weakness; yellow discoloration of the eyes or skin (jaundice).

AZATHIOPRINE

Available in: Tablets, injection
Available OTC? No **As Generic?** Yes
Drug Class: Immunosuppressant

▼ USAGE INFORMATION

WHY IT'S PRESCRIBED
To slow down or reduce the natural tendency of the immune system to reject organ transplants, and to treat rheumatoid arthritis and other conditions.

HOW IT WORKS
Azathioprine prevents the immune system from attacking transplanted organs and slows down immune cells that cause inflammation in joints and elsewhere.

▼ DOSAGE GUIDELINES

RANGE AND FREQUENCY
For transplant rejection—Tablet and injection: Initially, 3 to 5 mg per 2.2 lbs (1 kg) of body weight daily. With improvement the dose may be reduced to 1 to 2 mg per 2.2 lbs daily. For rheumatoid arthritis— Tablet: 1 mg per 2.2 lbs daily. This may be increased to not more than 2.5 mg per 2.2 lbs daily.

ONSET OF EFFECT
4 to 8 weeks.

DURATION OF ACTION
Suppression of the immune system may persist long after the drug is completely eliminated.

DIETARY ADVICE
Take it with food or immediately following a meal to reduce stomach irritation.

STORAGE
Store in a tightly sealed container in a dry place away from heat and direct light. Keep liquid form refrigerated, but do not allow it to freeze.

MISSED DOSE
For once-daily schedules: Do not take the missed dose. Take your next scheduled dose at the proper time and resume your regular dosage schedule. Do not double the next dose. For multiple-dose daily schedules: Take your missed dose as soon as you remember. If it is time for your next scheduled dose, take the two doses together and resume your regular dosage schedule. If you miss more than one dose in a day, call your doctor.

STOPPING THE DRUG
Take this drug as prescribed for the full length of treatment, even if you begin to feel better before the scheduled end of therapy.

PROLONGED USE
Prolonged use increases the risk of side effects and the possibility of cancer.

▼ PRECAUTIONS

Over 60: Adverse reactions may be more likely and more severe in older patients.

Driving and Hazardous Work: The use of azathioprine may impair your ability to perform such tasks safely.

Alcohol: Avoid alcohol.

Pregnancy: Do not use this drug if you are pregnant. It should not be used by either the male or the female partners if you are trying to become pregnant.

Breast Feeding: Azathioprine passes into breast milk; discontinue use while nursing.

Infants and Children: Azathioprine has not been shown to affect children differently than adults. Consult your pediatrician for advice.

Special Concerns: Infection is a great threat to people with suppressed immune systems. Azathioprine may lower your ability to resist infection by lowering the number of white blood cells in the blood. Do not receive any vaccinations without approval from your doctor. Avoid people with infections. Azathioprine may also suppress platelets (the blood components that control blood coagulation), and thus cause bleeding problems. Use care with scissors, nail clippers, nail files, razors, toothbrushes, dental floss, or toothpicks. Inform your dentist that you are taking azathioprine.

OVERDOSE
Symptoms: Unusual bleeding, increased susceptibility to infection.

What to Do: Call your doctor, emergency medical services (EMS), or the nearest poison control center immediately.

▼ INTERACTIONS

DRUG INTERACTIONS
Inform your doctor if you are taking allopurinol, ACE inhibitors, chlorambucil, corticosteroids, cotrimoxazole, cyclophosphamide, cyclosporine, mercaptopurine, or muromonab-CD3.

FOOD INTERACTIONS
No known food interactions.

DISEASE INTERACTIONS
Caution is advised when taking azathioprine. Consult your doctor if you have any of the following: chicken pox, shingles, gout, active infection, kidney or liver disease, or pancreatitis.

≡ SIDE EFFECTS ≡

SERIOUS
Rapid heartbeat; sudden fever or chills; back, side, muscle, or joint pain; unusual tiredness or weakness; cough or hoarseness; shortness of breath; black, tarry stools; blood in urine or stools; difficult or painful urination; severe or sudden stomach pain with nausea, vomiting, or diarrhea; red spots, red patches, or blisters on skin; unusual bleeding or bruising; abrupt or sudden, unusual feeling of discomfort or illness. These may be signs of serious infection, bleeding emergencies, or gastrointestinal problems. Seek immediate medical assistance.

COMMON
Moderate nausea and vomiting, loss of appetite.

LESS COMMON
Liver problems, skin rash, sores in mouth, stomach pain, swelling of feet or lower legs, shortness of breath.

AZELASTINE

Available in: Nasal spray
Available OTC? No   **As Generic?** No
Drug Class: Histamine (H1) blocker

| BRAND NAME |
| Astelin |

▼ USAGE INFORMATION

WHY IT'S PRESCRIBED
To treat or relieve symptoms of hay fever (allergic rhinitis).

HOW IT WORKS
Azelastine blocks the effects of histamine, a naturally occurring substance within the body that causes swelling, itching, sneezing, watery eyes, hives, and other symptoms of allergic reaction.

▼ DOSAGE GUIDELINES

RANGE AND FREQUENCY
2 sprays per nostril, not to exceed 2 times per day.

ONSET OF EFFECT
Within 1 to 3 hours.

DURATION OF ACTION
12 hours.

DIETARY ADVICE
No special restrictions.

STORAGE
Store upright in a tightly sealed container away from heat, moisture, and direct light. Do not allow the medication to freeze.

MISSED DOSE
Take it as soon as you remember. If it is near the time for the next dose, skip the missed dose and resume your regular dosage schedule. Do not double the next dose.

STOPPING THE DRUG
Take it as prescribed for the full treatment period, even if you start to feel better before the scheduled end of therapy.

PROLONGED USE
Azelastine is a relatively new medication. Safety and effectiveness during prolonged use have yet to be established.

▼ PRECAUTIONS

Over 60:
No special problems are expected.

Driving and Hazardous Work:
Azelastine may cause drowsiness. Do not drive or engage in hazardous work until you determine how the medication affects you.

Alcohol:
No specific restrictions, though alcohol may increase the drug's sedative effects in some patients.

Pregnancy:
Adequate studies of azelastine use during pregnancy have not been done. Before taking it, tell your doctor if you are pregnant or plan to become pregnant. Discuss with your doctor the relative risks and benefits of using this drug during pregnancy.

Breast Feeding:
Azelastine may pass into breast milk; caution is advised. Consult your doctor for specific advice.

Infants and Children:
The safety and effectiveness of azelastine use by children under the age of 12 have not been determined.

Special Concerns:
If the pump has not been used for 3 days or more, it should be reprimed with at least 2 sprays or until a fine mist appears. To avoid the possible spread of infection, this medicine should be used by one person only. Before using this medication, blow your nose gently. When inhaling the nasal spray, keep your head upright and sniff briskly while spraying.

OVERDOSE
Symptoms: No cases of overdose have been reported.

What to Do: An overdose of azelastine is unlikely to occur or to be life-threatening. However, if someone takes a much larger dose than prescribed or accidentally ingests the medication, call your doctor, emergency medical services (EMS), or the nearest poison control center right away.

▼ INTERACTIONS

DRUG INTERACTIONS
No drug interactions have been reported. Azelastine may, however, increase the depressant effects of alcohol, sedatives, tranquilizers, pain-killers, barbiturates, or other antihistamines on the central nervous system. Consult your doctor for specific advice.

FOOD INTERACTIONS
No food interactions have been reported.

DISEASE INTERACTIONS
No disease interactions have been reported.

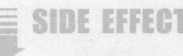
SIDE EFFECTS

SERIOUS
No serious side effects are associated with the use of azelastine.

COMMON
Bitter taste in the mouth, drowsiness, headache, unexpected weight gain.

LESS COMMON
Nasal burning, sore throat, dry mouth, sneezing, nausea, fatigue, dizziness, nosebleeds.

AZITHROMYCIN

Available in: Capsules, tablets, powder, injection
Available OTC? No   **As Generic?** No
Drug Class: Azalide antibiotic

▼ USAGE INFORMATION

WHY IT'S PRESCRIBED
To treat various bacterial infections, particularly of the sinuses, throat, and respiratory tract (such as bronchitis and pneumonia); infections of the ear; venereal disease due to chlamydial and chancroid infection; skin infections; and diarrhea associated with campylobacter and other bacteria that cause food poisoning. Also used to prevent and treat a tuberculosis-like disease known as Mycobacterium avium complex (MAC), which is common in people with advanced AIDS.

HOW IT WORKS
Azithromycin prevents bacterial cells from manufacturing specific proteins necessary for their survival.

▼ DOSAGE GUIDELINES

RANGE AND FREQUENCY
For bronchitis, strep throat, pneumonia, and skin infections: 500 mg (2 pills) taken in a single dose on the first day of treatment; then, 250 mg (1 pill) per day on days 2 through 5. For chlamydia and chancroid: 1,000 mg (4 pills) taken in a single one-time dose. To prevent MAC: 1,200 mg weekly. To treat MAC: 500 mg, twice a day.

ONSET OF EFFECT
Unknown.

DURATION OF ACTION
Unknown.

DIETARY ADVICE
Take capsules on an empty stomach, at least 1 hour before or 2 hours after eating. Tablets may be taken with or without food. Drink plenty of fluids (at least 2 to 3 quarts of water per day).

STORAGE
Store in a tightly sealed container away from heat and direct light.

MISSED DOSE
Take it as soon as you remember. If you miss a day entirely, skip the missed dose and resume your regular dosage schedule the next day. Do not double the next dose.

STOPPING THE DRUG
It is very important to take this drug as prescribed for the full treatment period, even if you begin to feel better before the scheduled end of therapy.

PROLONGED USE
For acute infections, treatment is usually complete after 5 days with capsules, and 1 day with the powdered form. For MAC prevention and treatment, therapy may be lifelong. Prolonged use may be associated with an increased risk of side effects.

▼ PRECAUTIONS

Over 60: Adverse reactions may be more likely and more severe.

Driving and Hazardous Work: The use of azithromycin should not impair your ability to perform such tasks safely.

Alcohol: Avoid alcohol while taking this drug.

Pregnancy: Adequate studies of the use of azithromycin during pregnancy have not been done; consult your doctor for advice.

Breast Feeding: It is not known if azithromycin passes into breast milk; consult your doctor for advice.

Infants and Children: The safety and effectiveness of azithromycin use in patients under 16 years of age have not been established, although no special problems are expected.

Special Concerns: Before taking any antibiotic, make sure you tell your doctor about allergies that you might have. If you are allergic to erythromycin, you are likely to be allergic to azithromycin. Azithromycin is useful only against bacteria that are susceptible to its effects. Therefore, it is important to tell your doctor if your condition has not improved, or instead has worsened, within a few days of starting the drug. The particular bacteria causing your illness may be resistant to azithromycin.

OVERDOSE
Symptoms: No cases of overdose have been reported.

What to Do: Emergency instructions not applicable.

▼ INTERACTIONS

DRUG INTERACTIONS
Other drugs may interact with azithromycin. Consult your doctor for specific advice if you are taking anticoagulants (such as warfarin), anticonvulsants (such as phenytoin and carbamazepine), antihistamines (especially terfenadine), and theophylline. Antacids that contain aluminum or magnesium can interfere with the absorption of azithromycin; separate the use of azithromycin and an antacid by at least 2 hours.

FOOD INTERACTIONS
Azithromycin capsules should be taken on an empty stomach.

DISEASE INTERACTIONS
Consult your doctor if you have a medical history that includes liver disease.

≡ SIDE EFFECTS ≡

SERIOUS
Breathing difficulty, fever, hives, itching, skin rash, swelling of face, mouth, lips, throat, or tongue, sweating, yellowish discoloration of the eyes or skin. These may be signs of a rare but potentially serious allergic reaction. Seek medical assistance immediately.

COMMON
No common side effects have been reported.

LESS COMMON
Nausea and vomiting, abdominal discomfort, diarrhea (generally mild), headache, dizziness.

BACAMPICILLIN HYDROCHLORIDE

Available in: Capsules, oral suspension
Available OTC? No   **As Generic?** No
Drug Class: Penicillin antibiotic

▼ USAGE INFORMATION

WHY IT'S PRESCRIBED
To treat a variety of bacterial infections, including those of the respiratory tract, gastrointestinal tract, urinary tract, and middle ear. Bacampicillin is effective only against infections caused by bacteria; it is ineffective against those caused by viruses, fungi, or other microorganisms.

HOW IT WORKS
Bacampicillin blocks the formation of bacterial cell walls, rendering bacteria unable to multiply and spread.

▼ DOSAGE GUIDELINES

RANGE AND FREQUENCY
Adults and children weighing 55 lbs or more: 400 to 800 mg every 12 hours (2 times a day). Children weighing less than 55 lbs: 5.7 to 11.4 mg per lb of body weight every 12 hours.

ONSET OF EFFECT
Unknown.

DURATION OF ACTION
Unknown.

DIETARY ADVICE
Tablets can be taken with or without food. The oral suspension should be taken on an empty stomach, at least 1 hour before or 2 hours after meals, with plenty of water.

STORAGE
Store in a tightly sealed container away from heat and direct light. The suspension can be refrigerated but should not be frozen.

MISSED DOSE
Take it as soon as you remember. If it is near the time for the next dose, skip the missed dose and resume your regular dosage schedule. Do not double the next dose.

STOPPING THE DRUG
Take it as prescribed for the full treatment period, even if you begin to feel better before the scheduled end of therapy. Stopping the drug prematurely may slow your recovery or lead to a rebound infection, also known as superinfection, in which the heartier strains of bacteria survive and multiply, leading to a more serious and drug-resistant infection.

PROLONGED USE
The prolonged use of any antibiotic will increase the risk of superinfection; caution is advised.

▼ PRECAUTIONS

Over 60: No special problems are expected.

Driving and Hazardous Work: Do not drive or engage in hazardous work until you determine how the medicine affects you.

Alcohol: No special precautions are necessary.

Pregnancy: Adequate studies of the use of penicillin antibiotics during pregnancy have not been done; however, no problems have been reported.

Breast Feeding: Bacampicillin may pass into breast milk and cause problems in the nursing infant; avoid use of this drug while nursing.

Infants and Children: No special problems are expected.

Special Concerns: Bacampicillin can cause false results on some urine sugar tests for patients with diabetes. Those who are prone to asthma, hay fever, hives, or allergies may be more likely to have an allergic reaction to a penicillin antibiotic. If severe diarrhea occurs as a side effect of this drug, do not take antidiarrheal medications; call your doctor.

OVERDOSE
Symptoms: Severe nausea, vomiting, diarrhea, muscle spasticity, seizures.

What to Do: Call your doctor, emergency medical services (EMS), or the nearest poison control center immediately.

▼ INTERACTIONS

DRUG INTERACTIONS
Consult your doctor for specific advice if you are taking aminoglycosides, ACE inhibitors, diuretics, potassium supplements or potassium-containing drugs, anticoagulants or other anticlotting drugs, nonsteroidal anti-inflammatory drugs, sulfinpyrazone, cholestyramine, colestipol, oral contraceptives, methotrexate, probenecid, allopurinol, or disulfiram.

FOOD INTERACTIONS
No known food interactions.

DISEASE INTERACTIONS
Consult your doctor if you have a history of allergies, asthma, congestive heart failure, gastrointestinal disorders (especially colitis associated with the use of antibiotics), infectious mononucleosis, or impaired kidney function.

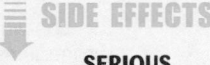
SIDE EFFECTS

SERIOUS
Irregular, rapid, or labored breathing, lightheadedness or sudden fainting, joint pain, fever, severe abdominal pain and cramping with watery or bloody stools, severe allergic reaction (marked by sudden swelling of the lips, tongue, face, or throat; breathing difficulty; severe rash, itching, or hives), unusual bleeding or bruising, yellowish tinge to eyes or skin. Call your doctor immediately.

COMMON
Rash, mild diarrhea, headache, sore tongue, sore mouth, vaginal discharge and itching, white patches in mouth.

LESS COMMON
Diminished urine output, chills, weakness, fatigue.

BACITRACIN

Available in: Ophthalmic ointment and solution; dermatologic (skin) ointment
Available OTC? Yes **As Generic?** Yes
Drug Class: Antibiotic

▼ USAGE INFORMATION

WHY IT'S PRESCRIBED
Dermatologic (skin) ointment is available over the counter for application to minor cuts and abrasions to prevent infection. Ophthalmic preparations are prescribed by a doctor for application to the eyelids or into the eye to treat early minor bacterial infections of the eyelids or conjunctiva (the mucous membranes that line the inner surface of the eyelids).

HOW IT WORKS
Hinders the ability of bacteria to manufacture cell walls, which causes cell death.

▼ DOSAGE GUIDELINES

RANGE AND FREQUENCY
Dermatologic ointment: Apply to a small cut or abrasion 2 times daily. Ophthalmic preparations: Apply to the eye 1 or more times daily.

ONSET OF EFFECT
Unknown.

DURATION OF ACTION
Unknown.

DIETARY ADVICE
No special restrictions.

STORAGE
Store in a tightly sealed container away from heat and direct light.

MISSED DOSE
Apply it as soon as you remember and resume your regular dosage schedule.

STOPPING THE DRUG
You can stop using the dermatologic ointment as soon as the cut or abrasion is sufficiently healed. The decision to stop using the ophthalmic preparation should be made by your doctor.

PROLONGED USE
Ongoing observation is needed when the ointment is used, to detect any possible overgrowth of bacterial organisms that are not susceptible to the drug (known as superinfection).

▼ PRECAUTIONS

Over 60: No special problems are expected.

Driving and Hazardous Work: Ophthalmic ointment may cloud vision; caution is advised.

Alcohol: No special precautions required.

Pregnancy: Before using bacitracin, tell your doctor if you are pregnant or plan to become pregnant.

Breast Feeding: Bacitracin may pass into breast milk. Consult your doctor for specific advice.

Infants and Children: No special problems are expected.

Special Concerns: Bacitracin preparations should not be used if you have a history of sensitivity or allergy to bacitracin or any of the other components in the ointment.

OVERDOSE
Symptoms: Severe eye pain, headache, rapid change in vision, sudden appearance of floating spots, acute redness of eye, pain on exposure to light, double vision, itching, burning, inflammation.

What to Do: Call your doctor, emergency medical services (EMS), or the nearest poison control center immediately.

▼ INTERACTIONS

DRUG INTERACTIONS
No other drugs should be applied topically when using bacitracin unless otherwise instructed by your doctor. Bacitracin has not been shown to have any significant interactions with orally taken medications.

FOOD INTERACTIONS
No known food interactions.

DISEASE INTERACTIONS
Caution is advised when using bacitracin. Consult your doctor if superinfection (see Prolonged Use) with nonsusceptible bacteria occurs during therapy, so appropriate treatment can be started immediately.

SIDE EFFECTS

SERIOUS
Dermatologic and ophthalmic ointment: Rare severe allergic reaction that may cause hives, breathing difficulty, or at the extreme, total closure of the airways with potentially fatal anaphylactic shock. Contact emergency medical services (EMS) immediately. Ophthalmic preparations only: Severe eye pain, headache, rapid change in vision, sudden appearance of floating spots, acute redness of eye, pain on exposure to light, double vision, itching, burning, inflammation. Call your doctor or ophthalmologist immediately.

COMMON
No common side effects have been reported.

LESS COMMON
Dermatologic ointment: Irritation or skin allergy at the site of application, marked by redness, burning, itching, or the development of a rash.

BACLOFEN

Available in: Tablets
Available OTC? No   **As Generic?** Yes
Drug Class: Muscle relaxant

▼ USAGE INFORMATION

WHY IT'S PRESCRIBED
To relax muscles and relieve the pain of muscle spasms and cramping. Chronic muscle spasms may be associated with disorders such as multiple sclerosis or spinal injuries. Baclofen has also been shown to improve urinary or fecal incontinence in patients with spinal cord injuries.

HOW IT WORKS
Baclofen appears to reduce the transmission of nerve impulses from the spinal cord to muscle tissue.

▼ DOSAGE GUIDELINES

RANGE AND FREQUENCY
To start, 5 mg, 3 times a day for 3 days. The dose may then be increased by 5 mg every 3 days until the desired response is attained. The maximum dose is 80 mg per day.

ONSET OF EFFECT
Varies from hours to weeks.

DURATION OF ACTION
Unknown.

DIETARY ADVICE
Take it with milk or food to reduce stomach upset.

STORAGE
Store in a tightly sealed container away from heat, moisture, and direct light.

MISSED DOSE
Take it as soon as you remember if it is within an hour of the scheduled dose. If more than an hour has passed, do not take the missed dose. Take your next scheduled dose at the proper time, and resume your regular dosage schedule. Do not double the next dose.

STOPPING THE DRUG
Do not stop taking this medication suddenly. Consult your doctor about reducing the doses gradually to avoid suffering from withdrawal symptoms such as hallucinations or seizures.

PROLONGED USE
Consult your doctor about reducing doses gradually after prolonged use.

▼ PRECAUTIONS

Over 60: Central nervous system side effects such as confusion, dizziness, and drowsiness are more likely in older persons.

Driving and Hazardous Work: This drug may cause drowsiness; avoid driving or engaging in hazardous work until you determine how the medicine affects you.

Alcohol: Avoid alcohol while taking this drug.

Pregnancy: Some animal studies have found that very large doses of baclofen can cause birth defects. Human studies have not been done. Before taking baclofen, tell your doctor if you are pregnant or are planning to become pregnant.

Breast Feeding: Baclofen passes into breast milk; caution is advised. Consult your doctor for specific advice.

Infants and Children: The safety and effectiveness of baclofen in children under age 12 have not been determined.

Special Concerns: Baclofen may cause dizziness, lightheadedness, or faintness when you rise from a sitting or lying position; avoid any sudden position changes. Some side effects may appear after stopping baclofen; if any of the following develop, call your doctor immediately: hallucinations; seizures; confusion or changes in mental state; increase in muscle spasms, cramping, or tightness; unusual restlessness or nervousness.

OVERDOSE
Symptoms: Blurred or loss of vision, drowsiness, loss of consciousness, muscle weakness, twitching, seizures, slowed breathing, vomiting.

What to Do: Call your doctor, emergency medical services (EMS), or the nearest poison control center immediately.

▼ INTERACTIONS

DRUG INTERACTIONS
Consult your doctor for specific advice if you are taking an antidepressant, an MAO inhibitor, a tranquilizer, a sedative, a barbiturate, another muscle relaxant, or a narcotic pain reliever.

FOOD INTERACTIONS
No known food interactions.

DISEASE INTERACTIONS
Caution is advised when taking baclofen. Consult your doctor if you have a history of any of the following: stroke, diabetes mellitus, a mental or emotional problem, epilepsy, or kidney disease.

⇊ SIDE EFFECTS ⇊

SERIOUS
Chest pain, bloody or dark urine, skin rash or itching, hallucinations, fainting, depression or changes in mood, ringing or buzzing in the ears. Call your doctor.

COMMON
Dizziness, drowsiness, weakness (especially muscle weakness), fatigue, nausea, headache, insomnia.

LESS COMMON
Muscle or joint pain; numbness or tingling in hands or feet; unsteadiness, clumsiness, trembling, or other muscle control problems; stomach pain or discomfort; diarrhea; constipation; false sense of well-being (euphoria); loss of appetite; sexual problems in males; swelling of ankles; frequent urge to urinate or uncontrolled urination; difficult or painful urination or decreased urine output; unexpected weight gain; unusual excitability.

BECAPLERMIN

Available in: Topical gel
Available OTC? No   **As Generic?** No
Drug Class: Topical recombinant human growth factor

▼ USAGE INFORMATION

WHY IT'S PRESCRIBED
To treat diabetic ulcers that develop on the lower legs.

HOW IT WORKS
Becaplermin is a genetically engineered form of a naturally occurring human platelet-derived growth factor. It helps heal ulcers by attracting and promoting the growth of cells involved in wound repair and the formation of new tissue.

▼ DOSAGE GUIDELINES

RANGE AND FREQUENCY
Apply a thin, continuous layer (approximately 1/16 of an inch in thickness) of becaplermin, as directed by your doctor, to the affected area once a day. Cover the treated area with a saline-moistened dressing and leave in place for 12 hours. The dressing should then be removed and the area rinsed with water or saline to remove any residual gel. Cover the area again with a second saline-moistened dressing (without the gel) for the rest of the day. Your doctor will tell you how much becaplermin to apply to the affected area and how to apply it.

ONSET OF EFFECT
Unknown.

DURATION OF ACTION
Unknown.

DIETARY ADVICE
Becaplermin can be applied without regard to meals.

STORAGE
Keep refrigerated, but do not allow it to freeze. Discard unused portions after the expiration date.

MISSED DOSE
If you miss a dose on one day, resume your regular treatment regimen the next day, following your doctor's instructions on the amount of gel to apply.

STOPPING THE DRUG
The decision to stop taking the drug should be made in consultation with your doctor.

PROLONGED USE
Consult your doctor if the ulcer does not shrink in size by 30% after 10 weeks or complete healing has not occurred after 20 weeks.

▼ PRECAUTIONS

Over 60: No special problems are expected.

Driving and Hazardous Work: The use of becaplermin should not impair your ability to engage in such tasks safely.

Alcohol: No special precautions are necessary.

Pregnancy: Adequate human studies have not been done. Before using becaplermin, tell your doctor if you are pregnant or plan to become pregnant.

Breast Feeding: Becaplermin may be absorbed into the bloodstream and pass into breast milk; caution is advised. Consult your doctor for specific advice.

Infants and Children: Not recommended for use by children under age 16.

Special Concerns: Wash your hands thoroughly before and after applying becaplermin. Do not allow the tip of the tube to touch the ulcer, your finger, or any other surface. Becaplermin should be applied in a carefully measured quantity each day. Your doctor will teach you how to determine the correct amount based on the size of the ulcer area. The calculated amount of gel should be squeezed onto a clean measuring surface (for example, wax paper). Becaplermin should then be transferred to the affected area using an applicator, such as a clean cotton swab or a tongue depressor. The amount of becaplermin to be applied should be recalculated at weekly or biweekly intervals by your doctor. Becaplermin should be used together with a good ulcer-care program, including a strict non-weight-bearing program.

OVERDOSE
Symptoms: No cases of overdose have been reported.

What to Do: An overdose with becaplermin is unlikely. If someone applies a much larger dose than prescribed or accidentally ingests the gel, call your doctor.

▼ INTERACTIONS

DRUG INTERACTIONS
Consult your doctor if you are applying any other topical medication to the affected area.

FOOD INTERACTIONS
No known food interactions.

DISEASE INTERACTIONS
You should not apply becaplermin if you have any cancerous or other unusual growths at the affected area. Consult your doctor for specific advice.

≡ SIDE EFFECTS ≡

SERIOUS
No serious side effects have been reported.

COMMON
Irritation at the site of application.

LESS COMMON
No less-common side effects have been reported.

BECLOMETHASONE INHALANT AND NASAL

Available in: Nasal inhaler, oral inhalation
Available OTC? No   **As Generic?** No
Drug Class: Respiratory corticosteroid

▼ USAGE INFORMATION

WHY IT'S PRESCRIBED
To treat bronchial asthma; to treat allergic rhinitis (seasonal and perennial allergies such as hay fever); to prevent recurrence of nasal polyps after they have been removed surgically.

HOW IT WORKS
Respiratory corticosteroids such as beclomethasone primarily reduce or prevent chronic inflammation of the lining of the airways (the underlying cause of asthma), reduce the allergic response to inhaled allergens, and inhibit the secretion of mucus within airways.

▼ DOSAGE GUIDELINES

RANGE AND FREQUENCY
Adults and teenagers— Nasal inhaler: 1 or 2 inhalations in each nostril, 1 or 2 times a day. Oral inhalation: 2 inhalations, 3 or 4 times a day. For severe asthma: 12 to 16 inhalations daily (maximum of 20 inhalations per day). Children ages 6 to 12— Nasal inhaler: 1 inhalation in each nostril, 1 to 3 times a day. Oral inhalation: 1 to 2 inhalations, 3 or 4 times a day. Maximum of 10 inhalations per day.

ONSET OF EFFECT
Within 5 to 7 days; it may take 3 weeks for the full effect to occur.

DURATION OF ACTION
6 hours or more.

DIETARY ADVICE
Use it before or after meals.

STORAGE
Store away from fire and direct light.

MISSED DOSE
Take it as soon as you remember. However, if it is near the time for the next dose, skip the missed dose and resume your regular dosage schedule. Do not double the next dose.

STOPPING THE DRUG
Take it as prescribed for the full treatment period, even if you begin to feel better before the scheduled end of the therapy.

PROLONGED USE
Consult your doctor about the need for periodic medical examinations and laboratory tests if you must take this drug for a prolonged period.

▼ PRECAUTIONS

Over 60: No special problems are expected.

Driving and Hazardous Work: The use of beclomethasone should not impair your ability to perform such tasks safely.

Alcohol: No special precautions are necessary.

Pregnancy: Nasal or inhaled steroids have not been reported to cause birth defects if taken during pregnancy. Before using such drugs, tell your doctor if you are pregnant or plan to become pregnant.

Breast Feeding: Beclomethasone may pass into breast milk; caution is advised. Consult your doctor for advice.

Infants and Children: It has not been established whether beclomethasone is safe and effective in young children.

Special Concerns: Inhaled steroids will not help an asthma attack in progress. Inhaled steroids can lower resistance to yeast infections of the mouth, throat, or voice box. To prevent yeast infections, gargle or rinse your mouth with water after each use; do not swallow the water. Know how to use the inhaler effectively; read and follow the directions that come with the device. Before you have surgery, tell the doctor or dentist that you are using a steroid.

OVERDOSE
Symptoms: No specific ones have been reported.

What to Do: An overdose of beclomethasone is unlikely to be life-threatening. However, if someone takes a much larger dose than prescribed, call your doctor, emergency medical services (EMS), or the nearest poison control center immediately.

▼ INTERACTIONS

DRUG INTERACTIONS
Consult your doctor for specific advice if you are taking systemic corticosteroids, other inhaled corticosteroids, or any drugs that suppress the immune system.

FOOD INTERACTIONS
No known food interactions.

DISEASE INTERACTIONS
Consult your doctor if you have any of the following: a lung disease such as tuberculosis; an infection of the mouth, nose, sinuses, throat, or lungs; a herpes infection of the eye; or any other untreated infection.

≡ SIDE EFFECTS ≡

SERIOUS
No serious side effects are associated with the use of beclomethasone.

COMMON
Nasal form: Nosebleeds or bloody nasal secretions, nasal burning or irritation, sore throat. Oral inhalation: Sore throat, white patches in the mouth or throat, hoarseness.

LESS COMMON
Eye pain, watering eyes, gradual decrease of vision, stomach pain and digestive disturbances.

BENAZEPRIL HYDROCHLORIDE

BRAND NAME

Lotensin

Available in: Tablets
Available OTC? No **As Generic?** No
Drug Class: Angiotensin-converting enzyme (ACE) inhibitor

▼ USAGE INFORMATION

WHY IT'S PRESCRIBED
To control high blood pressure; to treat congestive heart failure; to treat patients with left ventricular dysfunction (damage to the pumping chamber of the heart); and to minimize further kidney damage in diabetics with mild kidney disease.

HOW IT WORKS
Angiotensin-converting enzyme (ACE) inhibitors block an enzyme that produces angiotensin, a naturally occurring substance that causes blood vessels to constrict. As a result, ACE inhibitors relax blood vessels (causing them to widen), which lowers blood pressure and so decreases the workload of the heart.

▼ DOSAGE GUIDELINES

RANGE AND FREQUENCY
If you are not also taking a diuretic (water pill), 10 mg once a day to start, increased to 20 to 80 mg a day in 1 or 2 doses. If you are taking a diuretic, 5 mg per day.

ONSET OF EFFECT
60 to 90 minutes.

DURATION OF ACTION
Up to 24 hours.

DIETARY ADVICE
Take it on an empty stomach, about 1 hour before mealtime. Follow your doctor's dietary advice (such as low-salt or low-cholesterol restrictions) to improve control over high blood pressure and heart disease. Avoid high-potassium foods like bananas and citrus fruits and juices, unless you are also taking medications, such as diuretics, that lower potassium levels.

STORAGE
Store in a tightly sealed container away from heat and direct light.

MISSED DOSE
Take it as soon as you remember. If it is near the time for the next dose, skip the missed dose and resume your regular dosage schedule. Do not double the next dose.

STOPPING THE DRUG
Do not stop taking this drug abruptly, as this may cause potentially serious health problems. Dosage should be reduced gradually, according to your doctor's instructions.

PROLONGED USE
See your doctor regularly for examinations and tests if you must take this medicine for a prolonged period. Remember that benazepril helps control high blood pressure but does not cure it. Lifelong therapy may be necessary.

▼ PRECAUTIONS

Over 60: Adverse reactions may be more likely and more severe in older patients.

Driving and Hazardous Work: Avoid such activities until you determine how the medication affects you.

Alcohol: Consume alcohol only in moderation since it may increase the effect of the drug and cause an excessive drop in blood pressure.

Pregnancy: Tell your doctor before taking this medication if you are pregnant or plan to become pregnant. Use of this drug during the last 6 months of pregnancy may cause severe defects, even death, in the fetus.

Breast Feeding: Benazepril passes into breast milk; if possible, avoid using the drug while nursing.

Infants and Children: Benazepril is generally not prescribed for children; benefits must be weighed against risks. Consult your pediatrician for specific advice.

OVERDOSE
Symptoms: None reported.

What to Do: While overdose is unlikely, call your doctor, emergency medical services (EMS), or the nearest poison control center immediately if you suspect that someone has taken a much larger dose than prescribed.

▼ INTERACTIONS

DRUG INTERACTIONS
Consult your doctor if you are taking diuretics (especially potassium-sparing diuretics), potassium supplements or drugs containing potassium (check ingredient labels), lithium, anticoagulants (such as warfarin), indomethacin or other anti-inflammatory drugs, or any over-the-counter drugs (especially cold remedies and diet pills).

FOOD INTERACTIONS
Avoid low-salt milk and salt substitutes. Many of these products contain potassium.

DISEASE INTERACTIONS
Consult your doctor if you have systemic lupus erythematosus or if you have had a prior allergic reaction to ACE inhibitors. This medication should be used with caution by patients with severe kidney disease or renal artery stenosis (narrowing of one or both of the arteries that supply blood to the kidneys).

≡ SIDE EFFECTS ≡

SERIOUS
Fever and chills, sore throat and hoarseness, sudden difficulty breathing or swallowing, swelling of the face, mouth, or extremities, impaired kidney function (ankle swelling, decreased urination), confusion, yellow discoloration of the eyes or skin (indicating liver disorder), intense itching, chest pain or palpitations, abdominal pain. Serious side effects are very rare; contact your doctor immediately.

COMMON
Dry, persistent cough.

LESS COMMON
Dizziness or fainting, skin rash, numbness or tingling in the hands, feet, or lips, unusual fatigue or muscle weakness, nausea, drowsiness, loss of taste, headache.

BENZOCAINE

Available in: Cream, ointment, aerosol spray, dental paste, lozenges, solution
Available OTC? Yes   **As Generic?** No
Drug Class: Anesthetic

BRAND NAMES

Americaine Topical Anesthetic First Aid Ointment, Anbesol, Baby Orabase, Baby Orajel, Benzodent, Children's Chloraseptic Lozenges, Dent-Zel-Ite, Dentapaine, Hurricane, Num-Zit Lotion or Gel, Numzident, Orabase-B with Benzocaine, Orajel, Oratect Gel, Rid-A-Pain, SensoGARD Canker Sore Relief, Spec-T Sore Throat Anesthetic

▼ USAGE INFORMATION

WHY IT'S PRESCRIBED
To relieve minor pain and itching of the skin caused by mild burns, bites, cuts, abrasions, and contact dermatitis (skin inflammation caused by contact with an irritant such as poison ivy, or by an allergic response to certain metals or other substances). Dental forms of benzocaine are used to treat pain caused by toothache, teething, cold sores, canker sores, dentures, or other dental appliances.

HOW IT WORKS
Benzocaine interferes with the ability of certain nerves to conduct electrical signals, which blocks the transmission of nerve impulses that carry pain messages.

▼ DOSAGE GUIDELINES

RANGE AND FREQUENCY
Skin cream, ointment, aerosol spray: Apply to affected area 3 or 4 times a day as needed. Dental paste: Apply as needed. Lozenges: 1 lozenge dissolved in the mouth every 2 hours as needed. Aerosol dental solution: 1 or 2 sprays of at least 1 second each, taken as needed.

ONSET OF EFFECT
Within minutes.

DURATION OF ACTION
Unknown.

DIETARY ADVICE
Forms applied to skin: Can be taken without regard to diet. Oral and dental forms: Do not eat or drink anything for 1 hour after using medicine.

STORAGE
Store in a tightly sealed container away from heat and direct light.

MISSED DOSE
Take it as soon as you remember. If it is near the time for the next dose, skip the missed dose and resume your regular dosage schedule. Do not double the next dose.

STOPPING THE DRUG
It is advisable to take the medication as prescribed for the full treatment period.

However, you may stop taking the drug before the scheduled end of therapy if you are feeling better.

PROLONGED USE
For skin pain or discomfort: Check with your doctor if the condition does not improve within 7 days. For dental pain: If used temporarily for a toothache, arrange for proper dental treatment as soon as possible. For sore throat: Check with your doctor if pain lasts more than 2 days.

▼ PRECAUTIONS

Over 60: Skin: No information is available. Dental use: Adverse reactions may be more likely and more severe in older patients.

Driving and Hazardous Work: No special precautions are necessary.

Alcohol: No special precautions are necessary.

Pregnancy: Benzocaine has not been reported to cause problems in pregnancy.

Breast Feeding: No problems are expected.

Infants and Children: Dental paste can be used in teething babies 4 months and older. Use of other forms of benzocaine is not recommended for children under 2 unless prescribed by your doctor.

Special Concerns: Do not swallow the dental form unless your doctor has instructed you to do so.

OVERDOSE
Symptoms: Both skin and dental forms: Blurred or double vision; confusion; convulsions; dizziness or lightheadedness; drowsiness; feeling hot, cold, or numb; headache; increased sweating; ringing or buzzing in ears; shivering or trembling; slow or irregular heartbeat; trouble breathing; anxiety, nervousness, or restlessness; pale skin; unusual fatigue.

What to Do: Call your doctor, emergency medical services (EMS), or the nearest poison control center immediately.

▼ INTERACTIONS

DRUG INTERACTIONS
With dental benzocaine, consult your doctor for specific advice if you are taking cholinesterase inhibitors or sulfonamides.

FOOD INTERACTIONS
No known food interactions.

DISEASE INTERACTIONS
Consult your doctor if you have any other condition affecting the mouth or skin.

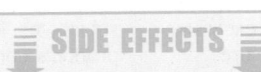

SIDE EFFECTS

SERIOUS
Skin: Severe allergic reaction, producing large, red, hive-like swellings on the skin. Dental use: Large swellings in the mouth or throat. Call your doctor immediately.

COMMON
No common side effects are associated with the skin product or the dental product.

LESS COMMON
Contact dermatitis (skin irritation), causing mild burning, stinging, swelling, itching, redness, or tenderness not present before treatment; hives in or around the mouth.

BENZOYL PEROXIDE

Available in: Lotion, cream, gel, pads, cleansing bar, facial mask, stick
Available OTC? Yes **As Generic?** Yes
Drug Class: Acne drug

▼ USAGE INFORMATION

WHY IT'S PRESCRIBED
To treat mild to moderate acne. In more severe cases benzoyl peroxide may be used in conjunction with other acne treatments, such as antibiotics, retinoic acid preparations, and sulfur- or salicylic-acid-containing medications. It may also be used to treat pressure sores and other skin disorders.

HOW IT WORKS
Benzoyl peroxide slowly releases oxygen, which has an antibacterial effect (bacteria are a primary cause of acne). It also causes peeling and drying of skin, which helps to eliminate blackheads and whiteheads.

▼ DOSAGE GUIDELINES

RANGE AND FREQUENCY
For the cream, gel, lotion or stick form of benzoyl, first wash the affected area of skin with medicated soap and water. Pat dry gently with a towel; apply enough medicine to cover the affected area and rub in gently once or twice a day. For the shave cream form, wet the area to be shaved, apply a small amount of the cream, rub over the entire area, shave, then rinse the area and pat it dry. Check with your doctor about using aftershave lotions. If you have a fair complexion, start with a single daily application at bedtime. Keep the medicine away from eyes, nose, and mouth.

ONSET OF EFFECT
1 to several weeks.

DURATION OF ACTION
Up to 24 hours.

DIETARY ADVICE
This medication may be used without regard to diet.

STORAGE
Store in a tightly sealed container away from heat and direct light.

MISSED DOSE
If you miss an application, apply it as soon as you remember.

STOPPING THE DRUG
Although benzoyl peroxide can be discontinued when acne improves, stopping usually leads to a recurrence of acne.

PROLONGED USE
Check with your doctor if you do not see improvement within 4 to 6 weeks. Other medications may be necessary to control acne and to prevent permanent scarring.

▼ PRECAUTIONS

Over 60: No special problems are expected.

Driving and Hazardous Work: No special warnings.

Alcohol: No special warnings.

Pregnancy: Problems in pregnancy have not been documented, but the manufacturer recommends that the medicine should not be used by pregnant women unless it is considered essential.

Breast Feeding: Benzoyl peroxide may pass into breast milk. Ask your doctor about its use during breast feeding.

Infants and Children: Studies on this medicine have been done only with teenagers and adults, so there is no specific information about its use with other age groups. Nonetheless, no special side effects or problems are expected in children over 12. No studies have been done in children under 12. Use and dose must be determined by a doctor.

OVERDOSE
Symptoms: Overapplication to the skin may cause burn-ing, itching, scaling, swelling, or redness.

What to Do: Discontinue the drug and consult your doctor. If this drug is accidentally ingested, call your doctor, emergency medical services (EMS), or the nearest poison control center immediately.

▼ INTERACTIONS

DRUG INTERACTIONS
Use of this medicine with skin-peeling agents such as salicylic acid, sulfur, tretinoin, or resorcinol can cause excessive skin irritation. Consult your doctor if you take an oral contraceptive, or if you are using any other prescription or nonprescription medication for acne, or if you use medicated cosmetics or abrasive skin cleaners.

FOOD INTERACTIONS
See below.

DISEASE INTERACTIONS
A history of allergy to cinnamon and foods containing benzoic acid increases the chances of developing an allergic skin rash to benzoyl peroxide. Be sure to notify your doctor if you have either of these allergies. Consult your doctor if you have any skin condition other than acne before using benzoyl peroxide.

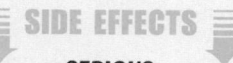

SIDE EFFECTS

SERIOUS
Allergic reaction causing burning, blistering, crusting, itching, severe redness, and swelling of skin. Contact your doctor right away.

COMMON
Mild dryness and peeling of skin.

LESS COMMON
Excessive dryness, unusual feeling of warmth or heat, mild stinging, redness, irritation. This medicine may cause a rash or intensify sunburn in areas of the skin exposed to sunlight or ultraviolet light; avoid excessive sun exposure and tell your doctor if a skin reaction occurs.

BENZPHETAMINE

BRAND NAME

Didrex

Available in: Tablets
Available OTC? No   **As Generic?** Yes
Drug Class: Appetite suppressant

▼ USAGE INFORMATION

WHY IT'S PRESCRIBED
For short-term use in a weight reduction program.

HOW IT WORKS
Benzphetamine reduces appetite by acting on the satiety center in the brain.

▼ DOSAGE GUIDELINES

RANGE AND FREQUENCY
To start, 25 to 50 mg once a day. Usually taken in midmorning or midafternoon. The dose can be increased up to 150 mg per day, taken in 3 doses, if necessary and if the patient can tolerate this dosage without severe side effects. The magnitude of the increased weight loss associated with benzphetamine is a fraction of a pound a week, with the weight loss greatest in the first weeks of therapy.

ONSET OF EFFECT
Within 1 to 2 hours.

DURATION OF ACTION
Up to 4 hours.

DIETARY ADVICE
Take the drug 1 hour before or 2 hours after meals, in midmorning or midafternoon. The last dose should be taken at least 4 to 6 hours before bedtime, since this medicine may cause insomnia.

STORAGE
Store in a tightly sealed container away from heat, moisture, and direct light.

MISSED DOSE
If you miss a dose, take it if you remember within 2 hours. However, if more than 2 hours have passed, skip the missed dose and return to your regular schedule. Do not double the next dose.

STOPPING THE DRUG
Take it as prescribed for the full treatment period. The decision to stop taking the drug should be made in consultation with your physician.

PROLONGED USE
The dose should be reduced with prolonged use. Prolonged use may cause drug dependence. The maximum recommended duration of therapy is 8 to 12 weeks.

▼ PRECAUTIONS

Over 60: Adverse reactions and side effects may be more common in older persons.

Driving and Hazardous Work: Don't drive or engage in hazardous work until you determine how the medicine affects you. It may cause dizziness or blurred vision.

Alcohol: Drink in strict moderation if at all while using this drug.

Pregnancy: Benzphetamine should not be taken during pregnancy because it may harm the fetus. A reliable form of birth control should be used while taking this medicine.

Breast Feeding: Benzphetamine passes into breast milk. It should not be taken while breast feeding.

Infants and Children: Benzphetamine should not be used in children under the age of 12.

OVERDOSE
Symptoms: Overactivity, irritability, trembling, insomnia, rapid heartbeat, confusion, hallucinations, convulsions, coma.

What to Do: Call your doctor, emergency medical services (EMS), or the nearest poison control center immediately.

▼ INTERACTIONS

DRUG INTERACTIONS
Benzphetamine should not be used with any other central nervous stimulant drug. It may decrease the effect of drugs for high blood pressure and increase the effect of antidepressants. Caution is necessary when urinary acidifiers or alkalizers are taken with benzphetamine. Avoid MAO inhibitors. Vitamin C supplements increase excretion and therefore decrease the effectiveness of this drug.

FOOD INTERACTIONS
Avoid beverages containing caffeine since they may increase the drug's effect of stimulating the central nervous system.

DISEASE INTERACTIONS
This medicine should not be taken by persons with advanced arteriosclerosis, moderate to severe high blood pressure, hyperthyroidism, or glaucoma. It should not be given to persons with a history of drug abuse. For people with diabetes, taking this medicine may affect the amount of insulin or oral antidiabetic medicines that must be taken.

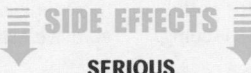
SIDE EFFECTS

SERIOUS
Mental depression, nausea or vomiting, abdominal pain, trembling, overactivity, rapid heartbeat, confusion, hallucinations, convulsions, coma, highly elevated blood pressure. Call your doctor at once.

COMMON
Irritability, nervousness, insomnia, mood changes including elation, euphoria, or a false sense of well-being.

LESS COMMON
Irregular or pounding heartbeat, difficulties with urination; call your doctor at once. Blurred vision, dry mouth, unpleasant or metallic taste in the mouth, decreased sexual ability, increased sweating, diarrhea, headache. Notify your doctor if such symptoms persist.

BENZTROPINE MESYLATE

Available in: Capsules, injection
Available OTC? No   **As Generic?** Yes
Drug Class: Antiparkinsonism drug

▼ USAGE INFORMATION

WHY IT'S PRESCRIBED
To treat Parkinson's disease or the adverse effects of some central nervous system drugs, which produce Parkinson-like symptoms or affect muscle control.

HOW IT WORKS
The exact mechanism of action is unknown, but it is believed to help increase the release of certain neurological chemicals that improve control over muscle movement.

▼ DOSAGE GUIDELINES

RANGE AND FREQUENCY
For Parkinson's disease: 0.5 to 6 mg per day in 1 dose at bedtime. For drug-induced Parkinson reactions: 1 to 4 mg per day either in 1 dose or 2 to 3 doses. For drug-induced nervous system effects: 1 to 4 mg per day in 1 to 3 doses.

ONSET OF EFFECT
Within 1 to 2 hours.

DURATION OF ACTION
Up to 24 hours.

DIETARY ADVICE
Benztropine can be taken with food to reduce stomach irritation.

STORAGE
Store this medicine in a tightly sealed container away from heat and direct light.

MISSED DOSE
If you miss a dose, take it as soon as you remember unless the next scheduled dose is to be taken within 2 hours. In that case, skip the missed dose and resume your normal schedule. Do not double the next dose.

STOPPING THE DRUG
Do not stop taking benztropine suddenly. If therapy is to be discontinued, dosage should be reduced gradually, according to your doctor's instructions.

PROLONGED USE
Prolonged use of this drug may increase pressure in the eye and thus increase the risk of glaucoma, especially in older persons.

▼ PRECAUTIONS

Over 60: Side effects may be more common in older persons. Smaller starting doses are advisable.

Driving and Hazardous Work: Avoid driving and hazardous work until you determine if the drug causes drowsiness.

Alcohol: Alcohol should be avoided or used with caution because it may increase the sedative effects of the drug.

Pregnancy: Benztropine may affect the unborn child's intestinal tract. Do not use the drug while pregnant.

Breast Feeding: It is not known whether benztropine passes into breast milk. Do not use the drug while breast feeding.

Infants and Children: Not generally prescribed for children under the age of 3. Your doctor must determine the exact dosage for older children.

Special Concerns: Eye pressure should be measured regularly because of the risk of glaucoma. Limit physical activity in hot weather.

OVERDOSE
Symptoms: Clumsiness, drowsiness, fast or slow heartbeat, flushed skin, breathing difficulty, seizures, loss of consciousness, muscle weakness, inability to sweat, uncoordinated movement.

What to Do: Call your doctor, emergency medical services (EMS), or the nearest poison control center immediately.

▼ INTERACTIONS

DRUG INTERACTIONS
The activity of benztropine can affect or be affected by many drugs. Talk to your doctor about any drug you are taking, especially phenothiazines, tricyclic antidepressants, and amantadine.

FOOD INTERACTIONS
None are expected.

DISEASE INTERACTIONS
Consult your doctor if you have glaucoma, high blood pressure, heart disease, impaired liver function, kidney disease, or myasthenia gravis.

SIDE EFFECTS

SERIOUS
Unusually rapid or slow heartbeat, heart palpitations, abnormal behavior, confusion, bowel obstruction. Call your doctor immediately.

COMMON
Constipation. It can be reduced by drinking more fluids and eating high-fiber foods.

LESS COMMON
Restlessness, irritability, disorientation, headache, sleepiness, depression, muscle weakness, eye sensitivity to light, dry mouth, heartburn, nausea, vomiting, difficulty swallowing, increased body temperature, decreased sweating.

BETA-CAROTENE

Available in: Capsules, tablets
Available OTC? Yes **As Generic?** Yes
Drug Class: Dietary supplement

▼ USAGE INFORMATION

WHY IT'S PRESCRIBED
Beta-carotene is a natural source of vitamin A. While most Americans get sufficient amounts of vitamin A in their diet, beta-carotene may be prescribed as a dietary supplement for people with certain medical conditions that increase the need for the vitamin. Such conditions include cystic fibrosis, long-term chronic illness, chronic diarrhea, and intestinal malabsorption. A profound deficiency of vitamin A (which occurs very rarely) can lead to night blindness. It may also lead to skin problems, dry eyes and eye infections, and slowed growth. Beta-carotene may also be prescribed in larger doses to reduce the severity of photosensitive reactions (heightened sensitivity to sunlight) that occur in patients with a rare inherited disorder known as erythopoietic protoporphyria. Beta-carotene is an antioxidant that has been prescribed to prevent atherosclerosis and coronary heart disease, but beta-carotene supplements did not reduce the incidence of heart attacks in three large clinical trials.

HOW IT WORKS
Approximately half of ingested beta-carotene is converted to vitamin A in the intestine. The rest is absorbed unchanged and is stored in various tissues, especially fat.

▼ DOSAGE GUIDELINES

RANGE AND FREQUENCY
As a dietary supplement— Adults and teenagers: 6 to 15 mg a day. Children: 3 to 6 mg a day. To treat erythopoietic porphyria— 30 to 300 mg a day.

ONSET OF EFFECT
Unknown.

DURATION OF ACTION
Unknown.

DIETARY ADVICE
It is best taken with meals.

STORAGE
Store in a tightly sealed container away from heat, moisture, and direct light. Do not refrigerate beta-carotene, and keep it from freezing.

MISSED DOSE
There is no danger in doubling the next dose if you miss a scheduled dose.

▼ SIDE EFFECTS

SERIOUS
No serious side effects are associated with beta-carotene.

COMMON
Yellowing of the palms, hands, or soles of feet, and, in some cases, the face.

LESS COMMON
No less common side effects are associated with the use of beta-carotene.

STOPPING THE DRUG
Take it as prescribed. If beta-carotene is prescribed for a specific medical condition, the decision to stop taking it should be made in consultation with your physician.

PROLONGED USE
No known problems.

▼ PRECAUTIONS

Over 60: No special precautions are warranted.

Driving and Hazardous Work: No precautions are necessary.

Alcohol: No special precautions are necessary.

Pregnancy: Beta-carotene has not been studied in pregnant women, but no problems with fertility or pregnancy have been reported in women taking up to 30 mg of beta-carotene a day. The effects of higher daily doses are unknown.

Breast Feeding: Beta-carotene may pass into breast milk, although problems have not been documented with the intake of normal recommended amounts. Consult your doctor for advice.

Infants and Children: No problems have been reported with the intake of recommended amounts of beta-carotene.

Special Concerns: Beta-carotene is found in carrots, dark-green leafy vegetables such as spinach and lettuce, tomatoes, sweet potatoes, broccoli, cantaloupe, and winter squash. Be sure to eat a proper, balanced diet to obtain adequate amounts of beta-carotene from foods. Some fat is needed so that the body can absorb beta-carotene. Beta-carotene is safer than vitamin A because high doses of vitamin A can be harmful. If high levels of vitamin A are present, less beta-carotene is converted to vitamin A by the body.

OVERDOSE
Symptoms: None have been reported.

What to Do: An overdose of beta-carotene is unlikely to be dangerous. Emergency instructions do not apply.

▼ INTERACTIONS

DRUG INTERACTIONS
Consult your doctor for specific advice if you are taking cholestyramine or colestipol (cholesterol-lowering drugs), mineral oil, neomycin (an antibiotic), or vitamin E.

FOOD INTERACTIONS
No known food interactions.

DISEASE INTERACTIONS
If you have any medical problems, consult your doctor before taking beta-carotene. Large doses of beta-carotene may cause complications in patients with liver disease or kidney disease.

BETAMETHASONE SYSTEMIC

Available in: Syrup, tablets, extended-release tablets, injection, rectal solution
Available OTC? No   **As Generic?** Yes
Drug Class: Corticosteroid

BRAND NAME

Celestone

▼ USAGE INFORMATION

WHY IT'S PRESCRIBED
To treat numerous conditions that involve inflammation (a response by body tissues, producing redness, warmth, swelling, and pain). Such conditions include arthritis, allergic reactions, asthma, some skin diseases, multiple sclerosis flare-ups, and other autoimmune diseases. Also prescribed to treat deficiency of natural steroid hormones.

HOW IT WORKS
Betamethasone mimics the effects of the body's corticosteroids. It depresses the synthesis, release, and activity of inflammation-producing chemicals. It also suppresses immune system activity.

▼ DOSAGE GUIDELINES

RANGE AND FREQUENCY
Adults— Syrup or tablets: 600 micrograms (mcg) to 7.2 mg a day, as a single dose or in divided doses. Extended-release tablets: 2 to 6 mg a day to start, then as ordered by your doctor. Injection: Up to 9 mg a day. Rectal solution: 5 mg, given as an enema at night. Consult pediatrician for children's dosage.

ONSET OF EFFECT
Within 1 hour. It may take 2 to 4 days for full effect.

DURATION OF ACTION
More than 3 days for oral forms; 24 hours or more for other forms.

DIETARY ADVICE
Take it with food or milk to minimize stomach upset. Your doctor may recommend a special diet.

STORAGE
Store in a tightly sealed container away from heat, moisture, and direct light.

MISSED DOSE
Take it as soon as you remember. If you take several doses a day and it is close to the next dose, double the next dose. If you take 1 dose a day and you do not remember until the next day, skip the missed dose and do not double the next dose.

STOPPING THE DRUG
With long-term therapy, do not stop taking the drug abruptly; the dosage should be decreased gradually.

PROLONGED USE
See your doctor regularly for tests and examinations. Long-term use may lead to cataracts, diabetes, hypertension, or osteoporosis.

▼ PRECAUTIONS

Over 60: Adverse reactions may be more likely and more severe in older patients.

Driving and Hazardous Work: Do not drive or engage in hazardous work until you determine how the medicine affects you.

Alcohol: May cause stomach problems; avoid alcohol unless your doctor approves occasional moderate drinking.

Pregnancy: Overuse during pregnancy can retard the child's growth and cause other developmental problems. Consult your physician.

Breast Feeding: Do not use while nursing.

Infants and Children: Betamethasone may retard the normal growth and development of bone and other tissues. Consult your doctor for advice.

Special Concerns: Avoid immunizations with live vaccines if possible. This drug can lower your resistance to infection. Patients undergoing long-term therapy should wear a medical-alert bracelet. Call your doctor if you develop a fever.

OVERDOSE
Symptoms: Fever, muscle or joint pain, nausea, dizziness, fainting, difficulty breathing. Prolonged overuse: Moonface, obesity, unusual hair growth, acne, loss of sexual function, muscle wasting.

What to Do: Seek medical assistance immediately.

▼ INTERACTIONS

DRUG INTERACTIONS
Consult your doctor for specific advice if you are taking aminoglutethimide, antacids, barbiturates, carbamazepine, griseofulvin, mitotane, phenylbutazone, phenytoin, primidone, rifampin, injectable amphotericin B, oral antidiabetes agents, insulin, digitalis drugs, diuretics, or medications that contain potassium or sodium.

FOOD INTERACTIONS
Avoid excess sodium.

DISEASE INTERACTIONS
Consult your doctor if you have a history of bone disease, chicken pox, measles, gastrointestinal disorders, diabetes, recent serious infection, tuberculosis, glaucoma, heart disease, hypertension, liver or kidney disorders, high blood cholesterol, overactive or underactive thyroid, myasthenia gravis, or lupus.

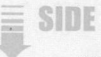

SIDE EFFECTS

SERIOUS
Vision problems, frequent urination, increased thirst, rectal bleeding, blistering skin, confusion, hallucinations, paranoia, euphoria, depression, mood swings, redness and swelling at injection site. Call your doctor immediately.

COMMON
Increased appetite, indigestion, nervousness, insomnia, greater susceptibility to infections, increased blood pressure, slowed healing of wounds, unusual weight gain, easy bruising, fluid retention.

LESS COMMON
Change in skin color, dizziness, headache, increased sweating, unusual growth of body or facial hair, increased blood sugar, peptic ulcers, adrenal insufficiency, muscle weakness, cataracts, glaucoma, osteoporosis.

BETAMETHASONE TOPICAL

Available in: Cream, gel, lotion, ointment, aerosol, foam
Available OTC? No   **As Generic?** Yes
Drug Class: Topical corticosteroid

▼ USAGE INFORMATION

WHY IT'S PRESCRIBED
To treat skin rashes and inflammation.

HOW IT WORKS
Topical betamethasone appears to interfere with the formation of natural substances within the body that are directly responsible for the process of inflammation, which produces swelling, redness, and itching.

▼ DOSAGE GUIDELINES

RANGE AND FREQUENCY
Apply sparingly as a thin film, 2 (sometimes 3) times a day, only to the specific areas where needed. Wash or soak the affected area prior to application, as this may improve absorption of the drug. Foam is for use on the scalp.

ONSET OF EFFECT
Rapid, but may take 24 to 48 hours to see effect.

DURATION OF ACTION
Unknown.

DIETARY ADVICE
No special restrictions.

STORAGE
Store in a tightly sealed container away from heat and direct light.

MISSED DOSE
Apply it as soon as you remember. If it is near the time for the next dose, skip the missed dose and resume your regular dosage schedule as prescribed.

STOPPING THE DRUG
Take as prescribed for the full treatment period, even if you begin to feel better before the scheduled end of therapy.

PROLONGED USE
Avoid prolonged use, particularly near the eyes, on the face in general, on the genital or rectal regions, or in the folds of the skin (for example, underneath the breasts).

≡ SIDE EFFECTS ≡

SERIOUS
Serious side effects from the use of topical betamethasone are rare.

COMMON
Burning, itching, irritation, redness, dryness, acne, stinging and cracking of skin, numbness or tingling in the extremities in 0.5% to 1% of patients. Risk of such reactions is higher with lotion and gel and lower in ointment and cream. (Products vary in potency from one brand to another; higher-potency products are more likely to cause side effects.)

LESS COMMON
Blistering and pus near hair follicles, unusual bleeding or easy bruising, darkening or prominence of small surface veins, increased susceptibility to infection.

▼ PRECAUTIONS

Over 60: Side effects may be more likely and more severe in older patients; therapy with topical corticosteroids should be limited.

Driving and Hazardous Work: No special precautions are necessary.

Alcohol: No special precautions are necessary.

Pregnancy: Should not be used for prolonged periods in pregnant women or in women trying to become pregnant.

Breast Feeding: Although problems have not been documented, caution is advised. Do not apply to breasts prior to nursing. Consult your doctor for specific advice.

Infants and Children: It should not be used for more than 2 weeks on children and adolescents, unless otherwise directed by your doctor. Do not use tight-fitting diapers or plastic pants on children when treating skin irritation in the diaper area.

Special Concerns: Wash your hands thoroughly after application. Do not wrap the treated area with bandages or tight-fitting clothing unless otherwise instructed by your doctor. Doing so may cause skin infections to worsen; corticosteroid treatment may need to be discontinued to treat infections, then resumed later. Note that topical betamethasone is not a treatment for acne, burns, infections, or disorders of pigmentation.

OVERDOSE

Symptoms: No specific ones have been reported.

What to Do: An overdose of a topical corticosteroid is unlikely to be life-threatening. However, in the event of accidental ingestion or an apparent overdose, call a doctor, emergency medical services (EMS), or the nearest poison control center right away.

▼ INTERACTIONS

DRUG INTERACTIONS
Do not mix topical betamethasone with other products, especially alcohol-containing preparations (which include colognes, aftershave, and many moisturizer lotions), since this may cause dryness and irritation, or increase the risk of an allergic reaction.

FOOD INTERACTIONS
Potassium supplements may decrease this drug's effects. Avoid foods high in sodium.

DISEASE INTERACTIONS
Caution is advised when taking this drug. Consult your doctor if you have any of the following: cataracts; diabetes mellitus; glaucoma; infection, sores, or ulcerations of the skin; infection at another site in your body; or tuberculosis.

BETAMETHASONE/CLOTRIMAZOLE

Available in: Cream
Available OTC? No   **As Generic?** Yes
Drug Class: Topical antifungal

▼ USAGE INFORMATION

WHY IT'S PRESCRIBED
To treat fungal infections of the skin.

HOW IT WORKS
Clotrimazole prevents fungal organisms from manufacturing the vital proteins they require for growth and function. Betamethasone dipropionate is a steroid; it interferes with the formation of natural substances within the body that are directly responsible for the process of inflammation, which produces swelling, redness, and pain. The use of these two effective medications in combination for skin infections appears to hasten recovery sooner than use of clotrimazole alone. This medication is only effective for infections caused by fungal organisms. It will not work for bacterial or viral infections.

▼ DOSAGE GUIDELINES

RANGE AND FREQUENCY
Adults and children older than 12 years of age: Apply and massage a sufficient amount of cream to the affected site twice daily for 2 to 4 weeks. This combination drug contains a high-potency topical steroid that should not be used in skin creases or with bandages (occlusive dressing) unless closely supervised by your doctor.

ONSET OF EFFECT
Clotrimazole begins killing susceptible fungi shortly after contact. The effects may not be noticeable for several days or weeks.

DURATION OF ACTION
Unknown.

DIETARY ADVICE
Drink plenty of fluids.

STORAGE
Store in a tightly sealed container away from heat and direct light. Keep away from moisture and extremes in temperature.

MISSED DOSE
Apply it as soon as you remember. If it is near the time for the next dose, skip the missed dose and resume your regular dosage schedule. Do not double the next dose or apply an excessively thick film of topical medication to compensate for a missed dose.

STOPPING THE DRUG
Apply as prescribed for the full treatment period, even if the fungal infection appears to be eradicated before the scheduled end of therapy. Unfortunately, it can be difficult to assess when the drug has achieved its desired effect since it suppresses redness and inflammation of the skin before the infection is completely clear; recurrence of fungal infection owing to inadequate length of therapy is a significant risk.

PROLONGED USE
Therapy with this medication should not exceed 4 weeks.

▼ PRECAUTIONS

Over 60: Adverse reactions may be more likely and more severe in older patients.

Driving and Hazardous Work: No special precautions are necessary.

Alcohol: No special precautions are necessary.

Pregnancy: Not recommended during pregnancy.

Breast Feeding: Betamethasone dipropionate/clotrimazole may pass into breast milk; caution is advised. Consult your doctor for advice.

Infants and Children: Not recommended for use by children under age 12.

Special Concerns: Avoid contact with eyes. Wash hands thoroughly after application. Tell your doctor if your condition has not improved within a few days of starting the medication. As with any other antifungal, betamethasone dipropionate/clotrimazole is useful only against organisms that are vulnerable to its effects. Therefore, it is important to tell your doctor if your condition has not improved—or has worsened—within a few days of starting betamethasone dipropionate/clotrimazole. The particular organism causing your illness may be resistant to this medication.

OVERDOSE
Symptoms: No specific ones have been reported.

What to Do: An overdose is unlikely to be life-threatening. However, if someone applies a much larger dose than prescribed or ingests the medication, call your doctor, emergency medical services (EMS), or the nearest poison control center immediately.

▼ INTERACTIONS

DRUG INTERACTIONS
No specific drug interactions have been documented.

FOOD INTERACTIONS
No known food interactions.

DISEASE INTERACTIONS
Consult your physician if you have ever experienced an allergic reaction to any topical medication, or undesirable reactions to any steroid or steroid-containing preparation.

SIDE EFFECTS

SERIOUS
Blistering or ulceration of the skin; blistering of the lips, nose, and mouth.

COMMON
Brief burning or irritation after application; peeling.

LESS COMMON
Severe burning, itching, swelling, increased redness, or any increased discomfort developing at the application site that was not present prior to therapy; dry skin; pus or inflammation at base of hair follicles; change in skin color at site of application; acne.

BETAXOLOL OPHTHALMIC

Available in: Ophthalmic solution, suspension
Available OTC? No   **As Generic?** No
Drug Class: Antiglaucoma drug; ophthalmic beta-blocker

▼ USAGE INFORMATION

WHY IT'S PRESCRIBED
To treat glaucoma.

HOW IT WORKS
Glaucoma, a sight-threatening disorder, occurs when aqueous humor (the fluid inside the eye) cannot drain properly, resulting in an increase in pressure within the eyeball (known as intraocular pressure). Increased intraocular pressure (IOP) can damage the optic nerve and lead to a gradually progressive loss of vision. Betaxolol decreases the production of aqueous humor, thereby reducing intraocular pressure.

▼ DOSAGE GUIDELINES

RANGE AND FREQUENCY
1 or 2 drops of 0.5% solution or 0.25% suspension twice a day.

ONSET OF EFFECT
30 minutes.

DURATION OF ACTION
12 hours or more.

DIETARY ADVICE
No special restrictions or recommendations.

STORAGE
Store in a tightly sealed container away from heat, moisture, and direct light. Do not allow the medicine to freeze.

MISSED DOSE
Apply the missed dose as soon as you remember. If it is near the time for the next dose, skip the missed dose and resume your regular dosage schedule. Do not double the next dose.

STOPPING THE DRUG
The decision to stop taking the drug should be made by your doctor. Gradual discontinuation rather than a sudden stop may be required.

PROLONGED USE
Consult your doctor about the need for periodic ophthalmological examinations to check intraocular pressure (the pressure within the eyeball).

▼ PRECAUTIONS

Over 60: Adverse reactions may be more likely and more severe in older patients.

Driving and Hazardous Work: Exercise caution until you determine how the drug affects your vision.

Alcohol: Alcohol should be used with caution.

Pregnancy: Ophthalmic betaxolol has not been shown to cause birth defects in animals; human studies have not been done. Before taking it, tell your doctor if you are pregnant or planning to become pregnant.

Breast Feeding: Ophthalmic betaxolol may pass into breast milk; caution is advised. Consult your doctor for specific advice.

Infants and Children: Not recommended for use by children under age 12.

Special Concerns: To use the eye drops, first wash your hands. Tilt your head back. Gently apply pressure to the inside corner of the eyelid and with the index finger of the same hand, pull downward on the lower eyelid to make a space. Drop the medicine into this space and close your eye. Apply pressure for 1 or 2 minutes while keeping the eye closed without blinking. Then wash your hands again. Make sure the tip of the dropper does not touch your eye, finger, or any other surface. Betaxolol may make your eyes more sensitive to sunlight. If this occurs, wear sunglasses or avoid bright light as necessary. Shake the suspension well before using.

OVERDOSE
Symptoms: Double vision, slow pulse, dizziness and weakness caused by low blood pressure, unusual fatigue, drowsiness, seizures, hallucinations, loss of consciousness.

What to Do: An overdose of this drug is unlikely to be life-threatening. If a large volume of the medicine enters the eyes, flush with water. If someone accidentally ingests it, seek medical assistance immediately.

▼ INTERACTIONS

DRUG INTERACTIONS
It is not recommended to use two ophthalmic beta-blockers at the same time. Special concern is warranted in people taking antidiabetic drugs, since ophthalmic betaxolol may mask symptoms of low blood sugar. Other drugs may interact with ophthalmic betaxolol. Tell your doctor if you are using any other prescription or over-the-counter medication.

FOOD INTERACTIONS
No known food interactions.

DISEASE INTERACTIONS
Caution is advised when taking ophthalmic betaxolol. Consult your doctor if you have any of the following conditions: diabetes, hypoglycemia, heart disease, high blood pressure, lung disorders, irregular heartbeat, or an overactive thyroid gland.

SIDE EFFECTS

SERIOUS
Palpitations, trouble breathing, dizziness and weakness caused by low blood pressure. Call your doctor right away.

COMMON
Temporary eye irritation, tearing, eye inflammation, burning, swelling.

LESS COMMON
Blurred vision, poor night vision, and increased sensitivity to light; headache; insomnia; sinus irritation; odd or bitter taste in the mouth.

BETAXOLOL ORAL

Available in: Tablets
Available OTC? No   **As Generic?** No
Drug Class: Beta-blocker

▼ USAGE INFORMATION

WHY IT'S PRESCRIBED
To treat high blood pressure (hypertension).

HOW IT WORKS
Betaxolol slows the rate and force of contraction of the heart by blocking certain nerve impulses, thus reducing blood pressure.

▼ DOSAGE GUIDELINES

RANGE AND FREQUENCY
To start, 10 mg, once a day. Dose may be increased to a maximum of 20 mg per day.

ONSET OF EFFECT
Within 1 hour.

DURATION OF ACTION
24 hours or more.

DIETARY ADVICE
This medication can be used without regard to diet.

STORAGE
Store in a tightly sealed container away from heat and direct light.

MISSED DOSE
Take the missed dose as soon as possible. If it is within 8 hours of the next dose, skip the missed dose and resume your regular dosage schedule. Do not double the next dose.

STOPPING THE DRUG
Take it as prescribed for the full treatment period even if you begin to feel better before the scheduled end of therapy. Lifelong therapy with betaxolol may be necessary. Do not stop taking the medication suddenly, as this may result in potentially serious medical consequences. Dose must be tapered gradually.

PROLONGED USE
Consult your doctor about the need for periodic examinations or laboratory studies to check blood pressure, heart function, kidney function, and blood sugar levels.

▼ PRECAUTIONS

Over 60: Adverse reactions may be more likely and more severe in older patients. Lower doses may be warranted, and frequent measurement of blood pressure is important.

Driving and Hazardous Work: Use caution when driving or engaging in hazardous work until you determine how the medication affects you.

Alcohol: Drink in careful moderation if at all. Alcohol may interact with the drug and cause a dangerous drop in blood pressure.

Pregnancy: Betaxolol has caused birth defects in animals; adequate human studies have not been done. Use of this drug should be avoided during the first three months of pregnancy if possible, and during labor and delivery, because of possible damaging effects on the newborn baby.

Breast Feeding: Betaxolol may pass into breast milk; caution is advised. Consult your doctor for advice.

Infants and Children: The safety and effectiveness of this drug for children under the age of 12 have not been established. If it is used, the child should have periodic tests for low blood glucose (sugar) levels.

OVERDOSE
Symptoms: Double vision, unusually slow or rapid heartbeat, severe dizziness or fainting, poor circulation in the hands (bluish skin), breathing difficulty, seizures.

What to Do: Call your doctor, emergency medical services (EMS), or the nearest poison control center immediately.

▼ INTERACTIONS

DRUG INTERACTIONS
Consult your doctor for specific advice if you are taking calcium channel blockers, ACE inhibitors, insulin or any other diabetes drug, antihistamines, other drugs for high blood pressure, nonsteroidal anti-inflammatory drugs, barbiturates, or clonidine.

FOOD INTERACTIONS
No known food interactions.

DISEASE INTERACTIONS
Betaxolol should be used with caution in people with diabetes, especially insulin-dependent diabetes, since the drug may mask symptoms of hypoglycemia. Consult your doctor if you have any of the following: heart disease, hay fever, asthma, chronic bronchitis, hypoglycemia, an overactive thyroid gland, impaired liver function, or impaired kidney function.

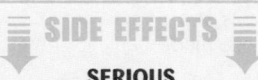

SIDE EFFECTS

SERIOUS
Shortness of breath, wheezing; irregular or slow heartbeat (50 beats per minute or less); pain or feelings of tightness or pressure in the chest; swelling of the ankles, feet, and lower legs; mental depression. If you experience such symptoms, stop taking betaxolol and call your doctor immediately.

COMMON
Dizziness or lightheadedness, especially when rising suddenly to a standing position, rapid heartbeat or palpitations, decreased sexual ability, frequent headaches.

LESS COMMON
Anxiety, irritability, nervousness; constipation; diarrhea; dry, sore eyes; itching; nausea or vomiting; nightmares or intensely vivid dreams; numbness, tingling, or other unusual sensations in the fingers, toes, or scalp.

BETHANECHOL CHLORIDE

Available in: Tablets, injection
Available OTC? No **As Generic?** Yes
Drug Class: Cholinergic

▼ USAGE INFORMATION

WHY IT'S PRESCRIBED
To treat bladder or urinary tract disorders that make urination difficult. To help initiate urination after surgery.

HOW IT WORKS
Bethanechol strengthens the ability of bladder muscles to contract, facilitating urination.

▼ DOSAGE GUIDELINES

RANGE AND FREQUENCY
Tablets— Adults: 10 to 50 mg, 3 or 4 times a day. Children: 0.6 mg per 2.2 lbs (1 kg) of body weight, in 3 to 4 doses a day. Injection— Adults: 2.5 to 5 mg injected under the skin 3 or 4 times a day. Children: 0.2 mg per 2.2 lbs of body weight per day, injected 3 to 4 times a day, as determined by your pediatrician.

ONSET OF EFFECT
30 to 90 minutes.

DURATION OF ACTION
Up to 6 hours.

DIETARY ADVICE
Take this medicine on an empty stomach with liquid 1 hour before or 2 hours after meals to avoid nausea and vomiting.

STORAGE
Store in a tightly sealed container away from heat and direct light.

MISSED DOSE
Take it as soon as you remember. If it is near the time for the next dose, skip the missed dose and resume your regular dosage schedule. Do not double the next dose.

STOPPING THE DRUG
It may not be necessary to take this drug for the entire prescribed course of treatment. Follow your doctor's instructions about discontinuing the medicine.

PROLONGED USE
No problems expected.

▼ PRECAUTIONS

Over 60: Adverse reactions and side effects may be more severe in older persons.

Driving and Hazardous Work: Determine if the drug causes dizziness, lightheadedness or blurred vision before driving or doing hazardous work. Danger increases if you drink alcohol or take a medicine that affects alertness, such as an antihistamine, a tranquilizer, a pain medicine, a sedative, or a narcotic.

Alcohol: Alcohol intake should be limited to 1 or 2 drinks a day because it can add to the diminished alertness caused by this medicine. Consult your doctor about the exact amount of alcohol you can consume.

Pregnancy: Animal and human studies have not been done. Consult your doctor about taking bethanechol if you are pregnant or plan to become pregnant.

Breast Feeding: It is not known whether bethanechol passes into breast milk. Consult your doctor about taking it if you are nursing.

Infants and Children: Use of bethanechol by infants and children requires close medical supervision.

Special Concerns: Bethanechol interferes with diagnostic laboratory studies of pancreas and liver function. While undergoing treatment with this drug, be cautious when standing up suddenly, as dizziness and lightheadedness are common side effects.

OVERDOSE
Symptoms: Abdominal discomfort, salivation, flushing of the skin, sweating, nausea, vomiting.

What to Do: Call your doctor, emergency medical services (EMS), or the nearest poison control center immediately.

▼ INTERACTIONS

DRUG INTERACTIONS
Consult your doctor if you are taking bethanechol at the same time that you are taking any prescription or nonprescription drugs, especially anticholinergics, ganglionic blockers, nitrates, procainamide, quinidine, or other cholinergic drugs.

FOOD INTERACTIONS
None expected.

DISEASE INTERACTIONS
Consult your doctor if you have low blood pressure, any blood vessel problem, a weakened bladder wall, any urinary tract problem, any digestive problem, an overactive thyroid (hyperthyroidism), asthma, seizures, or Parkinson's disease.

⯬ SIDE EFFECTS ⯮

SERIOUS
Difficulty breathing, wheezing, severe or persistent abdominal cramps, diarrhea. Call your doctor at once.

COMMON
Dizziness or lightheadedness. This can be minimized by getting up slowly from a sitting or lying position.

LESS COMMON
Headache, blurred vision, nausea, stomach discomfort, excessive urge to urinate.

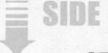

BIOTIN

BRAND NAMES

Bio-tin, Coenzyme R,
Other generic names:
Vitamin H, Vitamin Bw

Available in: Capsules, tablets
Available OTC? Yes **As Generic?** Yes
Drug Class: Vitamin

▼ USAGE INFORMATION

WHY IT'S PRESCRIBED
Biotin is a vitamin found naturally in various foods (see Dietary Advice for more information). While most people get sufficient amounts of it in their diet, biotin may be prescribed as a dietary supplement for people on inadequate or unusual diets or with medical conditions that increase the need for it. Such conditions include a genetic deficiency of the enzyme (biotinidase) needed by the body to utilize biotin, intestinal malabsorption, seborrheic dermatitis in infancy, and an inability to absorb biotin as a result of surgical removal of the stomach. Biotin deficiency may lead to dermatitis, hair loss, high blood cholesterol levels, and heart problems.

HOW IT WORKS
Biotin is one of the B vitamins necessary for the formation of glucose and fatty acids, and for the metabolism of amino acids and carbohydrates. B vitamins are particularly crucial to the proper functioning of the cardiovascular and nervous systems.

▼ DOSAGE GUIDELINES

RANGE AND FREQUENCY
No recommended daily allowances (RDAs) have been established for biotin. The following daily intakes are advised. Adults and teenagers: 30 to 100 micrograms (mcg). Children ages 7 to 10 years: 30 mcg. Children ages 4 to 6 years: 25 mcg daily. Birth to 3 years: 10 to 20 mcg.

ONSET OF EFFECT
Unknown.

DURATION OF ACTION
Unknown.

DIETARY ADVICE
Biotin can be taken with or between meals. Foods that contain biotin include cauliflower, liver, salmon, carrots, bananas, cereals, yeast, and soy flour. Biotin content is reduced when food is cooked or preserved.

STORAGE
Store in a tightly sealed container away from heat, moisture, and direct light.

MISSED DOSE
Take it as soon as you remember.

STOPPING THE DRUG
If you are taking biotin for a vitamin deficiency or medical problem, take it as prescribed for the full treatment period.

PROLONGED USE
When biotin is prescribed to overcome a deficiency, periodic monitoring of biotin levels in the blood may be required.

▼ PRECAUTIONS

Over 60: No problems are expected in older persons taking recommended doses of biotin.

Driving and Hazardous Work: The use of biotin should not impair your ability to perform such tasks safely.

Alcohol: No special precautions are necessary.

Pregnancy: No problems are expected with the intake of recommended doses of biotin during pregnancy.

Breast Feeding: No problems are expected with the intake of recommended doses of biotin during breast feeding.

Infants and Children: No problems are expected with recommended doses.

Special Concerns: Some drastic weight-reducing diets may may not supply enough biotin. Consult your doctor for specific advice. Biotin is generally available as part of a multivitamin complex.

OVERDOSE
Symptoms: No cases of overdose have been reported.

What to Do: Emergency instructions not applicable.

▼ INTERACTIONS

DRUG INTERACTIONS
There are no known drug interactions associated with biotin.

FOOD INTERACTIONS
No known food interactions.

DISEASE INTERACTIONS
None reported.

≣ SIDE EFFECTS ≣

SERIOUS
No serious side effects are associated with recommended doses of biotin. However, check with your doctor if you notice anything unusual while you are taking it.

COMMON
No common side effects are associated with recommended doses.

LESS COMMON
No less-common side effects have been reported.

BIPERIDEN

Available in: Tablets, injection
Available OTC? No   **As Generic?** Yes
Drug Class: Antiparkinsonism drug

▼ USAGE INFORMATION

WHY IT'S PRESCRIBED
To treat Parkinson's disease or the side effects of certain drugs that act on the central nervous system and produce Parkinson-like symptoms, including slowed movement, stiffness, and loss of balance.

HOW IT WORKS
The exact mechanism of action is unknown, but biperiden is believed to help increase the release of certain neurological chemicals that improve control over movement.

▼ DOSAGE GUIDELINES

RANGE AND FREQUENCY
Tablets: For Parkinson's disease, 2 mg, 3 or 4 times per day, to a maximum of 16 mg per day. For side effects of other drugs, 2 mg, 1 to 3 times per day. If you have difficulty swallowing the tablet, it can be crushed. Injection: 2 mg up to 4 times per day, injected into a muscle or vein. The maximum dose should not exceed 10 mg per day.

ONSET OF EFFECT
Within 1 hour.

DURATION OF ACTION
6 to 12 hours with tablets; 1 to 8 hours after injection.

DIETARY ADVICE
Take this medicine with or immediately after meals unless your doctor orders otherwise.

STORAGE
Store in a tightly sealed container away from heat and direct light.

MISSED DOSE
If you miss a dose, take it as soon as you remember unless it is within 2 hours of the next dose. In that case, skip the missed dose and return to your regular schedule. Do not double the next dose.

STOPPING THE DRUG
Do not stop taking the drug suddenly. If therapy is to be discontinued, the dosage should be reduced gradually, according to your doctor's instructions, to avoid a withdrawal reaction.

PROLONGED USE
Your doctor should test your progress regularly so that the dose can be adjusted if necessary.

▼ PRECAUTIONS

Over 60: Side effects may be more common in older persons. A reduced dose may be necessary. This medicine can aggravate symptoms of an enlarged prostate gland and cause impaired thinking, hallucinations, and nightmares in older persons.

Driving and Hazardous Work: Determine how this medicine affects you before engaging in such activities.

Alcohol: Alcohol intake should be avoided because this medicine increases its effects.

Pregnancy: Do not use this drug while pregnant.

Breast Feeding: Do not use this drug while breast feeding.

Infants and Children: Safety and effectiveness have not been established for infants and children.

Special Concerns: Pay careful attention to dental hygiene, since biperiden tends to decrease salivation, which can promote the development of cavities and other dental problems.

OVERDOSE
Symptoms: Agitation, anxiety, restlessness, disorientation, hallucinations, blurred vision, fast pulse, difficulty swallowing, and difficulty urinating.

What to Do: Call your doctor, emergency medical services (EMS), or the nearest poison control center immediately.

▼ INTERACTIONS

DRUG INTERACTIONS
Tell your doctor about any other drugs you are taking, especially amantadine, digoxin, any drug for mental illness, antidepressants, or antacids. This medicine can decrease the activity of phenothiazines (mood-altering drugs used in the treatment of psychiatric disorders).

FOOD INTERACTIONS
No known food interactions.

DISEASE INTERACTIONS
Glaucoma, seizures, an irregular pulse, a bowel obstruction, or an enlarged prostate may make it impossible for you to take this medicine.

 SIDE EFFECTS

SERIOUS
Retention of urine (decreased urine output), confusion, disorientation.

COMMON
Blurred vision, drowsiness, agitation, dry mouth, constipation, urine retention. Constipation can be avoided by increasing the intake of fluids and high-fiber foods. Dry mouth can be relieved by cool drinks, sugarless gum, or hard candy.

LESS COMMON
Restlessness, irritability or unusual feeling of well-being, dizziness, tremor, stomach upset, nausea.

BISACODYL

Available in: Tablets, powder, suppositories
Available OTC? Yes   **As Generic?** Yes
Drug Class: Stimulant laxative

▼ USAGE INFORMATION

WHY IT'S PRESCRIBED
To relieve short-term constipation or to clear the bowel before rectal or bowel examination, surgery, or childbirth.

HOW IT WORKS
Bisacodyl increases the volume of fluid in the intestines to stimulate passage of the stool. It also acts on the smooth muscle of the intestine to increase contractions.

▼ DOSAGE GUIDELINES

RANGE AND FREQUENCY
For constipation— Adults and teenagers: Tablets: 10 to 15 mg at bedtime. Children age 6 and older: 5 mg before breakfast. Swallow tablets whole; do not chew. For medical examination— Adults and teenagers: Up to 30 mg orally, or 10 mg given rectally before examination. Children age 6 and older: 5 mg orally or rectally, before breakfast.

ONSET OF EFFECT
Tablets: Within 6 to 12 hours. Suppositories: Within 15 to 60 minutes.

DURATION OF ACTION
Variable.

DIETARY ADVICE
Take the tablet on an empty stomach for rapid effect. Increase intake of fluids and dietary fiber.

STORAGE
Store in a tightly sealed container away from heat, moisture, and direct light.

MISSED DOSE
Take the missed dose as soon as you remember, unless it is almost time for your next dose. In that case, skip the missed dose and resume your regular dosage schedule. Do not double the next dose.

STOPPING THE DRUG
Take it as prescribed for the full treatment period. However, you may stop taking the drug if you are feeling better before the scheduled end of the therapy.

PROLONGED USE
Do not use this medicine for more than one week unless your doctor prescribes it.

▼ PRECAUTIONS

Over 60: Excessive use of this drug by an older person can cause loss of body fluid leading to weakness and lack of coordination.

Driving and Hazardous Work: Do not drive or engage in hazardous work until you determine how the medicine affects you.

Alcohol: Avoid alcohol while taking this drug.

Pregnancy: Bisacodyl is not usually used during pregnancy, except immediately before delivery. Consult your doctor for advice.

Breast Feeding: Bisacodyl may pass into breast milk. Consult your doctor for specific advice.

Infants and Children: Do not give this medicine to a child under 6 without your doctor's approval. Do not give this medicine to a child who refuses to have a bowel movement. It may result in a painful bowel movement, which will make the child resist even more.

Special Concerns: Remember that chronic use of bisacodyl or any laxative can lead to laxative dependence. You should consume adequate amounts of fiber in your diet, sources of which include bran or whole-grain cereals, fruit, and vegetables.

**OVERDOSE
Symptoms:** Weakness, increased sweating, lower abdominal pain, muscle cramps, irregular heartbeat.

What to Do: An overdose of bisacodyl is unlikely to be life-threatening. However, if someone takes a much larger dose than prescribed, seek medical assistance right away.

▼ INTERACTIONS

DRUG INTERACTIONS
Be sure to tell your doctor about any other drugs you are taking, especially antacids. Do not take an antacid within 2 hours of taking this drug.

FOOD INTERACTIONS
Do not drink milk within 2 hours of taking this drug.

DISEASE INTERACTIONS
Caution is advised when taking bisacodyl. Consult your doctor if you have very severe constipation, severe pain in the stomach or lower abdomen, cramping, bloating, nausea, or unexplained rectal bleeding. Failure to produce a bowel movement or the presence of rectal bleeding may indicate a serious medical condition.

SIDE EFFECTS

SERIOUS
Severe stomach pain, laxative dependence. Call your doctor immediately.

COMMON
Abdominal cramping, burning sensation in the rectum (with suppository), diarrhea.

LESS COMMON
Nausea; vomiting; muscle weakness; rectal pain, bleeding, burning, or itching. If you have a sudden change in bowel habits that lasts longer than 2 weeks, consult your doctor.

BISMUTH SUBSALICYLATE

Available in: Tablets, oral suspension
Available OTC? Yes   **As Generic?** Yes
Drug Class: Antidiarrheal/antacid

▼ USAGE INFORMATION

WHY IT'S PRESCRIBED
To treat heartburn, acid indigestion, diarrhea, and duodenal ulcers, and to help prevent traveler's diarrhea.

HOW IT WORKS
Bismuth subsalicylate stimulates the passage of fluid and electrolytes across the wall of the intestinal tract, and binds or neutralizes the toxins of some bacteria, rendering them nontoxic. It decreases intestinal inflammation and increases the activity of intestinal muscles and lining.

▼ DOSAGE GUIDELINES

RANGE AND FREQUENCY
Adults— For acid indigestion or mild diarrhea: 2 tablets or 2 tablespoons of liquid every 30 to 60 minutes, to a maximum of 16 doses daily of the regular-strength drug for no more than 2 days. Children ages 9 to 12— 1 tablet or 1 tablespoon every 30 to 60 minutes, to a maximum of 8 doses daily of the regular-strength drug for no more than 2 days. Children ages 6 to 9— 2 teaspoons every 30 to 60 minutes, to a maximum of 16 doses daily of the regular-strength drug for no more than 2 days. Children under age 3— Consult your pediatrician. Tablets are not recommended for children under the age of 9.

ONSET OF EFFECT
Within 30 to 60 minutes.

DURATION OF ACTION
Unknown.

DIETARY ADVICE
A mild diet is recommended when recovering from diarrhea. Bananas, rice, applesauce, and plain toast are good choices. Be sure to get plenty of fluids.

STORAGE
Store in a tightly sealed container away from heat and direct light. Keep liquid forms of bismuth subsalicylate refrigerated, but do not allow the medicine to freeze.

MISSED DOSE
Take it as soon as you remember. If it is near the time for the next dose, skip the missed dose and resume your regular dosage schedule. Do not double the next dose.

STOPPING THE DRUG
Take it as prescribed for the full treatment period. However, you may stop taking the drug if you feel better before the scheduled end of therapy.

PROLONGED USE
Prolonged use of this medicine may cause constipation. Consult your physician if relief is not achieved within two days.

▼ PRECAUTIONS

Over 60: Adverse reactions may be more likely and more severe in older patients.

Driving and Hazardous Work: Do not drive or engage in hazardous work until you determine how this medicine affects you.

Alcohol: Alcohol intake should be limited.

Pregnancy: Regular use of this medicine late in pregnancy may harm the fetus or cause delivery problems. Consult your doctor about taking it if you are pregnant or plan to become pregnant.

Breast Feeding: Bismuth subsalicylate passes into breast milk; avoid or discontinue use while nursing.

Infants and Children: Consult your doctor before giving this medicine to a child or teenager who has or is recovering from chicken pox or flu.

Special Concerns: Do not take bismuth subsalicylate if you are allergic to aspirin or another salicylate, an anticoagulant, or a medicine for diabetes or gout. Do not swallow tablets whole. They should be crushed, chewed, or allowed to dissolve in the mouth.

OVERDOSE
Symptoms: Seizures, confusion, rapid or deep breathing, hearing loss or ringing or buzzing in the ears, severe excitability or nervousness, severe drowsiness, loss of consciousness.

What to Do: Call your doctor, emergency medical services (EMS), or the nearest poison control center immediately.

▼ INTERACTIONS

DRUG INTERACTIONS
Consult your doctor for specific advice if you are taking anticoagulants, aspirin and other salicylates, oral diabe-tes medicine, heparin, pro-benecid, thrombolytic agents, oral tetracycline, or sulfinpyrazone.

FOOD INTERACTIONS
No known food interactions.

DISEASE INTERACTIONS
Caution is advised when using bismuth subsalicylate. Before taking this drug, tell your doctor if you have a history of allergies, diabetes, kidney disease, dehydration, stomach ulcers, dysentery, gout, or a bleeding problem.

SIDE EFFECTS

SERIOUS
Ringing in the ears. Call your doctor immediately.

COMMON
Black stools, darkening of the tongue.

LESS COMMON
Nausea, vomiting (with high doses), abdominal pain, increased sweating, muscle weakness, hearing loss, thirst, confusion, dizziness, vision problems, trouble breathing. Discontinue the medicine and call your physician right away.

BISOPROLOL FUMARATE

Available in: Tablets
Available OTC? No **As Generic?** No
Drug Class: Beta-blocker

▼ USAGE INFORMATION

WHY IT'S PRESCRIBED
To control hypertension (high blood pressure).

HOW IT WORKS
Bisoprolol slows the rate and force of contraction of the heart by blocking certain nerve impulses, thus reducing blood pressure.

▼ DOSAGE GUIDELINES

RANGE AND FREQUENCY
Starting dose is 5 mg once a day, or 2.5 mg once a day for those with kidney or liver problems. If necessary, it may be increased gradually to 20 mg once a day. Maximum dose is 20 mg per day.

ONSET OF EFFECT
Within 1 to 4 hours.

DURATION OF ACTION
24 hours.

DIETARY ADVICE
Take this drug at mealtime or immediately afterward.

STORAGE
Store in a tightly sealed container away from heat and direct light.

MISSED DOSE
If you miss a dose, take it as soon as you remember unless it is almost time for your next dose. In that case, skip the missed dose and return to your regular schedule. Do not double the next dose.

STOPPING THE DRUG
Do not stop taking this drug without consulting your doctor. It may be necessary to reduce the dosage gradually to prevent adverse effects.

PROLONGED USE
Ask your doctor about the need for medical examinations or laboratory studies of your heart, blood pressure, kidney function, and blood sugar. Monitor your blood pressure often.

▼ PRECAUTIONS

Over 60: Adverse reactions and side effects may be more common in older persons.

Driving and Hazardous Work: Determine how bisoprolol affects you before driving or engaging in any hazardous activities.

Alcohol: Drink in careful moderation if at all. Alcohol may interact with the drug and cause a dangerous drop in blood pressure.

Pregnancy: Be sure to notify your doctor promptly if you are pregnant or plan to become pregnant. Use bisoprolol during pregnancy only if the expected benefits outweigh the possible risks.

Breast Feeding: Bisoprolol passes into breast milk. Do not use it while you are breast feeding.

Infants and Children: Your pediatrician must determine the correct dose for a child.

Special Concerns: Prior to any dental or medical procedure or test, be sure to tell the doctor or dentist that you are taking bisoprolol. This drug may mask exercise-induced chest pain (angina). Ask your doctor for advice on a safe exercise program. Dress warmly in cold weather.

OVERDOSE
Symptoms: Asthmalike attacks (wheezing, breathlessness), very slow pulse, extreme shortness of breath associated with congestive heart failure.

What to Do: Call your doctor, emergency medical services (EMS), or the nearest poison control center immediately.

▼ INTERACTIONS

DRUG INTERACTIONS
Consult your doctor if you are taking any other blood pressure drug or beta-blocker. Be sure to check with your doctor before taking any over-the-counter medication, especially diet aids or cold preparations, as these may contain ingredients that can interact adversely with bisoprolol.

FOOD INTERACTIONS
None are expected, unless you are allergic to certain foods, as this medicine may cause allergic reactions to be more severe.

DISEASE INTERACTIONS
Bisoprolol should be used with caution in people with diabetes, especially insulin-dependent diabetes, since the drug may mask symptoms of hypoglycemia. Consult your doctor if you have a medical history of heart disease, asthma, blood vessel (vascular) disease, or thyroid disease. Diabetic patients must monitor their blood glucose (sugar) levels closely.

▤ SIDE EFFECTS ▤

SERIOUS
Shortness of breath, wheezing; irregular or slow heartbeat (50 beats per minute or less); pain or feelings of tightness or pressure in the chest; swelling of the ankles, feet, and lower legs; mental depression. If you experience such symptoms, stop taking bisoprolol and call your doctor immediately.

COMMON
Dizziness or lightheadedness, especially when rising suddenly to a standing position; rapid heartbeat or palpitations; decreased sexual ability; unusual fatigue, weakness, or drowsiness; insomnia.

LESS COMMON
Anxiety, irritability, nervousness; constipation; diarrhea; dry, sore eyes; itching; nausea or vomiting; nightmares or intensely vivid dreams; numbness, tingling, or other unusual sensations in the fingers, toes, or scalp.

BISOPROLOL FUMARATE/HYDROCHLOROTHIAZIDE

Available in: Tablets
Available OTC? No   **As Generic?** No
Drug Class: Beta-blocker/thiazide diuretic

▼ USAGE INFORMATION

WHY IT'S PRESCRIBED
To control hypertension (high blood pressure).

HOW IT WORKS
Bisoprolol, a beta-blocker, blocks certain nerve impulses to various parts of the body, which accounts for its many effects. For example, it reduces the rate and force of the heart's contractions (which helps to lower blood pressure), decreases the heart's oxygen requirement (which helps prevent angina) and helps stabilize heart rhythm. Hydrochlorothiazide (HCTZ), a diuretic, increases the excretion of salt and water in the urine. By reducing the overall amount of fluid in the body, diuretics reduce pressure within the blood vessels.

▼ DOSAGE GUIDELINES

RANGE AND FREQUENCY
Tablets contain 6.25 mg HCTZ and 2.5, 5, or 10 mg bisoprolol. Therapy is initiated with the lowest dose and may be increased at 1 week intervals to 2 tablets with 10 mg bisoprolol once a day.

ONSET OF EFFECT
Within 1 to 4 hours.

DURATION OF ACTION
Up to 24 hours.

DIETARY ADVICE
No special restrictions.

STORAGE
Store in a tightly sealed container away from heat, moisture, and direct light.

MISSED DOSE
If you miss a dose on one day, resume your regular dosage schedule the next day. Do not double the next dose.

STOPPING THE DRUG
The decision to stop taking the drug should be made in consultation with your physician. Do not stop taking this drug abruptly; your doctor will gradually decrease your dose before stopping completely.

PROLONGED USE
Bisoprolol/hydrochlorothi-azide can control high blood pressure, but cannot cure it. Lifelong therapy may be necessary. See your doctor regularly for tests and examinations if you must take this drug for a prolonged period of time.

▼ PRECAUTIONS

Over 60: Adverse reactions, especially dizziness, lightheadedness, and reduced tolerance to cold, may be more likely and more severe in older patients.

Driving and Hazardous Work: Do not drive or engage in hazardous work until you determine how the medicine affects you.

Alcohol: Drink in careful moderation if at all. Alcohol may interact with the bisoprolol component and cause a dangerous drop in blood pressure.

Pregnancy: Beta-blockers and thiazide diuretics may cause problems during pregnancy. Before taking this medication, tell your doctor if you are pregnant or plan to become pregnant.

Breast Feeding: This drug passes into breast milk; caution is advised. Consult your doctor for specific advice.

Infants and Children: Adequate studies have not been done on the use of this drug in children. No special problems are expected. Consult your pediatrician for advice.

Special Concerns: In addition to taking this medicine, follow your doctor's instructions on weight control and diet for reduction of blood pressure.

OVERDOSE
Symptoms: Slow heartbeat, severe dizziness or fainting, difficulty breathing, bluish-colored fingernails or palms of hands, seizures.

What to Do: Call your doctor, emergency medical services (EMS), or the nearest poison control center immediately.

▼ INTERACTIONS

DRUG INTERACTIONS
Do not take with other beta-blockers. Consult your doctor for specific advice if you are taking any other antihypertensive medications, oral diabetes medications, insulin, digitalis drugs, cholestyramine, colestipol, clonidine, lithium, nonsteroidal anti-inflammatory drugs, MAO inhibitors, rifampin, narcotic analgesics, or skeletal muscle relaxants.

FOOD INTERACTIONS
Avoid foods high in sodium.

DISEASE INTERACTIONS
Do not use if you have a history of bronchospasm. Consult your doctor if you have any of the following: bronchial asthma, emphysema, slow heartbeat, heart or blood vessel disease, diabetes mellitus, congestive heart failure, gout, kidney disease, liver disease, depression, parathyroid disease, or an overactive thyroid (hyperthyroidism).

SIDE EFFECTS

SERIOUS
Slow heartbeat, difficulty breathing, mental depression, cold hands and feet, swelling of ankles, feet, or lower legs. Call your doctor immediately.

COMMON
Dizziness or lightheadedness, decreased sexual ability, drowsiness, insomnia, fatigue, diarrhea.

LESS COMMON
Anxiety, loss of appetite, upset stomach, nervousness or excitability, constipation, numbness and tingling in the fingers and toes, stuffy nose.

BITOLTEROL MESYLATE

Available in: Aerosol inhaler
Available OTC? No **As Generic?** No
Drug Class: Bronchodilator/sympathomimetic

▼ USAGE INFORMATION

WHY IT'S PRESCRIBED
Bitolterol is used to dilate air passages in the lungs that have become narrowed as a result of disease or inflammation. It is used in the treatment of asthma and chronic obstructive pulmonary disease (COPD).

HOW IT WORKS
Bitolterol widens constricted airways in the lungs by relaxing the smooth muscles that surround the bronchial passages.

▼ DOSAGE GUIDELINES

RANGE AND FREQUENCY
To treat bronchial asthma and bronchospasm; use it when needed to relieve breathing difficulty: 1 or 2 inhalations at an interval of 1 to 3 minutes, with a third inhalation 2 to 3 minutes later if needed. To prevent bronchospasm: Usually 2 inhalations every 8 hours, with a maximum dose of 2 inhalations every 4 hours or 3 inhalations every 6 hours; actual dosage and administration schedule must be determined by a doctor for each patient. Specific written directions from your doctor should be followed carefully. Rinse your mouth after each dose. Rinse and dry inhaler after each use.

ONSET OF EFFECT
Within 5 minutes.

DURATION OF ACTION
From 5 to 8 hours.

DIETARY ADVICE
Excessive intake of coffee or other caffeine-containing beverages should be avoided.

STORAGE
Store in a tightly sealed container away from heat and direct light.

MISSED DOSE
Skip the missed dose and resume your regular dosage schedule. Do not double the next dose.

SIDE EFFECTS

SERIOUS
This drug may become ineffective if used too often, resulting in more-severe breathing difficulty that does not improve. Signs include persistent wheezing, coughing, or shortness of breath; confusion; bluish color to lips or fingernails; inability to speak. Other side effects include chest pain or heaviness; irregular, racing, fluttering, or pounding heartbeat; lightheadedness; fainting; severe weakness; severe headache.

COMMON
Changes in blood pressure causing headache, blurred vision, weakness.

LESS COMMON
Nervousness, throat irritation, nausea.

STOPPING THE DRUG
It may not be necessary to finish the recommended course of therapy. Consult your doctor.

PROLONGED USE
Therapy may require months or years. Excessive use may result in temporary loss of effectiveness.

▼ PRECAUTIONS

Over 60: Adverse reactions may be more likely and more severe in older patients.

Driving and Hazardous Work: Be cautious about driving or doing hazardous work until you determine if excessive nervousness or dizziness occurs.

Alcohol: No special precautions are necessary.

Pregnancy: Adequate studies have not been done; the benefits must be weighed against potential risks. Consult your doctor for specific advice.

Breast Feeding: Bitolterol can pass into breast milk; breast feeding should be avoided while taking bitolterol.

Infants and Children: Safety and effectiveness of bitolterol for children under the age of 12 have not been established.

Special Concerns: Call your doctor if you cannot breathe properly 1 hour after using bitolterol or if your breathing problem worsens. Do not let the spray from the inhaler get in your eyes. Discontinue use and contact your doctor if you notice an unusual smell or taste when using this product. Use of this medicine is a disqualification for piloting an aircraft.

OVERDOSE
Symptoms: Tremor, nausea, vomiting, rapid or irregular pulse.

What to Do: Call your doctor immediately.

▼ INTERACTIONS

DRUG INTERACTIONS
Use of MAO inhibitors may cause an excessive increase in blood pressure and heart stimulation. If you are also using a steroid inhaler, take bitolterol first and then wait about 15 minutes before using the steroid inhaler. This allows bitolterol to open air passages, increasing the effectiveness of the steroid.

FOOD INTERACTIONS
Excessive intake of coffee or other caffeine-containing beverages should be avoided.

DISEASE INTERACTIONS
Before taking bitolterol, consult your doctor if you have a circulatory disorder, heart disease, diabetes, epilepsy, or an overactive thyroid.

BRIMONIDINE TARTRATE

BRAND NAME

Alphagan

Available in: Ophthalmic solution
Available OTC? No   **As Generic?** No
Drug Class: Antiglaucoma agent

▼ USAGE INFORMATION

WHY IT'S PRESCRIBED
To treat glaucoma.

HOW IT WORKS
Glaucoma, a sight-threatening disorder, occurs when aqueous humor (fluid inside the eye) cannot drain properly, causing increased pressure within the eyeball (intraocular pressure). Increased eye pressure can damage the optic nerve and lead to a gradually progressive loss of vision. Brimonidine decreases the production of aqueous humor and promotes its outflow, thereby reducing intraocular pressure.

▼ DOSAGE GUIDELINES

RANGE AND FREQUENCY
1 drop of brimonidine in each eye 3 times a day at 8-hour intervals.

ONSET OF EFFECT
Within 60 minutes.

DURATION OF ACTION
8 hours or more.

DIETARY ADVICE
No special restrictions.

STORAGE
Store in a tightly sealed container away from heat, moisture, and direct light. Do not allow the medicine to freeze.

MISSED DOSE
Apply it as soon as you remember. If it is near the time for the next dose, skip the missed dose and resume your regular dosage schedule. Do not double the next dose.

STOPPING THE DRUG
The decision to stop using the drug should be made by your doctor.

PROLONGED USE
You should see your doctor regularly for tests and examinations as part of glaucoma follow-up if you take this drug for a prolonged period.

▼ PRECAUTIONS

Over 60: Adverse reactions may be more likely and more severe in older patients.

Driving and Hazardous Work: Do not drive or engage in hazardous work until you determine how the drug affects your vision.

Alcohol: Use alcohol with caution.

Pregnancy: In animal studies, brimonidine caused impaired fetal circulation. Human studies have not been done. Before you take brimonidine, tell your doctor if you are pregnant or are planning to become pregnant.

Breast Feeding: Brimonidine may pass into breast milk; caution is advised. Consult your doctor for advice.

Infants and Children: The safety and effectiveness of brimonidine in infants and children have not been established.

Special Concerns: To use the eye drops, first wash your hands. Tilt your head back. Gently apply pressure to the inside corner of the eyelid and with the index finger of the same hand, pull downward on the lower eyelid to make a space. Drop the medicine into this space and close your eye. Apply pressure for 1 or 2 minutes while keeping the eye closed without blinking. Then wash your hands again. Make sure the tip of the dropper does not touch your eye, finger, or any other surface. Bromonidine may make your eyes more sensitive to sunlight. If this occurs, wear sunglasses or avoid bright light as comfort dictates.

OVERDOSE
Symptoms: No specific ones have been reported.

What to Do: An overdose of brimonidine is unlikely to be life-threatening. However, if someone takes a much larger dose than prescribed or accidentally ingests the medicine, call your doctor, emergency medical services (EMS), or the nearest poison control center immediately.

▼ INTERACTIONS

DRUG INTERACTIONS
Consult your doctor for advice if you are taking MAO inhibitors, tricyclic antidepressants, central nervous system depressants, beta-blockers, antihypertensives, or digitalis drugs (such as digoxin).

FOOD INTERACTIONS
No known food interactions.

DISEASE INTERACTIONS
Caution is advised when taking brimonidine. Consult your doctor if you have cardiovascular disease, kidney disease, liver disease, depression, cerebral or coronary insufficiency, Raynaud's phenomenon, orthostatic hypotension, or thromboangiitis obliterans.

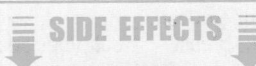
SIDE EFFECTS

SERIOUS
Fainting. Call your doctor immediately.

COMMON
Burning or stinging of the eyes, fatigue, dry mouth, eye discomfort, drowsiness.

LESS COMMON
Excess tear production, redness of eyes or inner lining of the eyelids, headache, swelling of eye or eyelid, eye ache or pain, blurring or other changes in vision, dizziness, mental depression, insomnia, muscle pain or weakness, nausea, increased blood pressure, vomiting, anxiety, pounding heartbeat, change in taste, crusting in corner of eye or on eyelid, discoloration of eyeball, paleness of inner lining of eyelid, dry eyes, sensitivity of eyes to light.

BRINZOLAMIDE

Available in: Ophthalmic suspension
Available OTC? No **As Generic?** No
Drug Class: Antiglaucoma agent; carbonic anhydrase inhibitor

▼ USAGE INFORMATION

WHY IT'S PRESCRIBED
To treat glaucoma or ocular hypertension (a glaucoma-like condition).

HOW IT WORKS
Glaucoma and ocular hypertension, both sight-threatening disorders, occur when poor drainage of aqueous humor (the fluid inside the front part of the eye) increases the pressure within the eyeball (known as intraocular pressure). Increased intraocular pressure can damage the optic nerve and lead to a gradual loss of vision. By inhibiting the activity of the enzyme carbonic anhydrase, brinzolamide decreases the production of aqueous humor, and so reduces intraocular pressure.

▼ DOSAGE GUIDELINES

RANGE AND FREQUENCY
Adults and teenagers:
1 drop in affected eye(s)
3 times per day.

ONSET OF EFFECT
Unknown.

DURATION OF ACTION
Unknown.

DIETARY ADVICE
No special restrictions.

STORAGE
Store in a tightly sealed container away from heat, moisture, and direct light. Do not refrigerate or allow it to freeze.

MISSED DOSE
Apply it as soon as you remember. If it is near the time for the next dose, skip the missed dose and resume your regular dosage schedule. Do not double the next dose.

STOPPING THE DRUG
The decision to stop using the drug should be made by your doctor.

PROLONGED USE
Schedule regular eye examinations with your doctor to be sure the drug is controlling the glaucoma or ocular hypertension.

▼ PRECAUTIONS

Over 60: No special problems are expected.

Driving and Hazardous Work: Do not drive or engage in hazardous work until you determine how the medicine affects your vision.

Alcohol: No special precautions are necessary.

Pregnancy: One animal study found that very high doses of this drug caused birth defects. Human studies have not been done. Before using this medicine, tell your doctor if you are pregnant or plan to become pregnant.

Breast Feeding: It is not known whether brinzolamide passes into breast milk; caution is advised. Consult your doctor for specific advice about whether to use a different medicine or to stop breast feeding.

Infants and Children: Safety and dosage guidelines for children have not been established. Brinzolamide should be given to infants and children only under close medical supervision.

Special Concerns: To use the eye drops, first wash your hands. Tilt your head back. Gently apply pressure to the inside corner of the eyelid and with the index finger of the same hand, pull downward on the lower eyelid to make a space. Drop the medicine into this space and close your eye. Apply pressure for 1 or 2 minutes while keeping the eye closed without blinking. Then wash your hands again. Make sure that the tip of the dropper does not touch your eye, finger, or any other surface.

OVERDOSE

Symptoms: No specific ones have been reported.

What to Do: An overdose of brinzolamide is unlikely to be life-threatening. If a large volume enters the eye, flush with water. If someone accidentally ingests the medicine, call your doctor, emergency medical services (EMS), or the nearest poison control center immediately.

▼ INTERACTIONS

DRUG INTERACTIONS
Wait 10 minutes before administering any other eye medicine. Brinzolamide should not be used in conjunction with oral carbonic anhydrase inhibitors. People allergic to sulfa-type drugs should not use brinzolamide.

FOOD INTERACTIONS
No known food interactions.

DISEASE INTERACTIONS
Do not use this medication if you have severe kidney impairment. Use with caution if you have liver disease.

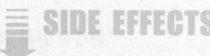

≡ SIDE EFFECTS ≡

SERIOUS
Severe generalized reactions involving the skin, liver, and blood cells. Discontinue using the medication and call your doctor immediately if signs of serious reaction occur.

COMMON
Burning, stinging, or discomfort in the eye or blurred vision when drug is administered; bitter taste in mouth.

LESS COMMON
Eye pain, severe or continued tearing, nausea.

BROMOCRIPTINE MESYLATE

BRAND NAME
Parlodel

Available in: Tablets, capsules
Available OTC? No **As Generic?** Yes
Drug Class: Ergot alkaloid

▼ USAGE INFORMATION

WHY IT'S PRESCRIBED
To treat hyperprolactinemia, a disorder caused by overproduction of the hormone prolactin. Hyperprolactinemia may occur by itself or in association with a tumor (prolactinoma) in the pituitary gland. The disorder causes abnormal production and persistent leakage of breast milk (in either men or women), infertility and cessation of menstrual periods in women, and testicular shrinkage and impotence in men. In some cases bromocriptine may be used to treat acromegaly (overproduction of growth hormone, causing enlargement of the hands, feet, jawbone, and internal organs). It is also used to treat Parkinson's disease.

HOW IT WORKS
Bromocriptine blocks the pituitary from releasing the hormone prolactin, which is involved in the regulation of the menstrual cycle, reproduction, and milk production.

Similarly, it blocks the pituitary from releasing growth hormone. The drug activates certain chemical receptor sites in brain cells to reduce Parkinson's symptoms.

▼ DOSAGE GUIDELINES

RANGE AND FREQUENCY
For hyperprolactinemia: Starting with 1.25 to 2.5 mg a day, the dose is increased by 1.25 mg a day at 3- to 7-day intervals until the desired therapeutic effect is achieved. Maintenance dose is 1.25 to 15 mg in divided doses, 2 or 3 times a day. For acromegaly: 1.25 to 30 mg a day in divided doses, 2 or 3 times a day. For Parkinson's disease: Starting with 1.25 to 2.5 mg a day, the dose is increased by 2.5 mg a day at 14- to 28-day intervals, to a maximum of 100 mg a day in divided doses, 2 or 3 times a day.

ONSET OF EFFECT
From 30 to 90 minutes. Full effects become apparent after a few weeks of therapy.

DURATION OF ACTION
For hyperprolactinemia and acromegaly: 8 hours. For Parkinson's disease: 12 to 18 hours.

DIETARY ADVICE
For best results, bromocriptine should be taken with food or milk.

STORAGE
Store in a dry place away from heat and direct light. Discard the medicine if it becomes outdated.

MISSED DOSE
If you miss a dose, take it if you remember within 2 hours. After that, wait for the next dose and return to your regular schedule. Do not double the next dose.

STOPPING THE DRUG
Complete the prescribed dose even though symptoms diminish or disappear. Consult your doctor before discontinuing this drug.

PROLONGED USE
Prolonged use at doses greater than 50 mg per day may cause uncontrolled movements of face, mouth, tongue, arms, or legs (a condition known as tardive dyskinesia). Consult your doctor if such symptoms occur.

▼ PRECAUTIONS

Over 60: Adverse reactions and side effects may be more common in older persons.

Driving and Hazardous Work: Do not drive or engage in hazardous work until you determine how bromocriptine affects you.

Alcohol: Bromocriptine reduces the body's tolerance to alcohol.

Pregnancy: If you are pregnant or plan to become pregnant, tell your doctor before taking this drug.

Breast Feeding: Bromocriptine should not be used when nursing because it reduces breast milk production.

Infants and Children: Not recommended for anyone under the age of 15.

OVERDOSE
Symptoms: Severe dizziness and weakness, nausea, and vomiting.

What to Do: Call your doctor immediately.

▼ INTERACTIONS

DRUG INTERACTIONS
Consult your doctor for specific advice if you are taking any of the following drugs that may interact with bromocriptine: blood pressure medication, an oral contraceptive, erythromycin, a phenothiazine, an MAO inhibitor, progestin, levodopa, or a rauwolfia alkaloid.

FOOD INTERACTIONS
None are expected.

DISEASE INTERACTIONS
Consult your doctor if you have any of the following: diabetes, epilepsy, heart disease, lung disease, a peptic ulcer, or high blood pressure. Also tell your doctor if you plan to have surgery, including dental surgery, within 2 months.

≡ SIDE EFFECTS ≡

SERIOUS
Seizures, chest pain, severe nausea and vomiting, headache and blurred vision caused by high blood pressure, wet cough and shortness of breath caused by fluid in the lungs. Consult your doctor immediately.

COMMON
Dizziness, weakness, and fainting caused by low blood pressure; nasal congestion and headache; abdominal cramping or pain.

LESS COMMON
Confusion, fatigue, nervousness, depression, ringing in the ears, dry mouth, blurred vision, hallucinations, hair loss, anemia, impotence, constipation, or diarrhea.

BROMPHENIRAMINE MALEATE

Available in: Capsules, tablets, extended-release tablets, elixir, injection
Available OTC? Yes   **As Generic?** Yes
Drug Class: Antihistamine

▼ USAGE INFORMATION

WHY IT'S PRESCRIBED
To prevent or relieve symptoms of hay fever, other allergies, itching skin, or hives.

HOW IT WORKS
Brompheniramine blocks the effects of histamine, a substance in the body that causes swelling, itching, sneezing, watery eyes, hives, and other symptoms of allergic reaction.

▼ DOSAGE GUIDELINES

RANGE AND FREQUENCY
Capsules, tablets, elixir— Adults and teenagers: 4 mg every 4 to 6 hours. Children ages 6 to 12: 2 mg every 4 to 6 hours. Children ages 2 to 6: 1 mg every 4 to 6 hours. Extended-release tablets— Adults: 8 mg every 8 to 12 hours, or 12 mg every 12 hours. Children age 6 and older: 8 or 12 mg every 12 hours. Injection— Adults and teenagers: 10 mg under the skin or into a vein or muscle every 8 to 12 hours. Children younger than

age 12: 0.125 mg per 2.2 lbs (1 kg) of body weight, under the skin or into a vein or muscle 3 or 4 times a day.

ONSET OF EFFECT
15 to 60 minutes.

DURATION OF ACTION
3 to 6 hours for regular form; 8 to 12 for extended-release tablets.

DIETARY ADVICE
Take it with food or milk to minimize stomach upset.

STORAGE
Store in a tightly sealed container away from heat and direct light.

MISSED DOSE
Take it as soon as you remember. If it is near the time for the next dose, skip the missed dose and resume your regular dosage schedule. Do not double the next dose.

STOPPING THE DRUG
Take as prescribed for the full treatment period. However, you may stop if you feel better before the scheduled end of therapy, or take as needed.

PROLONGED USE
No special concerns.

▼ PRECAUTIONS

Over 60: Older persons are more sensitive to antihistamine side effects, particularly confusion, dizziness, drowsiness, restlessness, irritability, nightmares, and dry mouth, nose, and throat.

Driving and Hazardous Work: Brompheniramine can make you feel tired and lessen your concentration. Avoid driving or engaging in hazardous work until you determine how the drug affects you.

Alcohol: Alcohol increases the likelihood and the severity of side effects like drowsiness and confusion.

Pregnancy: Studies in animals suggest that brompheniramine has no adverse effect on fetal development, but human studies have not been done. Before taking this drug, tell your doctor if you are pregnant or are planning to become pregnant.

Breast Feeding: Brompheniramine passes into breast milk; avoid or discontinue use while breast feeding.

Infants and Children: Brompheniramine should be given to children age 6 and under only as directed by a pediatrician.

Special Concerns: Do not break, crush, or chew the capsules or the extended-release tablets.

OVERDOSE
Symptoms: Seizures, loss of consciousness, hallucinations, severe drowsiness.

What to Do: The patient should be made to vomit immediately, using ipecac syrup. If he or she is unconscious, the patient should be taken to a hospital emergency room immediately.

▼ INTERACTIONS

DRUG INTERACTIONS
MAO inhibitors can increase the sedative effects of brompheniramine. Central nervous system depressants such as alcohol, sedatives, or narcotics should be taken only if approved by a doctor.

FOOD INTERACTIONS
No known food interactions.

DISEASE INTERACTIONS
Before taking brompheniramine, consult your doctor if you wear contact lenses or you have glaucoma, prostate enlargement, difficulty with urination, or dryness of the mouth or eyes.

 SIDE EFFECTS

SERIOUS
Bleeding problems; small, red pinpoints on the skin; fever; extreme fatigue; bleeding ulcers in the rectum, mouth, and vagina; reduced white blood cell count (rare).

COMMON
Drowsiness; unusual excitability; dry mouth, nose, or throat. Symptoms of drowsiness tend to subside after a few days' use as your body adjusts to the drug.

LESS COMMON
Vision changes, loss of appetite, dizziness, painful or difficult urination, less tolerance for contact lenses.

BUDESONIDE

Available in: Nasal inhalant, oral inhalation, inhalation powder
Available OTC? No   **As Generic?** No
Drug Class: Respiratory corticosteroid

▼ USAGE INFORMATION

WHY IT'S PRESCRIBED
To treat the symptoms of allergic rhinitis (seasonal and perennial allergies, such as hay fever) and to prevent recurrence of nasal polyps after surgical removal.

HOW IT WORKS
Respiratory corticosteroids such as budesonide primarily reduce or prevent inflammation of the lining of the airways, reduce the allergic response to inhaled allergens, and inhibit the secretion of mucus within the airways.

▼ DOSAGE GUIDELINES

RANGE AND FREQUENCY
Nasal inhalant: 2 sprays (32 micrograms [mcg] each) in each nostril in the morning and evening or 4 sprays in each nostril in the morning. Oral inhalation: 200 to 800 mcg (1 to 4 inhalations), 2 times a day. Highest dose for children is 400 mcg (2 inhalations), 2 times a day. The dose may be increased or decreased as determined by your doctor, based on the patient's response.

ONSET OF EFFECT
Usually within several days; it may take 3 weeks for the full effect to occur.

DURATION OF ACTION
Up to 12 hours.

DIETARY ADVICE
Budesonide can be taken without regard to diet.

STORAGE
Store in a dry place away from heat and light, out of the reach of children.

MISSED DOSE
Take the missed dose if you remember within an hour. Otherwise, skip the missed dose and return to your regular schedule. Do not double the next dose.

STOPPING THE DRUG
Nasal inhalant: No problems expected. Oral inhalation: Do not discontinue without consulting your doctor. Gradual reduction in dosage may be required.

PROLONGED USE
Consult with your doctor about the need for periodic physical examinations and laboratory tests.

▼ PRECAUTIONS

Over 60: No special problems are expected.

Driving and Hazardous Work: Budesonide should not affect your ability to perform such tasks safely.

Alcohol: No special precautions are necessary.

Pregnancy: Nasal or inhaled steroids have not been reported to cause birth defects if taken during pregnancy. Before using such drugs, tell your doctor if you are pregnant or plan to become pregnant.

Breast Feeding: This drug may pass into breast milk. Consult your doctor about use of either form during breast feeding.

Infants and Children: Nasal form: Should be used only under close medical supervision. Oral form: Large doses may make children more susceptible to infectious disease. Long-term use may affect the adrenal glands.

Special Concerns: Inhaled steroids will not help an asthma attack in progress. Inhaled steroids can lower resistance to yeast infections of the mouth, throat, or voice box. To prevent yeast infections, gargle or rinse your mouth with water after each use; do not swallow the water. Know how to use the inhalant properly; read and follow the directions that come with the device. Before you have surgery, tell the doctor or dentist that you are using a steroid.

OVERDOSE
Symptoms: No specific symptoms.

What to Do: Call your doctor, emergency medical services (EMS), or the nearest poison control center if you have any reason to suspect an overdose.

▼ INTERACTIONS

DRUG INTERACTIONS
Consult your doctor for specific advice if you are taking systemic corticosteroids, other inhaled corticosteroids, or any medications that suppress the immune system.

FOOD INTERACTIONS
No known food interactions.

DISEASE INTERACTIONS
Consult your doctor if you have any other medical problem, particularly glaucoma, a herpes infection of the eye, a history of tuberculosis, liver disease, an underactive thyroid, or osteoporosis.

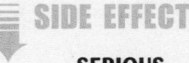
SIDE EFFECTS

SERIOUS
No serious side effects are associated with budesonide.

COMMON
Nasal inhalant: Nosebleeds or bloody nasal secretions, nasal burning or irritation, sore throat. Oral inhalation: Sore throat, white patches in mouth or throat, hoarseness.

LESS COMMON
Eye pain, watering eyes, gradual decrease of vision, stomach pain and digestive disturbances.

BUMETANIDE

Available in: Tablets, injection
Available OTC? No   **As Generic?** Yes
Drug Class: Loop diuretic

▼ USAGE INFORMATION

WHY IT'S PRESCRIBED
To reduce the accumulation of fluid (containing salts and water) that leads to edema (swelling) and breathlessness in patients with heart disease, cirrhosis of the liver, and kidney disease. Bumetanide may also be used to help control high blood levels of potassium.

HOW IT WORKS
Loop diuretics work on a specific portion of the kidney (the loop of Henle) to increase the excretion of both water and sodium in the urine.

▼ DOSAGE GUIDELINES

RANGE AND FREQUENCY
0.5 to 6 mg per day, usually taken in the morning; may be increased to 2 to 3 doses a day, as needed.

ONSET OF EFFECT
This drug begins eliminating excess water within 1 to 2 hours.

DURATION OF ACTION
Up to 4 hours.

DIETARY ADVICE
Bumetanide can be taken with or after meals to reduce stomach irritation.

STORAGE
Store in a tightly sealed container away from heat and direct light.

MISSED DOSE
If you miss a dose, take it as soon as you remember unless it is almost time for the next dose. In that case, skip the missed dose and return to your regular schedule. Do not double the next dose.

STOPPING THE DRUG
Take it as prescribed for the full treatment period, even if you begin to feel better before the scheduled end of therapy. The decision to stop taking the drug should be made by your doctor.

PROLONGED USE
Prolonged use of bumetanide requires regular examinations by your doctor, since it may lead to imbalances of sodium, potassium, magnesium, and body fluid.

▼ PRECAUTIONS

Over 60: No special problems are expected.

Driving and Hazardous Work: No special precautions are necessary.

Alcohol: No special precautions are necessary.

Pregnancy: Adequate studies of using this drug during pregnancy have not been done. Before taking this drug, tell your doctor if you are pregnant or plan to become pregnant. If diuretic treatment is warranted, other drugs are preferred.

Breast Feeding: This drug may pass into breast milk. Consult your doctor about its use while nursing.

Infants and Children: This drug is not generally prescribed for children. Its safety and effectiveness for anyone under the age of 18 have not been established.

Special Concerns: You may have to take a potassium supplement or consume foods or fluids high in potassium while taking this drug. To prevent disruption of sleep, avoid taking this drug in the evening.

OVERDOSE
Symptoms: Severe fatigue, weakness, lethargy, confusion, muscle cramps, nausea, vomiting, weak and rapid pulse, loss of consciousness.

What to Do: Call your doctor, emergency medical services (EMS), or the nearest poison control center immediately.

▼ INTERACTIONS

DRUG INTERACTIONS
Consult your doctor about any other drugs you are taking, particularly antibiotics, other blood pressure medications (especially ACE inhibitors), analgesics (pain relievers), lithium, cortisone-related drugs, digitalis drugs, or any nonsteroidal anti-inflammatory drug (NSAID).

FOOD INTERACTIONS
No food interactions have been documented.

DISEASE INTERACTIONS
Caution is advised when taking bumetanide. Consult your doctor if you have any of the following: diabetes, gout, a hearing problem, or a recent heart attack.

≣ SIDE EFFECTS ≣
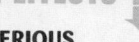

SERIOUS
Rapid or irregular heartbeat, dry mouth, increased thirst, mood or mental changes, muscle cramps or pain, nausea or vomiting, unusual fatigue, black and tarry stools, buzzing or ringing in ears, hearing loss, skin rash. Call your doctor immediately.

COMMON
Muscle cramps. Fluid depletion can cause dizziness when the patient rises from a sitting or lying position, as well as thirst and constipation. Minor potassium depletion can cause mild weakness and rapid or irregular heartbeat.

LESS COMMON
Gout, increased blood sugar (glucose) levels, hearing loss.

BUPROPION HYDROCHLORIDE

BRAND NAMES

Wellbutrin, Wellbutrin-SR (for depression), Zyban (for smoking cessation)

Available in: Tablets, extended-release tablets
Available OTC? No   **As Generic?** No
Drug Class: Antidepressant/smoking deterrent

▼ USAGE INFORMATION

WHY IT'S PRESCRIBED
To relieve symptoms of major depression. Bupropion is also used as a nicotine-free agent to help stop smoking. It should be used as a part of a comprehensive smoking cessation program carried out under the supervision of your doctor.

HOW IT WORKS
While the exact mechanism of action of bupropion is not known, it appears to help balance the levels of neurotransmitters (brain chemicals) that are thought to be linked to mood, emotions, and mental state. Unlike other smoking cessation medications, bupropion does not contain nicotine. It is believed that bupropion's effects on brain chemistry help to curb the desire for nicotine and enhance the patient's ability to abstain from smoking.

▼ DOSAGE GUIDELINES

RANGE AND FREQUENCY
Depression (Wellbutrin)— Adults: To start, 100 mg twice a day. Dosage may be increased to 450 mg a day. No more than 150 mg should be taken within 4 hours. Older adults: To start, 75 or 100 mg twice a day. Children: Dosages must be determined by your doctor. Smoking cessation (Zyban)— Adults: For the first 3 days of treatment, 150 mg a day. Dosage may then be increased to 150 mg, 2 times a day. The doses should be taken at least 8 hours apart. Do not take more than 300 mg per day. You should not stop smoking until you have been taking Zyban for 1 week. Treatment generally lasts 7 to 12 weeks.

ONSET OF EFFECT
1 to 3 weeks.

DURATION OF ACTION
Unknown.

DIETARY ADVICE
Bupropion can be taken with food to reduce stomach irritation. The tablet should be swallowed whole, because it has a bitter taste and can produce an unpleasant numbing sensation inside of the mouth.

STORAGE
Store in a tightly sealed container away from heat, moisture, and direct light.

MISSED DOSE
Take it as soon as you remember, unless your next scheduled dose is within the next 4 hours (8 hours for smoking cessation). If so, do not take the missed dose. Take your next scheduled dose at the proper time and resume your regular dosage schedule. Do not double the next dose.

STOPPING THE DRUG
Depression: Take it as prescribed for the full treatment period, even if you begin to feel better before the scheduled end of therapy. Discontinuing the drug abruptly may produce unpleasant withdrawal symptoms. Dosage should be reduced gradually according to your doctor's instructions. The decision to stop taking the drug should be made in consultation with your doctor. Smoking cessation: If you have not made significant progress toward abstinence by the end of the seventh week of treatment, consult your doctor. Treatment should probably be discontinued. You do not need to gradually decrease the dose before stopping.

PROLONGED USE
Depression: The usual course of therapy lasts 6 months to 1 year; some patients benefit from additional therapy. Smoking cessation: Treatment generally lasts 7 to 12 weeks.

▼ PRECAUTIONS

Over 60: Dosage may be decreased because of age-related decline in liver or kidney function.

Driving and Hazardous Work: Use caution until you determine how the medication affects you. Drowsiness or lightheadedness can occur.

Alcohol: Alcohol increases the risk of seizures. It is recommended to abstain from alcohol or to drink very little while taking bupropion. If you regularly drink a lot of alcohol and then suddenly stop, this may also increase your chance of having a seizure; gradual tapering of alcohol is recommended.

Pregnancy: Bupropion has not caused birth defects in animals. Adequate human studies have not been done. Bupropion is not recommended while you are pregnant. Before taking it, tell your doctor if you are pregnant or plan to become pregnant.

Breast Feeding: Bupropion passes into breast milk; avoid or discontinue using it while nursing.

Infants and Children: Adequate studies in children have not been done. Bupropion is not recommended for use by children under age 18.

≡ SIDE EFFECTS ≡

SERIOUS
When treating depression: Hallucinations, heartbeat irregularities, confusion, skin rash, insomnia, severe headache, excitement or agitation, seizures. Call your doctor immediately. Smoking cessation: None reported.

COMMON
When treating depression: Nausea or vomiting, constipation, unusual weight loss, dry mouth, loss of appetite, dizziness, increased sweating, trembling or shaking. Smoking cessation: Dry mouth, insomnia.

LESS COMMON
When treating depression: Fever or chills, concentration difficulties, drowsiness, fatigue, change in or blurred vision, unusual feeling of euphoria, hostility or anger. Smoking cessation: Mild rash, tremor.

Special Concerns: This is a potentially dangerous drug, especially if taken in excess. Antidepressants should not be within easy reach of suicidal patients. To prevent insomnia, take the last dose several hours before bedtime. When taking bupropion for smoking cessation, it is advised to continue smoking through the first week of treatment. Set a target date to stop smoking no later than the second week of therapy. Continuing to smoke beyond the designated date reduces your chances of successfully quitting. You may use a nicotine transdermal patch (see Nicotine) while taking Zyban, but consult your doctor before initiating such therapy. The combination of nicotine and bupropion increases the risk of hypertension; blood pressure should be monitored regularly throughout treatment. Zyban should be regarded as but one part of a comprehensive treatment program that includes counseling, socal support, and regular contact with your doctor. The goal of therapy with Zyban is complete abstinence from cigarettes. Do not chew, divide, or crush the tablets or extended-release tablets.

OVERDOSE

Symptoms: Hallucinations, seizures, rapid heartbeat, chest pain, breathing difficulty, loss of consciousness. Few cases of overdose associated with treatment for smoking cessation have been reported. Some of the symptoms experienced include vomiting, blurred vision, light-headedness, confusion, lethargy, nausea, jitteriness, hallucinations, drowsiness, and seizures.

What to Do: Call your doctor, emergency medical services (EMS), or the nearest poison control center immediately.

▼ INTERACTIONS

DRUG INTERACTIONS

Bupropion should not be taken if you are taking other medicines containing bupropion or within 14 days of taking an MAO inhibitor. Consult your doctor for advice if you are taking loxapine, tricyclic antidepressants, phenothiazines, clozapine, molindone, fluoxetine, thioxanthenes, haloperidol, lithium, trazodone, maprotiline, levodopa, or theophylline.

FOOD INTERACTIONS

No known food interactions.

DISEASE INTERACTIONS

Bupropion should not be taken if you have a history of seizures, anorexia nervosa, or bulimia. Caution is advised when taking bupropion. Consult your doctor if you have any of the following: a tumor of the brain or spinal cord, heart disease, or head injury. Since the liver and kidneys work together to remove bupropion from the body, a lower dose may be prescribed for patients with impaired liver or kidney function.

BUSPIRONE HYDROCHLORIDE

Available in: Tablets
Available OTC? No **As Generic?** No
Drug Class: Antianxiety drug

▼ USAGE INFORMATION

WHY IT'S PRESCRIBED
To treat anxiety.

HOW IT WORKS
Buspirone affects the activity of specific brain chemicals (dopamine and especially serotonin) that are profoundly linked to mood, emotions, and mental state. Unlike many other medications used to treat anxiety disorders, buspirone has no muscle relaxant or sedative effects, and does not appear to lead to physical dependence.

▼ DOSAGE GUIDELINES

RANGE AND FREQUENCY
To start, 5 mg, 3 times per day (for a total of 15 mg a day). Can be increased to 60 mg a day, taken in divided doses every 6 to 8 hours.

ONSET OF EFFECT
May take 1 to 2 weeks to attain the full therapeutic benefit of buspirone.

DURATION OF ACTION
8 hours or more.

DIETARY ADVICE
No special restrictions.

STORAGE
Store in a tightly sealed container away from heat, moisture, and direct light.

MISSED DOSE
If you miss a dose, take it as soon as you remember. If it is near the time for your next dose, skip the missed dose and resume your regular dosage schedule. Do not double the next dose.

STOPPING THE DRUG
The decision to stop taking buspirone should be made in consultation with your doctor.

PROLONGED USE
No known problems.

▼ PRECAUTIONS

Over 60: Adverse side effects and reactions may be more common and more severe in older patients.

Driving and Hazardous Work: The use of buspirone may impair your ability to drive or perform hazardous tasks safely. The danger increases if you drink alcohol or take other medications that can affect alertness, such as antihistamines, painkillers, or mind-altering drugs.

Alcohol: Avoid alcohol while using this medication.

Pregnancy: No problems are expected, but adequate studies of buspirone use during pregnancy have not been done. Consult your doctor if you are pregnant or plan to become pregnant.

Breast Feeding: Buspirone can pass into breast milk. Avoid taking it if possible or refrain from breast feeding.

Infants and Children: The safety and effectiveness of buspirone have not been established for anyone under the age of 18.

Special Concerns: Before you undergo surgery requiring anesthesia, be sure to notify the surgeon that you take buspirone.

OVERDOSE
Symptoms: Severe drowsiness, dizziness, nausea and vomiting, constricted (pinpoint) pupils.

What to Do: Call your doctor, emergency medical services (EMS), or the nearest poison control center immediately.

▼ INTERACTIONS

DRUG INTERACTIONS
Other drugs may interact with buspirone. Consult your doctor for specific advice if you take any of the following: antihistamines, barbiturates, MAO inhibitors, muscle relaxants, narcotics, sedatives, or other tranquilizers.

FOOD INTERACTIONS
None expected.

DISEASE INTERACTIONS
Use of buspirone may cause complications in patients with liver or kidney disease, since these organs work together to remove the medication from the body.

≡ SIDE EFFECTS ≡

SERIOUS
No serious side effects have been directly associated with the use of buspirone.

COMMON
Dizziness or lightheadedness, nausea, paradoxical increase in nervousness or excitability, restlessness, headache.

LESS COMMON
Blurred vision, impaired ability to concentrate, drowsiness, dry mouth, difficulty sleeping, muscle cramps or spasms, fatigue or weakness, ringing in the ears, dreams that are unusual, disturbing, or vivid.

BUSULFAN

Available in: Tablets
Available OTC? No   **As Generic?** No
Drug Class: Alkylating agent

▼ USAGE INFORMATION

WHY IT'S PRESCRIBED
To treat certain forms of chronic leukemia (myeloid, myelocytic, and granulocytic leukemias). Busulfan slows the progress of these cancers, eases symptoms, and generally improves the condition of the patient, but it does not cure the disease. It is also used in conjunction with the transplanting of bone marrow to treat other forms of cancer.

HOW IT WORKS
Leukemia, in its many varieties, is a cancer marked by overproduction and abnormal formation of white blood cells, which are made in the bone marrow. Busulfan interferes with the growth and function of all cells, including the cells of the bone marrow. By interfering with bone marrow function, busulfan slows the production of the abnormal white blood cells.

▼ DOSAGE GUIDELINES

RANGE AND FREQUENCY
From 4 to 8 mg a day, as ordered by your doctor, until the desired response occurs.

ONSET OF EFFECT
Begins to take effect in 1 to 2 weeks.

DURATION OF ACTION
Up to 24 hours.

DIETARY ADVICE
Swallow tablet with liquid after a light meal. Avoid sweet or fatty foods. Do not drink fluids with meals. Drink extra fluids between meals.

STORAGE
Store in a tightly sealed container away from heat and direct light.

MISSED DOSE
Take it as soon as you remember. If it is near the time for the next dose, skip the missed dose and resume your regular dosage schedule. Do not double the next dose.

STOPPING THE DRUG
Stop taking this medicine only on your doctor's advice.

PROLONGED USE
Careful, continuous patient monitoring is needed during prolonged use.

▼ PRECAUTIONS

Over 60: No special precautions are warranted.

Driving and Hazardous Work: Determine whether this drug affects your alertness and physical abilities before you drive or engage in hazardous activities.

Alcohol: Do not consume alcohol while you take this medicine.

Pregnancy: Busulfan may cause birth defects; it is best to use some method of birth control while you are taking this medicine. Inform your doctor at once if you become pregnant during therapy.

Breast Feeding: It is not known whether this medicine passes into breast milk. Breast feeding is generally not recommended while taking busulfan.

Infants and Children: This medicine is not expected to cause problems or side effects in children that are different from those it causes in adults.

Special Concerns: Busulfan can increase the risk of infection because it reduces the number of white blood cells in your body. Try to avoid contact with people who have infections. The medicine can also reduce blood levels of platelets, cells that are necessary for clotting. Be careful when using a toothbrush, dental floss, or toothpick, and be careful to avoid cutting yourself when you use a knife, razor, or other sharp instrument.

OVERDOSE
Symptoms: Bleeding, chills, fever, fatigue, fainting, loss of consciousness.

What to Do: Seek emergency medical assistance immediately; call emergency medical services (EMS) or go to a hospital emergency room.

▼ INTERACTIONS

DRUG INTERACTIONS
Avoid any OTC product that contains aspirin, since it increases the danger of bleeding; carefully read ingredient labels of nonprescription drugs. Tell your doctor about any other drug you are taking, including an anticoagulant, any other anticancer drug, antithyroid medication, antibiotics, and antiviral medication.

FOOD INTERACTIONS
Avoid sweet or fatty foods.

DISEASE INTERACTIONS
Consult your doctor if you have any other medical problem, such as a history of seizures, chicken pox (or recent exposure to someone with chicken pox), shingles, gout, kidney stones, any head injury, or any infection.

≡ SIDE EFFECTS ≡

SERIOUS
Signs of unusual bleeding, including black, tarry, or bloody stools; blood in the urine; bright red, pinpointlike dots on the skin; unusual bruising; excessive gum bleeding; uncontrolled bleeding. Seizures are associated with higher doses. Consult your doctor at once.

COMMON
Increased pigmentation (darkening) of the skin; menstrual irregularities or absent periods.

LESS COMMON
Joint pain; shortness of breath; dizziness; sudden, unexpected loss of weight or appetite; lip or mouth sores; swelling in legs, ankles, and feet; nausea and vomiting; diarrhea; unusual fatigue or weakness.

BUTALBITAL/ACETAMINOPHEN/CAFFEINE

BRAND NAMES

Amaphen, Anolor-300, Anoquan, Arcet, Butace, Dolmar, Endolor, Esgic, Esgic-Plus, Ezol, Femcet, Fioricet, Isocet, Isopap, Medigesic, Pacaps, Pharmagesic, Repan, Tencet, Triad, Two-Dyne, Zebutal

Available in: Capsules, tablets
Available OTC? No   **As Generic?** Yes
Drug Class: Nonnarcotic analgesic

▼ USAGE INFORMATION

WHY IT'S PRESCRIBED
To treat headaches when non-prescription pain relievers are ineffective.

HOW IT WORKS
Butalbital, a barbiturate, acts on the central nervous system to cause sedation. Acetaminophen (APAP) appears to interfere with the action of prostaglandins, naturally occurring substances in the body that cause inflammation and make nerves more sensitive to pain impulses. Caffeine, a stimulant, is believed to enhance the effectiveness of pain relievers.

▼ DOSAGE GUIDELINES

RANGE AND FREQUENCY
1 or 2 tablets every 4 hours as needed. If your medication contains 325 or 500 mg of acetaminophen per capsule or tablet, do not take more than 6 pills a day. If your medication contains 650 mg of acetaminophen per capsule or tablet, do not take more than 4 pills a day.

ONSET OF EFFECT
Unknown.

DURATION OF ACTION
Up to 4 hours.

DIETARY ADVICE
Take this medicine with milk or meals to minimize stomach upset.

STORAGE
Store in a tightly sealed container away from heat, moisture, and direct light.

MISSED DOSE
If your doctor has directed you to take this medication on a regular schedule, take it as soon as you remember. If it is near the time for the next dose, skip the missed dose and resume your regular dosage schedule. Do not double the next dose.

STOPPING THE DRUG
You should take it as prescribed for the full treatment period, but you may stop taking the drug if you are feeling better before the scheduled end of therapy. This medication should never be stopped abruptly after long-term regular use.

PROLONGED USE
Barbiturates such as butalbital can cause physical dependence. Taking too much acetaminophen may cause liver damage.

▼ PRECAUTIONS

Over 60: Adverse reactions may be more likely and more severe in older patients.

Driving and Hazardous Work: The use of this medicine may impair your ability to perform such tasks safely.

Alcohol: Avoid alcohol.

Pregnancy: Before taking this medicine, tell your doctor if you are pregnant or plan to become pregnant.

Breast Feeding: This medicine passes into breast milk; do not use while nursing.

Infants and Children: Not recommended for use by children under age 12.

Special Concerns: The medicine works best if you take it at the first sign of a headache. Do not take the medicine if it has a strong vinegary odor. If you do not feel better 1 hour after taking this medication, call your doctor. Do not take a larger dose.

OVERDOSE
Symptoms: Difficulty breathing, excessive perspiration, impaired mental state, loss of consciousness, agitation or nervousness.

What to Do: Call your doctor, emergency medical services (EMS), or the nearest poison control center immediately.

▼ INTERACTIONS

DRUG INTERACTIONS
Consult your doctor for specific advice if you are taking antihistamines, antidepressants, antipsychotic drugs, muscle relaxants, other narcotic pain relievers, sleep medications, tranquilizers, or anticoagulants.

FOOD INTERACTIONS
No known food interactions.

DISEASE INTERACTIONS
Consult your doctor if you have any of the following: asthma, mental depression, heart disease, a blood disorder, an overactive thyroid gland, a kidney or liver disorder, or a history of alcoholism or drug abuse.

SIDE EFFECTS

SERIOUS
Shallow breathing, dizziness, weakness, confusion, blood in urine or stools, unusual bleeding or bruising, bleeding or crusting sores on lips, hives, muscle cramps, chest pain, white spots on the tongue, sore throat, pinpoint red spots on skin, fever, itchiness, rash, persistent or recurrent pain before next scheduled dose, swollen or painful glands, vomiting, yellow discoloration of skin or gums. Also swelling of the eyelids, lips, tongue, or face; red, thickened, or scaly skin. Call your physician immediately.

COMMON
Abdominal pain, dizziness, nausea or vomiting, mild stomach pain, lightheadedness, drowsiness.

LESS COMMON
Mental depression.

BUTALBITAL/ACETAMINOPHEN/CAFFEINE/CODEINE

BRAND NAMES

Amaphen with Codeine #3, Fioricet with Codeine

Available in: Capsules, tablets
Available OTC? No   **As Generic?** Yes
Drug Class: Opioid (narcotic) analgesic

▼ USAGE INFORMATION

WHY IT'S PRESCRIBED
To treat tension headaches when nonprescription pain relievers prove ineffective.

HOW IT WORKS
Butalbital, a barbiturate, acts on the central nervous system to cause sedation. Acetaminophen (APAP) appears to interfere with the action of prostaglandins, naturally occurring substances in the body that cause inflammation and make nerves more sensitive to pain impulses. Caffeine, a stimulant, is believed to enhance the effectiveness of pain relievers. Codeine, a narcotic, is believed to block pain signals to the brain and spinal cord.

▼ DOSAGE GUIDELINES

RANGE AND FREQUENCY
1 or 2 tablets or capsules every 4 hours. Do not take more than 6 pills a day.

ONSET OF EFFECT
Unknown.

DURATION OF ACTION
Unknown.

DIETARY ADVICE
This medication should be taken with food or water.

STORAGE
Store in a tightly sealed container away from heat, moisture, and direct light.

MISSED DOSE
If your doctor has directed you to take this drug on a regular schedule, take it as soon as you remember. If it is near the time for the next dose, skip the missed dose and resume your regular dosage schedule. Do not double the next dose.

STOPPING THE DRUG
Take it as prescribed for the full treatment period, but you may stop taking the drug if you are feeling better before the scheduled end of therapy. This medicine should never be stopped abruptly after long-term regular use.

PROLONGED USE
Narcotic drugs, such as codeine, and barbiturates, such as butalbital, can cause physical dependence. Taking too much acetaminophen may cause liver damage.

▼ PRECAUTIONS

Over 60: Adverse reactions may be more likely and more severe in older patients.

Driving and Hazardous Work: Do not drive or engage in hazardous work until you determine how the medicine affects you.

Alcohol: Avoid alcohol.

Pregnancy: Components of this medication have caused birth defects in animals. Taking the drug late in pregnancy may cause drug dependence in the unborn child. Tell your doctor if you are pregnant or plan to become pregnant before you take this drug.

Breast Feeding: Components of this medicine pass into breast milk; discontinue use while breast feeding.

Infants and Children: Not recommended for use by children under age 12.

Special Concerns: Tell any doctor or dentist whom you consult that you are taking this medicine. It works best if taken at the first sign of a headache. Tell your doctor if you begin having headaches more frequently than before you started using this drug. Check with your doctor if the medicine stops working as well as it did at the outset of therapy. This may be a sign of drug dependence. Do not increase the dose to attain better pain relief.

OVERDOSE
Symptoms: Drowsiness, confusion, nausea, vomiting, abnormal heartbeat, insomnia, slowed or suppressed breathing, trembling, loss of consciousness.

What to Do: Call your doctor, emergency medical services (EMS), or the nearest poison control center immediately.

▼ INTERACTIONS

DRUG INTERACTIONS
Consult your doctor for specific advice if you are taking beta-blockers, estrogens, felodipine, griseofulvin, nifedipine, theophylline, warfarin, carbamazepine, sulfinpyrazone, tranquilizers, sedatives, or tricyclic antidepressants.

FOOD INTERACTIONS
No known food interactions. A high-fiber diet is recommended because the medicine may cause constipation.

DISEASE INTERACTIONS
Consult your doctor if you have any of the following: asthma, liver disease, kidney disease, diabetes, mental depression, an overactive thyroid, porphyria, heart disease, or a history of alcohol or drug abuse.

SIDE EFFECTS

SERIOUS
Chest pains; muscle or joint pain; sores or ulcers in mouth; swelling of face, lips, or eyelids; yellow discoloration of eyes or skin; sore throat with or without fever. Call your doctor immediately.

COMMON
Drowsiness, dizziness, shortness of breath, lightheadedness, constipation, confusion, nausea, and vomiting.

LESS COMMON
Skin rash or hives.

BUTALBITAL/ASPIRIN/CAFFEINE

Available in: Capsules, tablets
Available OTC? No   **As Generic?** Yes
Drug Class: Nonnarcotic analgesic

▼ USAGE INFORMATION

WHY IT'S PRESCRIBED
To treat headaches or migraines.

HOW IT WORKS
Butalbital, a barbiturate, acts on the central nervous system to cause sedation. Aspirin appears to interfere with the action of prostaglandins, naturally occurring substances in the body that cause inflammation and make nerves more sensitive to pain impulses. Caffeine is believed to enhance the effectiveness of pain relievers.

▼ DOSAGE GUIDELINES

RANGE AND FREQUENCY
1 or 2 capsules or tablets every 4 hours. Do not take more than 6 pills a day.

ONSET OF EFFECT
Within 1 hour.

DURATION OF ACTION
4 hours.

DIETARY ADVICE
Take this drug with food or a full glass of water to avoid stomach irritation.

STORAGE
Store in a tightly sealed container away from heat, moisture, and direct light.

MISSED DOSE
If your doctor has directed you to take this drug on a regular schedule, take it as soon as you remember. If it is near the time for the next dose, skip the missed dose and resume your regular dosage schedule. Do not double the next dose.

STOPPING THE DRUG
Take it as prescribed for the full treatment period, but you may stop taking the drug if you are feeling better before the scheduled end of therapy. This drug should never be stopped abruptly after long-term regular use.

PROLONGED USE
Prolonged use may result in physical dependence and may cause kidney damage. Periodic kidney function tests are recommended. Prolonged use may make exposure to cold weather more hazardous.

▼ PRECAUTIONS

Over 60: Adverse reactions may be more likely and more severe in older patients.

Driving and Hazardous Work: Do not drive or engage in hazardous work until you determine how the medicine affects you.

Alcohol: Avoid alcohol.

Pregnancy: Taking this medicine late in pregnancy may cause drug dependence in the unborn child. Before you take it, tell your doctor if you are pregnant or are planning to become pregnant.

Breast Feeding: Butalbital and aspirin pass into breast milk; avoid or discontinue use while nursing.

Infants and Children: Consult your doctor before giving this medicine to anyone under age 18 who has a viral illness, especially chicken pox or influenza. The aspirin may cause a serious illness called Reye's syndrome.

Special Concerns: Tell any doctor or dentist whom you consult that you are taking this medicine. It works best if taken at the first sign of a headache. Tell your doctor if you begin having headaches more frequently than before you started using it, or if the drug stops working as well as it did at the outset of therapy. This may be a sign of drug dependence. Do not try to get better pain relief by increasing the dose. Do not take the drug if it has a strong vinegary odor.

OVERDOSE
Symptoms: Deep sleep, weak pulse, ringing in ears, nausea, vomiting, dizziness, deep and rapid breathing, convulsions, loss of consciousness.

What to Do: Call your doctor, emergency medical services (EMS), or the nearest poison control center immediately.

▼ INTERACTIONS

DRUG INTERACTIONS
Consult your doctor for advice if you are taking acetazolamide, gout medicines, beta-blockers, anticoagulants, methotrexate, narcotic pain relievers, nonsteroidal anti-inflammatory drugs, oral contraceptives, oral diabetes medicines, steroid medicines, tranquilizers, or valproic acid.

FOOD INTERACTIONS
No known food interactions.

DISEASE INTERACTIONS
Consult your doctor if you have any of the following: stomach or duodenal ulcers, asthma, epilepsy, anemia, gout, or a history of alcohol or drug abuse. Use of this drug may cause complications in patients with liver or kidney disease, since these organs work together to remove the medication from the body.

≣ SIDE EFFECTS ≣

SERIOUS
Difficulty breathing, tightness in chest, coughing, or wheezing; sores or white spots in mouth; bluish discoloration, flushing, or redness of skin; stuffy nose; pinpoint pupils; fever; swollen eyelids, face, lips, or tongue; difficulty swallowing; crusting or bleeding sores on lips; sore throat; burning, tenderness, or peeling of skin. Call your physician immediately.

COMMON
Drowsiness, dizziness, heartburn.

LESS COMMON
Insomnia, nightmares, headache, constipation, increased sweating, unusual fatigue.

BUTALBITAL/ASPIRIN/CAFFEINE/CODEINE PHOSPHATE

Available in: Capsules, tablets
Available OTC? No   **As Generic?** Yes
Drug Class: Opioid (narcotic) analgesic

▼ USAGE INFORMATION

WHY IT'S PRESCRIBED
To treat tension headaches or migraines.

HOW IT WORKS
Butalbital, a barbiturate, acts on the central nervous system to relieve pain. Aspirin appears to interfere with the action of prostaglandins, naturally occurring substances in the body that cause inflammation and make nerves more sensitive to pain impulses. Caffeine is believed to enhance the effectiveness of pain relievers. Codeine, a narcotic, is believed to block pain signals to the brain.

▼ DOSAGE GUIDELINES

RANGE AND FREQUENCY
1 or 2 capsules or tablets every 4 hours. Do not take more than 6 pills a day.

ONSET OF EFFECT
Within 1 hour.

DURATION OF ACTION
4 hours.

DIETARY ADVICE
This medicine should be taken with food or water to minimize stomach irritation.

STORAGE
Store in a tightly sealed container away from heat, moisture, and direct light.

MISSED DOSE
Take it as soon as you remember. If it is near the time for the next dose, skip the missed dose and resume your regular dosage schedule. Do not double the next dose.

STOPPING THE DRUG
You should take this medication as prescribed for the full treatment period, but you may stop taking it if you are feeling better before the scheduled end of therapy. This drug should never be stopped abruptly after long-term regular use.

PROLONGED USE
Narcotic drugs, such as codeine, and barbiturates, such as butalbital, can cause physical dependence. Prolonged use can cause kidney dysfunction.

≣ SIDE EFFECTS ≣

SERIOUS
Wheezing, tightness in chest, pinpoint pupils, yellowish discoloration of the skin and eyes, easy bruising, vomiting blood, sore throat, fever, mouth sores, difficult urination, hearing loss, blood in urine. Call your doctor immediately.

COMMON
Drowsiness, dizziness, lightheadedness, flushed face, depression, increased urination.

LESS COMMON
Insomnia, nightmares, headache, constipation, increased sweating, unusual fatigue.

▼ PRECAUTIONS

Over 60: Adverse reactions may be more likely and more severe in older patients.

Driving and Hazardous Work: Do not drive or engage in hazardous work until you determine how the medicine affects you.

Alcohol: Avoid alcohol.

Pregnancy: Taking the medicine late in pregnancy may cause drug dependence in the unborn child. Before you take this medicine, tell your doctor if you are pregnant or plan to become pregnant.

Breast Feeding: Do not use while nursing.

Infants and Children: This medicine is generally not prescribed for children under age 12. Consult your doctor before giving it to anyone under age 18 who has a viral illness, especially chicken pox or influenza. The aspirin may cause a serious illness called Reye's syndrome.

Special Concerns: Tell any doctor or dentist whom you consult that you are taking this medicine. The drug works best if taken at the first sign of a headache. Tell your doctor if you begin having headaches more frequently than before you started using this medicine. Check with your doctor if the medicine stops working as well as it did at the outset of therapy. Do not try to get better pain relief by increasing the dose. Do not take this drug if it has a strong, vinegary odor.

▼ OVERDOSE

Symptoms: Ringing in ears, slow and weak pulse, deep sleep, dizziness, nausea, vomiting, hallucinations, deep and rapid breathing, convulsions, loss of consciousness.

What to Do: Call your doctor, emergency medical services (EMS), or the nearest poison control center immediately.

▼ INTERACTIONS

DRUG INTERACTIONS
Consult your doctor for specific advice if you are taking acetazolamide, gout medicines, beta-blockers, anticoagulants, methotrexate, narcotic pain relievers, nonsteroidal anti-inflammatory drugs, oral contraceptives, oral diabetes medicines, steroid medicines, tranquilizers, or valproic acid.

FOOD INTERACTIONS
No known food interactions.

DISEASE INTERACTIONS
Consult your doctor if you have any of the following: stomach or duodenal ulcers, asthma, epilepsy, anemia, gout, or a history of alcohol or drug abuse. Use of this drug may cause complications in patients with liver or kidney disease, since these organs work together to remove the medication from the body.

BUTENAFINE HYDROCHLORIDE

BRAND NAME

Mentax

Available in: Cream
Available OTC? No   **As Generic?** No
Drug Class: Topical antifungal

▼ USAGE INFORMATION

WHY IT'S PRESCRIBED
To treat tinea pedis (athlete's foot), a fungal infection.

HOW IT WORKS
Butenafine prevents fungal organisms from producing vital substances required for their growth and function. This drug is effective only for infections caused by fungal organisms. It will not work for bacterial or viral infections.

▼ DOSAGE GUIDELINES

RANGE AND FREQUENCY
Apply it to the affected area either twice a day for 7 days or once a day for 4 weeks, in accordance with your doctor's instructions.

ONSET OF EFFECT
Unknown.

DURATION OF ACTION
Unknown.

DIETARY ADVICE
No special restrictions.

STORAGE
Store in a tightly sealed container away from heat, moisture, and direct light. Do not allow the cream to freeze.

MISSED DOSE
Apply butenafine as soon as you remember. If it is near the time for the next dose, skip the missed dose and resume your regular dosage schedule. Do not double the next dose or apply an excessively thick film of topical medication to compensate for a missed dose.

STOPPING THE DRUG
Apply as prescribed for the full treatment period, even if the fungal infection appears to be eradicated before the scheduled end of therapy. Unfortunately, it can be difficult to assess when the drug has achieved its desired effect since it suppresses redness and inflammation of the skin before the infection is completely clear; recurrence of fungal infection owing to inadequate length of therapy is a significant risk.

PROLONGED USE
If your skin problem does not improve or instead becomes worse after 4 weeks of treatment, consult your doctor.

▼ PRECAUTIONS

Over 60: No special problems are expected.

Driving and Hazardous Work: The use of butenafine should not impair your ability to perform such tasks safely.

Alcohol: No special precautions are necessary.

Pregnancy: Adequate human studies have not been done. Before taking butenafine, tell your physician if you are pregnant or plan to become pregnant.

Breast Feeding: It is not known whether butenafine passes into breast milk; caution is advised. Consult your doctor for specific advice.

Infants and Children: The safety and effectiveness of butenafine use by children below the age of 12 have not been determined. Use of the medication in patients 12 to 16 years of age has not caused any problems and has been effective.

Special Concerns: Butenafine is intended for external use only. Wash your hands after butenafine is applied to the affected area. Contact with the eyes, nose, and mouth should be avoided. If you apply butenafine after bathing or showering, dry the affected area thoroughly first. Do not use a tight-fitting dressing unless your physician tells you to do so. Do not use butenafine for any condition other than the one for which it was prescribed. As with any antifungal, butenafine is useful only against organisms that are vulnerable to its effects. Therefore, it is important to tell your doctor if your condition has not improved—or instead has worsened—within a few days of starting butenafine. The particular organism causing your illness may be resistant to this drug.

OVERDOSE
Symptoms: No cases of overdose have been reported.

What to Do: An overdose of butenafine is unlikely to be life-threatening. However, if someone uses a much larger dose than prescribed or ingests the medicine, seek medical assistance immediately.

▼ INTERACTIONS

DRUG INTERACTIONS
Consult your doctor for specific advice if you are taking allylamine antifungal drugs. Also tell your doctor if you are taking any other prescription or over-the-counter drugs.

FOOD INTERACTIONS
No known food interactions.

DISEASE INTERACTIONS
Caution is advised when taking butenafine. Consult your doctor if you have any other medical condition.

SIDE EFFECTS

SERIOUS
There are no serious side effects associated with the use of butenafine.

COMMON
Burning, stinging, irritation, itching, redness, swelling, or blistering at the site of application.

LESS COMMON
There are no less-common side effects associated with the use of butenafine.

BUTOCONAZOLE NITRATE

Available in: Vaginal cream
Available OTC? Yes **As Generic?** No
Drug Class: Antifungal

▼ USAGE INFORMATION

WHY IT'S PRESCRIBED
To treat fungal (yeast) infections of the vagina.

HOW IT WORKS
Butoconazole prevents fungal organisms from producing vital substances required for growth and function. This drug is effective only for infections caused by fungal organisms. It will not work for bacterial or viral infections.

▼ DOSAGE GUIDELINES

RANGE AND FREQUENCY
Nonpregnant women and teenagers: 5 g (1 applicatorful) of cream inserted with an applicator into the vagina at bedtime for 3 consecutive days. Pregnant women and teenagers: After third month, 5 g (1 applicatorful) of cream inserted with an applicator into the vagina at bedtime for 6 consecutive days.

ONSET OF EFFECT
Unknown.

DURATION OF ACTION
Unknown.

DIETARY ADVICE
Butoconazole can be applied without regard to diet.

STORAGE
Store in a tightly sealed container away from heat, moisture, and direct light. Do not allow it to freeze.

MISSED DOSE
Insert it as soon as you remember. If it is near the time for the next dose, skip the missed dose and resume your regular dosage schedule.

STOPPING THE DRUG
Take the medicine as directed for the full treatment period, even if you begin to feel better before the scheduled end of therapy. Recurrence of the infection is likely if you stop before the full treatment period is complete.

PROLONGED USE
Butoconazole is generally prescribed for short-term therapy (3 to 6 days).

▼ PRECAUTIONS

Over 60: No special problems are expected.

Driving and Hazardous Work: The use of butoconazole should not impair your ability to perform such tasks safely.

Alcohol: No special precautions are necessary.

Pregnancy: Studies on the use of butoconazole during the first 3 months (trimester) of pregnancy have not been done. No adverse effects while using it during the second or third trimesters have been reported.

Breast Feeding: No problems are expected. Consult your doctor about using this medicine while nursing.

Infants and Children: Studies on the use of butoconazole in children have not been done. Consult your pediatrician for specific advice.

Special Concerns: The drug may be used with oral contraceptives and antibiotic therapy. Sanitary napkins should be used to prevent staining of clothing. The affected area should be kept cool and dry. The patient should wear loose-fitting cotton clothing and freshly laundered cotton underwear or pantyhose with a cotton crotch. Avoid underwear made from nonventilating materials. Do not sit for a long time in a wet bathing suit. Avoid feminine hygiene sprays. Wash daily with unscented soap and dry thoroughly with a clean towel. Tampons should not be used during therapy. The patient's sexual partner should wear a condom during intercourse and should consult a doctor if penile redness, itching, or discomfort occurs. Do not stop using this medicine during your menstrual period. After urination or a bowel movement, cleanse by wiping the area from front to back to prevent reinfection.

OVERDOSE
Symptoms: An overdose with butoconazole is unlikely.

What to Do: If someone should swallow a large amount of the medicine, call your doctor, emergency medical services (EMS), or the nearest poison control center immediately.

▼ INTERACTIONS

DRUG INTERACTIONS
Tell your doctor if you are using any other vaginal prescription or over-the-counter medication.

FOOD INTERACTIONS
No food interactions have been reported.

DISEASE INTERACTIONS
No disease interactions have been reported.

≡ SIDE EFFECTS ≡

SERIOUS
Vaginal itching, burning, discharge, or irritation not present prior to treatment. Call your doctor as soon as possible.

COMMON
No common side effects are associated with the use of butoconazole.

LESS COMMON
Headache, stomach cramps or pain, irritation or burning of sexual partner's penis.

BUTORPHANOL TARTRATE

Available in: Nasal spray
Available OTC? No   **As Generic?** No
Drug Class: Opioid (narcotic) analgesic

▼ USAGE INFORMATION

WHY IT'S PRESCRIBED
To relieve headaches, postoperative pain, or other pain for which a narcotic analgesic is necessary.

HOW IT WORKS
Butorphanol blocks pain impulses at specific sites in the brain and spinal cord.

▼ DOSAGE GUIDELINES

RANGE AND FREQUENCY
Spray once into one nostril only. Do not spray into both nostrils unless directed by physician. Dose may be repeated in 60 to 90 minutes, and every 4 to 6 hours if needed.

ONSET OF EFFECT
Within 15 minutes.

DURATION OF ACTION
4 to 5 hours.

DIETARY ADVICE
No special restrictions.

STORAGE
Store in a tightly sealed container away from heat, moisture, and direct light.

MISSED DOSE
Not applicable; butorphanol should not be taken on a routine schedule.

STOPPING THE DRUG
You may stop taking the drug if you are feeling better, but butorphanol should never be stopped abruptly after long-term regular use.

PROLONGED USE
The effects of long-term use are unknown. This drug could be habit-forming. Consult your doctor regularly during prolonged use.

▼ PRECAUTIONS

Over 60: Adverse reactions, particularly dizziness, may be more likely and more severe in older persons.

Driving and Hazardous Work: Do not drive or engage in hazardous work until you determine how the medicine affects you.

Alcohol: Avoid alcohol because it can further dull alertness and slow reflexes.

Pregnancy: Before taking butorphanol, discuss with your doctor the relative risks and benefits of using this drug while pregnant.

Breast Feeding: Butorphanol may pass into breast milk; caution is advised. Consult your doctor for advice.

Infants and Children: Butorphanol is not recommended for use by children under the age of 18.

Special Concerns: When you first use this medicine, get up slowly from a sitting or lying position to avoid dizziness. Tell any doctor or dentist whom you consult that you are using butorphanol. Do not increase or decrease the dosage without consulting your doctor. When using a new bottle of butorphanol, point the bottle away from you and pump about 3 times to start the pump. Each time you use the spray, wipe the tip with a clean tissue or cloth. Every 3 or 4 days, rinse the tip with warm water and wipe the tip for about 15 seconds, then dry. To administer a dose of butorphanol, first blow your nose gently. Hold your head forward a little, put the spray tip in the nostril, and aim for the back. Close the other nostril by pressing with one finger. After the spray, tilt your head back for a few seconds. Do not blow your nose.

OVERDOSE
Symptoms: Irregular heartbeat; difficulty breathing; seizures; cold, clammy skin; loss of consciousness; pinpoint pupils of eyes; severe drowsiness, restlessness, weakness, dizziness, or nervousness.

What to Do: Call your doctor, emergency medical services (EMS), or the nearest poison control center immediately.

▼ INTERACTIONS

DRUG INTERACTIONS
The following drugs may interact with butorphanol: tranquilizers, sleeping pills, barbiturates, antihistamines, heart drugs, oral diabetes drugs, and antidepressants. Consult your doctor for specific advice about any drug you are taking.

FOOD INTERACTIONS
None expected.

DISEASE INTERACTIONS
Tell your doctor if you have had a heart attack or a head injury or if you have heart disease, a respiratory disease, a kidney problem, a liver problem, or a history of alcohol or drug abuse.

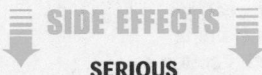
SIDE EFFECTS

SERIOUS
Shallow or slow breathing, sinus congestion, changes in mental state, nosebleeds, fever, sneezing, runny nose, blurred or distorted vision, ear pain, bronchitis, itching, hallucinations, difficulty urinating, skin rash, fainting. Call your doctor immediately.

COMMON
Headache, sedation, dizziness, insomnia, nose irritation, confusion, dry mouth, nausea, vomiting, constipation, loss of appetite, clammy skin, unpleasant taste in mouth.

LESS COMMON
Nervousness, unusual dreams, sluggishness, agitation, euphoria, floating sensation, trembling, stomach pain.

CAFFEINE

Available in: Tablets, extended-release capsules
Available OTC? Yes   **As Generic?** Yes
Drug Class: Central nervous system stimulant

▼ USAGE INFORMATION

WHY IT'S PRESCRIBED
To restore mental alertness.

HOW IT WORKS
Caffeine acts as a stimulant to all levels of the central nervous system.

▼ DOSAGE GUIDELINES

RANGE AND FREQUENCY
Tablets: 100 to 200 mg; repeat after 3 or 4 hours if needed. Extended-release capsules: 200 to 250 mg; can be repeated after 3 or 4 hours if needed. Citrated caffeine: 65 to 325 mg, 3 times a day as needed. Take no more than 1,000 mg a day.

ONSET OF EFFECT
Unknown.

DURATION OF ACTION
Unknown.

DIETARY ADVICE
Take it with food to minimize stomach upset.

STORAGE
Store in a tightly sealed container away from heat and direct light. Keep away from moisture and extremes in temperature.

MISSED DOSE
Take it as soon as you remember. If it is near the time for the next dose, skip the missed dose and resume your regular dosage schedule. Do not double the next dose.

STOPPING THE DRUG
The decision to stop taking the drug should be made by your doctor.

PROLONGED USE
Caffeine is not intended for prolonged use.

▼ PRECAUTIONS

Over 60: No special problems are expected.

Driving and Hazardous Work: The use of caffeine should not impair your ability to perform such tasks safely.

Alcohol: No special precautions are necessary.

Pregnancy: Large doses can cause miscarriage, delay the growth of the fetus, or cause problems with the heart rhythm of the fetus. No more than 300 mg of caffeine (the amount in 3 cups of coffee) should be consumed daily during pregnancy.

Breast Feeding: Caffeine passes into breast milk; caution is advised. Consult your doctor for specific advice.

Infants and Children: Caffeine is not recommended for use by children under the age of 12.

Special Concerns: To prevent insomnia, do not take caffeine or caffeine-containing beverages too close to bedtime. After you stop taking caffeine, you may experience anxiety, dizziness, headache, irritability, muscle tension, nausea, nervousness, stuffy nose, and unusual fatigue. Consult your doctor if you suffer from any of these symptoms.

OVERDOSE

Symptoms: Stomach or abdominal pains, agitation, anxiety, excitement, restlessness, confusion, delirium, seizures. A very large overdose can cause an irregular heartbeat; seeing zig-zag flashes of light; frequent urination; increased sensitivity to touch; muscle twitching; nausea and vomiting, sometimes with blood; insomnia; and ringing in the ears.

What to Do: An overdose of caffeine is unlikely to be life-threatening. However, if someone takes a much larger dose than directed, call your doctor, emergency medical services (EMS), or the nearest poison control right away.

▼ INTERACTIONS

DRUG INTERACTIONS
Call your doctor for specific advice if you are taking central nervous system stimulants; MAO inhibitors; amantadine; ciprofloxacin and norfloxacin (antibiotics); cold, sinus, hay fever, or allergy medications; asthma medicine; pemoline; amphetamines; nabilone; methylphenidate; or chlophedianol.

FOOD INTERACTIONS
Do not drink large amounts of caffeine-containing beverages like coffee, tea, soft drinks, cocoa, or chocolate milk.

DISEASE INTERACTIONS
Caution is advised when taking caffeine. Consult your doctor if you have any of the following: anxiety, panic attacks, heart disease, high blood pressure, agoraphobia (fear of open places), or insomnia. Use of caffeine may cause complications in patients with liver disease, since this organ works to remove the medication from the body.

SIDE EFFECTS

SERIOUS
Diarrhea, insomnia, dizziness, rapid heartbeat, severe nausea, vomiting, irritability, unusual agitation, tremors. Call your doctor immediately.

COMMON
Mild nausea or jitters.

LESS COMMON
There are no less-common side effects associated with the use of caffeine.

CALAMINE

BRAND NAME
Calamox

Available in: Lotion, ointment
Available OTC? Yes   **As Generic?** Yes
Drug Class: Topical anti-itching agent; astringent

▼ USAGE INFORMATION

WHY IT'S PRESCRIBED
To relieve the itching, pain, and discomfort of skin irritations, such as those caused by poison ivy, poison oak, and poison sumac. Calamine will also dry the oozing and weeping of skin eruptions caused by poison ivy, poison oak, and poison sumac.

HOW IT WORKS
The exact mechanism of action is unknown; calamine appears to have natural soothing properties.

▼ DOSAGE GUIDELINES

RANGE AND FREQUENCY
Apply calamine to the affected area of skin as often as needed. To use the lotion, shake it well to start. Then moisten a wad of cotton with the lotion and use the cotton to apply the lotion to the affected area of skin. Allow the lotion to dry on the skin. To use the ointment, gently rub just enough ointment into the skin to lightly cover the affected area.

ONSET OF EFFECT
Within 1 hour.

DURATION OF ACTION
Unknown.

DIETARY ADVICE
Calamine can be used without regard to diet.

STORAGE
Store in a tightly sealed container away from heat and direct light. Do not refrigerate or allow medication to freeze.

MISSED DOSE
If you are using calamine on a fixed schedule, apply the missed dose as soon as you remember. If it is close to the next dose, skip the missed dose and resume your regular dosage schedule. Do not use more lotion or ointment than necessary.

STOPPING THE DRUG
Take it as prescribed for the full treatment period. However, you may stop taking the drug if you are feeling better before the scheduled end of therapy.

PROLONGED USE
Call your doctor if your condition does not improve or gets worse after 7 days of treatment.

≡ SIDE EFFECTS ≡

SERIOUS
No serious side effects are associated with calamine.

COMMON
No common side effects are associated with calamine.

LESS COMMON
Rash, irritation, or sensitivity of the treated area that was not present prior to beginning therapy. Call your doctor promptly if such symptoms persist.

▼ PRECAUTIONS

Over 60: No special problems have been documented in older patients.

Driving and Hazardous Work: Use of calamine should not impair your ability to perform such tasks safely.

Alcohol: No special precautions are necessary.

Pregnancy: No problems during pregnancy have been documented.

Breast Feeding: Calamine may be used safely while nursing; no problems that affect the baby during breast feeding have been documented.

Infants and Children: Studies on the use of calamine on infants and children have not been done; however, no pediatric-specific problems have been documented.

Special Concerns: Calamine is for external use only. Do not swallow it. Do not use calamine on the eyes or mucous membranes, such as the inside of the mouth, nose, genitals, or anal area. Ingestion of calamine has been reported to cause gastritis (inflammation of the stomach lining) and vomiting. Milk or antacids may be used to treat gastritis.

OVERDOSE
Symptoms: None.

What to Do: No emergency instructions are applicable, since no cases of overdose have been reported. However, if someone accidentally ingests calamine, seek medical assistance right away.

▼ INTERACTIONS

DRUG INTERACTIONS
No drug interactions with calamine have been reported. However, you should tell your doctor if you are using any other prescription or over-the-counter medication to treat the same area of skin as calamine.

FOOD INTERACTIONS
No known food interactions.

DISEASE INTERACTIONS
No disease interactions with calamine have been documented. However, tell your doctor if you have any other skin condition.

CALCIPOTRIENE

Available in: Cream, ointment, scalp solution
Available OTC? No   **As Generic?** No
Drug Class: Vitamin D analog

▼ USAGE INFORMATION

WHY IT'S PRESCRIBED
Cream and ointment are used to treat mild to moderate psoriasis in adults. Scalp solution is used to treat chronic, moderately severe psoriasis of the scalp.

HOW IT WORKS
Calcipotriene is a synthetic form of vitamin D. It appears to slow excessive growth of skin cells; however, the exact mechanism of action is unknown.

▼ DOSAGE GUIDELINES

RANGE AND FREQUENCY
Cream and ointment: Apply a thin layer to the affected area once or twice daily and rub in evenly. Do not apply to the face. Scalp solution: Comb through the hair to remove scaly debris. Apply calcipotriene only to the lesions and rub in evenly. Do not allow the solution to spread to the forehead or other unaffected areas. Wash hands thoroughly after use.

ONSET OF EFFECT
Within 24 hours.

DURATION OF ACTION
Unknown.

DIETARY ADVICE
Calcipotriene can be used without regard to diet.

STORAGE
Store in a tightly sealed container away from heat, moisture, and direct light. Do not allow it to freeze. Keep the scalp solution away from open flame.

MISSED DOSE
Apply it as soon as you remember.

STOPPING THE DRUG
The decision to stop taking the drug should be made in consultation with your doctor.

PROLONGED USE
Treatment periods, depending on the severity of the psoriasis, generally last 8 weeks but have been approved to continue for up to 1 year.

▼ PRECAUTIONS

Over 60: Adverse reactions may be more likely and more severe in older patients.

Driving and Hazardous Work: The use of calcipotriene should not impair your ability to perform such tasks safely.

Alcohol: No special precautions are necessary.

Pregnancy: Adequate human studies have not been done. Before taking calcipotriene, tell your doctor if you are pregnant or plan to become pregnant.

Breast Feeding: Calcipotriene may pass into breast milk; caution is advised. Consult your doctor for specific advice.

Infants and Children: Not recommended for use by children under age 12.

OVERDOSE
Symptoms: Small amounts of the medication are absorbed through the skin. Symptoms of an overdose are due to elevated levels of blood calcium (hypercalcemia). Early symptoms of hypercalcemia: Constipation (especially in children), diarrhea, dry mouth, increased thirst and frequency of urination, persistent headache, loss of appetite, metallic taste, nausea and vomiting, unusual fatigue. Advanced symptoms: Bone and muscle pain, irregular heartbeat, persistent itching, extreme drowsiness, mental changes. Severe calcium toxicity may be fatal.

What to Do: Call your doctor, emergency medical services (EMS), or the nearest poison control center immediately.

▼ INTERACTIONS

DRUG INTERACTIONS
No known drug interactions.

FOOD INTERACTIONS
No known food interactions.

DISEASE INTERACTIONS
You should not take calcipotriene if you have high blood levels of calcium (hypercalcemia) or evidence of vitamin D toxicity.

≡ SIDE EFFECTS ≡

SERIOUS
No serious side effects have been reported in association with the use of calcipotriene.

COMMON
Temporary burning, tingling, and stinging; rash; peeling. Consult your doctor if these symptoms persist.

LESS COMMON
Skin irritation, dry skin, worsening of psoriasis, thinning of the skin, darkening of the skin.

CALCITONIN — SALMON

Available in: Injection, nasal spray
Available OTC? No   **As Generic?** No
Drug Class: Hormone/bone resorption inhibitor

BRAND NAMES
Calcimar, Miacalcin

▼ USAGE INFORMATION

WHY IT'S PRESCRIBED
To treat Paget's disease, a disorder in which bone tissue is broken down and restored too rapidly, resulting in bone fragility and in some cases malformation; to prevent bone loss in women with postmenopausal osteoporosis; to treat abnormally high blood calcium levels; to treat osteoporosis resulting from hormonal disturbances, drug therapy, and immobilization; to relieve compression of nerves that may occur with Paget's disease of bone.

HOW IT WORKS
Calcitonin blocks the bone-mineral-absorbing activity of the osteoclasts (bone cells), increases calcium excretion by the kidneys, and slows bone resorption (the speed at which bone is broken down before it is replaced).

▼ DOSAGE GUIDELINES

RANGE AND FREQUENCY
Injection— For Paget's disease: 100 international units (IU)

injected under the skin once a day to start. The dosage may be reduced depending on results. To prevent post-menopausal bone loss: 100 IU injected into muscle or under the skin once a day, once every other day, or 3 times a week. For excessive blood calcium: 1.8 IU per lb of body weight injected every 12 hours to start. Dose may be increased or decreased by your doctor. Nasal spray— 200 IU (1 spray) a day delivered in alternating nostrils, 1 spray a day.

ONSET OF EFFECT
Within 15 minutes.

DURATION OF ACTION
8 to 24 hours.

DIETARY ADVICE
If you are using this drug to lower blood calcium, your doctor may want you to follow a low-calcium diet. An injection is best administered at bedtime.

STORAGE
Store in a tightly sealed container away from heat and direct light.

SIDE EFFECTS

SERIOUS
Skin rash or hives. Call your doctor immediately.

COMMON
Diarrhea, loss of appetite, nausea or vomiting, stomach pain, pain and redness at injection site, flushing or redness of face, ears, hands, or feet.

LESS COMMON
Increased output of urine, headache, dizziness, pressure in the chest, breathing difficulty, stuffy nose, nasal bleeding or crusting, tingling of hands or feet, weakness, back pain, joint pain, chills.

MISSED DOSE
If you take 2 doses a day: Take the missed dose if you remember within 2 hours. If not, skip the missed dose and resume your regular dosage schedule. If you take 1 dose a day: Take the missed dose if you remember it the same day, then resume your regular dosage schedule. If you remember the next day, skip the missed dose and resume your regular dosage schedule. If you take one dose every other day: Take the missed dose if you remember the same day. Otherwise, take the dose the next day, skip a day and resume your regular dosage schedule. If you take 1 dose 3 times a week: Take the missed dose the next day, set each dose back a day for the rest of the week, then resume your regular dosage schedule. In no cases should you double the next dose.

STOPPING THE DRUG
The decision to stop taking the drug should be made by your doctor.

PROLONGED USE
Development of antibodies to the medicine may diminish its effectiveness over time.

▼ PRECAUTIONS

Over 60: Fluid balance should be monitored if the drug is given to reduce blood levels of calcium.

Driving and Hazardous Work: The use of calcitonin should not impair your ability to perform such tasks safely.

Alcohol: Avoid alcohol.

Pregnancy: In animal studies, large doses of calcitonin reduced birth weight. Before you take calcitonin, tell your doctor if you are pregnant or plan to become pregnant.

Breast Feeding: Calcitonin may pass into breast milk; caution is advised. Consult your doctor for specific advice.

Infants and Children: Studies of calcitonin use in infants and children have not been done. Consult your doctor for specific advice.

Special Concerns: You should not take calcitonin if you have a recently healed bone fracture.

OVERDOSE
Symptoms: No specific ones have been reported.

What to Do: An overdose of calcitonin is unlikely to be life-threatening. However, if someone takes a much larger dose than prescribed, call your doctor, emergency medical services (EMS), or the nearest poison control center.

▼ INTERACTIONS

DRUG INTERACTIONS
There are no known drug interactions.

FOOD INTERACTIONS
No known food interactions.

DISEASE INTERACTIONS
Caution is advised when taking calcitonin. Consult your doctor for specific advice if you have a kidney problem or a history of allergies.

CALCITRIOL

BRAND NAME

Rocaltrol

Available in: Capsules, oral solution
Available OTC? No   **As Generic?** No
Drug Class: Vitamin D analog

▼ USAGE INFORMATION

WHY IT'S PRESCRIBED
To treat abnormally low blood levels of calcium (hypocalcemia) in those with chronic kidney failure who are undergoing dialysis or who have other conditions resulting in low blood calcium, such as hypoparathyroidism (underactive parathyroid gland).

HOW IT WORKS
Vitamin D must be modified by both the liver and kidneys before it is fully active. Calcitriol, a synthetic form of active vitamin D, promotes the absorption and utilization of calcium and phosphorus in the body. This ensures that blood levels of these minerals are high enough to support the constant turnover of bone and to supply cells with the calcium needed to perform essential functions.

▼ DOSAGE GUIDELINES

RANGE AND FREQUENCY
Frequent blood tests to measure levels of calcium and phosphorus are required when calcitriol is first taken to determine the proper dose. For hypocalcemia in dialysis patients: Adults and children age 6 and over start at 0.25 micrograms (mcg) once a day. Dose may be gradually increased every 4 to 8 weeks to no more than 1 mcg a day. Maintenance dose is usually 0.25 mcg every other day up to 1.25 mcg daily. Children ages 1 to 5: 0.25 to 2 mcg once a day. For hypoparathyroidism: Adults and children age 6 and over start at 0.25 mcg once a day. Dose may be gradually increased every 2 to 4 weeks to no more than 0.5 to 2 mcg a day. Children ages 1 to 5: 0.25 to 0.75 mcg per 2.2 lbs (1 kg) once a day.

ONSET OF EFFECT
2 to 6 hours.

DURATION OF ACTION
3 to 5 days.

DIETARY ADVICE
No special advice.

STORAGE
Store in a tightly sealed container away from heat, moisture, and direct light.

SIDE EFFECTS

SERIOUS
Fatigue, headache, loss of appetite, metallic taste in mouth, nausea, vomiting, abdominal cramps, constipation or diarrhea, dizziness, drowsiness, dry mouth, ringing in ears, muscle pains, joint pains, irritability. Call your doctor immediately.

COMMON
No common side effects are associated with calcitriol.

LESS COMMON
No less-common side effects are associated with calcitriol.

MISSED DOSE
Take it as soon as you remember. If it is near the time for the next dose, skip the missed dose and resume your regular dosage schedule. Do not double the next dose.

STOPPING THE DRUG
The decision to stop taking the drug should be made by your doctor.

PROLONGED USE
See your doctor regularly for tests and examinations.

▼ PRECAUTIONS

Over 60: Adverse reactions may be more likely and more severe in older patients.

Driving and Hazardous Work: Do not drive or engage in hazardous work until you determine how the medicine affects you.

Alcohol: Avoid excessive amounts of alcohol.

Pregnancy: No problems have been reported with the recommended daily dose. However, during pregnancy, calcitriol may cause problems in the unborn child when taken in excess of the recommended dosage, especially if the mother develops hypercalcemia (high blood levels of calcium). Before taking it, tell your doctor if you are pregnant or plan to become pregnant.

Breast Feeding: Calcitriol may pass into breast milk; extreme caution is advised. Some experts recommend that the mother not nurse while taking calcitriol. Consult your doctor.

Infants and Children: Calcitriol is not recommended for use by children under the age of 1. Consult your doctor.

OVERDOSE
Symptoms: Symptoms are due to the resulting hypercalcemia. Early symptoms: Constipation (especially in children), diarrhea, dry mouth, increased thirst and frequency of urination, persistent headache, loss of appetite, metallic taste, nausea and vomiting, unusual fatigue. Advanced symptoms: Bone and muscle pain, irregular heartbeat, persistent itching, extreme drowsiness, mental changes.

What to Do: Call your doctor if such symptoms occur. If someone accidentally ingests an extremely large dose, seek medical assistance right away.

▼ INTERACTIONS

DRUG INTERACTIONS
Consult your doctor for specific advice if you are taking antacids, cardiac glycosides, cholestyramine, colestipol, mineral oil, phenobarbital, phenytoin, primidone, thiazide diuretics, other forms of vitamin D, or calcium.

FOOD INTERACTIONS
No known food interactions.

DISEASE INTERACTIONS
Consult your doctor if you have blood vessel disease, heart disease, hypercalcemia, hypervitaminosis D, hypoparathyroidism, kidney disease, hyperphosphatemia, or sarcoidosis.

CALCIUM

Available in: Capsules, oral suspension, tablets, chewable tablets, liquid
Available OTC? Yes **As Generic?** Yes
Drug Class: Antihypocalcemic; dietary supplement; antacid

▼ USAGE INFORMATION

WHY IT'S PRESCRIBED
To ensure adequate calcium intake in those who do not get sufficient amounts by diet alone. Calcium is essential to many body functions, including the transmission of nerve impulses, the regulation of muscle contraction and relaxation (including of the heart), blood clotting, and various metabolic activities. Calcium is also necessary for maintaining strong bones and is commonly prescribed to prevent and treat postmenopausal osteoporosis (bone thinning). Vitamin D, which aids in the absorption of calcium from the intestine, is often prescribed along with calcium supplements to prevent or treat osteoporosis. (Indeed, some calcium supplement tablets contain vitamin D.) Calcium is also prescribed for individuals with persistently low blood calcium levels (hypocalcemia) caused, for example, by low levels of parathyroid hormone (hypoparathyroidism).

HOW IT WORKS
Calcium supplements compensate for inadequate dietary intake of this essential mineral. Forms of supplements available include calcium carbonate (the most common and inexpensive), calcium citrate (the best absorbed, but relatively expensive), calcium phosphate, calcium lactate, and calcium gluconate. Because calcium carbonate and phosphate supplements are difficult to absorb, other calcium products are preferable for individuals with low gastric (stomach) acid secretion.

▼ DOSAGE GUIDELINES

RANGE AND FREQUENCY
Optimal daily calcium intakes— Ages 0 to 6 months: 210 mg. Ages 6 months to 1 year: 270 mg. Ages 1 to 3 years: 500 mg. Ages 4 to 8 years: 800 mg. Ages 9 to 18 years: 1,300 mg. Ages 19 to 50 years: 1,000 mg. Age 51 and older: 1,200. For pregnant or breast-feeding women, under 19 years: 1,300 mg; ages 19 to 50 years: 1,000 mg. Be sure to include dietary calcium as well as the supplements in your total daily intake. It is important to realize that calcium itself constitutes only a fraction of any calcium-containing pill. For example, calcium accounts for only 40% of the weight of a calcium carbonate tablet. Thus, a 500 mg tablet of calcium carbonate provides only 200 mg of calcium.

ONSET OF EFFECT
Unknown.

DURATION OF ACTION
For as long as the supplement is taken.

DIETARY ADVICE
Calcium carbonate and calcium phosphate supplements are best absorbed if taken 60 to 90 minutes after meals. Take with 1 full glass (8 oz) of water or juice. Follow all special dietary guidelines as recommended by your doctor.

STORAGE
Store in a tightly sealed container away from heat, moisture, and direct light.

MISSED DOSE
If you are taking calcium supplements on a regular basis and miss a dose, take it as soon as you remember, then resume your regular dosage schedule.

STOPPING THE DRUG
The decision to stop taking calcium supplements should be made in consultation with your doctor.

PROLONGED USE
Adverse effects are more likely to occur if supplements are taken in doses greater than 2,000 to 2,500 mg a day for a long period of time. Your doctor should regularly check your blood calcium levels if you are taking calcium supplements to treat low blood calcium (hypocalcemia).

▼ PRECAUTIONS

Over 60: No special problems are expected.

Driving and Hazardous Work: Calcium supplements should have no effect on your ability to perform such tasks safely.

Alcohol: To ensure proper absorption of calcium, consume alcohol in moderation only (no more than 2 drinks per day).

Pregnancy: It is crucial to receive enough calcium during pregnancy and to maintain those levels throughout pregnancy, preferably through diet alone. However, excessive calcium intake during pregnancy may be harmful to

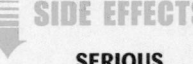

SIDE EFFECTS

SERIOUS
Serious side effects are associated with excessively high doses (see Overdose).

COMMON
No common side effects are associated with recommended doses of calcium.

LESS COMMON
Constipation, diarrhea, drowsiness, loss of appetite, dry mouth, and muscle weakness are some of the symptoms that could result if blood levels of calcium are too high (hypercalcemia).

the mother or fetus and should be avoided.

Breast Feeding: Excessive amounts of this supplement taken while nursing may be harmful to the mother or infant and should be avoided.

Infants and Children: No special problems expected.

OVERDOSE

Symptoms: Early symptoms: Constipation (especially in children), diarrhea, dry mouth, increased thirst and frequency of urination, persistent headache, loss of appetite, metallic taste, nausea and vomiting, unusual fatigue. Advanced symptoms: Bone and muscle pain, irregular heartbeat, persistent itching, extreme drowsiness, mental changes. Severe calcium toxicity may be fatal.

What to Do: Call your doctor, emergency medical services (EMS), or the nearest poison control center immediately.

▼ INTERACTIONS

DRUG INTERACTIONS
Consult your doctor for specific advice if you are taking other calcium-containing preparations, cellulose sodium phosphate, digitalis drugs, etidronate, gallium nitrate, phenytoin, or tetracycline antibiotics. Combined use of calcium supplements with thiazide diuretics or vitamin D may lead to excessively high calcium levels.

FOOD INTERACTIONS
Excessive protein consumption can increase the excretion of calcium in the urine. In meals preceding calcium consumption, avoid spinach and rhubarb (high in oxalic acid), and bran and whole cereals (high in phytic acid), since these substances may interfere with calcium absorption.

DISEASE INTERACTIONS
Consult your doctor if you have frequent episodes of diarrhea, any stomach or intestinal problems, heart disease, sarcoidosis, kidney disease, or kidney stones.

CANDESARTAN CILEXETIL

Available in: Tablets
Available OTC? No   **As Generic?** No
Drug Class: Antihypertensive/angiotensin II antagonist

▼ USAGE INFORMATION

WHY IT'S PRESCRIBED
To control high blood pressure. This drug appears to have the same benefits as the class of antihypertensive medications known as "ACE inhibitors," without producing the common side effect (experienced by as many as 30% of patients) of a dry cough. Candesartan may be used by itself or in conjunction with other antihypertensive medications.

HOW IT WORKS
Candesartan blocks the effects of angiotensin II, a naturally occurring substance that causes blood vessels to narrow. Candesartan causes the blood vessels to dilate, thereby lowering blood pressure and decreasing the workload of the heart.

▼ DOSAGE GUIDELINES

RANGE AND FREQUENCY
To start, 16 mg once a day when used as the only drug to treat hypertension. Usual maintenance dose is 8 to 32 mg daily, taken once a day or divided into 2 doses.

ONSET OF EFFECT
Within 2 weeks.

DURATION OF ACTION
Up to 24 hours.

DIETARY ADVICE
No special restrictions, unless your doctor has advised a low-sodium diet or other dietary modifications to help you control your blood pressure.

STORAGE
Store in a tightly sealed container away from heat, moisture, and direct light.

MISSED DOSE
Take it as soon as you remember. If it is near the time for the next dose, skip the missed dose and resume your regular dosage schedule. Do not double the next dose.

STOPPING THE DRUG
Take it as prescribed for the full treatment period. The decision to stop taking the drug should be made in consultation with your physician.

PROLONGED USE
Lifelong therapy may be necessary. However, if you do modify certain health habits (for example, increasing exercise or losing weight), a reduced dose may be possible under a physician's supervision.

▼ PRECAUTIONS

Over 60: No special problems are expected.

Driving and Hazardous Work: Do not drive or engage in hazardous work until you determine how the medicine affects you.

Alcohol: No special precautions are necessary.

Pregnancy: Candesartan should not be used by pregnant women. Discontinue taking the drug as soon as possible when pregnancy is detected and discuss treatment alternatives with your doctor.

Breast Feeding: Candesartan may pass into breast milk; caution is advised. Consult your doctor for advice.

Infants and Children: The safety and effectiveness of use in children have not been established.

Special Concerns: Candesartan may cause excessively low blood pressure with dizziness or lightheadedness, which is most noticeable when you change position. This may lead to fainting, falls, and injury. Sit or lie down immediately if you feel dizzy or lightheaded. This side effect may be worsened by alcohol, hot weather, dehydration, salt depletion from diuretic use, fever, prolonged standing, prolonged sitting, or exercise.

OVERDOSE

Symptoms: Few cases of overdose have been reported. However, if you take a much larger dose than prescribed, you may experience fainting, dizziness, or weak pulse that might be very slow or very fast.

What to Do: Call your doctor, emergency medical services (EMS), or the nearest poison control center immediately.

▼ INTERACTIONS

DRUG INTERACTIONS
No drug interactions have yet been observed with candesartan. Consult your doctor for specific advice if you are taking any other medication, especially other drugs for high blood pressure. Candesartan can be taken together with diuretics or other medications for high blood pressure, if your doctor approves.

FOOD INTERACTIONS
No known food interactions.

DISEASE INTERACTIONS
Patients with moderate to severe liver or kidney disease are advised to exercise caution when taking candesartan.

≡ SIDE EFFECTS ≡

SERIOUS
No serious side effects are associated with the use of candesartan. (In clinical trials, the incidence of adverse effects was not significantly greater with the medication than with a placebo.)

COMMON
No common side effects are associated with the use of candesartan.

LESS COMMON
Headache, dizziness, back pain, upper respiratory tract infection, sore throat, and nasal congestion.

CAPECITABINE

	BRAND NAME
	Xeloda

Available in: Tablets
Available OTC? No   **As Generic?** No
Drug Class: Antineoplastic (anticancer) agent

▼ USAGE INFORMATION

WHY IT'S PRESCRIBED
To treat advanced (metastatic) breast cancer. Capecitabine is used for secondary treatment when other therapies have not produced adequate results. Your oncologist will determine if capecitabine is appropriate for your condition.

HOW IT WORKS
By interfering with essential phases of cell division in cancer cells, capecitabine prevents them from multiplying. The drug may cause side effects by affecting other kinds of cells in the body.

▼ DOSAGE GUIDELINES

RANGE AND FREQUENCY
2,500 mg per square meter of body surface in 2 divided doses (12 hours apart) a day. Capecitabine is taken in 3-week cycles: 2 weeks on and 1 week off. Your oncologist will determine the proper dosage and how many cycles of treatment are needed.

ONSET OF EFFECT
Unknown.

DURATION OF ACTION
Unknown.

DIETARY ADVICE
Take with water within 30 minutes after the end of a meal (breakfast and dinner).

STORAGE
Store at room temperature in a tightly sealed container away from heat, moisture, and direct light.

MISSED DOSE
It is imperative to try not to miss a dose. If you do miss a dose, skip the missed dose and resume your regular dosage schedule. Do not double the next dose. If you miss more than one dose, contact your oncologist.

STOPPING THE DRUG
Take it as prescribed for the full treatment period. The decision to stop taking the drug should be made by your oncologist.

PROLONGED USE
See your oncologist regularly if you must take this drug for a prolonged period.

▼ PRECAUTIONS

Over 60: Severe gastrointestinal side effects may be more likely and more severe in patients 80 years of age and older.

Driving and Hazardous Work: Do not drive or engage in hazardous work until you determine how the medicine affects you.

Alcohol: No special precautions are necessary.

Pregnancy: Avoid becoming pregnant while taking this drug. Tell your doctor at once if you become pregnant while taking capecitabine.

Breast Feeding: Capecitabine may pass into breast milk; avoid nursing while taking this medication.

Infants and Children: The safety and effectiveness of the use of capecitabine in children under the age of 18 have not been determined.

Special Concerns: Take the medication in the combination prescribed by your oncologist for the morning and evening doses.

OVERDOSE
Symptoms: Nausea, vomiting, diarrhea, stomach irritation and bleeding, fatigue, and paleness.

What to Do: Call your oncologist, emergency medical services (EMS), or the nearest poison control center immediately.

▼ INTERACTIONS

DRUG INTERACTIONS
Do not take leucovorin or fluorouracil if you are taking capecitabine. Consult your oncologist for advice if you are taking folic acid or anticoagulants (such as warfarin).

FOOD INTERACTIONS
No known food interactions.

DISEASE INTERACTIONS
Consult your oncologist if you have a history of heart disease. Patients with liver or kidney disease should be carefully monitored by their doctor while taking capecitabine.

▼ SIDE EFFECTS

SERIOUS
Fever greater than 100.5°F; severe diarrhea, nausea, and vomiting; loss of or decreased appetite; pain, redness, swelling and sores in the mouth and throat; pain, numbness, tingling, swelling, and redness of the palms of the hands or soles of the feet (hand-and-foot syndrome). Stop taking the drug and call your oncologist immediately.

COMMON
Abdominal pain, constipation, dehydration, rash, dry or itchy skin, weakness, headache, drowsiness, dizziness, mild fever.

LESS COMMON
Numerous less common side effects can occur; consult your doctor if you are concerned about any adverse or unusual reactions you experience while taking this drug.

CAPSAICIN

BRAND NAMES

Axsain, Zostrix

Available in: Cream
Available OTC? Yes   **As Generic?** Yes
Drug Class: Analgesic

▼ USAGE INFORMATION

WHY IT'S PRESCRIBED
To relieve neuralgia—pain in the nerve endings near the surface of the skin. Capsaicin is commonly prescribed for neuralgia associated with shingles, an acutely painful condition caused by infection with the varicella zoster virus, the same organism that causes chicken pox. Capsaicin is also used to relieve mild to moderate arthritis, diabetic neuropathy (pain caused by nerve cell damage that occurs as a complication of diabetes), and postoperative pain.

HOW IT WORKS
When applied topically, capsaicin (a derivative of hot peppers) appears to reduce the amount of a natural chemical known as substance P, which is present in painful joints. Substance P is believed to be involved in two processes central to arthritis: the release of enzymes that produce inflammation and the transmission of pain impulses from the joints to the central nervous system. By blocking the production and release of substance P, capsaicin can reduce the pain associated with arthritis as well as dampen the transmission of pain messages to the brain.

▼ DOSAGE GUIDELINES

RANGE AND FREQUENCY
Apply a small amount to the affected area up to 4 times a day. Do not apply to broken or irritated skin. If the use of a bandage is recommended, do not apply it too tightly.

ONSET OF EFFECT
Therapeutic pain response is usually achieved in 1 to 2 weeks but may take as long as 4 weeks.

DURATION OF ACTION
Up to 6 hours.

DIETARY ADVICE
This medication can be used without regard to diet.

STORAGE
Store in a tightly sealed container away from heat and direct light.

MISSED DOSE
Apply it as soon as you remember. If it is near the time for the next dose, skip the missed dose and resume your regular dosage schedule. Do not double the next dose.

STOPPING THE DRUG
Pain relief will last only as long as capsaicin is used regularly. If you discontinue using the medication and the pain returns, it is safe to resume treatment.

PROLONGED USE
No special problems are expected. Burning and stinging sensations upon application frequently subside with prolonged use. If your condition worsens or does not improve after 1 month, discontinue using capsaicin and consult your doctor.

▼ PRECAUTIONS

Over 60: No special problems are expected.

Driving and Hazardous Work: No speical problems are expected.

Alcohol: No special precautions are necessary.

Pregnancy: No problems have been reported.

Breast Feeding: No problems are expected.

Infants and Children: Not recommended for use on children under the age of 2. No problems are expected in older children.

Special Concerns: You may not be able to use capsaicin if you are allergic to it or if you have ever had an allergic reaction to hot peppers. Wash your hands thoroughly after applying the cream; if you are using it for arthritis of the hands, wait 30 minutes before washing. It can cause a burning sensation if even small amounts get into the eyes or on other sensitive areas of the body. If you wear contact lenses, be especially cautious. If it does get into your eyes, flush them with water. On other sensitive areas of the body, wash the area with warm (but not hot) soapy water. After applying capsaicin cream, avoid contact with children and pets until you have thoroughly washed your hands.

OVERDOSE
Symptoms: No cases of overdose have been reported.

What to Do: An overdose is unlikely to be life-threatening. However, if someone applies a much larger dose than prescribed, suffers adverse side effects, or accidentally ingests it, call your doctor or the nearest poison control center for advice.

▼ INTERACTIONS

DRUG INTERACTIONS
Capsaicin may alter the action of some drugs or trigger unwanted side effects. Consult your doctor about any other drugs that you take, including over-the-counter medications.

FOOD INTERACTIONS
None are known.

DISEASE INTERACTIONS
Consult your doctor if you have broken or irritated skin, or conditions that may result in broken skin, on the area to be treated.

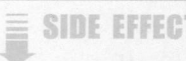

SIDE EFFECTS

SERIOUS
No serious side effects are associated with capsaicin.

COMMON
Stinging or burning sensation when cream is applied. This should subside with regular use, as your body adjusts to the medication.

LESS COMMON
Skin redness; coughing, sneezing, or shortness of breath if dried residues of the drug are inhaled.

CAPTOPRIL

Available in: Tablets
Available OTC? No **As Generic?** Yes
Drug Class: Angiotensin-converting enzyme (ACE) inhibitor

▼ USAGE INFORMATION

WHY IT'S PRESCRIBED
To control high blood pressure; to treat congestive heart failure (CHF); to treat patients with left ventricular dysfunction (damage to the pumping chamber of the heart); and to minimize further kidney damage in people with diabetes who have mild kidney disease.

HOW IT WORKS
Angiotensin-converting enzyme (ACE) inhibitors block an enzyme that produces angiotensin, a naturally occurring substance that causes blood vessels to constrict and stimulates production of the adrenal hormone, aldosterone, which promotes sodium retention in the body. As a result, ACE inhibitors relax blood vessels (causing them to widen) and reduces sodium retention, which lowers blood pressure and so decreases the workload of the heart.

▼ DOSAGE GUIDELINES

RANGE AND FREQUENCY
Adults— For high blood pressure: 12.5 to 150 mg, 2 or 3 times a day. For CHF: 6.25 to 100 mg, 2 or 3 times a day. For left ventricular dysfunction: 6.25 to 50 mg, 3 times a day. For kidney problems associated with diabetes: 25 mg, 3 times a day. Children— Consult your pediatrician.

ONSET OF EFFECT
15 to 60 minutes.

DURATION OF ACTION
6 to 12 hours.

DIETARY ADVICE
Take it on an empty stomach, about 1 hour before mealtime. Follow your doctor's dietary advice (such as low-salt or low-cholesterol restrictions) to improve control over high blood pressure and heart disease. Avoid high-potassium foods like bananas and citrus fruits and juices, unless you are also taking medications, that lower potassium levels.

STORAGE
Store in a tightly sealed container away from heat and direct light.

MISSED DOSE
Take it as soon as you remember. If it is near the time for the next dose, skip the missed dose and resume your regular dosage schedule. Do not double the next dose.

STOPPING THE DRUG
Do not stop taking this drug abruptly, as this may cause potentially serious health problems. Dosage should be reduced gradually, according to your doctor's instructions.

PROLONGED USE
See your doctor regularly for examinations and tests if you must take this medicine for a prolonged period. Remember that captopril helps control high blood pressure but does not cure it. Lifelong therapy may be necessary.

▼ PRECAUTIONS

Over 60: Adverse reactions may be more likely and more severe in older patients.

Driving and Hazardous Work: Avoid such activities until you determine how the medication affects you.

Alcohol: Alcohol may increase the effect of the drug and cause an excessive drop in blood pressure. Consult your doctor for advice.

Pregnancy: Captopril should not be used during the final 6 months of pregnancy. Notify your doctor right away if you become pregnant.

Breast Feeding: If possible, avoid using captopril while nursing.

Infants and Children: Captopril is only prescribed for children when other means of controlling hypertension fail; benefits must be weighed against risks.

OVERDOSE
Symptoms: Dizziness or fainting; weak, rapid pulse; nausea, vomiting; chest pain.

What to Do: Call your doctor, emergency medical services (EMS), or the nearest poison control center immediately.

▼ INTERACTIONS

DRUG INTERACTIONS
Consult your doctor if you are taking diuretics (especially potassium-sparing diuretics), potassium supplements or drugs containing potassium, lithium, anticoagulants, anti-inflammatory drugs, or over-the-counter drugs (especially cold remedies and diet pills).

FOOD INTERACTIONS
Avoid low-salt milk and salt substitutes. Many of these products contain potassium.

DISEASE INTERACTIONS
Consult your doctor if you have systemic lupus erythematosus or if you have had a prior allergic reaction to ACE inhibitors. This medication should be used with caution by patients with severe kidney disease or renal artery stenosis (narrowing of one or both of the arteries that supply blood to the kidneys).

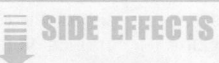

SIDE EFFECTS

SERIOUS
Fever and chills; sore throat and hoarseness; sudden difficulty breathing or swallowing; swelling of the face, mouth, or extremities; impaired kidney function (ankle swelling, decreased urination); confusion; yellow discoloration of the eyes or skin (indicating liver disorder); intense itching; chest pain or palpitations; abdominal pain. Serious side effects are very rare; contact your doctor immediately.

COMMON
Dry, persistent cough.

LESS COMMON
Dizziness or fainting; skin rash; numbness or tingling in the hands, feet, or lips; unusual fatigue or muscle weakness; nausea; drowsiness; loss of taste; headache.

CARBAMAZEPINE

Available in: Oral suspension, tablets, extended-release tablets and capsules
Available OTC? No   **As Generic?** Yes
Drug Class: Anticonvulsant/analgesic

▼ USAGE INFORMATION

WHY IT'S PRESCRIBED
To control certain types of seizures due to epilepsy. Also to treat facial pain in those with trigeminal neuralgia (tic douloureux).

HOW IT WORKS
Carbamazepine appears to inhibit neurons from firing repeatedly and uncontrollably (which causes seizures).

▼ DOSAGE GUIDELINES

RANGE AND FREQUENCY
Adults: 600 to 2,000 mg a day, in 3 or 4 divided doses. Children: 9 to 18 mg per lb of body weight, in 3 or 4 divided doses. Some patients require higher doses. A low dose should be used initially, then gradually increased if needed. The extended-release forms may be given twice a day.

ONSET OF EFFECT
Several hours or longer.

DURATION OF ACTION
Maximum effectiveness: 12 hours or longer; effectiveness then gradually decreases.

DIETARY ADVICE
Take with food to lessen the chance of stomach upset.

STORAGE
Store in a tightly sealed container away from heat, moisture, and direct light.

MISSED DOSE
Take it as soon as you remember. If it is near the time for the next dose, skip the missed dose and resume your regular dosage schedule. Do not double the next dose, unless advised to do so by your doctor. Call your doctor if you miss more than a full day's worth of doses.

STOPPING THE DRUG
Never stop this drug abruptly; seizures may occur. Your doctor will taper the dose over many weeks.

PROLONGED USE
Therapy may last several years or longer. Some side effects may diminish after a few weeks of therapy.

▼ PRECAUTIONS

Over 60: Older patients may require lower doses to minimize side effects.

Driving and Hazardous Work: Avoid such tasks until you determine how the medication affects you.

Alcohol: May contribute to excessive drowsiness.

Pregnancy: This drug increases the risk of birth defects. However, seizures during pregnancy also increase the risks to the fetus. Discuss potential risks and benefits with your doctor. Folate supplementation is advised starting 1 to 2 months before conception and continuing throughout pregnancy. Vitamin K1 may be needed during the last 4 weeks of pregnancy.

Breast Feeding: This drug passes into breast milk, although at low levels. Consult your doctor for advice.

Infants and Children: Behavioral side effects are more likely to be seen in children.

Special Concerns: The generic form is not recommended. Do not change the brand you are taking without consulting your doctor. Your doctor may suggest you carry an ID card or bracelet saying that you take this drug.

OVERDOSE
Symptoms: Confusion, double vision, seizures, extreme drowsiness, loss of consciousness, poor muscle control, spasms, tremors, walking difficulty, abnormal heartbeat, slow or irregular breathing.

What to Do: Seek medical assistance immediately.

▼ INTERACTIONS

DRUG INTERACTIONS
Carbamazepine may interact with many drugs, including other anticonvulsants (clonazepam, ethosuximide, primidone, valproic acid, phenytoin, and phenobarbital), anticoagulants, certain anti-infectives (erythromycin, doxycycline, troleandomycin, isoniazid), oral contraceptives, cimetidine, corticosteroids, danazol, diltiazem, lithium, nicotinamide, propoxyphene, theophylline, thyroid hormones, verapamil.

FOOD INTERACTIONS
No known food interactions.

DISEASE INTERACTIONS
Special caution is advised in those with lupus; heart, kidney, or liver disease; diabetes; or glaucoma.

SIDE EFFECTS

SERIOUS
Fever, sore throat, swollen glands, point-like rash, blistering or peeling, easy bruising, pallor, weakness, confusion, lethargy, or seizures may be a sign of a potentially fatal blood reaction (aplastic anemia). Call your doctor at once.

COMMON
Drowsiness, rash, itching, increased sensitivity of the skin to sunlight, dizziness, blurred vision, incoordination, nausea, vomiting, stomach pain or upset, diarrhea, constipation, loss of appetite, dry or inflamed mouth.

LESS COMMON
Impaired speech; involuntary movements of the face, limbs, or tongue; tingling or numbness in the extremities; depression; agitation; psychosis; talkativeness; abnormal eye movements; ringing in the ears; heart rhythm abnormalities; impotence; hair loss; or excessive hair growth. There are numerous additional potential side effects.

CARBENICILLIN INDANYL SODIUM

BRAND NAMES

Geocillin, Geopen

Available in: Tablets, injection
Available OTC? No   **As Generic?** Yes
Drug Class: Penicillin antibiotic

▼ USAGE INFORMATION

WHY IT'S PRESCRIBED
To treat bacterial infections, especially those of the prostate and urinary tract. Carbenicillin is effective only against infections caused by bacteria; it is ineffective against those caused by viruses, fungi, or other microorganisms.

HOW IT WORKS
Carbenicillin blocks the formation of bacterial cell walls, rendering bacteria unable to multiply and spread.

▼ DOSAGE GUIDELINES

RANGE AND FREQUENCY
Tablets— Adults and teenagers: 382 to 764 mg every 6 hours. Children: Consult your pediatrician. Injection— The dose is determined based on patient's body weight and other variables.

ONSET OF EFFECT
Unknown.

DURATION OF ACTION
Unknown.

DIETARY ADVICE
Carbenicillin should be taken on an empty stomach, at least 1 hour before or 2 hours after meals, with plenty of water. Patients with high blood pressure who follow a sodium-restricted diet should be aware that carbenicillin tablets contain a significant amount of salt.

STORAGE
Store in a tightly sealed container away from heat and direct light.

MISSED DOSE
Take it as soon as you remember. If it is within 2 hours of the next dose, skip the missed dose and resume your regular dosage schedule. Do not double the next dose.

STOPPING THE DRUG
Take it as prescribed for the full treatment period, even if you begin to feel better before the scheduled end of therapy. Stopping the drug prematurely may slow your recovery or lead to a rebound infection, also known as superinfection, in which the heartier strains of bacteria survive and multiply, leading to a more serious and drug-resistant infection.

PROLONGED USE
Prolonged use of any antibiotic increases the risk of superinfection; caution is advised.

▼ PRECAUTIONS

Over 60: No special problems are expected.

Driving and Hazardous Work: Do not drive or engage in hazardous work until you determine how the medicine affects you.

Alcohol: No special precautions are necessary.

Pregnancy: Adequate studies of the use of penicillin antibiotics during pregnancy have not been done; however, no problems have been reported.

Breast Feeding: Carbenicillin may pass into breast milk and cause problems in the nursing infant; avoid use while nursing.

Infants and Children: No special problems are expected.

Special Concerns: Carbenicillin can cause false results on some urine sugar tests for patients with diabetes. Those who are prone to asthma, hay fever, hives, or allergies may be more likely to have an allergic reaction to a penicillin antibiotic. If severe diarrhea occurs as a side effect of this drug, do not take antidiarrheal medications; call your doctor.

OVERDOSE
Symptoms: Seizures may occur with very high doses; overdose is nonetheless unlikely.

What to Do: If you have reason to suspect an overdose, seek medical assistance immediately.

▼ INTERACTIONS

DRUG INTERACTIONS
Consult your doctor for specific advice if you are taking aminoglycosides, ACE inhibitors, diuretics, potassium supplements or potassium-containing medications, anticoagulants or other anti-clotting drugs, nonsteroidal anti-inflammatory drugs, sulfinpyrazone, cholestyramine, colestipol, oral contraceptives, methotrexate, or probenecid.

FOOD INTERACTIONS
No known food interactions.

DISEASE INTERACTIONS
Consult your doctor if you have a history of allergies, asthma, bleeding disorders (such as hemophilia), congestive heart failure, gastrointestinal disorders (especially colitis associated with the use of antibiotics), high blood pressure, or impaired kidney function.

▼ SIDE EFFECTS

SERIOUS
Irregular, rapid, or labored breathing; lightheadedness or sudden fainting; joint pain; fever; severe abdominal pain and cramping with watery or bloody stools; severe allergic reaction (marked by sudden swelling of the lips, tongue, face, or throat; breathing difficulty; skin rash, itching, or hives); unusual bleeding or bruising; yellowish tinge to eyes or skin. Call your doctor immediately.

COMMON
Mild rash, mild diarrhea, nausea, vomiting, headache, vaginal discharge and itching, pain or white patches in the mouth or on the tongue.

LESS COMMON
Diminished urine output, chills, weakness, fatigue.

CARISOPRODOL

BRAND NAMES

Rela, Soma, Vanadom

Available in: Tablets
Available OTC? No   **As Generic?** Yes
Drug Class: Muscle relaxant

▼ USAGE INFORMATION

WHY IT'S PRESCRIBED
Skeletal muscle relaxants are used to relieve stiffness and discomfort caused by severe sprains and strains, muscle spasms, or other muscle problems. They may be prescribed in conjunction with other treatment methods, such as physical therapy.

HOW IT WORKS
Muscle relaxants such as carisoprodol depress activity in the central nervous system, which in turn interferes with the transmission of nerve impulses from the spinal cord to the muscles.

▼ DOSAGE GUIDELINES

RANGE AND FREQUENCY
Adults and teenagers: 350 mg, 3 to 4 times a day. Children ages 5 to 12: 6.25 mg per 2.2 lbs (1 kg) of body weight 4 times a day.

ONSET OF EFFECT
30 minutes.

DURATION OF ACTION
4 to 6 hours.

DIETARY ADVICE
Be sure to eat a well-balanced diet; the healing of injured tissue increases the body's protein and calorie requirements. To avoid dry mouth, maintain adequate fluid intake and suck on ice chips.

STORAGE
Store in a tightly sealed container in a dry place away from heat and direct light.

MISSED DOSE
Take it as soon as you remember. If it is within 2 hours of the next dose, skip the missed dose and resume your regular dosage schedule. Do not double the next dose.

STOPPING THE DRUG
This medication should be taken as prescribed for the full treatment period. Do not stop taking carisoprodol abruptly.

PROLONGED USE
Therapy with carisoprodol ranges from several days to weeks. Prolonged use may be associated with an increased risk of side effects.

▼ PRECAUTIONS

Over 60: Adverse reactions to medications such as carisoprodol may be more likely and more severe in older patients.

Driving and Hazardous Work: Carisoprodol may impair your ability to drive or perform hazardous work.

Alcohol: Avoid alcohol while taking this medication because it may compound the sedative effect and may cause liver damage.

Pregnancy: Adequate studies of carisoprodol during pregnancy have not been done; discuss the relative risks and benefits with your doctor.

Breast Feeding: Breast feeding is not recommended during therapy.

Infants and Children: No special problems have been documented; consult your pediatrician for advice.

Special Concerns: Carisoprodol will intensify the effect that alcohol, sedatives, and other central nervous system depressants have on the brain. It is not a substitute for other safe, nonmedical therapies for muscle stiffness, including rest, gentle guided exercise, and physical therapy.

OVERDOSE
Symptoms: Excessive drowsiness or difficulty awakening, even when being shaken or pinched; confusion; weakness; slowed breathing; coma.

What to Do: Call emergency medical services (EMS) or the nearest poison control center immediately.

▼ INTERACTIONS

DRUG INTERACTIONS
Consult your doctor for specific advice if you are taking antihistamines and decongestants, antidepressants, sedatives, tranquilizers, sleep aids, pain medication, barbiturates, or seizure medication.

FOOD INTERACTIONS
No known food interactions.

DISEASE INTERACTIONS
Caution is advised when taking carisoprodol. Consult your doctor if you have a history of any of the following: allergies, drug abuse or dependence, kidney disease, liver disease, porphyria, epilepsy, or any other seizure disorder.

≡ SIDE EFFECTS ≡

SERIOUS
Fainting; palpitations or rapid heartbeat; fever; hives or severe swelling of face, lips, or tongue along with shortness of breath, chest tightness, or wheezing (indicating a potentially life-threatening allergic reaction); depression. Seek medical help immediately.

COMMON
Drowsiness, dizziness, dry mouth.

LESS COMMON
Inability to pass urine; sores on lips, ulcers in mouth; abdominal cramps or pain; clumsiness; unsteady gait; confusion; constipation; diarrhea; excitability, nervousness, restlessness, or irritability; flushing or redness of face; headache; heartburn; hiccups; muscle weakness; nausea and vomiting; trembling; insomnia or fitful sleep; burning, red eyes; stuffy nose.

CARMUSTINE

BRAND NAMES

BCNU, BiCNU

Available in: Injection
Available OTC? No   **As Generic?** Yes
Drug Class: Alkylating agent

▼ USAGE INFORMATION

WHY IT'S PRESCRIBED
To treat brain, liver, and gastrointestinal cancers, in addition to lymphomas (cancers of the lymphatic system).

HOW IT WORKS
Carmustine interferes with the growth of cancer cells by preventing them from reproducing. The drug may also affect the growth and development of normal cells in the body, resulting in unpleasant side effects.

▼ DOSAGE GUIDELINES

RANGE AND FREQUENCY
Adults and children: The dose of carmustine depends on the type of tumor, the patient's body weight, and whether other chemotherapy drugs are being used. Your oncologist (cancer specialist) will determine the proper dose.

ONSET OF EFFECT
Almost immediately following injection.

DURATION OF ACTION
Unknown.

DIETARY ADVICE
Maintain optimal food and fluid intake. Calorie, protein, and vitamin needs increase in patients with cancer. Good nutrition is essential to cope with the demands of chemotherapy.

STORAGE
Refrigerate.

MISSED DOSE
Inform your oncologist as soon as possible.

STOPPING THE DRUG
The decision to stop administering carmustine must be made by your doctor.

PROLONGED USE
Use beyond 1 to 2 days is not recommended.

▼ PRECAUTIONS

Over 60: Adverse reactions may be more likely and more severe.

Driving and Hazardous Work: The use of this drug may impair your ability to drive or operate machinery safely, or perform hazardous work.

Alcohol: Avoid alcohol.

Pregnancy: Carmustine may cause birth defects. Persons of childbearing years should take steps to prevent pregnancy during therapy.

Breast Feeding: Not recommended during therapy.

Infants and Children: Consult your pediatrician.

Special Concerns: Patients with cancer are very often weakened by their illness, by poor nutrition, and by the effects of chemotherapy, radiation, and surgery. These patients are more likely to experience undesirable side effects of a medication. In addition, these side effects may be more pronounced. Follow directions very carefully for all medication that you are taking. Read and understand all potential side effects and drug interactions. Infection is the single greatest threat to people receiving chemotherapy. Carmustine may lower your ability to resist infection by lowering the number of white blood cells in the blood. Therefore, do not receive any vaccinations without your doctor's approval. Avoid people with infections. Inform your doctor immediately if you have fever, chills, diarrhea, or a cough. Shortness of breath may develop many years after initial treatment in children or adolescents who receive higher doses.

OVERDOSE
Symptoms: No cases of overdose have been reported.

What to Do: Although not likely to occur, if you are concerned about the possibility of an overdose of carmustine, contact your doctor.

▼ INTERACTIONS

DRUG INTERACTIONS
Consult your doctor for specific advice if you are taking amphotericin B, thyroid medications, azathioprine, chloramphenicol, colchicine, flucytosine, ganciclovir, interferon, plicamycin, or zidovudine (AZT).

FOOD INTERACTIONS
None are known.

DISEASE INTERACTIONS
Consult your doctor if you have any of the following: chicken pox (or recent exposure to someone with it), shingles, an infection, kidney disease, liver disease, or lung disease.

≡ SIDE EFFECTS ≡

SERIOUS
Black or tarry stools; blood-tinged (pink or maroon) urine or stools; cough or shortness of breath; fever and chills; lower back pain or pain in flanks; painful, difficult urination; small, red spots on the skin; bleeding from gums, nose, or other unusual places; easy bruising. These side effects may mean that normal blood cells and special blood-clotting cells have been affected, or that normal immune cells have been affected and an infection is developing somewhere in your body. See your doctor right away if any of these symptoms occur.

COMMON
Nausea and vomiting, weakness, fatigue, loss of appetite, pain or redness at injection site (tell your nurse immediately if this happens while the drug is being administered).

LESS COMMON
Decreased urination, edema (swelling) of the feet and ankles, diarrhea, dizziness, skin discoloration at injection site, skin rash or itching, difficulty swallowing, difficulty walking, hair loss.

CARTEOLOL HYDROCHLORIDE OPHTHALMIC

Available in: Ophthalmic solution
Available OTC? No   **As Generic?** No
Drug Class: Antiglaucoma drug; ophthalmic beta-blocker

▼ USAGE INFORMATION

WHY IT'S PRESCRIBED
To treat glaucoma.

HOW IT WORKS
Glaucoma, a sight-threatening disorder, occurs when aqueous humor (the fluid inside the eye) cannot drain properly, causing an increase in pressure within the eyeball (known as intraocular pressure). Increased intraocular pressure can damage the optic nerve and lead to a gradually progressive loss of vision. Carteolol decreases the production of aqueous humor, thereby reducing intraocular pressure.

▼ DOSAGE GUIDELINES

RANGE AND FREQUENCY
1 drop twice a day.

ONSET OF EFFECT
30 to 60 minutes.

DURATION OF ACTION
From 6 to 8 hours.

DIETARY ADVICE
Can be applied without regard to dietary habits or schedule.

STORAGE
Store in a tightly sealed container away from heat, moisture, and direct light.

MISSED DOSE
Apply it as soon as you remember. If it is near the time for the next dose, skip the missed dose and resume your regular dosage schedule. Do not double the next dose.

STOPPING THE DRUG
The decision to stop using the drug should be made by your doctor.

PROLONGED USE
Eye examinations should be done regularly as part of glaucoma follow-up.

▼ PRECAUTIONS

Over 60: Adverse reactions may be more likely and more severe in older patients.

Driving and Hazardous Work: Do not drive or engage in hazardous work until you determine how the medicine affects your vision.

Alcohol: Use with caution.

Pregnancy: Adequate human studies have not been completed. Before taking ophthalmic carteolol, tell your doctor if you are pregnant or plan to become pregnant.

Breast Feeding: Ophthalmic carteolol may pass into breast milk; caution is advised. Consult your doctor for advice.

Infants and Children: Adverse reactions may be more likely and more severe in children.

Special Concerns: To use the eye drops, first wash your hands. Tilt your head back. Gently apply pressure to the inside corner of the eyelid and with the index finger of the same hand, pull downward on the lower eyelid to make a space. Drop the medicine into this space and close your eye. Apply pressure for 1 or 2 minutes while keeping the eye closed without blinking. Then wash your hands again. Make sure the tip of the dropper does not touch your eye, finger, or any other surface. Carteolol may make your eyes more sensitive to sunlight. If this occurs, wear sunglasses or avoid bright light as comfort dictates. Before you have any kind of surgery, emergency treatment, or dental treatment, tell the doctor or dentist that you are taking ophthalmic carteolol.

OVERDOSE
Symptoms: Nervousness, chest pain, confusion, hallucinations, coughing, wheezing, drowsiness, dizziness, irregular or pounding heartbeat, insomnia, fatigue.

What to Do: If a large volume of the drug enters the eyes, flush with water. If the medication is accidentally ingested, seek medical assistance right away.

▼ INTERACTIONS

DRUG INTERACTIONS
It is not recommended to use two ophthalmic beta-blockers at the same time. Special caution is warranted in people taking antidiabetic drugs, since ophthalmic carteolol may mask symptoms of low blood sugar. Other drugs may interact with ophthalmic carteolol. Tell your doctor if you are using any other prescription or over-the-counter medication.

FOOD INTERACTIONS
No known food interactions.

DISEASE INTERACTIONS
Do not use ophthalmic carteolol if you have asthma, chronic obstructive pulmonary disease (COPD), or heart rhythm irregularities. Caution is advised when taking ophthalmic carteolol. Consult your doctor if you have any of the following: hay fever, chronic bronchitis, diabetes, low blood sugar, heart disease, blood vessel disease, myasthenia gravis, or an overactive thyroid. Use of this drug may cause complications in patients with liver or kidney disease, since these organs work together to remove the medication from the body.

SIDE EFFECTS

SERIOUS
Palpitations, breathing difficulty, dizziness and weakness caused by low blood pressure. Call your doctor right away.

COMMON
Temporary eye irritation, tearing, eye inflammation, burning, swelling.

LESS COMMON
Blurred vision, poor night vision, and increased sensitivity to light; headache; insomnia; sinus irritation; odd or bitter taste in the mouth.

CARTEOLOL HYDROCHLORIDE ORAL

Available in: Tablets
Available OTC? No **As Generic?** No
Drug Class: Beta-blocker

▼ USAGE INFORMATION

WHY IT'S PRESCRIBED
To treat high blood pressure (hypertension).

HOW IT WORKS
By blocking actions of the sympathetic nervous system, carteolol reduces the rate and force of the heartbeat, thus lowering blood pressure.

▼ DOSAGE GUIDELINES

RANGE AND FREQUENCY
To treat high blood pressure: 2.5 mg once a day, increased to 5 to 10 mg per day if needed. (Dosage schedule for persons with impaired kidney function: 2.5 mg once every 1, 2, or 3 days as needed.)

ONSET OF EFFECT
Three weeks of therapy may be needed for the full effect of the drug to occur.

DURATION OF ACTION
24 hours.

DIETARY ADVICE
Most effective when taken at least 1 hour before or 2 hours after eating.

STORAGE
Store in a tightly sealed container away from heat and direct light.

MISSED DOSE
Take it as soon as you remember. If it is within 8 hours of the next dose, skip the missed dose and resume your regular dosage schedule. Do not double the next dose.

STOPPING THE DRUG
The decision to stop taking the drug should be made in consultation with your doctor. Gradual reduction of the dose over a 2 to 3 week period is generally necessary; stopping the drug abruptly may cause potentially serious medical consequences.

PROLONGED USE
Prolonged use may weaken the heart.

▼ PRECAUTIONS

Over 60: Adverse reactions may be more likely and more severe in older patients. Treatment usually begins with small doses that are increased gradually by your doctor to avoid an excessive reduction in blood pressure.

Driving and Hazardous Work: Do not drive or engage in hazardous work until you determine how the medicine affects you.

Alcohol: Drink in careful moderation if at all. Alcohol may interact with the drug and cause a dangerous drop in blood pressure.

Pregnancy: No birth defects were found in animal studies. Adequate studies in pregnant human patients have not been done. Before taking carteolol, notify your doctor if you are pregnant or plan to become pregnant.

Breast Feeding: Carteolol may pass into breast milk; caution is advised. Consult your doctor for advice.

Infants and Children: The safety and effectiveness of carteolol use in children under 12 have not been determined. It should be used only under close medical supervision.

Special Concerns: Be cautious about exposure to very hot or very cold weather conditions. Heavy exercise or exertion can cause excessive fatigue, muscle cramping, or dangerous increases in your blood pressure.

OVERDOSE

Symptoms: Slow heartbeat, severe dizziness, fainting, fast or irregular heartbeat, difficulty breathing, bluish-colored fingernails or palms, seizures.

What to Do: Call your doctor, emergency medical services (EMS), or the nearest poison control center immediately.

▼ INTERACTIONS

DRUG INTERACTIONS
Consult your doctor for specific advice if you are taking other drugs for high blood pressure, reserpine, theophylline, amiodarone, clonidine, diltiazem, epinephrine, ergot preparations, fluvoxamine, insulin, nifedipine, oral antidiabetic agents, phenothiazines, nonsteroidal anti-inflammatory drugs, or indomethacin.

FOOD INTERACTIONS
No known food interactions.

DISEASE INTERACTIONS
Use of carteolol may cause complications in patients with liver or kidney disease, since these organs work together to remove the medication from the body. Carteolol should be used with caution in people with diabetes, especially insulin-dependent diabetes, since the drug may mask the symptoms of hypoglycemia. Also consult your doctor if you have any of the following disorders: congestive heart failure, coronary artery disease, allergic rhinitis (seasonal allergies), asthma, chronic bronchitis, hyperthyroidism, myasthenia gravis, or blood vessel (vascular) disease.

≡ SIDE EFFECTS ≡

SERIOUS
Shortness of breath, wheezing; irregular or slow heartbeat (50 beats per minute or less); pain or feelings of tightness or pressure in the chest; swelling of the ankles, feet, and lower legs; mental depression. Call your doctor right away.

COMMON
Dizziness or lightheadedness, especially when rising rapidly to a standing position; rapid heartbeat or palpitations; decreased sexual ability; unusual fatigue, weakness, or drowsiness; muscle cramps; insomnia.

LESS COMMON
Anxiety, irritability, nervousness; constipation; diarrhea; dry, sore eyes; itching; nausea or vomiting; nightmares or intensely vivid dreams; numbness, tingling, or other unusual sensations in the fingers, toes, or scalp.

CARVEDILOL

Available in: Tablets
Available OTC? No   **As Generic?** No
Drug Class: Beta-blocker

▼ USAGE INFORMATION

WHY IT'S PRESCRIBED
To treat mild to moderate congestive heart failure (CHF) in conjunction with digitalis, diuretics, or ACE inhibitors. Also used to treat high blood pressure.

HOW IT WORKS
It is not known how carvedilol improves CHF and lowers blood pressure.

▼ DOSAGE GUIDELINES

RANGE AND FREQUENCY
Dosages must be tailored individually to each patient, using the following guidelines as starting points. For CHF: Initially, 3.125 mg twice a day for 2 weeks. For patients weighing less than 187 lbs, maximum daily dose is 25 mg twice a day. For patients weighing more than 187 lbs, maximum daily dose is 50 mg twice a day. For high blood pressure: Initially, 6.25 mg twice a day for 7 to 14 days. Maximum daily dose is 50 mg.

ONSET OF EFFECT
Within 1 to 2 hours.

DURATION OF ACTION
Unknown.

DIETARY ADVICE
Take it with food to reduce the risk of potentially dangerous drop in blood pressure. Follow your doctor's dietary guidelines.

STORAGE
Store in a tightly sealed container away from heat, moisture, and direct light.

MISSED DOSE
Take it as soon as you remember. If it is within 4 hours of the next scheduled dose, skip the missed dose and resume your regular dosage schedule. Do not double the next dose.

STOPPING THE DRUG
This drug should not be stopped suddenly, as this may lead to angina and possibly a heart attack in patients with advanced heart disease. Slow reduction of dosage over a period of 1 to 2 weeks is advised.

PROLONGED USE
Regular visits to your doctor are needed to evaluate the drug's ongoing, long-term effectiveness.

▼ PRECAUTIONS

Over 60: Many elderly patients are more sensitive to the drug than younger persons. Smaller doses and frequent blood pressure checks may be warranted.

Driving and Hazardous Work: Use caution in such activities until you determine how the drug affects you.

Alcohol: Alcohol may interact with the drug and cause a dangerous drop in blood pressure.

Pregnancy: Discuss with your doctor the relative risks and benefits of using this drug while pregnant.

Breast Feeding: Trace amounts of this drug can be found in breast milk; however, adverse effects in infants have not been documented. Consult your doctor for specific advice.

Infants and Children: Not recommended.

Special Concerns: Use of the drug should be considered but one element of a comprehensive therapeutic program that includes weight control, smoking cessation, regular exercise, and a healthy (low-salt, low-fat) diet.

OVERDOSE
Symptoms: Unusually slow heartbeat, severe dizziness or fainting, vomiting, breathing difficulty, seizures.

What to Do: Call your doctor, emergency medical services (EMS), or the nearest poison control center immediately.

▼ INTERACTIONS

DRUG INTERACTIONS
Inform your doctor if you are taking amphetamines, oral antidiabetic agents, insulin, asthma medication, calcium channel blockers, clonidine, guanabenz, allergy shots, MAO inhibitors, reserpine, cyclosporine, other beta-blockers, or any over-the-counter medicine.

FOOD INTERACTIONS
None reported.

DISEASE INTERACTIONS
Carvedilol should be used with caution by people with diabetes, especially insulin-dependent diabetes, since the drug may mask symptoms of hypoglycemia. Consult your doctor for specific advice if you have allergies or asthma; heart or blood vessel disease (including peripheral vascular disease); hyperthyroidism; irregular (slow) heartbeat; a history of mental depression; myasthenia gravis; psoriasis; respiratory problems, such as bronchitis or emphysema; or kidney or liver disease.

 SIDE EFFECTS

SERIOUS
Shortness of breath, wheezing; irregular or slow heartbeat (50 beats per minute or less); pain or feelings of tightness or pressure in the chest; swelling of the ankles, feet, and lower legs; mental depression. If you experience such symptoms, call your doctor immediately.

COMMON
Dizziness or lightheadedness, especially when rising suddenly to a standing position; decreased sexual ability; unusual fatigue, weakness, or drowsiness; insomnia; diarrhea; nausea or vomiting.

LESS COMMON
Anxiety, irritability, nervousness; constipation; dry, sore eyes; itching; nightmares or intensely vivid dreams; numbness, tingling, or other unusual sensations in the fingers, toes, or scalp.

CASTOR OIL

Available in: Oral solution
Available OTC? Yes   **As Generic?** Yes
Drug Class: Stimulant laxative

▼ USAGE INFORMATION

WHY IT'S PRESCRIBED
For short-term relief of constipation.

HOW IT WORKS
Castor oil stimulates muscle contractions in the wall of the bowel. These contractions promote the passage of stool.

▼ DOSAGE GUIDELINES

RANGE AND FREQUENCY
The dose will be different for different products. A typical dose is 15 to 60 ml for adults and teenagers. Castor oil should be taken early in the day because the laxative effect is unpredictable and might otherwise interfere with a full night's sleep.

ONSET OF EFFECT
Within 2 to 6 hours.

DURATION OF ACTION
Variable.

DIETARY ADVICE
Laxatives may contain a large amount of sodium or sugar. Regular bowel movements are more likely with a diet that contains an adequate amount of liquid (6 to 8 full 8-oz glasses per day), whole-grain products and bran, fruit, and vegetables.

STORAGE
Store in a tightly sealed container away from heat, moisture, and direct light. Keep the liquid form refrigerated, but do not allow it to freeze.

MISSED DOSE
If you are on a prescribed dosage schedule, take a missed dose as soon as you remember, unless the time for your next scheduled dose is within the next 2 hours. If so, do not take the missed dose. Take your next scheduled dose at the proper time, and resume your regular dosage schedule. Do not double the next dose.

STOPPING THE DRUG
Take it as prescribed for the full treatment period. However, you may stop taking the drug if you are feeling better before the scheduled end of the therapy.

PROLONGED USE
Do not use castor oil for more than 3 to 5 days without informing your physician. Prolonged, excessive use of castor oil may be associated with an increased risk of side effects, including laxative dependence.

▼ PRECAUTIONS

Over 60: Adverse reactions may be more likely and more severe in older patients.

Driving and Hazardous Work: Do not drive or engage in hazardous work until you determine how the medicine affects you.

Alcohol: Avoid alcohol when using this medication.

Pregnancy: Castor oil may cause premature contractions and so should be avoided in pregnant women.

Breast Feeding: Castor oil may be used by nursing mothers.

Infants and Children: Do not give laxatives to children under 6 years of age unless prescribed by a physician.

Special Concerns: Occasional missed bowel movements do not constitute constipation; do not use castor oil under such circumstances. Persistent constipation or difficulty in passing stool is serious and requires evaluation.

OVERDOSE
Symptoms: No cases of overdose with castor oil have been reported.

What to Do: An overdose of castor oil is unlikely to be life-threatening. However, if someone takes a much larger dose than prescribed, contact a physician.

▼ INTERACTIONS

DRUG INTERACTIONS
Do not take a prescription medication within 2 hours of taking a laxative (either before or after), since this may diminish the effects of the prescription drug. Consult your doctor for specific advice if you are taking digitalis drugs or a diuretic.

FOOD INTERACTIONS
No known food interactions.

DISEASE INTERACTIONS
Caution is advised when taking castor oil. Do not use any laxative if you have any of the following: stomach or abdominal pain, especially if accompanied by fever; cramping; abdominal swelling or bloating; nausea or vomiting. Consult your doctor if you have any of the following problems: abdominal pain and fever, rectal bleeding, ostomy (an artificial surgical opening in the body to allow the release of urine or feces), diabetes, heart or kidney disease, or high blood pressure.

SIDE EFFECTS

SERIOUS
Confusion, irregular heartbeat, muscle cramps. Call your doctor immediately.

COMMON
Laxative dependence, skin rashes, stomach cramps, belching, diarrhea, nausea.

LESS COMMON
Fatigue or weakness.

CEFACLOR

Available in: Capsules, oral suspension
Available OTC? No   **As Generic?** Yes
Drug Class: Cephalosporin antibiotic

▼ USAGE INFORMATION

WHY IT'S PRESCRIBED
To treat a variety of bacterial infections, including those of the nose, tonsils, and throat, skin and soft tissues, genito-urinary tract, and the respiratory tract. Cefaclor is effective only against infections caused by bacteria; it is ineffective against those caused by viruses, fungi, or other microorganisms.

HOW IT WORKS
Cefaclor prevents bacteria from forming cell walls.

▼ DOSAGE GUIDELINES

RANGE AND FREQUENCY
Adults and teenagers: 250 to 500 mg every 8 hours. Children 1 month to 12 years: 20 mg per 2.2 lbs (1 kg) of body weight a day in divided doses every 8 hours. It can be given every 12 hours for ear infection or sore throat.

ONSET OF EFFECT
30 to 60 minutes.

DURATION OF ACTION
1 to 2 hours.

DIETARY ADVICE
Cefaclor may be taken on a full or empty stomach, but taking it with food will reduce stomach irritation.

STORAGE
Store in a tightly sealed container away from heat, moisture, and direct light. Keep liquid form refrigerated, but do not allow it to freeze.

MISSED DOSE
Take it as soon as you remember. This will help keep a constant level of medication in your system. If it is near the time for the next dose, skip the missed dose and resume your regular dosage schedule. Do not double the next dose.

STOPPING THE DRUG
Take it as prescribed for the full treatment period, even if you begin to feel better before the scheduled end of therapy. Stopping cefaclor prematurely may slow your recovery or lead to a rebound infection, also known as superinfection, in which the heartier strains of bacteria survive and multiply, leading to a more serious and drug-resistant infection. When taking this drug to treat a streptococcal (strep) infection, it is particularly important to take it for the entire treatment period. Serious heart and kidney problems can develop later if the drug is discontinued prematurely.

PROLONGED USE
Cefaclor is generally prescribed for short-term therapy (10 to 14 days). Use of cefaclor beyond this period increases the risk of adverse effects and superinfection.

▼ PRECAUTIONS

Over 60: Adverse reactions may be more likely and more severe in older patients.

Driving and Hazardous Work: Do not drive or engage in hazardous work until you determine how the medicine affects you.

Alcohol: Avoid alcohol.

Pregnancy: Adequate studies of cephalosporin use in pregnant women have not been done. Before taking cefaclor, tell your physician if you are pregnant or are planning to become pregnant.

Breast Feeding: Cefaclor passes into breast milk; caution is advised. Consult your doctor for specific advice.

Infants and Children: This drug may be used by children 1 month and older. Consult your pediatrician for advice.

Special Concerns: People who are allergic to penicillin may have equally serious allergic reactions to cephalosporin antibiotics, such as cefaclor. This drug is useful only against bacteria that are susceptible to its effects, not against colds, flu, or other viral infections. If your condition has not improved within a few days of starting cefaclor, or instead has worsened, tell your doctor.

▼ OVERDOSE

Symptoms: Seizures, severe abdominal pain, bloody diarrhea, vomiting.

What to Do: Call your doctor, emergency medical services (EMS), or the nearest poison control center immediately.

▼ INTERACTIONS

DRUG INTERACTIONS
Consult your doctor for specific advice if you are taking carbenicillin injection, heparin, divalproex, anticoagulants, sulfinpyrazone, dipyridamole, pentoxifylline, plicamycin, ticarcillin, probenecid, or valproic acid.

FOOD INTERACTIONS
No known food interactions.

DISEASE INTERACTIONS
Caution is advised when taking cefaclor. Consult your doctor if you have a history of kidney disease or colitis.

≡ SIDE EFFECTS ≡

SERIOUS
Severe allergic reaction (breathing difficulties, confusion, hives, itching, swelling of the face or throat, sweating, and lightheadedness), severe stomach pain and cramps, fever, severe, sometimes bloody diarrhea. Call your doctor immediately.

COMMON
Mild diarrhea or stomach cramps, sore mouth or tongue, nausea and vomiting.

LESS COMMON
Vaginal itching or unusual discharge, anemia, rash, decreased white blood cell count causing increased susceptibility to infection.

CEFADROXIL

BRAND NAMES

Duricef, Ultracef

Available in: Capsules, tablets, oral suspension
Available OTC? No   **As Generic?** Yes
Drug Class: Cephalosporin antibiotic

▼ USAGE INFORMATION

WHY IT'S PRESCRIBED
To treat a variety of bacterial infections, including those of the throat, skin and soft tissues, and the genitourinary tract. Cefadroxil is effective only against infections caused by bacteria; it is ineffective against those caused by viruses, fungi, or other microorganisms.

HOW IT WORKS
Cefadroxil prevents bacteria from forming protective cell walls necessary for survival.

▼ DOSAGE GUIDELINES

RANGE AND FREQUENCY
Adults and teenagers: 500 mg every 12 hours, or 1 to 2 g once a day. Children: 15 mg per 2.2 lbs (1 kg) of body weight every 12 hours, or 30 mg per 2.2 lbs once a day.

ONSET OF EFFECT
12 hours.

DURATION OF ACTION
20 to 22 hours.

DIETARY ADVICE
Cefadroxil may be taken on a full or empty stomach, but taking it with food will reduce stomach irritation.

STORAGE
Store in a tightly sealed container away from heat, moisture, and direct light. Keep liquid form refrigerated, but do not allow it to freeze.

MISSED DOSE
Take it as soon as you remember. This will help keep a constant level of medication in your system. If it is near the time for the next dose, skip the missed dose and resume your regular dosage schedule. Do not double the next dose.

STOPPING THE DRUG
Take it as prescribed for the full treatment period, even if you begin to feel better before the scheduled end of therapy. Stopping cefadroxil prematurely may slow your recovery or lead to a rebound infection, also known as superinfection, in which the heartier strains of bacteria survive and multiply, leading to a more serious and drug-resistant infection. When taking this drug to treat a streptococcal (strep) infection, it is particularly important to take it for the entire treatment period. Serious heart and kidney problems can develop later if the drug is discontinued prematurely.

PROLONGED USE
Cefadroxil is generally prescribed for short-term therapy (10 to 14 days). Use of cefadroxil beyond this period increases the risk of adverse effects and superinfection.

▼ PRECAUTIONS

Over 60: Adverse reactions may be more likely and more severe in older patients.

Driving and Hazardous Work: Do not drive or engage in hazardous work until you determine how the medicine affects you.

Alcohol: Avoid alcohol.

Pregnancy: Adequate studies of cephalosporin use in pregnant women have not been done. Before taking cefadroxil, tell your doctor if you are or plan to become pregnant.

Breast Feeding: Cefadroxil passes into breast milk; caution is advised. Consult your doctor for specific advice.

Infants and Children: This drug may be used by children age 1 and older. Consult your pediatrician for advice.

Special Concerns: People who are allergic to penicillin may have equally serious allergic reactions to cephalosporin antibiotics, such as cefadroxil. This drug is useful only against bacteria that are susceptible to its effects, not against colds, flu, or other viral infections. If your condition has not improved within a few days of starting cefadroxil, or instead has worsened, tell your doctor.

OVERDOSE
Symptoms: Seizures, severe abdominal pain, bloody diarrhea, vomiting.

What to Do: Call your doctor, emergency medical services (EMS), or the nearest poison control center immediately.

▼ INTERACTIONS

DRUG INTERACTIONS
Consult your doctor for specific advice if you are taking carbenicillin injection, heparin, divalproex, anticoagulants, sulfinpyrazone, dipyridamole, pentoxifylline, plicamycin, ticarcillin, probenecid, or valproic acid.

FOOD INTERACTIONS
No known food interactions.

DISEASE INTERACTIONS
Caution is advised when taking cefadroxil. Consult your doctor if you have a history of kidney disease or colitis.

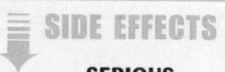 SIDE EFFECTS

SERIOUS
Severe allergic reaction (breathing difficulties, confusion, hives, itching, swelling of the face or throat, sweating, and lightheadedness), severe stomach pain and cramps, fever, severe, sometimes bloody diarrhea. Call your doctor immediately.

COMMON
Mild diarrhea or stomach cramps, sore mouth or tongue, nausea and vomiting.

LESS COMMON
Vaginal itching or discharge, anemia, rash, decreased white blood cell count causing increased susceptibility to infection, decreased blood platelets causing increased risk of bleeding problems.

CEFAMANDOLE NAFATE

Available in: Injection
Available OTC? No **As Generic?** Yes
Drug Class: Cephalosporin antibiotic

▼ USAGE INFORMATION

WHY IT'S PRESCRIBED
To treat a variety of serious bacterial infections, including those of the lung, genitourinary tract, blood, bones, joints, skin, and other organs. Cefamandole nafate is effective only against infections caused by bacteria; it is ineffective against those caused by viruses, fungi, or other microorganisms. Cephalosporins, such as cefamandole nafate, are prescribed when other antibiotics are not sufficient to treat the infection.

HOW IT WORKS
Cefamandole nafate prevents bacteria from forming protective cell walls.

▼ DOSAGE GUIDELINES

RANGE AND FREQUENCY
Adults and teenagers: 500 to 1,000 mg (2,000 mg for life-threatening infections) every 4 to 8 hours, injected into a vein or muscle. Children 1 month to 12 years: 8.3 to 33.3 mg per 2.2 lbs (1 kg) of body weight every 4 to 8 hours into a vein or muscle.

ONSET OF EFFECT
Into a vein: Immediate. Into a muscle: 30 to 120 minutes.

DURATION OF ACTION
Into a vein: 1 hour. Into a muscle: 2 hours.

DIETARY ADVICE
Eat 4 oz of yogurt or drink 4 oz of buttermilk a day to protect against intestinal superinfection. Drink plenty of fluids.

STORAGE
Not applicable; the dose is administered only at a health care facility.

MISSED DOSE
Not applicable; the dose is administered by a health care professional.

STOPPING THE DRUG
The decision to stop taking cefamandole nafate should be made by your doctor.

PROLONGED USE
Cefamandole nafate is generally prescribed for short-term therapy (10 to 14 days). Use beyond this period increases the risk of adverse effects and superinfection, a subsequent infection caused by heartier, drug-resistant strains of bacteria.

▼ PRECAUTIONS

Over 60: Adverse reactions may be more likely and more severe in older patients.

Driving and Hazardous Work: Not applicable; the dose is administered only in a health care institution.

Alcohol: Avoid alcohol.

Pregnancy: Adequate studies of cephalosporin use in pregnant women have not been done. Before taking cefamandole nafate, tell your doctor if you are pregnant or plan to become pregnant.

Breast Feeding: Cefamandole nafate passes into breast milk; caution is advised. Consult your doctor for advice.

Infants and Children: This drug may be used by children 1 month and older. Consult your pediatrician for advice.

Special Concerns: People who are allergic to penicillin may have equally serious allergic reactions to cephalosporin antibiotics, such as cefamandole nafate. This drug is useful only against bacteria that are susceptible to its effects, not against colds, flu, or other viral infections. If your condition has not improved within a few days of starting cefamandole nafate, or instead has worsened, tell your doctor.

OVERDOSE
Symptoms: An overdose of cefamandole nafate is unlikely to occur.

What to Do: Emergency instructions not applicable.

▼ INTERACTIONS

DRUG INTERACTIONS
Consult your doctor for advice if you are taking carbenicillin injection, heparin, divalproex, anticoagulants, sulfinpyrazone, dipyridamole, pentoxifylline, plicamycin, ticarcillin, probenecid, medications containing alcohol, or valproic acid.

FOOD INTERACTIONS
No known food interactions.

DISEASE INTERACTIONS
Caution is advised when taking cefamandole nafate. Consult your doctor if you have a history of kidney disease, bleeding disorders, or colitis.

 SIDE EFFECTS

SERIOUS
Severe allergic reaction (breathing difficulties, confusion, hives, swelling of the face or throat, sweating, and light-headedness), severe stomach pain and cramps, fever, severe, sometimes bloody diarrhea, unusual bleeding or bruising. Call your doctor immediately.

COMMON
Mild diarrhea or stomach cramps, sore mouth or tongue, nausea and vomiting.

LESS COMMON
Vaginal itching or discharge, pain at site of injection, rash, decreased white blood cell count causing increased susceptibility to infection, decreased blood platelets causing increased risk of bleeding problems.

CEFAZOLIN SODIUM

Available in: Injection
Available OTC? No   **As Generic?** Yes
Drug Class: Cephalosporin antibiotic

▼ USAGE INFORMATION

WHY IT'S PRESCRIBED
To treat a variety of moderately severe bacterial infections, including those of the heart, lung, genitourinary tract, bones, joints, skin and soft tissue, and blood. Cefazolin sodium is effective only against infections caused by bacteria; it is ineffective against those caused by viruses, fungi, or other microorganisms. Cephalosporins, such as cefazolin sodium, are prescribed when other antibiotics are not sufficient to treat the infection. It is also used prior to some surgeries to prevent infection.

HOW IT WORKS
Cefazolin sodium prevents bacteria from forming protective cell walls.

▼ DOSAGE GUIDELINES

RANGE AND FREQUENCY
Adults and teenagers: 250 to 1,500 mg every 6 to 8 hours into a vein. Children 1 month to 12 years: 6.25 to 25 mg per 2.2 lbs (1 kg) of body weight every 6 hours, or 8.3 to 33.3 mg per 2.2 lbs every 8 hours into a vein.

ONSET OF EFFECT
Immediate.

DURATION OF ACTION
4 hours.

DIETARY ADVICE
Eat 4 oz of yogurt or drink 4 oz of buttermilk a day to protect against intestinal superinfection. Drink plenty of fluids.

STORAGE
Not applicable; the dose is administered only at a health care facility.

MISSED DOSE
Not applicable; the dose is administered by a health care professional.

STOPPING THE DRUG
The decision to stop taking the drug should be made by your doctor.

PROLONGED USE
Cefazolin sodium is generally prescribed for short-term therapy (10 to 14 days). Use beyond this period increases the risk of adverse effects and superinfection, a subsequent infection caused by heartier, drug-resistant strains of bacteria.

▼ PRECAUTIONS

Over 60: Adverse reactions may be more likely and more severe in older patients.

Driving and Hazardous Work: Not applicable; the dose is administered only in a health care institution.

Alcohol: Avoid alcohol.

Pregnancy: Adequate studies of cephalosporin use in pregnant women have not been done. Before taking cefazolin sodium, tell your doctor if you are pregnant or plan to become pregnant.

Breast Feeding: Cefazolin sodium passes into breast milk; caution is advised. Consult your doctor for advice.

Infants and Children: This drug may be used by children 1 month and older. Consult your pediatrician for advice.

Special Concerns: People who are allergic to penicillin may have equally serious allergic reactions to cephalosporin antibiotics. Cefazolin sodium is useful only against bacteria that are susceptible to its effects and will not work against colds, flu, or other viral infections. If your condition has not improved within a few days of starting cefazolin sodium, or instead has worsened, tell your doctor.

▼ OVERDOSE

Symptoms: An overdose of cefazolin sodium is unlikely.

What to Do: Emergency instructions not applicable.

▼ INTERACTIONS

DRUG INTERACTIONS
Consult your doctor for specific advice if you are taking carbenicillin injection, heparin, divalproex, anticoagulants, sulfinpyrazone, dipyridamole, pentoxifylline, plicamycin, ticarcillin, probenecid, or valproic acid.

FOOD INTERACTIONS
No known food interactions.

DISEASE INTERACTIONS
Caution is advised when taking cefazolin. Consult your doctor if you have a history of kidney disease or colitis.

 SIDE EFFECTS

SERIOUS
Severe allergic reaction (breathing difficulties, confusion, itching, hives, swelling of the face or throat, sweating, and lightheadedness), severe stomach pain and cramps, fever, severe, sometimes bloody diarrhea. Call your doctor immediately.

COMMON
Mild diarrhea or stomach cramps, sore mouth or tongue, nausea and vomiting.

LESS COMMON
Vaginal itching or unusual discharge, pain or itching at the site of injection.

CEFEPIME

Available in: Injection
Available OTC? No   **As Generic?** No
Drug Class: Cephalosporin antibiotic

▼ USAGE INFORMATION

WHY IT'S PRESCRIBED
To treat a variety of moderate to serious bacterial infections, including those of the ear, nose, tonsils, and throat, skin and soft tissues, genitourinary tract, and the respiratory tract. Cefepime is effective only against infections caused by bacteria; it is ineffective against those caused by viruses, fungi, or other microorganisms. Cephalosporins, such as cefepime, are prescribed when other antibiotics are not sufficient to treat the infection.

HOW IT WORKS
Cefepime prevents bacteria from forming cell walls.

▼ DOSAGE GUIDELINES

RANGE AND FREQUENCY
Adults and teenagers— Mild to moderate urinary tract infections: 500 to 1,000 mg every 12 hours. Severe urinary tract infections: 2,000 mg every 12 hours. Moderate to severe pneumonia: 1,000 to 2,000 mg every 12 hours. Moderate to severe skin infections: 2,000 mg every 12 hours. Injections are usually into a vein. For mild to moderate urinary tract infections, cefepime may be administered into a muscle. Children age 2 months to 16 years and weighing less than 40 kg: 50 mg per 2.2 lbs (1 kg) of body weight every 12 hours. The dose should not exceed the recommended adult dose.

ONSET OF EFFECT
Immediate.

DURATION OF ACTION
Unknown.

DIETARY ADVICE
Eat 4 oz of yogurt or drink 4 oz of buttermilk a day to protect against intestinal superinfection. Drink plenty of fluids.

STORAGE
Not applicable; the dose is administered only at a health care facility.

MISSED DOSE
Not applicable; the dose is administered by a health care professional.

STOPPING THE DRUG
The decision to stop taking the drug should be made by your doctor.

PROLONGED USE
Cefepime is generally prescribed for short-term therapy (10 to 14 days). Use of cefepime beyond this period increases the risk of adverse effects and superinfection, a subsequent infection caused by heartier, drug-resistant bacteria.

▼ PRECAUTIONS

Over 60: Adverse reactions may be more likely and more severe in older patients.

Driving and Hazardous Work: Not applicable; the dose is administered only in a health care institution.

Alcohol: Avoid alcohol.

Pregnancy: Adequate studies of cephalosporin use in pregnant women have not been done. Before taking cefepime, tell your doctor if you are pregnant or plan to become pregnant.

Breast Feeding: Cefepime passes into breast milk; caution is advised. Consult your doctor for specific advice.

Infants and Children: This drug is not recommended for use by children under 2 months of age.

Special Concerns: People who are allergic to penicillin may have equally serious allergic reactions to cephalosporin antibiotics, such as cefepime. This drug is useful only against bacteria that are susceptible to its effects. Cephalosporins will not work against colds, flu, or other viral infections. If your condition has not improved within a few days of starting cefepime, or instead has worsened, tell your doctor.

OVERDOSE
Symptoms: An overdose of cefepime is unlikely.

What to Do: Emergency instructions not applicable.

▼ INTERACTIONS

DRUG INTERACTIONS
Consult your doctor for specific advice if you are taking carbenicillin injection, heparin, divalproex, anticoagulants, sulfinpyrazone, dipyridamole, pentoxifylline, plicamycin, ticarcillin, probenecid, or valproic acid.

FOOD INTERACTIONS
No known food interactions.

DISEASE INTERACTIONS
Consult your doctor if you have a history of kidney disease, bleeding disorders, or colitis.

≡ SIDE EFFECTS ≡

SERIOUS
Severe allergic reaction (breathing difficulties, confusion, hives, swelling of the face or throat, sweating, and lightheadedness), severe stomach pain and cramps, fever, severe, sometimes bloody diarrhea, unusual bleeding or bruising. Call your doctor immediately.

COMMON
Mild diarrhea or stomach cramps, sore mouth or tongue, nausea and vomiting.

LESS COMMON
Vaginal itching or unusual discharge, pain at the site of injection, itching.

CEFIXIME

Available in: Tablets, oral suspension
Available OTC? No   **As Generic?** No
Drug Class: Cephalosporin antibiotic

▼ USAGE INFORMATION

WHY IT'S PRESCRIBED
To treat a variety of bacterial infections, including those of the ear, nose, tonsils, and throat, skin and soft tissues, genitourinary tract, and the respiratory tract. Cefixime is also used to treat gonorrhea. It is effective only against infections caused by bacteria; it is ineffective against those caused by viruses, fungi, or other microorganisms.

HOW IT WORKS
Cefixime prevents bacteria from forming protective cell walls necessary for survival.

▼ DOSAGE GUIDELINES

RANGE AND FREQUENCY
Adults and teenagers: 200 mg every 12 hours, or 400 mg once a day. Uncomplicated gonorrhea is treated with 400 mg, given in a one-time dose. Children 6 months to 12 years: 4 mg per 2.2 lbs (1 kg) of body weight every 12 hours, or 8 mg per 2.2 lbs once a day.

ONSET OF EFFECT
2 to 4 hours.

DURATION OF ACTION
6 to 18 hours.

DIETARY ADVICE
It may be taken with food to reduce stomach irritation.

STORAGE
Store in a tightly sealed container away from heat, moisture, and direct light. Oral suspension does not need to be refrigerated.

MISSED DOSE
Take it as soon as you remember. If it is near the time for the next dose, skip the missed dose and resume your regular dosage schedule. Do not double the next dose.

STOPPING THE DRUG
Take it as prescribed for the full treatment period, even if you begin to feel better before the scheduled end of therapy. Stopping cefixime prematurely may slow your recovery or lead to a rebound infection, also known as superinfection, in which the heartier strains of bacteria survive and multiply, leading to a more serious and drug-resistant infection. When taking this drug to treat a streptococcal (strep) infection, it is particularly important to take it for the entire treatment period. Serious heart and kidney problems can develop later if the drug is discontinued prematurely.

PROLONGED USE
Cefixime, when taken to treat gonorrhea, is prescribed as a one-time dose. For other bacterial infections, it is generally prescribed for short-term therapy (10 to 14 days). Use beyond this period increases the risk of adverse effects and superinfection.

▼ PRECAUTIONS

Over 60: Adverse reactions may be more likely and more severe in older patients.

Driving and Hazardous Work: Do not drive or engage in hazardous work until you determine how the medicine affects you.

Alcohol: Avoid alcohol.

Pregnancy: Adequate studies of cephalosporin use in pregnant women have not been done. Before taking cefixime, tell your doctor if you are pregnant or are planning to become pregnant.

Breast Feeding: Cefixime passes into breast milk; caution is advised. Consult your doctor for specific advice.

Infants and Children: May be used by children 6 months and older. Consult your pediatrician for specific advice.

Special Concerns: People who are allergic to penicillin may have equally serious allergic reactions to cephalosporin antibiotics, such as cefixime. It is useful only against bacteria that are susceptible to its effects, not against colds, flu, or other viral infections. If your condition has not improved within a few days of starting cefixime, or instead has worsened, tell your doctor.

OVERDOSE
Symptoms: Seizures, severe abdominal pain, bloody diarrhea, vomiting.

What to Do: Call your doctor, emergency medical services (EMS), or the nearest poison control center immediately.

▼ INTERACTIONS

DRUG INTERACTIONS
Consult your doctor for specific advice if you are taking carbenicillin injection, heparin, divalproex, anticoagulants, sulfinpyrazone, dipyridamole, pentoxifylline, plicamycin, ticarcillin, probenecid, or valproic acid.

FOOD INTERACTIONS
No known food interactions.

DISEASE INTERACTIONS
Consult your doctor if you have a history of kidney disease or colitis.

 SIDE EFFECTS

SERIOUS
Severe allergic reaction (breathing difficulties, confusion, hives, itching, swelling of the face or throat, sweating, and lightheadedness), severe stomach pain and cramps, fever, severe, sometimes bloody diarrhea. Call your doctor immediately.

COMMON
Mild diarrhea or stomach cramps, sore mouth or tongue, nausea and vomiting.

LESS COMMON
Vaginal itching or unusual discharge, decreased white blood cell count causing increased susceptibility to infection, decreased blood platelets causing increased risk of bleeding problems, itching.

CEFOTETAN DISODIUM

Available in: Injection
Available OTC? No **As Generic?** No
Drug Class: Cephalosporin antibiotic

▼ USAGE INFORMATION

WHY IT'S PRESCRIBED
To treat a variety of serious bacterial infections, including those of the lung, genitourinary tract, blood, bones, joints, skin and soft tissues, and other organs. Cefotetan disodium is also used to treat gonorrhea. It is effective only against infections caused by certain strains of bacteria; it is ineffective against those caused by viruses, fungi, or other microorganisms. Cephalosporins, such as cefotetan disodium, are prescribed when other antibiotics are not sufficient to treat the infection. Cefotetan disodium is also used in some cases prior to certain major surgical procedures in order to minimize the risk of infection.

HOW IT WORKS
Cefotetan disodium prevents bacteria from forming protective cell walls necessary for their survival.

▼ DOSAGE GUIDELINES

RANGE AND FREQUENCY
1 to 3 g into a vein or muscle every 12 hours.

ONSET OF EFFECT
Into a vein: Immediate. Into a muscle: 1 hour.

DURATION OF ACTION
6 to 9 hours.

DIETARY ADVICE
Eat 4 oz of yogurt or drink 4 oz of buttermilk a day to protect against intestinal superinfection. Drink plenty of fluids.

STORAGE
Not applicable; the dose is administered only at a health care facility.

MISSED DOSE
Not applicable; the dose is administered by a health care professional.

STOPPING THE DRUG
The decision to stop taking the drug should be made by your doctor.

PROLONGED USE
Cefotetan disodium is generally prescribed for short-term therapy (10 to 14 days). Use beyond this period increases the likelihood of adverse effects and superinfection, a subsequent infection caused by heartier, drug-resistant strains of bacteria.

▼ PRECAUTIONS

Over 60: Adverse reactions may be more likely and more severe in older patients.

Driving and Hazardous Work: Not applicable; the dose is administered only in a health care institution.

Alcohol: Avoid alcohol.

Pregnancy: Adequate studies of cephalosporin use in pregnant women have not been done. Before taking cefotetan disodium, tell your doctor if you are pregnant or plan to become pregnant.

Breast Feeding: Cefotetan disodium passes into breast milk; caution is advised. Consult your doctor for advice.

Infants and Children: This drug is not recommended for use by children under the age of 12.

Special Concerns: People who are allergic to penicillin may have equally serious allergic reactions to cephalosporin antibiotics, such as cefotetan disodium. This drug is useful only against bacteria that are susceptible to its effects, not against colds, flu, or other viral infections. If your condition has not improved within a few days of starting cefotetan disodium, or instead has worsened, tell your doctor.

OVERDOSE
Symptoms: An overdose of cefotetan disodium is unlikely.

What to Do: Emergency instructions not applicable.

▼ INTERACTIONS

DRUG INTERACTIONS
Consult your doctor for advice if you are taking carbenicillin injection, heparin, divalproex, anticoagulants, sulfinpyrazone, dipyridamole, pentoxifylline, plicamycin, ticarcillin, probenecid, medications containing alcohol, or valproic acid.

FOOD INTERACTIONS
No known food interactions.

DISEASE INTERACTIONS
Caution is advised when taking cefotetan disodium. Consult your doctor if you have a history of kidney disease, bleeding disorders, or colitis.

≡ SIDE EFFECTS ≡

SERIOUS
Severe allergic reaction (breathing difficulties, confusion, hives, swelling of the face or throat, sweating, and lightheadedness), severe stomach pain and cramps, fever, severe, sometimes bloody diarrhea, unusual bleeding or bruising. Call your doctor immediately.

COMMON
Mild diarrhea or stomach cramps, sore mouth or tongue, nausea and vomiting.

LESS COMMON
Vaginal discharge or itching, pain at site of injection, rash, decreased white blood cell count causing increased susceptibility to infection, decreased blood platelets causing increased risk of bleeding problems.

CEFPODOXIME PROXETIL

Available in: Oral suspension, tablets
Available OTC? No   **As Generic?** No
Drug Class: Cephalosporin antibiotic

▼ USAGE INFORMATION

WHY IT'S PRESCRIBED
To treat a variety of bacterial infections, including those of the ear, nose, and throat, skin and soft tissues, genitourinary tract, respiratory tract, and other organs. Cefpodoxime is also used to treat gonorrhea. It is effective only against infections caused by bacteria; it is ineffective against those caused by viruses, fungi, or other microorganisms.

HOW IT WORKS
Cefpodoxime prevents bacteria from forming protective cell walls.

▼ DOSAGE GUIDELINES

RANGE AND FREQUENCY
Adults and teenagers: 100 to 400 mg every 12 hours. Gonorrhea is treated with 200 mg, given in a one-time dose. Children 6 months to 12 years: 5 mg per 2.2 lbs (1 kg) of body weight every 12 hours.

ONSET OF EFFECT
Unknown.

DURATION OF ACTION
Approximately 6 hours.

DIETARY ADVICE
Take it with food to increase the absorption of the drug by the body.

STORAGE
Store in a tightly sealed container away from heat, moisture, and direct light. Keep liquid form refrigerated, but do not allow it to freeze.

MISSED DOSE
Take it as soon as you remember. This will help keep a constant level of medication in your system. If it is near the time for the next dose, skip the missed dose and resume your regular schedule. Do not double the next dose.

STOPPING THE DRUG
Take it as prescribed for the full treatment period, even if you begin to feel better before the scheduled end of therapy. Stopping the drug prematurely may slow your recovery or lead to a rebound infection, also known as superinfection, in which the heartier strains of bacteria survive and multiply, leading to a more serious and drug-resistant infection. When taking this drug to treat a streptococcal (strep) infection, it is particularly important to take it for the entire treatment period. Serious heart and kidney problems can develop later if it is discontinued prematurely.

PROLONGED USE
Cefpodoxime is generally prescribed for short-term therapy (10 to 14 days). Use of cefpodoxime beyond this period increases the risk of adverse effects and superinfection.

▼ PRECAUTIONS

Over 60: Adverse reactions may be more likely and more severe.

Driving and Hazardous Work: Avoid such activities until you determine how the medicine affects you.

Alcohol: Avoid alcohol.

Pregnancy: Adequate studies of cephalosporin use in pregnant women have not been done. Before taking cefpodoxime proxetil, tell your doctor if you are pregnant or plan to become pregnant.

Breast Feeding: Cefpodoxime proxetil passes into breast milk and may be hazardous to the nursing infant; caution is advised. Consult your doctor for advice.

Infants and Children: May be used in children 6 months and older. Consult your pediatrician for advice.

Special Concerns: People who are allergic to penicillin may have equally serious allergic reactions to cephalosporin antibiotics. Cefpodoxime is useful only against bacteria that are susceptible to its effects, not against colds, flu, or other viral infections. If your condition has not improved within a few days of starting the drug, or instead has worsened, notify your physician.

OVERDOSE
Symptoms: Seizures, severe abdominal pain, bloody diarrhea, vomiting.

What to Do: Call your doctor, emergency medical services (EMS), or the nearest poison control center immediately.

▼ INTERACTIONS

DRUG INTERACTIONS
Consult your doctor for specific advice if you are taking carbenicillin injection, heparin, divalproex, anticoagulants, sulfinpyrazone, dipyridamole, pentoxifylline, plicamycin, ticarcillin, probenecid, or valproic acid.

FOOD INTERACTIONS
No known food interactions.

DISEASE INTERACTIONS
Caution is advised when taking cefpodoxime proxetil. Consult your doctor if you have a history of kidney disease or colitis.

▬ SIDE EFFECTS ▬

SERIOUS
Severe allergic reaction (breathing difficulties, itching, hives, swelling of the face or throat, and sweating), severe stomach pain and cramps, fever, severe, sometimes bloody diarrhea. Call your doctor immediately.

COMMON
Mild diarrhea or stomach cramps, sore mouth or tongue, nausea and vomiting.

LESS COMMON
Vaginal itching or unusual discharge, rash, decreased white blood cell count causing increased susceptibility to infection, decreased blood platelets causing increased risk of bleeding problems.

CEFPROZIL

Available in: Oral suspension, tablets
Available OTC? No   **As Generic?** No
Drug Class: Cephalosporin antibiotic

BRAND NAME
Cefzil

▼ USAGE INFORMATION

WHY IT'S PRESCRIBED
To treat a variety of bacterial infections, including those of the ear, nose, tonsils, and throat, skin and soft tissues, and the respiratory tract. Cefprozil is effective only against infections caused by bacteria; it is ineffective against those caused by viruses, fungi, or other microorganisms.

HOW IT WORKS
Cefprozil prevents bacteria from forming protective cell walls necessary for survival.

▼ DOSAGE GUIDELINES

RANGE AND FREQUENCY
Adults and teenagers: 250 to 500 mg every 12 to 24 hours. Children ages 2 to 12: 7.5 mg per 2.2 lbs (1 kg) of body weight every 12 hours. Children 6 months to 12 years: 15 mg per 2.2 lbs every 12 hours.

ONSET OF EFFECT
Approximately 90 minutes.

DURATION OF ACTION
Unknown.

DIETARY ADVICE
It may be taken with food to reduce stomach irritation.

STORAGE
Store in a tightly sealed container away from heat, moisture, and direct light. Keep liquid form refrigerated, but do not allow it to freeze.

MISSED DOSE
Take it as soon as you remember. This will help keep a constant level of medication in your system. If it is near the time for the next dose, skip the missed dose and resume your regular dosage schedule. Do not double the next dose.

STOPPING THE DRUG
Take it as prescribed for the full treatment period, even if you begin to feel better before the scheduled end of therapy. Stopping cefprozil prematurely may slow your recovery or lead to a rebound infection, also known as superinfection, in which the heartier strains of bacteria survive and multiply, leading to a more serious and drug-resistant infection. When taking this drug to treat a streptococcal (strep) infection, it is particularly important to take it for the entire treatment period. Serious heart and kidney problems can develop later if it is discontinued prematurely.

PROLONGED USE
Cefprozil is generally prescribed for short-term therapy (10 to 14 days). Use of cefprozil beyond this period increases risks of adverse effects and superinfection.

▼ PRECAUTIONS

Over 60: Adverse reactions may be more likely and more severe in older patients.

Driving and Hazardous Work: Do not drive or engage in hazardous work until you determine how the medicine affects you.

Alcohol: Avoid alcohol.

Pregnancy: Adequate studies of cephalosporin use in pregnant women have not been done. Before taking cefprozil, tell your doctor if you are pregnant or are planning to become pregnant.

Breast Feeding: Cefprozil passes into breast milk; caution is advised. Consult your doctor for specific advice.

Infants and Children: Cefprozil may be used by children 6 months and older. Consult your pediatrician for specific advice.

Special Concerns: People who are allergic to penicillin may have equally serious allergic reactions to cephalosporin antibiotics, such as cefprozil. This drug is useful only against bacteria that are susceptible to its effects, not against colds, flu, or other viral infections. If your condition has not improved within a few days of starting cefprozil, or instead has worsened, tell your doctor.

OVERDOSE
Symptoms: Seizures, severe abdominal pain, bloody diarrhea, vomiting.

What to Do: Call your doctor, emergency medical services (EMS), or the nearest poison control center immediately.

▼ INTERACTIONS

DRUG INTERACTIONS
Consult your doctor for specific advice if you are taking carbenicillin injection, heparin, divalproex, anticoagulants, sulfinpyrazone, dipyridamole, pentoxifylline, plicamycin, ticarcillin, probenecid, or valproic acid.

FOOD INTERACTIONS
No known food interactions.

DISEASE INTERACTIONS
Caution is advised when taking cefprozil. Consult your doctor if you have a history of kidney disease, phenylketonuria, or colitis.

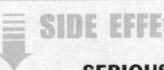

≡ SIDE EFFECTS ≡

SERIOUS
Severe allergic reaction (breathing difficulties, confusion, lightheadedness, itching, hives, swelling of the face or throat, and unusual sweating), severe stomach pain and cramps, fever, severe, sometimes bloody diarrhea. Call your doctor immediately.

COMMON
Mild diarrhea or stomach cramps, sore mouth or tongue, nausea and vomiting.

LESS COMMON
Vaginal itching or unusual discharge, decreased white blood cell count causing increased susceptibility to infection, decreased blood platelets causing increased risk of bleeding problems.

CEFUROXIME

BRAND NAMES
Ceftin, Kefurox, Zinacef

Available in: Tablets, injection, oral suspension
Available OTC? No   **As Generic?** Yes
Drug Class: Cephalosporin antibiotic

▼ USAGE INFORMATION

WHY IT'S PRESCRIBED
To treat a variety of bacterial infections, including those of the brain, ear, nose, tonsils, and throat, skin and soft tissues, genitourinary tract, respiratory tract, blood, bones, joints, and other organs. Cefuroxime also is used to treat gonorrhea and is given prior to some surgeries to prevent infection. It is effective only against susceptible infections caused by bacteria.

HOW IT WORKS
Cefuroxime prevents bacteria from forming cell walls.

▼ DOSAGE GUIDELINES

RANGE AND FREQUENCY
Adults and teenagers— Tablets: 125 to 500 mg every 12 hours for 5 to 10 days. Injection: 750 to 1,500 mg every 6 to 8 hours into a vein or muscle. Children 3 months to 12 years— Tablets: 125 mg every 12 hours for 10 days. Injection: 16.7 to 33.3 mg per 2.2 lbs (1 kg) of body weight every 8 hours into a vein or muscle. Oral suspension: 10 to 15 mg per 2.2 lbs every 12 hours for 10 days. Gonorrhea is treated with a one-time tablet dose of 1,000 mg or a one-time injected dose of 1,500 mg into a muscle. The injected dose is divided and administered at 2 separate sites on the body, along with a single 1,000 mg oral dose of probenecid.

ONSET OF EFFECT
Into a vein: Immediate. Into a muscle: 15 to 60 minutes. Oral forms: Unknown.

DURATION OF ACTION
5 to 8 hours.

DIETARY ADVICE
Tablets can be taken without regard to meals. Take oral suspension with food to increase the absorption of the drug by the body. Maintain normal fluid intake.

STORAGE
Store in a tightly sealed container away from heat, moisture, and direct light. Keep liquid form refrigerated, but do not allow it to freeze.

MISSED DOSE
Take it as soon as you remember. If it is near the time for the next dose, skip the missed dose and resume your regular dosage schedule. Do not double the next dose.

STOPPING THE DRUG
Take it as prescribed for the full treatment period. Stopping prematurely may slow your recovery or lead to a rebound infection, also known as superinfection, in which the heartier strains of bacteria survive and multiply, leading to a more serious and drug-resistant infection. When taking this drug to treat a streptococcal (strep) infection, it is particularly important to take it for the entire treatment period. Serious heart and kidney problems can develop later if the drug is discontinued prematurely.

PROLONGED USE
Cefuroxime is generally prescribed for short-term therapy (5 to 10 days). Use beyond this period increases risks of adverse effects and super-infection.

▼ PRECAUTIONS

Over 60: Adverse reactions may be more likely and more severe in older patients.

Driving and Hazardous Work: Do not drive or engage in hazardous work until you determine how the medicine affects you.

Alcohol: Avoid alcohol.

Pregnancy: Adequate studies of use during pregnancy have not been done. Consult your doctor for advice.

Breast Feeding: Cefuroxime passes into breast milk; caution is advised. Consult your doctor for advice.

Infants and Children: May be used by children 3 months and older. Consult your pediatrician for advice.

Special Concerns: Those who are allergic to penicillin may have equally serious allergic reactions to cephalosporin antibiotics. If your condition has not improved within a few days, or instead has worsened, tell your doctor. The tablets and the oral suspension can not be equally substituted for each other.

OVERDOSE
Symptoms: Seizures, severe abdominal pain, bloody diarrhea, vomiting.

What to Do: Seek medical assistance immediately.

▼ INTERACTIONS

DRUG INTERACTIONS
Consult your doctor for advice if you are taking carbenicillin injection, divalproex, anticoagulants, sulfinpyrazone, dipyridamole, pentoxifylline, plicamycin, ticarcillin, probenecid, or valproic acid.

FOOD INTERACTIONS
No known food interactions.

DISEASE INTERACTIONS
Consult your doctor if you have a history of kidney disease or colitis.

⧖ SIDE EFFECTS ⧖

SERIOUS
Severe allergic reaction (breathing difficulties, confusion, hives, swelling of the face or throat, and lightheadedness), severe stomach pain and cramps, fever, severe, sometimes bloody diarrhea. Call your doctor immediately.

COMMON
Mild diarrhea or stomach cramps, sore mouth or tongue, nausea and vomiting.

LESS COMMON
Vaginal itching or discharge, pain at site of injection, rash, decreased white blood cell count causing increased susceptibility to infection, decreased blood platelets causing increased risk of bleeding problems.

CELECOXIB

Available in: Capsules
Available OTC? No **As Generic?** No
Drug Class: Nonsteroidal anti-inflammatory drug (NSAID)/COX-2 inhibitor

▼ USAGE INFORMATION

WHY IT'S PRESCRIBED
To relieve pain, inflammation, and stiffness of osteoarthritis and rheumatoid arthritis.

HOW IT WORKS
By inhibiting the activity of the enzyme cyclooxygenase-2 (COX-2), celecoxib reduces the synthesis of prostaglandins that play a role in causing arthritis pain and inflammation. It does not inhibit the activity of COX-1, the enzyme involved in the synthesis of prostaglandins that help protect against stomach ulcers and other health problems.

▼ DOSAGE GUIDELINES

RANGE AND FREQUENCY
For osteoarthritis: 200 mg a day. For rheumatoid arthritis: 100 to 200 mg twice a day. To minimize potential gastrointestinal side effects, the lowest effective dose should be used for the shortest possible time.

ONSET OF EFFECT
Within 24 to 48 hours.

DURATION OF ACTION
Unknown.

DIETARY ADVICE
Celecoxib may be taken with or without food.

STORAGE
Store in a tightly sealed container away from heat, moisture, and direct light.

MISSED DOSE
Take it as soon as you remember. If it is near the time for the next dose, skip the missed dose and resume your regular dosage schedule. Do not double the next dose.

STOPPING THE DRUG
The decision to stop taking the drug should be made in consultation with your doctor.

PROLONGED USE
The risk of gastrointestinal side effects may be increased with extended use.

▼ PRECAUTIONS

Over 60: Adverse reactions may be more likely and more severe in older patients.

Driving and Hazardous Work: No special problems are expected.

Alcohol: Avoid alcohol when using this medication because it increases the risk of stomach irritation.

Pregnancy: Discuss with your doctor the relative risks and benefits of using this drug while pregnant. Do not use celecoxib during the last trimester.

Breast Feeding: Celecoxib may pass into breast milk; caution is advised. Consult your doctor for advice on whether to discontinue nursing or discontinue the drug.

Infants and Children: The safety and effectiveness of this drug have not been established for children under the age of 18.

OVERDOSE
Symptoms: No cases of overdose have been reported. Symptoms may include lethargy, drowsiness, nausea, vomiting, abdominal pain, black, tarry stools, breathing difficulty, and coma.

What to Do: If you suspect an overdose or if someone takes a much larger dose than prescribed, call your doctor, emergency medical services (EMS), or the nearest poison control center immediately.

▼ INTERACTIONS

DRUG INTERACTIONS
Do not take this drug with aspirin or any other NSAIDs without your doctor's approval. Consult your doctor if you are taking furosemide, ACE inhibitors, fluconazole, lithium, or warfarin.

FOOD INTERACTIONS
No known food interactions.

DISEASE INTERACTIONS
Celecoxib should not be taken by people who have experienced asthma, hives, or allergic-type reactions after taking aspirin or other NSAIDs. Consult your doctor if you have any of the following: bleeding problems, inflammation or ulcers of the stomach and intestines, asthma, high blood pressure, or heart failure. Use of celecoxib may cause complications in patients with liver or kidney disease, since these organs work together to remove the medication from the body.

SIDE EFFECTS

SERIOUS
Stomach ulcers. Black, tarry stools may signal stomach bleeding. Symptoms of liver disease (nausea, fatigue, lethargy, itching, yellowish discoloration of the eyes or skin, fluid retention). Call your doctor immediately.

COMMON
Indigestion, diarrhea, and mild abdominal pain.

LESS COMMON
Flatulence, mild swelling, sore throat, and upper respiratory tract infection.

CEPHALEXIN

Available in: Capsules, oral suspension, tablets
Available OTC? No   **As Generic?** Yes
Drug Class: Cephalosporin antibiotic

▼ USAGE INFORMATION

WHY IT'S PRESCRIBED
To treat a variety of bacterial infections, including those of the ear, nose, tonsils, and throat, bones, joints, skin and soft tissues, genitourinary tract, and respiratory tract. It is effective only against infections caused by bacteria; it is ineffective against those caused by viruses, fungi, or other microorganisms.

HOW IT WORKS
Cephalexin prevents bacteria from forming cell walls.

▼ DOSAGE GUIDELINES

RANGE AND FREQUENCY
Adults and teenagers: 250 to 500 mg every 6 to 12 hours. Children: 6.25 to 25 mg per 2.2 lbs (1 kg) of body weight every 6 hours, or 12.5 to 50 mg per kg every 12 hours.

ONSET OF EFFECT
1 hour.

DURATION OF ACTION
Unknown.

DIETARY ADVICE
Cephalexin may be taken on a full or empty stomach, but taking it with food will reduce stomach irritation.

STORAGE
Store in a tightly sealed container away from heat, moisture, and direct light. Keep liquid form refrigerated, but do not allow it to freeze.

MISSED DOSE
Take it as soon as you remember. This will help keep a constant level of medication in your system. If it is near the time for the next dose, skip the missed dose and resume your regular dosage schedule. Do not double the next dose.

STOPPING THE DRUG
Take it as prescribed for the full treatment period, even if you begin to feel better before the scheduled end of therapy. Stopping cephalexin prematurely may slow your recovery or lead to a rebound infection, also known as superinfection, in which the heartier strains of bacteria survive and multiply, leading to a more serious and drug-resistant infection. When taking this drug to treat a streptococcal (strep) infection, it is particularly important to take it for the entire treatment period. Serious heart and kidney problems can develop later if it is discontinued prematurely.

PROLONGED USE
Cephalexin is generally prescribed for short-term therapy (10 to 14 days). Further use increases the risk of adverse effects and superinfection.

▼ PRECAUTIONS

Over 60: Adverse reactions may be more likely and more severe in older patients.

Driving and Hazardous Work: Do not drive or engage in hazardous work until you determine how the medicine affects you.

Alcohol: Avoid alcohol.

Pregnancy: Adequate studies of cephalosporin use in pregnant women have not been done. Before taking cephalexin, tell your doctor if you are pregnant or plan to become pregnant.

Breast Feeding: Cephalexin passes into breast milk; caution is advised. Consult your doctor for specific advice.

Infants and Children: Adequate studies of cephalexin use in children have not been done. Consult your doctor.

Special Concerns: People who are allergic to penicillin may have equally serious allergic reactions to cephalosporin antibiotics, such as cephalexin. This drug is useful only against bacteria that are susceptible to its effects, not against colds, flu, or other viral infections. If your condition has not improved within a few days of starting cephalexin, or instead has worsened, tell your doctor.

OVERDOSE
Symptoms: Seizures, severe abdominal pain, bloody diarrhea, vomiting.

What to Do: Call your doctor, emergency medical services (EMS), or the nearest poison control center immediately.

▼ INTERACTIONS

DRUG INTERACTIONS
Consult your doctor for specific advice if you are taking carbenicillin injection, heparin, divalproex, anticoagulants, sulfinpyrazone, dipyridamole, pentoxifylline, plicamycin, ticarcillin, probenecid, or valproic acid.

FOOD INTERACTIONS
No known food interactions.

DISEASE INTERACTIONS
Caution is advised when taking cephalexin. Consult your doctor if you have a history of kidney disease or colitis.

SIDE EFFECTS

SERIOUS
Severe allergic reaction (breathing difficulties, confusion, hives, itching, swelling of the face or throat, unusual sweating, and lightheadedness), severe stomach pain and cramps, fever, severe, sometimes bloody diarrhea. Call your doctor immediately.

COMMON
Mild diarrhea or stomach cramps, sore mouth or tongue, nausea and vomiting.

LESS COMMON
Vaginal itching or unusual discharge, rash, decreased white blood cell count causing increased susceptibility to infection, decreased blood platelets causing increased risk of bleeding problems.

CEPHRADINE

Available in: Oral suspension, capsules
Available OTC? No   **As Generic?** Yes
Drug Class: Cephalosporin antibiotic

▼ USAGE INFORMATION

WHY IT'S PRESCRIBED
To treat a variety of bacterial infections, including those of the ear, nose, tonsils, and throat, skin and soft tissues, genitourinary tract, and the respiratory tract. Cephradine is effective only against infections caused by bacteria; it is ineffective against those caused by viruses, fungi, or other microorganisms.

HOW IT WORKS
Cephradine prevents bacteria from forming cell walls.

▼ DOSAGE GUIDELINES

RANGE AND FREQUENCY
Oral suspension and capsules— Adults and teenagers: 250 to 500 mg every 6 hours, or 500 to 1,000 mg every 12 hours. Children: 6.25 to 25 mg every 6 hours.

ONSET OF EFFECT
1 hour.

DURATION OF ACTION
Unknown.

DIETARY ADVICE
Cephradine may be taken on a full or empty stomach, but taking it with food will reduce stomach irritation.

STORAGE
Store in a tightly sealed container away from heat, moisture, and direct light. Keep liquid form refrigerated, but do not allow it to freeze.

MISSED DOSE
Take it as soon as you remember. This will help keep a constant level of medication in your system. If it is near the time for the next dose, skip the missed dose and resume your regular dosage schedule. Do not double the next dose.

STOPPING THE DRUG
Take it as prescribed for the full treatment period, even if you begin to feel better before the scheduled end of therapy. Stopping cephradine prematurely may slow your recovery or lead to a rebound infection, also known as superinfection, in which the heartier strains of bacteria survive and multiply, leading to a more serious and drug-resistant infection. When taking this drug to treat a streptococcal (strep) infection, it is particularly important to take it for the entire treatment period. Serious heart and kidney problems can develop later if it is discontinued prematurely.

PROLONGED USE
Cephradine is generally prescribed for short-term therapy (10 to 14 days). Use of cephradine beyond this period increases the risk of adverse effects and superinfection.

▼ PRECAUTIONS

Over 60: Adverse reactions may be more likely and more severe in older patients.

Driving and Hazardous Work: Do not drive or engage in hazardous work until you determine how the medicine affects you.

Alcohol: Avoid alcohol.

Pregnancy: Adequate studies of cephalosporin use during pregnancy have not been done. Consult your doctor for specific advice.

Breast Feeding: Cephradine passes into breast milk; caution is advised. Consult your doctor for specific advice.

Infants and Children: Cephradine may be used by children age 1 and older. Consult your pediatrician for specific advice.

Special Concerns: People who are allergic to penicillin may have equally serious allergic reactions to cephalosporin antibiotics, such as cephradine. This drug is useful only against bacteria that are susceptible to its effects, not against colds, flu, or other viral infections. If your condition has not improved within a few days of starting cephradine, or instead has worsened, tell your doctor.

OVERDOSE
Symptoms: Seizures, severe abdominal pain, bloody diarrhea, vomiting.

What to Do: Call your doctor, emergency medical services (EMS), or the nearest poison control center immediately.

▼ INTERACTIONS

DRUG INTERACTIONS
Consult your doctor for specific advice if you are taking carbenicillin injection, heparin, divalproex, anticoagulants, sulfinpyrazone, dipyridamole, pentoxifylline, plicamycin, ticarcillin, probenecid, or valproic acid.

FOOD INTERACTIONS
No known food interactions.

DISEASE INTERACTIONS
Caution is advised when taking cephradine. Consult your doctor if you have a history of kidney disease or colitis.

SIDE EFFECTS

SERIOUS
Severe allergic reaction (breathing difficulties, confusion, hives, itching, swelling of the face or throat, sweating, and lightheadedness), severe stomach pain and cramps, fever, severe, sometimes bloody diarrhea. Call your doctor immediately.

COMMON
Mild diarrhea or stomach cramps, sore mouth or tongue, nausea and vomiting.

LESS COMMON
Vaginal itching or discharge.

CERIVASTATIN

Available in: Tablets
Available OTC? No **As Generic?** No
Drug Class: Antilipidemic (cholesterol-lowering agent)

▼ USAGE INFORMATION

WHY IT'S PRESCRIBED
To treat high cholesterol. It is usually prescribed after the first lines of treatment—including diet, weight loss, and exercise—fail to reduce total and low-density lipoprotein (LDL) cholesterol to acceptable levels.

HOW IT WORKS
Cerivastatin blocks the action of an enzyme required for the manufacture of cholesterol, thereby interfering with its formation. By lowering the amount of cholesterol in liver cells, cerivastatin increases the formation of receptors for LDL and thereby reduces blood levels of total and LDL cholesterol. In addition to lowering LDL cholesterol, cerivastatin also modestly reduces triglyceride levels and raises HDL (the so-called "good") cholesterol.

▼ DOSAGE GUIDELINES

RANGE AND FREQUENCY
Initial dose is 0.4 mg, taken once daily in the evening. The recommended dose for patients who have significant impairment of kidney function is 0.2 to 0.3 mg a day.

ONSET OF EFFECT
Unknown; the full effect occurs within 4 weeks.

DURATION OF ACTION
The effect persists for the duration of therapy.

DIETARY ADVICE
Cholesterol-lowering drugs are only one part of a total program that should include regular exercise and a healthy diet. The American Heart Association publishes a "Healthy Heart" diet, which is recommended.

STORAGE
Store in a tightly sealed container away from heat and direct light.

MISSED DOSE
This drug is prescribed to be taken once a day. If you miss a day, skip the missed dose and resume your regular dosage schedule. Do not double the next dose.

STOPPING THE DRUG
The decision to stop taking the drug should be made in consultation with your doctor. Once the medication is discontinued, blood cholesterol is likely to return to original elevated levels.

PROLONGED USE
Side effects are more likely with prolonged use. Your doctor will order blood tests to evaluate liver function at the outset of therapy and then periodically as the drug is continued.

▼ PRECAUTIONS

Over 60: No special problems are expected.

Driving and Hazardous Work: The use of cerivastatin should not impair your ability to perform such tasks safely.

Alcohol: No special precautions are necessary.

Pregnancy: Cerivastatin should not be used during pregnancy or by women who plan to become pregnant in the near future.

Breast Feeding: This drug is not recommended for women who are nursing.

Infants and Children: Long-term effects of cerivastatin in children have not been established. It is rarely used by young patients; consult your doctor.

Special Concerns: Important elements of treatment for high cholesterol include proper diet, weight loss, regular moderate exercise, and the avoidance of certain medications that may increase cholesterol levels. Because cerivastatin has potential side effects, it is important that you maintain a recommended healthy diet and that you follow your doctor's suggestions regarding other treatments.

OVERDOSE
Symptoms: Overdose is unlikely to occur.

What to Do: Emergency instructions not applicable.

▼ INTERACTIONS

DRUG INTERACTIONS
Consult your doctor if you are taking cyclosporine, gemfibrozil, niacin, antibiotics, especially erythromycin, or medications for fungus infections. All of these drugs may increase the risk of muscle inflammation (myositis) when taken with cerivastatin, and may lead to kidney failure.

FOOD INTERACTIONS
No known food interactions.

DISEASE INTERACTIONS
Consult your doctor if you have any of the following problems: liver, kidney, or muscle disease, or a medical history involving organ transplant, recent surgery, or alcohol abuse.

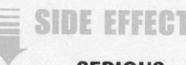 **SIDE EFFECTS**

SERIOUS
Fever, unusual or unexplained muscle aches and tenderness. Call your doctor right away.

COMMON
Side effects occur in only 1% to 2% of patients. Side effects of the statin class of drugs include constipation or diarrhea, dizziness, gas, headache, heartburn, nausea, skin rash, stomach pain, and rise in liver enzymes (detectable by your physician).

LESS COMMON
Sleeping difficulty.

CETIRIZINE

Available in: Tablets, syrup
Available OTC? No   **As Generic?** No
Drug Class: Histamine (H1) blocker

▼ USAGE INFORMATION

WHY IT'S PRESCRIBED
For symptomatic relief of perennial and seasonal allergies (including hay fever), itchy skin, and chronic hives.

HOW IT WORKS
Cetirizine blocks the effects of histamine, a naturally occurring substance within the body that causes swelling, itching, sneezing, watery eyes, hives, and other symptoms of allergic reaction.

▼ DOSAGE GUIDELINES

RANGE AND FREQUENCY
Adults and teenagers: 5 to 10 mg once a day. Do not increase the dose to obtain quicker relief of symptoms. A lower dose (no more than 5 mg a day) is recommended for patients with impaired kidney or liver function.

ONSET OF EFFECT
Within 20 to 40 minutes.

DURATION OF ACTION
Approximately 24 hours.

DIETARY ADVICE
Cetirizine can be taken without regard to diet.

STORAGE
Store in a tightly sealed container away from heat, moisture, and direct light. Do not allow the syrup to freeze.

MISSED DOSE
This drug is prescribed to be taken once a day. If you miss a day, skip the missed dose and resume your regular dosage schedule. Do not double the next dose.

STOPPING THE DRUG
Take it as prescribed for the full treatment period, even if you feel better before the scheduled end of therapy.

PROLONGED USE
Safety and effectiveness during prolonged use have yet to be established.

▼ PRECAUTIONS

Over 60: The dosage may need to be reduced in elderly patients, especially for those in whom kidney function is impaired.

Driving and Hazardous Work: Do not drive or engage in hazardous work until you determine how the medication affects you.

Alcohol: Avoid alcohol while taking this medication, since it can magnify side effects such as drowsiness and fatigue.

Pregnancy: Adequate human studies of the use of this drug during pregnancy have not been done; caution is advised. Before taking cetirizine, tell your doctor if you are pregnant or plan to become pregnant.

Breast Feeding: Cetirizine passes into breast milk; avoid or discontinue use while nursing.

Infants and Children: The safety and effectiveness of cetirizine use by children under the age of 12 have not been established.

Special Concerns: If cetirizine causes dry mouth as a side effect, use sugarless gum, sugarless sour hard candy, or ice chips for relief.

OVERDOSE
Symptoms: No cases of overdose have been reported.

What to Do: An overdose of cetirizine is unlikely to be life-threatening. However, if someone takes a much larger dose than prescribed, call your doctor, emergency medical services (EMS), or the nearest poison control center immediately.

▼ INTERACTIONS

DRUG INTERACTIONS
No significant drug interactions have been reported. Cetirizine may, however, increase the depressant effects of alcohol, sedatives, tranquilizers, painkillers, barbiturates, or other antihistamines on the central nervous system. Consult your doctor for specific advice.

FOOD INTERACTIONS
No food interactions have been reported.

DISEASE INTERACTIONS
Cetirizine blood levels may increase in patients with liver or kidney disease, since these organs work together to remove the medication from the body. Reduced doses may be required for such persons.

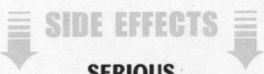

SIDE EFFECTS

SERIOUS
No serious side effects are associated with the use of cetirizine.

COMMON
Drowsiness, fatigue, headache, dry mouth.

LESS COMMON
Nausea and vomiting.

CEVIMELINE HYDROCHLORIDE

Available in: Capsules
Available OTC? No   **As Generic?** No
Drug Class: Cholinergic (muscarinic) agonist

▼ USAGE INFORMATION

WHY IT'S PRESCRIBED
To treat dry mouth in patients with Sjögren's syndrome.

HOW IT WORKS
Cevimeline stimulates the secretion of glands, such as salivary and sweat glands, and increases the tone of smooth muscle in the gastrointestinal and urinary tracts.

▼ DOSAGE GUIDELINES

RANGE AND FREQUENCY
Adults: 30 mg 3 times a day.

ONSET OF EFFECT
Unknown.

DURATION OF ACTION
Unknown.

DIETARY ADVICE
Cevimeline may be taken with or without food.

STORAGE
Store in a tightly sealed container away from heat, moisture, and direct light.

MISSED DOSE
Take it as soon as you remember. If it is near the time for the next dose, skip the missed dose and resume your regular dosage schedule. Do not double the next dose.

STOPPING THE DRUG
The decision to stop taking the drug should be made in consultation with your physician.

PROLONGED USE
See your doctor regularly for tests and examinations if you must take this drug for a prolonged period.

▼ PRECAUTIONS

Over 60: Adverse reactions may be more likely and more severe in older patients.

Driving and Hazardous Work: This drug can cause visual blurring, which may affect depth perception, night vision, and general vision. Do not drive or engage in hazardous work until you determine how the medicine affects you.

Alcohol: Avoid alcohol while taking this medication, as the diuretic effect of alcohol may aggravate your condition.

Pregnancy: No human tests have been done. However, discuss with your doctor the risks and benefits of using this drug while pregnant.

Breast Feeding: Cevimeline may pass into breast milk; caution is advised. Consult your doctor for advice on whether to discontinue nursing or discontinue the drug.

Infants and Children: The safety and effectiveness of this drug have not been established for children under the age of 18.

Special Concerns: Dehydration may result if you sweat excessively while taking cevimeline. Drink extra water and consult your doctor.

OVERDOSE
Symptoms: No cases of overdose have been reported.

What to Do: If you suspect an overdose or if someone takes a much larger dose than prescribed, call your doctor, emergency medical services (EMS), or the nearest poison control center immediately.

▼ INTERACTIONS

DRUG INTERACTIONS
Consult your doctor for specific advice if you are taking a beta-blocker.

FOOD INTERACTIONS
No known interactions.

DISEASE INTERACTIONS
Do not take cevimeline if you have uncontrolled asthma or if you have an eye condition, such as acute iritis or narrow-angle glaucoma, which may be aggravated by the drug's tendency to cause the pupil's to constrict. The drug should be used with caution in people with a history of kidney or gallbladder stones.

≡ SIDE EFFECTS ≡

SERIOUS
Serious side effects are rare, but may include: heartbeat irregularities, chest pain, increased bronchial secretions. Some of these side effects may be relevant only to those who have a history of heart problems or respiratory conditions (see Disease Interactions).

COMMON
Excessive sweating, nausea, runny nose.

LESS COMMON
Excessive salivation, weakness, sinusitis, upper respiratory infection, abdominal pain, urinary tract infection, coughing, vomiting, back pain, conjunctivitis, bronchitis, joint pain, fatigue, pain, insomnia, hot flushes.

CHARCOAL, ACTIVATED

BRAND NAMES

Actidose-Aqua,
CharcoAid 2000,
Charcocaps, Insta-Char
Aqueous, Liqui-Char,
Pediatric Aqueous
Insta-Char, Supercar

Available in: Oral suspension, powder, tablets, capsules
Available OTC? Yes   **As Generic?** Yes
Drug Class: Antidote

▼ USAGE INFORMATION

WHY IT'S PRESCRIBED
Used as an emergency antidote for treatment of poisonings by most drugs and chemicals; also used to relieve diarrhea or excess gas.

HOW IT WORKS
Activated charcoal prevents the absorption of certain kinds of drugs and chemicals by the body.

▼ DOSAGE GUIDELINES

RANGE AND FREQUENCY
For treatment of poisoning— Oral suspension and powder: Adults and teenagers: 25 to 100 grams (g). Children: 1 g per 2.2 lbs (1 kg) of body weight, or 25 to 50 g. Mix powder with water. Take 1 time only. For treatment of diarrhea— Capsules: Adults and children age 3 and older: 520 mg every 30 to 60 minutes, as needed. Do not take more than 4.16 g per day. For treatment of excess gas— Tablets and capsules: Adults and teenagers: 975 mg to 3.9 g, 3 times a day.

ONSET OF EFFECT
Immediate.

DURATION OF ACTION
Not applicable. Activated charcoal is not absorbed by the body.

DIETARY ADVICE
As an antidote: No special restrictions. To treat diarrhea: It is important to replace the fluid lost by your body and to eat a proper diet. During the first 24 hours, drink plenty of caffeine-free clear liquids like water, broth, ginger ale, and decaffeinated tea. During the second 24 hours you may eat bland foods, such as applesauce, bread, crackers, and oatmeal. Avoid caffeine, fried or spicy foods, bran, candy, fruits, and vegetables. These may worsen your condition.

STORAGE
Store in a tightly sealed container away from heat, moisture, and direct light. Premixed suspension can be stored for up to 1 year. Do not allow the liquid form of activated charcoal to freeze.

MISSED DOSE
As an antidote: Not applicable. To treat diarrhea or excess gas: Take it as soon as you remember. If it is near the time for the next dose, skip the missed dose and resume your regular dosage schedule. Do not double the next dose.

STOPPING THE DRUG
As an antidote: Not applicable. To treat diarrhea or excess gas: Take as prescribed for the full treatment period. However, you may stop taking the drug if you are feeling better before the scheduled end of therapy.

PROLONGED USE
As an antidote: Not applicable. To treat diarrhea: If diarrhea has not improved or if you have developed a fever after 2 days, call your doctor. To treat excess gas: If your condition has not improved after 3 to 4 days, call your doctor.

▼ PRECAUTIONS

Over 60: No special problems are expected.

Driving and Hazardous Work: The use of activated charcoal should not impair your ability to perform such tasks safely.

Alcohol: No special precautions are necessary.

Pregnancy: Activated charcoal has not been reported to cause problems in an unborn child. Consult your doctor for specific advice.

Breast Feeding: No problems have been reported.

Infants and Children: May be used in infants and children only under strict supervision by a doctor.

Special Concerns: Call your doctor, emergency medical services (EMS), or the nearest poison control center before administering activated charcoal. Charcoal will not be effective if you have been poisoned by swallowing alkalies (lye), petroleum products, strong acids, ethyl or methyl alcohol, iron, boric acid, or lithium. Activated charcoal will not prevent these poisons from being absorbed by the body. If inducing vomiting with ipecac syrup, do so 1 to 2 hours before administering activated charcoal.

OVERDOSE
Symptoms: None expected.

What to Do: Emergency procedures not applicable.

▼ INTERACTIONS

DRUG INTERACTIONS
Activated charcoal may decrease the absorption of any medicine taken within 2 hours of administration. Acetylcysteine and ipecac syrup can decrease the effectiveness of activated charcoal.

FOOD INTERACTIONS
Do not eat chocolate syrup, ice cream, or sherbet with activated charcoal. They will decrease the amount of poison the charcoal can absorb.

DISEASE INTERACTIONS
Caution is advised when taking activated charcoal if you also suffer from dysentery or dehydration.

≡ SIDE EFFECTS ≡

SERIOUS
Swelling or pain in stomach. If this symptom persists, call your doctor immediately.

COMMON
Black, tarry stools.

LESS COMMON
Nausea, constipation. Notify your doctor if any common or less-common side effects persist.

CHLORAL HYDRATE

Available in: Capsules, syrup
Available OTC? No   **As Generic?** Yes
Drug Class: Sedative/hypnotic

▼ USAGE INFORMATION

WHY IT'S PRESCRIBED
For the short-term treatment of insomnia. Chloral hydrate is being replaced by safer, more effective drugs for this purpose.

HOW IT WORKS
Drugs such as chloral hydrate depress activity in the central nervous system (brain and spinal cord), producing a mild sedative effect.

▼ DOSAGE GUIDELINES

RANGE AND FREQUENCY
Adults: 250 to 1,500 mg, 30 minutes before bedtime.

ONSET OF EFFECT
Within 30 minutes.

DURATION OF ACTION
From 4 to 8 hours.

DIETARY ADVICE
Both oral forms of chloral hydrate should be taken shortly after meals. They may be taken with a full glass of a liquid, such as water, fruit juice, or ginger ale, to improve flavor and minimize stomach upset.

STORAGE
Store in a tightly sealed container away from heat, moisture, and direct light. Avoid extremes in temperature.

MISSED DOSE
If it is near the time for the next dose, skip the missed dose and resume your regular dosage schedule. Do not double the next dose.

STOPPING THE DRUG
The dosage will be gradually reduced to prevent withdrawal effects.

PROLONGED USE
Chloral hydrate may be habit-forming. Prolonged use increases the risk of drug dependency.

▼ PRECAUTIONS

Over 60: Adverse reactions may be more likely and more severe in older patients.

Driving and Hazardous Work: Avoid such activities until you determine how this medication affects you.

Alcohol: Avoid alcohol while taking this drug.

≡ SIDE EFFECTS ≡

SERIOUS
Hallucinations, confusion, excitability, skin rash, hives. Stop taking the drug and call your doctor immediately.

COMMON
Nausea, vomiting, stomach pain or abdominal discomfort, hangover-like symptoms, drowsiness.

LESS COMMON
Diarrhea, loss of coordination, dizziness, lightheadedness.

Pregnancy: Adequate studies of the use of chloral hydrate during pregnancy have not been done. Before taking chloral hydrate, tell your doctor if you are pregnant or plan to become pregnant.

Breast Feeding: Chloral hydrate passes into breast milk; caution is advised. Consult your doctor for advice.

Infants and Children: Chloral hydrate should be used by children only under a doctor's supervision.

Special Concerns: Swallow the capsules whole. Do not chew them, since chloral hydrate has an unpleasant taste. Make sure your doctor has specifically indicated to your pharmacist both how many milligrams and how many capsules or teaspoonfuls you or your child should receive in a single dose.

OVERDOSE
Symptoms: Severe nausea, vomiting, or stomach pain; difficulty swallowing; severe drowsiness; continuing confusion; seizures; low body temperature; difficulty breathing or shortness of breath; irregular heartbeat; severe weakness; staggering; slurred speech.

What to Do: Call your doctor, emergency medical services (EMS), or the nearest poison control center immediately.

▼ INTERACTIONS

DRUG INTERACTIONS
The following drugs may interact with chloral hydrate. Consult your doctor for specific advice if you are taking anticoagulants, tricyclic antidepressants, or central nervous system depressants.

FOOD INTERACTIONS
No food interactions have been reported.

DISEASE INTERACTIONS
Caution is advised when taking chloral hydrate. Consult your doctor if you have any of the following: kidney or liver problems, ulcers or other intestinal problems, esophagitis, or sleep apnea.

CHLORAMBUCIL

Available in: Tablets
Available OTC? No   **As Generic?** No
Drug Class: Alkylating agent

▼ USAGE INFORMATION

WHY IT'S PRESCRIBED
To treat some types of cancer, especially leukemia and lymphoma (cancer of the lymphatic system). More specifically, chlorambucil is used to treat chronic lymphocytic leukemia (a type of leukemia caused by overproduction and abnormal formation of certain white blood cells important in the body's immune system) and Hodgkin's disease (a type of cancer affecting the lymphatic system, characterized by painless swelling of the lymph nodes).

HOW IT WORKS
Chlorambucil kills cancer cells by interfering with the activity of their genetic material, thus preventing the cells from reproducing. The drug may also affect the growth and development of normal cells in the body, resulting in unpleasant side effects.

▼ DOSAGE GUIDELINES

RANGE AND FREQUENCY
Initial dose: 0.1 to 0.2 mg per 2.2 lbs (1 kg) of body weight daily (approximately 4 to 10 mg per day) for 3 to 6 weeks. Maintenance dose will depend on white blood cell counts.

ONSET OF EFFECT
Within 3 to 4 weeks.

DURATION OF ACTION
Unknown.

DIETARY ADVICE
Swallow with liquid 2 hours after a light meal. Drink plenty of fluids between meals.

STORAGE
Store in a tightly sealed container away from heat and direct light.

MISSED DOSE
Take it as soon as you remember. If it is near the time for the next dose, skip the missed dose and resume your regular dosage schedule. Do not double the next dose.

STOPPING THE DRUG
The decision to stop taking chlorambucil should be made by your doctor.

PROLONGED USE
Consult with your doctor about the need for periodic medical exams and blood tests, since adverse reactions are more likely the longer the drug is used.

▼ PRECAUTIONS

Over 60: Adverse reactions may be more likely and severe in elderly patients.

Driving and Hazardous Work: Should not interfere with any activities requiring mental alertness.

Alcohol: Avoid alcohol.

Pregnancy: Chlorambucil may cause birth defects. Persons of childbearing years should take steps to prevent pregnancy when being treated with this medication.

Breast Feeding: Not recommended during therapy.

Infants and Children: No special problems are expected, although children with impaired kidney function may be at greater risk of having seizures while taking chlorambucil.

Special Concerns: Infection is the single greatest threat to people receiving chemotherapy. Chlorambucil may lower your ability to resist infection by lowering the number of white blood cells in the blood. Therefore, do not receive any vaccinations without doctor's approval. Avoid people with infections. Inform your doctor immediately if you have fever, chills, diarrhea, or a cough.

OVERDOSE
Symptoms: Fever, chills, unusual bleeding, seizures, agitation.

What to Do: Call your doctor, emergency medical services (EMS), or the nearest poison control center immediately.

▼ INTERACTIONS

DRUG INTERACTIONS
Consult your doctor for specific advice if you are taking amphotericin B (by injection), other antineoplastic (anticancer) drugs, antithyroid medications, chloramphenicol, colchicine or other antigout drugs, corticosteroid drugs, or immunosuppressant drugs (such as azathioprine, cyclosporine, ganciclovir, and interferon).

FOOD INTERACTIONS
Avoid consuming excess quantities of foods high in fat or sugar.

DISEASE INTERACTIONS
Caution is advised. Consult your doctor if you have any of the following: gout, a history of kidney stones, an active infection, recent exposure to chicken pox or shingles, liver or kidney problems.

▼ SIDE EFFECTS

SERIOUS
Black or tarry stools; blood-tinged (pink or maroon) urine or stools; cough or hoarseness; fever; chills; lower back pain or pain in flanks; painful, difficult urination; small, red spots on the skin; bleeding from gums, nose, or other unusual places; easy bruising; shortness of breath. These side effects may mean that normal blood cells and special blood-clotting cells have been affected, or that normal immune cells have been affected and an infection is developing somewhere in your body. See your doctor right away if any of these occur.

COMMON
Nausea and vomiting.

LESS COMMON
Painful joints, rash, itching, swelling of feet or lower legs (edema), changes in menstruation.

CHLORAMPHENICOL OPHTHALMIC AND OTIC

Available in: Ophthalmic solution and ointment, otic solution
Available OTC? No   **As Generic?** Yes
Drug Class: Antibiotic

▼ USAGE INFORMATION

WHY IT'S PRESCRIBED
To treat infections of the eye or of the ear canal.

HOW IT WORKS
Chloramphenicol inhibits the spread of bacteria by interfering with protein synthesis in bacterial cells, preventing them from multiplying.

▼ DOSAGE GUIDELINES

RANGE AND FREQUENCY
Ophthalmic solution: 1 drop every 1 to 4 hours. Ophthalmic ointment: Apply every 3 hours. Otic solution: 2 or 3 drops every 6 to 8 hours.

ONSET OF EFFECT
Unknown.

DURATION OF ACTION
Unknown.

DIETARY ADVICE
This drug can be used without regard to diet.

STORAGE
Store in a tightly sealed container away from heat, moisture, and direct light. Do not allow the medicine to freeze. You may refrigerate the otic solution.

MISSED DOSE
Apply it as soon as you remember. If it is near the time for the next dose, skip the missed dose and resume your regular dosage schedule. Do not double the next dose.

STOPPING THE DRUG
Use this drug as prescribed for the full treatment period, even if you begin to feel better before the scheduled end of therapy.

PROLONGED USE
You should see your doctor regularly for tests and examinations if you take this drug for a prolonged period.

▼ PRECAUTIONS

Over 60: No special problems are expected.

Driving and Hazardous Work: Do not drive or engage in hazardous work until you determine how the drug affects your vision.

Alcohol: Avoid alcohol.

Pregnancy: This medication has not been shown to cause birth defects or other problems during pregnancy. Before you use chloramphenicol, tell your doctor if you are pregnant or plan to become pregnant.

Breast Feeding: This drug has not been shown to cause problems in nursing babies.

Infants and Children: Do not use this drug on infants or children unless specifically directed by your physician.

Special Concerns: To use the eye drops or the ointment, first wash your hands. Tilt your head back. Gently apply pressure to the inside corner of the eyelid and with the index finger of the same hand, pull downward on the lower eyelid to make a space. Drop the medicine or put a short strip of ointment (about ⅓ inch long) into this space and close your eye. Apply pressure for 1 or 2 minutes while keeping the eye closed without blinking. To use the ear drops, lie down or tilt your head so the infected ear faces up. Gently pull the earlobe up and back for adults (down and back for children) to straighten the ear canal. Drop the medicine into the ear. Keep the ear facing upward for 1 to 2 minutes after inserting the drops to allow the medicine to reach the infection. You may insert a cotton ball to prevent the medicine from leaking out. Make sure the applicator for eye or ear drops does not touch your eye, ear, finger, or any other surface.

OVERDOSE
Symptoms: No specific symptoms have been reported.

What to Do: An overdose of ophthalmic or otic chloramphenicol is unlikely to be life-threatening. If a large volume enters the eye, flush with water. If a large volume enters the ear or someone accidentally ingests the medication, call your physician, emergency medical services (EMS), or the nearest poison control center immediately.

▼ INTERACTIONS

DRUG INTERACTIONS
Other drugs may interact with ophthalmic or otic chloramphenicol. Consult your doctor for specific advice if you are taking any other prescription or over-the-counter drug.

FOOD INTERACTIONS
No known food interactions.

DISEASE INTERACTIONS
Caution is advised when taking ophthalmic or otic chloramphenicol. Consult your doctor if you have a perforated eardrum (for otic solution) or any other medical condition.

SIDE EFFECTS

SERIOUS
Bone marrow depression is a rare complication of chloramphenicol use. Other serious side effects include pale skin, sore throat and fever, unusual bleeding or bruising, unusual fatigue, itching, redness, swelling, skin rash, and skin irritation. Stop using the medication and call your doctor immediately.

COMMON
No common side effects are associated with otic chloramphenicol. Ophthalmic chloramphenicol may delay healing of the surface layer of the cornea.

LESS COMMON
Stinging or burning sensation.

CHLORAMPHENICOL ORAL AND TOPICAL

Available in: Capsules, oral suspension, injection, cream
Available OTC? No   **As Generic?** Yes
Drug Class: Antibiotic

▼ USAGE INFORMATION

WHY IT'S PRESCRIBED
To treat serious infections caused by bacteria. Because of the risk of dangerous side effects, it is prescribed only when other less toxic antibiotics cannot be used.

HOW IT WORKS
Chloramphenicol works by killing bacteria or inhibiting their growth.

▼ DOSAGE GUIDELINES

RANGE AND FREQUENCY
Oral forms and injection— Adults and teenagers: 5.7 mg per lb of body weight, 4 times a day. Children: 5.7 mg per lb of body weight, 4 times a day, or 11.4 mg per lb, 2 times a day. Infants under 2 weeks: 2.8 mg per lb, 4 times a day. Cream— Apply to infected area of skin 3 or 4 times a day.

ONSET OF EFFECT
Unknown.

DURATION OF ACTION
Unknown.

DIETARY ADVICE
Oral forms work best when taken on an empty stomach, at least 1 hour before or 2 hours after meals, with a full glass of water.

STORAGE
Store in a tightly sealed container away from heat and direct light. Do not allow liquid forms to freeze.

MISSED DOSE
Take it as soon as you remember. If it is near the time for the next dose, skip the missed dose and resume your regular dosage schedule. Do not double the next dose.

STOPPING THE DRUG
Take the medicine as prescribed for the full treatment period, even if you begin to feel better before the scheduled end of therapy.

PROLONGED USE
You should see your doctor regularly for tests and examinations if you must take this medicine for a prolonged period of time.

▼ PRECAUTIONS

Over 60: In older patients it is not known whether chloramphenicol causes side effects different from or more severe than those in younger persons.

Driving and Hazardous Work: Do not drive or engage in hazardous work until you determine how the medicine affects you.

Alcohol: It is advisable to abstain from alcohol when fighting an infection.

Pregnancy: Chloramphenicol has not been shown to cause birth defects in humans. However, its use is not recommended in the weeks immediately before delivery because it can cause temporary adverse side effects in the newborn child. Consult your doctor before using this drug during pregnancy.

Breast Feeding: Chloramphenicol passes into breast milk; avoid or discontinue use while nursing.

Infants and Children: Adverse reactions may be more likely and more severe in newborn babies.

Special Concerns: Chloramphenicol may cause anemia, which may increase the risk of infections and other problems in the gums. Blood must be monitored frequently while using this medicine. Be careful when brushing and flossing. Delay dental work, if possible, until you have stopped taking chloramphenicol. Chloramphenicol may cause false results on blood sugar tests for people with diabetes. Use of chloramphenicol while you are receiving x-ray treatment can increase the risk of blood problems.

OVERDOSE
Symptoms: Nausea, vomiting, unpleasant taste in the mouth, diarrhea.

What to Do: An overdose of chloramphenicol is unlikely to be life-threatening, Nonetheless, call your doctor, emergency medical services (EMS), or the nearest poison control center immediately.

▼ INTERACTIONS

DRUG INTERACTIONS
Consult your doctor for specific advice if you are taking alfentanil, amphotericin B, antithyroid agents, azathioprine, chemotherapy drugs for cancer, colchicine, clindamycin, cyclophosphamide, ethotoin, erythromycins, oral antidiabetic agents, flucytosine, ganciclovir, interferon, mephenytoin, mercaptopurine, methotrexate, phenytoin, plicamycin, or zidovudine (AZT).

FOOD INTERACTIONS
No known food interactions.

DISEASE INTERACTIONS
Caution is advised when taking chloramphenicol. Consult your doctor if you have anemia or another blood disorder, liver disease, or if you are undergoing radiation therapy.

SIDE EFFECTS

SERIOUS
Pale or sickly appearance; sore throat; fever; unusual bruising or bleeding; unusual fatigue; confusion; delirium; headache; eye pain; blurring or loss of vision; weakness; numbness, tingling, or pain in hands or feet; skin rash; breathing difficulty. Call your doctor immediately.

COMMON
No common side effects are associated with the use of chloramphenicol.

LESS COMMON
Diarrhea, nausea, and vomiting.

CHLORDIAZEPOXIDE

BRAND NAME

Librium

Available in: Capsules, tablets, injection
Available OTC? No   **As Generic?** Yes
Drug Class: Benzodiazepine tranquilizer; antianxiety agent

▼ USAGE INFORMATION

WHY IT'S PRESCRIBED
To treat anxiety, muscle spasms, and alcohol withdrawal symptoms.

HOW IT WORKS
In general, chlordiazepoxide produces mild sedation by depressing activity in the central nervous system. In particular, the drug appears to enhance the effect of gamma-aminobutyric acid (GABA), a natural chemical that inhibits the firing of neurons and dampens the transmission of nerve signals, thus decreasing nervous excitation.

▼ DOSAGE GUIDELINES

RANGE AND FREQUENCY
For anxiety– Adults: 5 to 25 mg, 3 or 4 times per day. Patients older than 60 or those who have a chronic illness: Initial dose of 5 to 10 mg, 2 to 4 times per day. Dose may be increased by your doctor to a maximum of 25 mg, 2 to 3 times per day. For alcohol withdrawal– Initial dose is 50 to 100 mg, repeated as recommended by your doctor. Some patients will require up to 300 mg per day in the early stages of alcohol withdrawal. Your doctor will determine a daily maintenance dose once the early stages of withdrawal have passed.

ONSET OF EFFECT
Within 1 to 2 hours.

DURATION OF ACTION
Up to 48 hours.

DIETARY ADVICE
No special restrictions.

STORAGE
Store in a tightly sealed container away from heat, moisture, and direct light.

MISSED DOSE
Take it as soon as you remember. If it is near the time for the next dose, skip the missed dose and resume your regular dosage schedule. Do not double the next dose.

STOPPING THE DRUG
Do not stop taking the drug abruptly or without your doctor's approval. Dosage should be reduced gradually to prevent withdrawal symptoms, including seizures.

PROLONGED USE
This medication may slowly lose its effectiveness with prolonged use. You should see your doctor for periodic evaluation if you must take it for an extended time.

▼ PRECAUTIONS

Over 60: Adverse reactions may be more likely and more severe in older patients.

Driving and Hazardous Work: The use of this drug may impair your ability to perform such tasks safely.

Alcohol: Alcohol intake should be extremely moderate or stopped altogether while taking this drug.

Pregnancy: Use during pregnancy should be avoided if possible. Be sure to tell your doctor if you are pregnant or plan to become pregnant.

Breast Feeding: This drug passes into breast milk; do not take it while nursing.

Infants and Children: This drug is not recommended for use by children under age 6.

Special Concerns: Chlordiazepoxide use can lead to psychological or physical dependence. Never take more than the prescribed daily dose.

OVERDOSE
Symptoms: Extreme drowsiness, confusion, slurred speech, slow reflexes, poor coordination, staggering gait, tremor, slowed breathing, loss of consciousness.

What to Do: Call your doctor, emergency medical services (EMS), or the nearest poison control center immediately.

▼ INTERACTIONS

DRUG INTERACTIONS
Consult your doctor for specific advice if you are taking any drugs that depress the central nervous system; these include antihistamines, antidepressants or other psychiatric medications, barbiturates, sedatives, cough medicines, decongestants, and painkillers. Be sure your doctor knows about any over-the-counter drug you may take.

FOOD INTERACTIONS
None reported.

DISEASE INTERACTIONS
Consult your doctor if you have a history of alcohol or drug abuse, stroke or other brain disease, any chronic lung disease, hyperactivity, depression or other mental illness, myasthenia gravis, sleep apnea, epilepsy, porphyria, kidney disease, or liver disease.

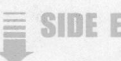

SIDE EFFECTS

SERIOUS
Difficulty concentrating, outbursts of anger, other behavior problems, depression, hallucinations, confusion, memory impairment, faintness, muscle weakness, skin rash or itching, sore throat, fever and chills, sores or ulcers in throat or mouth, unusual bruising or bleeding, extreme fatigue, yellow discoloration of the eyes or skin. Call your doctor immediately.

COMMON
Drowsiness, loss of coordination, unsteady gait, dizziness, lightheadedness, slurred speech.

LESS COMMON
Change in sexual desire or ability, constipation, false sense of well-being, nausea and vomiting, urinary problems, unusual fatigue.

CHLORDIAZEPOXIDE/AMITRIPTYLINE

Available in: Tablets
Available OTC? No   **As Generic?** Yes
Drug Class: Benzodiazepine tranquilizer; antianxiety agent/antidepressant

▼ USAGE INFORMATION

WHY IT'S PRESCRIBED
Chlordiazepoxide/amitriptyline is used to treat anxiety occurring simultaneously with depression.

HOW IT WORKS
Chlordiazepoxide depresses activity in the central nervous system, producing a mild sedative effect. Amitriptyline affects the activity of certain brain chemicals (serotonin and norepinephrine) that are linked to mood, emotions, and mental state.

▼ DOSAGE GUIDELINES

RANGE AND FREQUENCY
Adults: Initial dose is 5 mg of chlordiazepoxide and 12.5 mg of amitriptyline, or 10 mg of chlordiazepoxide and 25 mg of amitriptyline, 3 to 4 times daily. Some patients require higher doses, while some do well with lower doses. Your doctor will determine the correct dose.

ONSET OF EFFECT
The antianxiety and sedation effects occur within the first week of therapy. The antidepressant effect may require several weeks.

DURATION OF ACTION
Unknown.

DIETARY ADVICE
No special restrictions.

STORAGE
Store in a tightly sealed container away from heat, moisture, and direct light.

MISSED DOSE
Take it as soon as you remember. If it is near the time for the next dose, skip the missed dose and resume your regular dosage schedule. Do not double the next dose.

STOPPING THE DRUG
Discontinuing the drug abruptly may produce withdrawal symptoms. Dosage should be reduced gradually according to your doctor's instructions.

PROLONGED USE
Short-term therapy (8 weeks or less) is typical; do not take it for a longer period unless so advised by your doctor.

▼ PRECAUTIONS

Over 60: Adverse reactions may be more likely and more severe in older patients.

Driving and Hazardous Work: This drug can impair mental alertness and physical coordination. Adjust your activities accordingly.

Alcohol: Avoid alcohol while using this medication.

Pregnancy: Use during pregnancy should be avoided if possible. Be sure to tell your doctor if you are pregnant or plan to become pregnant.

Breast Feeding: Avoid or discontinue use while breast feeding.

Infants and Children: This drug combination is not recommended for use by infants and children.

Special Concerns: Use of this medication can lead to physical dependence. Never take more than the prescribed daily dose.

OVERDOSE
Symptoms: Confusion; convulsions; poor concentration; severe drowsiness, fatigue, or weakness (some patients will become unusually restless or agitated); dilated pupils; rapid or irregular heartbeat; rapid, shallow breathing, shortness of breath, or other breathing trouble; fever; hallucinations.

What to Do: Call your doctor, emergency medical services (EMS), or the nearest poison control center immediately.

▼ INTERACTIONS

DRUG INTERACTIONS
Consult your doctor for specific advice if you are taking sedatives, tranquilizers, or other medications that cause drowsiness; amphetamines or diet pills; asthma medication; prescription or over-the-counter decongestants; prescription or nonprescription medicine for colds, sinus problems, allergies, and hay fever; high blood pressure medication; thyroid medicine; or MAO inhibitors.

FOOD INTERACTIONS
None reported.

DISEASE INTERACTIONS
Consult your doctor if you have a history of alcohol or drug abuse, stroke or other brain disease, any chronic lung disease, glaucoma, hyperactivity, depression or other mental illness, myasthenia gravis, sleep apnea, epilepsy, porphyria, kidney disease, or liver disease.

SIDE EFFECTS

SERIOUS
Blurred vision, confusion, difficulty speaking or swallowing, eye pain, fainting, rapid or uneven heartbeat, hallucinations, poor balance, nervousness or restlessness, problems urinating, shakiness or trembling, shuffling walk, slowed movements, stiffness in the arms and legs.

COMMON
Dizziness, drowsiness, loss of coordination, poor balance, dry mouth, headache, increased appetite, nausea, fatigue or mild weakness, unpleasant taste in mouth or of food, unexpected weight gain.

LESS COMMON
Diarrhea, heartburn, increased sweating, vomiting, increased sensitivity to sunlight.

CHLORHEXIDINE GLUCONATE

BRAND NAMES

Dyna-Hex, Hibiclens, Hibiclens Antiseptic/ Antimicrobial Skin Cleanser, Peridex, Periogard

Available in: Skin cleanser, wound cleanser, oral rinse
Available OTC? No **As Generic?** No
Drug Class: Topical antiseptic; anti-infective

▼ USAGE INFORMATION

WHY IT'S PRESCRIBED
Skin or wound cleanser: To prevent infection. Oral rinse: To treat gingivitis (inflammation of the gums, marked by redness, tenderness, swelling, and bleeding of gum tissue).

HOW IT WORKS
On the skin, it reduces surface bacteria to prevent infection. In the mouth, chlorhexidine kills the bacteria that cause dental plaque and gingivitis. However, it cannot prevent plaque from forming, nor does it remove plaque that has already formed. Scrupulous brushing and flossing and regular visits to a dentist are still necessary.

▼ DOSAGE GUIDELINES

RANGE AND FREQUENCY
Skin cleanser: 5 ml (1 teaspoon) lathered for 30 seconds to 3 minutes and rinsed.

Oral rinse: average adult dose (individual dose may vary): 15 ml (1 capful), used as a mouthwash for 30 seconds, twice a day, after brushing and flossing teeth. Do not dilute the drug with water. Rinse your mouth thoroughly before use and be careful not to swallow any of the product. Do not rinse with water after using the medication.

ONSET OF EFFECT
Within 1 hour.

DURATION OF ACTION
Unknown.

DIETARY ADVICE
Do not eat or drink for 2 to 3 hours following treatment.

STORAGE
Store in a tightly sealed container away from heat and direct light. Do not allow the medication to freeze.

MISSED DOSE
Use as soon as you remember. If it is near the time for the next dose, skip the missed dose and resume your regular dosing schedule following the next brushing. Do not double the next dose.

STOPPING THE DRUG
Use for the full treatment period, unless directed otherwise by your doctor or dentist.

PROLONGED USE
See your doctor as recommended; see your dentist every 6 months for professional cleaning and evaluation of the progress of therapy.

▼ PRECAUTIONS

Over 60: No precautions.

Driving and Hazardous Work: No special precautions are necessary.

Alcohol: No special restrictions. Persons with a history of alcoholism, however, should not use chlorhexidine oral rinse since it contains a relatively high percentage of alcohol, which may trigger a relapse of alcohol abuse.

Pregnancy: Adequate human studies have not been done; consult your doctor.

Breast Feeding: No problems have been documented, but be sure your doctor knows if you are breast feeding.

Infants and Children: It is not commonly prescribed for patients under 18 years old; children may be most susceptible to side effects, especially those related to alcohol intoxication (oral rinse contains more than 10% alcohol).

Special Concerns: If the skin or wound being scrubbed with chlorhexidene appears to become infected, notify your doctor immediately. Do not allow the medication to come in contact with eyes or ears, since it may cause permanent injury. Do not use chlorhexidine if you have had a prior allergic reaction to it. Cosmetic dentistry may be used to treat discoloration of teeth.

OVERDOSE
Symptoms: Slurred speech, staggering, drowsiness or stupor, stomach upset, nausea (overdose is most likely to affect young or underweight patients).

What to Do: Call your doctor or EMS right away if anyone—especially a child—accidentally ingests more than 4 oz of chlorhexidine or exhibits the above symptoms.

▼ INTERACTIONS

DRUG INTERACTIONS
Do not use any other prescription or nonprescription medications for the area of the skin being treated or for the mouth without checking with your doctor or dentist.

FOOD INTERACTIONS
No known food interactions.

DISEASE INTERACTIONS
Do not take chlorhexidine gluconate if you have periodontal disease (various disorders of the bones of the jaw and other tissues surrounding and supporting the teeth).

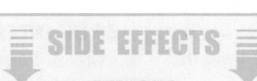

SIDE EFFECTS

SERIOUS
Rare severe allergic reaction with swelling, breathing difficulty, and even complete closure of the airways with potentially fatal anaphylactic shock. Seek medical assistance immediately.

COMMON
Staining (sometimes heavy) of the teeth, gums, dental fillings, dentures, and other oral surfaces (staining may be more pronounced in patients with greater preexisting plaque accumulation); alteration in taste perception (taste perception returns to normal when medicine is discontinued); paradoxical increase in plaque buildup on the teeth.

LESS COMMON
Irritation or allergy of the skin, gums, tongue, or other mouth surfaces with redness, burning, stinging, or rash; swollen glands in the neck or sides of the face.

CHLOROQUINE

Available in: Tablets, injection
Available OTC? No   **As Generic?** Yes
Drug Class: Anti-infective/antimalarial

▼ USAGE INFORMATION

WHY IT'S PRESCRIBED
To prevent and treat malaria caused by specific strains of plasmodia (the parasite that causes malaria) that are susceptible to chloroquine. (The drug is ineffective against other strains.) It is also used with another drug as a second line of therapy for hard-to-treat amebic (parasitic) liver abscess.

HOW IT WORKS
Chloroquine is poisonous to the malarial parasite.

▼ DOSAGE GUIDELINES

RANGE AND FREQUENCY
Tablets— For malaria prevention: 500 mg (300 mg base) once a week. For treatment of malaria: To start, 1,000 mg (600 mg base). Then, 500 mg (300 mg base), 6 to 8 hours after the first dose, and 500 mg once a day on the second and third days of treatment. To treat amebic liver abscess: To start, 250 mg (150 mg base), 4 times a day for 2 days. Then, 250 mg twice a day for at least 2 to 3 weeks. Injection— For treatment of malaria: 200 to 250 mg (160 to 200 mg base). If needed, the dose may be repeated after 6 hours, not to exceed 1,000 mg (800 mg base) in the first 24 hours. To treat amebic liver abscess: 200 to 250 mg a day for 10 to 12 days. (Note: All dosages are for adults and adolescents. Consult your pediatrician for children's doses.

ONSET OF EFFECT
Unknown.

DURATION OF ACTION
Unknown.

DIETARY ADVICE
Take it with food or milk to reduce stomach upset.

STORAGE
Store in a tightly sealed container away from heat, moisture, and direct light.

MISSED DOSE
If taking 1 or more doses a day, take it as soon as you remember. If it is near the time for the next dose, skip the missed dose and resume your regular dosage schedule. Do not double the next dose. If taking 1 weekly dose, take it as soon as possible, then resume regular schedule.

STOPPING THE DRUG
Take it as prescribed for the full treatment period.

PROLONGED USE
If you are taking this drug as a preventive, your doctor may want you to begin 1 to 2 weeks before you travel to an area where malaria is prevalent. Keep taking chloroquine while you are in the area and for 4 weeks after you leave.

▼ PRECAUTIONS

Over 60: Adverse reactions may be more likely and more severe.

Driving and Hazardous Work: Do not drive or engage in hazardous work until you determine how the medicine affects you.

Alcohol: No special precautions are necessary.

Pregnancy: The use of chloroquine is discouraged during pregnancy because of the risks it poses to the unborn child. However, in some cases it may be prescribed to prevent or treat malaria or amebic liver abscess, since the risks of these diseases are potentially more serious than those posed by the drug. Consult your doctor for advice.

Breast Feeding: Chloroquine passes into breast milk; extreme caution is advised. Consult your doctor.

Infants and Children: Extreme caution is necessary when used by children.

Special Concerns: If you take chloroquine once a week, take it on the same day every week. Malaria is spread by mosquitoes. Take appropriate precautions, such as using mosquito netting, to guard against being bitten by malaria-carrying mosquitoes.

OVERDOSE
Symptoms: Increased excitability, headache, drowsiness, seizures, vision changes, heartbeat irregularities, dizziness, fainting, respiratory and cardiac arrest.

What to Do: Seek medical assistance immediately.

▼ INTERACTIONS

DRUG INTERACTIONS
Consult your doctor for specific advice if you are taking magnesium salts, antacids, cimetidine, or penicillamine. The intradermal rabies vaccine may not be effective if chloroquine is being used at the time of vaccination.

FOOD INTERACTIONS
No known food interactions.

DISEASE INTERACTIONS
Consult your doctor for specific advice if you have a severe blood disorder, any eye disorder, liver disease, a severe nervous system disorder, G6PD deficiency, porphyria, or psoriasis.

 SIDE EFFECTS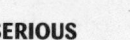

SERIOUS
Blurred or altered vision; blood problems, including low white blood cell count (sore throat, fever), anemia (fatigue, weakness), and low platelet count (easy bleeding and bruising). Such side effects are extremely rare; call your doctor immediately if they occur.

COMMON
No common side effects are associated with chloroquine.

LESS COMMON
Diarrhea, loss of appetite, headache, stomach cramps or pain, nausea or vomiting, itching, dizziness, fatigue, confusion, loss or bleaching of hair, skin rash. Also blue-black discoloration of skin, inside of mouth, or fingernails.

CHLOROTHIAZIDE

Available in: Tablets, oral suspension, injection
Available OTC? No   **As Generic?** Yes
Drug Class: Thiazide diuretic

▼ USAGE INFORMATION

WHY IT'S PRESCRIBED
To treat high blood pressure and conditions causing edema (swelling of body tissues resulting from excess salt and water retention).

HOW IT WORKS
Diuretics increase the excretion of salt and water in the urine. By reducing the overall fluid volume in the body, these drugs reduce blood volume and so reduce pressure within the blood vessels.

▼ DOSAGE GUIDELINES

RANGE AND FREQUENCY
Adults— For high blood pressure: 250 mg once a day. To reduce edema: 250 to 500 mg once a day, or 2 or 3 days a week.

ONSET OF EFFECT
2 hours after oral dose; 15 minutes after injection.

DURATION OF ACTION
6 to 12 hours.

DIETARY ADVICE
Tablets should be taken with food.

STORAGE
Store in a tightly sealed container away from heat and direct light. Keep the liquid form from freezing.

MISSED DOSE
Take it as soon as you remember. If it is near the time for the next dose, skip the missed dose and resume your regular dosage schedule. Do not double the next dose.

STOPPING THE DRUG
The decision to stop taking the drug should be made by your doctor.

PROLONGED USE
See your doctor regularly for examinations and tests if you must take this medicine for an extended period.

▼ PRECAUTIONS

Over 60: No special problems are expected.

≡ SIDE EFFECTS ≡

SERIOUS
Skin rash, hives, intense itching, swelling of the mouth and throat, breathing difficulty, serious heartbeat irregularities or palpitations, lightheadedness or dizziness, unusual bleeding or bruising. Call your doctor immediately.

COMMON
Potassium depletion may lead to heart palpitations and weakness. Fluid depletion may lead to dizziness, especially upon arising from a sitting or lying position.

LESS COMMON
Decreased sexual ability, increased sensitivity to sunlight, loss of appetite, gout, increased blood sugar (a problem for patients with diabetes).

Driving and Hazardous Work: No special precautions are necessary.

Alcohol: No special precautions are necessary.

Pregnancy: Chlorothiazide has caused birth defects in animals. Human studies have not been done. This medicine should not be taken during pregnancy unless recommended by your doctor. Other diuretics are preferred in pregnant women.

Breast Feeding: Chlorothiazide passes into breast milk; avoid or discontinue use during the first month of nursing.

Infants and Children: This drug generally is not prescribed for children.

Special Concerns: Chlorothiazide is usually taken once a day. To prevent it from interfering with sleep, take it in the morning (unless otherwise prescribed by your doctor). If you are taking it for high blood pressure, follow the diet and weight control measures recommended by your doctor. Avoid exposure to sunlight, use a sunblock, or wear protective clothing. This medicine may cause your body to lose potassium. Follow your doctor's instructions about eating potassium-rich foods or taking a potassium supplement.

OVERDOSE
Symptoms: Lethargy, dizziness, drowsiness, muscle weakness, cramps, heartbeat irregularities, fainting.

What to Do: Call your doctor, emergency medical services (EMS), or the nearest poison control center immediately.

▼ INTERACTIONS

DRUG INTERACTIONS
Consult your doctor for specific advice if you are taking anticoagulants, cholestyramine, colestipol, drugs for diabetes, nonsteroidal anti-inflammatory drugs, digitalis drugs, or lithium.

FOOD INTERACTIONS
No known food interactions.

DISEASE INTERACTIONS
Caution is advised when taking chlorothiazide. Consult your doctor if you have any of the following: diabetes, gout, lupus erythematosus, pancreatitis, heart disease, blood vessel disease, liver disease, or kidney disease.

CHLOROTRIANISENE

Available in: Capsules
Available OTC? No   **As Generic?** Yes
Drug Class: Female sex hormone

▼ USAGE INFORMATION

WHY IT'S PRESCRIBED
To relieve the symptoms of inoperable prostate cancer and ease some of the symptoms of menopause (hot flashes, sweating, chills, faintness). Chlorotrianisene may also be used to prevent breast engorgement following childbirth.

HOW IT WORKS
In women, chlorotrianisene supplements deficient natural levels of estrogen in the body. In men, the drug inhibits growth of cells in the prostate gland.

▼ DOSAGE GUIDELINES

RANGE AND FREQUENCY
For prostate cancer: 12 to 25 mg a day. For menopausal symptoms: 12 to 25 mg a day for 30 days or a cyclic regimen that requires 3 weeks on and 1 week off.

ONSET OF EFFECT
Unknown.

DURATION OF ACTION
24 hours.

DIETARY ADVICE
Take chlorotrianisene with or immediately following a meal to reduce nausea. If you have difficulty swallowing the capsule whole, open it and take it with liquid or food. Follow a low-sodium diet, since sodium causes your body to retain excess water.

STORAGE
Store in a tightly sealed container away from heat, moisture, and direct light.

MISSED DOSE
Take it as soon as you remember, unless the time for your next scheduled dose is within the next 12 hours. If so, skip the missed dose and resume your regular dosage schedule. Do not double the next dose.

STOPPING THE DRUG
Take it as prescribed for the full treatment period, even if you begin to feel better before the scheduled end of therapy. The decision to stop taking the drug should be made in consultation with your doctor.

PROLONGED USE
Prolonged use of chlorotrianisene may lead to an increased risk of uterine or breast cancer and growth of fibroid tumors of the uterus (a common benign tumor). Talk to your doctor about the need for follow-up medical examinations or laboratory tests including Pap smear, mammogram, and liver function tests.

▼ PRECAUTIONS

Over 60: Adverse reactions may be more likely and more severe in elderly patients.

Driving and Hazardous Work: This drug does not interfere with your ability to engage in such activities.

Alcohol: No special precautions are necessary.

Pregnancy: You should not use chlorotrianisene if you are pregnant or plan to become pregnant.

Breast Feeding: Chlorotrianisene is used to prevent breast engorgement and milk production following pregnancy; it should not be used by women wishing to nurse.

Infants and Children: Not prescribed for children.

Special Concerns: If you are on cyclic therapy (3 weeks on, 1 week off) for menopausal symptoms, some minor vaginal bleeding may occur during the week you are not taking the drug. This symptom is common and should diminish at the start of the next treatment cycle.

OVERDOSE
Symptoms: Nausea and vomiting, fluid retention, breast enlargement, abnormal vaginal bleeding.

What to Do: Call your doctor, emergency medical services (EMS), or the nearest poison control center immediately.

▼ INTERACTIONS

DRUG INTERACTIONS
Consult your doctor for advice if you are taking antidepressants, aspirin, barbiturates, bromocriptine, calcium supplements, corticosteroids, corticotropin, cyclosporine, dantrolene, nicotine, somatropin, tamoxifen, or warfarin.

FOOD INTERACTIONS
No known food interactions.

DISEASE INTERACTIONS
Caution is advised when taking chlorotrianisene. Consult your doctor if you have any of the following: a history of cancer of the breast or reproductive organs; a family history of breast cancer; breast lumps; heart or blood vessel disease; asthma; bone disease; gallbladder disease; liver or kidney problems; migraines; seizures; or phlebitis.

 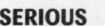 SIDE EFFECTS

SERIOUS
Profuse or abnormal vaginal bleeding, blood clots (pain, redness, swelling in arm, leg, or buttock), stroke (slurred speech, loss of sensation, blurry vision), chest pain, shortness of breath. Call your doctor immediately.

COMMON
Nausea, diarrhea, stomach cramps, loss of appetite, breast pain or tenderness. In men: Breast enlargement, reduction in the size of the testicles, diminished sex drive.

LESS COMMON
Rash, joint pain, lumps in breast, depression, dizziness, migraine headaches.

CHLORPHENIRAMINE MALEATE ORAL

Available in: Tablets, sustained-release capsules, syrup
Available OTC? Yes   **As Generic?** Yes
Drug Class: Antihistamine

▼ USAGE INFORMATION

WHY IT'S PRESCRIBED
To relieve the symptoms of hay fever and other allergies, and for itching skin and hives.

HOW IT WORKS
Chlorpheniramine maleate works by blocking the effects of histamine, a naturally occurring substance that causes swelling, itching, sneezing, watery eyes, hives, and other symptoms of allergic reaction.

▼ DOSAGE GUIDELINES

RANGE AND FREQUENCY
Tablets— Adults: 4 mg, 3 to 4 times per day as needed, for a maximum dose of 24 mg a day. Sustained-release capsules— 8 mg every 8 hours, or 12 mg every 12 hours, as needed. Syrup— Children ages 6 to 12: 2 mg, 3 to 4 times a day, not exceeding 12 mg a day. Children ages 2 to 6: 1 mg every 6 hours.

ONSET OF EFFECT
15 to 60 minutes.

DURATION OF ACTION
3 to 6 hours for regular form, 8 to 12 hours for sustained-release capsules.

DIETARY ADVICE
Chlorpheniramine maleate may be taken with food or milk to reduce stomach upset. Use sugarless gum, sugarless sour hard candy, or ice chips to ease dry mouth.

STORAGE
Store in a tightly sealed container away from heat and direct light.

MISSED DOSE
Take it as soon as you remember, up to 2 hours late. If it is more than 2 hours late, skip the missed dose and resume your regular dosage schedule. Do not double the next dose.

STOPPING THE DRUG
You should take it as prescribed for the full treatment period, but you may stop if you are feeling better before the scheduled end of therapy. Chlorpheniramine may be taken as needed.

PROLONGED USE
No special concerns.

▼ PRECAUTIONS

Over 60: Older persons are more sensitive to antihistamine side effects, particularly confusion, dizziness, drowsiness, restlessness, irritability, nightmares, and dry mouth, nose, and throat.

Driving and Hazardous Work: Do not drive or engage in hazardous work until you determine how the medicine affects you. Use of this drug is a disqualification for piloting aircraft.

Alcohol: Alcohol increases the likelihood and the severity of side effects like drowsiness and confusion.

Pregnancy: In animal studies, no birth defects have been reported. Studies of pregnant women have not been undertaken. Before taking this drug, tell your doctor if you are pregnant or are planning to become pregnant.

Breast Feeding: Chlorpheniramine passes into breast milk; avoid or discontinue use while nursing.

Infants and Children: This drug is not recommended for children under the age of 2.

Special Concerns: Do not break, crush, or chew sustained-release capsules.

OVERDOSE

Symptoms: Marked drowsiness, dilated and sluggish pupils, combativeness, excessive excitability, confusion, loss of coordination, weak pulse, seizures, loss of consciousness.

What to Do: Patient should be made to vomit immediately, using ipecac syrup. If the patient is unconscious, he or she should be taken to the nearest hospital emergency room right away.

▼ INTERACTIONS

DRUG INTERACTIONS
Consult your doctor for specific advice if you are taking anticholinergics, bepridil, medications containing alcohol, or MAO inhibitors.

FOOD INTERACTIONS
No known food interactions.

DISEASE INTERACTIONS
Before taking chlorpheniramine, consult your doctor if you wear contact lenses or if you have glaucoma, prostate enlargement, difficulty with urination, or dry mouth or eyes.

≡ SIDE EFFECTS ≡

SERIOUS
Bleeding problems; small red pinpoints on the skin; fever; extreme fatigue; bleeding ulcers in the rectum, mouth, and vagina; reduced count of white blood cells (rare).

COMMON
Drowsiness; unusual excitability; dry mouth, nose, or throat. Symptoms of drowsiness tend to subside after a few days' use as your body adjusts to the drug.

LESS COMMON
Vision changes, loss of appetite, dizziness, painful or difficult urination, less tolerance for contact lenses.

CHLORPROMAZINE HYDROCHLORIDE

BRAND NAME

Thorazine

Available in: Capsules, tablets, liquid concentrate, syrup, suppositories
Available OTC? No   **As Generic?** Yes
Drug Class: Neuroleptic; antipsychotic

▼ USAGE INFORMATION

WHY IT'S PRESCRIBED
To treat psychotic conditions such as schizophrenia. It can also be used to ease severe nausea and vomiting, and persistent hiccups.

HOW IT WORKS
Chlorpromazine inhibits activity of the brain chemical dopamine, thereby helping to prevent the overstimulation of specific nerve centers believed to be responsible for certain psychiatric disorders. The drug also suppresses activity in the trigger zones of the brain and gastrointestinal tract that govern the vomiting reflex and hiccupping.

▼ DOSAGE GUIDELINES

RANGE AND FREQUENCY
Dose, dosage form, and dosing schedule vary based on many factors, including patient's age, medical condition, body weight, tolerance of side effects, and overall response to the drug. Usual adult dose: Initially, 10 to 25 mg, 3 or 4 times a day. Your doctor may increase it as needed and tolerated; maximum dose may reach 200 mg a day for many, or even 800 mg a day for severely psychotic patients. Children: Consult your pediatrician.

ONSET OF EFFECT
For psychotic conditions: 4 to 6 weeks. For nausea and vomiting: 1 hour or less.

DURATION OF ACTION
Unknown.

DIETARY ADVICE
Take it with meals in order to reduce stomach upset.

STORAGE
Store in a tightly sealed container away from heat, moisture, and direct light.

MISSED DOSE
Take it as soon as you remember. However, if it is near the time for the next dose, skip the missed dose and resume your regular dosage schedule. Do not double the next dose.

STOPPING THE DRUG
Do not stop taking the drug abruptly or without your doctor's approval. Dosage should be reduced gradually by your doctor to prevent withdrawal symptoms.

PROLONGED USE
Prolonged use may lead to tardive dyskinesia (involuntary movements of the jaw, lips, and tongue). Consult your doctor about the need for follow-up evaluations and tests if you must take this drug for an extended period.

▼ PRECAUTIONS

Over 60: Adverse reactions, especially drowsiness and low blood pressure, are more common in elderly patients. A lower dose may be warranted.

Driving and Hazardous Work: The use of this drug may impair your ability to perform such tasks safely.

Alcohol: Avoid alcohol.

Pregnancy: Avoid using this drug if you are pregnant or plan to become pregnant.

Breast Feeding: Either avoid taking the drug if possible or refrain from breast feeding.

Infants and Children: This drug should not be used by infants and children younger than 2 years old. For older children, use it only under the care of your pediatrician.

OVERDOSE
Symptoms: Extreme drowsiness, heart rhythm irregularities, dry mouth, restlessness or agitation, seizures, unconsciousness.

What to Do: Call your doctor, emergency medical services (EMS), or the nearest poison control center immediately.

▼ INTERACTIONS

DRUG INTERACTIONS
Consult your doctor for specific advice if you are taking amantadine, high blood pressure medication, bromocriptine, deferoxamine, diuretics, levobunolol, heart medication, metoprolol, nabilone, other psychiatric drugs, pentamidine, pimozide, promethazine, trimeprazine, a thyroid agent, central nervous system depressants, epinephrine, lithium, levodopa, methyldopa, metoclopramide, metyrosine, pemoline, a rauwolfia alkaloid, or metrizamide.

FOOD INTERACTIONS
No known food interactions.

DISEASE INTERACTIONS
Consult your doctor if you have a history of alcohol abuse, any blood disorder, breast cancer, benign prostatic hyperplasia (BPH), epilepsy or seizures, glaucoma, heart, lung, or blood vessel disease, liver disease, Parkinson's disease, peptic ulcer, or urinary difficulty.

≡ SIDE EFFECTS ≡

SERIOUS
Extreme and persistent restlessness; uncontrolled movements, including tics, twitching, twisting movements, and muscle spasms in the face, neck, and back; loss of coordination and balance; shuffling gait; trembling, weakness, or stiffness in the extremities; difficulty swallowing or speaking; persistent, uncontrolled chewing, lip-smacking, or tongue movements; staring and absence of facial expression; fainting; difficulty urinating; increased skin sensitivity to the sun; skin rash; yellow discoloration of the eyes or skin (indicating a liver disorder).

COMMON
Constipation, decreased sweating, lightheadedness, dizziness or faintness, drowsiness, dry mouth.

LESS COMMON
Menstrual irregularities; sexual dysfunction; breast pain, swelling, or secretion; weight gain; blurred vision.

CHLORPROPAMIDE

Available in: Tablets
Available OTC? No **As Generic?** Yes
Drug Class: Antidiabetic agent/sulfonylurea

▼ USAGE INFORMATION

WHY IT'S PRESCRIBED
To help control mild to moderate non-insulin-dependent (type 2) diabetes mellitus in patients whose blood sugar cannot be adequately controlled by diet, weight loss, and exercise.

HOW IT WORKS
Chlorpropamide stimulates the release of additional insulin from the pancreas and makes the tissues of the body more responsive to insulin.

▼ DOSAGE GUIDELINES

RANGE AND FREQUENCY
Initially, 250 mg once a day. After 5 to 7 days, dose can be increased by 50 to 125 mg. It may be increased every 3 to 5 days, if needed, to a maximum dose of 750 mg a day. Adults over age 65: 100 to 125 mg each day, increased as described above.

ONSET OF EFFECT
Within 1 hour.

DURATION OF ACTION
Up to 60 hours.

DIETARY ADVICE
Take 1 dose daily, 30 minutes before breakfast; if stomach upset occurs, divide the daily amount into two equal doses and take them before your morning and evening meals. The tablet may be crushed. Follow the dietary guidelines given to you by your doctor, and restrict intake of sugar-containing snacks.

STORAGE
Store in a tightly sealed container away from heat and direct light.

MISSED DOSE
Take it as soon as you remember. If it is near the time for the next dose, skip the missed dose and resume your regular dosage schedule. Do not double the next dose.

STOPPING THE DRUG
Do not stop taking the medication without your doctor's approval. Take it as prescribed for the full treatment period, even if you begin to feel better.

PROLONGED USE
Prolonged use increases the risk of adverse effects. Periodic physical examinations and laboratory tests (blood and urine tests to monitor sugar levels) are needed.

▼ PRECAUTIONS

Over 60: Adverse reactions may be more likely and more severe in elderly patients.

Driving and Hazardous Work: Do not drive or engage in hazardous work until you determine how this medication affects you.

Alcohol: Avoid alcohol. Patients who consume alcohol while taking chlorpropamide are at risk for a severe reaction that may include nausea, vomiting, flushing, lightheadedness, headache, and shortness of breath.

Pregnancy: Avoid using chlorpropamide if you are pregnant or are planning to become pregnant.

Breast Feeding: Chlorpropamide passes into breast milk and may be harmful; avoid or discontinue use while nursing.

Infants and Children: Chlorpropamide is not recommended for infants and children.

OVERDOSE

Symptoms: Excessive hunger, nausea, anxiety, cool skin, cold sweats, drowsiness, rapid heartbeat, tingling of lips and tongue, weakness, unconsciousness, confusion, seizures.

What to Do: Call your doctor, emergency medical services (EMS), or the nearest poison control center immediately.

▼ INTERACTIONS

DRUG INTERACTIONS
Consult your doctor for specific advice if you are taking anabolic steroids or corticosteroids, allopurinol, aspirin and aspirin-containing cough, cold, and appetite-control drugs, anticoagulants, barbiturates, beta-blockers, calcium channel blockers, cimetidine, ranitidine, pentamidine, chloramphenicol, ciprofloxacin, cyclosporine, estrogens, ethanol, thiazide diuretics, fenfluramine, oral miconazole or ketoconazole, lithium, MAO inhibitors, probenecid, rifampin, selegiline or procarbazine, sulfinpyrazone, quinidine.

FOOD INTERACTIONS
No known food interactions.

DISEASE INTERACTIONS
Caution is advised when taking chlorpropamide. Consult your doctor if you have any of the following: malnutrition, heart problems, liver or kidney disease, thyroid disease, a severe infection, fever, or an underactive pituitary or adrenal gland.

SIDE EFFECTS

SERIOUS
Low blood sugar; perspiration or a cold sweat; restlessness; rapid pulse; anxious feeling; nausea; difficulty breathing; feelings of dizziness, weakness, or lightheadedness; poor coordination, slurred speech, confusion; sleepiness; seizures or convulsions; weakness of an arm, leg, or an entire side of the body; fainting. Contact your doctor immediately. Administer sugar-containing substances only if the patient is conscious and alert.

COMMON
Mild dizziness, diarrhea, frequent or unusual hunger, nausea, heartburn, itching, changes in taste, constipation, fluid retention, rash.

LESS COMMON
Fatigue, heightened skin sensitivity to light, yellowish tinge to skin and eyes, ringing in the ears.

CHLORTHALIDONE

Available in: Tablets
Available OTC? No   **As Generic?** Yes
Drug Class: Thiazide-like diuretic

▼ USAGE INFORMATION

WHY IT'S PRESCRIBED
To treat high blood pressure and conditions that cause edema (swelling of body tissues resulting from excess salt and water retention).

HOW IT WORKS
Diuretics increase the excretion of salt and water in the urine. By reducing the overall fluid volume in the body, these drugs reduce blood volume and so reduce pressure within the blood vessels.

▼ DOSAGE GUIDELINES

RANGE AND FREQUENCY
Adults: 25 to 100 mg once a day or every other day.

ONSET OF EFFECT
2 to 3 hours.

DURATION OF ACTION
2 to 3 days.

DIETARY ADVICE
Take it with food to avoid stomach upset.

STORAGE
Store in a tightly sealed container away from heat, moisture, and direct light.

MISSED DOSE
Take it as soon as you remember. However, if it is near the time for the next dose, skip the missed dose and resume your regular dosage schedule. Do not double the next dose.

STOPPING THE DRUG
Unless directed otherwise by your doctor, take this medication as prescribed for the full treatment period, even if you begin to feel better before the scheduled end of therapy.

PROLONGED USE
See your doctor regularly for examinations and tests, if you must take this medicine for an extended period.

▼ PRECAUTIONS

Over 60: Adverse reactions may be more likely and severe in older patients.

Driving and Hazardous Work: No special precautions are warranted.

Alcohol: Avoid alcohol while taking this drug.

Pregnancy: This medicine should not be taken during pregnancy unless recommended by your doctor.

Breast Feeding: Chlorthalidone passes into breast milk; avoid or discontinue use while nursing.

Infants and Children: Although chlorthalidone is rarely prescribed for children, no unusual side effects are expected. The dose must be determined by a pediatrician.

Special Concerns: Chlorthalidone is usually taken once a day. To prevent it from interfering with sleep, take it in the morning. If you are taking chlorthalidone for high blood pressure, follow the diet and weight control measures recommended by your doctor. Avoid exposure to sunlight, use a sunblock, or wear protective clothing. This medicine may cause your body to lose potassium. Follow your doctor's instructions about eating potassium-rich foods or taking a potassium supplement.

OVERDOSE
Symptoms: Fainting, lethargy, dizziness, drowsiness, confusion, gastrointestinal irritation.

What to Do: Call your doctor, emergency medical services (EMS), or the nearest poison control center immediately.

▼ INTERACTIONS

DRUG INTERACTIONS
Consult your doctor for specific advice if you are taking anticoagulants, cholestyramine, colestipol, drugs for diabetes, nonsteroidal anti-inflammatory drugs, digitalis drugs, or lithium.

FOOD INTERACTIONS
No significant food interactions have been reported.

DISEASE INTERACTIONS
Caution is advised when taking chlorthalidone. Consult your doctor if you have any of the following: diabetes mellitus, gout, lupus erythematosus, pancreatitis, diabetes, heart disease, blood vessel disease, liver disease, or kidney disease.

SIDE EFFECTS

SERIOUS
Skin rash, hives, intense itching, swelling of the mouth and throat, breathing difficulty, serious heartbeat irregularities or palpitations, lightheadedness or dizziness, unusual bleeding or bruising. Call your doctor immediately.

COMMON
Potassium depletion may lead to heart palpitations and weakness. Fluid depletion may lead to dizziness, especially upon arising from a sitting or lying position.

LESS COMMON
Decreased sexual ability, increased sensitivity to sunlight, loss of appetite, gout, increased blood sugar (a problem for patients with diabetes).

CHLORZOXAZONE

Available in: Caplets, tablets
Available OTC? No   **As Generic?** Yes
Drug Class: Muscle relaxant

▼ USAGE INFORMATION

WHY IT'S PRESCRIBED
Muscle relaxants are used to relieve stiffness and discomfort caused by severe sprains and strains, muscle spasms, or other muscle problems. They may be prescribed in conjunction with other treatment methods, such as physical therapy.

HOW IT WORKS
Muscle relaxants such as chlorzoxazone depress activity in the central nervous system, which in turn interferes with the transmission of nerve impulses from the spinal cord to the skeletal muscles.

▼ DOSAGE GUIDELINES

RANGE AND FREQUENCY
Adults: 250 to 750 mg, 3 or 4 times a day. The dosage can be reduced as improvement occurs.

ONSET OF EFFECT
15 to 30 minutes.

DURATION OF ACTION
Up to 4 hours.

DIETARY ADVICE
Take it with meals to lessen stomach upset. Be sure to eat a well-balanced diet; the healing of injured tissue increases the body's protein and calorie requirements. To avoid dry mouth, maintain adequate fluid intake and suck on ice chips if desired.

STORAGE
Store in a tightly sealed container away from heat, moisture, and direct light.

MISSED DOSE
Take it as soon as you remember. If it is near the time for the next dose, skip the missed dose and resume your regular dosage schedule. Do not double the next dose.

STOPPING THE DRUG
The decision to stop taking the drug should be made by your doctor. Gradual reduction of the dose may be necessary if you have taken the drug for a long time.

PROLONGED USE
Adult use should generally be limited to 10 days. Consult your doctor about the need for follow-up medical examinations or laboratory studies. Periodic liver tests are recommended during therapy.

▼ PRECAUTIONS

Over 60: Adverse reactions may be more likely and more severe in older patients.

Driving and Hazardous Work: Do not drive or engage in hazardous work until you determine how the medicine affects you.

Alcohol: Avoid alcohol while taking this drug because it may compound the sedative effect and may cause liver damage.

Pregnancy: Before taking chlorzoxazone, be sure to tell your doctor if you are pregnant or are planning to become pregnant.

Breast Feeding: Chlorzoxazone passes into breast milk; avoid or discontinue use while nursing.

Infants and Children: Not recommended for use by children under age 12.

Special Concerns: If your symptoms do not improve after 2 days of use, call your doctor. Use of chlorzoxazone should be accompanied by bed rest, physical therapy, and other measures to relieve discomfort. Do not take this drug if you are allergic to any skeletal muscle relaxant.

OVERDOSE
Symptoms: Nausea, vomiting, diarrhea, loss of appetite, headache, severe weakness, unusual increase in sweating, fainting, breathing difficulties, irritability, convulsions, feeling of paralysis, loss of consciousness.

What to Do: An overdose of chlorzoxazone is unlikely to be life-threatening, However, if someone takes a much larger dose than prescribed, seek medical assistance immediately.

▼ INTERACTIONS

DRUG INTERACTIONS
Tell your doctor if you are taking oral anticoagulant drugs, antidepressants, antihistamines, clozapine, dronabinol, any mind-altering medication, MAO inhibitors, other muscle relaxants, any narcotic, phenobarbital, sertraline, sleeping pills, or a tetracycline antibiotic.

FOOD INTERACTIONS
No known food interactions.

DISEASE INTERACTIONS
Use of this drug may cause complications in patients with liver or kidney disease, since these organs work together to remove the medication from the body.

≡ SIDE EFFECTS ≡

SERIOUS
Fainting; palpitations or rapid heartbeat; fever; hives or severe swelling of face, lips, or tongue along with shortness of breath, chest tightness, or wheezing (indicating a potentially life-threatening allergic reaction); mental depression; temporary loss of vision. Call your doctor right away.

COMMON
Drowsiness, dizziness, dry mouth.

LESS COMMON
Bruises, feeling of illness, excitability, stomach upset, discolored urine, bloody or black stools, hiccups.

CHOLESTYRAMINE

Available in: Powder
Available OTC? No   **As Generic?** Yes
Drug Class: Antilipidemic (cholesterol-lowering agent)

▼ USAGE INFORMATION

WHY IT'S PRESCRIBED
To reduce cholesterol in people with high blood levels of low-density lipoprotein (LDL), as part of a comprehensive treatment program that includes exercise and special diet. The drug is also used to relieve itching caused by high levels of bile acids in the blood, a problem associated with blockage of the bile ducts. Cholestyramine may also be used to prevent some types of diarrhea or to serve as an antidote to poisoning from or overdose of digitalis drugs.

HOW IT WORKS
Cholestyramine binds with bile acids in the intestine, forming an insoluble complex that is excreted in the feces. This process reduces the bile acids in the blood. In response to the lower levels of bile acids, the liver converts more cholesterol to bile acids. Consequently, the amount of cholesterol in liver cells declines, and the liver makes more LDL receptors. The resulting increased removal of LDL from the blood lowers LDL cholesterol.

▼ DOSAGE GUIDELINES

RANGE AND FREQUENCY
Initial dose is 4 g, 1 or 2 times a day. Maintenance dose is 8 to 24 g per day in 2 equally divided doses. Always mix the powder thoroughly with appropriate liquid (water or fruit juice; do not use carbonated beverages), and wait 10 to 15 minutes after mixing before drinking. Dosages are increased or decreased according to the individual's response.

ONSET OF EFFECT
Within 1 to 3 weeks.

DURATION OF ACTION
Cholestyramine's effects persist for 2 to 4 weeks after final dose.

DIETARY ADVICE
Follow all special dietary restrictions and guidelines as directed by your doctor.

STORAGE
Store in a tightly sealed container away from heat and direct light. Keep away from moisture.

MISSED DOSE
Take it as soon as you remember. However, if it is near the time for the next dose, skip the missed dose and resume your regular dosage schedule. Do not double the next dose.

STOPPING THE DRUG
The drug may be stopped after 1 to 3 months if the therapeutic effect is not adequate. The decision to stop taking the drug should be made by your doctor.

PROLONGED USE
Cholestyramine may be used safely for years; however, periodic evaluation of its effectiveness is necessary.

▼ PRECAUTIONS

Over 60: Adverse reactions (particularly constipation) are more likely and more severe in older patients.

Driving and Hazardous Work: No special precautions are necessary.

Alcohol: No special precautions are necessary.

Pregnancy: The effects on a fetus are unknown. Consult your doctor if you become or plan to become pregnant.

Breast Feeding: At very high doses cholestyramine may interfere with the absorption of vitamins A, D, E, and K, which may affect the nutritional intake of the nursing infant. Consult your doctor for specific advice.

Infants and Children: Prescribed for children only in rare circumstances. Follow doctor's instructions and dosage guidelines carefully in such cases.

Special Concerns: At very high doses cholestyramine may interfere with the absorption of fats and fat-soluble vitamins (vitamins A, D, E, and K); vitamin supplementation may be advised.

OVERDOSE
Symptoms: None reported.

What to Do: Emergency instructions not applicable.

▼ INTERACTIONS

DRUG INTERACTIONS
Cholestyramine may bind with other drugs and hinder their absorption. Therefore, take all other drugs 1 to 2 hours before or 4 hours after taking cholestyramine.

FOOD INTERACTIONS
No known food interactions.

DISEASE INTERACTIONS
Do not take this drug if you have had a prior allergic reaction to it. Do not take Questran Light if you have phenylketonuria. Use of cholestyramine may make the following conditions worse: gallstones, peptic ulcer, intestinal bleeding disorders, hemorrhoids, malabsorption, constipation.

≡ SIDE EFFECTS ≡

SERIOUS
Severe abdominal pain (a very rare reaction, indicating intestinal obstruction). Stop taking the drug and contact your doctor immediately.

COMMON
Constipation, heartburn, bloating, belching, abdominal discomfort, irritation of the anal area.

LESS COMMON
Hives, rash, gas, diarrhea, nausea, vomiting, gallstones.

CIDOFOVIR INTRAVENOUS

Available in: Intravenous injection
Available OTC? No   **As Generic?** No
Drug Class: Antiviral

▼ USAGE INFORMATION

WHY IT'S PRESCRIBED
To treat cytomegalovirus (CMV) retinitis (an eye infection) or other forms of CMV disease in patients with human immunodeficiency virus (HIV) infection. Cidofovir is given in combination with probenecid, a drug that enhances the effectiveness of antimicrobial medications.

HOW IT WORKS
Cidofovir interferes with the activity of enzymes needed for the replication of DNA in viral cells, thus preventing CMV from reproducing.

▼ DOSAGE GUIDELINES

RANGE AND FREQUENCY
For patients with normal kidney function: Initially, 5 mg per 2.2 lbs (1 kg) of body weight infused intravenously over a period of 60 minutes, once a week, for 2 consecutive weeks. Probenecid is also given at a dose of 2 g, 3 hours before infusion, followed by 1 g, 2 hours later, then again 8 hours later. Maintenance dose of cido-

fovir: 5 mg per kg once every 2 weeks. For patients with impaired kidney function: A reduced dose is necessary, as determined by your doctor.

ONSET OF EFFECT
Unknown.

DURATION OF ACTION
Unknown.

DIETARY ADVICE
Cidofovir can be given without regard to diet. Probenecid should be given after food intake. Drink plenty of fluids.

STORAGE
Not applicable; the dose is administered at a health care facility or by a home nurse.

MISSED DOSE
If you miss a dose for any reason, contact your doctor and arrange to receive treatment as soon as possible.

STOPPING THE DRUG
The decision to stop taking the drug should be made in consultation with your doctor.

PROLONGED USE
See your doctor regularly for tests and examinations if you

must take this medication for a prolonged period. See an ophthalmologist regularly for eye examinations.

▼ PRECAUTIONS

Over 60: Older patients are more likely to have impaired kidney function requiring an adjustment in dosage.

Driving and Hazardous Work: Do not drive or engage in hazardous work until you determine how the medicine affects you.

Alcohol: Avoid alcohol if liver function is impaired.

Pregnancy: Cidofovir has been shown to cause birth defects in animals. Human studies have not been done. This medication should be given during pregnancy only if potential benefits outweigh the risks to the unborn child.

Breast Feeding: It is unknown whether cidofovir passes into breast milk; however, women infected with HIV should not nurse, to avoid transmitting the virus to an uninfected child.

Infants and Children: The safety and effectiveness of cidofovir in children under 18 have not been established.

Special Concerns: The risk of severe nausea when probenecid is given can be reduced by taking an anti-nausea medication, such as diphenhydramine hydrochloride.

OVERDOSE
Symptoms: No cases of overdose have been reported.

What to Do: An overdose of cidofovir is unlikely to occur. Nonetheless, if you have any reason to suspect an overdose, call your physician, emergency medical services (EMS), or the nearest poison control center immediately.

▼ INTERACTIONS

DRUG INTERACTIONS
Other drugs may interact with cidofovir. Consult your doctor for specific advice if you are taking any other drug that can cause kidney damage, such as aminoglycosides, amphotericin B, foscarnet, nonsteroidal anti-inflammatory drugs, pentamidine, vancomycin, and zidovudine. A seven-day waiting period after use of such drugs is recommended before beginning therapy with cidofovir.

FOOD INTERACTIONS
No known food interactions, but side effects of probenecid are decreased when it is taken with food.

DISEASE INTERACTIONS
Consult your doctor if you have any condition that impairs kidney function.

  SIDE EFFECTS

SERIOUS
Kidney damage, causing decreased or increased urination, thirst, and shortness of breath. Impaired vision or other changes in vision may also develop. If such symptoms occur, call your doctor right away.

COMMON
Probenecid, which is given with cidofovir, may cause fever, chills, headache, rash, nausea, or vomiting.

LESS COMMON
Persistent weakness and fatigue or general loss of strength.

CILOSTAZOL

Available in: Tablets
Available OTC? No   **As Generic?** No
Drug Class: Phosphodiesterase type 3 inhibitor

▼ USAGE INFORMATION

WHY IT'S PRESCRIBED
To reduce symptoms of intermittent claudication (leg pain that is induced by walking and subsides after rest).

HOW IT WORKS
Intermittent claudication results from impaired blood supply to the legs. Although its precise mechanism of action is not clear, cilostazol appears to improve circulation by dilating blood vessels, especially those supplying the legs. Cilostazol also appears to inhibit the aggregation (clumping) of platelets and this reduces the formation of blood clots which can block arterial blood flow.

▼ DOSAGE GUIDELINES

RANGE AND FREQUENCY
100 mg 2 times a day.

ONSET OF EFFECT
From 2 to 12 weeks.

DURATION OF ACTION
Unknown.

DIETARY ADVICE
Take on an empty stomach at least 30 minutes before or 2 hours after a meal.

STORAGE
Store in a tightly sealed container away from heat, moisture, and direct light.

MISSED DOSE
Take it as soon as you remember. If it is near the time for the next dose, skip the missed dose and resume your regular dosage schedule. Do not double the next dose.

STOPPING THE DRUG
The decision to stop taking the drug should be made in consultation with your physician.

PROLONGED USE
The safety and effectiveness of cilostazol have not been determined beyond 24 weeks of use.

▼ PRECAUTIONS

Over 60: No special problems are expected.

Driving and Hazardous Work: Use caution when driving or engaging in hazardous work until you determine how the medicine affects you.

Alcohol: No special precautions are necessary.

Pregnancy: Adequate human studies have not been done. Before taking cilostazol, tell your doctor if you are pregnant or plan to become pregnant.

Breast Feeding: Cilostazol may pass into breast milk; caution is advised. Consult your doctor for advice on whether to discontinue nursing or discontinue the drug.

Infants and Children: Safety and effectiveness have not been established for children under age 18.

OVERDOSE
Symptoms: Few cases of overdose have been reported. However, if you take a much larger dose than prescribed, you may experience severe headache, diarrhea, dizziness or fainting, and heartbeat irregularities.

What to Do: Call your doctor, emergency medical services (EMS), or the nearest poison control center immediately.

▼ INTERACTIONS

DRUG INTERACTIONS
The following drugs may interact with cilostazol. Consult your doctor for advice if you are taking ketoconazole, itraconazole, fluconazole, miconazole, fluvoxamine, fluoxetine, nefazodone, sertraline, erythromycin and other macrolide antibiotics, omeprazole, diltiazem, or clopidogrel.

FOOD INTERACTIONS
Do not take cilostazol with grapefruit juice.

DISEASE INTERACTIONS
Do not take cilostazol if you have congestive heart failure of any severity.

▼ SIDE EFFECTS

SERIOUS
No serious side effects have been reported.

COMMON
Headache, heart palpitations, diarrhea, increased risk of infection.

LESS COMMON
Rapid heartbeat, abdominal pain, indigestion, flatulence, nausea, swelling of the extremities, dizziness, sore throat, runny nose.

CIMETIDINE

BRAND NAMES

Tagamet, Tagamet HB, Tagamet HB 200

Available in: Tablets, oral solution, oral suspension
Available OTC? Yes   **As Generic?** Yes
Drug Class: Histamine (H2) blocker

▼ USAGE INFORMATION

WHY IT'S PRESCRIBED
To treat ulcers of the stomach and duodenum, as well as other conditions, such as esophagitis (chronic inflammation of the esophagus), and gastroesophageal reflux (backwash of stomach acid into the esophagus, resulting in heartburn).

HOW IT WORKS
Cimetidine blocks the action of histamine (a compound produced in the body's cells), which in turn decreases the stomach's secretion of hydrochloric acid. Once stomach acid production is decreased, the body is better able to heal itself.

▼ DOSAGE GUIDELINES

RANGE AND FREQUENCY
For treatment of acute (symptomatic, bothersome) duodenal or gastric ulcers— Adults and teenagers: Various dosage schedules are used, including 300 mg, 4 times a day, with meals and at bedtime; 400 or 600 mg, 2 times a day; or 800 mg taken once daily at bedtime. For prevention of duodenal ulcers— Adults and teenagers: Usual dose is 300 mg, 2 times a day; another common dosage schedule is 400 mg taken once daily at bedtime. For treatment as needed of heartburn and acid indigestion— Adults and teenagers: 200 mg with water when symptoms start; another 200 mg may be taken within the next 24 hours, for a maximum of 400 mg in a 24-hour period. For treatment of gastroesophageal reflux disease— Adults: 800 to 1,600 mg a day, in 2 to 4 divided doses, for approximately 12 weeks.

ONSET OF EFFECT
Within 1 hour.

DURATION OF ACTION
At least 4 to 5 hours.

DIETARY ADVICE
Avoid foods that cause stomach irritation.

STORAGE
Store away from heat and direct light. Keep the liquid form from freezing.

MISSED DOSE
Take it as soon as you remember. If it is near the time for the next dose, skip the missed dose and resume your regular dosage schedule. Do not double the next dose.

STOPPING THE DRUG
Prescription-strength: Take it for the full treatment period, even if you begin to feel better before the scheduled end of therapy. Nonprescription-strength: Take as needed.

PROLONGED USE
Do not take nonprescription-strength cimetidine for more than 2 weeks unless told to do so by your physician.

▼ PRECAUTIONS

Over 60: Adverse reactions may be more likely and more severe in older patients.

Driving and Hazardous Work: Do not drive or engage in hazardous work until you determine how the medicine affects you.

Alcohol: Avoid alcohol.

Pregnancy: Avoid or discontinue use if you are pregnant or trying to become pregnant.

Breast Feeding: Cimetidine passes into breast milk; avoid or discontinue use while breast feeding.

Infants and Children: Not recommended for use by children under age 16.

Special Concerns: Avoid cigarette smoking because it may increase stomach acid secretion and thus worsen the disease. Do not take cimetidine if you have ever had an allergic reaction to a histamine (H2) blocker. If stomach pain becomes worse while you are using the drug, tell your doctor right away.

OVERDOSE
Symptoms: No symptoms have been reported.

What to Do: An overdose is unlikely to be life-threatening. However, if someone takes a much larger dose than directed, seek medical assistance right away.

▼ INTERACTIONS

DRUG INTERACTIONS
Consult your doctor for specific advice if you are taking aminophylline, anticoagulants, caffeine, metoprolol, oxtriphylline, phenytoin, propranolol, theophylline, tricyclic antidepressants, itraconazole, ketoconazole, metronidazole.

FOOD INTERACTIONS
Carbonated drinks, citrus fruits and juices, caffeine-containing beverages, and other acidic foods or liquids may irritate the stomach or interfere with the therapeutic action of cimetidine.

DISEASE INTERACTIONS
Patients with kidney or liver disease or weakened immune systems should not use cimetidine or should use it in smaller, limited doses under careful medical supervision.

SIDE EFFECTS

SERIOUS
Irregular heart rhythm (palpitations), slowed heartbeat, severe blood problems resulting in unusual bleeding, bruising, fever, chills, and increased susceptibility to infection. Call your doctor immediately.

COMMON
Headache, fatigue, drowsiness, dizziness, nausea, vomiting, abdominal pain, diarrhea.

LESS COMMON
Blurred vision, decreased sexual desire or function, swelling of breasts in males or females, temporary hair loss, hallucinations, depression, insomnia, skin rash, hives, or redness.

CIPROFLOXACIN OPHTHALMIC

Available in: Ophthalmic solution
Available OTC? No   **As Generic?** No
Drug Class: Fluoroquinolone antibiotic

▼ USAGE INFORMATION

WHY IT'S PRESCRIBED
To treat or prevent bacterial infections of the eye, such as conjunctivitis or keratitis (infection of the cornea). Often used to prevent infection while a corneal abrasion is healing.

HOW IT WORKS
Ciprofloxacin interferes with the action of certain enzymes necessary for bacteria to grow and multiply.

▼ DOSAGE GUIDELINES

RANGE AND FREQUENCY
Exact dosing depends on the nature of the infection and its response to treatment. Follow your doctor's instructions precisely. The following is an example of a typical dose for conjunctivitis. Adults and teenagers: 1 drop in eye every 2 hours for 2 days, then 1 drop every 4 hours for the next 5 days (administer during waking hours only).

ONSET OF EFFECT
Unknown.

DURATION OF ACTION
Unknown.

DIETARY ADVICE
No special restrictions.

STORAGE
Store in a tightly sealed container away from heat, moisture, and direct light. Do not refrigerate or allow the solution to freeze.

MISSED DOSE
Apply it as soon as you remember. If it is near the time for the next dose, skip the missed dose and resume your regular dosage schedule. Do not double the next dose.

STOPPING THE DRUG
Use this drug as prescribed for the full treatment period, even if you begin to feel better before the scheduled end of therapy.

PROLONGED USE
Prolonged use, as directed by your doctor, may be necessary for severe cases of infection. See your doctor regularly for tests and examinations if you take this drug for a prolonged period.

≡ SIDE EFFECTS ≡

SERIOUS
Nausea, blurry or decreased vision, skin rash, severe irritation or redness of the eye. Stop using the drug and call your doctor immediately.

COMMON
Burning or crusting in the eye or eyelid.

LESS COMMON
Redness of the edge of the eyelids, bad taste in mouth, tearing or itching of the eye, swelling of the eyelid, sensation of a foreign body in the eye, increased sensitivity of eyes to bright light.

▼ PRECAUTIONS

Over 60: Adverse reactions may be more likely and more severe in older patients.

Driving and Hazardous Work: Do not drive or engage in hazardous work until you determine how the medicine affects your vision.

Alcohol: No special precautions are necessary.

Pregnancy: Adequate human studies have not been done. Before taking ophthalmic ciprofloxacin, tell your doctor if you are pregnant or plan to become pregnant.

Breast Feeding: Ophthalmic ciprofloxacin may pass into breast milk; caution is advised. Ciprofloxacin taken orally has been found in trace amounts in breast milk. Consult your doctor for advice.

Infants and Children: This medication is not recommended for use by children under the age of 12.

Special Concerns: To use the eye drops, first wash your hands. Tilt your head back. Gently apply pressure to the inside corner of the eyelid and with the index finger of the same hand, pull downward on the lower eyelid to make a space. Drop the medicine into this space and close your eye. Apply pressure for 1 or 2 minutes while keeping the eye closed without blinking. Then wash your hands again. Make sure the tip of the dropper does not touch your eye, finger, or any other surface. If your symptoms do not improve or if they become worse, check with your doctor. You should not share your medication, towels, or washcloths with other people. Call your doctor if anyone else close to you develops similar symptoms.

OVERDOSE
Symptoms: No specific ones have been reported.

What to Do: An overdose of ophthalmic ciprofloxacin is unlikely to be life-threatening. However, if someone takes a much larger dose of the drug than prescribed or accidentally ingests the medicine, seek medical assistance right away.

▼ INTERACTIONS

DRUG INTERACTIONS
Other drugs may interact with ophthalmic ciprofloxacin. Consult your doctor for specific advice if you are taking any other prescription or over-the-counter medication.

FOOD INTERACTIONS
No known food interactions.

DISEASE INTERACTIONS
Caution is advised when taking ophthalmic ciprofloxacin. Consult your doctor if you have ever had an allergic reaction to ciprofloxacin or other fluoroquinolone antibiotics.

CIPROFLOXACIN SYSTEMIC

Available in: Tablets, oral suspension
Available OTC? No   **As Generic?** No
Drug Class: Fluoroquinolone antibiotic

▼ USAGE INFORMATION

WHY IT'S PRESCRIBED
To treat mild to severe bacterial infections, including those of the urinary tract, lower respiratory tract, bones and joints, and the skin. It is also used to treat certain sexually transmitted diseases (such as chancroid and gonorrhea), and diarrhea caused by bacterial infection.

HOW IT WORKS
Ciprofloxacin inhibits the activity of a bacterial enzyme (gyrase) that is necessary for proper DNA formation and replication. This fights infection by preventing bacteria cells from reproducing.

▼ DOSAGE GUIDELINES

RANGE AND FREQUENCY
250 to 750 mg every 12 hours (2 times a day), for 5 to 14 days, depending on kidney function and the infection being treated. Gonorrhea is usually treated with a one-time dose of 250 mg.

ONSET OF EFFECT
Varies depending on the infection being treated.

DURATION OF ACTION
Unknown.

DIETARY ADVICE
Be sure to drink plenty of fluids, but avoid milk and dairy derivatives.

STORAGE
Store in a tightly sealed container away from heat and direct light.

MISSED DOSE
Take it as soon as you remember. If it is near the time for the next dose, skip the missed dose and resume your regular dosage schedule. Do not double the next dose.

STOPPING THE DRUG
Take it as prescribed for the full treatment period, even if you begin to feel better before the scheduled end of therapy.

PROLONGED USE
See your doctor regularly for tests and examinations if you must take this medicine for a prolonged period.

▼ PRECAUTIONS

Over 60: No special problems are expected.

Driving and Hazardous Work: Do not drive or engage in hazardous work until you determine how the medicine affects you.

Alcohol: It is advisable to abstain from alcohol when fighting an infection.

Pregnancy: In some animal tests, ciprofloxacin has caused birth defects. Adequate studies in humans have not been done. It should be used during pregnancy only if potential benefits clearly justify the risks. Before you take ciprofloxacin, tell your doctor if you are pregnant or plan to become pregnant.

Breast Feeding: Ciprofloxacin passes into breast milk and may cause serious side effects in the nursing infant; use of the drug is discouraged when nursing.

Infants and Children: Ciprofloxacin is not recommended for use by persons under the age of 18, as it has been shown to interfere with bone development.

Special Concerns: If ciprofloxacin causes sensitivity to sunlight, stop taking the drug and try to avoid exposure to sunlight for the next 5 days; also wear protective clothing and use a sunblock. Ciprofloxacin should not be taken by patients whose work makes it impossible to avoid exposure to sunlight. It is important to drink plenty of fluids while taking this drug.

OVERDOSE
Symptoms: No specific ones have been reported.

What to Do: If you have any reason to suspect an overdose, call your doctor, emergency medical services (EMS), or the nearest poison control center.

▼ INTERACTIONS

DRUG INTERACTIONS
Consult your doctor for specific advice if you are taking aminophylline, antacids, didanosine, iron supplements, oxtriphylline, sucralfate, theophylline, warfarin, or zinc salts. Also tell your doctor if you are taking any other prescription or over-the-counter medication.

FOOD INTERACTIONS
The effects of caffeine may be magnified by this drug. Milk and dairy products can reduce blood levels of ciprofloxacin by as much as half.

DISEASE INTERACTIONS
Caution is advised when taking ciprofloxacin. Consult your doctor if you have any other medical condition. Use of ciprofloxacin can cause complications in patients with kidney disease, since this organ works to remove the medication from the body.

≡ SIDE EFFECTS ≡

SERIOUS
Serious reactions to ciprofloxacin are rare and include seizures, mental confusion, hallucinations, agitation, nightmares, depression, shortness of breath, unusual swelling in the face or extremities, and loss of consciousness. Also skin burning, redness, blisters, rash, or itching on exposure to sunlight. Call your doctor immediately.

COMMON
Increased sensitivity to sunlight (and increased risk of sunburn) for days following therapy.

LESS COMMON
Diarrhea, nausea and vomiting, stomach pain and upset, gas, headache, dizziness, insomnia, changes in taste perception, drowsiness, itching, dry mouth, unusual body aches or pains.

CISAPRIDE

BRAND NAMES

Propulsid, Propulsid
Quicksolv

Available in: Tablets, oral suspension
Available OTC? No   **As Generic?** No
Drug Class: Cholinergic (gastrointestinal stimulant)

▼ USAGE INFORMATION

WHY IT'S PRESCRIBED
To prevent and treat gastro-esophageal reflux disease—chronic heartburn caused by the backwash of stomach acid into the esophagus. Cisapride is also used to treat esophagitis (inflammation of the esophagus), dyspepsia (indigestion), and irritable bowel syndrome. Note: The FDA and the manufacturer of this drug jointly decided to remove it from the market due to safety concerns. It will be remain available to a select group of people that is to be determined by the manufacturer and the FDA. If you currently use this drug, do not stop taking it. You should however consult your doctor about alternative medications as soon as possible.

HOW IT WORKS
Cisapride accelerates the movement of liquids and solids through the digestive tract by stimulating the body's release of acetylcholine, which increases rhythmic contractions and digestive activity of the lower esophagus, stomach, and intestines.

▼ DOSAGE GUIDELINES

RANGE AND FREQUENCY
Your doctor will determine the proper dose.

ONSET OF EFFECT
Within 30 to 60 minutes.

DURATION OF ACTION
From 7 to 10 hours.

DIETARY ADVICE
Eat foods that are high in dietary fiber and be sure to consume plenty of fluids to avoid constipation.

STORAGE
Store in a tightly sealed container away from heat and direct light.

MISSED DOSE
Take the missed dose as soon as possible. However, if it is near the time for the next dose, skip the missed dose and resume your regular dosage schedule. Do not double the next dose.

STOPPING THE DRUG
Take it as prescribed for the full treatment period.

PROLONGED USE
Periodic evaluation by your physician is necessary.

▼ PRECAUTIONS

Over 60: Adverse reactions may be more likely and more severe in older patients.

Driving and Hazardous Work: The use of cisapride may make you drowsy. Do not drive or engage in hazardous work until you determine how this medication affects you.

Alcohol: Avoid alcohol while taking this drug, or consult your doctor for guidelines.

Pregnancy: If you are pregnant or planning to become pregnant, discuss with your physician whether the medication's benefits outweigh potential risks.

Breast Feeding: Cisapride passes into breast milk, although it is unknown if this poses any risks. Consult your doctor for specific advice.

Infants and Children: Safety and effectiveness have not been established for patients under 18 years of age. Consult your doctor for advice.

Special Concerns: This drug should not be used by patients taking certain medications (see Drug Interactions), since combining such drugs with cisapride has been shown to cause serious heart rhythm disturbances that can be fatal.

OVERDOSE
Symptoms: Retching; rumbling and gurgling noises from stomach; frequent urination or bowel movements; excess gas.

What to Do: If someone takes a much larger dose than prescribed call your doctor, emergency medical services (EMS), or the nearest poison control right away.

▼ INTERACTIONS

DRUG INTERACTIONS
Do not use cisapride if you are also taking antifungal drugs (such as ketoconazole), antibiotics (such as erythromycin), antiarrhythmics, antipsychotics, tetracyclic or tricyclic antidepressants, indinavir, ritonavir, or astemizole.

FOOD INTERACTIONS
Do not take cisapride with grapefruit juice.

DISEASE INTERACTIONS
Cisapride should not be taken if you have a history of any kind of heart problem, including congestive heart failure, ventricular arrhythmias, coronary artery disease, ischemic heart disease, clinically significant bradycardia, or prolonged QT intervals on your electrocardiogram; kidney failure; uncorrected electrolyte disturbances (such as hypokalemia and hypomagnesemia); respiratory failure; blockage, bleeding, or perforation of the gastrointestinal tract; or if you have had a prior allergic reaction to the drug.

▤ SIDE EFFECTS ▤

SERIOUS
Heart rhythm irregularities may occur. In rare cases seizures may occur when using cisapride in patients with a history of seizure disorders. Contact your doctor immediately if you experience either of these effects.

COMMON
Diarrhea (more likely with higher doses).

LESS COMMON
Abdominal cramps, headache, constipation, nausea, bloating, drowsiness. If such symptoms persist or interfere with daily activities, contact your doctor.

CITALOPRAM HYDROBROMIDE

Available in: Tablet, oral solution
Available OTC? No   **As Generic?** No
Drug Class: Selective serotonin reuptake inhibitor (SSRI) antidepressant

▼ USAGE INFORMATION

WHY IT'S PRESCRIBED
To treat symptoms of major depression.

HOW IT WORKS
Citalopram increases brain levels of serotonin, a chemical that is thought to be linked to mood, emotions, and mental state.

▼ DOSAGE GUIDELINES

RANGE AND FREQUENCY
To start, 20 mg once a day, taken in the morning or evening; dose may be gradually increased by your doctor to 40 mg a day.

ONSET OF EFFECT
Unknown.

DURATION OF ACTION
Unknown.

DIETARY ADVICE
No special restrictions.

STORAGE
Store in a tightly sealed container away from heat, moisture, and direct light.

MISSED DOSE
If you miss a dose on one day, do not double the dose the next day.

STOPPING THE DRUG
Take it as prescribed for the full treatment period even if you notice improvement. When it is time to stop therapy, your dosage will be tapered gradually by your doctor.

PROLONGED USE
Usual course of therapy for depression lasts 6 months to 1 year; some patients may benefit from additional therapy.

▼ PRECAUTIONS

Over 60:
Adverse reactions may be more likely and more severe in older patients. A lower dose may be warranted.

Driving and Hazardous Work:
Use caution when driving or engaging in hazardous work until you determine how the medicine affects you.

Alcohol:
Avoid alcohol.

Pregnancy:
Citalopram should be used during pregnancy only if the potential benefit justifies the potential risk to the fetus. Before you take this medicine, tell your doctor if you are pregnant or plan to become pregnant.

Breast Feeding:
Citalopram passes into breast milk; caution is advised. Consult your doctor for specific advice.

Infants and Children:
The safety and effectiveness of the use of citalopram in children under age 18 have not been established.

OVERDOSE
Symptoms: Dizziness, sweating, nausea, vomiting, trembling, drowsiness, rapid heartbeat.

What to Do: Call your doctor, emergency medical services (EMS), or the nearest poison control center immediately.

▼ INTERACTIONS

DRUG INTERACTIONS
Citalopram and MAO inhibitors should not be used within 14 days of each other. Very serious side effects, such as myoclonus (uncontrolled muscle spasms), hyperthermia (excessive rise in body temperature), and extreme stiffness may result. The following drugs may also interact with citalopram; consult your doctor if you are taking cimetidine, warfarin, lithium, carbamazepine, antifungals (such as ketoconazole, itraconazole, and fluconazole), erythromycin antibiotics, omeprazole, tricyclic antidepressants, or any prescription or over-the-counter drugs that depress the central nervous system (including antihistamines, barbiturates, sedatives, cough medicines, and decongestants).

FOOD INTERACTIONS
No known food interactions.

DISEASE INTERACTIONS
Caution is advised when taking citalopram, especially if you have heart disease or a seizure disorder. Use of citalopram may cause complications in patients with liver or kidney disease.

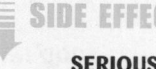

≡ SIDE EFFECTS ≡

SERIOUS
Chest pain, rapid or irregular heartbeat, lightheadedness or fainting. Call your doctor immediately.

COMMON
Delayed ejaculation (males), dry mouth, increased sweating, nausea, trembling, diarrhea, drowsiness, numbness, tingling, or prickling sensations.

LESS COMMON
Fatigue, fever, loss of appetite, agitation, nasal congestion, sinus infection, erectile dysfunction.

CLARITHROMYCIN

Available in: Tablets, oral suspension
Available OTC? No **As Generic?** No
Drug Class: Macrolide antibiotic

▼ USAGE INFORMATION

WHY IT'S PRESCRIBED
To treat various bacterial infections, including those of the sinuses, tonsils, and respiratory tract (such as bronchitis and pneumonia); ear infections; and venereal disease due to chlamydial infection. Clarithromycin may also be used to treat certain skin infections, Legionnaires' disease, Lyme disease, and peptic ulcers caused by the bacterium Helicobacter pylori. Also used to prevent and, when taken with other drugs, treat a tuberculosis-like disease known as Mycobacterium avium complex (MAC), which is common in people with advanced acquired immunodeficiency syndrome (AIDS).

HOW IT WORKS
Clarithromycin prevents bacterial cells from manufacturing specific proteins necessary for their survival.

▼ DOSAGE GUIDELINES

RANGE AND FREQUENCY
For bacterial infections— Usual adult dose: 250 to 500 mg every 12 hours, for 7 to 14 days. Children 6 months of age or older: 3.4 mg per lb of body weight, up to 500 mg every 12 hours for 10 days. To prevent MAC— 500 mg, 2 times a day. To treat MAC— 500 mg, 2 times a day in combination with other drugs.

ONSET OF EFFECT
Within 2 hours; full effect may occur in 2 to 5 days.

DURATION OF ACTION
Unknown.

DIETARY ADVICE
Clarithromycin may be taken with or without food. Drink plenty of liquids.

STORAGE
Store in a tightly sealed container away from heat, moisture, and direct light.

MISSED DOSE
Take it as soon as you remember. If it is near the time for the next dose, skip the missed dose and resume your regular dosing schedule. Do not double the next dose. If you are taking 2 doses a day, wait 5 to 6 hours before taking the next dose.

STOPPING THE DRUG
For acute infections, take it exactly as prescribed for the full treatment period, even if you feel better before the scheduled end of therapy. Therapy for prevention of MAC should be lifelong.

PROLONGED USE
You may become susceptible to infections caused by germs that are not responsive to clarithromycin. Also, severe drug-induced gastrointestinal problems may result from long-term use.

▼ PRECAUTIONS

Over 60: Older patients, especially those with kidney disease, may require a decrease in dose.

Driving and Hazardous Work: No special precautions are necessary.

Alcohol: No special precautions are necessary.

Pregnancy: Adequate studies of the use of this drug during pregnancy have not been done; discuss potential risks and benefits with your doctor.

Breast Feeding: It is not known if clarithromycin passes into breast milk; consult your doctor for advice.

Infants and Children: No special problems are expected.

OVERDOSE
Symptoms: Severe nausea, vomiting, diarrhea, abdominal discomfort.

What to Do: Call your doctor, emergency medical services (EMS), or the nearest poison control center immediately.

▼ INTERACTIONS

DRUG INTERACTIONS
This drug should not be taken by patients known to have had prior allergic reactions to erythromycins or other macrolide antibiotics. Do not take clarithromycin if you are taking astemizole, pimozide, or cisapride. Also, alert your doctor if you are taking any of the following drugs: carbamazepine, digoxin, theophylline, warfarin, rifabutin, rifampin, or zidovudine.

FOOD INTERACTIONS
No known food interactions.

DISEASE INTERACTIONS
Consult your doctor if you have a history of a blood disorder, liver disease, or any allergy.

≡ SIDE EFFECTS ≡

SERIOUS
Colitis (inflammation of the lower gastrointestinal tract, with symptoms including severe abdominal pain, watery or bloody stools, severe diarrhea, fever); liver toxicity (causing fever, nausea, vomiting, yellowish tinge to eyes or skin); allergic reaction (swelling of the lips, tongue, face, and throat, breathing difficulty, skin rash or hives); blood clotting disorders (causing unusual bleeding and bruising); confusion or change in behavior; heartbeat irregularities in patients with predisposing heart conditions. Such side effects are rare, but if they do occur, stop taking the drug and seek medical assistance immediately.

COMMON
No common side effects.

LESS COMMON
Changes in taste perception; mild abdominal pain or discomfort; mild diarrhea; mild nausea or vomiting; headache; oral thrush (fungal infections of the mouth or throat).

CLEMASTINE FUMARATE

Available in: Tablets, syrup, extended-release tablets and caplets
Available OTC? Yes   **As Generic?** Yes
Drug Class: Antihistamine

▼ USAGE INFORMATION

WHY IT'S PRESCRIBED
To prevent or relieve symptoms of hay fever and other allergies, and for itching skin and hives.

HOW IT WORKS
Clemastine blocks the effects of histamine, a naturally occurring substance within the body that causes swelling, itching, sneezing, watery eyes, hives, and other symptoms of allergic reactions.

▼ DOSAGE GUIDELINES

RANGE AND FREQUENCY
Adults and teenagers: 1.34 mg, 2 times a day (for hay fever), or 2.68 mg, 1 to 3 times a day (for hay fever or hives). Children ages 6 to 12: 0.67 mg (syrup) to 1.34 mg, 2 times a day.

ONSET OF EFFECT
15 minutes to 60 minutes.

DURATION OF ACTION
At least 12 hours.

DIETARY ADVICE
Take it with food, water, or milk to avoid stomach irritation. Drinking coffee or tea will help reduce drowsiness. Use sugarless gum, sugarless sour hard candy, or ice chips to ease dry mouth.

STORAGE
Store in a tightly sealed container away from heat and direct light.

MISSED DOSE
Take it as soon as you remember. If it is near the time for the next dose, skip the missed dose and resume your regular dosage schedule. Do not double the next dose.

STOPPING THE DRUG
You should take it as prescribed for the full treatment period, but you may stop if you are feeling better before the scheduled end of therapy. It may be taken as needed.

PROLONGED USE
No special problems are expected.

▼ PRECAUTIONS

Over 60: Adverse reactions may be more likely and more severe in older patients.

Driving and Hazardous Work: The use of clemastine may impair your ability to perform such tasks safely. Do not drive or engage in hazardous work until you determine how the medicine affects you.

Alcohol: Alcohol increases the likelihood and the severity of side effects like drowsiness and confusion.

Pregnancy: Animal studies with high doses of clemastine have found no birth defects. Human studies have not been done. Because the studies cannot rule out potential harm, the drug should be used during pregnancy only if it is clearly needed.

Breast Feeding: Clemastine passes into breast milk; do not use it while nursing.

Infants and Children: Children tend to be more sensitive to the effects of antihistamines. Symptoms of excitability, restlessness, and nightmares may occur.

Special Concerns: Tavist-D, a combination of clemastine fumarate and the decongestant phenylpropanolamine hydrochloride, is available to treat cold and allergy symptoms in adults and teenagers. (See also Phenylpropanolamine Hydrochloride.)

OVERDOSE
Symptoms: Hallucinations, seizures, drowsiness, lethargy, coma.

What to Do: Call your doctor, emergency medical services (EMS), or the nearest poison control center immediately. A conscious patient should be induced to vomit using ipecac syrup.

▼ INTERACTIONS

DRUG INTERACTIONS
Sleeping pills, sedatives, tranquilizers, MAO inhibitors, and antidepressants can increase the sedative effects of clemastine. Anticholinergics may further increase the likelihood that drying of the mucous membranes and urinary obstruction will occur as side effects.

FOOD INTERACTIONS
No known food interactions.

DISEASE INTERACTIONS
Consult your doctor if you have any of the following: asthma, enlarged prostate, difficult urination, glaucoma, sleep apnea, or dry mouth or eyes.

SIDE EFFECTS

SERIOUS
Confusion, hallucinations, convulsions, blurred vision, difficulty urinating (urinary obstruction).

COMMON
Drowsiness; nausea; thickening of mucus; dry mouth, nose, and throat; dizziness; disturbed coordination.

LESS COMMON
Chills, headache, fatigue, vomiting, restlessness, irritability, nasal congestion, profuse sweating, diarrhea, constipation.

CLINDAMYCIN

Available in: Capsules, oral solution, injection, topical forms, vaginal suppositories
Available OTC? No **As Generic?** Yes
Drug Class: Antibiotic

▼ USAGE INFORMATION

WHY IT'S PRESCRIBED
Orally and by injection, clindamycin is used to treat serious bacterial infections. Topically, it is used to treat acne and vaginal infections.

HOW IT WORKS
Clindamycin inhibits the synthesis of protein in bacterial organisms.

▼ DOSAGE GUIDELINES

RANGE AND FREQUENCY
For systemic infections (oral forms)– Adults and teenagers: 150 to 300 mg, 4 times a day. Children 1 month and older: See your pediatrician. For systemic infections (injection)– Your doctor will determine the appropriate dose. For acne (gel, solution, or suspension)– Adults and teenagers: Apply 2 times a day. Use and dose for children under 12 must be determined by your doctor. For vaginal infections (vaginal cream)– Non-pregnant adults and teenagers: 100 mg inserted in vagina once daily at bedtime for 3 or 7 days (7-day therapy is prescribed for pregnant patients). Dose for children must be determined by your doctor. For bacterial vaginal infections (vaginal suppositories)– Nonpregnant adults and teenagers: 1 suppository (containing 100 mg) inserted in vagina once daily at bedtime for 3 days.

ONSET OF EFFECT
Unknown.

DURATION OF ACTION
Unknown.

DIETARY ADVICE
Take the oral forms with food to minimize stomach upset. Take the capsule with water.

STORAGE
Store in a tightly sealed container away from heat, moisture, and direct light. Do not refrigerate the liquid forms, cream, or suppositories.

MISSED DOSE
Take it as soon as you remember. If it is near the time for the next dose, skip the missed dose and resume your regular dosage schedule. Do not double the next dose.

STOPPING THE DRUG
Take it as prescribed for the full treatment period.

PROLONGED USE
See your doctor regularly for tests and examinations if you must take this medicine for a prolonged period.

▼ PRECAUTIONS

Over 60: No special problems are expected.

Driving and Hazardous Work: No special problems are expected.

Alcohol: It is advisable to abstain from alcohol when fighting an infection.

Pregnancy: Consult your doctor before taking it during pregnancy.

Breast Feeding: Clindamycin may pass into breast milk; consult your doctor for specific advice.

Infants and Children: Adequate studies of clindamycin use by children have not been done, although no special problems are expected.

Special Concerns: Wash and dry the skin thoroughly before applying the gel, topical solution, or suspension. When using vaginal cream or suppository, avoid sexual intercourse. Clindamycin may weaken latex or rubber products, such as condoms and vaginal contraceptive diaphragms; use of such products is not recommended within 72 hours of the application of these forms. Do not use other vaginal products, such as tampons or douches, when using the suppositories.

OVERDOSE
Symptoms: None reported.

What to Do: If you have reason to suspect an overdose, call your doctor, emergency medical services (EMS), or the nearest poison control.

▼ INTERACTIONS

DRUG INTERACTIONS
Consult your doctor for advice if you are taking chloramphenicol, erythromycin, or any diarrhea medicine containing kaopectate or attapulgite.

FOOD INTERACTIONS
No known food interactions.

DISEASE INTERACTIONS
Consult your doctor if you have a history of kidney disease, liver disease, or intestinal or stomach disease, especially colitis. The vaginal suppositories should not be used if you have a history of enteritis, ulcerative colitis, or "antibiotic-associated" colitis.

SIDE EFFECTS

SERIOUS
For oral forms, injection, gel, solution, and suspension: Severe stomach or abdominal pains and cramps, weight loss, severe diarrhea, fever, sore throat, skin rash, itching, and redness, unusual bleeding or bruising. For vaginal cream and suppositories: Itching of genital area, pain during intercourse, whitish vaginal discharge, diarrhea, dizziness, headache, nausea, vomiting, stomach cramps or pain. Call your doctor right away.

COMMON
For oral forms: Mild diarrhea, nausea, vomiting, stomach pain. For gel, topical solution, and suspension: Dry, peeling, or scaly skin.

LESS COMMON
For oral forms: Itching of rectal or genital regions. For topical forms: Stomach pain, mild diarrhea, irritated or oily skin, stinging or burning skin, dizziness (cream and suppository), headache (cream and suppository).

CLOMIPHENE CITRATE

Available in: Tablets
Available OTC? No　**As Generic?** Yes
Drug Class: Antiestrogen

▼ USAGE INFORMATION

WHY IT'S PRESCRIBED
To stimulate the release of eggs by the ovaries (ovulation) in women who wish to become pregnant.

HOW IT WORKS
Clomiphene causes an increase in the level of the hormones that stimulate the ovary to release eggs.

▼ DOSAGE GUIDELINES

RANGE AND FREQUENCY
The usual dose is 50 mg once daily for 5 days, starting on the fifth day of the menstrual period. Women who do not have menstrual cycles can begin taking it on any convenient day. The dose may be increased gradually, up to a maximum of 250 mg a day. Clomiphene is usually prescribed for 3 to 4 menstrual cycles and is stopped if pregnancy is achieved during that time.

ONSET OF EFFECT
Ovulation occurs 7 to 10 days after the last day of clomiphene treatment. There may be considerable individual variation in this number, depending on the patient's sensitivity to clomiphene.

DURATION OF ACTION
Unknown.

DIETARY ADVICE
No special restrictions.

STORAGE
Store in a tightly sealed container away from heat and direct light.

MISSED DOSE
Take the missed dose as soon as you remember, unless the time for your next scheduled dose is within the next 2 hours. If so, take a double dose at the proper time, and resume your regular dosage schedule. Inform your doctor if you miss more than 1 day of treatment.

▼ SIDE EFFECTS

SERIOUS
Bloating, stomach or pelvic pain, changes in vision or unusual sensitivity to light, yellow discoloration of the eyes or skin (jaundice). Serious side effects with clomiphene are unusual. If any of these side effects develop, call your doctor immediately.

COMMON
Hot flashes, premenstrual syndrome (PMS). Multiple pregnancies (especially twin pregnancies) are more likely in women who use this drug.

LESS COMMON
Swelling, tenderness, or discomfort in the breasts; dizziness; headache; heavy menstrual periods or unexpected bleeding from the vagina; depression; nausea and vomiting; nervousness; restlessness; fatigue; insomnia.

STOPPING THE DRUG
To be effective, this medication should be taken as prescribed for the full treatment period. Do not stop taking clomiphene on your own.

PROLONGED USE
Do not take clomiphene for more than 5 days in each cycle unless otherwise instructed by your doctor. Clomiphene is usually prescribed for no more than 3 to 4 cycles; do not take it for more than 3 to 4 cycles without your doctor's approval.

▼ PRECAUTIONS

Over 60: Clomiphene is usually prescribed only for women of childbearing age.

Driving and Hazardous Work: Do not drive or engage in hazardous work until you determine how the medicine affects you.

Alcohol: Drink in strict moderation if at all.

Pregnancy: Clomiphene must not be used during pregnancy; discontinue use immediately if you become pregnant.

Breast Feeding: Clomiphene interferes with the production of breast milk and should not be used while nursing.

Infants and Children: Clomiphene should not be used by children.

Special Concerns: Use some means of monitoring ovulation (for example, by recording body temperature changes or by using a home urine ovulation test kit), as it is crucial to discontinue use of this drug when pregnancy occurs. See your doctor with each cycle and be examined before resuming clomiphene therapy. Remember to follow instructions concerning the frequency and timing of intercourse with your partner. Try to take clomiphene at the same time every day. Maintain a strict dosing schedule and try not to miss any doses. Remember that doses of clomiphene can be doubled if you miss one day.

OVERDOSE
Symptoms: No cases of overdose have been reported.

What to Do: If you are concerned about the possibility of an overdose of clomiphene, call your doctor, emergency medical services (EMS), or the nearest poison control center.

▼ INTERACTIONS

DRUG INTERACTIONS
None reported.

FOOD INTERACTIONS
No known food interactions.

DISEASE INTERACTIONS
Consult your doctor if you have any of the following conditions: large ovary, cyst on ovary, endometriosis or excessively painful menstrual periods, fibroids (growths on the uterus), phlebitis (painful inflammation of the veins, usually in the leg), liver disease, depression, or unusual vaginal bleeding.

CLOMIPRAMINE HYDROCHLORIDE

Available in: Capsules
Available OTC? No **As Generic?** Yes
Drug Class: Tricyclic antidepressant

▼ USAGE INFORMATION

WHY IT'S PRESCRIBED
To treat obsessive-compulsive disorder, depression, panic disorder, and chronic pain.

HOW IT WORKS
Clomipramine affects levels of a specific brain chemical (serotonin) that is thought to be linked to mood, emotions, and mental state.

▼ DOSAGE GUIDELINES

RANGE AND FREQUENCY
Adults: To start, 25 mg once a day; may be increased to 250 mg a day. Children age 10 and older: To start, 25 mg once a day; may be increased to 200 mg a day. Older adults: To start, 25 mg a day; may be increased gradually by your doctor.

ONSET OF EFFECT
1 to 6 weeks.

DURATION OF ACTION
Unknown.

DIETARY ADVICE
To lessen stomach upset, take with food, unless your doctor instructs otherwise. Increase intake of fiber and fluids.

STORAGE
Store in a tightly sealed container away from heat, moisture, and direct light.

MISSED DOSE
If you take a one-time daily bedtime dose, do not take a missed dose in the morning because it may cause drowsiness. Call your doctor. If you take more than 1 dose a day, take it as soon as you remember. If it is near the time for the next dose, skip the missed dose and resume your regular dosage schedule. Do not double the next dose.

STOPPING THE DRUG
Take as prescribed for the full treatment period, even if you begin to feel better before the scheduled end of therapy. The decision to stop taking the drug should be made in consultation with your doctor. The dosage should be gradually tapered when stopping.

PROLONGED USE
Usual course of therapy for depression lasts 6 months to 1 year; some patients may benefit from additional therapy. Usual course of therapy for obsessive-compulsive disorder lasts 1 year or more.

▼ PRECAUTIONS

Over 60: Adverse reactions, especially confusion, are more likely and more severe in older patients. A lower dose may be warranted.

Driving and Hazardous Work: Exercise caution until you determine how the medication affects you. Drowsiness, lightheadedness, or confusion can occur.

Alcohol: Avoid alcohol.

Pregnancy: Adequate human studies have not been done. Consult your doctor.

Breast Feeding: Do not use clomipramine while nursing.

Infants and Children: Not prescribed for children under the age of 10.

Special Concerns: This is a potentially dangerous drug, especially if taken in excess. Tricyclic antidepressants should not be within easy reach of suicidal patients. If dry mouth occurs, use sugarless gum or candy.

OVERDOSE
Symptoms: Difficulty breathing, severe fatigue, seizures, confusion, hallucinations, distractibility, dilated pupils, irregular heartbeat, fever.

What to Do: Call your doctor, emergency medical services (EMS), or the nearest poison control center immediately.

▼ INTERACTIONS

DRUG INTERACTIONS
Consult your doctor for specific advice if you are taking antithyroid agents, cimetidine, cisapride, clonidine, guanadrel, guanethidine, metrizamide, SSRI antidepressants, appetite suppressants, isoproterenol, ephedrine, epinephrine, amphetamines, phenylephrine, antipsychotic drugs, pimozide, methyldopa, metyrosine, metoclopramide, pemoline, promethazine, trimeprazine, rauwolfia alkaloids, MAO inhibitors, or any drugs that depress the central nervous system.

FOOD INTERACTIONS
No known food interactions.

DISEASE INTERACTIONS
Consult your doctor if you have any of the following: a history of alcohol abuse, difficulty urinating, asthma, bipolar disorder, high blood pressure, stomach or intestinal problems, glaucoma, overactive thyroid, enlarged prostate, schizophrenia, seizures, a blood disorder, or kidney, heart, or liver disease.

≡ SIDE EFFECTS ≡

SERIOUS
Confusion, sexual dysfunction, heartbeat irregularities, hallucinations, seizures, extreme fatigue or drowsiness, vision problems, breathing difficulty, constipation, staring and absence of facial expression, impaired concentration, difficult urination, fever, extreme and persistent restlessness, loss of coordination and balance, difficulty swallowing or speaking, dilated pupils, eye pain, fainting. Also trembling, weakness, and stiffness in the extremities, shuffling gait. Call your doctor as soon as possible.

COMMON
Drowsiness or dizziness, headache, dry mouth or unpleasant taste, fatigue, heightened sensitivity to light, weight gain, nausea, increased appetite.

LESS COMMON
Heartburn, insomnia, diarrhea, sweating, vomiting.

CLONAZEPAM

BRAND NAME

Klonopin

Available in: Tablets, wafer
Available OTC? No **As Generic?** Yes
Drug Class: Benzodiazepine tranquilizer; antianxiety agent

▼ USAGE INFORMATION

WHY IT'S PRESCRIBED
To control seizures; for relief of anxiety and panic attacks.

HOW IT WORKS
In general, clonazepam produces mild sedation by depressing activity in the central nervous system (the brain and spinal cord). In particular, clonazepam appears to enhance the effect of gamma-aminobutyric acid (GABA), a natural chemical that inhibits the firing of neurons and dampens the transmission of nerve signals, thus decreasing nervous excitation.

▼ DOSAGE GUIDELINES

RANGE AND FREQUENCY
Adults: Initial dose of 0.5 mg, 3 times a day. Patients with seizures may require significantly higher doses. Your doctor will determine the optimal dose. Maximum dose rarely exceeds 20 mg a day.

Children: Dose is based on age and body weight.

ONSET OF EFFECT
Within 1 to 2 hours.

DURATION OF ACTION
Less than 24 hours.

DIETARY ADVICE
No special restrictions.

STORAGE
Store in a tightly sealed container away from heat, moisture, and direct light.

MISSED DOSE
Take it as soon as you remember, unless your next scheduled dose is within the next 2 hours. If so, do not take the missed dose. Take your next scheduled dose at the proper time and resume your regular dosage schedule. Do not double the next dose.

STOPPING THE DRUG
Discontinuing the drug abruptly may produce withdrawal symptoms (sleep disruption, nervousness, irritability, diarrhea, abdominal cramps, muscle aches, memory impairment). Dosage should be reduced gradually according to your doctor's instructions.

PROLONGED USE
Short-term therapy (8 weeks or less) is typical; do not take it for a longer period unless so advised by your doctor.

▼ PRECAUTIONS

Over 60: Adverse reactions are more likely and more severe in older patients.

Driving and Hazardous Work: Clonazepam can impair mental alertness and physical coordination. Adjust your activities accordingly.

Alcohol: Alcohol must be avoided while taking this medication.

Pregnancy: Taking clonazepam during pregnancy is not recommended.

Breast Feeding: Clonazepam passes into breast milk and may be harmful to the infant; do not take it while nursing.

Infants and Children: This drug is rarely prescribed for young patients.

Special Concerns: Clonazepam use can lead to psychological or physical dependence. Never take more than the prescribed daily dose.

OVERDOSE
Symptoms: Extreme drowsiness, confusion, slurred speech, slow reflexes, poor coordination, staggering gait, tremor, slowed breathing, loss of consciousness.

What to Do: Call your doctor, emergency medical services (EMS), or the nearest poison control center immediately.

▼ INTERACTIONS

DRUG INTERACTIONS
Other drugs may interact with clonazepam. Consult your doctor for specific advice if you are taking any drugs that depress the central nervous system; these include antihistamines, antidepressants or other psychiatric medications, barbiturates, sedatives, cough medicines, decongestants, and painkillers. Be sure your doctor knows about any over-the-counter medication you may take.

FOOD INTERACTIONS
None reported.

DISEASE INTERACTIONS
Caution is advised when taking clonazepam. Consult your doctor if you have a history of alcohol or drug abuse, stroke or other brain disease, any chronic lung disease, hyperactivity, depression or other mental illness, myasthenia gravis, sleep apnea, epilepsy, porphyria, kidney disease, or liver disease.

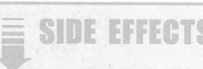

SIDE EFFECTS

SERIOUS
Difficulty concentrating, outbursts of anger, other behavior problems, depression, hallucinations, low blood pressure (causing faintness or confusion), memory impairment, muscle weakness, skin rash or itching, sore throat, fever and chills, sores or ulcers in throat or mouth, unusual bruising or bleeding, extreme fatigue, yellowish tinge to eyes or skin. Call your doctor immediately.

COMMON
Drowsiness, loss of coordination, unsteady gait, dizziness, lightheadedness, slurred speech.

LESS COMMON
Change in sexual desire or ability, constipation, false sense of well-being, nausea and vomiting, urinary problems, unusual fatigue.

CLONIDINE HYDROCHLORIDE

Available in: Tablets, skin patch
Available OTC? No   **As Generic?** Yes
Drug Class: Centrally acting antihypertensive

BRAND NAMES
Catapres, Catapres-TTS

▼ USAGE INFORMATION

WHY IT'S PRESCRIBED
To treat high blood pressure (hypertension).

HOW IT WORKS
Clonidine acts upon certain areas of the central nervous system (the brain and spinal cord) that regulate the activity of the heart and the smooth muscle tissue surrounding the arteries. It causes the blood vessels to relax and widen, which lowers blood pressure.

▼ DOSAGE GUIDELINES

RANGE AND FREQUENCY
Tablets— Adults: Initial dose is 0.1 mg, 2 times per day. Your doctor may increase this to 0.3 mg, 2 times per day. Most patients achieve adequate blood pressure control with 1 mg or less per day; maximum daily dose is 2.4 mg. Children: Pediatrician will determine proper dosage. Skin patch— The starting dose is one TTS-1 patch per week. Doses above two TTS-3 patches per week are usually not effective. The patch should be applied to a hair-less area of skin, ideally on the chest or upper arm. The skin must be free of rashes, blisters, or any form of skin disease.

ONSET OF EFFECT
Tablets: 30 to 60 minutes. Skin patch: 2 to 3 days.

DURATION OF ACTION
Tablets: Up to 8 hours. Skin patch: 7 days per patch, if patch is left in place as directed; otherwise, up to 8 hours from the time the patch is removed.

DIETARY ADVICE
Follow a healthy diet (low-salt, low-fat, low-cholesterol) as advised by your doctor to help control blood pressure and prevent heart disease.

STORAGE
Store in a tightly sealed container away from heat, moisture, and direct light.

MISSED DOSE
Take your missed dose as soon as you remember, unless the time for your next scheduled dose is within the next 2 hours. If so, do not take the missed dose. Take your next dose at the proper time and resume your regular dosage schedule. Do not take a double dose. If you miss more than 1 day of clonidine, inform your doctor.

STOPPING THE DRUG
Stopping clonidine abruptly can lead to a dangerous increase in blood pressure. Do not stop taking clonidine on your own, even if you are feeling better. Your doctor will gradually decrease your dose if necessary.

PROLONGED USE
Long-term use may be necessary and may lead to an increased risk of side effects.

▼ PRECAUTIONS

Over 60: Adverse reactions may be more likely and more severe in older patients.

Driving and Hazardous Work: This medication may cause dizziness and drowsiness; avoid potentially dangerous activities until you know how it affects you.

Alcohol: Avoid alcohol while taking this drug.

Pregnancy: Clonidine use is not recommended during pregnancy.

Breast Feeding: Clonidine passes into breast milk; consult your doctor for advice.

Infants and Children: This drug is not recommended for young patients.

Special Concerns: Blood pressure may rise significantly after missing a few doses.

Signs of dangerously high blood pressure are chest pain, dizziness, headache, blurred vision, confusion, restlessness, trembling of hands and fingers, anxiety, stomach pains, nausea, and vomiting. Make sure you have enough clonidine to last through weekends, vacations, or extended trips. Apply each skin patch to a different area of the chest or upper arm.

OVERDOSE
Symptoms: Low blood pressure, slow heartbeat, difficulty breathing, severe dizziness, confusion, weakness or faintness, tiny, constricted pupils.

What to Do: Call your doctor, emergency medical services (EMS), or the nearest poison control center immediately.

▼ INTERACTIONS

DRUG INTERACTIONS
Consult your doctor if you are taking beta-blockers or tricyclic antidepressants.

FOOD INTERACTIONS
No known food interactions.

DISEASE INTERACTIONS
Tell your doctor if you have any of the following problems: heart or blood vessel disease, including strokes and cardiac arrhythmias; skin disease, such as scleroderma (a concern with the skin patch only); kidney disease; mental depression; Raynaud's syndrome; or lupus.

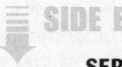

SIDE EFFECTS

SERIOUS
Serious side effects are less likely when clonidine is used as directed.

COMMON
Dry mouth, reduced saliva, drowsiness, dizziness, constipation. Also itching or skin irritation (with skin patch only).

LESS COMMON
Mental depression, swelling of feet and lower legs, pale or cold fingertips and toes, vivid dreams or nightmares. Also darkening of skin (skin patch only).

CLOPIDOGREL BISULFATE

Available in: Tablets
Available OTC? No   **As Generic?** No
Drug Class: Antiplatelet drug

▼ USAGE INFORMATION

WHY IT'S PRESCRIBED
To reduce the risk of recurrence of heart attack or stroke in patients diagnosed with severe arterial disease (atherosclerosis).

HOW IT WORKS
Heart attacks and strokes occur when a blood clot that forms in a narrowed portion of an artery blocks blood flow and thus cuts off the supply of oxygen and nutrients to the tissue that lies beyond the site of the clot. Clopidogrel can prevent heart attacks and strokes by preventing the aggregation (clumping) of platelets, a type of blood cell that initiates clot formation.

▼ DOSAGE GUIDELINES

RANGE AND FREQUENCY
75 mg once a day.

ONSET OF EFFECT
2 hours or more.

DURATION OF ACTION
Unknown.

DIETARY ADVICE
Clopidogrel can be taken with or without food.

STORAGE
Store in a tightly sealed container away from heat, moisture, and direct light.

MISSED DOSE
If you miss a dose on one day, do not double the dose the next day. Resume your regular dosage schedule.

STOPPING THE DRUG
Take it as prescribed for the full treatment period.

PROLONGED USE
Side effects are more likely with prolonged use.

≡ SIDE EFFECTS ≡

SERIOUS
Gastrointestinal bleeding, fainting, palpitations, extreme fatigue, shortness of breath, chest pain. Call your doctor immediately. In rare instances the drug can block production of white blood cells (a major component of the immune system), leading to potentially severe infections. Seek medical attention promptly at the first signs of infection, especially a high fever.

COMMON
Stomach pain, indigestion, diarrhea, skin rash, itching, flu-like symptoms, body aches or pain, headache, dizziness, joint pain, back pain, increased risk of upper respiratory infection.

LESS COMMON
General weakness, hernia, leg cramps, tingling and numbness in the limbs, vomiting, gout, arthritis, anxiety, insomnia, anemia, dermatitis and skin eruptions, bladder infection, cataract, conjunctivitis.

▼ PRECAUTIONS

Over 60: No special problems are expected.

Driving and Hazardous Work: The use of this drug should not impair your ability to perform such tasks safely.

Alcohol: No special precautions are necessary.

Pregnancy: Adequate human studies have not been done. Before taking clopidogrel, tell your doctor if you are pregnant or plan to become pregnant.

Breast Feeding: Clopidogrel passes into breast milk; extreme caution is advised. Consult your doctor for specific advice.

Infants and Children: The safety and effectiveness of clopidogrel use in infants and children have not been established.

Special Concerns: Before you schedule surgery, tell the surgeon or dentist that you are taking this drug.

OVERDOSE
Symptoms: No overdose symptoms have been reported.

What to Do: However, if a greatly excessive dose is taken, call your doctor, emergency medical services (EMS), or the nearest poison control center.

▼ INTERACTIONS

DRUG INTERACTIONS
Consult your doctor for specific advice if you are taking any of the following drugs that may interact with clopidogrel: aspirin or any other nonsteroidal anti-inflammatory drugs (NSAIDs), phenytoin, tamoxifen, tolbutamide, torsemide, fluvastatin, or warfarin.

FOOD INTERACTIONS
No known food interactions.

DISEASE INTERACTIONS
This drug should not be used if you have a peptic ulcer or a history of brain hemorrhage. Caution is advised when taking clopidogrel. Consult your doctor if you have a history of bleeding problems or if you develop bleeding problems while taking this drug. Use of clopidogrel may cause complications in patients with liver disease, since the liver inactivates the drug.

CLORAZEPATE DIPOTASSIUM

Available in: Tablets
Available OTC? No **As Generic?** Yes
Drug Class: Benzodiazepine tranquilizer; antianxiety agent

▼ USAGE INFORMATION

WHY IT'S PRESCRIBED
For relief of anxiety and panic attacks.

HOW IT WORKS
In general, clorazepate produces mild sedation by depressing activity in the central nervous system. In particular, clorazepate appears to enhance the effect of gamma-aminobutyric acid (GABA), a natural chemical that inhibits the firing of neurons and dampens the transmission of nerve signals, thus decreasing nervous excitation.

▼ DOSAGE GUIDELINES

RANGE AND FREQUENCY
For anxiety: Usual dose is 7.5 to 15 mg, 2 to 4 times a day. The dosage may be increased or decreased depending on an individual's response. Older adults are usually started at a total dose of 7.5 to 15 mg a day.

ONSET OF EFFECT
Within 1 to 2 hours.

DURATION OF ACTION
Less than 48 hours.

DIETARY ADVICE
No special restrictions.

STORAGE
Store in a tightly sealed container away from heat, moisture, and direct light.

MISSED DOSE
Take it as soon as you remember, unless the time for your next scheduled dose is within 2 hours. If so, skip the missed dose and resume your regular dosage schedule. Do not double the next dose.

STOPPING THE DRUG
Do not stop taking the drug abruptly, as this can cause withdrawal symptoms (seizures, sleep disruption, nervousness, irritability, diarrhea, abdominal cramps, muscle aches, memory impairment). Dosage should be reduced gradually as directed by your doctor.

PROLONGED USE
Clorazepate may slowly lose its effectiveness with prolonged use. See your doctor for periodic evaluation if you must take this drug for an extended time.

▼ PRECAUTIONS

Over 60: Adverse reactions may be more likely and more severe in older patients.

Driving and Hazardous Work: The use of clorazepate may impair your ability to perform such tasks safely.

Alcohol: Avoid alcohol.

Pregnancy: Avoid or discontinue use of this drug during pregnancy.

Breast Feeding: Do not take this drug while breast feeding.

Infants and Children: Not recommended for children under 9 years of age.

Special Concerns: Use of this drug can lead to psychological or physical dependence. Never take more than the prescribed daily dose.

OVERDOSE
Symptoms: Extreme drowsiness, confusion, slurred speech, slow reflexes, poor coordination, staggering gait, tremor, slowed breathing, loss of consciousness.

What to Do: Call your doctor, emergency medical services (EMS), or the nearest poison control center immediately.

▼ INTERACTIONS

DRUG INTERACTIONS
Consult your doctor for specific advice if you are taking any drugs that depress the central nervous system; these include antihistamines, antidepressants or other psychiatric medications, barbiturates, sedatives, cough medicines, decongestants, and painkillers. Be sure your doctor knows about any over-the-counter drug you may take.

FOOD INTERACTIONS
None are known.

DISEASE INTERACTIONS
Consult your doctor if you have a history of alcohol or drug abuse, stroke or other brain disease, any chronic lung disease, hyperactivity, depression or other mental illness, myasthenia gravis, sleep apnea, epilepsy, porphyria, kidney disease, or liver disease.

≡ SIDE EFFECTS ≡

SERIOUS
Difficulty concentrating, outbursts of anger, other behavior problems, depression, hallucinations, low blood pressure (causing faintness or confusion), memory impairment, muscle weakness, skin rash or itching, sore throat, fever and chills, sores or ulcers in throat or mouth, unusual bruising or bleeding, extreme fatigue, yellowish tinge to eyes or skin. Call your doctor immediately.

COMMON
Drowsiness, loss of coordination, unsteady gait, dizziness, lightheadedness, slurred speech.

LESS COMMON
Change in sexual desire or ability, constipation, false sense of well-being, nausea and vomiting, urinary problems, unusual fatigue.

CLOTRIMAZOLE

Available in: Topical cream, lotion, solution, oral lozenges, vaginal cream, tablets
Available OTC? Yes   **As Generic?** Yes
Drug Class: Antifungal

▼ USAGE INFORMATION

WHY IT'S PRESCRIBED
To treat fungal infections of the mouth and throat (thrush), vaginal area (yeast infection), and the skin, such as tinea corporis (ringworm), tinea cruris (jock itch), tinea pedis (athlete's foot), and pityriasis versicolor ("sun fungus," a fungal skin condition characterized by fine scaly patches of varying shapes, sizes, and colors).

HOW IT WORKS
Clotrimazole prevents fungal organisms from producing vital substances required for growth and function.

▼ DOSAGE GUIDELINES

RANGE AND FREQUENCY
Topical cream, lotion, solution (for skin infections)– Adults and children: Apply twice a day, in the morning and in the evening. Oral lozenges (to treat thrush)– Adults and children age 5 and older: Dissolve one 10 mg lozenge in mouth 5 times a day for 14 days. To prevent thrush: Adults and children age 5 and older: Dissolve one 10 mg lozenge in mouth 3 times a day. Vaginal cream (for yeast infections)– Adults and teenagers: At bedtime, insert vaginally with an applicator 50 mg of 1% cream for 6 to 14 nights, or 100 mg of 2% cream for 3 nights, or 500 mg of 10% cream for 1 night only. Vaginal tablets (for yeast infections)– Nonpregnant women and teenagers: At bedtime, insert one 100 mg tablet for 6 to 7 nights, or one 200 mg tablet for 3 nights, or one 500 mg tablet for 1 night only. Pregnant women and teenagers: At bedtime, insert one 100 mg tablet for 7 nights.

ONSET OF EFFECT
Unknown.

DURATION OF ACTION
Lozenges: 3 hours. Other forms: Unknown.

DIETARY ADVICE
No special restrictions.

STORAGE
Store in a tightly sealed container away from heat, moisture, and direct light. Do not allow it to freeze.

MISSED DOSE
Take it as soon as you remember. If it is near the time for the next dose, skip the missed dose and resume your regular dosage schedule. Do not double the next dose.

STOPPING THE DRUG
If you are using this drug by prescription, take it as prescribed for the full treatment period, even if you begin to feel better before the scheduled end of therapy. Recurrence of the infection is likely if you stop before the full treatment period is complete.

PROLONGED USE
Clotrimazole is generally prescribed for short-term therapy (1 to 14 days). Consult your doctor for further information.

▼ PRECAUTIONS

Over 60: No special problems are expected.

Driving and Hazardous Work: No special precautions are necessary.

Alcohol: No special precautions are necessary.

Pregnancy: Adequate studies on the use of clotrimazole during pregnancy have not been done; however, no problems have been reported. Consult your doctor for specific advice.

Breast Feeding: Clotrimazole may pass into breast milk; caution is advised. Consult your doctor for advice.

Infants and Children: Topical forms: No special warnings. Lozenges are not recommended for children younger than age 5. Vaginal forms: Not commonly prescribed for children under the age of 12.

Special Concerns: Do not chew or swallow lozenges. Clotrimazole lozenges may take 15 to 30 minutes to dissolve completely and are useless if swallowed.

OVERDOSE
Symptoms: An overdose with clotrimazole is unlikely.

What to Do: If someone should swallow a large amount of the medicine, call your doctor, emergency medical services (EMS), or the nearest poison control center immediately.

▼ INTERACTIONS

DRUG INTERACTIONS
No drug interactions have been reported.

FOOD INTERACTIONS
No food interactions have been reported.

DISEASE INTERACTIONS
No disease interactions have been reported.

⯐ SIDE EFFECTS ⯐

SERIOUS
Topical: Hives, skin rash, itching, burning, peeling, stinging, redness, or other skin irritation not present prior to treatment. Lozenge and vaginal: None reported.

COMMON
Topical: None reported. Lozenge (when swallowed): Diarrhea, stomach cramping or pain, nausea or vomiting. Vaginal: Vaginal burning, itching, discharge, or other irritation not present prior to treatment.

LESS COMMON
Topical and lozenge: None reported. Vaginal: Headache, stomach cramps or pain, irritation or burning of sexual partner's penis.

CLOZAPINE

Available in: Tablets
Available OTC? No   **As Generic?** Yes
Drug Class: Neuroleptic; antipsychotic

▼ USAGE INFORMATION

WHY IT'S PRESCRIBED
Clozapine is used to treat schizophrenia after other standard medications have proved inadequate.

HOW IT WORKS
Clozapine inhibits activity of the brain chemical dopamine, thereby helping to prevent the overstimulation of specific nerve centers in the brain believed to be responsible for certain psychiatric disorders.

▼ DOSAGE GUIDELINES

RANGE AND FREQUENCY
Adults: 12.5 mg, 1 to 2 times daily; may be increased gradually by your doctor to as much as 900 mg a day. Children: Consult your doctor.

ONSET OF EFFECT
Within 2 to 4 weeks. Full effect may not be seen until after 3 months of therapy.

DURATION OF ACTION
Unknown.

DIETARY ADVICE
No special restrictions.

STORAGE
Store in a tightly sealed container away from heat and direct light.

MISSED DOSE
Take it as soon as you remember, unless the time for the next scheduled dose is within the next 2 hours. If so, skip the missed dose and resume your regular dosage schedule with the next dose. Do not double the next dose.

STOPPING THE DRUG
Do not stop taking the drug abruptly or without your doctor's approval. Dose must be reduced gradually to prevent withdrawal symptoms from occurring.

PROLONGED USE
The risk of side effects may increase with long-term use of clozapine.

▼ PRECAUTIONS

Over 60: Adverse reactions may be more likely and more severe in older patients.

Driving and Hazardous Work: The use of clozapine may impair your ability to perform such tasks safely.

Alcohol: Avoid alcohol.

Pregnancy: Adequate studies on the use of clozapine during pregnancy have not been done. Consult your doctor for specific advice.

Breast Feeding: Clozapine passes into breast milk; do not use it while nursing.

Infants and Children: Safety and effectiveness of the use of clozapine in children under the age of 16 have not been established.

Special Concerns: Frequent blood tests are required while taking clozapine. This medication can cause a marked decrease in the level of white blood cells in the body. Clozapine prescriptions are sometimes filled only one week at a time, on the condition that the patient be given a blood test to check white cell count before the following week's medication is dispensed. Report symptoms of fever, chills, nausea, vomiting, diarrhea, painful urination, or cough to your doctor when taking this medication.

OVERDOSE
Symptoms: Confusion, restlessness, nervousness, severe drowsiness, hallucinations, fainting, unconsciousness, coma; unusual excitement or agitation; slow, deep breathing or rapid, shallow breathing, or breathing difficulty; increased salivation; rapid or irregular pulse.

What to Do: Call your doctor, emergency medical services (EMS), or the nearest poison control center immediately.

▼ INTERACTIONS

DRUG INTERACTIONS
Other drugs may interact with clozapine. Consult your doctor for specific advice if you are taking sleeping pills or sedatives, antidepressants, amphotericin B, anticancer drugs, thyroid medications, azathioprine, chlorambucil, chloramphenicol, colchicine, cyclophosphamide, flucytosine, haloperidol, interferon, lithium, mercaptopurine, methotrexate, plicamycin, zidovudine (AZT), cimetidine, or erythromycin.

FOOD INTERACTIONS
None reported.

DISEASE INTERACTIONS
Consult your doctor if you have a history of any type of blood disorder, enlarged prostate, difficult urination, stomach or intestinal disorder, heart or blood vessel disease, epilepsy or other seizure disorder, kidney disease, or liver disease.

 SIDE EFFECTS

SERIOUS
Signs of serious infection, including high fever, chills, and sweating, sores or ulcers in the mouth, unusual bruising or bleeding, severe fatigue or weakness. Other serious side effects include seizures, yellow discoloration of the eyes or skin, rapid or irregular heartbeat, severe dizziness, severe low blood pressure (which may cause lightheadedness and fainting, especially when getting up suddenly from sitting or lying positions), and hyperglycemia (elevated blood glucose levels), with symptoms including increased thirst, hunger, and urination. If you experience such symptoms, contact your doctor immediately.

COMMON
Increased salivation, dizziness, drowsiness, mild headache, constipation, nausea or vomiting, weight gain.

LESS COMMON
Abdominal pain, heartburn, sore throat, diarrhea, muscle aches, spasms, or weakness, loss of coordination.

COAL TAR

Available in: Cleansing bar, cream, gel, lotion, ointment, shampoo, liquid
Available OTC? Yes   **As Generic?** Yes
Drug Class: Antipsoriasis drug

BRAND NAMES

Alphosyl, Aquatar, Balnetar Therapeutic Tar Bath, Cutar Water Dispersible Emollient Tar, Denorex Medicated Shampoo, DHS Tar Shampoo, Doak Oil Therapeutic Bath Treatment, Doctar Hair & Scalp Shampoo and Conditioner, Estar, Exorex, Fototar, Ionil T Plus, Lavatar, Medotar, Pentrax Anti-Dandruff Tar Shampoo, Psorigel, PsoriNail Topical Solution, T/Derm Tar Emollient, T/Gel Therapeutic Shampoo, Taraphilic, Tarbonis, Tarpaste 'Doak', Tegrin, Tersa-Tar Soapless Tar Shampoo, Theraplex T Shampoo, Zetar

▼ USAGE INFORMATION

WHY IT'S PRESCRIBED
To treat skin conditions including dandruff, eczema, seborrheic dermatitis, and psoriasis.

HOW IT WORKS
Coal tar promotes softening, dissolution, and peeling of hard, scaly, roughened, or irregular surface skin. It also has antiseptic properties and fights fungal, bacterial, and parasitic organisms.

▼ DOSAGE GUIDELINES

RANGE AND FREQUENCY
Cleansing bar: Use 1 or 2 times a day as directed by your doctor. Cream: Apply to affected areas up to 4 times a day. Gel: Apply to affected areas 1 or 2 times a day. Lotion: Apply to affected areas as needed. Ointment: Apply to affected areas 2 or 3 times a day. Shampoo: Use once a day, once a week, or as directed by your doctor. Topical solution: Apply to skin or scalp or use in the bath, depending on product. Topical bath solution: Add appropriate amount to bath water; immerse yourself in the bath for 20 minutes. If you have any questions about its use, consult your doctor.

ONSET OF EFFECT
Unknown.

DURATION OF ACTION
Unknown.

DIETARY ADVICE
Coal tar can be used without regard to diet.

STORAGE
Store in a tightly sealed container away from heat and direct light. Do not allow liquid forms to freeze.

MISSED DOSE
Apply it as soon as you remember. If it is near the time for the next dose, skip the missed dose and resume your regular dosage schedule. Do not apply a double dose.

STOPPING THE DRUG
If you are applying coal tar by prescription, the decision to stop using it should be made by your doctor. If you are using the drug without a prescription, you may stop treatment whenever you choose.

PROLONGED USE
Do not use coal tar for longer than your physician prescribes.

▼ PRECAUTIONS

Over 60: Coal tar is not expected to cause different side effects or problems in older patients than it does in younger persons.

Driving and Hazardous Work: The use of coal tar should not impair your ability to perform such tasks safely.

Alcohol: No special restrictions apply.

Pregnancy: Studies of coal tar use during pregnancy have not been done in animals or humans. Before you use coal tar, tell your doctor if you are pregnant or plan to become pregnant.

Breast Feeding: It is not known if coal tar passes into breast milk. Consult your doctor for specific advice.

Infants and Children: Use and dose in infants and children must be determined by your doctor.

Special Concerns: For external use only. Keep coal tar away from the eyes. If you accidentally get some of the medicine in your eyes, flush them thoroughly with water. After applying coal tar, protect the treated area from sunlight for 72 hours, and be sure to remove all coal tar before being exposed to sunlight or using a sunlamp . Do not apply coal tar to infected, blistered, raw, or oozing areas of the skin.

OVERDOSE
Symptoms: None reported.

What to Do: Emergency instructions not applicable.

▼ INTERACTIONS

DRUG INTERACTIONS
Consult your doctor for specific advice if you are using tetracyclines, psoralens, or retinoids. Also tell your doctor if you are using any other prescription or over-the-counter medication.

FOOD INTERACTIONS
No known food interactions.

DISEASE INTERACTIONS
You should not use coal tar if you have had a prior allergic reaction to it.

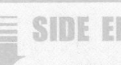
SIDE EFFECTS

SERIOUS
Skin irritation or rash not present before use of coal tar. Call your doctor immediately.

COMMON
Mild stinging, increased sensitivity to sunlight.

LESS COMMON
There are no less-common side effects associated with the use of coal tar.

CODEINE

Available in: Tablets, oral solution
Available OTC? No   **As Generic?** Yes
Drug Class: Opioid (narcotic) analgesic

▼ USAGE INFORMATION

WHY IT'S PRESCRIBED
To treat mild to moderate pain or to control a severe cough.

HOW IT WORKS
Narcotics such as codeine relieve pain by acting on specific areas of the spinal cord and brain that process pain signals from nerves throughout the body. Codeine dulls the cough reflex, which is why it may be used to treat certain coughs.

▼ DOSAGE GUIDELINES

RANGE AND FREQUENCY
Adults— For pain: 15 to 60 mg every 3 to 6 hours as needed. Usual dose is 30 mg. For cough: 10 to 20 mg every 3 to 6 hours as needed. Children— Oral solution: For pain: 0.5 mg per 2.2 lbs (1 kg) of body weight every 4 to 6 hours as needed. For cough: Age 2: 3 mg every 4 to 6 hours. Take no more than 12 mg a day. Age 3: 3.5 mg every 4 to 6 hours. Take no more than 14 mg a day. Age 4: 4 mg every 4 to 6 hours. Take no more than 16 mg a day. Age 5: 4.5 mg every 4 to 6 hours. Take no more than 18 mg a day. Ages 6 to 12: 5 to 10 mg every 4 to 6 hours. Take no more than 60 mg per day.

ONSET OF EFFECT
30 to 45 minutes.

DURATION OF ACTION
4 to 6 hours.

DIETARY ADVICE
Codeine is constipating; make sure your diet contains adequate amounts of fiber and vegetables.

STORAGE
Store in a tightly sealed container away from heat, moisture, and direct light.

MISSED DOSE
Take it as soon as you remember. If it is near the time for the next dose, skip the missed dose and resume your regular dosage schedule. Do not double the next dose.

STOPPING THE DRUG
You should take it as prescribed for the full treatment period, but you may stop taking the drug if you are feeling better before the scheduled end of therapy.

PROLONGED USE
Therapy varies, depending on the cause of the pain. Some patients require long-term narcotic therapy. Side effects may be more likely with prolonged use.

▼ PRECAUTIONS

Over 60: Adverse reactions may be more likely and more severe in older patients.

Driving and Hazardous Work: The use of codeine may impair your ability to perform such tasks safely.

Alcohol: Avoid alcohol.

Pregnancy: Adequate human studies have not been completed. Before taking codeine, tell your physician if you are pregnant or plan to become pregnant.

Breast Feeding: Codeine passes into breast milk; caution is advised. Consult your doctor for specific advice.

Infants and Children: Adverse reactions may be more likely and more severe in children.

Special Concerns: Codeine can cause physical dependence. Some patients may experience withdrawal symptoms when the medication is discontinued. These may include body aches, abdominal pain, stomach cramps, diarrhea, runny nose, gooseflesh, nervousness, agitation, sweating, yawning, loss of appetite, shivering, insomnia, dilated pupils, and weakness. Do not exceed recommended doses or increase the dose on your own.

OVERDOSE
Symptoms: Confusion; sleepiness; slurred speech; unconsciousness; small, pinpoint pupils; cold, clammy skin; slow breathing; seizures; severe drowsiness, weakness, or dizziness.

What to Do: Call your doctor, emergency medical services (EMS), or the nearest poison control center immediately.

▼ INTERACTIONS

DRUG INTERACTIONS
Consult your doctor for specific advice if you are taking carbamazepine or other medicine for seizures, barbiturates, sedatives, cough medicines, decongestants, antidepressants, other prescription pain medications, MAO inhibitors, naltrexone, rifampin, or zidovudine.

FOOD INTERACTIONS
None known.

DISEASE INTERACTIONS
Consult your doctor if you have any of the following: emotional illness; brain disorders or head injury; seizures; lung disease; prostate problems or other problems with urination; gallstones; colitis; heart, kidney, liver, or thyroid disease; or a history of alcohol or drug abuse.

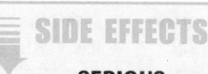

SIDE EFFECTS

SERIOUS
Serious side effects of codeine are indistinguishable from those of overdose: Confusion; sleepiness; slurred speech; unconsciousness; small, pinpoint pupils; cold, clammy skin; slow breathing; seizures; severe drowsiness, weakness, or dizziness.

COMMON
Mild dizziness or lightheadedness, nausea or vomiting, constipation, drowsiness, itching.

LESS COMMON
Headache, sweating, false sense of well-being (euphoria).

COLCHICINE

Available in: Tablets, injection
Available OTC? No **As Generic?** Yes
Drug Class: Antigout drug

▼ USAGE INFORMATION

WHY IT'S PRESCRIBED
To treat painful attacks of gout, as well as to prevent or reduce the frequency of such attacks. Oral colchicine is used for moderate attacks. Injectable colchicine is used for serious attacks or in patients who cannot take the tablets.

HOW IT WORKS
In gout, crystals of a chemical called monosodium urate are deposited in joints, where they cause inflammation and lead to the sharp, excruciating pain of a gout attack. Colchicine prevents inflammation that may result from the accumulation of monosodium urate crystals.

▼ DOSAGE GUIDELINES

RANGE AND FREQUENCY
For an acute attack: 0.5 to 1.2 mg immediately; then 0.5 or 0.6 mg every 1 or 2 hours, or 1 to 1.2 mg every 2 hours, to a maximum of 6 mg. Stop as soon as you achieve relief. For chronic gout or to prevent attacks: 0.5 or 0.6 mg, usually once a day. Not all patients require daily doses; some may take colchicine periodically. Consult your doctor.

ONSET OF EFFECT
6 to 12 hours.

DURATION OF ACTION
Unknown.

DIETARY ADVICE
No special restrictions.

STORAGE
Store in a tightly sealed container away from heat and direct light. Keep it away from moisture and extremes in temperature.

MISSED DOSE
Take it as soon as you remember. If it is near the time for the next dose, skip the missed dose and resume your regular dosage schedule. Do not double the next dose.

STOPPING THE DRUG
You may stop taking the drug if you are feeling better before the scheduled end of therapy. If it was prescribed for long-term use, however, do not stop without first consulting your doctor.

PROLONGED USE
Therapy for a severe attack is usually completed within 1 day. Do not take colchicine for a longer period without your doctor's approval.

▼ PRECAUTIONS

Over 60: Adverse reactions may be more likely and more severe in older patients.

Driving and Hazardous Work: Do not drive or engage in hazardous work until you determine how the medicine affects you.

Alcohol: Avoid alcohol.

Pregnancy: Avoid or discontinue this medication if you are pregnant or trying to become pregnant.

Breast Feeding: Colchicine passes into breast milk; avoid or discontinue use while nursing.

Infants and Children: Not recommended.

Special Concerns: Make sure you understand how to take this drug; colchicine treatments vary. Dosing schedules for an acute attack can be confusing. Read your label carefully; make sure you understand how many tablets constitute the correct dose. Many patients find it helpful to write the dosing plan on an index card and to carry a copy in a wallet or handbag.

Do not continue taking colchicine during an acute gout attack if you begin feeling nauseated, begin vomiting, or develop diarrhea. Call your doctor. Do not continue taking colchicine during an acute attack once you have taken 6 mg; if you still have not achieved relief after reaching this limit, call your doctor.

OVERDOSE
Symptoms: Fever; convulsions; confusion, disorientation, delirium; rapid or irregular breathing; sharp, burning pain in stomach; diarrhea, which may be bloody.

What to Do: Call emergency medical services (EMS), your doctor, or the nearest poison control center immediately.

▼ INTERACTIONS

DRUG INTERACTIONS
Consult your doctor for advice if you are taking phenylbutazone or drugs that may affect your bone marrow including anticonvulsants, certain antibiotics, and chemotherapy drugs for cancer.

FOOD INTERACTIONS
None are likely, but a low-purine diet is recommended to reduce the risk of gout attacks. Foods high in purines include anchovies, sardines, legumes, poultry, sweetbreads, liver, kidneys, and other organ meats.

DISEASE INTERACTIONS
Consult your doctor if you have heart, liver, or kidney disease; blood disorders; or gastrointestinal disorders, such as ulcers, colitis, and intestinal malabsorption.

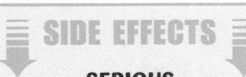
≡ SIDE EFFECTS ≡

SERIOUS
Allergic reactions, causing rash or hives, swelling of face, lips, tongue, eyelids, and throat; such reactions may interfere with breathing—seek medical help immediately. Unusual or persistent fevers, fatigue, chills, sore throat, bruising, or bleeding; these may be signs of serious anemia or suppression of the immune system.

COMMON
Diarrhea, vomiting, nausea, stomach pain.

LESS COMMON
Muscle weakness; numbness, tingling, or prickling in the hands and feet.

COLESTIPOL HYDROCHLORIDE

Available in: Powder, tablets
Available OTC? No **As Generic?** No
Drug Class: Antilipidemic (cholesterol-lowering agent)

▼ USAGE INFORMATION

WHY IT'S PRESCRIBED
To reduce cholesterol in people with high blood levels of low-density lipoprotein (LDL), as part of a comprehensive treatment program that includes exercise and special diet. The drug is also used to relieve itching caused by high levels of bile acids in the blood, a problem associated with blockage of the bile ducts. It may also be used to prevent some types of diarrhea or serve as an antidote to poisoning from or overdose of digitalis drugs.

HOW IT WORKS
Colestipol binds with bile acids in the intestine, forming an insoluble complex that is excreted in the feces. This process reduces the amount of bile acids in the blood. In response to the lower levels of bile acids, the liver converts more cholesterol to bile acids. As a consequence, the amount of cholesterol in liver cells declines, and the liver makes more receptors for LDL. The resulting increased removal of LDL from the blood lowers LDL cholesterol.

▼ DOSAGE GUIDELINES

RANGE AND FREQUENCY
Initial dose is 5 g, 1 or 2 times a day. Maintenance dose is 10 to 30 g, given in 2 equally divided doses. Always mix the powder thoroughly with appropriate liquid (water or fruit juice; do not use carbonated beverages) and wait 10 to 15 minutes after mixing before drinking. Doses are increased or decreased according to the individual's response.

ONSET OF EFFECT
Within 1 to 3 weeks.

DURATION OF ACTION
The drug's effects persist for 2 to 4 weeks after the final dose.

DIETARY ADVICE
Follow all special dietary restrictions and guidelines as directed by your doctor.

STORAGE
Store in a tightly sealed container away from heat, moisture, and direct light.

MISSED DOSE
Take as soon as you remember. However, if it is near the time for the next dose, skip the missed dose and resume your regular dosage schedule. Do not double the next dose.

STOPPING THE DRUG
The drug may be stopped after 1 to 3 months if the therapeutic effect is not adequate. The decision to stop taking the drug should be made by your doctor.

PROLONGED USE
Colestipol may be used safely for years; periodic evaluation of the drug's effectiveness is necessary.

▼ PRECAUTIONS

Over 60: Adverse reactions (particularly constipation) are more likely and more severe in older patients.

Driving and Hazardous Work: Colestipol should not impair your ability to perform such tasks safely.

Alcohol: No special precautions are necessary.

Pregnancy: Consult your doctor if you become or plan to become pregnant.

Breast Feeding: At very high doses colestipol may interfere with the absorption of vitamins A, D, E, and K, which may affect the nutritional intake of the nursing infant. Consult your doctor for specific advice.

Infants and Children: Prescribed for children only in rare circumstances. Follow doctor's instructions and dosage guidelines carefully in such cases.

Special Concerns: At very high doses, colestipol may interfere with the absorption of fats and fat-soluble vitamins (vitamins A, D, E, and K); vitamin supplementation may be advised.

OVERDOSE
Symptoms: None reported.

What to Do: Emergency instructions not applicable.

▼ INTERACTIONS

DRUG INTERACTIONS
Colestipol may bind with other drugs and hinder their absorption. Therefore, take all other drugs 1 to 2 hours before or 4 hours after taking colestipol.

FOOD INTERACTIONS
No known food interactions.

DISEASE INTERACTIONS
Do not take this drug if you have had a prior allergic reaction to it. Use of colestipol may make the following conditions worse: gallstones, peptic ulcer, intestinal bleeding disorders, hemorrhoids, malabsorption, constipation.

 SIDE EFFECTS

SERIOUS
Severe abdominal pain (a very rare reaction, indicating intestinal obstruction). Stop taking the drug and contact your doctor immediately.

COMMON
Constipation, heartburn, bloating, belching, abdominal discomfort, irritation of the anal area.

LESS COMMON
Hives, rash, gas, diarrhea, nausea, vomiting, gallstones.

COLISTIN/NEOMYCIN/HYDROCORTISONE

BRAND NAME

Coly-Mycin Otic

Available in: Otic suspension
Available OTC? No   **As Generic?** No
Drug Class: Antibiotic combination drug

▼ USAGE INFORMATION

WHY IT'S PRESCRIBED
To treat infections of the ear canal and other types of ear problems.

HOW IT WORKS
This drug is a combination of three active ingredients. Colistin and neomycin are both antibiotics that destroy infection-causing bacteria. Hydrocortisone is a steroid hormone that mimics the effects of the body's natural corticosteroids to help reduce redness and pain associated with specific ear problems.

▼ DOSAGE GUIDELINES

RANGE AND FREQUENCY
Adults: 4 drops in the affected ear, 3 or 4 times a day. Children: Up to 3 drops in the affected ear, 3 or 4 times a day.

ONSET OF EFFECT
Unknown.

DURATION OF ACTION
Unknown.

DIETARY ADVICE
No special restrictions.

STORAGE
Store in a tightly sealed container away from heat, moisture, and direct light. Do not allow it to freeze.

MISSED DOSE
Apply it as soon as you remember. If it is near the time for the next dose, skip the missed dose and resume your regular dosage schedule. Do not double the next dose.

STOPPING THE DRUG
Use it as prescribed for the full treatment period, even if you feel better before the scheduled end of therapy.

PROLONGED USE
Do not use this medication for more than 10 days unless directed otherwise by your doctor.

▼ PRECAUTIONS

Over 60:
No special problems are expected.

Driving and Hazardous Work:
The use of this medication should not impair your ability to perform such tasks safely.

Alcohol:
No special problems are expected, although it is generally advisable to abstain from alcohol when fighting an infection.

Pregnancy:
Problems related to the use of this preparation during pregnancy have not been reported. Consult your doctor before using this medication during pregnancy.

Breast Feeding:
When used as directed, this medication does not pass into breast milk. Consult your doctor for specific advice.

Infants and Children:
No studies on the use of this medication by children have been done. No special problems are expected.

Special Concerns:
Before applying this medication, clean the ear canal thoroughly and dry it with a sterile wipe. Tilt the head so that the affected ear is up. Adults should gently pull the earlobe up and back; for children, pull down and back. After the medicine is dropped into the ear canal, keep the ear facing up for 5 minutes (or 1 to 2 minutes for restless children). Your doctor may have further instructions on how to apply the medication.

OVERDOSE

Symptoms: No cases of overdose have been reported.

What to Do: An overdose of this medication is unlikely to be life-threatening. However, if someone takes a much larger dose than prescribed or accidentally ingests the medication, call your doctor, emergency medical services (EMS), or the nearest poison control center immediately.

▼ INTERACTIONS

DRUG INTERACTIONS
It is possible that other drugs may interact with colistin, neomycin, and hydrocortisone. Before you use this medication, tell your doctor if you are taking any other prescription or over-the-counter medication, especially any other kinds of ear drops.

FOOD INTERACTIONS
No known food interactions.

DISEASE INTERACTIONS
Caution is advised when taking this drug. Consult your doctor if you have herpes simplex infection or any other ear problem.

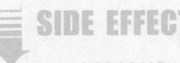

SIDE EFFECTS

SERIOUS
Skin rash, itching, redness, swelling, or other signs of irritation that were not present before therapy. Call your doctor immediately.

COMMON
No common side effects are associated with this drug.

LESS COMMON
There are no less-common side effects associated with the use of this drug.

CONTRACEPTIVES, ORAL AND INJECTION (PROGESTIN ONLY)

Available in: Tablets, injection
Available OTC? No   **As Generic?** No
Drug Class: Progestin (hormone)

▼ USAGE INFORMATION

WHY IT'S PRESCRIBED
To prevent pregnancy.

HOW IT WORKS
Progestin prevents a woman's egg from developing fully; it also causes changes in the uterine lining and the cervical secretions, making it difficult for sperm to reach the egg.

▼ DOSAGE GUIDELINES

RANGE AND FREQUENCY
Tablets: 75 micrograms (mcg) (Ovrette) or 350 mcg (Nor-QD, Miconor) every day beginning on the first day of the menstrual cycle. Injection (Depo-Provera): 150 mg injected into the upper arm or buttock every 13 weeks.

ONSET OF EFFECT
Tablets: Protection begins 3 weeks after first taking the medication. Injection: Immediate if the injection is given within 5 days of the menstrual period.

DURATION OF ACTION
Tablets: 24 hours. Injection: 13 weeks.

DIETARY ADVICE
Tablets can be taken with meals to prevent gastrointestinal upset.

STORAGE
Store in a tightly sealed container away from heat and direct light.

MISSED DOSE
Take the missed dose of the tablet as soon as you remember, resume your regular dosage, and use another birth control method for 2 days.

STOPPING THE DRUG
You may stop at any time you choose. This will naturally increase the likelihood of pregnancy unless another birth control method is employed.

PROLONGED USE
You should see your doctor for periodic examinations and laboratory tests if you use these contraceptives for a prolonged period.

▼ PRECAUTIONS

Over 60: Generally not used by older patients.

Driving and Hazardous Work: No special precautions are necessary.

Alcohol: No special precautions are necessary.

Pregnancy: Low-dose progestins for contraception have not been shown to cause problems later if pregnancy occurs.

Breast Feeding: Progestins pass into breast milk but have not been shown to cause problems. They are recommended for nursing mothers who wish to practice contraception.

Infants and Children: Progestin contraceptives have not caused problems in teenagers. Birth control methods that protect against sexually transmitted diseases are also recommended for them.

Special Concerns: No contraceptive method is perfect. If you suspect a pregnancy, call your doctor immediately. If you have any laboratory test, tell the health professional that you are using these contraceptives. Cigarette smoking or alcohol abuse can increase the risk of osteoporosis and may increase the risk of blood clots.

OVERDOSE
Symptoms: No specific ones have been reported.

What to Do: An overdose of these contraceptives is unlikely to be life-threatening. However, if someone takes a much larger dose than prescribed, call your doctor, emergency medical services (EMS), or the nearest poison control center immediately.

▼ INTERACTIONS

DRUG INTERACTIONS
The following drugs may interact with these contraceptives. Consult your doctor for specific advice if you are taking aminoglutethimide, carbamazepine, phenytoin, rifabutin, or rifampin.

FOOD INTERACTIONS
No known food interactions.

DISEASE INTERACTIONS
Caution is advised when taking these contraceptives. Consult your doctor if you have any of the following: asthma, epilepsy, heart problems, circulation problems, kidney disease, liver disease, migraine headaches, breast disease, bleeding problems, diabetes, high blood cholesterol, or central nervous system disorders, such as depression.

 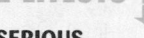
SIDE EFFECTS

SERIOUS
Changes in or cessation of menstrual bleeding, unexpected or increased flow of breast milk, mental depression, skin rash, loss of or change in speech, impaired coordination or vision, severe and sudden shortness of breath. Call your doctor immediately.

COMMON
Stomach pain, swelling of face, ankles, or feet, mild headache, mood changes, unusual fatigue, weight gain, pain or irritation at site of injection.

LESS COMMON
Acne, breast pain or tenderness, hot flashes, insomnia, loss of sexual desire, loss or gain of scalp hair or body hair, brown spots on skin.

CONTRACEPTIVES, ORAL (COMBINATION PRODUCTS)

Available in: Tablets
Available OTC? No   **As Generic?** Yes
Drug Class: Hormones, estrogen with progestins

▼ USAGE INFORMATION

WHY IT'S PRESCRIBED
To prevent pregnancy.

HOW IT WORKS
Such products stop a woman's egg from fully developing each month.

▼ DOSAGE GUIDELINES

RANGE AND FREQUENCY
For 21-day cycle: 1 tablet a day for 21 days. Skip 7 days; repeat the cycle. For 28-day cycle: 1 tablet a day for 28 days. Repeat cycle. Each package of pills has 21 active tablets only, or 21 active tablets and 7 placebos. When taking placebos or no tablets, menstruation should occur.

ONSET OF EFFECT
At least 7 days.

DURATION OF ACTION
As long as tablets are taken.

DIETARY ADVICE
Take it with food if stomach upset occurs.

STORAGE
Store in a tightly sealed container away from heat and direct light.

MISSED DOSE
If you miss the first tablet of a new cycle or 1 tablet during the cycle, take the missed tablet as soon as you remember and take the next tablet at the usual time. If you miss 2 tablets in a row in the first or second week, take 2 tablets the day you remember and 2 the next day, then resume normal dosage schedule and use another birth control method until the next cycle begins. If you miss 2 tablets during the third week or 3 tablets at any time, begin a new cycle on its scheduled starting day, but use another birth control method for 7 days into the new cycle.

STOPPING THE DRUG
You may stop at any time you choose after completing a full 21-day cycle of tablets.

PROLONGED USE
See your doctor at least every 6 months.

▼ PRECAUTIONS

Over 60: Generally not used by older persons.

Driving and Hazardous Work: No special precautions are necessary.

Alcohol: No special precautions are necessary.

Pregnancy: Discontinue use if you become pregnant or suspect that you might be pregnant.

Breast Feeding: Oral contraceptive hormones pass into breast milk; avoid or discontinue use while nursing.

Infants and Children: No special problems have been found in teenagers who use oral contraception.

Special Concerns: Limit your exposure to sunlight until you determine how this medication affects you. Smoking can reduce the effectiveness of oral contraceptives and increase the risk of potentially dangerous blood clots.

OVERDOSE
Symptoms: Unexplained vaginal bleeding.

What to Do: An overdose is unlikely to be life-threatening. However, if someone takes a much larger dose than prescribed, call your doctor, emergency medical services (EMS), or the nearest poison control center immediately.

▼ INTERACTIONS

DRUG INTERACTIONS
Consult your doctor for advice if you are taking: amiodarone, anabolic steroids, corticosteroids, androgens, anti-infectives, barbiturates, carbamazepine, carmustine, dantrolene, daunorubicin, disulfiram, divalproex, estrogens, etretinate, gold salts, griseofulvin, hydroxychloroquine, mercaptopurine, methotrexate, naltrexone, phenothiazines, phenylbutazone, phenytoin, plicamycin, primidone, rifabutin, rifampin, troleandomycin, theophylline, cyclosporine, or ritonavir.

FOOD INTERACTIONS
No known food interactions.

DISEASE INTERACTIONS
Consult your doctor if you have any of the following: endometriosis, fibroid tumors of the uterus, heart or circulation disease, a history of stroke, breast disease, cancer, gallbladder disease, high blood cholesterol, liver disease, mental depression, diabetes, epilepsy, or migraines.

☰ SIDE EFFECTS ☰

SERIOUS
Sudden, severe, or continuing stomach pain; sudden or severe headache or migraine; loss of coordination; loss of or change in vision; pains in chest, groin, or leg; sudden slurring of speech; weakness, numbness, or pain in an arm or leg; changes in uterine bleeding pattern; prolonged bleeding at menses; vaginal infection. Call your doctor immediately.

COMMON
Abdominal cramps or bloating; acne; breast pain, tenderness, or swelling; dizziness; nausea; swelling of ankles or feet; unusual fatigue; vomiting; absence of normal menstruation. Call your doctor if you do not have your period at the end of the cycle and before you start a new cycle.

LESS COMMON
Blotchy spots on skin, gain or loss of hair, increased sensitivity to sunlight, changes in sexual interest.

CORTISONE ORAL

BRAND NAME

Cortone Acetate

Available in: Tablets
Available OTC? No   **As Generic?** Yes
Drug Class: Corticosteroid

▼ USAGE INFORMATION

WHY IT'S PRESCRIBED
To treat numerous conditions that involve inflammation (a response by body tissues, producing redness, warmth, swelling, and pain). Such conditions include arthritis, allergic reactions, asthma, some skin diseases, multiple sclerosis flare-ups, and other autoimmune diseases. Also prescribed to treat deficiency of natural steroid hormones.

HOW IT WORKS
This hormone mimics the effects of the body's natural corticosteroids. It depresses the synthesis, release, and activity of inflammation-producing body chemicals. It also suppresses the activity of the immune system.

▼ DOSAGE GUIDELINES

RANGE AND FREQUENCY
Adults and teenagers: 25 to 300 mg a day, in 1 or several doses. Doses are individualized, depending on the condition being treated. The dose for children depends on body weight or size and must be determined by your doctor.

ONSET OF EFFECT
Variable.

DURATION OF ACTION
Variable.

DIETARY ADVICE
It can be taken with food or milk to minimize stomach upset. Your doctor may recommend a low-salt, high-potassium, high-protein diet.

STORAGE
Store in a tightly sealed container away from heat, moisture, and direct light.

MISSED DOSE
Take it as soon as you remember. If you take several doses a day and it is close to the next dose, double the next dose. If you take 1 dose a day and you do not remember until the next day, skip the missed dose and do not double the next dose.

STOPPING THE DRUG
With long-term therapy, do not stop taking the drug abruptly; the dosage should be decreased gradually.

PROLONGED USE
See your doctor regularly for tests and examinations. Long-term use may lead to cataracts, diabetes, hypertension, or osteoporosis.

▼ PRECAUTIONS

Over 60: Adverse reactions may be more likely and more severe in older patients.

Driving and Hazardous Work: Do not drive or engage in hazardous work until you determine how the medicine affects you.

Alcohol: May cause stomach problems; avoid unless your doctor approves occasional moderate drinking.

Pregnancy: Overuse during pregnancy can retard the child's growth and cause other developmental problems. Consult your physician.

Breast Feeding: Do not use while nursing.

Infants and Children: Cortisone may retard the normal growth and development of bone and other tissues. Consult your doctor for advice.

Special Concerns: Avoid immunizations with live vaccines if possible. Remember that this drug can lower your resistance to infection. Patients undergoing long-term therapy should wear a medical-alert bracelet. Call your doctor if you develop a fever.

OVERDOSE
Symptoms: Fever, muscle or joint pain, nausea, dizziness, fainting, breathing difficulty. Prolonged overuse: Moon-face, obesity, unusual hair growth, acne, loss of sexual function, muscle wasting.

What to Do: Call your doctor, emergency medical services (EMS), or the nearest poison control center immediately.

▼ INTERACTIONS

DRUG INTERACTIONS
Consult your doctor for specific advice if you are taking aminoglutethimide, antacids, barbiturates, carbamazepine, griseofulvin, mitotane, phenylbutazone, phenytoin, primidone, rifampin, injectable amphotericin B, oral antidiabetes agents, insulin, digitalis drugs, diuretics, or medications containing potassium or sodium.

FOOD INTERACTIONS
Avoid excess sodium.

DISEASE INTERACTIONS
Consult your doctor if you have a history of bone disease, chicken pox, measles, stomach or intestinal disorders, diabetes mellitus, recent serious infection, tuberculosis, glaucoma, heart disease, hypertension, liver or kidney disorders, high blood cholesterol, overactive or underactive thyroid, myasthenia gravis, or lupus.

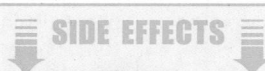
SIDE EFFECTS

SERIOUS
Vision problems, frequent urination, increased thirst, rectal bleeding, blistering skin, confusion, hallucinations, paranoia, euphoria, depression, mood swings, redness and swelling at injection site. Call your doctor immediately.

COMMON
Increased appetite, indigestion, nervousness, insomnia, greater susceptibility to infections, increased blood pressure, slow healing of wounds, weight gain, easy bruising, fluid retention.

LESS COMMON
Change in skin color, dizziness, headache, increased sweating, unusual growth of body or facial hair, increased blood sugar, peptic ulcers, adrenal insufficiency, muscle weakness, cataracts, glaucoma, osteoporosis.

COSYNTROPIN

BRAND NAME

Cortrosyn

Available in: Injection
Available OTC? No   **As Generic?** No
Drug Class: Hormone; diagnostic agent

▼ USAGE INFORMATION

WHY IT'S PRESCRIBED
The adrenal glands manufacture steroids and other substances that are vital for overall health and well-being. Cosyntropin is used for diagnostic purposes when the adrenal gland is suspected of not working properly. The injection of cosyntropin forms the basis of a very simple, safe, and reliable test, taking 30 to 60 minutes, that measures adrenal gland function.

HOW IT WORKS
Cosyntropin is a synthetic form of corticotropin, a naturally occurring substance that stimulates the adrenal gland to release the hormone cortisol. After the injection of cosyntropin, blood tests will be performed to measure whether or not your adrenal gland was properly stimulated to produce cortisol.

▼ DOSAGE GUIDELINES

RANGE AND FREQUENCY
Adults: 0.25 mg injected into a vein or into a muscle. Children 2 years of age or less: 0.125 mg injected into a vein or muscle.

ONSET OF EFFECT
Within 30 minutes.

DURATION OF ACTION
Several hours at most.

DIETARY ADVICE
You may be given special dietary instructions for the period prior to diagnostic testing. If not, maintain your usual food and fluid intake. Follow other dietary restrictions, if any, as recommended by your doctor.

STORAGE
Not applicable.

MISSED DOSE
Not applicable.

STOPPING THE DRUG
Not applicable. This medication is designed to be administered only once. Your doctor will determine if further injections are needed at a later date.

PROLONGED USE
Cosyntropin is never used for extended periods; it is generally administered on a one-time only basis.

▼ PRECAUTIONS

Over 60: Adverse reactions are not anticipated in older patients.

Driving and Hazardous Work: The use of cosyntropin should not impair your ability to perform such tasks safely.

Alcohol: Alcohol should be avoided during the day or two before diagnostic testing is scheduled.

Pregnancy: Cosyntropin may be used during pregnancy; consult your physician for specific recommendations.

Breast Feeding: It is not known if cosyntropin passes into breast milk. However, no serious problems have been documented.

Infants and Children: Cosyntropin may be used safely in children.

OVERDOSE
Symptoms: No specific ones have been reported.

What to Do: An overdose of cosyntropin is unlikely, since it is administered under the close supervision of your doctor. No cases of overdose have been documented.

▼ INTERACTIONS

DRUG INTERACTIONS
None known.

FOOD INTERACTIONS
None known.

DISEASE INTERACTIONS
None known.

SIDE EFFECTS

SERIOUS
No serious side effects are associated with cosyntropin.

COMMON
No common side effects are associated with cosyntropin, especially since it is used for diagnostic rather than therapeutic purposes.

LESS COMMON
It has not been established whether cosyntropin produces any minor or rare side effects. In an extremely few number of instances, it has been shown to cause mild allergy-like reactions (mild fever, nausea, vomiting, or skin irritation and redness at the site of injection).

CROMOLYN SODIUM INHALANT AND NASAL

Available in: Inhalation aerosol, inhalation solution, nasal solution
Available OTC? Yes   **As Generic?** Yes
Drug Class: Respiratory inhalant

▼ USAGE INFORMATION

WHY IT'S PRESCRIBED
To control, through regular use, chronic bronchial asthma; or it may be used preventively just prior to exposure to certain conditions or substances (allergens such as pollen and dust mites, as well as cold air, chemicals, exercise, or air pollution) that can trigger an acute asthma attack (bronchospasm).

HOW IT WORKS
Cromolyn sodium inhibits the release of histamine, a naturally occurring substance that causes swelling, itching, sneezing, watery eyes, hives, and other symptoms of allergic reaction, including those that occur in association with an asthma attack.

▼ DOSAGE GUIDELINES

RANGE AND FREQUENCY
Inhalation aerosol— To prevent asthma symptoms: Adults and children age 5 and older: 2 inhalations 4 times a day, 4 to 6 hours apart. To prevent bronchospasm: Adults and children age 5 and older: 2 inhalations at least 10 to 15 minutes before exercise or exposure. Inhalation solution— To prevent asthma symptoms: Adults and children 2 and older: 20 mg, 4 times a day, 4 to 6 hours apart. Nasal solution— For hay fever: Adults and children age 6 and older: 1 spray in each nostril 3 to 6 times a day.

ONSET OF EFFECT
Inhalation: Up to 4 weeks. Nasal: Unknown.

DURATION OF ACTION
Unknown.

DIETARY ADVICE
This medication should be taken 30 minutes before meals.

STORAGE
Store in a tightly sealed container away from heat and direct light.

MISSED DOSE
Take it as soon as you remember. If it is near the time for the next dose, skip the missed dose and resume your regular dosage schedule. Do not double the next dose.

STOPPING THE DRUG
The decision to stop taking cromolyn sodium should be made in consultation with your doctor.

PROLONGED USE
If your symptoms do not improve after 4 weeks, consult your doctor.

▼ PRECAUTIONS

Over 60: No special problems are expected in older patients.

Driving and Hazardous Work: No special problems are expected.

Alcohol: No special precautions are necessary.

Pregnancy: In animal studies, large doses of cromolyn sodium have caused a decrease in successful pregnancies and a decrease in fetal weight. Human studies have not been done. Before taking cromolyn sodium, tell your doctor if you are currently pregnant or plan to become pregnant.

Breast Feeding: It is not known whether cromolyn sodium passes into breast milk. Mothers who wish to breast feed while taking this drug should discuss the matter with their doctor.

Infants and Children: The inhalation form of cromolyn sodium has not been shown to cause special problems in children. The nasal form has not been studied in children. Consult your pediatrician for specific advice.

Special Concerns: Clean the inhaler and other devices at least once a week.

OVERDOSE
Symptoms: None reported.

What to Do: An overdose of cromolyn sodium is unlikely to be life-threatening. However, if someone takes a much larger dose than prescribed, call your doctor, emergency medical services (EMS), or the nearest poison control center immediately.

▼ INTERACTIONS

DRUG INTERACTIONS
Before taking cromolyn sodium, check with your doctor if you are using any other prescription or over-the-counter drug.

FOOD INTERACTIONS
No known food interactions.

DISEASE INTERACTIONS
Before taking cromolyn sodium, consult your physician if you are undergoing treatment for any medical condition.

 SIDE EFFECTS ▼

SERIOUS
Difficulty swallowing; hives; itching; swelling of face, lips, or eyelids; rash; nosebleeds. Call your doctor immediately.

COMMON
Inhalation: Throat irritation or dryness. Nasal: Increased sneezing; burning, stinging, or irritation in nose.

LESS COMMON
Nasal: Cough, headache, postnasal drip, unpleasant taste.

CROMOLYN SODIUM OPHTHALMIC

Available in: Ophthalmic solution
Available OTC? No   **As Generic?** No
Drug Class: Antiallergy agent

▼ USAGE INFORMATION

WHY IT'S PRESCRIBED
To treat eye disorders associated with seasonal allergies. Such disorders include conjunctivitis (inflammation of the mucous membranes that line the inner surface of the eyelids and whites of the eyes) and keratitis (inflammation of the cornea).

HOW IT WORKS
Cromolyn inhibits the body's release of certain allergy-related chemicals including histamine, a naturally occurring substance that causes swelling, itching, sneezing, watery eyes, hives, and other symptoms of an allergic reaction.

▼ DOSAGE GUIDELINES

RANGE AND FREQUENCY
Adults and children age 4 and older: 1 drop 4 to 6 times a day in regularly spaced intervals. Children up to age 4: Use and dosage must be determined by your doctor.

ONSET OF EFFECT
The effect might not be felt for several days or possibly several weeks.

DURATION OF ACTION
Unknown.

DIETARY ADVICE
This drug can be used without regard to diet.

STORAGE
Store in a tightly sealed container away from heat, moisture, and direct light. Do not allow it to freeze.

MISSED DOSE
Apply it as soon as you remember. If it is near the time for the next dose, skip the missed dose and resume your regular dosage schedule. Do not double the next dose.

STOPPING THE DRUG
Use this drug as prescribed for the full treatment period.

PROLONGED USE
You should see your doctor regularly for tests and examinations if you take this drug for a prolonged period. The therapy may last for as long as 6 weeks.

▼ PRECAUTIONS

Over 60: No special problems are expected.

Driving and Hazardous Work: The use of ophthalmic cromolyn should not impair your ability to perform such tasks safely.

Alcohol: No special precautions are necessary.

Pregnancy: Adequate human studies have not been completed. Before taking ophthalmic cromolyn, tell your doctor if you are pregnant or plan to become pregnant.

Breast Feeding: Ophthalmic cromolyn may pass into breast milk; caution is advised. Consult your doctor for specific advice.

Infants and Children: Use and dosage for infants and children under the age of 4 years must be determined by your doctor.

Special Concerns: To use the eye drops, first wash your hands. Tilt your head back. Gently apply pressure to the inside corner of the eyelid and with the index finger of the same hand, pull downward on the lower eyelid to make a space. Drop the medicine into this space and close your eye. Apply pressure for 1 or 2 minutes while keeping the eye closed without blinking. Then wash your hands again. Make sure the tip of the dropper does not touch your eye, finger, or any other surface. If your symptoms do not improve or if they become worse, check with your doctor.

OVERDOSE
Symptoms: No specific ones have been reported.

What to Do: An overdose of ophthalmic cromolyn is unlikely to be life-threatening. However, if someone takes a much larger dose of the drug than prescribed or accidentally ingests the medicine, call your doctor, emergency medical services (EMS), or the nearest poison control center.

▼ INTERACTIONS

DRUG INTERACTIONS
Other drugs may interact with ophthalmic cromolyn. Consult your doctor for specific advice if you are taking any other prescription or over-the-counter medication.

FOOD INTERACTIONS
No known food interactions.

DISEASE INTERACTIONS
Caution is advised when taking ophthalmic cromolyn. Consult your doctor if you have any other medical condition.

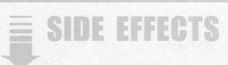

SIDE EFFECTS

SERIOUS
Rarely, ophthalmic cromolyn sodium causes a rash or redness around the eyes, swelling of the membrane covering the whites of the eyes, red or bloodshot eyes, or other eye irritation. Call your doctor immediately.

COMMON
Mild and temporary burning or stinging of the eyes.

LESS COMMON
Increased watering or itching of the eyes, dryness or puffiness around the eyes.

CYCLOBENZAPRINE

Available in: Tablets
Available OTC? No   **As Generic?** Yes
Drug Class: Muscle relaxant

▼ USAGE INFORMATION

WHY IT'S PRESCRIBED
To relieve painful, temporary muscle stiffness and spasms. It is not used for stiffness and spasms due to serious, chronic illnesses of the nervous system and muscles, such as spinal cord injury or cerebral palsy.

HOW IT WORKS
Cyclobenzaprine appears to work by decreasing nerve impulses from the brain and spinal cord that lead to tensing or tightening of muscles.

▼ DOSAGE GUIDELINES

RANGE AND FREQUENCY
Adults and teenagers 15 years of age and older: Usual dose is 10 mg, 3 times a day, which may be increased by your doctor to a maximum total dose of no more than 60 mg per day. Children and teenagers up to 15 years of age: Consult pediatrician.

ONSET OF EFFECT
Within 1 hour. The maximum effect may require 1 to 2 weeks of therapy.

DURATION OF ACTION
12 to 24 hours following a single dose.

DIETARY ADVICE
Dry mouth is a common complaint with muscle relaxants; maintain adequate fluid intake and suck on ice chips if desired.

STORAGE
Store in a tightly sealed container away from heat and direct light. Keep it away from moisture and extremes in temperature.

MISSED DOSE
Take it as soon as you remember. If it is near the time for the next dose, skip the missed dose and resume your regular dosage schedule. Do not double the next dose.

STOPPING THE DRUG
You should take it as prescribed for the full treatment period, but you may stop if you are feeling better before the scheduled end of therapy.

PROLONGED USE
Therapy with cyclobenzaprine is usually completed within 14 to 21 days. Do not take cyclobenzaprine for a longer period without your doctor's approval. Muscle pain and stiffness that does not improve within 14 to 21 days may require a more thorough evaluation.

▼ PRECAUTIONS

Over 60: Adverse reactions may be more likely and more severe in older patients.

Driving and Hazardous Work: The use of cyclobenzaprine may impair your ability to perform such tasks safely; use caution.

Alcohol: Avoid alcohol.

Pregnancy: Adequate studies of cyclobenzaprine use during pregnancy have not been done; discuss the relative risks and benefits with your doctor.

Breast Feeding: Cyclobenzaprine may pass into breast milk; caution is advised. Consult your doctor for advice.

Infants and Children: Cyclobenzaprine is not recommended for use by children under the age of 15.

Special Concerns: Cyclobenzaprine is not meant to be used as the only treatment for sore or stiff muscles. It should be accompanied by bed rest, physical therapy, and other measures to relieve discomfort, such as the application of heat or ice packs (as suggested by your physician).

OVERDOSE
Symptoms: Severe mental confusion, agitation, impaired concentration, difficulty walking or standing, dilated pupils, severe drowsiness, coma.

What to Do: Call emergency medical services (EMS), your doctor, or the nearest poison control center immediately.

▼ INTERACTIONS

DRUG INTERACTIONS
Consult your doctor for specific advice if you are taking sedatives, tranquilizers, or other medications that cause drowsiness (including alcohol); tricyclic antidepressants; or MAO inhibitors.

FOOD INTERACTIONS
No known food interactions.

DISEASE INTERACTIONS
Consult your doctor if you have a history of any of the following: glaucoma, difficult urination, prostate problems, heart disease, or overactive thyroid.

SIDE EFFECTS

SERIOUS
Unusual heartbeat (racing, pounding, or fluttering), confusion, seizures, hallucinations.

COMMON
Drowsiness, dry mouth, dizziness.

LESS COMMON
Fatigue or excessive tiredness, weakness, nausea, constipation, heartburn, unpleasant bitter or metallic taste in mouth, vision problems, headache, restlessness, nervousness, difficulty urinating, unusual bleeding or bruising.

CYCLOPENTOLATE

Available in: Ophthalmic solution
Available OTC? No   **As Generic?** No
Drug Class: Eye muscle relaxant, pupil enlarger

▼ USAGE INFORMATION

WHY IT'S PRESCRIBED
To dilate the pupils and temporarily paralyze certain structures within the eye. This is useful in eye examinations to help determine the proper prescription for eyeglasses or for other diagnostic procedures involving the eyes. It may also be needed before or after eye surgery.

HOW IT WORKS
Cyclopentolate relaxes the ciliary muscle, which controls the shape of the eye's lens as it focuses, and another eye muscle called the sphincter, which controls the narrowing and widening of the pupil. Relaxation of these muscles prevents the lens from focusing and widens the pupil. This allows the doctor to view the interior structures of the eye during an ophthalmologic procedure. And, by immobilizing the tiny structures within the eye, the drug prevents scarring of eye tissue and may alleviate eye pain.

▼ DOSAGE GUIDELINES

RANGE AND FREQUENCY
1 to 2 drops, applied 3 times a day or as needed as determined by your eye doctor.

ONSET OF EFFECT
Maximum effect occurs within 25 to 75 minutes.

DURATION OF ACTION
8 hours, although some effects may persist for up to several days.

DIETARY ADVICE
No special restrictions.

STORAGE
Store in a tightly sealed container away from heat, moisture, and direct light. Do not allow it to freeze.

MISSED DOSE
Apply it as soon as you remember. If it is near the time for the next dose, skip the missed dose and resume your regular dosage schedule. Do not double the next dose.

STOPPING THE DRUG
The decision to stop taking the drug should be made by your ophthalmologist.

PROLONGED USE
Not recommended for long-term therapy.

▼ PRECAUTIONS

Over 60: Adverse reactions may be more likely and more severe in older patients.

Driving and Hazardous Work: Do not drive or engage in hazardous work until you determine how the medicine affects your vision. Extreme caution should be observed for activities requiring sharp vision for close objects (less than an arm's length away).

Alcohol: No special precautions are necessary.

Pregnancy: Adequate studies have not been done. Inform your doctor if you are pregnant or are planning to become pregnant.

Breast Feeding: It is not known if cyclopentolate passes into breast milk; caution is advised. Consult your doctor for specific advice.

Infants and Children: Young children with blond hair or blue eyes may be more sensitive to the drug and may have an increased risk of side effects. Use with extreme caution. Infants should not eat for 4 hours following application of drops.

Special Concerns: To use the eye drops, first wash your hands. Tilt your head back. Gently apply pressure to the inside corner of the eyelid and with the index finger of the same hand, pull downward on the lower eyelid to make a space. Drop the medicine into this space and close your eye. Apply pressure for 1 or 2 minutes while keeping the eye closed without blinking. Then wash your hands again. Make sure that the tip of the dropper does not touch your eye, finger, or any other surface.

OVERDOSE
Symptoms: Drowsiness, hallucinations, memory problems, dry mouth, dry skin, restlessness, palpitations, dizziness and disorientation, delirium.

What to Do: Call your doctor, emergency medical services (EMS), or the nearest poison control center immediately.

▼ INTERACTIONS

DRUG INTERACTIONS
Consult your physician if you are taking any other prescription or over-the-counter drugs, especially those designed for use in the eyes.

FOOD INTERACTIONS
No known food interactions.

DISEASE INTERACTIONS
Consult your doctor if you have a history of glaucoma, Down syndrome, or spastic paralysis.

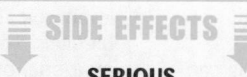

SIDE EFFECTS

SERIOUS
If absorbed into the bloodstream: Clumsiness or unsteadiness, confusion or changes in behavior, hallucinations, slurred speech, rapid or irregular pulse, flushing, fever, unusual fatigue, dizziness, unusually dry skin, skin rash, dry mouth; in infants, abdominal swelling. Seek medical assistance immediately.

COMMON
Eye irritation and redness not present prior to treatment, swelling of the eyelids, blurred vision, increased sensitivity to bright light.

LESS COMMON
There are no less-common side effects associated with the use of cyclopentolate.

CYCLOPHOSPHAMIDE

BRAND NAMES

Cytoxan, Neosar

Available in: Tablets, liquid for injection
Available OTC? No   **As Generic?** No
Drug Class: Antineoplastic (anticancer) agent; immunosuppressant

▼ USAGE INFORMATION

WHY IT'S PRESCRIBED
To treat a number of cancers, including malignant lymphoma, multiple myeloma, sarcoma, retinoblastoma, leukemia, breast cancer, and ovarian cancer. Cyclophosphamide is sometimes prescribed for other, noncancerous conditions, although this is done with extreme caution in light of the potentially serious side effects associated with it.

HOW IT WORKS
Cyclophosphamide kills cancer cells by interfering with the synthesis of their genetic material, which prevents malignant cells from multiplying.

▼ DOSAGE GUIDELINES

RANGE AND FREQUENCY
Adults— Oral dose for cancer: 1 to 5 mg for every 2.2 lbs (1 kg) of body weight, once a day, for 5 to 7 days every month. Injection: 40 to 60 mg a day, in divided doses, for 2 to 5 days, depending on the type of cancer treated. This drug should never be administered intravenously without additional intravenous fluids. The dosage may vary considerably, depending on the patient, the disease, and whether any other drugs are being taken. Children— Consult your pediatric oncologist.

ONSET OF EFFECT
2 to 3 hours.

DURATION OF ACTION
Unknown.

DIETARY ADVICE
Take it on an empty stomach; may be taken with small amounts of food or milk if stomach irritation occurs. Be sure to drink plenty of fluids.

STORAGE
Store the tablets in a tightly sealed container away from heat and light.

MISSED DOSE
Skip the missed dose and resume your regular dosage schedule. Do not double the next dose.

STOPPING THE DRUG
Continue taking this drug as prescribed, even if you experience side effects, such as nausea and vomiting. The decision to stop taking the medication should be made by your doctor.

PROLONGED USE
Prolonged use is associated with an increased risk of adverse effects. Consult your doctor about the need for periodic medical tests and examinations.

▼ PRECAUTIONS

Over 60: Side effects more common in older patients.

Driving and Hazardous Work: Avoid such activities until you determine how the medicine affects you.

Alcohol: Limit alcohol to moderate intake only.

Pregnancy: This drug can cause serious birth defects when taken by the mother or father. Use reliable birth control while taking this drug and for 4 months after therapy.

Breast Feeding: Use is not recommended while nursing.

Infants and Children: Cyclophosphamide can be used in children under close medical supervision.

Special Concerns: Watch for signs of infection, such as fever, sore throat, and fatigue. If your temperature rises above 100°F, call your doctor. To avoid urinary problems, drink a minimum of 3 quarts of water a day. Do not get vaccinated against bacteria or viruses while taking this drug.

OVERDOSE
Symptoms: Shortness of breath, palpitations, chest pain or discomfort, bloody urine, water retention, unusual weight gain, severe infection.

What to Do: Call emergency medical services (EMS) to receive evaluation and treatment in the closest emergency facility.

▼ INTERACTIONS

DRUG INTERACTIONS
Consult your doctor for specific advice if you are taking allopurinol or other gout medications, oral hypoglycemia drugs, clozapine, cyclosporine, digoxin or other antiarrhythmic drugs, other immunosuppressants, insulin, levamisole, lovastatin, phenobarbital, probenecid, sulfinpyrazone, or tiopronin.

FOOD INTERACTIONS
No known food interactions.

DISEASE INTERACTIONS
Consult your doctor if you have a recent history of chicken pox, shingles, gout, kidney stones, or infections. Use of this drug may cause complications in patients with liver or kidney disease, since these organs work together to remove the medication from the body.

⇊ SIDE EFFECTS ⇊

SERIOUS
Shortness of breath, chest tightness, chest or abdominal pain, persistent cough or hoarseness, fever and chills, pain in the lower back or sides, painful or difficult urination, tiny bright red dots on the skin, unusual bleeding or bruising, breathing difficulty, blood in the urine or stool. Call your doctor immediately should any of these occur.

COMMON
Nausea and vomiting, loss of appetite and weight, temporary hair loss, increased susceptibility to infections, loss of hearing or ringing in the ears, sterility in men (usually temporary), unusual fatigue, increased pigmentation in skin and fingernails, dizziness, confusion.

LESS COMMON
Diarrhea, stomach upset, flushing, skin rash, itching, or hives, rapid heartbeat, swelling in the feet or lower legs.

CYCLOSERINE

Available in: Capsules
Available OTC? No **As Generic?** No
Drug Class: Anti-infective/antitubercular agent

▼ USAGE INFORMATION

WHY IT'S PRESCRIBED
To treat active tuberculosis; used in conjunction with other antitubercular agents after use of the primary antitubercular agents, such as isoniazid, rifampin, ethambutol, pyrazinamide, and streptomycin, have proven ineffective.

HOW IT WORKS
Cycloserine kills tuberculosis bacteria by interfering with specific enzymes needed for the manufacture of cell walls.

▼ DOSAGE GUIDELINES

RANGE AND FREQUENCY
Adults and teenagers: To start, 250 mg every 12 hours for 2 weeks. If needed, your doctor may increase the dose to 250 mg every 6 to 8 hours; usually not more than 750 to 1,000 mg (6.8 mg per lb of body weight) a day. Children under age 12: 4.5 to 9 mg per lb per day. Cycloserine is taken in conjunction with other antitubercular agents. Vitamin B6 (pyridox-ine) should also be taken (at least 100 mg a day) to prevent nerve damage.

ONSET OF EFFECT
Unknown.

DURATION OF ACTION
Unknown.

DIETARY ADVICE
This medication may be taken with liquid or food to minimize stomach irritation.

STORAGE
Store in a tightly sealed container away from heat, moisture, and direct light.

MISSED DOSE
Take the drug as soon as you remember. This will help keep a constant level of medication in your system. If it is near the time for the next dose, skip the missed dose and resume your regular dosage schedule. Do not double the next dose.

STOPPING THE DRUG
Take it as prescribed for the full treatment period, even if you begin to feel better before the scheduled end of therapy. Treatment may continue for months or years. The decision to stop taking the drug should be made by your doctor.

PROLONGED USE
Consult your doctor about the need for having periodic medical examinations and laboratory tests.

▼ PRECAUTIONS

Over 60: Adverse reactions may be more likely and more severe in older patients. Smaller doses for shorter treatment periods may be warranted.

Driving and Hazardous Work: Do not drive or engage in hazardous work until you determine how the medicine affects you.

Alcohol: Avoid alcohol.

Pregnancy: No problems have been reported. In any case, tell your doctor if you are pregnant or plan to become pregnant before taking cycloserine.

Breast Feeding: Cycloserine may pass into breast milk; caution is advised. Consult your doctor for advice.

Infants and Children: Adequate studies of the use of cycloserine by children have not been done. Consult your pediatrician for advice.

Special Concerns: Before taking cycloserine, tell your doctor if you are depressed or have severe anxiety. Persons with a seizure disorder should not take cycloserine.

OVERDOSE
Symptoms: Seizures; drowsiness; confusion; dizziness; headache; extreme irritability; joint pain; psychosis; numbness, tingling, or prickling sensation in the hands or feet.

What to Do: Call your doctor, emergency medical services (EMS), or the nearest poison control center immediately.

▼ INTERACTIONS

DRUG INTERACTIONS
Ethionamide may interact with cycloserine. Consult your doctor for specific advice if you are taking it. Also tell your doctor if you are taking any other prescription or over-the-counter medication.

FOOD INTERACTIONS
No known food interactions.

DISEASE INTERACTIONS
Use of cycloserine may cause complications in patients with kidney disease, since the kidneys play a major role in removing the medication from the body. Caution is advised when taking cycloserine. Consult your doctor if you have any of the following: a seizure disorder, such as epilepsy; a history of alcohol abuse; mental depression; psychosis; or severe anxiety.

≡ SIDE EFFECTS ≡

SERIOUS
Dizziness, drowsiness, changes in mental state, depression, anxiety, suicidal thoughts, psychosis, confusion, nightmares, speech difficulties, increased irritability, muscle twitches, increased restlessness, skin rash, seizures. Call your doctor immediately.

COMMON
Headache; numbness, burning pain, prickling, tingling, or weakness in the hands or feet.

LESS COMMON
Abnormal heart rhythm, liver disease (hepatitis).

CYCLOSPORINE

Available in: Capsules, oral solution, injection
Available OTC? No   **As Generic?** No
Drug Class: Immunosuppressant

▼ USAGE INFORMATION

WHY IT'S PRESCRIBED
To slow down or reduce the natural tendency of the immune system to reject organ transplants. To treat severe rheumatoid arthritis or psoriasis that has not responded to other drug therapy.

HOW IT WORKS
Cyclosporine suppresses the functioning of the body's immune system. In this way it prevents the normal reaction against foreign substances or tissue that would otherwise cause the body to reject donor organs. Cyclosporine is also used to manage rheumatoid arthritis and psoriasis, as these disorders are classified as autoimmune diseases, that is, those in which the immune system inappropriately attacks healthy tissue.

▼ DOSAGE GUIDELINES

RANGE AND FREQUENCY
Your doctor will determine the correct dose based on a number of individual factors. During therapy, doses may be adjusted according to drug levels in the blood. The various brands of cyclosporine are not interchangeable.

ONSET OF EFFECT
Unknown.

DURATION OF ACTION
Unknown.

DIETARY ADVICE
Can be taken with food to avoid stomach upset. Oral solution can be taken with orange juice in a glass container, served at room temperature. Do not take cyclosporine with grapefruit juice.

STORAGE
Store in a tightly sealed container away from heat and direct light. Do not store the oral solution in the refrigerator. Injection: Not applicable.

MISSED DOSE
Take it as soon as you remember, up to 12 hours late. However, if more than 12 hours have elapsed since the time for the missed dose, skip the missed dose and resume your regular dosage schedule. Do not double the next dose.

STOPPING THE DRUG
The decision to stop taking cyclosporine should be made by your doctor.

PROLONGED USE
Prolonged use of cyclosporine may impair kidney function. Periodic exams and laboratory tests are required.

▼ PRECAUTIONS

Over 60: The dose must be adjusted for a possible decline in kidney function in older patients.

Driving and Hazardous Work: Do not drive or engage in hazardous work until you determine how the medicine affects you.

Alcohol: Avoid alcohol.

Pregnancy: Cyclosporine has been shown to cause serious birth defects in animals. Avoid this drug during pregnancy unless it is clearly needed.

Breast Feeding: Cyclosporine passes into breast milk; avoid or discontinue use while breast feeding.

Infants and Children: Cyclosporine has not been shown to affect children differently than adults.

Special Concerns: Avoid any immunizations except those approved by your doctor. Do not use plastic or wax-lined cups to take this medicine. Maintain good dental hygiene; this medication can cause gum problems. Cyclosporine can make you more sensitive to sunlight. Limit exposure until you determine how the drug affects you.

OVERDOSE
Symptoms: Yellowish tinge to the skin or eyes (jaundice), lethargy, confusion, swelling of body tissues.

What to Do: Call your doctor, emergency medical services (EMS), or the nearest poison control center immediately.

▼ INTERACTIONS

DRUG INTERACTIONS
Consult your doctor if you are taking androgens, cimetidine, danazol, diltiazem, diuretics, erythromycin, estrogens, other immunosuppressants, ketoconazole, statin (cholesterol-lowering) drugs, or virus vaccines. Many other drugs interact with cyclosporine. Consult your doctor before taking any new medicines, whether by prescription or over the counter.

FOOD INTERACTIONS
Do not take cyclosporine with grapefruit juice.

DISEASE INTERACTIONS
Consult your doctor if you have any of the following: chicken pox, shingles, high blood pressure, infection, a chronic gastrointestinal disorder, a blood disorder, kidney disease, or liver disease.

≡ SIDE EFFECTS ≡

SERIOUS
Frequent urge to urinate; fever or chills; yellow-tinged eyes and skin caused by liver problems; abnormal bleeding; fatigue; high blood pressure. Call your doctor immediately. Psoriasis patients formerly treated with other types of therapy (for example, ultraviolet light or methotrexate) are at increased risk of skin cancer; report any new skin lesion to your doctor immediately.

COMMON
Headache, tremor, unusual hair growth on body and face, swelling or bleeding of gums.

LESS COMMON
Nausea, vomiting, diarrhea, acne or oily skin, sinus inflammation or infection, leg cramps, enlargement and tenderness of the breasts in males (gynecomastia).

CYPROHEPTADINE HYDROCHLORIDE

BRAND NAMES

Periactin, Pyrohep

Available in: Syrup, tablets
Available OTC? No **As Generic?** Yes
Drug Class: Antihistamine; serotonin blocker

▼ USAGE INFORMATION

WHY IT'S PRESCRIBED
To prevent or relieve symptoms of rhinitis (inflammation of the mucous membranes of the nasal passages, often associated with hay fever and other seasonal allergies); skin itching and hives; and tissue swelling (angioedema). Cyproheptadine is also used as an appetite stimulant in patients with anorexia nervosa and to treat vascular headaches.

HOW IT WORKS
Cyproheptadine blocks the effects of histamine, a naturally occurring substance within the body that causes swelling, itching, sneezing, watery eyes, hives, and other symptoms of allergic reaction. It also blocks the brain chemical serotonin, and so may stimulate appetite and relieve the symptoms of vascular headaches.

▼ DOSAGE GUIDELINES

RANGE AND FREQUENCY
Adults and children over age 14: 4 mg every 8 hours. The dose may gradually be increased by your doctor.

Children ages 2 to 6: 2 mg every 8 to 12 hours. Children ages 6 to 14: 4 mg every 8 to 12 hours.

ONSET OF EFFECT
15 to 60 minutes.

DURATION OF ACTION
8 hours.

DIETARY ADVICE
Maintain your usual food and fluid intake. Increase fluid intake during persistent attacks, or if you have a fever or diarrhea.

STORAGE
Store in a tightly sealed container away from heat and direct light. Keep it away from moisture and extremes in temperature. Keep the liquid form refrigerated, but do not allow it to freeze.

MISSED DOSE
Take it as soon as you remember. However, if it is near the time for the next dose, skip the missed dose and resume your regular dosage schedule. Do not double the next dose.

STOPPING THE DRUG
Take it as prescribed for the full treatment period, but you may stop if you are feeling better before the scheduled end of therapy.

PROLONGED USE
Therapy with cyproheptadine may require days or weeks, depending on the severity of your allergies. Side effects may be more likely with prolonged use.

▼ PRECAUTIONS

Over 60: Adverse reactions may be more likely and more severe in older patients.

Driving and Hazardous Work: Because cyproheptadine may cause drowsiness, its use may impair your ability to perform hazardous tasks safely.

Alcohol: Avoid alcohol.

Pregnancy: Animal studies with high doses of cyproheptadine have found no birth defects. Human studies have not been done. Because the studies cannot rule out harm, the drug should be used during pregnancy only if it is clearly needed.

Breast Feeding: Cyproheptadine may pass into breast milk; caution is advised. Consult your doctor for advice.

Infants and Children: This drug is not recommended for use by children under 2 years of age.

Special Concerns: Children should be observed carefully for signs of side effects; they are more likely to develop serious complications from these medications, and younger children are often unable to describe changes in the way that they are feeling.

OVERDOSE
Symptoms: Hallucinations; convulsions; excitability or severe sedation; blurred vision; flushing or redness of skin; very dry, warm skin; wide, dilated pupils.

What to Do: Call your doctor, emergency medical services (EMS), or the nearest poison control center immediately.

▼ INTERACTIONS

DRUG INTERACTIONS
Consult your doctor for specific advice if you are taking medications containing alcohol or medications that may cause drowsiness, such as barbiturates, sedatives, cough medicines, other antihistamines, psychiatric medications (especially MAO inhibitors), and prescription pain medications.

FOOD INTERACTIONS
No known food interactions.

DISEASE INTERACTIONS
Consult your doctor if you have glaucoma or other visual disorders, prostate problems, or other problems urinating.

SIDE EFFECTS

SERIOUS
Confusion, hallucinations, seizures, restlessness, blurred vision, fainting, unusual or irregular pulse, wheezing.

COMMON
Dry mouth, dry nose, drowsiness (often transient).

LESS COMMON
Difficult urination, dizziness, increased sensitivity to sunlight, rash, weight gain, unusual excitement, irritability, or euphoria.

CYSTEAMINE BITARTRATE

BRAND NAME

Cystagon

Available in: Capsules
Available OTC? No   **As Generic?** No
Drug Class: Nephropathic cystinosis therapeutic agent

▼ USAGE INFORMATION

WHY IT'S PRESCRIBED
To treat the kidney-damaging form of cystinosis. People born without the ability to metabolize the amino acid cystine suffer from cystinosis, a rare inherited disorder characterized by the deposition and accumulation of cystine crystals throughout the body. These crystals cause considerable damage, particularly in the kidney. Kidney failure can occur by the age of 10 in untreated patients. Cysteamine prevents the accumulation of cystine crystals and is prescribed to prevent further kidney damage.

HOW IT WORKS
Cysteamine helps to convert cystine into less harmful chemical forms that can be removed from cells.

▼ DOSAGE GUIDELINES

RANGE AND FREQUENCY
Adults and teenagers weighing more than 110 pounds:

To start, 500 mg a day. Over a period of 4 to 6 weeks, your doctor will gradually increase the dose to a total of 2,000 mg per day, taken in 4 divided doses. Children up to age 12: Dose depends on weight and body surface area. White blood cell counts and cystine levels should be measured every 3 months until the proper dose is determined.

ONSET OF EFFECT
Unknown.

DURATION OF ACTION
As long as it is taken.

DIETARY ADVICE
Children or people who have difficulty swallowing the capsules may open them and sprinkle the contents onto food. Your doctor will recommend dietary and nutritional adjustments should kidney failure develop.

STORAGE
Store in a tightly sealed container away from heat, moisture, and direct light.

▼ SIDE EFFECTS

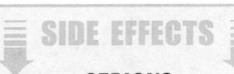

SERIOUS
Loss of appetite, fever, abdominal pain, nausea or vomiting, drowsiness, diarrhea, skin rash, confusion, dizziness, sore throat, mental depression, trembling, headache. Call your doctor as soon as possible. Side effects are most common when cysteamine is first started. Symptoms may improve when the drug is temporarily stopped or the dose is reduced.

COMMON
No common side effects are associated with the use of cysteamine.

LESS COMMON
Constipation, bad breath.

MISSED DOSE
Take it as soon as you remember, unless the time for your next scheduled dose is within the next 2 hours. If so, skip the missed dose and resume your regular dosage schedule. Do not double the next dose.

STOPPING THE DRUG
Continue to take the medicine as prescribed unless your doctor recommends that the dose be reduced or the drug be discontinued.

PROLONGED USE
Lifelong therapy with cysteamine bitartrate may be necessary.

▼ PRECAUTIONS

Over 60: No studies specifically on older patients have been done.

Driving and Hazardous Work: Do not drive or engage in hazardous work until you determine how the medicine affects you.

Alcohol: Avoid alcohol.

Pregnancy: Adequate human studies have not been done. Before taking cysteamine, tell your physician if you are pregnant or are planning to become pregnant.

Breast Feeding: It is not known whether cysteamine passes into breast milk; caution is advised. Consult your doctor for specific advice.

Infants and Children: Treatment should be started as soon as diagnosis of cystinosis is made. Your pediatri-

cian will determine the size and frequency of the dose.

Special Concerns: If you vomit your dose of cysteamine within 20 minutes of taking it, take the dose again. If you vomit again, do not repeat the dose. Wait until your next scheduled dose. If you vomit 20 minutes after taking the dose, do not repeat the dose.

OVERDOSE
Symptoms: An overdose is unlikely to occur or to be life-threatening.

What to Do: If you have any reason to suspect an overdose, call your doctor, emergency medical services (EMS), or the nearest poison control center.

▼ INTERACTIONS

DRUG INTERACTIONS
No drug interactions have been reported.

FOOD INTERACTIONS
No known food interactions.

DISEASE INTERACTIONS
The dose of cysteamine may need to be adjusted for patients with a medical history of seizures, blood problems, or any form of kidney disease.

DACARBAZINE

Available in: Injection
Available OTC? No **As Generic?** Yes
Drug Class: Antineoplastic (anticancer) agent

▼ USAGE INFORMATION

WHY IT'S PRESCRIBED
Dacarbazine is used for treatment of malignant melanoma (a type of skin cancer), Hodgkin's disease (a type of lymph node cancer), and occasionally sarcomas (uncommon cancers of the soft tissues).

HOW IT WORKS
Dacarbazine kills cancer cells by interfering with the synthesis of their genetic material, which prevents the cells from reproducing.

▼ DOSAGE GUIDELINES

RANGE AND FREQUENCY
The dose of dacarbazine depends on the type of tumor, patient weight, and whether other chemotherapy medicines are being used. Your oncologist (cancer specialist) will determine the proper dose.

ONSET OF EFFECT
Immediately after injection.

DURATION OF ACTION
Unknown.

DIETARY ADVICE
Maintain optimal food and fluid intake. Calorie, protein, and vitamin needs increase in patients with cancer. Good nutrition is essential to cope with the demands of chemotherapy.

STORAGE
Refrigerate, but do not allow it to freeze.

MISSED DOSE
Inform your oncologist if you miss a dose. Adjustments will be made depending on the other chemotherapy you receive.

STOPPING THE DRUG
The decision to stop dacarbazine must be made in consultation with your physician.

PROLONGED USE
Use beyond 5 to 10 days out of every 28 days in a chemotherapy cycle is not recommended.

▼ PRECAUTIONS

Over 60: Adverse reactions may be more likely and more severe in older patients.

Driving and Hazardous Work: The use of dacarbazine with other chemotherapy agents may impair your ability to perform such tasks safely.

Alcohol: Limit alcohol to moderate intake only.

Pregnancy: The use of chemotherapy during pregnancy could cause birth defects or fetal death. A reliable method of contraception is recommended while using this drug.

Breast Feeding: Dacarbazine passes into breast milk; you should avoid or discontinue use while breast feeding.

Infants and Children: Consult your pediatric oncologist.

Special Concerns: Dacarbazine may lower your ability to resist infection by reducing the number of white blood cells in the blood. Therefore, do not get vaccinated against bacteria or viruses without your doctor's approval. Avoid people with infections. Use care when shaving, trimming nails, or using sharp objects. Inform your doctor immediately if you have fever, chills, unusual bleeding or bruising, diarrhea, or a cough.

OVERDOSE
Symptoms: No specific information is available.

What to Do: If you are concerned about the possibility of an overdose of dacarbazine, call emergency medical services (EMS) to receive evaluation and treatment in the closest emergency facility.

▼ INTERACTIONS

DRUG INTERACTIONS
Consult your doctor if you are taking aspirin, ibuprofen, phenobarbital, phenytoin, amphotericin B, thyroid medications, azathioprine, chloramphenicol, colchicine, flucytosine, ganciclovir, interferon, plicamycin, or zidovudine.

FOOD INTERACTIONS
No known food interactions.

DISEASE INTERACTIONS
Consult your doctor if you have any of the following problems: chicken pox (or possible recent exposure to it), shingles, other infections elsewhere in your body, or kidney, liver, or lung disease.

SIDE EFFECTS

SERIOUS
Black, tarry, or bloody stools; blood-tinged (pink or maroon) urine; cough or hoarseness; fever; chills; lower back pain or pain in flanks; painful, difficult urination; tiny bright red spots on skin; bleeding from gums, nose, or other unusual places; easy bruising; shortness of breath. These side effects may mean that normal blood cells and special blood-clotting cells have been affected, or that normal immune cells have been affected and an infection is developing somewhere in your body. Contact your doctor immediately if any of these occur.

COMMON
Nausea, vomiting, weakness, loss of appetite. If pain or redness occurs at the injection site while dacarbazine is being administered, tell your physician or nurse immediately.

LESS COMMON
Flushing; unusual numbness or tingling of the face; flu-like symptoms (including muscle aches, fever, and joint pain) usually occurring about 7 days after treatment begins.

DALTEPARIN SODIUM

Available in: Injection
Available OTC? No   **As Generic?** No
Drug Class: Anticoagulant

▼ USAGE INFORMATION

WHY IT'S PRESCRIBED
To prevent or inhibit the formation of potentially dangerous blood clots within a blood vessel. Dalteparin is usually prescribed before major surgery, especially for prolonged operations that require general anesthesia. Those most likely to require the drug include patients who are over 40 years old, obese, immobile, suffering from a chronic debilitating disease, or who have had problems in the past with blood clots or who have a history of cancer.

HOW IT WORKS
Blood clotting (coagulation) is controlled by the interaction of many specialized proteins called coagulation factors. Dalteparin interferes with the normal functioning of several coagulation factors, thereby reducing the risk that a clot will form within a blood vessel. Anticoagulants, such as dalteparin, are often referred to as blood thinners.

▼ DOSAGE GUIDELINES

RANGE AND FREQUENCY
Adults: 2,500 international units injected under the skin once daily, beginning 1 to 2 hours prior to surgery, and continuing for 5 to 10 days afterward.

ONSET OF EFFECT
Rapid; within minutes.

DURATION OF ACTION
Therapeutic effect will persist for approximately 24 hours.

DIETARY ADVICE
Follow all of your doctor's dietary recommendations and other instructions carefully. Patients recovering from surgery require increased quantities of carbohydrates and proteins.

STORAGE
Not applicable; the dose is administered only at a health care facility.

MISSED DOSE
Hospital personnel will ensure that you are administered this medication on schedule.

STOPPING THE DRUG
The decision to stop taking the drug should be made by your doctor.

PROLONGED USE
Therapy with this medication is usually concluded within 5 to 10 days. Prolonged use may increase the risk of undesirable side effects.

▼ PRECAUTIONS

Over 60: Adverse reactions may be more likely and more severe in older patients.

Driving and Hazardous Work: Consult your doctor regarding the advisability of driving and performing hazardous work while taking an anticoagulant.

Alcohol: No special precautions are necessary.

Pregnancy: Adequate studies of the use of dalteparin during pregnancy have not been done; the drug should be used only if it is determined that benefits clearly outweigh potential risks. One form of dalteparin contains benzyl alcohol; this should not be used in pregnant women.

Breast Feeding: Dalteparin may pass into breast milk; caution is advised. Consult your doctor for specific advice.

Infants and Children: This drug is not recommended for use by children.

Special Concerns: Used properly, dalteparin prevents undesirable blood clots without seriously disrupting your ability to stop bleeding following minor injuries, scrapes, and bruises. Before taking this medication, be sure to inform your doctor if you have had any problem with unusual bleeding in the past. Occasionally, bleeding may occur internally and not be visible; primary symptoms are dizziness or weakness, especially when moving about or changing position. Keep in mind that such symptoms may occur following surgery for many reasons (use of pain medications or other drugs, or prolonged bed rest). It is important to tell your doctor about any changes in the way you are feeling during recovery period.

OVERDOSE
Symptoms: Unusual or uncontrolled bleeding, unusual bruising, weakness, or dizziness.

What to Do: Discontinue use and inform hospital personnel immediately.

▼ INTERACTIONS

DRUG INTERACTIONS
Consult your doctor if you are taking aspirin or other blood thinners.

FOOD INTERACTIONS
No known food interactions.

DISEASE INTERACTIONS
Caution is advised when taking dalteparin. Consult your doctor if you have allergies to pork or pork products, unusual bleeding or bruising, peptic ulcer, or high blood pressure, or if you have had recent surgery.

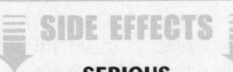

SIDE EFFECTS

SERIOUS
Easy or unusual bruising or bleeding, especially from the nose and gums, passage of black or tarry stools, vomiting or coughing of bright red blood, unusual weakness, dizziness.

COMMON
Pain or bruising at site of needle injection.

LESS COMMON
Shortness of breath, wheezing, breathing difficulty, confusion, hives, itching, rash, abdominal pain, facial swelling, sweating, weakness, lightheadedness (symptoms of anaphylaxis, a severe allergic reaction).

DANAZOL

Available in: Capsules
Available OTC? No   **As Generic?** No
Drug Class: Gonadotropin inhibitor

▼ USAGE INFORMATION

WHY IT'S PRESCRIBED
Danazol is used to treat endometriosis, fibrocystic breast disease, and a rare condition called hereditary angioedema, which causes abnormal swelling of body tissues.

HOW IT WORKS
Danazol blocks the production of the hormone estrogen by the ovaries. Without estrogen, endometrial tissue (the uterine lining) shrinks and becomes inactive. Subsequently, menstrual cycles cease, as do the hormone-related flare-ups of endometriosis and fibrocystic breast disease.

▼ DOSAGE GUIDELINES

RANGE AND FREQUENCY
Endometriosis: 100 to 400 mg, 2 times a day, beginning on the first day of menstrual flow. Treatment may take up to 6 months. Fibrocystic breast disease: 50 to 200 mg, 2 times a day, beginning on the first day of menstrual flow. Angioedema: 200 mg, 2 or 3 times a day. Increase in dosage may be necessary depending on results.

ONSET OF EFFECT
The full effect of danazol may take months to occur.

DURATION OF ACTION
Menstrual cycles return within 60 to 90 days after stopping danazol; breast discomfort due to fibrocystic disease may return within one year.

DIETARY ADVICE
Maintain your usual food and fluid intake. Increase fluids if you have a fever or diarrhea.

STORAGE
Store in a tightly sealed container away from heat and direct light. Keep away from moisture and extremes in temperature.

≡ SIDE EFFECTS ≡

SERIOUS
Yellow tinge in the eyes or skin (jaundice); headache, which may be accompanied by nausea, vomiting, and changes in vision; severe abdominal pain; fatigue; skin rashes, which may be extensive and involve the inside of the mouth and nose; unusual nosebleeds, vaginal bleeding, bleeding from gums, or other bruising and bleeding.

COMMON
Cessation of menstruation, irregular or unpredictable vaginal bleeding or spotting, decreased breast size, weight gain, edema (swelling due to fluid retention), flushing, sweating, vaginal dryness, acne.

LESS COMMON
Cataracts; pain or tingling in fingers; increased sensitivity to sunlight; increase in body hair; enlargement of clitoris; hoarseness, sore throat, or deepening of voice.

MISSED DOSE
Take it as soon as you remember. If it is near the time for the next dose, skip the missed dose and resume your regular dosage schedule. Do not double the next dose.

STOPPING THE DRUG
Take danazol as prescribed for the full treatment period, even if you begin to feel better before the scheduled end of therapy.

PROLONGED USE
Therapy with danazol is usually completed within 3 to 6 months, although it may be extended to 9 months if necessary. Prolonged use may be associated with an increased risk of side effects.

▼ PRECAUTIONS

Over 60: Adverse reactions may be more likely and more severe in older patients.

Driving and Hazardous Work: Do not drive or engage in hazardous work until you determine how the medicine affects you.

Alcohol: Drink alcohol only in moderation.

Pregnancy: Do not use danazol if you are pregnant.

Breast Feeding: Danazol must be avoided by women who are nursing.

Infants and Children: Danazol is not recommended for use by children.

Special Concerns: An effective method of contraception other than birth control pills (such as condoms or other barrier methods) should be used while taking danazol. Exposure of a fetus to danazol may lead to severe deformities. Be sure to report any unusual headache or change in vision to your physician. Some patients are treated successfully with one course of danazol; others require further treatments.

OVERDOSE
Symptoms: No specific ones have been reported.

What to Do: An overdose of danazol is unlikely to be life-threatening. However, if someone takes a much larger dose than prescribed, call your doctor, emergency medical services (EMS), or the nearest poison control center immediately.

▼ INTERACTIONS

DRUG INTERACTIONS
Consult your doctor for advice if you are taking anticoagulants (blood thinners).

FOOD INTERACTIONS
No known food interactions.

DISEASE INTERACTIONS
Consult your doctor if you have any of the following: heart or kidney disease; epilepsy or other seizure disorders; headaches, especially migraines; or any unexplained vaginal bleeding. Such conditions must be evaluated before starting danazol.

DANTROLENE SODIUM

Available in: Capsules, injection
Available OTC? No   **As Generic?** No
Drug Class: Muscle relaxant

▼ USAGE INFORMATION

WHY IT'S PRESCRIBED
To control recurrent muscle spasms and cramps, which may occur in association with multiple sclerosis, cerebral palsy, stroke, spinal cord injury, and other conditions. Dantrolene is sometimes used to prevent or control extremely high body temperature (malignant hyperthermia).

HOW IT WORKS
Calcium is necessary for muscle contraction; dantrolene directly interferes with the release of calcium in skeletal muscle tissue and thereby inhibits muscle cramping and spasms.

▼ DOSAGE GUIDELINES

RANGE AND FREQUENCY
For muscle spasms— Adults: 25 mg once a day to start, increased in 25 mg increments to 100 mg, 2 to 4 times a day, to a maximum of 400 mg a day. Children: 0.5 mg for each 2.2 lbs (1 kg) of body weight, 2 times a day to start; may be increased to a maximum of 100 mg, 4 times a day. For malignant hyperthermia: 4 to 8 mg for each 2.2 lbs of body weight in 3 or 4 doses a day.

ONSET OF EFFECT
1 to 2 weeks.

DURATION OF ACTION
Up to 24 hours.

DIETARY ADVICE
Capsules should be swallowed with milk or meals to prevent stomach upset.

STORAGE
Store in a tightly sealed container in a dry place away from heat and direct light.

MISSED DOSE
Take it if you remember within 2 hours. Otherwise, skip the missed dose and resume your regular dosage schedule. Do not double the next dose.

SIDE EFFECTS

SERIOUS
Seizures, yellowish tinge to eyes and skin (indicating serious liver inflammation), difficulty breathing caused by fluid in the lungs, unusual bleeding, blood in urine or stools, fever, severe diarrhea, weakness, rash, itching, hives. Call your doctor immediately.

COMMON
Muscle weakness, drowsiness, dizziness, headaches.

LESS COMMON
Nervousness, confusion, insomnia, hallucinations, rapid or irregular heartbeat, watery eyes, blood pressure changes, double vision, weight loss, constipation, cramps, difficulty swallowing, frequent urination, sensitivity to sunlight, sweating, unusual hair growth, muscle pain, chills.

STOPPING THE DRUG
The decision to stop taking the drug should be made by your doctor. Gradual reduction of the dose may be necessary if you have taken the drug for a long time.

PROLONGED USE
Tests that should be conducted periodically during prolonged use include blood counts, liver function studies, and G6PD tests.

▼ PRECAUTIONS

Over 60: Adverse reactions may be more likely and more severe.

Driving and Hazardous Work: Avoid such activites until you determine how the medicine affects you.

Alcohol: Avoid alcohol while taking this drug.

Pregnancy: Dantrolene has not been shown to cause birth defects in humans. Consult your doctor about its use during pregnancy.

Breast Feeding: Dantrolene passes into breast milk; avoid or discontinue use while breast feeding.

Infants and Children: This drug should be used in children only under close medical supervision.

Special Concerns: You may have trouble swallowing while taking dantrolene; take care to avoid choking. Follow your doctor's advice regarding rest and physical therapy.

OVERDOSE
Symptoms: Bloody urine, chest pains, shortness of breath, convulsions, loss of consciousness.

What to Do: Call your doctor, emergency medical services (EMS), or the nearest poison control center immediately.

▼ INTERACTIONS

DRUG INTERACTIONS
Consult your doctor for specific advice if you are taking acetaminophen, amiodarone, anabolic steroids, androgens, anti-infectives, antithyroid agents, calcium channel blockers (verapamil in particular), carbamazepine, central nervous system depressants, chloroquine, daunorubicin, disulfiram, divalproex, estrogens, etretinate, gold salts, hydroxychloroquine, mercaptopurine, methotrexate, methyldopa, naltrexone, oral contraceptives, phenothiazines, phenytoin, plicamycin, tricyclic antidepressants, or valproic acid.

FOOD INTERACTIONS
No known food interactions.

DISEASE INTERACTIONS
Caution is advised when taking dantrolene. Consult your doctor if you have any of the following: emphysema, asthma, bronchitis, another chronic lung disease, heart disease, or liver disease.

DELAVIRDINE

Available in: Tablets
Available OTC? No   **As Generic?** No
Drug Class: Antiviral

▼ USAGE INFORMATION

WHY IT'S PRESCRIBED
To treat HIV infection in combination with other drugs. While not a cure for HIV, it may suppress the replication of the virus and delay the progression of the disease.

HOW IT WORKS
Delavirdine interferes with the activity of enzymes needed for the replication of DNA in viral cells, thus preventing the human immunodeficiency virus (HIV) from reproducing.

▼ DOSAGE GUIDELINES

RANGE AND FREQUENCY
400 mg, 3 times a day. The tablets can be dissolved in water before being administered. Rinse the glass and drink the rinse water to be sure that the entire dose has been taken.

ONSET OF EFFECT
Unknown. With most antiretroviral drugs, an early response can be seen within the first few days of therapy, but the maximum effect may take 12 to 16 weeks.

DURATION OF ACTION
Unknown. Effects of the drug may be prolonged if delavirdine is used in combination with other effective drugs and the virus is maximally suppressed.

DIETARY ADVICE
No special restrictions.

STORAGE
Store in a tightly sealed container away from heat and direct light.

MISSED DOSE
Take it as soon as you remember. If it is near the time for the next dose, skip the missed dose and resume your regular dosage schedule. Do not double the next dose.

STOPPING THE DRUG
Take delavirdine every day, as prescribed. The decision to stop taking the drug should be made in consultation with your doctor.

PROLONGED USE
See your doctor regularly for tests and examinations for the duration of therapy.

▼ PRECAUTIONS

Over 60: A lower dose may be advised for older patients.

Driving and Hazardous Work: Do not drive or engage in hazardous work until you determine how the medicine affects you.

Alcohol: Avoid alcohol if liver function is impaired.

Pregnancy: Delavirdine has been shown to cause birth defects in animals. Nevertheless, it is increasingly being used with other antiretroviral drugs to treat pregnant HIV-infected women.

Breast Feeding: It is not known whether delavirdine passes into breast milk; however, women infected with HIV should not breast feed, to avoid transmitting the virus to an uninfected child.

Infants and Children: Safety and effectiveness of the use of this drug in children under 16 have not been established.

Special Concerns: Use of delavirdine does not eliminate the risk of passing the AIDS virus to other persons. Be sure to take appropriate preventive measures.

OVERDOSE
Symptoms: No cases of overdose have been reported.

What to Do: An overdose is unlikely to occur. Nonetheless, if you have any reason to suspect an overdose, seek medical assistance right away.

▼ INTERACTIONS

DRUG INTERACTIONS
Some drugs, when combined with delavirdine, may cause severe liver damage and so should not be taken. These drugs include certain nonsedating antihistamines, sedative hypnotic drugs, calcium channel blockers, ergot alkaloid preparations, amphetamines, and cisapride. Other drugs may interact with delavirdine, requiring changes in your drug regimen; consult your doctor for specific advice if you are taking any other prescription or over-the-counter medication, especially antacids, clarithromycin, fluoxetine, ketoconazole, phenytoin, phenobarbital, carbamazepine, rifabutin, rifampin, cimetidine, famotidine, nizatidine, ranitidine, didanosine, indinavir, ritonavir, nelfinavir, or saquinavir.

FOOD INTERACTIONS
No known food interactions.

DISEASE INTERACTIONS
No disease interactions have been reported.

SIDE EFFECTS

SERIOUS
Severe skin rash, fever, blistering, mouth sores, muscle or joint aches. Stop taking the medication and call your doctor immediately.

COMMON
Skin rash.

LESS COMMON
Abdominal cramps or pain, back or chest pain, chills, fatigue, lethargy, stiff neck, rapid breathing, migraine headache, fainting, loss of appetite, unusual gain or loss of weight, blood in stools, constipation or diarrhea, loss of appetite, gas, increased thirst, swollen or ulcerated tongue, leg cramps, swollen arms or legs, loss of coordination, amnesia, anxiety, decreased sexual function, depression, disorientation, dizziness, hallucinations, impaired concentration, insomnia, nightmares, restlessness, tremor, cough, breathing difficulty, hair loss, dry eyes, ear pain, ringing in ears, flank pain, blood in urine.

DESIPRAMINE HYDROCHLORIDE

Available in: Tablets
Available OTC? No **As Generic?** Yes
Drug Class: Tricyclic antidepressant

▼ USAGE INFORMATION

WHY IT'S PRESCRIBED
To relieve symptoms of major depression.

HOW IT WORKS
Desipramine affects levels of norepinephrine, a brain chemical that is thought to be linked to mood, emotions, and mental state.

▼ DOSAGE GUIDELINES

RANGE AND FREQUENCY
Adults: 100 to 200 mg once a day; may be increased to 300 mg a day. Older adults: 25 to 50 mg a day; may be increased to 150 mg a day.

ONSET OF EFFECT
1 to 6 weeks.

DURATION OF ACTION
Unknown.

DIETARY ADVICE
To lessen stomach upset, take with food, unless your doctor instructs otherwise. Increase your intake of fiber and fluids.

STORAGE
Store in a tightly sealed container away from heat, moisture, and direct light.

MISSED DOSE
If you take a one-time daily bedtime dose, do not take the missed dose in the morning because it may cause drowsiness. Call your doctor. If you take more than 1 dose a day, take it as soon as you remember. If it is near the time for the next dose, skip the missed dose and resume your regular dosage schedule. Do not double the next dose.

STOPPING THE DRUG
Take it as prescribed for the full treatment period, even if you begin to feel better before the scheduled end of therapy. The decision to stop taking desipramine should be made in consultation with your doctor. The dosage should be tapered gradually over a period of 5 to 7 days when stopping treatment.

PROLONGED USE
Usual course of therapy lasts 6 months to 1 year; some patients may benefit from additional therapy.

▼ PRECAUTIONS

Over 60: Adverse reactions may be more likely and more severe in older patients. A lower dose may be warranted.

Driving and Hazardous Work: Use caution when driving or engaging in hazardous work until you determine how the medication affects you. Drowsiness or lightheadedness can occur.

Alcohol: Avoid alcohol.

Pregnancy: Adequate studies have not been done. Consult your doctor for advice.

Breast Feeding: Desipramine passes into breast milk; do not use it while nursing.

Infants and Children: Not prescribed for children under age 16. Should not be prescribed for children, as unexplained deaths have occurred.

Special Concerns: This is a potentially dangerous drug, especially if taken in excess. Tricyclic antidepressants should not be within easy reach of suicidal patients.

OVERDOSE
Symptoms: Difficulty breathing, severe fatigue, seizures, confusion, hallucinations, distractibility, dilated pupils, irregular heartbeat, fever.

What to Do: Call your doctor, emergency medical services (EMS), or the nearest poison control center immediately.

▼ INTERACTIONS

DRUG INTERACTIONS
Consult your doctor for specific advice if you are taking antithyroid agents, cimetidine, cisapride, clonidine, guanadrel, guanethidine, metrizamide, appetite suppressants, isoproterenol, ephedrine, epinephrine, amphetamines, phenylephrine, antipsychotic drugs, pimozide, methyldopa, metyrosine, metoclopramide, pemoline, promethazine, trimeprazine, rauwolfia alkaloids, MAO inhibitors, or any drugs that depress the central nervous system.

FOOD INTERACTIONS
No known food interactions.

DISEASE INTERACTIONS
Consult your doctor if you have any of the following: a history of alcohol abuse, difficulty urinating, asthma, bipolar disorder, high blood pressure, stomach or intestinal problems, glaucoma, overactive thyroid, enlarged prostate, schizophrenia, seizures, a blood disorder, or kidney, heart, or liver disease.

≡ SIDE EFFECTS ≡

SERIOUS
Confusion, heartbeat irregularities, hallucinations, seizures, extreme fatigue or drowsiness, blurred or altered vision, breathing difficulty, constipation, impaired concentration, difficult urination, fever, extreme and persistent restlessness, loss of coordination and balance, difficulty swallowing or speaking, dilated pupils, eye pain, fainting. Also trembling, shaking, weakness, and stiffness in the extremities; shuffling gait. Call your doctor immediately.

COMMON
Drowsiness or dizziness, headache, dry mouth or unpleasant taste, fatigue, heightened sensitivity to light, weight gain, nausea, increased appetite.

LESS COMMON
Heartburn, difficulty sleeping, diarrhea, sweating, vomiting.

DESMOPRESSIN ACETATE

Available in: Injection, nasal solution, tablets
Available OTC? No   **As Generic?** Yes
Drug Class: Antidiuretic; antihemorrhagic

▼ USAGE INFORMATION

WHY IT'S PRESCRIBED
To treat diabetes insipidus, a relatively rare disorder characterized by excessive loss of water in the urine. Desmopressin is also used to help manage nighttime bedwetting. It may also be used to increase blood plasma levels of factor VIII, a crucial protein needed for clot formation. A deficiency of factor VIII may result in uncontrolled bleeding, the primary feature of hemophilia and a related disorder known as von Willebrand's disease type 1.

HOW IT WORKS
Desmopressin simulates the action of the hormone vasopressin, which helps the kidneys reabsorb water from urine, thus maintaining proper fluid balance. Helps to boost plasma levels of factor VIII.

▼ DOSAGE GUIDELINES

RANGE AND FREQUENCY
For diabetes insipidus— Injection: 2 to 4 mg, 1 or 2 times a day. Nasal solution: 1 to 2 sprays per day. Tablets: 0.1 to 0.8 mg, 2 times a day in divided doses. For bedwetting in patients age 6 and over— Tablets: 0.2 mg at bedtime. May be increased to 0.6 mg. For von Willebrand's type 1— Injection: 0.3 mg per 2.2 lbs (1 kg) of body weight per day. Lowest effective dose will be determined by the doctor based on the patient's response to the drug.

ONSET OF EFFECT
Within 1 hour.

DURATION OF ACTION
Injection or nasal spray: 12 to 24 hours. Tablets: Approximately 8 hours.

DIETARY ADVICE
Take it with or between meals.

STORAGE
Keep nasal or injectable forms refrigerated, but do not allow them to freeze. When traveling, these forms remain stable at room temperature for up to 3 weeks. Keep tablets at room temperature, away from heat and direct light.

MISSED DOSE
Take it as soon as you remember. If it is near the time for the next dose, skip the missed dose and resume your regular dosage schedule. Do not double the next dose.

STOPPING THE DRUG
The decision to stop taking the drug should be made by your doctor.

PROLONGED USE
No apparent problems with prolonged use of this drug.

▼ PRECAUTIONS

Over 60: Adverse reactions may be more likely and more severe in older patients.

Driving and Hazardous Work: Do not drive or engage in hazardous work until you determine how the medication affects you.

Alcohol: Drink alcohol only in moderation.

Pregnancy: Desmopressin has not been shown to cause birth defects in animals. While no adequate studies have been done in humans, the drug is presumed to be safe.

Breast Feeding: Desmopressin has not been shown to cause problems in nursing babies. Consult your doctor about its use if nursing.

Infants and Children: Adverse reactions may be more likely and more severe in children under age 18.

Special Concerns: Periodic laboratory tests are needed to check your fluid status. Desmopressin tablets used for bedwetting may be taken alone or in conjunction with other kinds of nonmedical therapy, such as behavioral conditioning.

OVERDOSE
Symptoms: Drowsiness, listlessness, headache, confusion, inability to urinate, unexpected weight gain or fluid retention.

What to Do: An overdose of desmopressin is unlikely to be life-threatening but can cause water intoxication (leading to symptoms above) and spasm of the blood vessels. If someone takes a much larger dose than prescribed, call your doctor, emergency medical services (EMS), or poison control center immediately.

▼ INTERACTIONS

DRUG INTERACTIONS
Large doses should be used with other "pressor" agents only with careful monitoring. Consult your doctor for advice if you are taking carbamazepine, chlorpropamide, demeclocycline, ethanol, fludrocortisone, heparin, lithium, norepinephrine, or tricyclic antidepressants.

FOOD INTERACTIONS
No known food interactions.

DISEASE INTERACTIONS
Consult your doctor if you have: seizures, migraine headaches, asthma, heart disease, blood vessel disease, congestive heart failure, or kidney disease.

SIDE EFFECTS

SERIOUS
Rare severe allergic reaction (skin rash, itching, wheezing, swelling of lips, tongue, and throat). In some cases water intoxication may occur, causing lethargy, nausea, vomiting, mental impairment, and in severe cases seizures or coma. Seek medical attention immediately.

COMMON
No common side effects are associated with the use of desmopressin.

LESS COMMON
Headache, flushing, nausea, abdominal cramps, and slight rise in blood pressure. Such symptoms are generally associated with excessive doses.

DEXAMETHASONE INHALANT AND NASAL

BRAND NAMES

Decadron Respihaler,
Dexacort Respihaler,
Dexacort Turbinaire

Available in: Oral inhalation, nasal spray
Available OTC? No   **As Generic?** No
Drug Class: Respiratory corticosteroid

▼ USAGE INFORMATION

WHY IT'S PRESCRIBED
To treat bronchial asthma; to treat allergic rhinitis (seasonal allergies such as hay fever); to prevent recurrence of nasal polyps after they have been removed surgically.

HOW IT WORKS
Respiratory corticosteroids such as dexamethasone primarily reduce or prevent inflammation of the lining of the airways, reduce the allergic response to inhaled allergens, and inhibit the secretion of mucus within the airways.

▼ DOSAGE GUIDELINES

RANGE AND FREQUENCY
Oral inhalation– Adults: To start, 3 inhalations 3 or 4 times a day; decreased as needed. Most patients respond to 2 inhalations 2 times a day. Children: 2 inhalations 3 or 4 times a day; decreased as needed. Most patients respond to 2 inhalations 2 times a day. Nasal spray– 2 sprays each nostril 3 times a day; decreased as needed.

ONSET OF EFFECT
Usually within 1 week; it may take 3 weeks for the full effect to occur.

DURATION OF ACTION
Unknown.

DIETARY ADVICE
No special restrictions.

STORAGE
Store in a tightly sealed container away from heat and direct light. Keep from getting cold; the medicine is less effective when cold.

MISSED DOSE
Take it as soon as you remember. However, if it is near the time for the next dose, skip the missed dose and resume your regular dosage schedule. Do not double the next dose.

STOPPING THE DRUG
The decision to stop taking the drug should be made by your doctor.

PROLONGED USE
Consult your doctor about the need for regular medical tests and examinations if you must take this drug for a prolonged period of time.

▼ PRECAUTIONS

Over 60: No special problems are expected.

Driving and Hazardous Work: The use of dexamethasone should not impair your ability to perform such tasks safely.

Alcohol: No special precautions are necessary.

Pregnancy: Nasal or inhaled steroids have not been reported to cause birth defects if taken during pregnancy. Before using such drugs, tell your doctor if you are pregnant or plan to become pregnant.

Breast Feeding: Dexamethasone may pass into breast milk; caution is advised. Consult your doctor for advice.

Infants and Children: Inhalation corticosteroids like dexamethasone have not been shown to cause different side effects or problems in children than they do in adults. Consult your doctor for specific advice.

Special Concerns: Inhaled steroids will not help an asthma attack in progress. Inhaled steroids can lower resistance to yeast infections of the mouth, throat, or voice box. To prevent yeast infections, gargle or rinse your mouth with water after each use; do not swallow the water. Know how to use the spray properly; read and follow the directions that come with the device. Before you have surgery, tell the doctor or dentist that you are using a steroid.

OVERDOSE
Symptoms: No specific ones have been reported.

What to Do: Call your doctor, emergency medical services (EMS), or the nearest poison control center right away if you have any reason to suspect an overdose.

▼ INTERACTIONS

DRUG INTERACTIONS
Consult your doctor for specific advice if you are taking systemic corticosteroids, other inhaled corticosteroids, or any medications that suppress the immune system.

FOOD INTERACTIONS
No known food interactions.

DISEASE INTERACTIONS
Caution is advised when taking dexamethasone. Consult your doctor if you have osteoporosis or a history of tuberculosis.

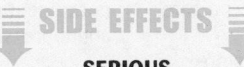
SIDE EFFECTS

SERIOUS
No serious side effects are associated with this drug.

COMMON
Nosebleeds or bloody nasal secretions, nasal burning or irritation, sore throat.

LESS COMMON
Eye pain, watering eyes, gradual decrease of vision, stomach pain and digestive disturbances.

DEXAMETHASONE OPHTHALMIC

Available in: Ophthalmic solution, suspension
Available OTC? No   **As Generic?** Yes
Drug Class: Corticosteroid

▼ USAGE INFORMATION

WHY IT'S PRESCRIBED
To control inflammation and prevent potentially permanent damage that may result from conditions that involve inflammation in the eye tissues.

HOW IT WORKS
Dexamethasone inhibits the release of natural substances that stimulate an inflammatory reaction.

▼ DOSAGE GUIDELINES

RANGE AND FREQUENCY
Solution or suspension: 1 or 2 drops in each eye up to 16 times a day.

ONSET OF EFFECT
Unknown.

DURATION OF ACTION
Unknown.

DIETARY ADVICE
This drug can be used without regard to diet.

STORAGE
Store in a tightly sealed container away from heat, moisture, and direct light. Do not allow it to freeze.

MISSED DOSE
Administer it as soon as you remember. If it is near the time for the next dose, skip the missed dose and resume your regular dosage schedule. Do not double the next dose.

STOPPING THE DRUG
Use this drug as prescribed for the full treatment period, even if symptoms improve before the scheduled end of the therapy.

PROLONGED USE
See your doctor regularly for tests and examinations if you must take this drug for a prolonged period.

▼ PRECAUTIONS

Over 60: No special problems are expected.

Driving and Hazardous Work: Avoid such activities until you determine how the medicine affects your vision.

Alcohol: No special precautions are necessary.

Pregnancy: Ophthalmic dexamethasone has caused birth defects in animals. Reliable human studies have not been done, but no human birth defects have been documented. Before you use this drug, tell your doctor if you are pregnant or plan to become pregnant.

Breast Feeding: This drug has not been reported to cause problems in nursing babies. Consult your doctor for specific advice.

Infants and Children: Children under age 2 may be especially sensitive to the effects of this drug.

Special Concerns: To use the eye drops, first wash your hands. Tilt your head back. Gently apply pressure to the inside corner of the eyelid and with the index finger of the same hand, pull downward on the lower eyelid to make a space. Drop the medicine into this space and close your eye. Apply pressure for 1 or 2 minutes while keeping the eye closed without blinking. Then wash your hands again. Make sure the tip of the dropper does not touch your eye, finger, or any other surface. If your symptoms do not improve in 5 to 7 days or if they become worse, check with your doctor. Wearing contact lenses while using this medication may increase the risk of infection. Your doctor may tell you not to wear contact lenses during and for a day or two after treatment.

OVERDOSE

Symptoms: When applied topically, an overdose of ophthalmic dexamethasone is very unlikely. Inadvertent oral ingestion, however, may cause fever, muscle weakness, nausea, loss of appetite, dizziness, fainting, or difficulty breathing.

What to Do: An overdose of this drug is unlikely to be life-threatening. However, if someone takes a much larger dose than prescribed or accidentally ingests the medicine, call your doctor, emergency medical services (EMS), or the nearest poison control center.

▼ INTERACTIONS

DRUG INTERACTIONS
Other drugs may interact with ophthalmic dexamethasone. Consult your doctor for specific advice if you are taking any other prescription or over-the-counter medication.

FOOD INTERACTIONS
No known food interactions.

DISEASE INTERACTIONS
Caution is advised when taking ophthalmic dexamethasone. Consult your doctor if you have any of the following: diabetes, herpes infection of the eye, glaucoma, cataracts, tuberculosis of the eye, or any other eye infection.

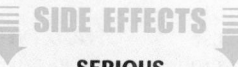

SIDE EFFECTS

SERIOUS
Decreased vision or blurring of vision (from cataract); eye pain, nausea, vomiting (from increased eye pressure); pain, redness, sensitivity to bright light, discharge (from eye infection). Call your doctor immediately if you experience any of these signs or symptoms. This drug may trigger a recurrence of herpes infection of the eye; mention any previous herpes infection to your doctor.

COMMON
No common side effects have been reported.

LESS COMMON
Burning, stinging, redness, or watering of eyes.

DEXAMETHASONE SYSTEMIC

Available in: Elixir, oral solution, tablets, injection
Available OTC? No   **As Generic?** Yes
Drug Class: Corticosteroid

▼ USAGE INFORMATION

WHY IT'S PRESCRIBED
To treat numerous conditions that involve inflammation (a response by body tissues, producing redness, warmth, swelling, and pain). Such conditions include arthritis, allergic reactions, asthma, some skin diseases, multiple sclerosis flare-ups, and other autoimmune diseases. Also prescribed to treat deficiency of natural steroid hormones.

HOW IT WORKS
This hormone mimics the effects of the body's natural corticosteroids. It depresses the synthesis, release, and activity of inflammation-producing body chemicals. It also suppresses the activity of the immune system.

▼ DOSAGE GUIDELINES

RANGE AND FREQUENCY
Adults and teenagers— Oral dosage: 25 to 300 mg a day, depending on condition, in 1 or several doses. Injection: 20 to 300 mg once a day, depending on condition. Children— Consult your doctor.

ONSET OF EFFECT
Within 2 hours of oral form, 1 hour of injection.

DURATION OF ACTION
More than 2 days for oral form; 6 days after injection.

DIETARY ADVICE
It can be taken with food or milk to minimize stomach upset. Your doctor may recommend a low-salt, high-potassium, high-protein diet.

STORAGE
Store in a tightly sealed container away from heat, moisture, and direct light.

MISSED DOSE
Take it as soon as you remember. If you take several doses a day and it is close to the next dose, double the next dose. If you take 1 dose a day and you do not remember until the next day, skip the missed dose and do not double the next dose.

STOPPING THE DRUG
With long-term therapy, do not stop taking the drug abruptly; the dosage should be decreased gradually.

PROLONGED USE
See your doctor regularly for tests and examinations. Long-term use may lead to cataracts, diabetes, hypertension, or osteoporosis.

▼ PRECAUTIONS

Over 60: Adverse reactions may be more likely and more severe in older patients.

Driving and Hazardous Work: Do not drive or engage in hazardous work until you determine how the medicine affects you.

Alcohol: May cause stomach problems; avoid it unless your physician approves occasional moderate drinking.

Pregnancy: Overuse during pregnancy can retard the child's growth and cause other developmental problems. Consult your physician.

Breast Feeding: Do not use while nursing.

Infants and Children: Dexamethasone may retard the normal growth and development of bone and other tissues. Consult your doctor.

Special Concerns: Avoid immunizations with live vaccines if possible. Remember that this drug can lower your resistance to infection. Patients undergoing long-term therapy should wear a medical-alert bracelet. Call your doctor if you develop a fever.

OVERDOSE
Symptoms: Fever, muscle or joint pain, nausea, dizziness, fainting, difficulty breathing. Prolonged overuse: Moon-face, obesity, unusual hair growth, acne, loss of sexual function, muscle wasting.

What to Do: Call your doctor, emergency medical services (EMS), or the nearest poison control center immediately.

▼ INTERACTIONS

DRUG INTERACTIONS
Consult your doctor for specific advice if you are taking aminoglutethimide, antacids, barbiturates, carbamazepine, griseofulvin, mitotane, phenylbutazone, phenytoin, primidone, rifampin, injectable amphotericin B, oral antidiabetes agents, insulin, digitalis drugs, diuretics, or medications containing potassium or sodium.

FOOD INTERACTIONS
Avoid excess sodium.

DISEASE INTERACTIONS
Consult your doctor if you have a history of bone disease, chicken pox, measles, gastrointestinal disorders, diabetes, recent serious infection, tuberculosis, glaucoma, heart disease, hypertension, liver or kidney disorders, high blood cholesterol, overactive or underactive thyroid, myasthenia gravis, or lupus.

SIDE EFFECTS

SERIOUS
Vision problems, frequent urination, increased thirst, rectal bleeding, blistering skin, confusion, hallucinations, paranoia, euphoria, depression, mood swings, redness and swelling at injection site. Call your doctor immediately.

COMMON
Increased appetite, indigestion, nervousness, insomnia, greater susceptibility to infections, increased blood pressure, slow healing of wounds, weight gain, easy bruising, fluid retention.

LESS COMMON
Change in skin color, dizziness, headache, increased sweating, unusual growth of body or facial hair, increased blood sugar, peptic ulcers, adrenal insufficiency, muscle weakness, cataracts, glaucoma, osteoporosis.

DEXAMETHASONE TOPICAL

Available in: Gel, aerosol solution, cream
Available OTC? No   **As Generic?** Yes
Drug Class: Topical corticosteroid

▼ USAGE INFORMATION

WHY IT'S PRESCRIBED
To treat skin rash and inflammation. Topical steroids come in many strengths; dexamethasone is a lower-strength steroid, which is safest and most appropriate for certain minor skin conditions.

HOW IT WORKS
Topical dexamethasone appears to interfere with the formation of natural substances within the body that are directly responsible for the process of inflammation, which produces swelling, redness, and pain.

▼ DOSAGE GUIDELINES

RANGE AND FREQUENCY
Gel (0.1% strength)– Apply 2 or 3 times daily. Aerosol (0.01% and 0.04% strength)– Adults: Apply 2 to 4 times daily. Children: 1 or 2 times daily. Cream (0.1% strength)– Adults: Apply 3 or 4 times daily. Children: once daily.

ONSET OF EFFECT
Soon after application. However, recognizable changes in your condition may take several days or more to develop.

DURATION OF ACTION
Unknown.

DIETARY ADVICE
No special restrictions.

STORAGE
Store in a tightly sealed container away from heat and direct light.

MISSED DOSE
Apply it as soon as you remember. If it is near the time for the next dose, skip the missed dose and resume your regular dosage schedule.

STOPPING THE DRUG
Take as prescribed for the full treatment period.

PROLONGED USE
Avoid prolonged use, particularly near the eyes, on the face, genital, or rectal areas, or in the folds of the skin.

▼ PRECAUTIONS

Over 60: Side effects may be more likely and more severe in elderly patients; therapy with topical corticosteroids should therefore be brief and infrequent.

Driving and Hazardous Work: The use of topical dexamethasone should not impair your ability to perform such tasks safely.

Alcohol: No special precautions are necessary.

Pregnancy: This drug should not be used for prolonged periods by pregnant women or women trying to become pregnant.

Breast Feeding: Although problems have not been documented, caution is advised. Do not apply to breasts prior to nursing. Consult your doctor for specific advice.

Infants and Children: It should not be used for more than 2 weeks on children and teenagers, unless otherwise directed by your doctor. Do not use tight-fitting diapers or plastic pants on children when treating skin irritation in the diaper area.

Special Concerns: Take care to avoid use of this medication around the eyes. Take care to apply only to the affected area. Note that dexamethasone is not a treatment for acne, burns, infections, or disorders of pigmentation. Do not bandage or wrap the medicated area of skin with any special dressings or coverings unless specifically told to do so by your doctor.

Applying special coverings may increase the chance of an undesirable interaction or side effect.

OVERDOSE
Symptoms: None known.

What to Do: An overdose of a topical corticosteroid is unlikely to be life-threatening. However, in the event of accidental ingestion or an apparent overdose, call your doctor, emergency medical services (EMS), or the nearest poison control center as soon as possible.

▼ INTERACTIONS

DRUG INTERACTIONS
Do not mix topical dexamethasone with other products, especially alcohol-containing preparations (which include colognes, aftershave, and many moisturizer lotions), since this may cause dryness and irritation, or increase the risk of an allergic reaction.

FOOD INTERACTIONS
Potassium supplements may decrease this drug's effects. Avoid foods high in sodium.

DISEASE INTERACTIONS
Consult your doctor if you have any of the following: cataracts; diabetes mellitus; glaucoma; infection, sores, or ulcerations of the skin; infection elsewhere in your body; or tuberculosis.

≡ SIDE EFFECTS ≡

SERIOUS
No serious side effects are associated with topical dexamethasone.

COMMON
Burning, itching, irritation, redness, dryness, acne, stinging and cracking of skin, numbness or tingling in the extremities. Such side effects are unlikely to occur except when topical dexamethasone is used with bandages or other occlusive dressings.

LESS COMMON
With prolonged use: Blistering and pus near hair follicles, unusual bleeding or bruising, darkening or prominence of small surface veins, increased susceptibility to infection.

DEXTROAMPHETAMINE SULFATE

Available in: Extended-release capsules, tablets
Available OTC? No **As Generic?** No
Drug Class: Central nervous system stimulant/amphetamine

▼ USAGE INFORMATION

WHY IT'S PRESCRIBED
To treat attention-deficit hyperactivity disorder, sometimes referred to as ADHD or simply hyperactivity. It is also used to treat narcolepsy (uncontrolled onset of sleep).

HOW IT WORKS
Dextroamphetamine activates nerve cells in the brain and spinal cord to increase motor activity and alertness and lessen drowsiness and fatigue. In hyperactivity disorders and narcolepsy, amphetamines improve mental focus and the ability to stay awake or concentrate.

▼ DOSAGE GUIDELINES

RANGE AND FREQUENCY
To treat ADHD— Adults: 5 to 60 mg a day. Children age 6 and older: To start, 5 mg, 1 or 2 times a day. Children ages 3 to 6: To start, 2.5 mg a day. To treat narcolepsy— Adults: 5 to 60 mg a day. Teenagers: To start, 10 mg once a day. Children ages 6 to 12: To start, 5 mg once a day.

ONSET OF EFFECT
Usually within 30 to 45 minutes for tablets, and somewhat later for extended-release capsules.

DURATION OF ACTION
In adults, 8 to 12 hours; in children, 6 to 10 hours. Extended-release capsules have a somewhat longer duration of action.

DIETARY ADVICE
Take it with liquid 30 to 45 minutes before meals. Avoid caffeinated beverages like tea, coffee, and some colas. Avoid vitamin C pills and acidic foods rich in vitamin C, such as fruit juices and other citrus products.

STORAGE
Store in a tightly sealed container away from heat, moisture, and direct light.

MISSED DOSE
Take it as soon as you remember. If it is near the time for the next dose, skip the missed dose and resume your regular dosage schedule. Do not double the next dose.

STOPPING THE DRUG
Take it as prescribed for the full treatment period, even if you begin to feel better before the scheduled end of therapy. The decision to stop taking the drug should be made by your doctor. The doctor may decrease your dosage gradually to reduce the possibility of withdrawal symptoms.

PROLONGED USE
Amphetamines can be habit-forming, and prolonged use may increase the risk of dependency.

▼ PRECAUTIONS

Over 60: Adverse reactions may be more likely and more severe in older patients.

Driving and Hazardous Work: Do not drive or engage in hazardous work until you determine how the medicine affects you.

Alcohol: Avoid alcohol.

Pregnancy: Adequate human studies have not been completed. Before taking dextroamphetamine, tell your doctor if you are pregnant or plan to become pregnant.

Breast Feeding: Dextroamphetamine passes into breast milk; caution is advised. Consult your doctor for advice.

Infants and Children: Not recommended for use by children under age 3.

Special Concerns: Take only as directed and do not increase the dose on your own. Remember that fatigue, excessive drowsiness, sleepiness, or depression while taking stimulants may mean an emergency situation is developing. Difficulty sleeping may be improved by taking the last scheduled dose several hours before bedtime.

OVERDOSE
Symptoms: Extreme restlessness, agitation, or bizarre behavior; panic; rapid breathing; confusion; high fever; hallucinations; seizures; coma.

What to Do: Call your doctor, emergency medical services (EMS), or the nearest poison control center immediately.

▼ INTERACTIONS

DRUG INTERACTIONS
Consult your doctor for specific advice if you are taking tricyclic antidepressants, caffeine, beta-blockers, digitalis drugs, central nervous system stimulants, meperidine, MAO inhibitors, sympathomimetic agents, or thyroid hormones.

FOOD INTERACTIONS
Citrus juices and caffeinated beverages and foods may interact with this drug.

DISEASE INTERACTIONS
Consult your doctor if you have any of the following: advanced blood vessel disease, heart disease, hyperthyroidism, hypertension, severe anxiety, Tourette's syndrome, glaucoma, or a history of drug abuse.

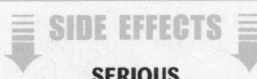

SIDE EFFECTS

SERIOUS
Irregular heartbeat, chest pain, increased blood pressure, skin rash, uncontrollable movements of arms and legs, mental changes, unusual weakness, very high fever. Call your doctor immediately.

COMMON
Mood changes, insomnia, drowsiness, restlessness.

LESS COMMON
Blurred vision, constipation, diarrhea, loss of appetite, headache, increased sweating, stomach cramps or pain, nausea or vomiting, changes in sexual desire or decreased sexual ability.

DEXTROMETHORPHAN

Available in: Capsules, lozenges, tablets, oral suspension, syrup
Available OTC? Yes **As Generic?** Yes
Drug Class: Cough suppressant

▼ USAGE INFORMATION

WHY IT'S PRESCRIBED
To relieve a dry or minimally productive cough (that is, a mild cough that rids the lungs of modest amounts of phlegm or mucus), commonly associated with allergies, colds, influenza, and certain lung disorders. This medicine is ideally useful when a mild or hacking cough would otherwise interrupt sleep or interfere with your daily activities.

HOW IT WORKS
Dextromethorphan works by directly reducing the sensitivity of the cough center—the part of the brain that responds to stimuli in the lower respiratory passages that irritate and trigger the cough reflex.

▼ DOSAGE GUIDELINES

RANGE AND FREQUENCY
Adults: 10 to 20 mg every 4 hours or 30 mg every 6 to 8 hours; 30 to 60 mg of extended-release liquid twice a day. Children 6 to 12: 5 to 10 mg every 4 hours or 30 mg of extended-release liquid twice a day. Children 2 to 6: 2.5 to 5 mg every 4 hours, or 7.5 mg every 6 to 8 hours, or 15 mg of the extended-release liquid twice a day. Children under 2: Dosage must be individualized.

ONSET OF EFFECT
15 to 30 minutes.

DURATION OF ACTION
Up to 6 hours.

DIETARY ADVICE
No special restrictions.

STORAGE
Store in a tightly sealed container away from heat, moisture, and direct light.

MISSED DOSE
Take it as soon as you remember. However, if it is near the time for the next dose, skip the missed dose and resume your regular dosage schedule. Do not double the next dose.

STOPPING THE DRUG
Take it as prescribed for the full treatment period. However, you may stop taking the drug if you are feeling better before the scheduled end of therapy. If the cough does not improve after 7 days, consult your doctor.

PROLONGED USE
No problems are expected.

▼ PRECAUTIONS

Over 60: Side effects may be more frequent and severe than in younger persons. Smaller doses for shorter periods may be needed. If this drug is used to control coughing, other treatment measures may be needed to liquefy any accumulation of thick mucus that may form in the bronchial tubes.

Driving and Hazardous Work: Determine whether it causes drowsiness or dizziness before you drive or engage in hazardous work.

Alcohol: Avoid alcohol while using this drug; it may increase the risk of sedation.

Pregnancy: Ask your doctor whether the benefits of the drug justify the possible risk to the fetus.

Breast Feeding: Dextromethorphan may pass into breast milk; caution is advised. Consult your doctor for specific advice about taking dextromethorphan while you are nursing.

Infants and Children: Doses for children under 2 must be individualized; consult your pediatrician.

Special Concerns: Do not take dextromethorphan to relieve a cough caused by asthma, emphysema, or smoking.

OVERDOSE
Symptoms: Nausea, vomiting, extreme drowsiness or dizziness, nervousness and agitation, extreme irritability or mood changes, hallucinations, blurred vision, uncontrollable eye movement, inability to urinate, confusion, loss of consciousness, or coma.

What to Do: Call your doctor, emergency medical services (EMS), or the nearest poison control center immediately.

▼ INTERACTIONS

DRUG INTERACTIONS
Taking a sedative or other depressant can increase the sedative effects of both drugs. Using doxepin increases the toxic effects of both drugs. Taking an MAO inhibitor can cause a high fever, disorientation, or loss of consciousness. Using quinidine increases the risk of experiencing side effects with dextromethorphan.

FOOD INTERACTIONS
No known food interactions.

DISEASE INTERACTIONS
Caution is advised when taking dextromethorphan. Consult your doctor if you have a history of asthma or impaired liver function.

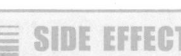
SIDE EFFECTS

SERIOUS
Serious side effects occur only in cases of overdose (see Overdose).

COMMON
No common side effects are associated with this drug.

LESS COMMON
Mild dizziness or sedation, nausea or vomiting, abdominal pain. Such symptoms are more likely to occur at the beginning of therapy and tend to diminish as your body becomes accustomed to taking the drug. Consult your doctor if they persist or interfere with daily activities.

DIAZEPAM

BRAND NAMES

Di-Tran, Diastat, Diazepam Intensol, Diazepm, T-Quil, Valium, Valrelease, Vazepam, X-O'Spaz, Zetran

Available in: Tablets, capsules, injection, rectal gel
Available OTC? No   **As Generic?** Yes
Drug Class: Benzodiazepine tranquilizer; antianxiety agent/muscle relaxant

▼ USAGE INFORMATION

WHY IT'S PRESCRIBED
To treat anxiety, panic attacks, and muscle spasms; also used in acute treatment of seizures.

HOW IT WORKS
In general, diazepam produces mild sedation by depressing activity in the central nervous system. In particular, diazepam appears to enhance the effect of gamma-aminobutyric acid (GABA), a natural chemical that inhibits the firing of neurons and dampens the transmission of nerve signals, thus decreasing nervous excitation.

▼ DOSAGE GUIDELINES

RANGE AND FREQUENCY
For anxiety— Adults: 2 to 10 mg, 4 times a day. Children: 1 to 2.5 mg, 3 or 4 times a day. For muscle spasms— 2 to 10 mg, 2 to 4 times a day. For treatment of seizures— Injection and rectal gel: Your doctor will determine the correct dosage.

ONSET OF EFFECT
30 minutes.

DURATION OF ACTION
Up to 48 hours.

DIETARY ADVICE
No special restrictions.

STORAGE
Store in a tightly sealed container away from heat, moisture, and direct light.

MISSED DOSE
Take the missed dose if you remember within 2 hours. If more than 2 hours, skip the missed dose and return to your regular schedule. Do not double the next dose.

STOPPING THE DRUG
Discontinuing the drug abruptly may produce withdrawal symptoms (seizures, sleep disruption, nervousness, irritability, diarrhea, abdominal cramps, muscle aches, memory impairment). Dosage should be reduced gradually according to your physician's instructions.

PROLONGED USE
Diazepam may slowly lose its effectiveness with prolonged use. You should see your doctor for periodic evaluation if you must take it for an extended time.

▼ PRECAUTIONS

Over 60: Dosage is often reduced because adverse reactions are more likely and may be more severe in older patients.

Driving and Hazardous Work: Diazepam can impair mental alertness and physical coordination. Adjust your activities accordingly.

Alcohol: Alcohol intake should be extremely moderate or stopped altogether while taking this drug.

Pregnancy: Use during pregnancy should be avoided if possible. Be sure to tell your doctor if you are pregnant or plan to become pregnant.

Breast Feeding: Diazepam passes into breast milk; do not take it while nursing.

Infants and Children: Diazepam should be used by children only under close medical supervision.

Special Concerns: Diazepam use can lead to psychological or physical dependence. Never take more than the prescribed daily dose. Your physician will teach you how to determine when it is appropriate and how to properly administer the rectal gel.

OVERDOSE
Symptoms: Extreme drowsiness, confusion, slurred speech, slow reflexes, poor coordination, staggering gait, tremor, slowed breathing, loss of consciousness.

What to Do: Call your doctor, emergency medical services (EMS), or the nearest poison control center immediately.

▼ INTERACTIONS

DRUG INTERACTIONS
Other drugs may interact with diazepam. Consult your doctor for advice if you are taking any drugs that depress the central nervous system; these include antihistamines, antidepressants or other psychiatric medications, barbiturates, sedatives, cough medicines, decongestants, and painkillers. Be sure your doctor knows about any over-the-counter drug you may take.

FOOD INTERACTIONS
None reported.

DISEASE INTERACTIONS
Do not take diazepam if you have acute narrow angle glaucoma. Consult your doctor if you have a history of alcohol or drug abuse, stroke or other brain disease, any chronic lung disease, hyperactivity, depression or other mental illness, myasthenia gravis, sleep apnea, epilepsy, porphyria, kidney disease, or liver disease.

≡ SIDE EFFECTS ≡

SERIOUS
Difficulty concentrating, outbursts of anger, other behavior problems, depression, hallucinations, low blood pressure (causing faintness or confusion), memory impairment, muscle weakness, skin rash or itching, sore throat, fever and chills, sores or ulcers in throat or mouth, unusual bruising or bleeding, extreme fatigue, yellowish tinge to eyes or skin. Call your doctor immediately.

COMMON
Drowsiness, loss of coordination, unsteady gait, dizziness, lightheadedness, slurred speech.

LESS COMMON
Change in sexual desire or ability, constipation, false sense of well-being, nausea and vomiting, urinary problems, unusual fatigue.

DIAZOXIDE

Available in: Capsules, injectable solution
Available OTC? No   **As Generic?** Yes
Drug Class: Glucose-elevating agent (capsules); antihypertensive (injection)

▼ USAGE INFORMATION

WHY IT'S PRESCRIBED
To correct low blood glucose levels (hypoglycemia) resulting from overproduction of insulin by the pancreas, which may occur when an insulin-producing pancreatic tumor cannot be removed by surgery or when a malignant insulin-producing tumor has spread.

HOW IT WORKS
Insulin, a hormone produced by the beta cells of the pancreas, lowers blood glucose (sugar) levels by increasing the uptake of glucose by muscles and reducing its release from the liver. Too much insulin causes blood glucose to drop to low levels. Diazoxide inhibits the release of insulin from the pancreas and thus helps to prevent blood glucose from falling to low levels.

▼ DOSAGE GUIDELINES

RANGE AND FREQUENCY
The dose is based on body weight and should be determined by your doctor. Adults, teenagers, and children: Starting at 1 mg per 2.2 lbs (1 kg) of body weight every 8 hours. Can be increased to 3 to 8 mg per 2.2 lbs in 2 or 3 doses a day. Newborn babies and infants: Starting at 3.3 mg per 2.2 lbs of body weight every 8 hours. Can be increased to 8 to 15 mg per 2.2 lbs (3.6 to 6.8 mg per lb) in 2 or 3 doses a day.

ONSET OF EFFECT
1 hour.

DURATION OF ACTION
8 hours.

DIETARY ADVICE
Can be taken with or between meals. A diet rich in carbohydrates may help to raise and maintain blood glucose levels.

STORAGE
Store in a dry place away from heat and light. Keep the solution from freezing.

MISSED DOSE
Take it as soon as you remember. If it is near the time for the next dose, skip the missed dose and go back to your regular dosage schedule. Do not double the next dose.

STOPPING THE DRUG
Do not stop taking diazoxide without first consulting your doctor.

PROLONGED USE
Close monitoring of blood sugar levels is necessary. Long-term side effects may include stiffening of limbs; shaking and trembling of hands and fingers; increased hair growth on forehead, back, arms, and legs.

▼ PRECAUTIONS

Over 60: Older persons are more likely to suffer from impaired kidney function and may therefore require a reduced dose.

Driving and Hazardous Work: Do not drive or engage in hazardous work until you determine how diazoxide affects you.

Alcohol: Follow your physician's instructions about alcohol use while taking this drug.

Pregnancy: Use of diazoxide during pregnancy may have adverse effects on the fetus. Consult your doctor if you are pregnant or plan to become pregnant.

Breast Feeding: It is not known whether diazoxide passes into breast milk. Consult your doctor about the drug's relative risks and benefits if you are breast feeding.

Infants and Children: Careful monitoring is required.

Special Concerns: Follow the special diet that your doctor gives you, and be sure to call your doctor if you experience edema (swelling, especially in the lower extremities), excessive rise in your blood glucose levels, or a drop in blood pressure.

OVERDOSE
Symptoms: An excessive rise in blood glucose can cause drowsiness, flushed skin, dry skin, increased urination, or unusual thirst (symptoms of diabetic ketoacidosis or hyperosmolar coma).

What to Do: Call your doctor immediately.

▼ INTERACTIONS

DRUG INTERACTIONS
Drugs that can affect or be affected by diazoxide include alpha- and beta-blockers, anticoagulants, antigout drugs, anticonvulsants, and thiazide diuretics.

FOOD INTERACTIONS
No known food interactions.

DISEASE INTERACTIONS
Your doctor must be aware of any other medical problems, especially angina, gout, heart disease, blood vessel disease, kidney disease, liver disease, or a recent stroke.

SIDE EFFECTS

SERIOUS
Excess sodium and water retention (edema), resulting in decreased urination, rapid weight gain (or bloating), swelling of feet or lower legs. In some cases this condition, if unchecked, may lead to congestive heart failure; call your doctor at once. A diuretic may be prescribed to counteract the edema, but the combination of diazoxide with a thiazide diuretic may further raise blood glucose levels. Attacks of gout may occur since diazoxide can raise uric acid levels.

COMMON
Rapid heartbeat.

LESS COMMON
Fever, rash, stiffness of arms or legs, unusual bleeding or bruising, constipation, loss of appetite, stomach pain, nausea and vomiting. With long-term use: growth of hair on forehead, back, arms, and legs.

DICLOFENAC OPHTHALMIC

Available in: Ophthalmic solution
Available OTC? No   **As Generic?** No
Drug Class: Nonsteroidal anti-inflammatory drug (NSAID)

▼ USAGE INFORMATION

WHY IT'S PRESCRIBED
To treat inflammation and eye problems that occur after cataract removal surgery. Also used to control eye pain after corneal refractive surgery (such as the increasingly popular radial keratotomy to correct nearsightedness).

HOW IT WORKS
Ophthalmic diclofenac inhibits the release of natural substances that stimulate inflammation and can cause pain in eye tissues.

▼ DOSAGE GUIDELINES

RANGE AND FREQUENCY
Adults: 1 drop in each affected eye 4 times a day, beginning 24 hours after surgery and continuing for the next 2 weeks. Children: Use and dosage must be determined by your doctor.

ONSET OF EFFECT
Unknown.

DURATION OF ACTION
Unknown.

DIETARY ADVICE
This medication can be used without regard to diet.

STORAGE
Store in a tightly sealed container away from heat and direct light. Do not refrigerate or allow to freeze.

MISSED DOSE
Apply it as soon as you remember. If it is near the time for the next dose, skip the missed dose and resume your regular dosage schedule. Do not double the next dose.

STOPPING THE DRUG
Use this drug as prescribed for the full treatment period, even if you begin to feel better before the scheduled end of therapy.

PROLONGED USE
You should see your doctor regularly for tests and examinations if you take this drug for a prolonged period.

▼ PRECAUTIONS

Over 60: No special problems are expected.

≡ SIDE EFFECTS ≡

SERIOUS
Rarely, ophthalmic diclofenac will cause bleeding in the eye, redness or swelling of the eye or eyelid not present before the start of therapy, or tearing or itching of the eye. Call your doctor immediately.

COMMON
Mild and temporary burning or stinging of eyes after application.

LESS COMMON
No less-common side effects are associated with the use of ophthalmic diclofenac.

Driving and Hazardous Work: The use of ophthalmic diclofenac should not impair your ability to perform such tasks safely.

Alcohol: No special precautions are necessary.

Pregnancy: Adequate human studies have not been completed. Before taking ophthalmic diclofenac, tell your doctor if you are pregnant or plan to become pregnant.

Breast Feeding: Ophthalmic diclofenac may pass into breast milk; caution is advised. Consult your doctor for specific advice.

Infants and Children: Use and dosage for infants and children must be determined by your doctor.

Special Concerns: To use the eye drops, first wash your hands. Tilt your head back. Gently apply pressure to the inside corner of the eyelid and with the index finger of the same hand, pull downward on the lower eyelid to make a space. Drop the medicine into this space and close your eye. Apply pressure for 1 or 2 minutes while keeping the eye closed without blinking. Then wash your hands again. Make sure the tip of the dropper does not touch your eye, finger, or any other surface. If your symptoms do not improve or if they become worse, check with your doctor. Ophthalmic diclofenac has caused severe eye irritation in some persons wearing soft contact lenses. Do not wear soft contact lenses while using this drug.

OVERDOSE
Symptoms: No specific ones have been reported.

What to Do: An overdose of ophthalmic diclofenac is unlikely to be life-threatening. However, if someone takes a much larger dose of the drug than prescribed or accidentally ingests the medicine, call your doctor, emergency medical services (EMS), or the nearest poison control center.

▼ INTERACTIONS

DRUG INTERACTIONS
Consult your doctor for advice if you are taking aspirin or another salicylate, diflunisal, etodolac, fenoprofen, floctafenine, flurbiprofen, ibuprofen, indomethacin, ketoprofen, ketorolac, meclofenamate, mefenamic acid, nabumetone, naproxen, oxyphenbutazone, phenylbutazone, piroxicam, sulindac, suprofen, tenoxicam, tiaprofenic acid, tolmetin, or zomepirac.

FOOD INTERACTIONS
No known food interactions.

DISEASE INTERACTIONS
Caution is advised when using ophthalmic diclofenac. Consult your doctor if you have hemophilia or any other bleeding problem.

DICLOFENAC SYSTEMIC

BRAND NAMES
Cataflam, Voltaren

Available in: Tablets, delayed-release tablets, suppositories
Available OTC? No   **As Generic?** Yes
Drug Class: Nonsteroidal anti-inflammatory drug (NSAID)

▼ USAGE INFORMATION

WHY IT'S PRESCRIBED
To treat mild to moderate pain and inflammation caused by tendinitis, arthritis, bursitis, gout, soft tissue injuries, migraine and other vascular headaches, menstrual cramps, and other conditions. When patients fail to respond to one NSAID, another may be tried. The greatest effectiveness often requires trial and error of several different NSAIDs.

HOW IT WORKS
NSAIDs work by interfering with the formation of prostaglandins, substances that cause inflammation and make nerves more sensitive to pain impulses. NSAIDs also have other modes of action that are less well understood.

▼ DOSAGE GUIDELINES

RANGE AND FREQUENCY
Adults— For osteoarthritis and rheumatoid arthritis: 50 mg, 2 or 3 times a day. Ankylosing spondylitis: 25 mg, 4 times a day, with another 25 mg at bedtime if needed. Menstrual pain: 50 mg, 3 times a day; an initial dose of 100 mg may be given.

ONSET OF EFFECT
Within 30 minutes.

DURATION OF ACTION
Up to 8 hours.

DIETARY ADVICE
Take it with food.

STORAGE
Store in a tightly sealed container away from heat, moisture, and direct light.

MISSED DOSE
Take it as soon as you remember. If it is near the time for the next dose, skip the missed dose and resume your regular dosage schedule. Do not double the next dose.

STOPPING THE DRUG
The decision to stop taking the medication should be made in consultation with your physician.

PROLONGED USE
Prolonged use can cause gastrointestinal problems, including ulceration and bleeding, kidney dysfunction, and liver inflammation. Consult your physician about the need for medical examinations and laboratory studies.

▼ PRECAUTIONS

Over 60: Because of the potentially greater consequences of gastrointestinal side effects, the dose of NSAIDs for older patients, especially those over age 70, is often cut in half.

Driving and Hazardous Work: Do not drive or engage in hazardous work until you determine how the medicine affects you.

Alcohol: Avoid alcohol when using this medication because it increases the risk of stomach irritation.

Pregnancy: Avoid or discontinue this drug if you are pregnant or plan to become pregnant.

Breast Feeding: Diclofenac passes into breast milk; avoid or discontinue use while breast feeding.

Infants and Children: Diclofenac may be used in exceptional circumstances; consult your pediatrician for specific advice.

Special Concerns: Because NSAIDs can inhibit blood coagulation, this drug should be discontinued at least 3 days prior to any surgery. Do not crush or chew the tablets.

OVERDOSE
Symptoms: Nausea, vomiting, severe headache, confusion, seizures.

What to Do: Call your doctor, emergency medical services (EMS), or the nearest poison control center immediately.

▼ INTERACTIONS

DRUG INTERACTIONS
Do not take this drug with aspirin or any other NSAIDs without your doctor's approval. In addition, consult your doctor if you are taking antihypertensives, steroids, anticoagulants, antibiotics, itraconazole or ketoconazole, plicamycin, penicillamine, valproic acid, phenytoin, cyclosporine, digitalis drugs, lithium, methotrexate, probenecid, triamterene, or zidovudine.

FOOD INTERACTIONS
No known food interactions.

DISEASE INTERACTIONS
Consult your doctor if you have any of the following: bleeding problems, inflammation or ulcers of the stomach and intestines, diabetes mellitus, systemic lupus erythematosus (SLE, lupus), anemia, asthma, epilepsy, Parkinson's disease, kidney stones, or a history of heart disease or alcohol abuse. Use of diclofenac may cause complications in patients with liver or kidney disease, since these organs work together to remove the medication from the body.

SIDE EFFECTS

SERIOUS
Shortness of breath or wheezing, with or without swelling of legs or other signs of heart failure; chest pain; peptic ulcer disease with vomiting of blood; black, tarry stools; decreasing kidney function. Call your doctor immediately.

COMMON
Nausea, vomiting, heartburn, diarrhea, constipation, headache, dizziness, sleepiness.

LESS COMMON
Ulcers or sores in mouth, depression, rashes or blistering of skin, ringing sound in the ears, unusual tingling or numbness of the hands or feet, seizures, blurred vision. Also elevated potassium levels, decreased blood counts; such problems can be detected by your doctor.

DICLOFENAC/MISOPROSTOL

Available in: Tablets
Available OTC? No   **As Generic?** No
Drug Class: Antirheumatic

▼ USAGE INFORMATION

WHY IT'S PRESCRIBED
To relieve the symptoms of osteoarthritis or rheumatoid arthritis in patients at high risk of developing peptic ulcers as a result of NSAID therapy.

HOW IT WORKS
Diclofenac, a nonsteroidal anti-inflammatory drug (NSAID), works by interfering with the formation of prostaglandins, substances that cause pain and inflammation. Ongoing NSAID therapy can irritate and damage the stomach lining, increasing the risk of peptic ulcers. Misoprostol, a synthetic prostaglandin, helps prevent ulcers and promotes healing by increasing the production of protective mucus and inhibiting the secretion of stomach acid.

▼ DOSAGE GUIDELINES

RANGE AND FREQUENCY
Osteoarthritis: 1 tablet of Arthrotec 50 (50 mg diclofenac/200 micrograms [mcg] misoprostol), 3 times a day. Rheumatoid arthritis: 1 tablet of Arthrotec 75 (75 mg diclofenac/200 mcg misoprostol), 3 to 4 times a day. Different doses may be warranted in some patients.

ONSET OF EFFECT
Unknown.

DURATION OF ACTION
Unknown.

DIETARY ADVICE
The drug should be taken with food to minimize stomach upset and diarrhea.

STORAGE
Store in a tightly sealed container away from heat, moisture, and direct light.

MISSED DOSE
Take it as soon as you remember. If it is near the time for the next dose, skip the missed dose and resume your regular dosage schedule. Do not double the next dose.

STOPPING THE DRUG
Take it as prescribed for the full treatment period.

PROLONGED USE
Side effects are more likely with prolonged use; regular follow-up visits with your doctor are important. To minimize the risk of an adverse effect, the lowest effective dose should be used for the shortest possible duration (misoprostol is generally not prescribed for longer than 4 weeks).

▼ PRECAUTIONS

Over 60: No special problems are expected.

Driving and Hazardous Work: Avoid such activities until you determine how the medicine affects you.

Alcohol: Avoid alcohol, as it may increase the risk of stomach irritation.

Pregnancy: This drug combination should not be used during pregnancy, because it may promote uterine contractions and bleeding, and can cause miscarriage. Before it can be prescribed, female patients are required to have had a negative pregnancy test within the previous 2 weeks. Therapy then begins only on the second or third day of the following menstrual period. Birth control should be used while taking this drug. If you suspect you are pregnant, stop taking the drug immediately and consult your doctor.

Breast Feeding: This drug passes into breast milk and may be harmful; avoid use while nursing.

Infants and Children: Not recommended for use by children under age 18.

OVERDOSE
Symptoms: Nausea, vomiting, severe headache, confusion, seizures, tremors, sleepiness, difficulty breathing, stomach pain, severe diarrhea, fever, extremely low blood pressure causing dizziness or fainting, palpitations, slow heartbeat.

What to Do: Call your doctor, emergency medical services (EMS), or the nearest poison control center immediately.

▼ INTERACTIONS

DRUG INTERACTIONS
The following drugs may interact with this drug: aspirin, digoxin, blood pressure medication, warfarin, methotrexate, cyclosporine, oral diabetes drugs, lithium, antacids, diuretics, or any over-the-counter drugs. Consult your doctor. To minimize the risk of diarrhea, avoid the use of magnesium-containing antacids.

FOOD INTERACTIONS
No known food interactions.

DISEASE INTERACTIONS
You should not take this medication if you have ever experienced breathing difficulty; hives; swelling of the face, tongue, or throat; or any other allergic reactions after taking aspirin or other NSAIDs. Caution is advised if you have a history of high blood pressure or asthma. Use of this drug may cause complications in patients with liver or kidney disease.

≡ SIDE EFFECTS ≡

SERIOUS
Irregular heartbeat, fainting, coma, seizures, yellowish tinge to eyes or skin, or pain or tenderness in the upper-right abdomen. Call your doctor immediately.

COMMON
Stomach pain or upset, diarrhea, indigestion, nausea, gas.

LESS COMMON
Fatigue, fever, tremor, dizziness, loss of appetite, breathing difficulty, persistent but unproductive urge to urinate or defecate, hemorrhoids, breast pain, painful menstruation, menstrual irregularities, hives, impotence, unexpected changes in weight, muscle and joint pain, mental depression, sleeping difficulty, nightmares or unusually vivid dreams, hallucinations, irritability, nervousness, bruising, skin rash, blurred or abnormal vision.

DICLOXACILLIN SODIUM

Available in: Capsules, liquid
Available OTC? No **As Generic?** Yes
Drug Class: Penicillin antibiotic

▼ USAGE INFORMATION

WHY IT'S PRESCRIBED
To treat bacterial infections, especially those of the skin or bone caused by penicillin-resistant staphylococcus bacteria. Dicloxacillin is ineffective against infections caused by viruses, fungi, or other microorganisms.

HOW IT WORKS
Dicloxacillin blocks the formation of bacterial cell walls, rendering bacteria unable to multiply and spread. Unlike other penicillin antibiotics, dicloxacillin is resistant to bacterial enzymes that chemically inactivate penicillins.

▼ DOSAGE GUIDELINES

RANGE AND FREQUENCY
Adults and children over 88 lbs: 125 to 250 mg every 6 hours, for a total dosage of 500 to 1,000 mg a day. Children under 88 lbs: Dose is determined by doctor, based on several factors. Usual dose is 1.4 to 2.8 mg per lb of body weight every 6 hours.

ONSET OF EFFECT
Unknown.

DURATION OF ACTION
Up to 6 hours.

DIETARY ADVICE
Take dicloxacillin on an empty stomach, 1 to 2 hours before or 2 to 3 hours after a meal, with a full glass of water.

STORAGE
Store capsules in a dry place away from heat and light. Refrigerate the liquid form, but do not allow it to freeze.

MISSED DOSE
Take it as soon as you remember. If you take 2 doses a day, take the next dose 5 to 6 hours later and go back to your regular schedule. If you take 3 or more doses a day, take the next dose 2 to 4 hours later, then go back to your regular schedule. Do not double the next dose.

STOPPING THE DRUG
Take it as prescribed for the full treatment period, even if you begin to feel better before the scheduled end of therapy. Stopping the drug prematurely may slow your recovery or lead to a rebound infection, also known as superinfection, in which the heartier strains of bacteria survive and multiply, leading to a more serious and drug-resistant infection.

PROLONGED USE
Prolonged use may make you more susceptible to infections that are resistant to penicillin; caution is advised.

▼ PRECAUTIONS

Over 60: No special problems are expected.

Driving and Hazardous Work: Usually not dangerous, since most hazardous reactions occur a few minutes after the drug is taken.

Alcohol: Alcohol may increase stomach irritation.

Pregnancy: Adequate studies of the use of penicillin antibiotics during pregnancy have not been done; however, no problems have been reported.

Breast Feeding: Dicloxacillin passes into breast milk and may cause diarrhea, fungal infections, and allergic reactions in nursing infants; avoid use while nursing.

Infants and Children: No special problems are expected.

Special Concerns: Dicloxacillin can cause false results on some urine sugar tests for patients with diabetes. Those who are prone to asthma, hay fever, hives, or allergies may be more likely to have an allergic reaction to a penicillin antibiotic. If severe diarrhea occurs as a side effect of this drug, do not take antidiarrheal medications; call your doctor.

OVERDOSE
Symptoms: Severe diarrhea, nausea, vomiting, seizures.

What to Do: Call your doctor, emergency medical services (EMS), or the nearest poison control center immediately.

▼ INTERACTIONS

DRUG INTERACTIONS
Consult your doctor for specific advice if you are taking aminoglycosides, ACE inhibitors, diuretics, potassium supplements or potassium-containing drugs, anticoagulants or other anti-clotting drugs, nonsteroidal anti-inflammatory drugs, sulfinpyrazone, cholestyramine, colestipol, oral contraceptives, methotrexate, probenecid, or rifampin.

FOOD INTERACTIONS
No known food interactions.

DISEASE INTERACTIONS
Consult your doctor if you have a history of allergies, asthma, congestive heart failure, gastrointestinal disorders (especially colitis associated with the use of antibiotics), or impaired kidney function.

≡ SIDE EFFECTS ≡

SERIOUS
Irregular, rapid, or labored breathing, lightheadedness or sudden fainting, joint pain, fever, severe abdominal pain and cramping with watery or bloody stools, severe allergic reaction (marked by sudden swelling of the lips, tongue, face, or throat; breathing difficulty; skin rash, itching, or hives), unusual bleeding or bruising, yellowish tinge to eyes or skin. Call your doctor immediately.

COMMON
Mild rash, mild diarrhea, nausea, vomiting, headache, vaginal discharge and itching, pain or white patches in the mouth or on the tongue.

LESS COMMON
Diminished urine output, chills, weakness, fatigue.

DICYCLOMINE HYDROCHLORIDE

Available in: Tablets, syrup, capsules, injection
Available OTC? No   **As Generic?** Yes
Drug Class: Antidiarrheal/antispasmodic

▼ USAGE INFORMATION

WHY IT'S PRESCRIBED
To treat irritable bowel syndrome, and to reduce spasms of the digestive system, bladder, and urethra.

HOW IT WORKS
Dicyclomine slows bowel action and reduces production of stomach acid.

▼ DOSAGE GUIDELINES

RANGE AND FREQUENCY
Oral forms– Adults and teenagers: 10 to 20 mg, 3 or 4 times a day. Children age 2 and older: 5 to 10 mg, 3 or 4 times a day. Children ages 6 months to 2 years: 5 to 10 mg of the syrup 3 or 4 times a day. Injection– Adults and teenagers: 20 mg into a muscle every 4 to 6 hours. Children: Consult a pediatrician for advice.

ONSET OF EFFECT
Unknown.

DURATION OF ACTION
Unknown.

DIETARY ADVICE
Take this medicine 30 to 60 minutes before meals and bedtime unless your doctor directs otherwise. Bedtime dose should be given at least 2 hours after the last meal of the day.

STORAGE
Store in a tightly sealed container away from heat, moisture, and direct light. Keep liquid forms of the drug refrigerated, but do not allow them to freeze.

MISSED DOSE
Take it as soon as you remember, unless the time for your next scheduled dose is within the next 2 hours. If so, skip the missed dose and resume your regular dosage schedule. Do not double the next dose.

STOPPING THE DRUG
Take it as prescribed for the full treatment period. However, you may stop taking the drug if you are feeling better before the scheduled end of therapy. The doctor may want you to reduce the amount you take gradually.

PROLONGED USE
Prolonged use can cause chronic constipation and fecal impaction. Consult your doctor immediately.

SIDE EFFECTS

SERIOUS
No serious side effects are associated with dicyclomine.

COMMON
Headache; dizziness; constipation; dry mouth, nose, throat, or skin; difficulty urinating; heart palpitations.

LESS COMMON
Drowsiness, decreased sweating, confusion, nervousness, rapid pulse, blurred vision, nausea, vomiting.

▼ PRECAUTIONS

Over 60: Adverse reactions may be more likely and more severe in older patients.

Driving and Hazardous Work: Do not drive or engage in hazardous work until you determine how the drug affects you. The use of dicyclomine disqualifies you from piloting an aircraft.

Alcohol: No special precautions are necessary.

Pregnancy: Consult your doctor about taking dicyclomine if you are pregnant or plan to become pregnant.

Breast Feeding: Dicyclomine passes into breast milk and decreases milk production. Avoid taking this medicine or discontinue breast feeding while you take it. Consult your doctor about maintaining milk flow if you breast feed.

Infants and Children: Give dicyclomine to infants and children only under close medical supervision.

Special Concerns: Tell any other doctor or dentist whom you consult that you take dicyclomine. Strenuous exercise, hot baths, or saunas while you take this medicine can make you dizzy or faint.

OVERDOSE
Symptoms: Blurred vision, dilated pupils, dizziness, rapid pulse, hot, dry skin, slurred speech, confusion, nausea, headache, loss of consciousness.

What to Do: Call your doctor, emergency medical services (EMS), or the nearest poison control center immediately.

▼ INTERACTIONS

DRUG INTERACTIONS
Consult your doctor about any other medicines you are taking, especially antacids, antihistamines, narcotic pain relievers, antiarrhythmic drugs, drugs for Parkinson's disease, antidepressants, or antipsychotic drugs (such as phenothiazines). Large doses of vitamin C can reduce the effect of dicyclomine. Potassium supplements can increase the risk of an intestinal ulcer. Nitrates and nitrites can increase internal pressure of the eye.

FOOD INTERACTIONS
No known food interactions.

DISEASE INTERACTIONS
You may not be able to take dicyclomine if you have intestinal problems, heart disease, bleeding problems, glaucoma, chronic bronchitis, an enlarged prostate, a hernia, liver disease, kidney disease, a fever, brain damage (in children), an overactive thyroid, or urinary problems.

DIDANOSINE (DIDEOXYINOSINE; DDI)

Available in: Tablets, powder for solution
Available OTC? No   **As Generic?** No
Drug Class: Antiviral

▼ USAGE INFORMATION

WHY IT'S PRESCRIBED
To treat HIV infection. While not a cure for HIV, this drug may suppress the replication of the virus and delay the progression of the disease.

HOW IT WORKS
Didanosine (also known as dideoxyinosine or ddI) interferes with the activity of enzymes needed for the replication of DNA in viral cells.

▼ DOSAGE GUIDELINES

RANGE AND FREQUENCY
Tablets– Adults and teenagers weighing 132 lbs or more: 200 mg every 12 hours. Adults and teenagers weighing less than 132 lbs: 125 mg every 12 hours. Children: Dose may range from 25 to 100 mg every 8 to 12 hours. Tablets must be chewed or dissolved in water or apple juice. Always take 2 tablets at the same time; there is not enough medicine in a single tablet to ensure adequate absorption. Powder (dissolved in water)– Adults and teenagers weighing 132 lbs or more: 250 mg every 12 hours. Adults and teenagers weighing less than 132 lbs: 167 mg every 12 hours. Children (a special pediatric formulation is used): Dose may range from 31 to 125 mg every 8 to 12 hours. Didanosine is sometimes given once a day, using the full dose (400 mg in adults).

ONSET OF EFFECT
Unknown.

DURATION OF ACTION
Unknown.

DIETARY ADVICE
Didanosine should be taken on an empty stomach, at least 1 hour before or 2 hours after eating. If you are on a low-salt diet, be aware that this drug contains high quantities of sodium.

STORAGE
Store tablets in a dry place away from heat and direct light. The mixed solution may be refrigerated, but do not allow it to freeze.

MISSED DOSE
If it is near the time for the next dose, skip the missed dose and resume your regular dosage schedule. Do not double the next dose.

STOPPING THE DRUG
The decision to stop taking the drug should be made in consultation with your physician.

PROLONGED USE
See your doctor regularly for tests and examinations.

▼ PRECAUTIONS

Over 60: No special problems are expected.

Driving and Hazardous Work: Do not drive or engage in hazardous work until you determine how the medicine affects you.

Alcohol: Avoid alcohol if liver function is impaired. Heavy alcohol use can increase the risk of pancreatitis, an uncommon side effect of didanosine.

Pregnancy: While didanosine has been shown to cause birth defects in animals, it is increasingly being used in combination with other antiretroviral drugs to treat pregnant HIV-infected women.

Breast Feeding: Women infected with HIV should not breast-feed.

Infants and Children: Safety and effectiveness for children under 6 months have not been established.

Special Concerns: Use of didanosine does not eliminate the risk of passing the AIDS virus to other persons. Be sure to take appropriate preventive measures.

OVERDOSE
Symptoms: Seizures, severe nausea, severe vomiting, extreme fatigue or weakness, unusual bleeding or bruising, clumsiness, involuntary eye movement.

What to Do: Seek medical assistance immediately.

▼ INTERACTIONS

DRUG INTERACTIONS
Consult your doctor for specific advice if you are taking antibiotic or anti-infective drugs, antidepressants, antifungals, antimalarial drugs, antiparkinson's agents, blood pressure medication, cancer drugs, diuretics, estrogens, lithium, nitrous oxide, phenytoin, or zalcitabine.

FOOD INTERACTIONS
Food can interfere with the absorption of didanosine.

DISEASE INTERACTIONS
You may not be able to take didanosine if you have had pancreatitis (inflammation of the pancreas), hepatitis (liver inflammation), other liver or kidney problems, high blood pressure, blood disorders, gout, swollen ankles, or numbness and tingling in the hands or feet.

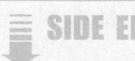

SIDE EFFECTS

SERIOUS
Nerve damage causing numbness, tingling, prickling, or pain in the hands and feet; pancreatitis (inflammation of the pancreas) causing abdominal pain, nausea, and vomiting. Call your doctor immediately.

COMMON
Temporary toxicity of the central nervous system causing headache, anxiety, irritability, restlessness, or sleep disruption; gastrointestinal disturbances, including stomach pain, gas, nausea, vomiting, and diarrhea; dry mouth.

LESS COMMON
Swollen hands or legs, shortness of breath, yellow discoloration of the eyes or skin, rash, itch, weakness, vision problems, muscle aches or spasms, muscle wasting, pain, pneumonia, cough, hair loss.

DIETHYLPROPION HYDROCHLORIDE

Available in: Tablets, extended-release tablets
Available OTC? No   **As Generic?** Yes
Drug Class: Sympathomimetic; central nervous system stimulant

▼ USAGE INFORMATION

WHY IT'S PRESCRIBED
Diethylpropion is used to suppress appetite in obese patients. It is used in conjunction with a strict diet, and should never be prescribed as the sole method of achieving weight loss. This drug is indicated for patients with an initial body mass index (BMI) of 30 or greater (see Special Concerns for information on BMI calculation).

HOW IT WORKS
It is believed the appetite-control center for the body may be found in a part of the brain called the hypothalamus. Diethylpropion probably affects the transmission of nerve impulses in this region.

▼ DOSAGE GUIDELINES

RANGE AND FREQUENCY
Oral tablet: 25 mg, 3 times per day before meals. Oral extended-release tablet: 75 mg, once a day, taken at mid-morning.

ONSET OF EFFECT
Within a few hours.

DURATION OF ACTION
Regular tablets: 4 hours. Extended-release: 12 hours.

DIETARY ADVICE
Take this medication one hour before meals. Significant weight loss will not occur without carefully adhering to a strict diet as outlined by your physician or nutritionist.

STORAGE
Store in a tightly sealed container away from heat and direct light. Keep away from moisture and extremes in temperature.

MISSED DOSE
Take it as soon as you remember. If it is near the time for the next dose, skip the missed dose and resume your regular dosage schedule. Do not double the next dose.

STOPPING THE DRUG
Take as prescribed for the full treatment period. Your dose may need to be reduced gradually to prevent withdrawal effects or a rebound increase in appetite.

PROLONGED USE
This drug is usually prescribed for several weeks. Side effects may become more likely over this period of time. Prolonged use may result in mental or physical dependence.

▼ PRECAUTIONS

Over 60: Adverse reactions may be more likely and more severe in older patients, especially with drugs that act on the central nervous system.

Driving and Hazardous Work: Do not drive or engage in hazardous activities until you determine how the drug affects you.

Alcohol: Avoid alcohol.

Pregnancy: Avoid or discontinue diethylpropion if you are pregnant or trying to become pregnant.

Breast Feeding: Diethylpropion passes into breast milk; avoid or discontinue usage while nursing.

Infants and Children: Not recommended for use by children under age 12.

Special Concerns: The appetite suppressant effect of this drug may diminish after a few weeks. This is known as drug tolerance, and you should inform your physician. Do not increase the dose. The BMI can be calculated by dividing your weight in pounds by your height in inches squared, and then multiplying by 705.

OVERDOSE
Symptoms: Extreme restlessness, tremor or shaking, confusion, hallucinations, coma, extreme fear or panic, rapid breathing, violent behavior, nausea, vomiting, fainting.

What to Do: Call emergency medical services (EMS), your doctor, or the nearest poison control center immediately.

▼ INTERACTIONS

DRUG INTERACTIONS
Consult your doctor for specific advice if you are taking amantadine; amphetamines, medications for hyperactivity, or other drugs for appetite control; caffeine; chlophedianol; asthma medication; prescription and nonprescription decongestants or medicine for colds, sinus problems, or seasonal allergies, such as hay fever (including nose drops or sprays); methylphenidate; nabilone; pemoline; or an MAO inhibitor.

FOOD INTERACTIONS
Avoid food or beverages containing caffeine.

DISEASE INTERACTIONS
Consult your doctor if you have a history of alcohol or drug abuse; diabetes mellitus; glaucoma; heart disease; blood vessel disease, especially of the arteries; strokes or "mini strokes" (transient ischemic attacks); high blood pressure; mental illness; or thyroid or kidney disease. An increased frequency of seizures has been reported in patients with epilepsy.

▼ SIDE EFFECTS

SERIOUS
Chest pain; severe dizziness; headache (especially if associated with nausea or vomiting); convulsions; rash; racing, pounding, or fluttering heartbeat.

COMMON
Lightheadedness; irritability or nervousness, difficulty falling asleep, exaggerated feelings of well-being or confidence (euphoria), increased heartbeat, palpitations, increased blood pressure.

LESS COMMON
Persistent or unusual fever, chills, sore throat, or cough; persistent or unusual bruising or bleeding; gastrointestinal problems.

DIETHYLSTILBESTROL (DES)

Available in: Tablets, injection
Available OTC? No **As Generic?** Yes
Drug Class: Antineoplastic (anticancer) agent; hormone treatment

▼ USAGE INFORMATION

WHY IT'S PRESCRIBED
To slow the progress of advanced breast and prostate cancers.

HOW IT WORKS
Diethylstilbestrol is a form of the hormone estrogen. It can block the action of certain other hormones that promote tumor growth; this in turn will slow the progress of the cancer.

▼ DOSAGE GUIDELINES

RANGE AND FREQUENCY
Tablet— For breast cancer: 15 mg once a day. For prostate cancer: 1 to 3 mg a day; dose may be decreased to 1 mg a day. Injection— 500 mg a day. The dose may be increased to 1 g per day, then lowered to 250 to 500 mg once a week.

ONSET OF EFFECT
Unknown.

DURATION OF ACTION
Unknown.

DIETARY ADVICE
Drink plenty of fluids.

STORAGE
Store in a tightly sealed container away from heat and direct light.

MISSED DOSE
Take it as soon as you remember. If it is close to the time for the next dose, skip the missed dose and resume your regular dosage schedule. Do not double the next dose.

STOPPING THE DRUG
The decision to stop taking diethylstilbestrol should be made in consultation with your doctor.

PROLONGED USE
You should see your doctor regularly for tests and examinations if you take this drug for a prolonged period.

▼ PRECAUTIONS

Over 60: No extra problems or side effects are expected in older patients as compared with younger persons.

Driving and Hazardous Work: Do not drive or engage in hazardous work until you determine how the medicine affects you.

Alcohol: Avoid alcohol.

Pregnancy: Diethylstilbestrol can cause birth defects and should never be taken during pregnancy.

Breast Feeding: Not recommended while taking diethylstilbestrol.

Infants and Children: Diethylstilbestrol is not recommended for use in infants and children.

Special Concerns: Diethylstilbestrol may cause tenderness, swelling, or bleeding of the gums. Brush and floss your teeth regularly and see your dentist regularly. Patients who take DES may be at increased risk for cancer.

OVERDOSE

Symptoms: Loss of appetite, nausea, vomiting, abdominal cramps, diarrhea, vaginal bleeding.

What to Do: Call your doctor, emergency medical services (EMS), or the nearest poison control center immediately.

▼ INTERACTIONS

DRUG INTERACTIONS
Consult your doctor for specific advice if you are taking acetaminophen, amiodarone, anabolic steroids, androgens, anti-infective medications, antithyroid agents, carbamazepine, carmustine, chloroquine, dantrolene, daunorubicin, disulfiram, divalproex, etretinate, gold salts, hydroxychloroquine, mercaptopurine, methotrexate, methyldopa, naltrexone, oral contraceptives, phenothiazines, phenytoin, plicamycin, tamoxifen, valproic acid, bromocriptine, or cyclosporine.

FOOD INTERACTIONS
No known food interactions.

DISEASE INTERACTIONS
Caution is advised when taking diethylstilbestrol. Consult your doctor if you have a history of blood clots, changes in vaginal bleeding, endometriosis, fibroid tumors of the uterus, gallbladder disease or gallstones, jaundice, liver disease, porphyria, blood clots, heart or circulatory disease, stroke, high blood pressure, diabetes mellitus, asthma, kidney disease, liver disease, or depression.

⇊ SIDE EFFECTS ⇊

SERIOUS
Breast pain or increased breast size (in both men and women), swelling of feet and lower legs, rapid weight gain, irregular vaginal bleeding, painful menstrual periods, breast lumps, pain in stomach, side, or abdomen, jerky muscle movements, yellowish tinge to eyes or skin (jaundice), sudden or severe headache, loss of coordination, loss of or change in vision, pain in chest, groin, or leg, sudden shortness of breath, slurred speech, weakness or numbness in arm or leg. Notify your doctor promptly.

COMMON
Bloating of or cramps in stomach, loss of appetite, nausea, rash, freckles on the face.

LESS COMMON
Abnormal hair loss or growth, joint pain, depression, dizziness, headache, problems with contact lenses, change in level of sexual desire, vomiting, diarrhea.

DIFLUNISAL

Available in: Tablets
Available OTC? No **As Generic?** Yes
Drug Class: Nonsteroidal anti-inflammatory drug (NSAID)

▼ USAGE INFORMATION

WHY IT'S PRESCRIBED
To treat mild to moderate pain and inflammation caused by tendinitis, arthritis, bursitis, gout, soft tissue injuries, migraine and other vascular headaches, menstrual cramps, and other conditions. When patients fail to respond to one NSAID, another may be tried. The greatest effectiveness often requires trial and error of several different NSAIDs.

HOW IT WORKS
NSAIDs work by interfering with the formation of prostaglandins, naturally occurring substances in the body that cause inflammation and make nerves more sensitive to pain impulses. NSAIDs also have other modes of action that are less well understood.

▼ DOSAGE GUIDELINES

RANGE AND FREQUENCY
Adults and teenagers: 500 to 1,000 mg a day in 2 divided doses. Adults over age 65: 250 to 500 mg a day in 2 divided doses.

ONSET OF EFFECT
Within 1 hour; 3 weeks of regular use may be required for maximum effect.

DURATION OF ACTION
8 to 12 hours.

DIETARY ADVICE
Take with food; maintain your usual food and fluid intake.

STORAGE
Store in a tightly sealed container away from heat, moisture, and direct light.

MISSED DOSE
Take it as soon as you remember. If it is near the time for the next dose, skip the missed dose and resume your regular dosage schedule. Do not double the next dose.

STOPPING THE DRUG
The decision to stop taking the drug should be made in consultation with your physician.

PROLONGED USE
Prolonged use can cause gastrointestinal problems, including ulceration and bleeding, kidney dysfunction, and liver inflammation. Consult your physician about the need for medical examinations and laboratory studies.

▼ PRECAUTIONS

Over 60: Because of the potentially greater consequences of gastrointestinal side effects, the dose of NSAIDs for older patients, especially those over age 70, is often cut in half.

Driving and Hazardous Work: Do not drive or engage in hazardous work until you determine how this drug affects you.

Alcohol: Avoid alcohol when using this medication because it increases the risk of stomach irritation.

Pregnancy: Avoid or discontinue this drug if you are pregnant or plan to become pregnant.

Breast Feeding: Diflunisal passes into breast milk; avoid or discontinue use while breast feeding.

Infants and Children: Diflunisal is not generally prescribed for children under the age of 12, but may be used in exceptional circumstances; consult your doctor.

Special Concerns: Because NSAIDs can interfere with blood coagulation, this drug should be stopped at least 3 days prior to any surgery.

OVERDOSE
Symptoms: Nausea, vomiting, severe headache, confusion, seizures.

What to Do: Call your doctor, emergency medical services (EMS), or the nearest poison control center immediately.

▼ INTERACTIONS

DRUG INTERACTIONS
Do not take this drug with aspirin or any other NSAIDs without your doctor's approval. In addition, consult your doctor if you are taking antihypertensives, steroids, anticoagulants, antibiotics, itraconazole or ketoconazole, plicamycin, penicillamine, valproic acid, phenytoin, cyclosporine, digitalis drugs, lithium, methotrexate, probenecid, triamterene, or zidovudine.

FOOD INTERACTIONS
No known food interactions.

DISEASE INTERACTIONS
Caution is advised when taking diflunisal. Consult your doctor if you have any of the following: bleeding problems, inflammation or ulcers of the stomach and intestines, diabetes mellitus, lupus, anemia, asthma, epilepsy, Parkinson's disease, kidney stones, or a history of heart disease or alcohol abuse. Use of diflunisal may cause complications in patients with liver or kidney disease, since these organs work together to remove the medication from the body.

 SIDE EFFECTS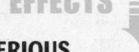

SERIOUS
Shortness of breath or wheezing, with or without swelling of legs or other signs of heart failure; chest pain; peptic ulcer disease with vomiting of blood; black, tarry stools; decreasing kidney function. Call your doctor immediately.

COMMON
Nausea, vomiting, heartburn, diarrhea, constipation, headache, dizziness, sleepiness.

LESS COMMON
Ulcers or sores in mouth, depression, rashes or blistering of skin, ringing sound in the ears, unusual tingling or numbness of the hands or feet, seizures, blurred vision. Also elevated potassium levels, decreased blood counts; such problems can be detected by your doctor.

DIGITOXIN

Available in: Tablets
Available OTC? No **As Generic?** Yes
Drug Class: Digitalis drug (cardiac glycoside)

▼ USAGE INFORMATION

WHY IT'S PRESCRIBED
To treat congestive heart failure and atrial arrhythmias (heart rhythm irregularities). Because this drug carries potentially serious risks, it is seldom prescribed in current medical practice.

HOW IT WORKS
Digitalis drugs such as digitoxin enhance and strengthen the force of the heart's contractions, and thus help to regulate the rate and the rhythm of the heartbeat.

▼ DOSAGE GUIDELINES

RANGE AND FREQUENCY
Adults: Initial dose is 0.2 mg, 2 times a day for 4 days. Maintenance dosage ranges from 0.05 to 0.3 mg, taken once a day. Children: Dosage must be determined by your pediatrician. Dosages for all patients must be closely regulated by frequently checking drug levels in the blood.

ONSET OF EFFECT
30 minutes to 2 hours.

DURATION OF ACTION
3 to 4 days.

DIETARY ADVICE
Take it on an empty stomach at the same time every day. Taking digitoxin with food can decrease the absorption rate and peak concentration.

STORAGE
Store in a tightly sealed container away from heat, moisture, and direct light.

MISSED DOSE
Take it as soon as you remember. However, if it is within 12 hours of the next scheduled dose, skip the missed dose and resume your regular dosage schedule. Do not double the next dose.

STOPPING THE DRUG
Many patients must take digitoxin for extended periods. Do not stop taking digitoxin unless your doctor advises you to do so.

SIDE EFFECTS

SERIOUS
Heartbeat irregularities that may be life-threatening and cause dizziness, palpitations, shortness of breath, sweating, or fainting. Other serious side effects include hallucinations, confusion, and mental changes; extreme drowsiness; and visual disturbances, such as double vision or seeing colored halos around objects. Call your doctor right away.

COMMON
Weakness, fatigue, blurred vision, nausea, agitation, erectile dysfunction, male breast enlargement.

LESS COMMON
Headache, vertigo, numbness or tingling sensation, overall feeling of illness, increased sensitivity of eyes to light, diarrhea, vomiting.

PROLONGED USE
Prolonged use requires your doctor's careful supervision and periodic assessments of the continued need to take the drug. Blood levels of digitoxin must be measured at regular intervals to ensure proper dosing.

▼ PRECAUTIONS

Over 60: Underweight or frail older persons may require a lower maintenance dose.

Driving and Hazardous Work: Digitoxin may cause drowsiness or vision changes. Do not drive or engage in hazardous work until you determine how it affects you.

Alcohol: No interactions are expected.

Pregnancy: Human studies have not been done. In animal studies, no birth defects have been reported. Digitoxin should be used during pregnancy only if your doctor says it is clearly needed.

Breast Feeding: Digitoxin passes into breast milk. The nursing infant should be monitored carefully. Stop using the drug or discontinue breast feeding if adverse effects develop.

Infants and Children: The dosage for infants and children must be determined by your pediatrician.

Special Concerns: You should carry a card that says you are taking digitoxin. Do not take over-the-counter antacids or cold or allergy remedies without consulting your doctor. Digitoxin causes impotence and enlarged breasts in a third of the men who take it. Mental changes induced by the drug may be mistaken for psychosis or senility.

OVERDOSE
Symptoms: Heart palpitations, abdominal pain, diarrhea, nausea, vomiting, very slow pulse.

What to Do: Call your doctor, emergency medical services (EMS), or the nearest poison control center immediately.

▼ INTERACTIONS

DRUG INTERACTIONS
Numerous drugs interact with digitoxin and may alter blood levels of the drug, leading to toxicity. Consult your doctor for specific advice if you are taking any drug, especially airway-opening drugs (bronchodilators); antacids; antibiotics, such as neomycin or tetracycline; anticholinergic drugs, such as atropine; cholesterol-lowering drugs; diuretics; steroids; indomethacin; or any other heart drug.

FOOD INTERACTIONS
Ask your doctor about the advisability of eating high-potassium foods.

DISEASE INTERACTIONS
Consult your doctor if you have any other medical condition, especially lung disease, kidney disease, or poor thyroid function.

DIGOXIN

Available in: Tablets, capsules, elixir
Available OTC? No **As Generic?** Yes
Drug Class: Digitalis drug (cardiac glycoside)

▼ USAGE INFORMATION

WHY IT'S PRESCRIBED
To treat congestive heart failure and atrial arrhythmias (heart rhythm irregularities).

HOW IT WORKS
Digitalis drugs such as digoxin enhance and strengthen the force of the heart's contractions, and help to regulate the rate and the rhythm of the heartbeat.

▼ DOSAGE GUIDELINES

RANGE AND FREQUENCY
Adults: Initial dose is 0.5 mg. Maintenance dosage, starting the next day, ranges from 0.125 to 0.25 mg a day (rarely more) taken once a day. Periodic blood tests are necessary to determine the proper dose. Children: Consult your doctor.

ONSET OF EFFECT
30 minutes to 2 hours.

DURATION OF ACTION
3 to 4 days.

DIETARY ADVICE
Take it on an empty stomach, at the same time every day. Taking digoxin with food can decrease the absorption rate and the peak concentration.

STORAGE
Store in a tightly sealed container away from heat, moisture, and direct light.

MISSED DOSE
Take it as soon as you remember. If it is within 12 hours of the next scheduled dose, skip the missed dose and resume your regular dosage schedule. Do not double the next dose.

STOPPING THE DRUG
Do not stop taking it unless your doctor advises otherwise. Abrupt discontinuation can cause serious heart problems. Most patients take digoxin for an extended period or for the rest of their lives.

PROLONGED USE
Prolonged use requires your doctor's supervision and periodic assessments of the continued need to take the drug. Blood levels of digoxin must be measured at regular intervals to ensure proper dosing.

▼ PRECAUTIONS

Over 60: Underweight or frail older persons may require a lower maintenance dose.

Driving and Hazardous Work: Digoxin may cause drowsiness or vision changes. Do not drive or engage in hazardous work until you determine how it affects you.

Alcohol: No interactions are expected.

Pregnancy: Human studies have not been done. In animal studies, no birth defects have been reported. Digoxin should be used during pregnancy only if your doctor decides it is clearly needed.

Breast Feeding: Digoxin passes into breast milk. The nursing infant should be monitored carefully. Stop using the drug or discontinue breast feeding if adverse effects develop.

Infants and Children: The dosage for infants and children must be determined by your pediatrician.

Special Concerns: You should carry a card that says you are taking digoxin. Do not take over-the-counter antacids or cold or allergy remedies without consulting your doctor. Digoxin causes

impotence and enlarged breasts in a third of the men who take it. Mental changes induced by the drug may be mistaken for psychosis or senility.

OVERDOSE
Symptoms: Heart palpitations, abdominal pain, diarrhea, nausea, vomiting, very slow pulse.

What to Do: Call your doctor, emergency medical services (EMS), or the nearest poison control center immediately.

▼ INTERACTIONS

DRUG INTERACTIONS
Numerous drugs interact with digoxin and may alter blood levels of the drug, leading to toxicity. Consult your doctor for specific advice if you are taking any medications, especially antiarrhythmic drugs, such as quinidine or procainamide; airway-opening drugs (bronchodilators); antacids; antibiotics, such as neomycin or tetracycline; anticholinergic drugs, such as atropine; cholesterol-lowering drugs; diuretics (water pills); steroids; indomethacin; or any other heart drug.

FOOD INTERACTIONS
Ask your doctor about the advisability of eating high-potassium foods.

DISEASE INTERACTIONS
Tell your doctor if you have any other medical condition, especially lung disease, kidney disease, or poor thyroid function.

≡ SIDE EFFECTS ≡

SERIOUS
Heartbeat irregularities causing dizziness, palpitations, shortness of breath, sweating, or fainting. Other serious side effects include hallucinations, confusion, and mental changes; extreme drowsiness; visual disturbances, such as double vision or seeing colored halos around objects; weakness, fatigue, blurred vision; nausea; or agitation. Call your doctor immediately.

COMMON
Erectile dysfunction, male breast enlargement. Notify your doctor if such symptoms occur.

LESS COMMON
Headache, vertigo, numbness or tingling sensation, overall feeling of illness, sensitivity of eyes to light, diarrhea, vomiting. Call your doctor if such symptoms persist.

DIHYDROERGOTAMINE MESYLATE

Available in: Injection, nasal spray
Available OTC? No   **As Generic?** No
Drug Class: Antimigraine/antiheadache drug

▼ USAGE INFORMATION

WHY IT'S PRESCRIBED
To treat migraine headaches. This drug is ineffective against other kinds of pain or headaches, and because of its potential for serious side effects, it is prescribed only when other treatments have proven ineffective.

HOW IT WORKS
It reduces throbbing pain by constricting the walls of the blood vessels that carry blood in the brain. It may also depress activity in certain areas in the brain, directly suppressing headache pain. Because this drug may cause constriction of blood vessels throughout the body, serious side effects may result from lack of sufficient blood supply to various organ systems.

▼ DOSAGE GUIDELINES

RANGE AND FREQUENCY
Injection: 1 mg per injection, up to 2 mg per attack, with at least 1 or 2 hours between injections. Maximum weekly dosage is 6 mg. Lie down in a quiet, dark room after the injection. Nasal spray: 1 spray (0.5 mg) in each nostril. Fifteen minutes later, an additional 1 spray should be administered in each nostril for a total of 4 sprays (2 mg). Maximum daily dosage is 3 mg; maximum weekly dosage is 4 mg. Do not sniff following administration. The nasal spray should stay in the nose so that it can be absorbed into the bloodstream through the lining of the nose. This drug works best when taken at the first sign of a migraine headache; it should not be taken preventively.

ONSET OF EFFECT
Injection: Intravenous: Within 5 minutes. Intramuscular: Within 15 to 30 minutes. Nasal spray: Unknown.

DURATION OF ACTION
Injection: About 8 hours. Nasal spray: Unknown.

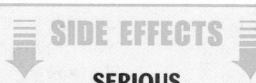

SIDE EFFECTS

SERIOUS
Blurred vision, headaches, chest pain, pale, cold, bluish-colored hands or feet, numbness or tingling in fingers and toes, gangrene. Such symptoms may indicate inadequate blood circulation owing to excessive blood vessel constriction. Other serious side effects include rapid or slow heartbeat, itching, weakness in legs, muscle pain, severe anxiety or confusion, and excess water retention. Seek medical attention immediately.

COMMON
Constipation, reduced sweating, dizziness or lightheadedness, drowsiness.

LESS COMMON
Nausea, vomiting.

DIETARY ADVICE
Do not fast or skip meals; this may trigger a migraine. Try to eat at least three meals a day, at the same times each day. Avoid foods that contain preservatives, monosodium glutamate (MSG), and large amounts of caffeine or salt.

STORAGE
Store in a tightly sealed container away from moisture, heat, and direct light. Do not refrigerate or freeze the spray.

MISSED DOSE
Not applicable.

STOPPING THE DRUG
Headaches may get worse if you stop using this drug. Consult your doctor.

PROLONGED USE
Prolonged use can lead to addiction or tolerance to this medicine. Consult your doctor if the usual dose fails to relieve headaches or if the frequency or severity of headaches increases.

▼ PRECAUTIONS

Over 60: Side effects may be more likely and more severe.

Driving and Hazardous Work: Exercise caution until you determine how this drug affects you.

Alcohol: Limit intake of alcohol, as it may increase the constriction of blood vessels caused by this drug.

Pregnancy: This medicine should not be used during pregnancy because it can cause a miscarriage or serious damage to the fetus.

Breast Feeding: This drug passes into breast milk and can cause vomiting, diarrhea, convulsions, or other untoward effects in nursing infants; avoid using.

Infants and Children: Consult your pediatrician.

OVERDOSE
Symptoms: Seizures, nausea, vomiting, stomach pain or bloating, unusually rapid or slow heartbeat, severe headache, dizziness, drowsiness, constipation, shortness of breath, excitability.

What to Do: Call your doctor, emergency medical services (EMS), or the nearest poison control center immediately.

▼ INTERACTIONS

DRUG INTERACTIONS
Do not take within 24 hours of taking a "triptan" migraine drug. Do not take this drug if you are taking an over-the-counter or prescription allergy or cold remedy. Consult your doctor for specific advice if you are taking any other medicine, especially erythromycin, nicotine, insulin, or a beta-blocker.

FOOD INTERACTIONS
Caffeine and salt intake should be limited.

DISEASE INTERACTIONS
Tell your doctor if you are overly sensitive to this drug or other ergot derivatives or if you have any other condition, especially hypertension, a blood vessel condition, any infection, or a liver, heart, or kidney problem.

DILTIAZEM HYDROCHLORIDE

Available in: Tablets, extended-release capsules, injection
Available OTC? No   **As Generic?** Yes
Drug Class: Calcium channel blocker

▼ USAGE INFORMATION

WHY IT'S PRESCRIBED
To relieve and control angina (chest pain associated with heart disease), to reduce high blood pressure, and to correct heartbeat irregularities (cardiac arrhythmia).

HOW IT WORKS
Diltiazem interferes with the movement of calcium into heart muscle cells and the smooth muscle cells in the walls of the arteries. This action relaxes blood vessels (causing them to widen), which lowers blood pressure, increases the blood supply to the heart, and decreases the heart's overall workload.

▼ DOSAGE GUIDELINES

RANGE AND FREQUENCY
Tablets (for chest pain)— 30 mg, 3 or 4 times a day to start, increased to 40 to 60 mg, 3 or 4 times a day. Extended-release capsules (for high blood pressure)— 120 to 240 mg a day taken in 1 or 2 divided doses. (For heartbeat irregularities, dilti-azem is administered by injection by a health care professional.)

ONSET OF EFFECT
Tablets: 30 to 60 minutes. Extended-release capsules: 2 to 3 hours.

DURATION OF ACTION
Tablets: 6 to 8 hours. Extended-release capsules: 10 to 14 hours.

DIETARY ADVICE
Diltiazem is best taken before meals or at bedtime.

STORAGE
Store tablets and capsules in a tightly sealed container away from heat, moisture, and direct light.

MISSED DOSE
Take it as soon as you remember. However, if it is near the time for the next dose, skip the missed dose and resume your regular dosage schedule. Do not double the next dose.

STOPPING THE DRUG
Do not stop taking this drug suddenly, as this may cause potentially serious health problems. If therapy is to be discontinued, dosage should be reduced gradually, according to doctor's instructions.

PROLONGED USE
No unusual side effects are expected with prolonged use.

▼ PRECAUTIONS

Over 60: Weakness, dizziness, and fainting are more likely in older persons.

Driving and Hazardous Work: Diltiazem can cause dizziness or drowsiness. Do not drive or engage in hazardous work until you determine how the medicine affects you.

Alcohol: Use alcohol with caution because it may increase the effect of the drug and cause an excessive drop in blood pressure.

Pregnancy: Birth defects have occurred in animal studies. Adequate human studies have not been done. Avoid this drug during the first 3 months of pregnancy and take it during the last 6 months only if your doctor says it is clearly needed.

Breast Feeding: Diltiazem passes into breast milk; avoid or discontinue use while breast feeding.

Infants and Children: Usually not prescribed; the safety and effectiveness of diltiazem for children under the age of 12 have not been established.

Special Concerns: It is important to brush and floss your teeth and see your dentist regularly, since using diltiazem may promote dental problems. This medication may make you sensitive to sunlight.

OVERDOSE
Symptoms: Heart block causing unusual shortness of breath; fatigue, excessive dizziness, fainting.

What to Do: Call your doctor, emergency medical services (EMS) or the nearest poison control center immediately.

▼ INTERACTIONS

DRUG INTERACTIONS
Consult your doctor for specific advice if you are taking aspirin, beta-blockers, digitalis preparations, carbamazepine, cyclosporine, digoxin, lithium, oral diabetes agents, phenytoin, rifampin, cimetidine, fluvoxamine, or ranitidine.

FOOD INTERACTIONS
Avoid excessive salt intake.

DISEASE INTERACTIONS
Consult your doctor if you have any of the following: kidney disease, liver disease, high blood pressure, or any kind of heart or blood vessel disease.

≡ SIDE EFFECTS ≡

SERIOUS
Irregular or slow heartbeat, shortness of breath, and fatigue caused by heart failure. Call a doctor immediately.

COMMON
Headache, drowsiness, swelling of feet and ankles, constipation, nausea, sudden weight gain, fatigue.

LESS COMMON
Dizziness, weakness, depression, nervousness, insomnia, confusion, slow pulse, vomiting, diarrhea, excessive urination, itch, sensitivity to sunlight, yellowish tinge to eyes or skin due to liver failure, skin rash, overgrowth of the gums.

DIMENHYDRINATE

Available in: Capsules, tablets, elixir, syrup, injection, suppositories
Available OTC? Yes **As Generic?** Yes
Drug Class: Antihistamine

▼ USAGE INFORMATION

WHY IT'S PRESCRIBED
To relieve nausea and vomiting and to treat or prevent motion sickness.

HOW IT WORKS
Dimenhydrinate directly inhibits the stimulation of certain nerves in the brain and inner ear to suppress nausea, vomiting, dizziness, and vertigo.

▼ DOSAGE GUIDELINES

RANGE AND FREQUENCY
Capsules, tablets, liquids– Adults: 50 to 100 mg every 4 to 6 hours. Children ages 6 to 12: 25 to 50 mg every 6 to 8 hours. Children ages 2 to 6: 12.5 to 25 mg every 6 to 8 hours. Injection– Adults: 50 mg into a vein every 4 hours. Children: 1.25 mg per 2.2 lbs (1 kg) of body weight into a vein or muscle every 6 hours. Suppositories– Adults: 50 to 100 mg every 6 to 8 hours. Children over age 12: 50 mg every 8 to 12 hours. Children ages 8 to 12: 25 to 50 mg every 8 to 12 hours. Children ages 6 to 8: 12.5 to 25 mg every 8 to 12 hours. To prevent motion sickness, take this drug at least 30 minutes, and preferably 1 to 2 hours, before traveling.

ONSET OF EFFECT
Oral: Within 20 to 30 minutes. Injection: 2 to 20 minutes. Suppositories: 30 to 45 minutes.

DURATION OF ACTION
3 to 6 hours.

DIETARY ADVICE
This drug can be taken with food or milk to minimize gastrointestinal distress.

STORAGE
Store in a tightly sealed container in a dry place away from heat and direct light.

MISSED DOSE
Take it as soon as you remember. However, if it is near the time for the next dose, skip the missed dose and resume your regular dosage schedule. Do not double the next dose.

STOPPING THE DRUG
You should take it as prescribed for the full treatment period, but you may stop if you are feeling better before the scheduled end of therapy.

PROLONGED USE
Take this drug only as long as it is needed.

▼ PRECAUTIONS

Over 60: Older persons are more sensitive to the effects of dimenhydrinate. Dizziness, drowsiness, confusion, difficult or painful urination, and other side effects are more likely to occur.

Driving and Hazardous Work: Do not drive or engage in hazardous work until you determine how the medicine affects you.

Alcohol: Avoid alcohol.

Pregnancy: Animal studies with high doses of dimenhydrinate have found no birth defects. Human studies have not been done. Because the studies cannot rule out harm, the drug should be used during pregnancy only if it is clearly needed.

Breast Feeding: Dimenhydrinate may pass into breast milk; caution is advised; avoid or discontinue use while breast feeding.

Infants and Children: The safety and efficacy of this drug in children under 2 years of age (age 6 for the suppository form) have not been established. Older children are especially sensitive to the drug's side effects.

Special Concerns: Children should be observed carefully for signs of side effects; they are more likely to develop serious complications from these medications, and younger children are often unable to describe changes in the way that they are feeling.

OVERDOSE
Symptoms: Seizures, hallucinations, drowsiness, difficulty breathing, unconsciousness.

What to Do: An overdose of dimenhydrinate is unlikely to be life-threatening. However, if someone takes a much larger dose than prescribed, call your doctor, emergency medical services (EMS), or the nearest poison control center immediately.

▼ INTERACTIONS

DRUG INTERACTIONS
Consult your doctor for specific advice if you are taking any narcotic pain relievers, sedatives, tranquilizers, antidepressants, antibiotics, aspirin, barbiturates, cisplatin, diuretics, or theophylline.

FOOD INTERACTIONS
No known food interactions.

DISEASE INTERACTIONS
Caution is advised when taking dimenhydrinate. Consult your doctor if you have glaucoma or an enlarged prostate.

SIDE EFFECTS

SERIOUS
No serious side effects are associated with this drug.

COMMON
Drowsiness.

LESS COMMON
Headache, blurred vision, palpitations, loss of coordination, dry mouth, low blood pressure causing dizziness and weakness, ringing in ears.

DIPHENHYDRAMINE HYDROCHLORIDE

Available in: Capsules, elixir, syrup, tablets, injection
Available OTC? Yes   **As Generic?** Yes
Drug Class: Antihistamine

▼ USAGE INFORMATION

WHY IT'S PRESCRIBED
To relieve hay fever symptoms, itching skin and hives, motion sickness, nonproductive cough due to cold or hay fever, and sleeping difficulty; also used to treat symptoms of Parkinson's disease.

HOW IT WORKS
It blocks the effects of histamine, a naturally occurring substance that causes swelling, itching, sneezing, and watery eyes. In patients with Parkinson's disease, it decreases tremors and muscle stiffness.

▼ DOSAGE GUIDELINES

RANGE AND FREQUENCY
For hay fever symptoms— Capsules, elixir, syrup, tablets: Adults and teenagers: 25 to 50 mg every 4 to 6 hours. Children younger than age 6: 6.25 to 12.5 mg every 4 to 6 hours. Children ages 6 to 12: 12.5 to 25 mg every 4 to 6 hours. Injection: Adults: 10 to 50 mg into a vein or muscle. Children: 1.25 mg per 2.2 lbs (1 kg) of body weight into a muscle 4 times a day. For nausea, vomiting and dizziness— Capsules, elixir, syrup, tablets: Adults: 25 to 50 mg every 4 to 6 hours. Children: 1 to 1.5 mg per 2.2 lbs every 4 to 6 hours. Injection: Adults: 10 mg into a vein or muscle. May be increased to 25 to 50 mg every 2 to 3 hours. Children: 1 to 1.5 mg per 2.2 lbs every 6 hours. For Parkinson's disease— Capsules, elixir, syrup, tablets: Adults: 25 mg, 3 times a day. Doctor may gradually increase dose. Injection: Adults: 10 to 50 mg into a vein or muscle. Children: 1.25 mg per 2.2 lbs into a muscle, 4 times a day. As a sedative— Capsules, elixir, syrup, tablets: Adults: 50 mg 20 to 30 minutes before bedtime. For cough— Liquid: Adults and teenagers: 25 mg every 4 to 6 hours. Children ages 2 to 6: 6.25 mg (½ teaspoon) every 4 to 6 hours. Children ages 6 to 12: 12.5 mg (1 teaspoon) every 4 to 6 hours.

ONSET OF EFFECT
After capsules, elixir, syrup, or tablets: 15 minutes. Injection: Unknown.

DURATION OF ACTION
6 to 8 hours.

DIETARY ADVICE
Take diphenhydramine with food or milk to reduce gastrointestinal distress.

STORAGE
Store in a dry place away from heat and direct light. Prevent liquid forms from freezing.

MISSED DOSE
Take it as soon as you remember. If it is near the time for the next dose, skip the missed dose and resume your regular dosage schedule. Do not double the next dose.

STOPPING THE DRUG
Stop taking this drug and call your doctor if it is not effective after 5 days.

PROLONGED USE
No special problems have been reported.

▼ PRECAUTIONS

Over 60: Adverse reactions may be more likely and more severe.

Driving and Hazardous Work: Do not drive or engage in hazardous work until you determine how the medicine affects you. Use of this drug is a disqualification for piloting aircraft.

Alcohol: Alcohol may increase the likelihood and severity of side effects, such as drowsiness and mental confusion.

Pregnancy: No birth defects have been reported in animals. Studies of pregnant women have found no significant increase in birth defects.

Breast Feeding: Diphenhydramine passes into breast milk; avoid or discontinue use while nursing.

Infants and Children: This drug is not recommended for children under the age of 2.

Special Concerns: Children should be observed carefully for signs of side effects; they are more likely to develop serious complications, and younger children are often unable to describe changes in the way that they are feeling.

OVERDOSE
Symptoms: Marked drowsiness, dilated and unreactive pupils, fever, excitability, breathing interruptions, combativeness, mental confusion, loss of coordination, weak pulse, seizures, loss of consciousness.

What to Do: Call your doctor, emergency medical services (EMS), or the nearest poison control center immediately.

▼ INTERACTIONS

DRUG INTERACTIONS
Consult your doctor for specific advice if you are taking anticholinergics, alcohol, disopyramide, central nervous system depressants, or MAO inhibitors.

FOOD INTERACTIONS
No known food interactions.

DISEASE INTERACTIONS
Consult your doctor if you have a history of severe respiratory disease, glaucoma, urinary obstruction, or prostate enlargement.

▬ SIDE EFFECTS ▬

SERIOUS
No serious side effects are associated with this drug.

COMMON
Drowsiness, dry mouth, nausea, thickening of mucus.

LESS COMMON
Confusion, difficult urination, blurred vision.

DIPHENOXYLATE HYDROCHLORIDE/ATROPINE SULFATE

BRAND NAMES

Lofene, Logen, Lomocot, Lomotil, Lonox, Vi-Atro

Available in: Liquid, tablet
Available OTC? No **As Generic?** Yes
Drug Class: Antidiarrheal

▼ USAGE INFORMATION

WHY IT'S PRESCRIBED
To relieve severe diarrhea and intestinal cramps.

HOW IT WORKS
This medication blocks nerve activity in the intestinal tract, which reduces propulsive contractions (peristalsis) and diminishes intestinal secretions.

▼ DOSAGE GUIDELINES

RANGE AND FREQUENCY
Adults and teenagers: 5 mg (2 tablets or 2 teaspoons), 3 or 4 times a day. Your doctor may reduce the dose when diarrhea starts to be controlled. Children: Consult your pediatrician.

ONSET OF EFFECT
Within 45 to 60 minutes.

DURATION OF ACTION
3 to 4 hours.

DIETARY ADVICE
The tablet should be taken with liquid or food to reduce stomach irritation. A mild diet is recommended when recovering from diarrhea. Bananas, rice, applesauce, and plain toast are good choices. Be sure to get plenty of fluids.

STORAGE
Store in a tightly sealed container away from heat, moisture, and direct light. Keep the liquid form from freezing.

MISSED DOSE
Take it as soon as you remember. If it is near the time for the next dose, skip the missed dose and resume your regular dosage schedule. Do not double the next dose.

STOPPING THE DRUG
Continue taking the medicine until at least 24 to 36 hours after diarrhea has stopped. Consult with your doctor if the diarrhea does not stop after 2 days or if you develop a fever.

PROLONGED USE
Diphenoxylate and atropine may be habit-forming if larger doses are taken for a long time. Ask your doctor about the need for follow-up medical examinations or laboratory studies to check liver function if you must take this medication for a prolonged period of time.

▼ PRECAUTIONS

Over 60: Adverse reactions may be more likely and more severe in older patients.

Driving and Hazardous Work: Do not drive or engage in hazardous work until you determine how the medicine affects you.

Alcohol: Avoid alcohol while taking this medicine.

Pregnancy: If you are pregnant or plan to become pregnant, consult your doctor; discuss whether the benefits justify the possible risks to the unborn child.

Breast Feeding: This drug passes into breast milk; caution is advised. Consult your doctor for specific advice.

Infants and Children: Not recommended for use by children under the age of 2. For children over 2, use the drug only under a doctor's supervision.

Special Concerns: During the first 24 hours, drink plenty of caffeine-free clear liquids such as broth, ginger ale, and decaffeinated tea. During the second 24 hours you may eat bland foods such as applesauce, bread, toast, crackers, rice, and oatmeal. Avoid caffeine, fried or spicy foods, bran, candy, fruits, and vegetables. They can make your condition worse.

OVERDOSE

Symptoms: Drowsiness, dizziness, and weakness caused by low blood pressure; seizures; slow or arrested breathing; blurred vision; reddened face; dryness of the mouth; unusual behavior.

What to Do: Call your doctor, emergency medical services (EMS), or the nearest poison control center immediately.

▼ INTERACTIONS

DRUG INTERACTIONS
The following drugs may interact with the combination of diphenoxylate and atropine. Consult your doctor for specific advice if you are taking antibiotics; central nervous system depressants; MAO inhibitors; naltrexone; or anticholinergic medicines to reduce stomach acid, spasms, or cramps.

FOOD INTERACTIONS
No known food interactions.

DISEASE INTERACTIONS
Caution is advised when taking this drug. Before starting, consult your doctor if you have liver problems, Down's syndrome, ulcerative colitis, Crohn's disease, glaucoma, chronic lung disease (such as emphysema), heart disease, a history of alcohol or drug abuse, an enlarged prostate, gallbladder disease or gallstones, high blood pressure, an underactive or overactive thyroid, kidney disease, dysentery, myasthenia gravis, or intestinal or urinary tract blockage.

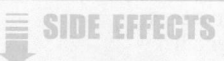

SIDE EFFECTS

SERIOUS
Swelling of the hands, feet, face, lips or throat; severe stomach pain accompanied by nausea and vomiting. Call your doctor immediately.

COMMON
Dizziness, dry mouth, sedation.

LESS COMMON
Drowsiness, lethargy, headache, restlessness, mental depression, fast pulse, enlarged pupils, nausea, vomiting, abdominal discomfort, loss of appetite, slowed breathing, rash, itching, inability to urinate.

DIPHTHERIA, TETANUS TOXOIDS, AND PERTUSSIS VACCINE (DTP)

Available in: Injection
Available OTC? No   **As Generic?** Yes
Drug Class: Vaccine

▼ USAGE INFORMATION

WHY IT'S PRESCRIBED
The DTP vaccine is used as a combination immunizing agent to prevent three serious childhood diseases—diphtheria, tetanus, and pertussis. Diphtheria can cause difficulty breathing, pneumonia, nerve damage, heart problems, and possibly death. Tetanus (lockjaw) can cause severe muscle spasms. Pertussis (whooping cough) causes severe bouts of coughing that can interfere with breathing. Pertussis can also cause long-lasting bronchitis, pneumonia, seizures, and brain damage, and can lead to death.

HOW IT WORKS
The DTP vaccine stimulates the body's immune system to produce protective antibodies against diphtheria, tetanus, and pertussis.

▼ DOSAGE GUIDELINES

RANGE AND FREQUENCY
Children 2 months to 7 years: 0.5 ml injected into muscle 4 to 8 weeks apart for 3 doses, followed by a fourth 0.5 ml dose injected into a muscle 1 year later, usually at 15 to 18 months of age. A fifth dose (booster) may be administered at 4 to 6 years of age. Persons over 7 years of age should not receive the whole-cell pertussis vaccine.

ONSET OF EFFECT
Unknown.

DURATION OF ACTION
Up to 10 years.

DIETARY ADVICE
The vaccine can be administered without regard to diet.

STORAGE
Not applicable; the dose is administered only at a health care facility.

MISSED DOSE
If your child misses a scheduled vaccination, contact your pediatrician.

STOPPING THE DRUG
The full schedule of injections should be followed unless a medical problem intervenes.

PROLONGED USE
No special problems are expected.

▼ PRECAUTIONS

Over 60: This vaccine is not intended for use by older persons.

Driving and Hazardous Work: Not applicable.

Alcohol: Not applicable.

Pregnancy: This vaccine is not intended for women of childbearing age.

Breast Feeding: This vaccine is not intended for women of childbearing age.

Infants and Children: Not recommended for use by children over age 7.

Special Concerns: Anyone over the age of 7 should receive a vaccine that contains tetanus and diphtheria toxoids, but not whole-cell pertussis vaccine. Older persons should receive the diphtheria and tetanus booster injections every 10 years for life. Your doctor may want the child to take 1 or more doses of acetaminophen or another medicine that helps prevent fever after receiving the DTP injection. Consult your doctor for specific advice. DTP should not be given to a child who has had a previous serious adverse reaction to a DTP vaccination.

OVERDOSE
Symptoms: Not applicable.

What to Do: No cases of overdose have been reported.

▼ INTERACTIONS

DRUG INTERACTIONS
The following drugs may interact with DTP. Consult your doctor for specific advice if your child is taking an anticoagulant or a drug that suppresses the immune system. DTP can be given with vaccines for other diseases, but should not be given within 3 days of influenza vaccine.

FOOD INTERACTIONS
No known food interactions.

DISEASE INTERACTIONS
Consult your doctor if your child has any of the following: a brain disease, a central nervous system disorder, epilepsy, a fever, muscle spasms, or seizures.

≡ SIDE EFFECTS ≡

SERIOUS
Fever of 105°F or more, seizures, collapse, difficulty breathing or swallowing, hives, unusual irritability, temporary loss of consciousness or awareness. Call your doctor as soon as possible.

COMMON
Fever between 100.4°F and 102.2°F, sometimes accompanied by loss of appetite, drowsiness, vomiting, and fretfulness; redness, swelling, lump, pain, or tenderness at the site of the injection.

LESS COMMON
Fever between 102.2°F and 104°F and skin rash.

DIPIVEFRIN

BRAND NAME

Propine

Available in: Ophthalmic solution
Available OTC? No   **As Generic?** Yes
Drug Class: Antiglaucoma agent

▼ USAGE INFORMATION

WHY IT'S PRESCRIBED
To treat glaucoma.

HOW IT WORKS
Glaucoma, a sight-threatening disorder, occurs when the aqueous humor (the fluid inside the eye) cannot drain properly, causing an increase in pressure within the eyeball (intraocular pressure). The increased eye pressure can damage the optic nerve and lead to a gradually progressive loss of vision. Dipivefrin is converted in the eye to epinephrine, which decreases the production of aqueous humor and increases its outflow.

▼ DOSAGE GUIDELINES

RANGE AND FREQUENCY
To start, 1 drop in each eye every 12 hours. The dose may be changed based on patient's response.

ONSET OF EFFECT
Within 30 minutes.

DURATION OF ACTION
12 hours or more.

DIETARY ADVICE
No special restrictions.

STORAGE
Store in a tightly sealed container away from heat, moisture, and direct light. Do not allow the medicine to freeze.

MISSED DOSE
Apply it as soon as you remember. If it is near the time for the next dose, skip the missed dose and resume your regular dosage schedule. Do not double the next dose.

STOPPING THE DRUG
The decision to stop using the drug should be made by your doctor.

PROLONGED USE
See your doctor regularly for tests and examinations if you must take this drug for a prolonged period.

▼ PRECAUTIONS

Over 60:
No special problems are expected.

Driving and Hazardous Work:
The use of dipivefrin should not impair your ability to perform such tasks safely.

Alcohol: No special precautions are necessary.

Pregnancy: Dipivefrin has not caused birth defects in animals. Human studies have not been done. Before you take dipivefrin, tell your doctor if you are pregnant or plan to become pregnant.

Breast Feeding: Dipivefrin may pass into breast milk; caution is advised. Consult your doctor for advice.

Infants and Children: No special precautions.

Special Concerns: Dipivefrin should not be used by people with closed-angle glaucoma. To use the eye drops, first wash your hands. Tilt your head back. Gently apply pressure to the inside corner of the eyelid and with the index finger of the same hand, pull downward on the lower eyelid to make a space. Drop the medicine into this space and close your eye. Apply pressure for 1 or 2 minutes while keeping the eye closed without blinking. Then wash your hands again. Make sure the tip of the dropper does not touch your eye, finger, or any other surface. If you are taking the medicine with the compliance cap (C Cap), make sure that the number 1 or the correct day of the week appears in the window of the cap before using the eye drops for the first time. After every dose, rotate the bottle until the cap clicks to the position that tells you the next dose.

OVERDOSE
Symptoms: Rapid or irregular heartbeat.

What to Do: An overdose of dipivefrin is unlikely to be life-threatening. If a large volume enters the eyes, flush with water. If someone accidentally ingests the medicine, call your doctor, emergency medical services (EMS), or the nearest poison control center.

▼ INTERACTIONS

DRUG INTERACTIONS
Other drugs may interact with dipivefrin. Consult your doctor for specific advice if you are taking tricyclic antidepressants, maprotiline, nomifensine, ophthalmic beta-blockers, digitalis drugs, or systemic sympathomimetics.

FOOD INTERACTIONS
No known food interactions.

DISEASE INTERACTIONS
Caution is advised when taking dipivefrin. Consult your doctor if you have closed-angle glaucoma or aphakia (absence of part or all of the lens of the eye).

SIDE EFFECTS

SERIOUS
Fast or irregular heartbeat. Call your doctor immediately.

COMMON
In people who have had prior cataract surgery, this drug may cause swelling at the center of the retina that can lead to (in most cases) reversible vision impairment.

LESS COMMON
Increased sensitivity of eyes to light; burning, stinging, or other eye irritation.

DIPYRIDAMOLE

Available in: Tablet, injection
Available OTC? No   **As Generic?** Yes
Drug Class: Antiplatelet drug

▼ USAGE INFORMATION

WHY IT'S PRESCRIBED
To prevent blood clots during recovery from heart valve replacement surgery; to reduce frequency and intensity of angina attacks (chest pain associated with heart disease).

HOW IT WORKS
Dipyridamole is believed to increase blood levels of adenosine, a metabolic product that causes blood vessels to expand and prevents platelets, a type of blood cell, from adhering to one another to form a clot.

▼ DOSAGE GUIDELINES

RANGE AND FREQUENCY
Tablets: 75 to 100 mg, 4 times a day, given with an anticoagulant such as warfarin, to prevent blood clots. If at all possible, when dipyridamole is taken with warfarin, the injectable form of dipyridamole should be avoided; injection (when necessary) is administered under doctor's supervision. Aspirin may also be used with dipyridamole, as the two drugs have a synergistic anticoagulant effect.

ONSET OF EFFECT
About 10 minutes; 3 months of continual use is needed for the full effect to occur.

DURATION OF ACTION
About 6 hours.

DIETARY ADVICE
Take this medication 1 hour before or 2 hours after meals. Swallow the tablet with 6 to 8 ounces of water.

STORAGE
Store in a tightly sealed container in a dry place away from heat and direct light.

MISSED DOSE
Take it as soon as you remember. However, if it is near the time for the next dose, skip the missed dose and resume your regular dosage schedule as prescribed. Do not double the next dose.

STOPPING THE DRUG
Take as prescribed for the full treatment period.

PROLONGED USE
If you must use dipyridamole for a prolonged period, consult your doctor about the possible need for follow-up medical examinations or laboratory studies.

▼ PRECAUTIONS

Over 60: Older patients should start with smaller doses. Otherwise, no special problems are expected.

Driving and Hazardous Work: Dipyridamole may cause dizziness. Do not drive or engage in hazardous work until you determine how the medicine affects you.

Alcohol: Avoid alcohol while taking this medication because it may lower blood pressure excessively.

Pregnancy: Dipyridamole has not been reported to cause birth defects. Consult your doctor about its use during pregnancy.

Breast Feeding: While dipyridamole passes into breast milk, it has not been reported to cause problems in nursing babies. Consult your doctor for specific advice about its use while nursing.

Infants and Children: Dipyridamole is not recommended for use by children under 12.

Special Concerns: If your doctor tells you to take dipyridamole with aspirin, take only the amount of aspirin that is prescribed. Tell any doctor or dentist whom you consult that you are taking dipyridamole.

OVERDOSE
Symptoms: Dizziness and weakness caused by extremely low blood pressure (hypotension).

What to Do: Discontinue taking the drug. An overdose of dipyridamole is unlikely to be life-threatening; however, if someone takes a much larger dose than prescribed, call your doctor, emergency medical services (EMS), or the nearest poison control center immediately.

▼ INTERACTIONS

DRUG INTERACTIONS
Consult your doctor for specific advice if you are taking anticoagulants (such as warfarin, aspirin, and ticlopidine), valproic acid, or any non-steroidal anti-inflammatory drug (NSAID), such as indomethacin.

FOOD INTERACTIONS
Taking dipyridamole within 1 hour of eating will decrease the body's absorption of the drug. When possible, take dipyridamole on an empty stomach.

DISEASE INTERACTIONS
Caution is advised when taking dipyridamole. Consult your doctor if you have low blood pressure or liver disease or if you are recovering from a heart attack.

 SIDE EFFECTS

SERIOUS
Dizziness and weakness caused by low blood pressure (hypotension). Call your doctor.

COMMON
Headache, nausea, rash.

LESS COMMON
Vomiting, diarrhea, flushing, itching, chest pain, liver problems causing nausea, vomiting, yellow-tinged eyes and skin, swelling, bloating.

DIRITHROMYCIN

Available in: Tablets
Available OTC? No   **As Generic?** No
Drug Class: Macrolide antibiotic

▼ USAGE INFORMATION

WHY IT'S PRESCRIBED
To treat bronchitis, some types of pneumonia such as Legionnaires' disease, skin infections, and tonsillitis or other throat infections such as strep throat. Dirithromycin is effective only against infections caused by bacteria; it is ineffective against those caused by viruses (for example, colds and flu), fungi, or other microorganisms.

HOW IT WORKS
Dirithromycin prevents bacterial cells from manufacturing specific proteins necessary for their survival.

▼ DOSAGE GUIDELINES

RANGE AND FREQUENCY
Adults and children age 12 and over: 500 mg, once a day for 5 to 14 days (depending on the condition being treated). It is recommended that this medication be taken at the same time every day.

ONSET OF EFFECT
Within 2 hours; full effect may occur in 2 to 5 days.

DURATION OF ACTION
From 30 to 50 hours.

DIETARY ADVICE
Take this medicine with food or within 1 hour of eating. Drink plenty of fluids.

STORAGE
Store in a tightly sealed container away from moisture, heat, and direct light.

MISSED DOSE
Take it as soon as you remember, up to 12 hours late. However, if more than 12 hours have passed, skip the missed dose and resume your regular dosage schedule. Do not double the next dose.

STOPPING THE DRUG
Take this drug for the full treatment period, even if you begin to feel better before the scheduled end of therapy.

PROLONGED USE
Prolonged use is not recommended. Your doctor will discontinue the medicine once the infection is cured. Unnecessary or prolonged use of any antibiotic may promote infection by microorganisms that are resistant to the drug's effects. This is known as "superinfection."

▼ PRECAUTIONS

Over 60: No special problems are expected.

Driving and Hazardous Work: Do not drive or engage in hazardous work until you determine how dirithromycin affects you.

Alcohol: No special precautions are necessary.

Pregnancy: Adequate studies of the use of dirithromycin during pregnancy have not been done; discuss the potential risks and benefits with your doctor.

Breast Feeding: It is not known if dirithromycin passes into breast milk; consult your doctor for advice.

Infants and Children: This drug should be given to children under 12 only under close medical supervision.

Special Concerns: Tell any doctor or dentist you consult that you are taking this medicine. Before taking dirithromycin, tell your doctor if you are allergic to any other drug, especially an antibiotic.

OVERDOSE
Symptoms: No cases of dirithromycin overdose have been reported. Symptoms would most likely include diarrhea, nausea, vomiting, and heartburn.

What to Do: An overdose of dirithromycin is unlikely to be life-threatening. However, if someone takes a much larger dose than prescribed, contact a doctor or the nearest poison control center for advice.

▼ INTERACTIONS

DRUG INTERACTIONS
This drug should not be taken by patients known to have had prior allergic reactions to erythromycins or other macrolide antibiotics. Also, consult your doctor for specific advice if you are taking any other drugs, especially allergy drugs, antacids or histamine (H2) blockers, anticoagulants, antiarrhythmics, seizure drugs, cholesterol-lowering drugs, digitalis drugs, ergotamine, bromocriptine, cyclosporine, or valproate.

FOOD INTERACTIONS
No known food interactions.

DISEASE INTERACTIONS
Consult your doctor if you have a blood or liver disorder or any allergy.

▽ SIDE EFFECTS ▽

SERIOUS
Colitis (inflammation of the lower gastrointestinal tract, with symptoms including severe abdominal pain or cramping, watery or bloody stools, severe diarrhea, fever); liver toxicity (causing fever, nausea, vomiting, yellowish tinge to eyes or skin); allergic reaction (swelling of the lips, tongue, face, and throat, breathing difficulty, skin rash or hives); blood clotting disorders (causing unusual bleeding, bruising, and tiny bright red spots on the skin). Such side effects are rare, but if they do occur, stop taking dirithromycin and seek medical assistance immediately.

COMMON
No common side effects are associated with the use of dirithromycin.

LESS COMMON
Dizziness, stomach upset or discomfort, mild diarrhea, mild nausea and vomiting, headache, unusual fatigue.

DISOPYRAMIDE

Available in: Capsules, extended-release capsules, tablets
Available OTC? No   **As Generic?** Yes
Drug Class: Antiarrhythmic

▼ USAGE INFORMATION

WHY IT'S PRESCRIBED
To control abnormal or irregular heart rhythms (cardiac arrhythmias).

HOW IT WORKS
It slows the activity of the heart's natural pacemaker and delays the transmission of electrical impulses through the heart muscle, thus stabilizing heartbeat.

▼ DOSAGE GUIDELINES

RANGE AND FREQUENCY
Adults weighing more than 110 lbs: 150 mg capsules every 6 hours; 300 mg extended-release capsules every 12 hours. Dosage must be individualized for adults weighing less than 110 lbs. Children age 12 to 18: 6 to 15 mg for every 2.2 lbs (1 kg) of body weight daily; ages 4 to 12: 10 to 15 mg per 2.2 lbs daily; ages 1 to 4: 10 to 20 mg per 2.2 lbs of body weight daily; under 1 year: 10 to 30 mg per 2.2 lbs daily. Doses are divided into equal amounts and taken every 6 hours. Initial doses should be smaller in patients suffering from impaired left ventricular function.

ONSET OF EFFECT
30 minutes to 3.5 hours.

DURATION OF ACTION
Up to 8.5 hours (longer in patients with impaired kidney function).

DIETARY ADVICE
Can be taken with or between meals.

STORAGE
Store in a tightly sealed container in a dry place away from heat and direct light.

MISSED DOSE
Take it as soon as you remember. However, if it is within 4 hours of the next dose, skip the missed dose and return to your regular dosage schedule as prescribed. Do not double the next dose.

STOPPING THE DRUG
The decision to stop taking the drug should be made by your doctor.

PROLONGED USE
Prolonged use requires supervision and periodic evaluation by your doctor.

▼ PRECAUTIONS

Over 60: Adverse reactions (especially dry mouth and difficulty urinating) may be more likely and more severe in older patients. Dosage reduction may be required.

Driving and Hazardous Work: Avoid such activities until you determine how the medicine affects you.

Alcohol: Avoid alcohol.

Pregnancy: Before taking this medicine, tell your doctor if you are pregnant or plan to become pregnant. Discuss with your doctor whether the benefits of taking disopyramide justify the possible risk to the unborn child.

Breast Feeding: Disopyramide passes into breast milk; avoid or discontinue use while nursing.

Infants and Children: Children using this drug should do so only under close medical supervision.

Special Concerns: Try to take disopyramide exactly at the times prescribed. An alarm clock may be needed for nighttime doses. Tell your doctor if you have had an unfavorable reaction to any other antiarrhythmic drug.

OVERDOSE
Symptoms: Heartbeat irregularities, severe drop in blood pressure, loss of consciousness, breathing difficulty.

What to Do: Call your doctor, emergency medical services (EMS), or the nearest poison control center immediately.

▼ INTERACTIONS

DRUG INTERACTIONS
Consult your doctor if you are taking other antiarrhythmics, anticholinergics, anticoagulants, insulin, drugs for high blood pressure, cisapride, nimodipine, phenobarbital, phenytoin, pimozide, propafenone, or rifampin.

FOOD INTERACTIONS
No known food interactions.

DISEASE INTERACTIONS
Caution is advised when taking disopyramide. Consult your doctor if you have any of the following: heart disease or heart block, diabetes mellitus, enlarged prostate, glaucoma, myasthenia gravis, kidney or liver disease.

≡ SIDE EFFECTS ≡

SERIOUS
Chest pain, shortness of breath, irregular or rapid heartbeat (palpitations), fainting, sudden weight gain, swelling of fingers or ankles, anxiety. Call your doctor immediately if such symptoms arise.

COMMON
Dizziness, faintness, weakness caused by low blood pressure, blurred vision, constipation, dry eyes, dry nose, dry mouth. Consult your doctor if such symptoms persist.

LESS COMMON
Depression, agitation, fatigue, muscle weakness, decreased urination, nausea, vomiting, severe loss of appetite and weight, abdominal pain, difficulty urinating, yellow-tinged eyes and skin, low blood sugar causing drowsiness, headache, cold sweats, nervousness, confusion, skin rash.

DISULFIRAM

Available in: Tablets
Available OTC? No   **As Generic?** Yes
Drug Class: Alcoholism control drug

▼ USAGE INFORMATION

WHY IT'S PRESCRIBED
To help treat chronic alcoholism.

HOW IT WORKS
Disulfiram interferes with the activity of the liver enzyme that processes and metabolizes alcohol, causing an accumulation of a chemical known as "acetaldehyde." A buildup of acetaldehyde in the body leads to a severely unpleasant reaction, including nausea and vomiting. Thus, while not a cure for alcoholism, disulfiram is a deterrent to alcohol consumption.

▼ DOSAGE GUIDELINES

RANGE AND FREQUENCY
Initial dose: 250 to 500 mg a day in a single dose in the morning or evening. Maintenance dose: 125 to 500 mg once a day. Treatment with disulfiram should not start until at least 12 hours after consumption of an alcoholic beverage.

ONSET OF EFFECT
1 to 2 hours.

DURATION OF ACTION
Effects usually last 3 to 4 days but may persist for up to 2 weeks.

DIETARY ADVICE
Take it with or after meals to decrease stomach irritation.

STORAGE
Store in a tightly sealed container away from heat, moisture, and direct light.

MISSED DOSE
Take it as soon as you remember. If it is within 12 hours of the next dose, skip the missed dose and return to your normal schedule. Do not double the next dose.

STOPPING THE DRUG
The decision to stop taking the drug should be made in consultation with your physician.

PROLONGED USE
Use of disulfiram on a regular schedule for several months is needed to see if alcohol consumption is deterred. Use should continue until permanent self-control is achieved. Periodic tests of liver function should be done. Gradual reduction of doses may be required when disulfiram has been taken for a prolonged period of time.

▼ PRECAUTIONS

Over 60: Adverse reactions may be more likely and more severe in older patients.

Driving and Hazardous Work: Do not drive or engage in hazardous work until you determine how the medication affects you.

Alcohol: This medication should never be taken by anyone with alcohol in the bloodstream.

Pregnancy: Studies have indicated that disulfiram may lead to birth defects; however, alcohol abuse may lead to births defects as well. Ask your doctor if the possible benefits justify the risk to the unborn baby.

Breast Feeding: It is not known whether disulfiram passes into breast milk. Consult your doctor for advice.

Infants and Children: Not recommended for use by children under age 12.

Special Concerns: Check all liquids that you drink or rub on your skin for the presence of alcohol. Disulfiram may interfere with sexual performance in men. Tell your doctor if you plan to have surgery under general anesthesia while taking disulfiram.

OVERDOSE
Symptoms: Loss of memory, behavior disturbances, confusion, headaches, lethargy, increased blood pressure, nausea, vomiting, stomach pain, diarrhea, unsteady walk, temporary paralysis.

What to Do: Call your doctor, emergency medical services (EMS), or the nearest poison control center immediately.

▼ INTERACTIONS

DRUG INTERACTIONS
Other drugs may interact with disulfiram. Consult your doctor if you are taking anticoagulants, anticonvulsants, antidepressants (especially amitriptyline), barbiturates, cephalosporin antibiotics, clozapine, fluoxetine, guanethidine, guanfacine, isoniazid, leucovorin, methyprion, metronidazole, paraldehyde, sedatives, or sertraline.

FOOD INTERACTIONS
Any food prepared with alcohol, including sauces, fermented vinegar, marinades, or desserts, can produce the unpleasant reaction characteristic of disulfiram.

DISEASE INTERACTIONS
Caution is advised when taking disulfiram. Consult your doctor if you have any of the following: diabetes mellitus, epilepsy, kidney disease, liver disease, low thyroid function, lung disease, or a history of psychosis.

SIDE EFFECTS

SERIOUS
Confusion and disorientation, severe skin rash, seizures, neuritis (nerve inflammation causing pain, numbness, or paralysis), low thyroid function, decrease or increase in blood pressure, carpal tunnel syndrome. Call your doctor if such symptoms arise.

COMMON
Drowsiness.

LESS COMMON
Eye pain, vision changes, abdominal discomfort, throbbing headache, mood change, numbness in hands and feet, decreased sexual ability in men, unpleasant taste in mouth, offensive breath and body odor.

DOCUSATE

Available in: Capsules, tablets, liquid, syrup
Available OTC? Yes   **As Generic?** Yes
Drug Class: Stool softener

▼ USAGE INFORMATION

WHY IT'S PRESCRIBED
To prevent constipation (but not to treat existing constipation). Recommended for persons who should not strain during defecation, such as those recovering from rectal or heart surgery, or women who experience constipation after childbirth.

HOW IT WORKS
Docusate draws liquid into stools, forming a softer mass.

▼ DOSAGE GUIDELINES

RANGE AND FREQUENCY
Adults and teenagers: 50 to 500 mg once a day until bowel movements return to normal. Children ages 6 to 12: 40 to 140 mg once a day. Liquid forms should be mixed with milk or fruit juice.

ONSET OF EFFECT
Within 24 to 72 hours.

DURATION OF ACTION
Up to 72 hours.

DIETARY ADVICE
Add high-fiber foods like bran and fresh fruits and vegetables to your diet. Drink at least 6 glasses (8 oz each) of water or other liquids a day to help soften stools.

STORAGE
Store in a tightly sealed container away from heat, moisture, and direct light.

MISSED DOSE
Take it as soon as you remember. If it is near the time for the next dose, skip the missed dose and resume your regular dosage schedule. Do not double the next dose.

STOPPING THE DRUG
Take it as prescribed for the full treatment period. However, you may stop taking the drug if you are feeling better and normal bowel function has returned before the scheduled end of therapy.

PROLONGED USE
Docusate should not be taken for more than 1 week unless you are under your doctor's supervision. Be aware that overuse can make you dependent on it and may cause damage to the nerves, muscles, and other tissues of the bowel and lead to vitamin and mineral deficiency.

▼ PRECAUTIONS

Over 60: No special problems are expected.

Driving and Hazardous Work: The use of docusate should not impair your ability to perform such tasks safely.

Alcohol: No special precautions are necessary.

Pregnancy: Before taking docusate, tell your doctor if you are pregnant or plan to become pregnant.

Breast Feeding: No special problems are expected if you take docusate while nursing.

Infants and Children: Do not give docusate to children under age 6 unless it is prescribed by your doctor.

Special Concerns: Do not take mineral oil while you are taking docusate.

OVERDOSE
Symptoms: Weakness, sweating, muscle cramps, irregular heartbeat.

What to Do: An overdose of docusate is unlikely to be life-threatening. However, if someone takes a much larger dose than prescribed, call your doctor, emergency medical services (EMS), or the nearest poison control center immediately.

▼ INTERACTIONS

DRUG INTERACTIONS
A number of drugs may interact with docusate if they are ingested at or near the time it is taken. Consult your doctor for specific advice if you are taking any other oral drug within 2 hours before or after taking docusate.

FOOD INTERACTIONS
No known food interactions.

DISEASE INTERACTIONS
This drug cannot be used by people with intestinal obstruction or appendicitis. Symptoms of these conditions include vomiting, abdominal rigidity and tenderness, and fever. Call your doctor or emergency medical services (EMS) immediately if you suspect you may be suffering from intestinal obstruction or appendicitis.

≡ SIDE EFFECTS ≡

SERIOUS
Severe cramping. Stop taking the drug and call your doctor immediately.

COMMON
Diarrhea, mild abdominal cramps.

LESS COMMON
Throat irritation, laxative dependence. Consult your doctor if you cannot maintain normal bowel habits without docusate for more than 2 weeks.

DONEPEZIL

Available in: Tablets
Available OTC? No   **As Generic?** No
Drug Class: Acetylcholinesterase inhibitor

BRAND NAME
Aricept

▼ USAGE INFORMATION

WHY IT'S PRESCRIBED
To treat mild to moderate Alzheimer's disease.

HOW IT WORKS
Donepezil prevents the breakdown of acetylcholine, a brain chemical crucial to memory. Acetylcholine deficiency is thought to result in memory loss associated with Alzheimer's disease.

▼ DOSAGE GUIDELINES

RANGE AND FREQUENCY
To start, 5 mg at bedtime. The dose may be increased after 4 to 6 weeks to 10 mg at bedtime.

ONSET OF EFFECT
Unknown.

DURATION OF ACTION
Unknown.

DIETARY ADVICE
No special restrictions.

STORAGE
Store in a tightly sealed container away from heat, moisture, and direct light.

MISSED DOSE
Skip the missed dose and resume your regular dosage schedule. Do not double the next dose.

STOPPING THE DRUG
The decision to stop taking the drug should be made by your doctor.

PROLONGED USE
No problems are expected with long-term use.

▼ PRECAUTIONS

Over 60: No special problems are expected.

Driving and Hazardous Work: Do not drive or engage in hazardous work until you determine how the medicine affects you.

Alcohol: Avoid alcohol while using this medication.

Pregnancy: In some animal studies, large doses of donepezil were shown to cause problems. Before you take donepezil, tell your doctor if you are pregnant or plan to become pregnant.

Breast Feeding: It is not known whether donepezil passes into breast milk; caution is advised. Consult your doctor for specific advice.

Infants and Children: Donepezil is not intended for use in children.

Special Concerns: Before you have any surgery or dental or emergency treatment, tell the doctor or dentist in charge that you are taking donepezil. Donepezil will not cure Alzheimer's disease and will not stop the disease from getting worse, but it will improve cognitive ability of some patients.

OVERDOSE
Symptoms: Seizures, severe nausea, slow heartbeat, increased muscle weakness, vomiting, greatly increased sweating, greatly increased watering of the mouth, weak pulse, irregular breathing, enlargement of the pupils of the eyes.

What to Do: Call your doctor, emergency medical services (EMS), or the nearest poison control center immediately.

▼ INTERACTIONS

DRUG INTERACTIONS
The following drugs may interact with donepezil. Consult your doctor for specific advice if you are taking carbamazepine, dexamethasone, ketoconazole, phenobarbital, phenytoin, quinidine, or rifampin. Also tell your doctor if you are taking any other prescription or over-the-counter medication.

FOOD INTERACTIONS
No known food interactions.

DISEASE INTERACTIONS
Caution is advised when taking donepezil. Consult your doctor if you have any of the following: asthma, chronic obstructive pulmonary disease, urinary difficulties, heart disease, liver disease, a seizure disorder, stomach ulcers, or blockage of the urinary tract.

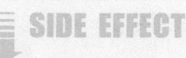 SIDE EFFECTS

SERIOUS
No serious side effects are associated with the use of donepezil.

COMMON
Nausea, vomiting, diarrhea, headache, dizziness, fatigue, insomnia.

LESS COMMON
Vivid or unusual dreams, drowsiness, depression, loss of appetite, unusual bleeding or bruising, fainting, muscle cramps, frequent urination, joint pain, stiffness, or swelling.

DORNASE ALFA

Available in: Inhalation solution
Available OTC? No   **As Generic?** No
Drug Class: Cystic fibrosis drug

▼ USAGE INFORMATION

WHY IT'S PRESCRIBED
To make breathing easier and help prevent lung infections in patients with cystic fibrosis. It is used in conjunction with other cystic fibrosis drugs, such as antibiotics, bronchodilators, and anti-inflammatory agents.

HOW IT WORKS
The mucus in the lungs of people with cystic fibrosis contains large amounts of DNA; this makes the mucus much thicker than normal. Dornase alfa breaks down the DNA, making the mucus less sticky and easier to cough up.

▼ DOSAGE GUIDELINES

RANGE AND FREQUENCY
Adults and children age 5 and older: 2.5 mg in a nebulizer once a day. Selected patients may require 2 daily doses. Use only the following nebulizers and compressors: Hudson T Up-draft II disposable jet nebulizer with the Pulmo-Aide compressor, Marquest Acorn II disposable jet nebulizer with the Pulmo-Aide compressor, or the PARI LC Jet+ nebulizer with the PARI PRONEB compressor.

SIDE EFFECTS

SERIOUS
Chest pain. Call your doctor immediately.

COMMON
Sore throat, voice changes, such as hoarseness.

LESS COMMON
Skin rash; redness, itching, swelling, pain, or other symptoms of eye irritation.

ONSET OF EFFECT
Lung function tests improve significantly within 3 days to 1 week. Reduction in respiratory tract infections may occur over the course of weeks to months.

DURATION OF ACTION
The drug is effective only when it is used daily.

DIETARY ADVICE
No special restrictions.

STORAGE
Refrigerate the drug in its protective foil pouch, away from heat, moisture, and direct light. Do not allow it to freeze. Discard the drug if it is cloudy or discolored.

MISSED DOSE
Take it as soon as you remember. If it is near the time for the next dose, skip the missed dose and resume your regular dosage schedule. Do not double the next dose.

STOPPING THE DRUG
Take it as prescribed for the full treatment period, even if you begin to feel better before the scheduled end of therapy. The decision to stop taking the drug should be made in conjunction with your doctor.

PROLONGED USE
Prolonged use requires periodic evaluation of response and possible dose adjustment by your doctor. It is expected that dornase alfa will be used for a prolonged period.

▼ PRECAUTIONS

Over 60: No special problems are expected.

Driving and Hazardous Work: The use of this medication should not impair your ability to perform such tasks safely.

Alcohol: No special precautions are necessary.

Pregnancy: Adequate human studies have not been done. Before taking dornase alfa, tell your doctor if you are pregnant or plan to become pregnant.

Breast Feeding: Dornase alfa may pass into breast milk; caution is advised. Consult your doctor for specific advice concerning the relative risks and benefits of using this drug while breast feeding.

Infants and Children: Dornase alfa is not recommended for use by children under the age of 5.

Special Concerns: Breathe only through the mouth while using the nebulizer. A nose clip can help. Use the mouthpiece provided with the nebulizer. Do not use a face mask because less medicine will get into the lungs. If you begin coughing during treatment, turn off the nebulizer taking care not to spill the drug. You can resume treatment when coughing stops. Do not dilute dornase alfa or use other medicines in the nebulizer.

OVERDOSE
Symptoms: An overdose of dornase alfa is unlikely to occur and unlikely to be life-threatening.

What to Do: If you have any reason to suspect an overdose, call your doctor, emergency medical services (EMS), or the nearest poison control center.

▼ INTERACTIONS

DRUG INTERACTIONS
Do not use this medication if you are allergic to Chinese hamster ovary cells. No other drug interactions are known.

FOOD INTERACTIONS
No known food interactions.

DISEASE INTERACTIONS
No disease interactions have been reported.

DORZOLAMIDE HYDROCHLORIDE

Available in: Ophthalmic solution
Available OTC? No   **As Generic?** No
Drug Class: Antiglaucoma agent; carbonic anhydrase inhibitor

▼ USAGE INFORMATION

WHY IT'S PRESCRIBED
To treat glaucoma.

HOW IT WORKS
Glaucoma, a sight-threatening disorder, occurs when aqueous humor (the fluid inside the eye) cannot drain properly, resulting in an increase in pressure within the eyeball (known as intraocular pressure). Increased intraocular pressure can damage the optic nerve and lead to a gradually progressive loss of vision. Dorzolamide inhibits the activity of the enzyme carbonic anhydrase, which is needed in the production of aqueous humor. In this way the drug reduces intraocular pressure.

▼ DOSAGE GUIDELINES

RANGE AND FREQUENCY
Adults and teenagers: 1 drop in each eye 3 times per day.

ONSET OF EFFECT
Unknown.

DURATION OF ACTION
8 hours.

DIETARY ADVICE
No special restrictions.

STORAGE
Store in a tightly sealed container away from heat, moisture, and direct light. Do not refrigerate or allow to freeze.

MISSED DOSE
Apply it as soon as you remember. If it is near the time for the next dose, skip the missed dose and resume your regular dosage schedule. Do not double the next dose.

STOPPING THE DRUG
The decision to stop using the drug should be made by your doctor.

PROLONGED USE
Schedule regular eye examinations with your doctor to be sure the drug is controlling the glaucoma.

▼ PRECAUTIONS

Over 60: No special problems are expected.

Driving and Hazardous Work: Do not drive or engage in hazardous work until you determine how the medicine affects your vision.

Alcohol: No special precautions are necessary.

Pregnancy: One animal study found that very high doses of this drug caused birth defects. Human studies have not been done. Before using this medicine, tell your doctor if you are pregnant or plan to become pregnant.

Breast Feeding: Dorzolamide may pass into breast milk; caution is advised. Consult your doctor for specific advice about whether to use a different medicine or to stop breast feeding.

Infants and Children: Safety and dosage for children have not been established. Dorzolamide should be given to infants and children only under close medical supervision.

Special Concerns: To use the eye drops, first wash your hands. Tilt your head back. Gently apply pressure to the inside corner of the eyelid and with the index finger of the same hand, pull downward on the lower eyelid to make a space. Drop the medicine into this space and close your eye. Apply pressure for 1 or 2 minutes while keeping the eye closed without blinking. Then wash your hands again. Make sure that the tip of the dropper does not touch your eye, finger, or any other surface.

OVERDOSE
Symptoms: No specific ones have been reported.

What to Do: An overdose of dorzolamide is unlikely to be life-threatening. If a large volume enters the eye, flush with water. If someone accidentally ingests the medicine, call your doctor, emergency medical services (EMS), or the nearest poison control center immediately.

▼ INTERACTIONS

DRUG INTERACTIONS
Wait 10 minutes before administering any other eye medicine. Dorzolamide should not be used in conjunction with eye medications containing silver, such as silver nitrate. People allergic to sulfa-type drugs should not use dorzolamide.

FOOD INTERACTIONS
No known food interactions.

DISEASE INTERACTIONS
Use of dorzolamide may cause complications in patients with liver disease or kidney disease, since these organs work together to remove the medication from the body.

≡ SIDE EFFECTS ≡

SERIOUS
Allergic reaction causing redness, itching, and swelling of the eyelid; continued or severe sensitivity to light; feeling that something is in the eye. Call your doctor immediately.

COMMON
Burning, stinging, or discomfort in the eye when drug is administered; bitter taste in mouth.

LESS COMMON
Eye pain, severe or continued tearing, nausea or vomiting, blood in urine.

DOXAZOSIN MESYLATE

Available in: Tablets
Available OTC? No   **As Generic?** No
Drug Class: Antihypertensive; BPH therapy agent

▼ USAGE INFORMATION

WHY IT'S PRESCRIBED
To treat mild to moderate high blood pressure; to ease urinary tract symptoms due to benign prostatic hyperplasia (BPH)—that is, noncancerous enlargement of the prostate gland, which is extremely common among men over the age of 50. Note: Findings from a major clinical trial indicate that doxazosin is associated with an unacceptably high incidence of cardiovascular complications. The American Academy of Cardiology has since recommended that physicians reconsider the use of doxazosin in the treatment of their hypertensive patients on a case-by-case basis.

HOW IT WORKS
For high blood pressure, the drug relaxes and widens blood vessels so blood passes through them more easily. For prostate enlargement, it relaxes muscles in the prostate and the opening of the bladder. Note that doxazosin will not shrink the prostate; symptoms may worsen and surgery may eventually be required.

▼ DOSAGE GUIDELINES

RANGE AND FREQUENCY
For high blood pressure, initial dose is 1 mg taken once a day. It can be increased gradually to a maximum of 16 mg a day. For prostate enlargement, initial dose is 1 mg taken once a day, which may be gradually increased to a maximum of 12 mg a day.

ONSET OF EFFECT
For high blood pressure: 1 to 2 hours. For prostate enlargement: 1 to 2 weeks.

DURATION OF ACTION
For high blood pressure: 24 hours. For prostate enlargement: Unknown.

DIETARY ADVICE
No special restrictions.

STORAGE
Store in a tightly sealed container away from heat, moisture, and direct light.

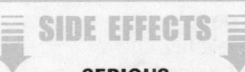

SIDE EFFECTS

SERIOUS
Irregular heartbeat. Call your doctor immediately. Another serious but rare side effect is priapism, a condition characterized by a prolonged or painful erection (lasting more than 4 hours).

COMMON
Dizziness, drowsiness.

LESS COMMON
Headache, weakness, palpitations, rapid pulse, pain and tingling sensations in the fingers or toes, diarrhea or constipation, runny nose, rash or itchy skin, muscle or joint pain, headache, mental depression.

MISSED DOSE
Take it as soon as you remember. If it is near the time for the next dose, skip the missed dose and resume your regular dosage schedule. Do not double the next dose.

STOPPING THE DRUG
Take it as prescribed for the full treatment period, even if you feel better before the scheduled end of therapy.

PROLONGED USE
Consult your doctor about the need for follow-up medical examinations and laboratory studies if you must take doxazosin for a prolonged period.

▼ PRECAUTIONS

Over 60: Adverse reactions may be more likely and more severe in older patients. Dose should be increased slowly in patients over 60.

Driving and Hazardous Work: Do not drive or engage in hazardous work until you determine how the medicine affects you.

Alcohol: Alcohol should be avoided while taking this medicine because it may cause an excessive drop in blood pressure.

Pregnancy: In animal studies, very high doses of doxazosin damaged the fetus. Before taking this medicine, tell your doctor if you are pregnant or plan to become pregnant.

Breast Feeding: Doxazosin may pass into breast milk; caution is advised. Consult your doctor for advice.

Infants and Children: This drug is not recommended for use by children.

Special Concerns: The first dose is likely to cause dizziness or lightheadedness. Take the drug at night and get out of bed slowly the next day. Be cautious while exercising and during hot weather. Tell your doctor whether you will have surgery requiring general anesthesia, including dental surgery, within the next 2 months.

OVERDOSE
Symptoms: Cold, sweaty skin, rapid pulse, weakness, loss of consciousness.

What to Do: Call your doctor, emergency medical services (EMS), or the nearest poison control center immediately.

▼ INTERACTIONS

DRUG INTERACTIONS
Consult your doctor for specific advice if you are taking amphetamines, other antihypertensive drugs, nonsteroidal anti-inflammatory drugs (NSAIDs), estrogen, or sympathomimetic drugs.

FOOD INTERACTIONS
No known food interactions.

DISEASE INTERACTIONS
Use of doxazosin may cause complications in patients with liver or kidney disease, since these organs work together to remove the medication from the body. Also, consult your doctor if you have coronary artery disease, impaired blood circulation to the brain, or mental depression.

DOXEPIN HYDROCHLORIDE

Available in: Capsules, oral solution
Available OTC? No   **As Generic?** Yes
Drug Class: Tricyclic antidepressant

▼ USAGE INFORMATION

WHY IT'S PRESCRIBED
To relieve symptoms of major depression.

HOW IT WORKS
Doxepin affects levels of serotonin, norepinephrine, and acetylcholine, brain chemicals that are thought to be linked to mood, emotions, and mental state.

▼ DOSAGE GUIDELINES

RANGE AND FREQUENCY
Adults: To start, 25 mg, 3 times a day; may be increased to 150 mg a day. Older adults: To start, 25 to 50 mg a day; the dose may be increased gradually by your doctor.

ONSET OF EFFECT
1 to 6 weeks.

DURATION OF ACTION
Unknown.

DIETARY ADVICE
To lessen stomach upset, take it with food, unless your doctor instructs otherwise. Increase intake of fiber and fluids. When taking the oral solution, dilute doxepin in half a glass of water, milk, or fruit juice, but not grapefruit juice. Do not take this drug with a carbonated beverage.

STORAGE
Store in a tightly sealed container away from heat, moisture, and direct light. Do not allow liquid form to freeze.

MISSED DOSE
If you take a one-time daily bedtime dose, do not take a missed dose in the morning because it may cause drowsiness. Call your doctor. If you take more than 1 dose a day, take it as soon as you remember. If it is near the time for the next dose, skip the missed dose and resume your regular dosage schedule. Do not double the next dose.

STOPPING THE DRUG
Take as prescribed for the full treatment period, even if you begin to feel better before the scheduled end of therapy. The decision to stop taking the drug should be made in consultation with your doctor.

PROLONGED USE
The usual course of therapy lasts 6 months to 1 year; some patients benefit from additional therapy.

▼ PRECAUTIONS

Over 60: Adverse reactions, especially confusion and urination difficulty, may be more likely and more severe in older patients. Your doctor may prescribe a lower dose.

Driving and Hazardous Work: Use caution when driving or engaging in hazardous work until you determine how the medication affects you. Drowsiness or lightheadedness can occur.

Alcohol: Avoid alcohol.

Pregnancy: Adequate human studies have not been done. Consult your doctor for specific advice.

Breast Feeding: Doxepin passes into breast milk; do not use it while nursing. Doxepin has been found to cause drowsiness in the infant.

Infants and Children: This drug is not prescribed for children under age 6.

Special Concerns: This is a potentially dangerous drug, especially if taken in excess. Tricyclic antidepressants should not be within easy reach of suicidal patients. If dry mouth occurs, use sugarless gum or candy.

OVERDOSE
Symptoms: Difficulty breathing, severe fatigue, seizures, confusion, hallucinations, dilated pupils, irregular heartbeat, fever, impaired ability to concentrate.

What to Do: Call your doctor, emergency medical services (EMS), or the nearest poison control center immediately.

▼ INTERACTIONS

DRUG INTERACTIONS
Consult your doctor for specific advice if you are taking antithyroid agents, cimetidine, cisapride, clonidine, guanadrel, guanethidine, metrizamide, appetite suppressants, isoproterenol, ephedrine, epinephrine, amphetamines, phenylephrine, antipsychotic drugs, pimozide, methyldopa, metyrosine, metoclopramide, pemoline, promethazine, trimeprazine, rauwolfia alkaloids, MAO inhibitors, or any drugs that depress the central nervous system.

FOOD INTERACTIONS
No known food interactions.

DISEASE INTERACTIONS
Consult your doctor if you have any of the following: a history of alcohol abuse, difficulty urinating, asthma, bipolar disorder, high blood pressure, stomach or intestinal problems, glaucoma, overactive thyroid, enlarged prostate, schizophrenia, seizures, a blood disorder, or kidney, heart, or liver disease.

≡ SIDE EFFECTS ≡

SERIOUS
Confusion, heartbeat irregularities, hallucinations, seizures, extreme fatigue or drowsiness, blurred or altered vision, breathing difficulty, constipation, impaired concentration, difficult urination, fever, extreme and persistent restlessness, loss of coordination and balance, difficulty swallowing or speaking, dilated pupils, eye pain, fainting. Also trembling, shaking, weakness, and stiffness in the extremities; shuffling gait. Call your doctor immediately.

COMMON
Drowsiness or dizziness, headache, dry mouth or unpleasant taste, fatigue, heightened sensitivity to light, weight gain, nausea, increased appetite.

LESS COMMON
Heartburn, sleeping difficulty, diarrhea, increased sweating, vomiting.

DOXYCYCLINE

Available in: Capsules, delayed-release capsules, liquid, tablets
Available OTC? No **As Generic?** Yes
Drug Class: Tetracycline antibiotic

▼ USAGE INFORMATION

WHY IT'S PRESCRIBED
To treat infections caused by bacteria or protozoa (tiny single-celled organisms), including certain sexually transmitted diseases (such as chlamydia, gonorrhea, and syphilis), urinary tract infections, and Lyme disease. Also used to prevent and treat malaria and to treat acne.

HOW IT WORKS
Doxycycline kills bacteria and protozoa by inhibiting their manufacture of proteins necessary for their survival.

▼ DOSAGE GUIDELINES

RANGE AND FREQUENCY
For bacterial or protozoal infections— Adults and children over 100 lbs: 100 mg every 12 hours (twice a day) on the first day of therapy, followed by 100 to 200 mg a day. Usual dose for children under 99 lbs: 1 mg per lb of body weight in 2 doses on first day, followed by 1 to 2 mg per lb per day in 1 single or 2 divided doses. For gonorrhea— Adults and children over 100 lbs: 200 mg to start, then 100 mg, 2 times a day for 3 days. For prevention of malaria— Adults and teenagers: 100 mg once a day, starting 1 or 2 days prior to travel, and for 4 weeks after return from a high-risk area. Children ages 8 to 12: 0.9 mg per lb with the same dosage schedule as adults.

ONSET OF EFFECT
Up to 5 days for infection.

DURATION OF ACTION
Several days.

DIETARY ADVICE
Take with a full glass of water.

STORAGE
Store in a tightly sealed container away from heat, moisture, and direct light.

MISSED DOSE
Take it as soon as you remember. If it is near the time for the next dose, skip the missed dose and resume your regular dosage schedule. Do not double the next dose.

STOPPING THE DRUG
Take it as prescribed for the full treatment period even if you feel better before the scheduled end of therapy.

PROLONGED USE
Prolonged use may make you more susceptible to infections caused by microorganisms resistant to this antibiotic. Some patients will need periodic monitoring of blood, liver, and kidney function.

▼ PRECAUTIONS

Over 60: Itching in the genital and anal areas may be more common among patients over 60.

Driving and Hazardous Work: No special warnings.

Alcohol: Avoid alcohol when fighting an infection.

Pregnancy: Studies of pregnant women indicate that this drug can cause discoloration and impaired development of teeth as well as other birth defects. Avoid using doxycycline during pregnancy.

Breast Feeding: Not recommended during therapy.

Infants and Children: Doxycycline should not be used in children younger than 8 years old since it can cause permanent tooth staining.

Special Concerns: To avoid heartburn, do not take capsules or tablets within 1 hour of bedtime. If you take the liquid form, use a specially marked spoon to measure the dose accurately. Do not take outdated capsules or tablets. If this drug causes increased sensitivity to sunlight, use sunscreen when outdoors to prevent sunburn.

OVERDOSE
Symptoms: Nausea, vomiting, diarrhea, difficulty swallowing.

What to Do: An overdose is unlikely to be life-threatening. However, if someone takes a much larger dose than prescribed, call your doctor, emergency medical services (EMS), or the nearest poison control center immediately.

▼ INTERACTIONS

DRUG INTERACTIONS
Consult your doctor for specific advice if you are taking any other antibiotics, antacids, warfarin, antiviral drugs, bismuth salicylate, calcium supplements, cefixime, cholestyramine, oral contraceptives, desmopressin, digitalis drugs, etretinate, lithium, mineral supplements, sodium bicarbonate, or tiopronin.

FOOD INTERACTIONS
Dairy products can decrease absorption of this drug. Take it 2 hours after or 1 hour before consuming milk or another dairy product. Avoid meats and iron-fortified cereals for 2 hours before and after taking doxycycline.

DISEASE INTERACTIONS
Consult your doctor if you have a history of kidney disease, liver disease, lupus, or myasthenia gravis.

 SIDE EFFECTS

SERIOUS
Chest pain; increased pressure in the head, causing confusion, sleepiness, and headache; allergic reaction causing severe headache, vision changes, itching, swelling, wheezing, or difficulty breathing; severe rash; severe abdominal pain and diarrhea. Call your doctor immediately.

COMMON
Stomach upset, nausea, mild diarrhea, increased sensitivity to sunlight, increased skin pigmentation, vaginal yeast infection, thrush (oral fungal infection).

LESS COMMON
Sore throat, tongue irritation, loss of appetite, colitis, inflamed anus or genitals, tooth discoloration, pain and swelling of legs.

DRONABINOL

Available in: Capsules
Available OTC? No **As Generic?** No
Drug Class: Antiemetic; appetite stimulant

▼ USAGE INFORMATION

WHY IT'S PRESCRIBED
To prevent nausea and vomiting caused by cancer drugs, and to stimulate the appetite of AIDS patients.

HOW IT WORKS
The exact mechanism of action is unknown. Dronabinol may inhibit the centers of the brain that govern the vomiting reflex.

▼ DOSAGE GUIDELINES

RANGE AND FREQUENCY
For nausea and vomiting: 5 mg per square meter of body surface, 1 to 3 hours before chemotherapy is given. The same dose can be taken every 2 to 4 hours after chemotherapy for 4 to 6 doses a day. To stimulate appetite: 2.5 mg twice a day, before lunch and dinner. The dose can be reduced to 2.5 mg taken once in the evening. Maximum dose (if necessary) is up to 20 mg a day, taken in divided doses.

ONSET OF EFFECT
Unknown.

DURATION OF ACTION
From 4 to 6 hours. Appetite stimulation may last 24 hours or longer.

DIETARY ADVICE
For nausea and vomiting control, take it between meals. As an appetite stimulant, take it before lunch and before dinner.

STORAGE
Store in a tightly sealed container away from heat, moisture, and direct light. Keep the medication refrigerated, but do not allow it to freeze.

MISSED DOSE
Take it as soon as you remember. If it is near the time for the next dose, skip the missed dose and resume your regular dosage schedule. Do not double the next dose.

STOPPING THE DRUG
The decision to stop taking the drug should be made by your doctor. Withdrawal effects such as insomnia, irritability, sweating, loss of appetite, and hot flashes may follow abrupt termination. These effects will dissipate over the subsequent 24 hours.

PROLONGED USE
Prolonged use increases the risk of side effects and drug dependence.

▼ PRECAUTIONS

Over 60: Adverse reactions may be more likely and more severe in older patients. Older patients should be watched carefully when they take this medicine because of dronabinol's effects on the mind. Changes in mental state due to dronabinol use should not be mistaken for those caused by conditions such as Alzheimer's disease.

Driving and Hazardous Work: Do not drive or engage in hazardous work until you determine how the medicine affects you.

Alcohol: Avoid alcohol.

Pregnancy: Adequate human studies have not been completed. Before taking dronabinol, tell your doctor if you are pregnant or plan to become pregnant.

Breast Feeding: Dronabinol passes into breast milk; avoid or discontinue its use while nursing.

Infants and Children: Dronabinol is not recommended for use by children under age 12 or children with AIDS cachexia.

Special Concerns: Be aware that dronabinol is a derivative of the principal active substance in marijuana and has a high potential for abuse. Prior allergic reaction to marijuana, marijuana by-products, or

sesame oil may rule out use of dronabinol.

OVERDOSE
Symptoms: Confusion, slurred speech, red eyes, hallucinations, change in perceptions of taste, sound, touch, smell, or sight, drastic mood changes, rapid, pounding heartbeat, difficulty urinating, nervousness, dry mouth, loss of coordination, fainting, or dizziness.

What to Do: If someone takes a much larger dose of dronabinol than prescribed, call your doctor, emergency medical services (EMS), or the nearest poison control center right away.

▼ INTERACTIONS

DRUG INTERACTIONS
Other drugs may interact with dronabinol. Consult your doctor for specific advice if you are taking anticonvulsants, antidepressants, antihistamines, barbiturates, clozapine, ethinamate, fluoxetine, leucovorin, narcotics, theophylline, muscle relaxants, or any central nervous system depressant.

FOOD INTERACTIONS
No known food interactions.

DISEASE INTERACTIONS
Caution is advised when taking dronabinol. Consult your doctor if you have any of the following: heart disease, high blood pressure, a history of alcohol or drug abuse, schizophrenia, or manic depression (bipolar disorder).

≣ SIDE EFFECTS ≣

SERIOUS
Hallucinations, severe mood changes, irritability, euphoria.

COMMON
Dizziness, drowsiness, poor coordination, trouble thinking.

LESS COMMON
Depression, anxiety, nervousness, headache, hallucinations, blurred vision, rapid heartbeat, frequent or difficult urination, convulsions, dry mouth.

DYPHYLLINE

Available in: Elixir, tablets
Available OTC? No   **As Generic?** No
Drug Class: Bronchodilator/xanthine

▼ USAGE INFORMATION

WHY IT'S PRESCRIBED
To prevent or treat acute bronchial asthma or episodes of breathing difficulty associated with chronic bronchitis and emphysema.

HOW IT WORKS
Dyphylline is a mild bronchodilator, similar in effect to drugs like theophylline and aminophylline. It relaxes the smooth muscle tissue surrounding the bronchial passages, helping to widen the airways and aid breathing.

▼ DOSAGE GUIDELINES

RANGE AND FREQUENCY
Adults: Dose is based on individual body weight, usually 15 mg per 2.2 lbs (1 kg), or 6.8 mg per lb, up to 4 times a day. Children: Consult pediatrician for appropriate dose.

ONSET OF EFFECT
Rapid.

DURATION OF ACTION
Unknown.

DIETARY ADVICE
Best when taken on an empty stomach at least 1 hour before or 2 hours after eating. However, it may be taken with meals to minimize the incidence of stomach irritation or upset.

STORAGE
Store in a tightly sealed container away from heat and direct light.

MISSED DOSE
Take it as soon as you remember. However, if it is near the time for the next dose, skip the missed dose and resume your regular dosage schedule. Do not double the next dose.

STOPPING THE DRUG
The decision to stop taking the drug should be made in consultation with your doctor.

PROLONGED USE
Therapy with this medication may require months or years. See your doctor regularly for tests and examinations if you must take the medication for a prolonged period.

▼ PRECAUTIONS

Over 60: Adverse reactions may be more likely and more severe in older patients.

Driving and Hazardous Work: Do not drive or engage in hazardous work until you determine how the medicine affects you.

Alcohol: No special precautions are necessary.

Pregnancy: Adequate studies of the use of dyphylline during pregnancy have not been done. Discuss the relative risks and benefits with your doctor.

Breast Feeding: Dyphylline passes into breast milk, although no adverse consequences have been reported. Consult your doctor for specific advice.

Infants and Children: The safety and effectiveness of dyphylline use by children have not been established; other medications are generally preferred.

OVERDOSE
Symptoms: Persistent and severe abdominal pain, confusion or changes in mental state, seizures, dark or bloody vomit, rapid or irregular heartbeat, nervousness, restlessness, trembling.

What to Do: Call your doctor, emergency medical services (EMS), or the nearest poison control center immediately.

▼ INTERACTIONS

DRUG INTERACTIONS
Other drugs may interact with dyphylline. Consult your doctor for specific advice if you are taking beta-blockers (including ophthalmic beta-blocker preparations used to treat glaucoma), probenecid, or other xanthine-derivative medications, such as theophylline or aminophylline.

FOOD INTERACTIONS
Your doctor may suggest that you restrict your consumption of foods and beverages containing caffeine (including chocolate), since caffeine may heighten dyphylline's stimulating effects to the central nervous system.

DISEASE INTERACTIONS
You should not use dyphylline if you have had a prior allergic reaction to xanthine-derivative drugs such as theophylline or aminophylline. Consult your doctor if you have active gastritis (inflammation of the stomach lining) or a history of peptic ulcer or impaired kidney function.

▼ SIDE EFFECTS

SERIOUS
No serious side effects are associated with dyphylline when used at recommended doses (see Overdose).

COMMON
No common side effects are associated with dyphylline.

LESS COMMON
Heartburn, nausea, vomiting, rapid heartbeat, headache, increased urine output, nervousness, trembling, difficulty.

ECONAZOLE NITRATE

Available in: Cream
Available OTC? No   **As Generic?** No
Drug Class: Antifungal

▼ USAGE INFORMATION

WHY IT'S PRESCRIBED
To treat fungal infections of the skin, such as tinea corporis (ringworm), tinea cruris (jock itch), tinea pedis (athlete's foot), and pityriasis versicolor ("sun fungus," a skin condition characterized by fine scaly patches of varying shapes, sizes, and colors).

HOW IT WORKS
Econazole prevents fungal organisms from producing vital substances required for growth and function. This drug is effective only for infections caused by fungal organisms. It will not work for bacterial or viral infections.

▼ DOSAGE GUIDELINES

RANGE AND FREQUENCY
Apply to affected area 1 to 2 times a day. When twice a day, apply it in the morning and the evening. Athlete's foot is usually treated for 1 month; jock itch, ringworm, and sun fungus, for 2 weeks.

ONSET OF EFFECT
Unknown.

DURATION OF ACTION
Unknown.

DIETARY ADVICE
Econazole can be applied without regard to diet.

STORAGE
Store in a tightly sealed container away from heat, moisture, and direct light. Do not allow it to freeze.

MISSED DOSE
Apply it as soon as you remember. However, if it is near the time for the next application, skip the missed dose and resume your regular dosage schedule.

STOPPING THE DRUG
Use it as prescribed for the full treatment period, even if you begin to feel better before the scheduled end of therapy. Recurrence of the infection is likely if you stop before the full treatment period is complete.

PROLONGED USE
Notify your doctor if no improvement occurs after 2 weeks for jock itch, ringworm, and sun fungus, or after 4 weeks for athlete's foot.

▼ PRECAUTIONS

Over 60: No special problems are expected.

Driving and Hazardous Work: The use of econazole should not impair your ability to perform such tasks safely.

Alcohol: No special precautions are necessary.

Pregnancy: Before using econazole, tell your doctor if you are pregnant or plan to become pregnant. Econazole should be used in the first trimester only if the doctor says it is essential to your health, and it should be used in the last two trimesters only if it is clearly needed.

Breast Feeding: Econazole may pass into breast milk; caution is advised. Consult your doctor for specific advice.

Infants and Children: No special problems are expected. Consult your pediatrician for specific advice.

Special Concerns: Avoid allowing econazole to come into contact with the eyes. If using the medication for jock itch, do not wear underwear that is tight or made from synthetic materials; wear loose-fitting cotton underwear. If using econazole for athlete's foot, dry your feet carefully after bathing and wear clean cotton socks with sandals or well-ventilated shoes. Before applying the medication, wash the affected area with soap and warm water and dry thoroughly. Econazole may stain your clothing.

OVERDOSE
Symptoms: An overdose of econazole is unlikely.

What to Do: If someone should swallow a large amount of econazole, call your doctor, emergency medical services (EMS), or the nearest poison control center immediately.

▼ INTERACTIONS

DRUG INTERACTIONS
Consult your doctor for specific advice if you are taking topical corticosteroids. They may inhibit the antifungal effect of econazole.

FOOD INTERACTIONS
No food interactions have been reported.

DISEASE INTERACTIONS
No disease interactions have been reported.

≡ SIDE EFFECTS ≡

SERIOUS
No serious side effects are associated with econazole.

COMMON
No common side effects are associated with econazole.

LESS COMMON
Itching, burning, stinging, skin redness, or other irritation not present prior to treatment.

EFAVIRENZ

Available in: Capsules
Available OTC? No   **As Generic?** No
Drug Class: Antiviral/reverse transcriptase inhibitor

▼ USAGE INFORMATION

WHY IT'S PRESCRIBED
To treat human immunodeficiency virus (HIV) infection in combination with other drugs. While not a cure for HIV, such drugs may suppress the replication of the virus and delay the progression of the disease.

HOW IT WORKS
Efavirenz prevents HIV from reproducing in two ways. A metabolite of the drug inhibits the activity of an enzyme needed for the replication of DNA in viral cells. The metabolite is also incorporated into viral DNA and terminates the formation of the complete DNA.

▼ DOSAGE GUIDELINES

RANGE AND FREQUENCY
Adults: To start, 600 mg once a day. The drug must be taken in combination with other drugs for HIV to delay the development of resistant strains of the virus. For the first 2 to 4 weeks of therapy, take the daily dose at bedtime to improve tolerability of certain side effects (such as dizziness, drowsiness, and impaired concentration). Children: Consult your doctor.

ONSET OF EFFECT
Unknown. With most antiretroviral drugs, an early response can be seen within the first few days of therapy, but the maximum effect may take 12 to 16 weeks.

DURATION OF ACTION
Unknown. Effects of the drug may be prolonged when efavirenz is used in combination with other effective drugs and the virus is maximally suppressed.

DIETARY ADVICE
Efavirenz should be taken with plenty of water or other liquid. It may also be taken with a low-fat meal.

STORAGE
Store at room temperature in a tightly sealed container away from heat, moisture, and direct light.

MISSED DOSE
Take it as soon as you remember. If it is near the time for the next dose, skip the missed dose and resume your regular dosage schedule. Do not double the next dose. It is especially important to take efavirenz on schedule to assure constant, proper blood levels of the drug.

STOPPING THE DRUG
The decision to stop taking the drug should be made in consultation with your doctor.

PROLONGED USE
See your doctor regularly for tests and examinations.

▼ PRECAUTIONS

Over 60: No special problems are expected.

Driving and Hazardous Work: Do not drive or engage in hazardous work until you determine how the medicine affects you.

Alcohol: Alcohol may raise the blood concentration of the drug.

Pregnancy: Efavirenz has been shown to cause birth defects in animals. Human studies have not been done. This medication should be given during pregnancy only if potential benefits outweigh the risks to the unborn child.

Breast Feeding: Women infected with HIV should not breast feed, to avoid transmitting the virus to an uninfected child.

Infants and Children: Your pediatrician will determine the appropriate dosage based on your child's weight. Call your doctor immediately if you notice rash or any other side effects while your child is taking efavirenz.

Special Concerns: Use of efavirenz does not eliminate the risk of passing the AIDS virus to other persons. You should take appropriate preventive measures.

OVERDOSE
Symptoms: Increased severity of common side effects.

What to Do: Call your doctor, emergency medical services (EMS), or the nearest poison control center immediately.

▼ INTERACTIONS

DRUG INTERACTIONS
Do not take efavirenz with astemizole, cisapride, midazolam, triazolam, or ergot medications (migraine drugs). Dose adjustments may be necessary if taking indinavir, saquinavir, or clarithromycin. Consult your doctor before taking this medication with warfarin, rifampin, rifabutin, or oral contraceptives.

FOOD INTERACTIONS
Do not take efavirenz with high-fat meals.

DISEASE INTERACTIONS
Consult your doctor if you have a history of mental illness or drug or alcohol abuse. This drug should be used with caution in patients with impaired liver function or risk factors for liver disease.

SIDE EFFECTS

SERIOUS
Severe depression, mood changes, confusion. Call your doctor immediately.

COMMON
Dizziness, difficulty sleeping, fatigue, impaired concentration, unusual dreams, stomach upset, fever, cough, vomiting, diarrhea. Rash is also common; although the rash usually goes away without a change in treatment, sometimes it may be serious. If you develop a rash, call your doctor immediately.

LESS COMMON
Numerous less common side effects can occur; consult your doctor if you are concerned about any adverse or unusual reactions you experience while taking this drug.

EMEDASTINE DIFUMARATE

BRAND NAME

Emadine

Available in: Ophthalmic solution
Available OTC? No   **As Generic?** No
Drug Class: Histamine (H1) blocker

▼ USAGE INFORMATION

WHY IT'S PRESCRIBED
For short-term therapy of eye itching caused by seasonal allergic conjunctivitis (inflammation of the mucous membranes that line the inner surface of the eyelids and whites of the eyes).

HOW IT WORKS
Emedastine blocks the effects of histamine, a naturally occurring substance within the body that causes swelling, itching, sneezing, watery eyes, and other symptoms associated with allergic reactions.

▼ DOSAGE GUIDELINES

RANGE AND FREQUENCY
Instill 1 drop in the affected eye(s) up to 4 times a day.

ONSET OF EFFECT
Unknown.

DURATION OF ACTION
Unknown.

DIETARY ADVICE
Emedastine can be used without regard to diet.

STORAGE
Store in a tightly sealed container away from heat, moisture, and direct light. Do not allow it to freeze.

MISSED DOSE
Apply it as soon as you remember. If it is near the time for the next dose, skip the missed dose and resume your regular dosage schedule. Do not double the next dose.

STOPPING THE DRUG
You may stop using emedastine whenever you choose.

PROLONGED USE
Emedastine is prescribed for short-term use only.

▼ PRECAUTIONS

Over 60: No special problems are expected.

Driving and Hazardous Work: Do not drive or engage in hazardous work until you determine how the medicine affects you.

Alcohol: No special precautions are necessary.

Pregnancy: No adequate human studies have been done. Before taking emedastine, tell your doctor if you are pregnant or plan to become pregnant.

Breast Feeding: Emedastine may pass into breast milk; caution is advised. Consult your doctor for advice.

Infants and Children: Not recommended for use by children under age 3.

Special Concerns: To use the eyedrops, first wash your hands. Tilt your head back. Gently apply pressure to the inside corner of the eyelid and with the index finger of the same hand, pull downward on the lower eyelid to make a space. Drop the medicine into this space and close your eye. Apply pressure for 1 or 2 minutes while keeping the eye closed without blinking. Then wash your hands again. Make sure the tip of the dropper does not touch your eye, finger, or any other surface. You should not wear a contact lens if your eye is red. Emedastine should not be used to treat contact-lens-related irritation. If you wear soft contact lenses and your eyes are not red, wait at least 10 minutes after instilling the drops before inserting your contact lenses.

OVERDOSE
Symptoms: Drowsiness and general feelings of illness have been reported following unintentional oral intake of the drug.

What to Do: An overdose with emedastine is unlikely to be life-threatening. However, if someone accidentally ingests the medicine, seek emergency medical attention immediately.

▼ INTERACTIONS

DRUG INTERACTIONS
None reported.

FOOD INTERACTIONS
None reported.

DISEASE INTERACTIONS
None reported.

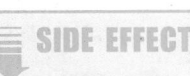 SIDE EFFECTS

SERIOUS
No serious side effects are associated with emedastine.

COMMON
Headache.

LESS COMMON
Bad taste in the mouth, abnormal dreams, eye dryness, blurred vision, burning or stinging of the eye, tearing, runny nose, skin rash, weakness.

ENALAPRIL MALEATE

Available in: Tablets
Available OTC? No   **As Generic?** No
Drug Class: Angiotensin-converting enzyme (ACE) inhibitor

▼ USAGE INFORMATION

WHY IT'S PRESCRIBED
To control high blood pressure; to treat congestive heart failure; to treat patients with left ventricular dysfunction (damage to the pumping chamber of the heart); and to minimize further kidney damage in diabetic patients with mild kidney disease.

HOW IT WORKS
Angiotensin-converting enzyme (ACE) inhibitors block an enzyme that produces angiotensin, a naturally occurring substance that causes blood vessels to constrict and stimulates production of the adrenal hormone, aldosterone, which promotes sodium retention in the body. As a result, ACE inhibitors relax blood vessels (causing them to widen) and reduces sodium retention, which lowers blood pressure and so decreases the workload of the heart.

▼ DOSAGE GUIDELINES

RANGE AND FREQUENCY
2.5 to 40 mg a day, taken 1 or 2 times a day.

ONSET OF EFFECT
Within 1 hour.

DURATION OF ACTION
Up to 24 hours.

DIETARY ADVICE
Take enalapril on an empty stomach, about 1 hour before mealtime. Follow your doctor's dietary advice (such as low-salt or low-cholesterol restrictions) to improve control over high blood pressure and heart disease. Avoid high-potassium foods like bananas and citrus fruits and juices, unless you are also taking medications, such as diuretics, that lower potassium levels.

STORAGE
Keep in a tightly sealed container in a cool, dry place.

MISSED DOSE
Take it as soon as you remember. If it is near the time for the next dose, skip the missed dose and resume your regular dosage schedule. Do not double the next dose.

STOPPING THE DRUG
Do not stop taking this drug abruptly, as this may cause potentially serious health problems. Dosage should be reduced gradually, according to your doctor's instructions.

PROLONGED USE
See your doctor regularly for exams and tests if you must take this medicine for a prolonged period. Enalapril helps control high blood pressure but does not cure it. Lifelong therapy may be necessary.

▼ PRECAUTIONS

Over 60: Some elderly patients may be more sensitive to the effects of this drug; smaller doses may be warranted.

Driving and Hazardous Work: Do not drive or engage in hazardous work until you determine how the medicine affects you.

Alcohol: Alcohol may increase the effect of the drug and cause an excessive drop in blood pressure.

Pregnancy: Enalapril use is not recommended, especially during the final 6 months of pregnancy. If you become pregnant, notify your doctor as soon as possible.

Breast Feeding: Trace amounts of enalapril can be found in breast milk; however, adverse effects in infants have not been documented. Consult your doctor.

Infants and Children: Benefits of enalapril use by children must be weighed against risks. Consult your pediatrician for specific advice.

OVERDOSE
Symptoms: No specific ones have been reported.

What to Do: While overdose is unlikely, call your doctor, emergency medical services (EMS), or the nearest poison control center immediately if you suspect that someone has taken a much larger dose than prescribed.

▼ INTERACTIONS

DRUG INTERACTIONS
Consult your doctor if you are taking diuretics (especially potassium-sparing diuretics), potassium supplements or drugs containing potassium, lithium, anticoagulants, anti-inflammatory drugs, or over-the-counter drugs (especially cold remedies and diet pills).

FOOD INTERACTIONS
Avoid low-salt milk and salt substitutes. Many of these products contain potassium.

DISEASE INTERACTIONS
Consult your doctor if you have lupus or if you have had a prior allergic reaction to ACE inhibitors. This drug should be used with caution by patients with severe kidney disease or renal artery stenosis (narrowing of one or both of the arteries that supply blood to the kidneys).

≡ SIDE EFFECTS ≡

SERIOUS
Fever and chills; sore throat and hoarseness; sudden difficulty breathing or swallowing; swelling of the face, mouth, or extremities; impaired kidney function (ankle swelling, decreased urination); confusion; yellow discoloration of the eyes or skin (indicating liver disorder); intense itching; chest pain or palpitations; abdominal pain. Serious side effects are very rare; contact your doctor immediately.

COMMON
Dry, persistent cough.

LESS COMMON
Dizziness or fainting; skin rash; numbness or tingling in the hands, feet, or lips; unusual fatigue or muscle weakness; nausea; drowsiness; loss of taste; headache; unusual dreams.

ENALAPRIL MALEATE/DILTIAZEM MALATE

Available in: Extended-release tablets
Available OTC? No   **As Generic?** No
Drug Class: ACE inhibitor/calcium channel blocker combination

▼ USAGE INFORMATION

WHY IT'S PRESCRIBED
As a secondary treatment for high blood pressure. It is prescribed when blood pressure is not adequately controlled by either enalapril or diltiazem alone and for those taking both drugs separately.

HOW IT WORKS
Angiotensin-converting enzyme (ACE) inhibitors, such as enalapril, block an enzyme that produces angiotensin, a naturally occurring substance that causes blood vessels to constrict, and stimulates production of the adrenal hormone, aldosterone, which promotes sodium retention in the body. This relaxes blood vessels (causing them to widen) and reduces sodium retention. Diltiazem, a calcium channel blocker, interferes with the movement of calcium into heart muscle cells and smooth muscle cells in the walls of the arteries. Their combined action causes blood vessels to relax, lowering blood pressure and decreasing the workload of the heart.

▼ DOSAGE GUIDELINES

RANGE AND FREQUENCY
Adults: 1 to 4 tablets, each containing 5 mg enalapril and 180 mg diltiazem, in a single dose per day.

ONSET OF EFFECT
Unknown.

DURATION OF ACTION
Unknown.

DIETARY ADVICE
Take this drug on an empty stomach, about 1 hour before mealtime. Avoid high-potassium foods like bananas and citrus fruits and juices, unless you are also taking drugs that lower potassium levels.

STORAGE
Store in a tightly sealed container away from heat, moisture, and direct light.

MISSED DOSE
If you miss a dose on one day, do not double the dose the next day.

STOPPING THE DRUG
Do not stop taking this drug abruptly, as this may cause potentially serious health problems. Dosage should be reduced gradually.

PROLONGED USE
See your doctor regularly for tests and examinations.

▼ PRECAUTIONS

Over 60: Adverse reactions may be more likely and more severe.

Driving and Hazardous Work: Exercise caution until you determine how the medicine affects you.

Alcohol: Alcohol may increase the effect of the drug and cause an excessive drop in blood pressure.

Pregnancy: This drug can cause injury and even death in the developing fetus. See your doctor and stop using the drug as soon as possible if pregnancy is detected.

Breast Feeding: Diltiazem passes into breast milk; avoid use while nursing.

Infants and Children: Safety has not been established for children under age 12.

Special Concerns: Diltiazem may promote dental problems.

OVERDOSE
Symptoms: None reported. However, heart block (causing shortness of breath), fatigue, dizziness, fainting, and low blood pressure have been attributed to enalapril and diltiazem when taken alone.

What to Do: If someone takes a much larger dose than prescribed, seek medical assistance right away.

▼ INTERACTIONS

DRUG INTERACTIONS
Consult your doctor if you are taking aspirin, beta-blockers, digitalis drugs, carbamazepine, cyclosporine, lithium, oral antidiabetic agents, phenytoin, rifampin, cimetidine, fluvoxamine, ranitidine, diuretics (especially potassium-sparing diuretics), drugs or supplements containing potassium, anticoagulants, anti-inflammatory drugs, or any over-the-counter drugs.

FOOD INTERACTIONS
Avoid excessive salt intake. Avoid low-salt milk and salt substitutes. Many of these products contain potassium.

DISEASE INTERACTIONS
Consult your doctor if you have lupus or if you have had a prior allergic reaction to ACE inhibitors. This drug should not be used by patients with sick sinus syndrome or heart block (unless a pacemaker is in place), or by those with low blood pressure or history of acute heart attack with lung congestion. It should be used cautiously by patients with congestive heart failure, liver disease, severe kidney disease, or renal artery stenosis (narrowing of one or both of the arteries that supply blood to the kidneys).

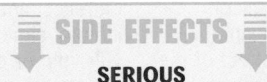

SIDE EFFECTS

SERIOUS
Fever and chills; sore throat and hoarseness; sudden difficulty breathing or swallowing; swelling of the face, mouth, or extremities; ankle swelling, decreased urination; confusion; yellow discoloration of the eyes or skin; intense itching; chest pain or palpitations; irregular or slow heartbeat, shortness of breath, and fatigue; abdominal pain. Serious side effects are very rare; contact your doctor immediately.

COMMON
Headache; drowsiness; swelling of feet and ankles; constipation; nausea; weight gain; fatigue; dry, persistent cough.

LESS COMMON
Dizziness or fainting; weakness; depression; nervousness; insomnia; vomiting; diarrhea; excessive urination; skin rash; sensitivity to sunlight; overgrowth of gums; numbness or tingling in hands, feet, or lips; loss of taste.

ENALAPRIL MALEATE/FELODIPINE

Available in: Tablets
Available OTC? No   **As Generic?** No
Drug Class: ACE inhibitor/calcium channel blocker combination

▼ USAGE INFORMATION

WHY IT'S PRESCRIBED
To control hypertension (high blood pressure).

HOW IT WORKS
Angiotensin-converting enzyme (ACE) inhibitors such as enalapril block an enzyme that produces angiotensin, a naturally occurring substance that causes blood vessels to constrict and stimulates production of the adrenal hormone, aldosterone, which promotes sodium retention in the body. As a result, ACE inhibitors relax blood vessels (causing them to widen) and reduces sodium retention. Felodipine, a calcium channel blocker, interferes with the movement of calcium into heart muscle cells and the smooth muscle cells in the walls of the arteries. As a result of the combined action of enalapril and felodipine, blood vessels relax, which lowers blood pressure and thereby decreases the workload of the heart.

▼ DOSAGE GUIDELINES

RANGE AND FREQUENCY
To start, 5 mg once a day. The dose may be increased or decreased gradually by your doctor to 2.5 to 10 mg once a day, as needed. The recommended initial dose for older patients is 2.5 mg a day.

ONSET OF EFFECT
Unknown.

DURATION OF ACTION
Unknown.

DIETARY ADVICE
Enalapril maleate/felodipine is best taken without food. The drug can, however, be taken with grapefruit juice.

STORAGE
Store in a tightly sealed container away from heat, moisture, and direct light.

MISSED DOSE
Take it as soon as you remember. If it is near the time for the next dose, skip the missed dose and resume your regular dosage schedule. Do not double the next dose.

STOPPING THE DRUG
The decision to stop taking the drug should be made by your doctor.

PROLONGED USE
See your doctor periodically for tests and examinations.

▼ PRECAUTIONS

Over 60: No special problems are expected.

Driving and Hazardous Work: Avoid such activities until you determine how this medication affects you.

Alcohol: Consume alcohol only in moderation since it may increase the effect of the drug and cause an excessive drop in blood pressure. Consult your doctor for advice.

Pregnancy: Adequate studies have not been done. Before taking this drug, tell your doctor if you are pregnant or plan to become pregnant.

Breast Feeding: This drug passes into breast milk. Discuss with your doctor the relative risks and benefits of using it while nursing.

Infants and Children: The safety and effectiveness of enalapril with felodipine use by infants and children have not been established.

Special Concerns: Enalapril with felodipine is not recommended as the first treatment when high blood pressure is diagnosed. It may be prescribed after other medications have proved unsatisfactory. Before you undergo surgery, tell the doctor or dentist in charge that you are taking this drug.

OVERDOSE
Symptoms: No cases of overdose have been reported.

What to Do: If someone takes a much larger dose than prescribed, call your doctor, emergency medical services (EMS), or the nearest poison control right away.

▼ INTERACTIONS

DRUG INTERACTIONS
Consult your doctor for specific advice if you are taking diuretics, antihypertensives, lithium, cimetidine, anticonvulsants, or other over-the-counter or prescription medications.

FOOD INTERACTIONS
No known food interactions.

DISEASE INTERACTIONS
Caution is advised when taking enalapril with felodipine. Consult your doctor if you have congestive heart failure (CHF) or any other medical condition. Use of this drug may cause complications in patients with liver or kidney disease, since these organs work together to remove the medication from the body.

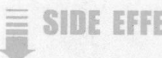 SIDE EFFECTS

SERIOUS
Serious side effects are very rare. They include fever and chills; sore throat and hoarseness; sudden difficulty breathing or swallowing; swelling of the face, mouth, or extremities; worsening kidney function (ankle swelling, decreased urination); confusion; jaundice (yellowish tinge to eyes or skin, indicating liver problems); intense itching; chest pain or heart palpitations; abdominal pain; irregular or slow heartbeats; low blood pressure (causing dizziness or faintness). Call your doctor immediately.

COMMON
Mild swelling of arms and legs, fatigue, mild headache, dizziness, cough, flushed skin.

LESS COMMON
Fainting, dry mouth, constipation or diarrhea, gas, nausea, vomiting, rectal pain, gout, neck pain, joint swelling, nervousness, insomnia, sleepiness, skin rash, increased eye pressure, impotence, hot flashes.

ENALAPRIL/HYDROCHLOROTHIAZIDE (HCTZ)

Available in: Tablets
Available OTC? No   **As Generic?** No
Drug Class: Angiotensin-converting enzyme (ACE) inhibitor/diuretic

▼ USAGE INFORMATION

WHY IT'S PRESCRIBED
To control high blood pressure; to treat congestive heart failure (CHF); to treat patients with left ventricular dysfunction (damage to the pumping chamber of the heart); and to minimize further kidney damage in patients with diabetes who have mild kidney disease.

HOW IT WORKS
Angiotensin-converting enzyme (ACE) inhibitors such as enalapril block an enzyme that produces angiotensin, a naturally occurring substance that causes blood vessels to constrict and stimulates production of the adrenal hormone, aldosterone, which promotes sodium retention in the body. As a result, ACE inhibitors relax blood vessels (causing them to widen) and reduces sodium retention, which lowers blood pressure and so decreases the workload of the heart. Hydro-chlorothiazide (HCTZ), a diuretic, increases sodium and water in the urine output. By reducing the overall fluid volume in the body, diuretics reduce blood volume and so reduce blood pressure.

▼ DOSAGE GUIDELINES

RANGE AND FREQUENCY
Adults: 1 to 2 tablets containing 10 mg enalapril and 25 mg hydrochlorothiazide a day.

ONSET OF EFFECT
Within 1 hour.

DURATION OF ACTION
24 hours.

DIETARY ADVICE
Take on an empty stomach, about 1 hour before mealtime. Follow your doctor's dietary advice (such as low-salt or low-cholesterol restrictions) to improve control over high blood pressure and heart disease.

STORAGE
Store in a tightly sealed container away from heat and direct light.

MISSED DOSE
Take it as soon as you remember. If it is near the time for the next dose, skip the missed dose and resume your regular dosage schedule. Do not double the next dose.

STOPPING THE DRUG
Do not stop taking this drug abruptly, as this may cause potentially serious health problems. Dosage should be reduced gradually, according to your doctor's instructions.

PROLONGED USE
See your doctor regularly for examinations and tests if you must take this medication for a prolonged period. Lifelong therapy may be necessary.

▼ PRECAUTIONS

Over 60: Adverse reactions may be more likely and more severe in older patients.

Driving and Hazardous Work: Do not drive or engage in hazardous work until you determine how the medicine affects you.

Alcohol: Alcohol may increase the effect of the drug and cause an excessive drop in blood pressure. Consult your doctor for advice.

Pregnancy: Before taking this drug, tell your doctor if you are pregnant or plan to become pregnant. Use of this drug during the last 6 months of pregnancy may cause severe defects, or death, in the fetus.

Breast Feeding: Enalapril may pass into breast milk; caution is advised. Consult your doctor for specific advice.

Infants and Children: Children may be especially sensitive to the effects of enalapril. Consult your doctor.

OVERDOSE
Symptoms: Overdose has not been reported; symptoms might include dizziness, faintness, or confusion.

What to Do: While overdose is unlikely, call your doctor, emergency medical services (EMS), or the nearest poison control center immediately if you suspect that someone has taken a much larger dose than prescribed.

▼ INTERACTIONS

DRUG INTERACTIONS
Consult your doctor for specific advice if you are taking cholestyramine, colestipol, digitalis drugs, lithium, potassium-containing medicines or supplements, or any over-the-counter drug (especially cold remedies and diet pills).

FOOD INTERACTIONS
Avoid low-salt milk and salt substitutes. Many of these products contain potassium.

DISEASE INTERACTIONS
Consult your doctor if you have lupus or if you have had a prior allergic reaction to ACE inhibitors. This drug should be used with caution by patients with severe kidney disease or renal artery stenosis (narrowing of one or both of the arteries that supply blood to the kidneys).

≣ SIDE EFFECTS ≣

SERIOUS
Fever and chills; sore throat and hoarseness; sudden difficulty breathing or swallowing; swelling of the face, mouth, or extremities; impaired kidney function (ankle swelling, decreased urination); confusion; yellow discoloration of the eyes or skin (indicating liver disorder); intense itching; chest pain or palpitations; abdominal pain. Serious side effects are very rare; contact your doctor immediately.

COMMON
Dry, persistent cough.

LESS COMMON
Dizziness or fainting; skin rash; numbness or tingling in the hands, feet, or lips; change in color of the hands from white to blue to red (Raynaud's phenomenon) in cold weather; unusual fatigue or muscle weakness; nausea; drowsiness; loss of taste; headache; unusual dreams.

ENOXACIN

BRAND NAME

Penetrex

Available in: Tablets
Available OTC? No   **As Generic?** No
Drug Class: Fluoroquinolone antibiotic

▼ USAGE INFORMATION

WHY IT'S PRESCRIBED
To treat bacterial urinary tract infections, including gonorrhea.

HOW IT WORKS
Enoxacin inhibits the activity of a bacterial enzyme (gyrase) that is necessary for proper DNA formation and replication. This prevents bacteria cells from reproducing.

▼ DOSAGE GUIDELINES

RANGE AND FREQUENCY
For uncomplicated urinary tract infections: 200 mg every 12 hours for 7 days. For severe or complicated urinary tract infections: 400 mg every 12 hours for 14 days. For gonorrhea: 400 mg in a one-time dose. For persons with kidney impairment, doses may be decreased by half.

ONSET OF EFFECT
Varies depending on the infection being treated.

DURATION OF ACTION
Unknown.

DIETARY ADVICE
Take with a full glass of water on an empty stomach, 1 hour before or 2 hours after a meal. Drink plenty of fluids.

STORAGE
Store in a tightly sealed container away from heat, moisture, and direct light.

MISSED DOSE
Take it as soon as you remember. If it is near the time for the next dose, skip the missed dose and resume your regular dosage schedule. Do not double the next dose.

STOPPING THE DRUG
Take it as prescribed for the full treatment period.

PROLONGED USE
There are no documented problems with prolonged use, but if you must take this drug for an extended period, see your physician regularly.

▼ PRECAUTIONS

Over 60: No special problems are expected.

Driving and Hazardous Work: Do not drive or engage in hazardous work until you determine how the medicine affects you.

Alcohol: It is advisable to abstain from alcohol when fighting an infection.

Pregnancy: In some animal tests, enoxacin has caused birth defects. Adequate studies in humans have not been done. It should be used during pregnancy only if potential benefits clearly justify the risks. Before you take enoxacin, tell your doctor if you are pregnant or plan to become pregnant.

Breast Feeding: Enoxacin passes into breast milk and may cause serious side effects in the nursing infant; use of the drug is discouraged when nursing.

Infants and Children: Not recommended for use by persons under age 18, as it has been shown to interfere with bone development.

Special Concerns: If enoxacin causes sensitivity to sunlight, stop taking the drug and try to avoid exposure to sunlight for the next 5 days; also wear protective clothing and use a sunblock. Enoxacin should not be taken by patients whose work makes it impossible to stay out of the sun. Avoid smoking. Do not take this medicine if you are allergic to any quinolone antibiotic. You should avoid people who have an active infection. Refrain from strenuous physical activity while taking this medicine. Be sure to drink at least 8 glasses of water a day while taking enoxacin.

OVERDOSE
Symptoms: No specific ones have been reported.

What to Do: If you have any reason to suspect an overdose, call your doctor, emergency medical services (EMS), or the nearest poison control center.

▼ INTERACTIONS

DRUG INTERACTIONS
Consult your doctor for specific advice if you are taking aminophylline, antacids, didanosine, iron supplements, oxtriphylline, sucralfate, theophylline, warfarin, or zinc salts. Also tell your doctor if you are taking any other prescription or over-the-counter medication.

FOOD INTERACTIONS
The effects of caffeine may be magnified by this drug.

DISEASE INTERACTIONS
Do not use enoxacin if you have a history of hypersensitivity, tendinitis, or tendon rupture associated with the use of enoxacin or any other quinolone antibiotic. Consult your doctor if you have any other medical condition. Use of enoxacin can cause complications in patients with kidney disease, since this organ works to remove the medication from the body.

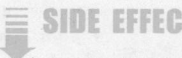

SIDE EFFECTS

SERIOUS
Serious reactions are rare and include seizures, confusion, hallucinations, agitation, nightmares, depression, shortness of breath, unusual swelling in the face or extremities, decreased urine output, and loss of consciousness. Also skin burning, redness, blisters, rash, or itching on exposure to sunlight. Call your doctor immediately.

COMMON
Increased sensitivity to sunlight (and increased risk of sunburn) for days following therapy.

LESS COMMON
Diarrhea, nausea and vomiting, stomach pain and upset, gas, headache, dizziness, restlessness, insomnia, changes in taste perception, drowsiness, itching, dry mouth, unusual body aches or pains.

ENOXAPARIN SODIUM INJECTION

Available in: Injection
Available OTC? No **As Generic?** No
Drug Class: Anticoagulant

▼ USAGE INFORMATION

WHY IT'S PRESCRIBED
To prevent blood clots in the legs after hip or knee replacement surgery, or for other conditions where blood clots could pose a problem.

HOW IT WORKS
Enoxaparin forms a complex with certain natural body chemicals that prevent clot formation; it also decreases the activity of chemicals that cause clot formation. The combined effect reduces the speed at which blood may coagulate and thus prevents blood clots from developing.

▼ DOSAGE GUIDELINES

RANGE AND FREQUENCY
To prevent blood clots after surgery: 30 mg injected under the skin every 12 hours for 7 to 10 days. It must not be administered intramuscularly or intravenously. Rotate the site of injections from abdomen to thighs to upper arms. After injection, do not massage the site of the injection. Watch for signs of bruising or bleeding at injection sites. Children: Consult your pediatrician for proper dosage.

ONSET OF EFFECT
Within 30 minutes to 3 hours.

DURATION OF ACTION
Up to 24 hours.

DIETARY ADVICE
Injections can be delivered regardless of diet or meal schedule.

STORAGE
Store in a tightly sealed container away from heat and direct light. Do not refrigerate or allow to freeze (for instance, in the trunk of a car during wintertime).

MISSED DOSE
Take it as soon as you remember. If it is near the time for the next dose, skip the missed dose and resume your regular dosage schedule. Do not double the next dose.

STOPPING THE DRUG
The decision to stop taking the drug should be made by your doctor.

PROLONGED USE
Enoxaparin should be used only for the period recommended by your doctor.

▼ PRECAUTIONS

Over 60: Older patients may be more susceptible to bleeding during therapy.

Driving and Hazardous Work: Do not drive or engage in hazardous work until you determine how the medicine affects you.

Alcohol: Alcohol should be avoided while taking this medicine.

Pregnancy: Enoxaparin does not appear to cross the placenta. No birth defects have been found in animal studies. Human studies have not been conducted.

Breast Feeding: It is not known if enoxaparin passes into breast milk. Use caution. Consult your doctor for specific advice.

Infants and Children: There is no information about the safety and efficacy of enoxaparin in infants and children. Consult your doctor for specific advice.

Special Concerns: Place used syringes in a disposable, puncture-proof container or follow your doctor's instructions on discarding them. Be sure to tell all doctors and dentists whom you consult that you are using enoxaparin. Before taking enoxaparin, tell your doctor if you have recently given birth, injured your head or body, or had surgery, including dental surgery. Tell your doctor if you are allergic to substances such as pork, preservatives, or dyes.

OVERDOSE
Symptoms: Bleeding complications (such as uncontrolled hemorrhaging).

What to Do: Stop taking the drug, and call your doctor, emergency medical services (EMS), or the nearest poison control center immediately.

▼ INTERACTIONS

DRUG INTERACTIONS
Consult your doctor for specific advice if you are taking aspirin or any other salicylate; inflammation or pain medicine; or drugs that lower blood platelet count, such as famotidine, plicamycin, sulfinpyrazone, ticlopidine, valproic acid, anagrelide, or any other anticoagulant.

FOOD INTERACTIONS
No known food interactions.

DISEASE INTERACTIONS
Caution is advised when taking enoxaparin. Consult your doctor if you have any of the following: blood disease, heart disease, high blood pressure, kidney disease, liver disease, a heart infection, or an ulcer.

≡ SIDE EFFECTS ≡

SERIOUS
Extreme fatigue; abnormal bleeding; bleeding gums; arm or leg bruises; purple or red spots on skin; nosebleeds; black, tarry stools; blood in urine; vomiting of blood. Seek medical assistance immediately.

COMMON
There are no common side effects associated with the use of enoxaparin.

LESS COMMON
Nausea, fever, increased menstrual bleeding, confusion, swelling, pain or redness at injection site.

ENTACAPONE

Available in: Tablets
Available OTC? No   **As Generic?** No
Drug Class: Antiparkinsonism drug/COMT inhibitor

▼ USAGE INFORMATION

WHY IT'S PRESCRIBED
To treat Parkinson's disease, in conjunction with standard levodopa/carbidopa therapy, in patients who have begun to be less responsive to levodopa and experience worsening symptoms between doses, a phenomenon known as "end-of-dose wearing-off."

HOW IT WORKS
When used with levodopa/carbidopa, entacapone sustains higher levels of levodopa in the blood. Entacapone increases blood levels of levodopa by blocking the action of catechol-O-methyltransferase (COMT), one of the enzymes responsible for breaking down levodopa, before it reaches its receptors in the brain. Levodopa raises the amount of dopamine available in the brain; dopamine plays an essential role in smooth movement of muscles and is deficient in patients with Parkinson's disease.

▼ DOSAGE GUIDELINES

RANGE AND FREQUENCY
Adults: 200 mg in conjunction with each levodopa/carbidopa dose, up to a maximum of 8 times a day (1600 mg a day). Entacapone must be administered with levodopa/carbidopa as entacapone has no antiparkinsonian effect of its own. Patients may require a decrease in their daily dosage of levodopa upon beginning entacapone therapy.

ONSET OF EFFECT
Unknown.

DURATION OF ACTION
Unknown.

DIETARY ADVICE
Entacapone can be taken without regard to meals.

STORAGE
Store in a tightly sealed container away from heat, moisture, and direct light.

MISSED DOSE
Take it as soon as you remember. If it is near the time for the next dose, skip the missed dose and resume your regular dosage schedule. Do not double the next dose.

STOPPING THE DRUG
Take it as prescribed for the full treatment period. The decision to stop taking the drug should be made in consultation with your physician. Abrupt discontinuation, without a gradual reduction in dose, may increase the risk of adverse effects.

PROLONGED USE
Since Parkinson's disease is a chronic condition, lifelong therapy with entacapone is likely to be required. No special problems are expected.

▼ PRECAUTIONS

Over 60: No specific problems for older people have been reported.

Driving and Hazardous Work: Do not drive or engage in hazardous work until you determine how the medicine affects you.

Alcohol: No special warnings.

Pregnancy: Adequate human studies have not been done. Before taking entacapone, tell your doctor if you are or are planning to become pregnant. Discuss with your doctor the risks and benefits of using this drug while pregnant.

Breast Feeding: Entacapone may pass into breast milk; caution is advised. Consult your doctor for advice.

Infants and Children: Not applicable. No potential use for entacapone has been identified in children.

Special Concerns: Entacapone may be combined with either the immediate or sustained-release forms of levodopa/carbidopa.

OVERDOSE
Symptoms: An overdose with entacapone is unlikely. However, diarrhea and abdominal pain may occur with an excessive dose.

What to Do: If someone takes a much larger dose than prescribed, call your doctor, emergency medical services (EMS), or the nearest poison control immediately.

▼ INTERACTIONS

DRUG INTERACTIONS
Consult your doctor for specific advice if you are taking any of the following drugs: MAO inhibitor antidepressants (such as phenelzine sulfate or tranylcypromine sulfate, but not selegiline), isoproterenol, epinephrine, norepinephrine, dopamine, dobutamine, bitolterol, probenecid, cholestyramine, and some antibiotics (erythromycin, rifampicin, ampicillin, and chloramphenicol).

FOOD INTERACTIONS
No known food interactions.

DISEASE INTERACTIONS
Entacapone should be used with caution in people with liver disease, bile duct obstruction, or low blood pressure.

 SIDE EFFECTS

SERIOUS
Dizziness, lightheadedness, or fainting, especially when rising from a sitting or lying position, owing to a sudden drop in blood pressure (orthostatic hypotension). Such symptoms, in addition to nausea, are more common at the beginning of therapy. Hallucinations may also occur and require discontinuation of therapy.

COMMON
Slowed movement, nausea, quirky involuntary muscle movements that may contort the body, discolored urine, abdominal pain, diarrhea.

LESS COMMON
Increased sweating, back pain, anxiety, agitation, drowsiness, vomiting, constipation, dry mouth, indigestion, flatulence, shortness of breath, fatigue, weakness.

EPHEDRINE

BRAND NAMES

Ephedrine Sulfate, Kondon's Nasal, Pretz-D, Vicks Vatronol

Available in: Capsules, injection
Available OTC? Yes **As Generic?** Yes
Drug Class: Adrenergic bronchodilator

▼ USAGE INFORMATION

WHY IT'S PRESCRIBED
To relieve bronchial asthma, to decrease nasal and lower respiratory congestion, and to suppress allergic reactions. Ephedrine commonly appears in combination with other drugs in such brand name products as Broncholate, Bronkotuss Expectorant, Quelidrine Cough Formula, and Rynatuss.

HOW IT WORKS
Ephedrine prevents cells from releasing histamine, a naturally occurring substance that causes swelling, itching, sneezing, watery eyes, hives, and other symptoms of allergic reaction. It also relaxes the smooth muscle surrounding the bronchial tubes, widening the airways, and causes constriction of blood vessels in the nose, which helps to open the nasal passages.

▼ DOSAGE GUIDELINES

RANGE AND FREQUENCY
Capsules— Adults: 25 to 50 mg every 3 or 4 hours, if needed. Children: 3 mg per 2.2 lbs (1 kg) of body weight per day, in 4 to 6 divided doses. Injection— Adults: 1 dose of 12.5 to 25 mg injected into a muscle, a vein, or under the skin. A second dose may be administered if approved by your doctor. Children: 3 mg per 2.2 lbs of body weight a day, in 4 to 6 divided doses.

ONSET OF EFFECT
Capsules: 15 to 60 minutes. Injection: 10 to 20 minutes.

DURATION OF ACTION
Capsules: 3 to 5 hours. Injection: 30 minutes to 1 hour after 25 to 50 mg dose.

DIETARY ADVICE
Swallow capsules with water and drink plenty of fluids.

STORAGE
Store in a dry place in a tightly sealed container away from heat and direct light. Keep injection form refrigerated, but do not allow it to freeze. Do not use injection if the liquid is cloudy or unclear.

MISSED DOSE
Take it if you remember within 2 hours. If not, skip the missed dose and resume your normal dosage schedule. Do not double the next dose.

STOPPING THE DRUG
You may stop taking this drug at your own discretion. Consult your doctor.

PROLONGED USE
This drug may lose its effectiveness if taken on a continuous basis for 3 to 4 days. Men with an enlarged prostate gland may have difficulty urinating.

▼ PRECAUTIONS

Over 60: Adverse reactions may be more likely and more severe in older patients. Small doses are advisable until your individual response to the drug has been evaluated.

Driving and Hazardous Work: Ephedrine may cause dizziness. Do not drive or engage in hazardous work until you determine how it affects you.

Alcohol: No special precautions are necessary.

Pregnancy: Consult your doctor; benefits must clearly outweigh risks.

Breast Feeding: Ephedrine passes into breast milk and may be harmful to the child; do not use it while nursing.

Infants and Children: Use caution. Ask your doctor if the benefits of ephedrine justify possible risk to the child.

Special Concerns: Ephedrine can cause insomnia. Take the last dose at least 2 hours before bedtime. Before you take ephedrine, tell your doctor if you will have surgery requiring general anesthesia, including dental surgery, within 2 months.

OVERDOSE
Symptoms: Severe anxiety, convulsions, trouble breathing, coma, confusion, delirium, rapid and irregular pulse, muscle tremors.

What to Do: Call your doctor, emergency medical services (EMS), or the nearest poison control center immediately.

▼ INTERACTIONS

DRUG INTERACTIONS
Consult your doctor for specific advice if you are taking tricyclic antidepressants, high blood pressure medication, beta-blockers, dextrothyroxine, digitalis drugs, ergot-containing preparations, furazolidone, guanadrel, guanethidine, heart medication, methyldopa, MAO inhibitors, nitrates, phenothiazines, pseudoephedrine, rauwolfia alkaloids, sympathomimetic drugs, terazosin, theophylline, or any nonprescription drug for a cough, cold, allergy, or asthma.

FOOD INTERACTIONS
No known food interactions.

DISEASE INTERACTIONS
Caution is advised when taking ephedrine. Consult your doctor if you have any of the following: enlarged prostate, high blood pressure, history of seizures, diabetes, Parkinson's disease, or an overactive thyroid gland.

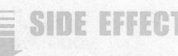

SIDE EFFECTS

SERIOUS
Irregular heartbeats, hallucinations with high doses, shortness of breath. Call your doctor.

COMMON
Nervousness, rapid heartbeat, paleness, insomnia.

LESS COMMON
Dizziness, loss of appetite, nausea, vomiting, muscle cramps, headache, difficult or painful urination.

EPINEPHRINE HYDROCHLORIDE

Available in: Inhalation aerosols and solutions, injection, eye drops
Available OTC? Yes   **As Generic?** Yes
Drug Class: Bronchodilator/sympathomimetic; antiglaucoma agent

▼ USAGE INFORMATION

WHY IT'S PRESCRIBED
To treat bronchial asthma, emphysema, and other lung diseases. Epinephrine is also a primary treatment for anaphylaxis; that is, hypersensitive (allergic) reaction to drugs or other substances. It may also be used to treat nasal congestion, to prolong the action of anesthetics, and to treat cardiac arrest. The ophthalmic form of the drug is used to treat glaucoma.

HOW IT WORKS
Epinephrine widens constricted airways in the lungs by relaxing smooth muscles that surround bronchial passages. It also raises blood pressure by constricting small blood vessels, increases the heart rate and strength of heart contractions, and decreases fluid pressure in the eye.

▼ DOSAGE GUIDELINES

RANGE AND FREQUENCY
It may be used when needed to relieve breathing difficulty. For adults and children 4 years of age or older with asthma— Inhaled aerosol: 200 micrograms (mcg) to 275 mcg (1 puff), repeated if needed after 1 or 2 minutes, with doses taken at least 3 hours apart. Inhalation solution: 1 puff of 1% solution repeated after 1 or 2 minutes, if needed. Injection: 0.2 to 1 mg, increased if needed. For open-angle glaucoma— 1 or 2 drops of 1% or 2% solution, once or twice daily.

ONSET OF EFFECT
Inhalation: Within 5 minutes.
Injection: 1 to 5 minutes.

DURATION OF ACTION
Inhalation: 1 to 3 hours.
Injection: 1 to 4 hours.

DIETARY ADVICE
No special concerns.

STORAGE
Store in a tightly sealed container, away from heat, moisture, and direct light.

MISSED DOSE
Take your missed dose as soon as you remember, unless the time for your next scheduled dose is within the next 2 hours, in which case skip the missed dose. Take your next scheduled dose at the proper time and resume your regular dosage schedule. Do not take a double dose.

STOPPING THE DRUG
Take the drug exactly as prescribed. Contact your doctor if you do not respond to the strength of the dosage you have been given.

PROLONGED USE
Tolerance to epinephrine may develop with prolonged use.

▼ PRECAUTIONS

Over 60: Adverse reactions may be more likely and more severe in older patients.

Driving and Hazardous Work: Do not drive or engage in hazardous work until you determine how the medicine affects you.

Alcohol: It may increase the excretion of epinephrine in the urine.

Pregnancy: Benefits of taking the drug must outweigh the potential risks; consult your doctor for specific advice.

Breast Feeding: Epinephrine passes into the breast milk. Consult your doctor for specific advice.

Infants and Children: They may be especially sensitive to epinephrine; fainting by children with asthma taking the drug has been reported.

Special Concerns: Do not use without a prescription, unless your problem has been diagnosed as asthma.

Take aerosol doses exactly as directed; overuse has caused sudden death. Keep the injectable form ready for use at all times, along with phone numbers of your doctor and the local emergency room.

OVERDOSE
Symptoms: Chest discomfort, chills or fever, seizures, dizziness, irregular heartbeat, trouble breathing.

What to Do: Call your doctor, emergency medical services (EMS), or the nearest poison control center immediately.

▼ INTERACTIONS

DRUG INTERACTIONS
Consult your doctor for specific advice if you are taking anesthetics, tricyclic antidepressants, antidiabetic agents, antihypertensives or diuretics, beta-blockers, digitalis drugs, ergoloid mesylates, maprotiline, ergotamine, or MAO inhibitors.

FOOD INTERACTIONS
Avoid any foods that have previously triggered an allergic reaction or asthma attack.

DISEASE INTERACTIONS
The benefits of taking the drug need to be weighed against the potential risks if you have any of the following conditions: organic brain damage, diabetes mellitus, Parkinson's disease, heart or blood vessel disease, or overactive thyroid.

SIDE EFFECTS

SERIOUS
Bluish color of skin, severe dizziness, flushing, and difficulty breathing may indicate an allergic reaction to sulfites in the medication. Contact your doctor immediately.

COMMON
Dry mouth and throat, trembling, headaches. Check with your doctor if these symptoms continue or become bothersome.

LESS COMMON
Eye pain or headache from using eye drops.

EPOETIN ALFA

Available in: Injection
Available OTC? No   **As Generic?** No
Drug Class: Antianemia drug

▼ USAGE INFORMATION

WHY IT'S PRESCRIBED
For treating severe anemia due to impaired production of erythropoietin (a hormone that stimulates the bone marrow to produce red blood cells), which may occur with chronic kidney disease, in anemic cancer patients receiving chemo-therapy, and anemic HIV-infected patients taking zidovudine.

HOW IT WORKS
Epoetin alfa stimulates the production of red blood cells in the bone marrow, replacing the hormone erythropoietin, which is depleted in patients suffering from renal (kidney) failure, or who have diseases or take medications that suppress the body's natural erythropoietin production.

▼ DOSAGE GUIDELINES

RANGE AND FREQUENCY
Average dosage range for adults and teenagers: 23 to 68 units per lb of body weight, 3 times a week. May be increased by 11 units per lb every 4 weeks or more, up to 90 units per lb, to produce the desired effect. Once that has been achieved, the dose should be adjusted downward at 4-week intervals to achieve the lowest effective maintenance dose.

ONSET OF EFFECT
Within 2 to 6 weeks.

DURATION OF ACTION
In the presence of impaired erythropoietin production, the drug must be given at least several times per week to maintain its effect.

DIETARY ADVICE
Patients may require iron supplements, but these should be taken only on the advice of a doctor; other vitamins may also be recommended to aid in the manufacture of red blood cells. Patients with kidney problems or high blood pressure are often on restricted diets, which need to be reinforced with vitamin supplementation.

STORAGE
Keep epoetin alfa refrigerated, but do not allow it to freeze.

MISSED DOSE
Take it as soon as you remember. If it is near the time for the next dose, skip the missed dose and resume your regular dosage schedule. Do not double the next dose.

STOPPING THE DRUG
Take the drug as prescribed for the full treatment period, in accordance with your doctor's instructions.

PROLONGED USE
Comply with schedules for proper dosage and administration, dialysis, blood tests, and blood pressure tests set by your doctor. If you are performing dialysis at home and self-administering epoetin alfa, follow your doctor's orders carefully and report changes outside of guidelines the doctor has given to you.

▼ PRECAUTIONS

Over 60: Adverse reactions may be more likely and more severe in older patients.

Driving and Hazardous Work: Avoid such activities in the first 90 days of treatment when seizures are most likely to occur.

Alcohol: No special problems are expected.

Pregnancy: Consult your doctor about whether benefits outweigh the potential risk to the unborn child.

Breast Feeding: Epoetin alfa may pass into breast milk; caution is advised. Consult your doctor for advice.

Infants and Children: Epoetin alfa is safe for use in children.

Special Concerns: Be sure to follow you doctor's advice, including dietary recommendations and dialysis prescriptions, even if you begin to feel better while taking the drug. Epoetin alfa will correct only anemia, not kidney disease or other medical problems that may be present.

OVERDOSE
Symptoms: Headache, weakness, flushing, dizziness, seizures, chest pain.

What to Do: Call your doctor, emergency medical services (EMS), or the nearest poison control center immediately.

▼ INTERACTIONS

DRUG INTERACTIONS
No known drug interactions.

FOOD INTERACTIONS
No known food interactions.

DISEASE INTERACTIONS
High blood pressure (hypertension) must be controlled before this drug is used. Also, advise your doctor if you have a history of blood clotting disorders, heart or blood vessel disease, blood disorders such as sickle cell anemia, or bone problems.

≣ SIDE EFFECTS ≣

SERIOUS
Chest pain; convulsions; shortness of breath; rapid heartbeat; headache; swelling in the face, hands, and lower extremities; vision problems; unexplained weight gain. Such symptoms are due to an inappropriate elevation of the number of red cells; check with your doctor immediately if such symptoms occur.

COMMON
Influenza-like symptoms, bone pain, burning at the injection site, fatigue. Such symptoms tend to occur at the beginning of therapy but usually diminish as your body adjusts to the medicine. Notify your doctor if such side effects persist or interfere with normal activities.

LESS COMMON
Skin rash, hives.

ERGOLOID MESYLATES

Available in: Capsules, sublingual tablets, oral solution
Available OTC? No   **As Generic?** Yes
Drug Class: Psychotherapeutic agent

▼ USAGE INFORMATION

WHY IT'S PRESCRIBED
To treat decline in mental capacity due to dementia (progressive breakdown of mental function).

HOW IT WORKS
The exact way in which ergoloid mesylates work has not been established.

▼ DOSAGE GUIDELINES

RANGE AND FREQUENCY
1 to 2 mg, 3 times a day. Maximum dose: 12 mg daily.

ONSET OF EFFECT
Unknown.

DURATION OF ACTION
Unknown.

DIETARY ADVICE
When taking the sublingual form of the medication, do not eat, drink, or smoke while the tablet is dissolving under your tongue; do not chew, swallow, or crush it either.

STORAGE
Store in a tightly sealed container away from heat, moisture, and direct light. Keep the oral solution form of the drug refrigerated, but do not allow it to freeze.

MISSED DOSE
Take it as soon as you remember. However, if it is near the time for the next dose, skip the missed dose and resume your regular dosage schedule. Do not double the next dose.

STOPPING THE DRUG
The decision to stop taking ergoloid mesylates should be made in consultation with your doctor.

PROLONGED USE
Regular evaluation by your doctor is necessary to determine whether or not there are initial and continuing therapeutic benefits from taking ergoloid mesylates; the medication's effectiveness may not be apparent for several weeks or even months.

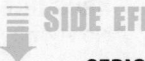
SIDE EFFECTS

SERIOUS
No serious side effects are associated with the recommended dosage of ergoloid mesylates.

COMMON
There are no common side effects.

LESS COMMON
At the recommended dosage, side effects are usually rare and remit when therapy is discontinued. Check with your doctor if the following symptoms appear: drowsiness, slow heartbeat, dizziness or lightheadedness when getting up from a sitting or lying position (orthostatic hypotension), skin rash, stomach pain, sensitivity of eyes to sunlight, soreness under the tongue (from sublingual tablet) that does not go away.

▼ PRECAUTIONS

Over 60: No special precautions are necessary.

Driving and Hazardous Work: Do not drive or engage in hazardous work until you determine how the medicine affects you.

Alcohol: Avoid alcohol. Be aware that some over-the-counter cough, cold, and allergy medications contain alcohol; check ingredient labels carefully.

Pregnancy: Studies of the use of ergoloid mesylates during pregnancy have not been done. Consult your doctor for specific advice.

Breast Feeding: Studies of the use of ergoloid mesylates in breast-feeding women have not been done. Consult your doctor for advice.

Infants and Children: Ergoloid mesylates are not prescribed for children.

Special Concerns: The therapeutic benefit of ergoloid mesylates in treating dementia is a matter of controversy. Some doctors believe it may be helpful; others do not.

OVERDOSE
Symptoms: Headache, blurred vision, dizziness, fainting, nausea or vomiting, stomach cramps, flushing, nasal congestion.

What to Do: Call your doctor, emergency medical services (EMS), or the nearest poison control center immediately.

▼ INTERACTIONS

DRUG INTERACTIONS
Other drugs may interact with ergoloid mesylates. Consult your doctor for specific advice if you are taking any other prescription or over-the-counter medication.

FOOD INTERACTIONS
No known food interactions.

DISEASE INTERACTIONS
The benefits of the drug should be weighed against possible risks for patients with the following conditions: bradycardia (slow heartbeat), low blood pressure, or liver disease. Ergoloid mesylates are not used to treat acute or chronic psychosis.

ERGOTAMINE/BELLADONNA ALKALOIDS/PHENOBARBITAL

BRAND NAME

Bellergal-S

Available in: Extended-release tablets
Available OTC? No   **As Generic?** No
Drug Class: Antimigraine/antiheadache drug

▼ USAGE INFORMATION

WHY IT'S PRESCRIBED
Used to prevent vascular headaches (those involving the blood vessels to the brain), such as migraines and cluster headaches. Also used to ease symptoms of menopause, such as hot flashes, sweating, restlessness, and insomnia, usually in women for whom estrogen replacement therapy has been ruled out.

HOW IT WORKS
The above conditions are believed to be caused, in part, by overactivity in the autonomic nervous system, the part that controls involuntary body functions like heart rate, sweating, and digestion. The combination of ergotamine, belladonna alkaloids, and phenobarbital helps to balance and calm this part of the nervous system, thus reducing various kinds of physical distress.

▼ DOSAGE GUIDELINES

RANGE AND FREQUENCY
Adults: 1 tablet in the morning and 1 in the evening. Children: Consult pediatrician. Tablet must be taken whole.

ONSET OF EFFECT
Unknown.

DURATION OF ACTION
Unknown.

DIETARY ADVICE
No special concerns.

STORAGE
Store in a tightly sealed container, away from heat, moisture, and direct light.

MISSED DOSE
Skip the missed dose and then resume your regular dosage schedule. Do not double the next dose.

STOPPING THE DRUG
The decision to stop taking the drug should be made by your doctor. Discontinue the drug in gradually diminishing doses, according to your doctor's instructions, to minimize the risk of withdrawal symptoms.

PROLONGED USE
Prolonged use at high doses may produce some degree of physical dependence due to the barbiturate, phenobarbital, and may increase the risk of blood circulation problems.

▼ PRECAUTIONS

Over 60: Adverse reactions may be more likely and more severe in older patients.

Driving and Hazardous Work: Do not drive or engage in hazardous work until you determine how the drug affects you.

Alcohol: Avoid alcohol.

Pregnancy: Do not take the drug combination during pregnancy. Consult your doctor if you become or plan to become pregnant.

Breast Feeding: The drug combination passes into breast milk; avoid or discontinue use while nursing.

Infants and Children: Adverse reactions may be more likely and more severe.

Special Concerns: Avoid smoking, since it may increase the risk of side effects associated with impaired blood circulation. Dress warmly if you have blood circulation problems (most common among elderly patients).

OVERDOSE
Symptoms: Convulsions; severe diarrhea, nausea, vomiting, stomach pain bloating; severe dizziness, drowsiness, or weakness; rapid or slow heartbeat; shortness of breath; unusual excitement.

What to Do: Call your doctor, emergency medical services (EMS), or the nearest poison control center immediately.

▼ INTERACTIONS

DRUG INTERACTIONS
Do not take this drug if you are taking naratriptan, sumatriptan, or zolmitriptan. Consult your doctor for advice if you are taking antacids, anticoagulants, anticholinergics, carbamazepine, central nervous system depressants, diarrhea medication, digitalis drugs, ketoconazole, MAO inhibitors, other ergot medications, oral contraceptives, potassium chloride, or tricyclic antidepressants.

FOOD INTERACTIONS
No known food interactions.

DISEASE INTERACTIONS
Consult your doctor if you have any of the following: chronic lung disease such as asthma or emphysema, difficult urination, urinary tract blockage, Down syndrome, enlarged prostate, heart, kidney, or liver disease, blood vessel disease or recent surgery on blood vessels, severe high blood pressure, infection, intestinal conditions, overactive thyroid, porphyria, glaucoma, severe dry mouth, severe itching. In children: brain damage, hyperactivity, spastic paralysis.

SIDE EFFECTS

SERIOUS
Severe anxiety or confusion; change in vision; chest pain; pale, cold, bluish-colored hands or feet; pain in arms, legs, or lower back; red blisters on hands or feet; gangrene. Seek medical attention immediately.

COMMON
Constipation; swelling of face, fingers, feet, or lower legs; reduced sweating; dizziness or lightheadedness; drowsiness; dry mouth, nose, throat, or skin.

LESS COMMON
Blurred vision; unusual weakness; increased sensitivity of eyes to bright light; diarrhea, nausea, or vomiting; skin rash or itching of skin; sore throat and fever; unusual bruising or bleeding; weakness in legs; yellow discoloration of the eyes or skin; difficulty urinating; difficulty in swallowing; unusual excitability; loss of memory.

ERYTHROMYCIN ETHYLSUCCINATE/SULFISOXAZOLE

Available in: Oral suspension
Available OTC? No **As Generic?** Yes
Drug Class: Erythromycin antibiotic

▼ USAGE INFORMATION

WHY IT'S PRESCRIBED
To treat middle ear infections in children.

HOW IT WORKS
Erythromycin prevents bacterial cells from manufacturing specific proteins necessary for their survival; sulfisoxazole prevents bacteria from utilizing folic acid, a vitamin essential to both cell growth and reproduction.

▼ DOSAGE GUIDELINES

RANGE AND FREQUENCY
Children weighing more than 100 lbs: 2 teaspoons (10 ml) 4 times a day for 10 days. Children weighing 53 to 100 lbs: 1 1/2 tsps (7.5 ml) 4 times a day for 10 days. Children weighing 35 to 53 lbs: 1 tsp (5 ml) 4 times a day for 10 days. Children weighing 18 to 35 lbs: 1/2 tsp (2.5 ml) 4 times a day for 10 days. Children under 18 lbs: The dose must be determined by your pediatrician.

ONSET OF EFFECT
Unknown.

DURATION OF ACTION
Unknown.

DIETARY ADVICE
Give it 1 hour before or 2 hours after meals with a full glass of water. If it causes stomach upset, it can be taken with milk or food. Increase patient's fluid intake.

STORAGE
Store in a tightly sealed container away from heat and direct light. Refrigerate but do not freeze.

MISSED DOSE
Give it as soon as you remember. If it is close to the time for the next dose, skip the missed dose and resume the regular dosage schedule. Do not double the next dose.

STOPPING THE DRUG
Give the medicine as prescribed for the full treatment period, even if the child begins to feel better before the scheduled end of therapy.

PROLONGED USE
Your child should see a doctor regularly for tests and examinations if this medicine is prescribed for a prolonged period. Bacteria that are resistant to this medication may develop with long-term use.

▼ PRECAUTIONS

Over 60: This medication is not intended for use by older persons.

Driving and Hazardous Work: This medication should not impair mental alertness or physical coordination.

Alcohol: Not applicable; this drug is for children.

Pregnancy: Adequate studies of the use of this drug during pregnancy have not been done; consult your doctor for specific advice if there is any chance that the patient could become pregnant.

Breast Feeding: Not applicable; the drug is for children.

Infants and Children: This medicine is not recommended for children under 2 months of age.

Special Concerns: If the medicine causes sensitivity to sunlight, take preventive measures: patients should use sunscreens, wear protective clothing, and avoid exposure to sunlight.

OVERDOSE
Symptoms: Severe nausea, vomiting, diarrhea, dizziness, headache, drowsiness, fever, loss of consciousness.

What to Do: Overdose is not likely, but if symptoms occur, call your doctor, emergency medical services (EMS), or the nearest poison control center immediately.

▼ INTERACTIONS

DRUG INTERACTIONS
This drug may interact with acetaminophen, acetohydroxamic acid, alfentanil, amiodarone, aminophylline, oral antidiabetics, carbamazepine, carmustine, chloramphenicol, chloroquine, cholesterol-lowering drugs, dantrolene, dapsone, daunorubicin, divalproex, estrogens, ethotoin, etretinate, gold salts, hydroxychloroquine, lincomycin, methenamine, mephenytoin, methotrexate, mercaptopurine, methyldopa, naltrexone, nitrofurantoin, oral contraceptives, phenytoin, plicamycin, primaquine, procainamide, quinidine, quinine, sulfoxone, or vitamin K. Consult your doctor for advice.

FOOD INTERACTIONS
Avoid caffeinated beverages or food.

DISEASE INTERACTIONS
Consult your doctor if the patient has any of the following: anemia or another blood problem, G6PD deficiency, kidney disease, liver disease, hearing loss, or porphyria.

≣ SIDE EFFECTS ≣

SERIOUS
Skin rash, itching, aching joints and muscles, difficulty swallowing, pale skin or red, blistered, peeling, or loose skin, sore throat and fever, unusual bleeding or bruising, unusual fatigue, yellowish tinge to the eyes or skin, blood in urine, darkened urine, pain in lower back, pain while urinating, pale stools, stomach pain, swollen neck, increased sensitivity to sunlight. Call your doctor immediately.

COMMON
Stomach or abdominal discomfort and cramps, diarrhea, loss of appetite, nausea, vomiting.

LESS COMMON
Sore tongue or mouth.

ERYTHROMYCIN OPHTHALMIC

Available in: Ophthalmic ointment
Available OTC? No   **As Generic?** Yes
Drug Class: Antibiotic

▼ USAGE INFORMATION

WHY IT'S PRESCRIBED
To treat infections of the eye; to treat inflammation of the edges of the eyelids (blepharitis); to prevent some eye infections in newborn babies (neonatal conjunctivitis and ophthalmia neonatorum).

HOW IT WORKS
Erythromycin kills bacteria by interfering with the genetic material of bacterial cells, thereby preventing them from multiplying.

▼ DOSAGE GUIDELINES

RANGE AND FREQUENCY
Adults and children— For eye infections: Apply ointment to the affected eye up to 6 times a day, as directed by your doctor. For blepharitis: Apply once a day immediately before bedtime after performing standard eyelid hygiene measures as directed by your doctor. To prevent eye infections in newborns— Ointment is applied once, shortly after birth.

ONSET OF EFFECT
Unknown.

DURATION OF ACTION
Unknown.

DIETARY ADVICE
This medication can be used without regard to diet.

STORAGE
Store in a tightly sealed container away from heat, moisture, and direct light. Do not allow it to freeze.

MISSED DOSE
Apply it as soon as you remember. If it is near the time for the next dose, skip the missed dose and resume your regular dosage schedule. Do not double the next dose.

STOPPING THE DRUG
Use it as prescribed for the full treatment period, even if you feel better before the scheduled end of therapy.

PROLONGED USE
You should see your doctor regularly for tests and examinations if you take this drug for a prolonged period.

▼ PRECAUTIONS

Over 60: No special problems are expected.

Driving and Hazardous Work: Do not drive or engage in hazardous work until you determine how the medicine affects your vision.

Alcohol: No special precautions are necessary.

Pregnancy: Erythromycin has not been shown to cause birth defects or other problems during pregnancy. Before using erythromycin, tell your doctor if you are pregnant or are planning to become pregnant.

Breast Feeding: Erythromycin has not been shown to cause problems in nursing babies.

Infants and Children: No special precautions.

Special Concerns: To use the ointment, first wash your hands. Tilt your head back. Gently apply pressure to the inside corner of the eyelid and with the index finger of the same hand, pull downward on the lower eyelid to make a space. Put a short strip of ointment (about ⅓ inch long) into this space and close your eye. Apply pressure for 1 or 2 minutes while keeping the eye closed without blinking. Then wash your hands again. Make sure that the tip of the applicator does not touch your eye, finger, or any other surface. If your symptoms do not improve in a few days or if they become worse, check with your doctor. Do not use this drug if you have a history of allergy to azithromycin, clarithromycin, erythromycin, or lincomycin.

OVERDOSE
Symptoms: No specific ones.

What to Do: If someone accidentally ingests the medicine, call your doctor, emergency medical services (EMS), or the nearest poison control center immediately.

▼ INTERACTIONS

DRUG INTERACTIONS
Other drugs may interact with ophthalmic erythromycin. Consult your doctor for specific advice if you are taking any other prescription or over-the-counter medication.

FOOD INTERACTIONS
No known food interactions.

DISEASE INTERACTIONS
Caution is advised when taking ophthalmic erythromycin. Consult your doctor if you have any other medical condition.

▬ SIDE EFFECTS ▬

SERIOUS
Eye irritation, redness, swelling, or itching that was not present before therapy. Stop using the medication and call your doctor immediately.

COMMON
Blurred vision for up to 30 minutes following application.

LESS COMMON
There are no less-common side effects associated with ophthalmic erythromycin.

ERYTHROMYCIN SYSTEMIC

Available in: Capsules, tablets, oral suspension, injection
Available OTC? No   **As Generic?** Yes
Drug Class: Erythromycin antibiotic

▼ USAGE INFORMATION

WHY IT'S PRESCRIBED
To treat bacterial infections, including throat infections, pneumonia, Legionnaires' disease, chlamydia, and diphtheria. It is also prescribed to prevent strep infections that may damage heart valves in susceptible patients (for example, those with a history of rheumatic fever or heart valve replacement) who are allergic to penicillin.

HOW IT WORKS
Erythromycin prevents bacterial cells from manufacturing specific proteins necessary for their survival.

▼ DOSAGE GUIDELINES

RANGE AND FREQUENCY
To treat infections— Adults and teenagers: 250 to 800 mg, 2 to 4 times a day. Children: 3.4 to 12.5 mg per lb of body weight, 2 to 4 times a day. To prevent strep infections— Adults and teenagers: 1 to 1.6 g before dental appointment or surgery; 500 to 800 mg, 6 hours later. Children: 1.7 to 11.4 mg per lb of body weight before dental appointment or surgery; 4.5 mg per lb of body weight 6 hours later.

ONSET OF EFFECT
Immediate after injection; unknown for oral forms.

DURATION OF ACTION
Unknown.

DIETARY ADVICE
This drug is best taken on an empty stomach, at least 1 hour before or 2 hours after meals, with a full glass of water. If it causes stomach upset, it can be taken with food or milk.

STORAGE
Store in a tightly sealed container away from heat and direct light. Refrigerate liquid form but do not freeze.

MISSED DOSE
Take it as soon as you remember. If it is near the time for the next dose, skip the missed dose and resume your regular dosage schedule. Do not double the next dose.

STOPPING THE DRUG
Take it as prescribed for the full treatment period.

PROLONGED USE
You should see your doctor regularly for tests and examinations, including those to evaluate liver function, if this medicine is taken for a prolonged period.

▼ PRECAUTIONS

Over 60: Older patients may be at higher risk of experiencing hearing loss as a side effect.

Driving and Hazardous Work: No special warnings.

Alcohol: No special warnings.

Pregnancy: Erythromycin has been shown to cause liver damage in some pregnant women. It has not been shown to cause birth defects or other problems in babies. Before taking erythromycin, tell your doctor if you are pregnant or plan to become pregnant.

Breast Feeding: Erythromycin passes into breast milk; caution is advised. Consult your doctor for specific advice.

Infants and Children: No special problems expected.

Special Concerns: Consult your doctor if your symptoms do not improve, or instead become worse, after a few days of therapy.

OVERDOSE
Symptoms: Severe nausea, vomiting, abdominal pain, diarrhea, dizziness, loss of hearing.

What to Do: Call your doctor, emergency medical services (EMS), or the nearest poison control center immediately.

▼ INTERACTIONS

DRUG INTERACTIONS
Do not use erythromycin if you are taking astemizole or cisapride. Consult your doctor for specific advice if you are taking acetaminophen, amiodarone, anabolic steroids, androgens, antibiotics, azithromycin, carbamazepine, carmustine, chloramphenicol, chloroquine, clarithromycin, cyclosporine, dantrolene, daunorubicin, disulfiram, divalproex, estrogens, etretinate, gold salts, hydroxychloroquine, lincomycin, methotrexate, mercaptopurine, methyldopa, naltrexone, oral contraceptives, phenothiazines, phenytoin, plicamycin, theophylline, valproic acid, warfarin, tacrolimus, disopyramide, lovastatin, or bromocriptine.

FOOD INTERACTIONS
No known food interactions.

DISEASE INTERACTIONS
Use of this drug is not advised in patients with a history of heart rhythm disorders, kidney disease, liver disease, or hearing problems. Consult your doctor.

SIDE EFFECTS

SERIOUS
Fever, nausea, skin reddening or itching, severe stomach pain, yellow discoloration of the eyes or skin, fainting, slow or irregular heartbeat in patients with predisposing heart conditions, breathing difficulty, persistent or severe diarrhea, abdominal pain, temporary deafness. Also pain, swelling, or redness at injection site. Although serious side effects are rare, call your doctor immediately.

COMMON
Stomach cramps and abdominal discomfort, diarrhea, nausea, vomiting.

LESS COMMON
Soreness of mouth or tongue, vaginal itching or discharge.

ESTAZOLAM

Available in: Tablets
Available OTC? No   **As Generic?** Yes
Drug Class: Benzodiazepine tranquilizer

▼ USAGE INFORMATION

WHY IT'S PRESCRIBED
To treat insomnia.

HOW IT WORKS
In general, estazolam produces a mild sedative effect by depressing activity in the central nervous system (the brain and spinal cord). In particular, estazolam appears to enhance the effect of gamma-aminobutyric acid (GABA), a natural chemical that inhibits the firing of neurons and dampens the transmission of nerve signals, thus decreasing nervous excitation.

▼ DOSAGE GUIDELINES

RANGE AND FREQUENCY
Adults: 1 or 2 mg taken at bedtime.

ONSET OF EFFECT
Unknown.

DURATION OF ACTION
Unknown.

DIETARY ADVICE
No special restrictions.

STORAGE
Store in a tightly sealed container away from heat and direct light.

MISSED DOSE
Take it as soon as you remember, unless it is late at night. Do not take the medicine unless your schedule permits a full night's sleep.

STOPPING THE DRUG
The decision to stop taking the drug should be made in consultation with your doctor. Stopping it abruptly may cause withdrawal symptoms.

PROLONGED USE
Estazolam can lead to psychological or physical dependence. Short-term therapy (8 weeks or less) is typical; do not take it for a longer period unless so advised by your doctor. Never take more than the prescribed daily dose.

▼ PRECAUTIONS

Over 60: Adverse reactions are more likely and more severe in older patients. A lower dose may be warranted.

Driving and Hazardous Work: Estazolam can impair mental alertness and physical coordination. Adjust your activities accordingly.

Alcohol: Avoid alcohol while taking this medication.

Pregnancy: Estazolam should not be used during the first 3 months (first trimester) of pregnancy and only with great caution and close medical supervision later in pregnancy. Overuse of estazolam during pregnancy may cause drug dependence in the unborn child.

Breast Feeding: Estazolam passes into breast milk; do not take it while nursing.

Infants and Children: Safety and effectiveness have not been determined for children under age 18.

Special Concerns: Estazolam use can lead to psychological or physical dependence.

OVERDOSE
Symptoms: Extreme drowsiness, confusion, slurred speech, slow reflexes, poor coordination, staggering gait, tremor, slowed breathing, loss of consciousness.

What to Do: Call your doctor, emergency medical services (EMS), or the nearest poison control center immediately.

▼ INTERACTIONS

DRUG INTERACTIONS
Other drugs may interact with estazolam. Consult your doctor for specific advice if you are taking any drugs that depress the central nervous system; these include antihistamines, antidepressants or other psychiatric medications, barbiturates, sedatives, cough medicines, decongestants, and painkillers. Be sure your doctor knows about any over-the-counter medication you may take.

FOOD INTERACTIONS
None reported.

DISEASE INTERACTIONS
Caution is advised when taking estazolam. Consult your doctor if you have a history of alcohol or drug abuse, stroke or other brain disease, any chronic lung disease, hyperactivity, depression or other mental illness, myasthenia gravis, sleep apnea, epilepsy, porphyria, kidney disease, or liver disease.

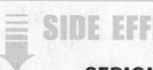

SIDE EFFECTS

SERIOUS
Difficulty concentrating, outbursts of anger, other behavior problems, depression, seizures, hallucinations, low blood pressure (causing faintness or confusion), memory impairment, muscle weakness, skin rash or itching, sore throat, fever and chills, sores or ulcers in throat or mouth, unusual bruising or bleeding, extreme fatigue, yellowish tinge to eyes or skin. Call your doctor immediately.

COMMON
Drowsiness, loss of coordination, unsteady gait, dizziness, lightheadedness, slurred speech.

LESS COMMON
Change in sexual desire or ability, constipation, false sense of well-being, nausea and vomiting, urinary problems, unusual fatigue.

ESTRADIOL

Available in: Tablets, skin patch, vaginal cream, injection
Available OTC? No   **As Generic?** Yes
Drug Class: Female sex hormone

▼ USAGE INFORMATION

WHY IT'S PRESCRIBED
To provide estrogen when the body does not produce enough; to treat carefully selected cases of advanced breast cancer; to reduce risk of osteoporosis after menopause; to ease unpleasant symptoms of menopause, including vaginal dryness; to prevent breast engorgement following childbirth; to ease symptoms of advanced prostate cancer.

HOW IT WORKS
In women, estradiol replaces deficient natural levels of estrogen in the body. In men, the hormone inhibits growth of cells in the prostate gland.

▼ DOSAGE GUIDELINES

RANGE AND FREQUENCY
To treat breast cancer: 10 mg, 3 times a day. For postmenopausal vaginal dryness or prevention of osteoporosis: 1 to 2 mg a day of oral form, or 10 to 20 mg injected every 4 weeks, or 1 Estraderm, Alora, or Vivelle patch (0.05 mg) 2 times a week or 1 Climara patch weekly. A progestin should also be taken for 10 to 14 days in each month of use, except in women who have had a hysterectomy. To relieve postmenopausal vaginal dryness using intravaginal estrogen creams: To start, ½ to 1 applicatorful daily and tapered to 1 applicatorful 1 to 3 times weekly. To treat menopausal symptoms: 1 to 5 mg injected every 3 to 4 weeks. To prevent breast engorgement after childbirth: 10 to 25 mg injected in a muscle at the time of delivery. To treat prostate cancer: 1 to 2 mg, 3 times daily.

ONSET OF EFFECT
Within 1 hour.

DURATION OF ACTION
Up to 24 hours.

DIETARY ADVICE
No special restrictions.

STORAGE
Keep in a tightly sealed container away from heat and direct light.

MISSED DOSE
Take the missed dose as soon as you remember. If it is near time for the next dose, skip the missed dose and resume your regular dosage schedule. Do not double the next dose.

STOPPING THE DRUG
The decision to stop taking the drug should be made in consultation with your doctor.

PROLONGED USE
May increase the risk of endometrial cancer and perhaps breast cancer. Consult your doctor about periodic examinations and other measures to help prevent these diseases.

▼ PRECAUTIONS

Over 60: No special problems are expected.

Driving and Hazardous Work: Do not drive or engage in hazardous work until you determine how the medicine affects you.

Alcohol: No special warnings.

Pregnancy: Not recommended during pregnancy; estrogens have been shown to cause birth defects in animals and humans.

Breast Feeding: Do not use estradiol while nursing.

Infants and Children: Not recommended for use by young patients in whom bone growth is not complete.

Special Concerns: Swelling or bleeding of gums may occur; see your dentist regularly. Do not apply a patch to the same site more than once a week.

OVERDOSE
Symptoms: Nausea, unexpected vaginal bleeding.

What to Do: An overdose is unlikely to occur. However, if someone takes a much larger dose than prescribed, seek immediate medical assistance.

▼ INTERACTIONS

DRUG INTERACTIONS
Consult your doctor for specific advice if you are taking acetaminophen, amiodarone, anticonvulsants, anti-infective drugs, antithyroid agents, carmustine, chloroquine, dantrolene, daunorubicin, gold salts, divalproex, etretinate, hydroxychloroquine, mercaptopurine, methotrexate, oral contraceptives, methyldopa, naltrexone, phenothiazines, plicamycin, steroids, bromocriptine or cyclosporine.

FOOD INTERACTIONS
No known food interactions.

DISEASE INTERACTIONS
You should not take estradiol if you have blood clot disorders, breast cancer, any hormone-dependent cancer, or abnormal genital bleeding.

⩵ SIDE EFFECTS ⩵

SERIOUS
For men being treated for prostate cancer: Sudden or severe headache; loss of coordination; sudden changes in vision; pains in chest, groin, or leg; shortness of breath; slurring of speech; weakness or numbness in arm or leg. For women: Breast pain or enlargement, swelling of legs and feet, rapid weight gain. Call your doctor immediately.

COMMON
Abdominal bloating, stomach cramps, loss of appetite, skin irritation at site of patch.

LESS COMMON
Diarrhea, dizziness, headaches, discomfort when wearing contact lenses, decreased sexual desire in men, increased sexual desire in women, vomiting.

ESTRAMUSTINE PHOSPHATE SODIUM

BRAND NAME

Emcyt

Available in: Capsules
Available OTC? No   **As Generic?** No
Drug Class: Antineoplastic (anticancer) agent

▼ USAGE INFORMATION

WHY IT'S PRESCRIBED
To treat some types of prostate cancer.

HOW IT WORKS
Estramustine is a combination of two drugs: a form of estrogen (estradiol) and mechlorethamine (nitrogen mustard). It is uncertain precisely how the drug works, but it appears to kill cancer cells by interfering with the synthesis of their genetic material and blocking the activity of hormones and proteins that certain types of prostate tumors need in order to grow.

▼ DOSAGE GUIDELINES

RANGE AND FREQUENCY
10 to 16 mg per 2.2 lbs (1 kg) of body weight daily in 3 or 4 doses.

ONSET OF EFFECT
Unknown.

DURATION OF ACTION
Unknown.

DIETARY ADVICE
Best taken with water 1 hour before or 2 hours after meals. Milk, milk products, or calcium-rich foods should not be taken simultaneously.

STORAGE
Store in a tightly sealed container away from heat and direct light.

MISSED DOSE
Take it as soon as you remember. If it is near the time for the next dose, skip the missed dose and resume your regular dosage schedule. Do not double the next dose.

STOPPING THE DRUG
The decision to stop taking the drug should be made in consultation with your doctor.

PROLONGED USE
You should see your doctor regularly for tests and examinations if you take this drug for a prolonged period.

▼ PRECAUTIONS

Over 60: Side effects tend to occur more commonly in patients over 60.

Driving and Hazardous Work: Do not drive or engage in hazardous work until you determine how the medicine affects you.

Alcohol: Avoid alcohol while taking this drug.

Pregnancy: Estramustine can cause birth defects if the father is taking it at the time of conception. Before taking estramustine, tell your doctor if you intend to have children; while taking it, a reliable barrier method of birth control is advised.

Breast Feeding: Not applicable for this drug.

Infants and Children: Estramustine is not intended for use in infants and children.

Special Concerns: If you vomit shortly after taking a dose of estramustine, ask your doctor if you should take the dose again or wait for the next scheduled dose. During and after treatment with estramustine, do not get immunized against bacteria or viruses without your doctor's approval. Avoid persons who have recently taken oral polio vaccine. If you must be close to them, consider wearing a protective mask that covers both the nose and mouth.

▼ OVERDOSE

Symptoms: Severe and exaggerated side effects (see Side Effects).

What to Do: Call your doctor, emergency medical services (EMS), or the nearest poison control center immediately.

▼ INTERACTIONS

DRUG INTERACTIONS
Consult your doctor for specific advice if you are taking acetaminophen, amiodarone, anabolic steroids, androgens, antibiotics, antithyroid agents, carbamazepine, carmustine, chloroquine, dantrolene, disulfiram, divalproex, estrogens, etretinate, gold salts, hydrochloroquine, mercaptopurine, methyldopa, naltrexone, phenothiazines, phenytoin, plicamycin, or valproic acid.

FOOD INTERACTIONS
See dietary advice.

DISEASE INTERACTIONS
Caution is advised when taking estramustine. Consult your doctor if you have: asthma, epilepsy, mental depression, migraine headaches, kidney disease, history of blood clots, history of stroke, a recent heart attack, shingles, diabetes, gallbladder disease, heart or blood vessel disease, liver disease, or a stomach ulcer.

 SIDE EFFECTS

SERIOUS
Black, tarry stools; blood in urine or stools; cough or hoarseness; fever or chills; severe or sudden headaches; sudden loss of coordination; pain in lower back or side; pain in chest, groin, or leg; painful urination; red spots on skin; sudden shortness of breath; sudden slurred speech; unusual bleeding or bruising; sudden changes in vision; weakness or numbness in arm or leg; skin rash; or fever. Call your doctor or emergency medical services (EMS) immediately.

COMMON
Breast tenderness or enlargement, swelling of feet or lower legs, decreased sexual desire, diarrhea, nausea, general weakness.

LESS COMMON
Insomnia, vomiting.

ESTROGENS, CONJUGATED

Available in: Tablets, injection, vaginal cream
Available OTC? No   **As Generic?** Yes
Drug Class: Female sex hormone

▼ USAGE INFORMATION

WHY IT'S PRESCRIBED
To provide estrogen after the menopause, when the body produces too little; to treat carefully selected cases of advanced breast cancer; to reduce risk of osteoporosis after meno-pause; to ease unpleasant symptoms of menopause, including vaginal dryness; to prevent breast engorgement following child-birth; or to ease symptoms of advanced prostate cancer.

HOW IT WORKS
In women, conjugated estrogens replace deficient natural levels of estrogen in the body. In men, estrogens inhibit growth of cells in the prostate gland.

▼ DOSAGE GUIDELINES

RANGE AND FREQUENCY
Usual adult dose is taken in cycles, with no dosing on certain days of the month. Women must also take a progestin 10 to 14 days in each month of use, except those who have had a hysterectomy (these women may take estrogen daily). To treat breast cancer in men or post-menopausal women: 10 mg, 3 times a day for 3 months or more. To prevent bone loss from osteoporosis: 0.3 to 1.25 mg a day. To ease symptoms of menopause: 0.625 to 1.25 mg a day. To treat prostate cancer: 1.25 to 2.5 mg a day.

ONSET OF EFFECT
Unknown.

DURATION OF ACTION
Unknown.

DIETARY ADVICE
Conjugated estrogens may be taken with food to reduce stomach upset.

STORAGE
Store in a tightly sealed container away from heat, moisture, and direct light. Keep it away from extremes in temperature. Keep the liquid form refrigerated, but do not allow it to freeze.

MISSED DOSE
Take it as soon as you remember. If it is near the time for the next dose, skip the missed dose and resume your regular dosage schedule. Do not double the next dose.

STOPPING THE DRUG
The decision to stop taking the drug should be made by your doctor.

PROLONGED USE
Prolonged use of estrogens has been reported to increase the risk of endometrial cancer and perhaps of breast cancer. Consult your doctor about the need for periodic examinations and other measures to screen for these diseases.

▼ PRECAUTIONS

Over 60: No special problems are expected.

Driving and Hazardous Work: Use of this hormone should not impair your ability to perform such tasks safely.

Alcohol: No special warnings.

Pregnancy: Do not use if you are pregnant. Estrogen use in pregnant women has been associated with birth defects.

Breast Feeding: Talk to your doctor about whether the benefits of the therapy outweigh the potential harm to the nursing infant.

Infants and Children: Should be used with caution by children, as the drug may interfere with bone growth.

OVERDOSE
Symptoms: Nausea, unexpected vaginal bleeding.

What to Do: An overdose of estrogen is unlikely to be life-threatening. However, if someone takes a much larger dose than prescribed, call your doctor, emergency medical services (EMS), or the nearest poison control center immediately.

▼ INTERACTIONS

DRUG INTERACTIONS
Other drugs may interact with estrogens. Consult your doctor if you are taking anticoagulants, anticonvulsants, antidiabetic drugs, thyroid hormones, tricyclic antidepressants, barbiturates, tranquilizers, cyclo-sporine, corticosteroids, corticotropin, tamoxifen, rifampin, carbamazepine, or bromocriptine.

FOOD INTERACTIONS
Calcium supplements used with estrogen may increase calcium absorption. Vitamin C may increase the effects of estrogen.

DISEASE INTERACTIONS
You should not take conjugated estrogens if you have thrombophlebitis, thromboembolitis, breast cancer, any hormone-dependent cancer, or abnormal genital bleeding. Consult your doctor if you have any of the following: a history of liver disease, heart attack, stroke, a blood clotting disorder, gallbladder disease or gallstones, or if you smoke tobacco heavily.

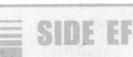
SIDE EFFECTS

SERIOUS
Women: Breast pain or enlargement, swelling of legs and feet, rapid weight gain. Men being treated for prostate cancer: Sudden or severe headache; loss of coordination; sudden changes in vision; pains in chest, groin, or leg; sudden shortness of breath; slurred speech; weakness or numbness in arm or leg. Call your doctor immediately.

COMMON
Abdominal bloating or cramps, loss of appetite, breast tenderness.

LESS COMMON
Diarrhea, dizziness, headaches, discomfort when wearing contact lenses, decreased sexual desire in men, increased sexual desire in women, vomiting.

ESTROGENS, CONJUGATED/MEDROXYPROGESTERONE ACETATE

Available in: Tablets
Available OTC? No   **As Generic?** No
Drug Class: Female sex hormones

▼ USAGE INFORMATION

WHY IT'S PRESCRIBED
To provide estrogen after the menopause, when the body produces too little; to reduce the risk of osteoporosis; to ease unpleasant symptoms of menopause, including hot flashes and vaginal dryness; and to treat atrophy (wasting) of the vulva or vagina. Estrogen also protects women against coronary artery disease.

HOW IT WORKS
Estrogen protects against osteoporosis by diminishing the loss of bone that results from estrogen deficiency. Conjugated estrogens replace deficient levels of natural estrogen in women. When given alone to menopausal women, estrogen increases the risk of excessive growth of the uterine lining, which can lead to endometrial cancer. Medroxyprogesterone (a type of progestin) given in conjunction with estrogen nearly eliminates this risk.

▼ DOSAGE GUIDELINES

RANGE AND FREQUENCY
1 tablet, taken once a day. Prempro contains 0.625 mg of estrogen (Premarin) and 2.5 mg of medroxyprogesterone (MPA). Premphase contains 0.625 mg Premarin and 5 mg of MPA.

ONSET OF EFFECT
Unknown.

DURATION OF ACTION
As long as the product is taken.

DIETARY ADVICE
Take it with food to reduce stomach upset.

STORAGE
Store in a tightly sealed container away from heat, moisture, and direct light.

MISSED DOSE
If you miss a dose on one day, do not double the dose the next day. Resume your regular dosage schedule.

≡ SIDE EFFECTS ≡

SERIOUS
The most serious side effect is a modest increase in the incidence of breast cancer among women taking estrogen, especially for a long time (10 years or longer). Other side effects requiring your doctor's attention include swelling of legs and feet, rapid weight gain, abnormal menstrual bleeding, mental depression, and skin rash.

COMMON
Nausea, breast tenderness, headache, abdominal pain.

LESS COMMON
Change in appetite, vomiting, stomach cramps or bloating, change in blood pressure, dizziness, nervousness, insomnia, sleepiness, increase or decrease in weight, fatigue, backache.

STOPPING THE DRUG
The decision to stop taking this hormone combination should be made in consultation with your doctor.

PROLONGED USE
You should be reevaluated at 3-month to 6-month intervals by your doctor to determine whether or not continued treatment is necessary.

▼ PRECAUTIONS

Over 60: No special problems are expected.

Driving and Hazardous Work: Use of this hormone combination should not impair your ability to perform such tasks safely.

Alcohol: No special warnings.

Pregnancy: Do not use this hormone combination if you are or are planning to become pregnant. Estrogen use in pregnant women has been associated with birth defects.

Breast Feeding: Do not use this hormone combination if you are nursing.

Infants and Children: Not recommended for use by children.

Special Concerns: When this hormone combination is being used in the management or prevention of osteoporosis, regular weight-bearing exercise and good nutrition are important.

OVERDOSE
Symptoms: No serious ill effects have been reported following an overdose. However, nausea, vomiting, and withdrawal bleeding may occur when extremely large doses are ingested.

What to Do: An overdose is unlikely. However, if someone takes a much larger dose than prescribed, seek medical attention.

▼ INTERACTIONS

DRUG INTERACTIONS
Other drugs may interact with this hormone combination. Consult your doctor if you are taking anticoagulants, anticonvulsants, antidiabetic drugs, thyroid hormones, tricyclic antidepressants, barbiturates, tranquilizers, cyclosporine, corticosteroids, corticotropin, tamoxifen, rifampin, carbamazepine, or bromocriptine.

FOOD INTERACTIONS
Estrogen may increase calcium absorption from calcium supplements. Vitamin C may increase the effects of estrogen.

DISEASE INTERACTIONS
You should not take this hormone combination if you have thrombophlebitis, breast cancer, any hormone-dependent cancer, or abnormal vaginal bleeding. Consult your doctor if you have a history of any of the following: liver disease, heart attack, diabetes mellitus, stroke, a blood clotting disorder, thromboembolic disease, gallbladder disease or gallstones, liver disease, or if you smoke cigarettes heavily.

ESTROPIPATE

BRAND NAMES

Ogen, Ortho-Est

Available in: Tablets, vaginal cream
Available OTC? No   **As Generic?** Yes
Drug Class: Female sex hormone

▼ USAGE INFORMATION

WHY IT'S PRESCRIBED
To provide estrogen when the body does not produce enough; to treat selected cases of advanced breast cancer; to reduce risk of osteoporosis after menopause; to ease unpleasant symptoms of menopause, including vaginal dryness; to ease symptoms of advanced prostate cancer.

HOW IT WORKS
In women, estropipate replaces deficient natural levels of estrogen in the body. In men, it inhibits the growth of cells in the prostate gland.

▼ DOSAGE GUIDELINES

RANGE AND FREQUENCY
For vaginal skin conditions: 0.625 to 5 mg a day of oral form or 2 to 4 grams a day of vaginal cream. For treating menopausal symptoms: 1.25 to 2.5 mg a day of oral form, 3 weeks on, 1 week off. To prevent osteoporosis: 0.625 mg of oral form daily for 25 days of a 31-day cycle. A progestin must also be taken for 10 to 14 days in each

month of use, except in women who have had a hysterectomy.

ONSET OF EFFECT
Within 1 hour.

DURATION OF ACTION
Up to 24 hours.

DIETARY ADVICE
This medicine can be taken without regard to meals.

STORAGE
Keep in a tightly sealed container away from heat and direct light.

MISSED DOSE
Take the missed dose as soon as you remember. If it is near time for the next dose, skip the missed dose and resume your regular dosage schedule. Do not double the next dose.

STOPPING THE DRUG
The decision to stop taking the drug should be made by your doctor.

PROLONGED USE
Prolonged use of estrogens has been reported to increase the risk of endometrial cancer and perhaps breast cancer.

Endometrial cancer is largely prevented by using estropipate in sequence with a progestin. Consult your doctor about the need for periodic examinations and other measures to help detect and prevent these diseases.

▼ PRECAUTIONS

Over 60: No special problems are expected.

Driving and Hazardous Work: Do not drive or engage in hazardous work until you determine how the medicine affects you.

Alcohol: No special warnings.

Pregnancy: Estrogens have been shown to cause birth defects in humans. Before taking estropipate, be sure to tell your doctor if you are pregnant or plan to become pregnant.

Breast Feeding: Estropipate passes into breast milk; avoid using it while nursing.

Infants and Children: This medicine is not recommended for use by children in whom bone growth is not complete.

Special Concerns: Swelling or bleeding of the gums may occur. See your dentist regularly. You should have a Pap test every 6 to 12 months while taking estropipate. Avoid excessive exposure to sunlight until you determine how the drug affects you.

OVERDOSE
Symptoms: Nausea, unexpected vaginal bleeding.

What to Do: An overdose of estropipate is unlikely to be life-threatening. However, if someone takes a much larger dose than prescribed, call your doctor, emergency medical services (EMS), or the nearest poison control center.

▼ INTERACTIONS

DRUG INTERACTIONS
Consult your doctor for specific advice if you are taking acetaminophen, amiodarone, anabolic steroids, androgens, anti-infective drugs, antithyroid agents, bromocriptine, carbamazepine, carmustine, chloroquine, cyclosporine, dantrolene, daunorubicin, disulfiram, divalproex, etretinate, gold salts, hydroxychloroquine, mercaptopurine, methotrexate, methyldopa, naltrexone, oral contraceptives, phenothiazines, phenytoin, plicamycin, or valproic acid.

FOOD INTERACTIONS
No known food interactions.

DISEASE INTERACTIONS
You should not take estropipate if you have thrombophlebitis, thromboembolitis, a history of breast cancer, any hormone-dependent cancer, or abnormal genital bleeding.

 SIDE EFFECTS

SERIOUS
Breast pain or enlargement, swelling of legs and feet, rapid weight gain. Call your doctor immediately.

COMMON
Stomach bloating, lower abdominal cramps, loss of appetite.

LESS COMMON
Diarrhea, dizziness, headaches, discomfort when wearing contact lenses, increased sexual desire in women, vomiting, unusual sensitivity to sunlight.

ETANERCEPT

Available in: Injection
Available OTC? No   **As Generic?** No
Drug Class: Biologic response modifier

▼ USAGE INFORMATION

WHY IT'S PRESCRIBED
To reduce the signs and symptoms of moderate to severe active rheumatoid arthritis. Etanercept is prescribed for patients who have not responded adequately to one or more antirheumatic drugs. It may also be used in combination with methotrexate in patients who have not responded adequately to methotrexate alone.

HOW IT WORKS
Etanercept works by binding with tumor necrosis factor (TNF), a key protein involved in the inflammatory process. Etanercept reduces inflammation by blocking the interaction of TNF with its receptors on cells.

▼ DOSAGE GUIDELINES

RANGE AND FREQUENCY
Adults: 25 mg, twice a week as a subcutaneous (under the skin) injection. Children: See your pediatrician for the appropriate dosage.

ONSET OF EFFECT
Within 1 to 2 weeks.

DURATION OF ACTION
As long as the drug is taken, but studies have only lasted for 6 months.

DIETARY ADVICE
May be taken without regard to diet.

STORAGE
Keep etanercept refrigerated, but do not allow it to freeze. If not administered immediately after preparing (reconstituting), etanercept may be stored in the vial in the refrigerator for up to 6 hours.

MISSED DOSE
Take it as soon as you remember. If it is near the time for the next dose, skip the missed dose and resume your regular dosage schedule. Do not double the next dose.

STOPPING THE DRUG
The decision to stop taking the medication should be made in consultation with your doctor.

PROLONGED USE
No special problems are expected.

▼ PRECAUTIONS

Over 60: No special problems are expected.

Driving and Hazardous Work: The use of etanercept should not impair your ability to perform such tasks safely.

Alcohol: Alcohol may accentuate the side effect of dizziness.

Pregnancy: Adequate human studies have not been done. Before taking etanercept, tell your doctor if you are pregnant or plan to become pregnant.

Breast Feeding: Etanercept may pass into breast milk; caution is advised. Consult your doctor for advice on whether to discontinue nursing or discontinue the drug.

Infants and Children: Not recommended for use by children under age 4.

Special Concerns: Your doctor should instruct you on how to prepare and administer the injection of etanercept before you attempt to do it yourself. Follow your doctor's instructions about selecting and rotating injection sites. Sites for self-injection are the arms, stomach, and thighs. The first injection should be administered under the supervision of your doctor. Other antirheumatic medications may be continued during treatment with etanercept. Consult your doctor for advice.

OVERDOSE
Symptoms: No cases of overdose have been reported.

What to Do: An overdose with etanercept is unlikely. If someone takes a much larger dose than prescribed, call your doctor.

▼ INTERACTIONS

DRUG INTERACTIONS
Avoid live-virus vaccines. No other medications should be added to solutions containing etanercept. Adequate studies involving interactions with other drugs have not been done. Consult your doctor for specific advice.

FOOD INTERACTIONS
No known food interactions.

DISEASE INTERACTIONS
Etanercept should be used with caution in patients with any active infection, including chronic or localized infections, or who are immunosuppressed.

  SIDE EFFECTS

SERIOUS
There are no serious side effects associated with the use of etanercept.

COMMON
Itching, redness, pain, or swelling at the site of injection; upper respiratory infection.

LESS COMMON
Headache, nasal congestion, dizziness, sore throat, cough, general weakness, abdominal discomfort, rash, runny nose.

ETHACRYNIC ACID (ETHACRYNATE)

BRAND NAMES
Edecrin, Edecrin Sodium

Available in: Tablets, injection
Available OTC? No   **As Generic?** No
Drug Class: Loop diuretic

▼ USAGE INFORMATION

WHY IT'S PRESCRIBED
To reduce fluid (salt and water) accumulation that leads to edema (swelling) and breathlessness in patients who have heart disease, cirrhosis of the liver, and kidney disease.

HOW IT WORKS
Loop diuretics work on a specific portion of the kidney (the loop of Henle) to increase the excretion of water and salts (including potassium) in urine.

▼ DOSAGE GUIDELINES

RANGE AND FREQUENCY
Adults— Ethacrynic acid (oral dose): 50 to 200 mg a day. Ethacrynate sodium (injection): 50 mg injected into a vein every 2 to 6 hours as needed.

ONSET OF EFFECT
Within 30 minutes after an oral dose; within 5 minutes after intravenous injection.

DURATION OF ACTION
Oral dose lasts 6 to 8 hours; intravenous, 2 hours.

DIETARY ADVICE
Ethacrynic acid may cause depletion of potassium; your doctor may want you to eat high-potassium foods (such as bananas, tomatoes, and citrus fruits) or take potassium supplements. Take the drug with food or milk to minimize stomach upset.

STORAGE
Store in a tightly sealed container away from heat, moisture, and direct light.

MISSED DOSE
Take it as soon as you remember. If it is near the time for the next dose, skip the missed dose and resume your regular dosage schedule. Do not double the next dose.

STOPPING THE DRUG
Take it as prescribed for the full treatment period, even if you begin to feel better before the scheduled end of therapy.

PROLONGED USE
Your doctor will schedule regular checkups to determine the medication's effect on your body, and adjust the dosage and dosing frequency. After a maintenance dose is established, diuretic therapy may continue for intermittent periods alternating with periods not using the drug.

▼ PRECAUTIONS

Over 60: No special precautions are warranted.

Driving and Hazardous Work: No special precautions are warranted.

Alcohol: Alcohol should be avoided or used with caution because it may increase the effect of antihypertensive drugs and cause an excessive drop in blood pressure.

Pregnancy: This drug is not usually prescribed during pregnancy. Other diuretics are preferred.

Breast Feeding: It is not known whether the drug is excreted in milk; consult your doctor for specific advice.

Infants and Children: Although ethacrynic acid is rarely prescribed for children, no unusual side effects are expected. The dose must be determined by a pediatrician.

Special Concerns: To prevent sleep disruption, avoid taking this medicine in the evening. You may be advised to increase potassium in your diet or take a potassium supplement while taking a diuretic.

OVERDOSE
Symptoms: Weakness, lethargy, dizziness, nausea, vomiting, leg muscle cramps.

What to Do: Call your doctor, emergency medical services (EMS), or the nearest poison control center immediately.

▼ INTERACTIONS

DRUG INTERACTIONS
Consult your doctor if you are taking any of the following: ACE inhibitors, aminoglycosides, cisplatin, digitalis drugs, lithium, nonsteroidal anti-inflammatory drugs, salicylates, or thiazide diuretics.

FOOD INTERACTIONS
No known food interactions.

DISEASE INTERACTIONS
Consult your doctor if you have any of the following conditions: diabetes, gout, hearing problems, pancreatitis, recent heart attack, kidney or liver disease, or lupus.

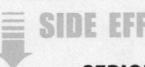

SIDE EFFECTS

SERIOUS
Mood or mental changes, nausea or vomiting, unusual fatigue, black and tarry stools, skin rash. Call your doctor immediately.

COMMON
Muscle cramps or pain. Potassium depletion may lead to heart palpitations and weakness. Fluid depletion may lead to thirst, dry mouth, constipation, and dizziness, especially upon arising from a sitting or lying position.

LESS COMMON
Buzzing or ringing in ears, loss of hearing (particularly after intravenous treatment), diarrhea, loss of appetite, gout, increased blood sugar (a problem for diabetic patients).

ETHCHLORVYNOL

BRAND NAME

Placidyl

Available in: Capsules
Available OTC? No **As Generic?** Yes
Drug Class: Sedative

▼ USAGE INFORMATION

WHY IT'S PRESCRIBED
Used as short-term therapy for insomnia; however, other medications are generally preferred.

HOW IT WORKS
The exact mechanism of action is unknown; ethchlorvynol appears to depress the central nervous system in a manner similar to that of barbiturates.

▼ DOSAGE GUIDELINES

RANGE AND FREQUENCY
Adults: 500 to 1,000 mg at bedtime.

ONSET OF EFFECT
30 to 60 minutes.

DURATION OF ACTION
5 hours.

DIETARY ADVICE
Take ethchlorvynol with milk or food to minimize temporary dizziness or unsteadiness that may result from the body's rapid absorption of the medication.

STORAGE
Store in a tightly sealed container away from heat, moisture, and direct light.

MISSED DOSE
Ethchlorvynol is generally prescribed for once-daily use at bedtime. If you are unable to take it on a particular night, resume your regular scheduled dose the following night.

STOPPING THE DRUG
The decision to stop taking the drug should be made in consultation with your doctor. Generally, therapy lasts no more than 1 week.

PROLONGED USE
Ethchlorvynol should not be prescribed for a period exceeding 1 week, as the body will build up tolerance to the drug, and physical and psychological dependence may develop. Patients abruptly stopping the drug after prolonged use may experience withdrawal symptoms (seizures, delirium, perceptual distortions, agitation, tremors) as late as 9 days after ending therapy. A gradual, progressive reduction of dosage over a period of days or weeks is recommended for patients who have become dependent on ethchlorvynol.

▼ PRECAUTIONS

Over 60: Older patients may be more sensitive to the effects of ethchlorvynol and so should take the smallest effective dose.

Driving and Hazardous Work: The use of this drug may impair your ability to perform such tasks safely.

Alcohol: Avoid alcohol.

Pregnancy: Ethchlorvynol should not be used during the first 2 trimesters (6 months) of pregnancy. Discuss with your doctor the relative risks and benefits of using this drug during the final 3 months (third trimester) of pregnancy.

Breast Feeding: Ethchlorvynol may pass into breast milk. Consult your doctor for specific advice.

Infants and Children: Not recommended for persons under the age of 18.

Special Concerns: Ethchlorvynol may become habit forming. Use only as directed by your doctor. Never take more than the prescribed dose and do not use the drug for a longer period than prescribed.

OVERDOSE
Symptoms: Severe nausea, vomiting, or stomach pain; difficulty swallowing; severe drowsiness; continuing confusion; seizures; low body temperature; difficulty breathing or shortness of breath; irregular heartbeat; severe weakness; staggering; slurred speech.

What to Do: Call your doctor, emergency medical services (EMS), or the nearest poison control center immediately.

▼ INTERACTIONS

DRUG INTERACTIONS
Consult your doctor for specific advice if you are taking barbiturates or other central nervous system depressants, tricyclic antidepressants, MAO inhibitors, or anticoagulants.

FOOD INTERACTIONS
No known food interactions.

DISEASE INTERACTIONS
Your physician should know if you have any of the following conditions: impaired kidney or liver function, a history of alcohol or drug abuse, mental depression, or porphyria.

 SIDE EFFECTS

SERIOUS
Unusual bleeding or bruising; unusual excitement, nervousness, or restlessness; skin rash or hives; yellowish tinge to eyes or skin (jaundice); itching; darkening of urine; pale stools. Call your doctor immediately.

COMMON
Blurred vision, nausea or vomiting, indigestion, bitter or unusual aftertaste, numbness in the face, abdominal pain, dizziness or lightheadedness, unusual fatigue or weakness.

LESS COMMON
Unsteady gait or loss of coordination, confusion, daytime sleepiness. Check with your doctor promptly if such symptoms persist.

ETHINYL ESTRADIOL

Available in: Tablets
Available OTC? No **As Generic?** Yes
Drug Class: Anticancer estrogen

▼ USAGE INFORMATION

WHY IT'S PRESCRIBED
To provide estrogen when the body does not produce enough (hypogonadism); to treat carefully selected cases of advanced breast cancer; to reduce risk of osteoporosis after menopause; to ease unpleasant symptoms of menopause, including vaginal dryness; to ease symptoms of advanced prostate cancer.

HOW IT WORKS
In women, ethinyl estradiol replaces deficient natural levels of estrogen in the body. In men, it inhibits the growth of cells in the prostate gland.

▼ DOSAGE GUIDELINES

RANGE AND FREQUENCY
For female hypogonadism: 0.05 mg, 1 to 3 times a day for 25 days per month (in conjunction with 10 to 14 days of a progestin, except in women who have had a hysterectomy), for 3 to 6 months. For breast cancer: 1 mg, 3 times a day. For menopausal symptoms: 0.02 to 0.05 mg a day. For prostate cancer: 0.15 to 2 mg a day.

ONSET OF EFFECT
Within 8 hours.

DURATION OF ACTION
Up to 24 hours.

DIETARY ADVICE
This drug can be taken with or immediately after meals to reduce nausea.

STORAGE
Store in a tightly sealed container away from heat and direct light.

MISSED DOSE
Take it as soon as you remember. However, if it is near the time for the next dose, skip the missed dose and resume your regular dosage schedule. Do not double the next dose.

STOPPING THE DRUG
The decision to stop taking the drug should be made by your doctor.

SIDE EFFECTS

SERIOUS
Breast pain or enlargement; swelling of feet and lower legs; rapid weight gain; changes in vaginal bleeding; lumps in or discharge from the breast; visual disturbances; sharp pains in stomach, side, or abdomen; uncontrolled muscle movements; yellowish tinge of eyes or skin (jaundice). Call your doctor immediately.

COMMON
Stomach bloating, lower abdominal cramping and discomfort, loss of appetite.

LESS COMMON
Dizziness, diarrhea, headaches, unusual increase in sexual desire, vomiting, problems with contact lenses.

PROLONGED USE
Women who take ethinyl estradiol for more than 5 years to treat menopausal symptoms may be at increased risk for endometrial cancer. Consult your doctor about the need for discontinuing the drug temporarily. Although the drug may cause menstrual bleeding, it does not restore fertility.

▼ PRECAUTIONS

Over 60: No special problems are expected.

Driving and Hazardous Work: The use of ethinyl estradiol may impair your ability to perform such tasks safely. Do not drive or engage in hazardous work until you determine how the medication affects you.

Alcohol: No special precautions are necessary.

Pregnancy: Drugs of this class have caused serious birth defects in animals and humans. Ethinyl estradiol should not be taken if you are pregnant or are planning to become pregnant.

Breast Feeding: Ethinyl estradiol passes into breast milk; avoid or discontinue use while nursing.

Infants and Children: Not recommended for use by children and adolescents whose bone growth is not complete.

Special Concerns: Ethinyl estradiol may cause dental bleeding and excessive gingival (gum) growth. See your dentist regularly. Nausea may occur in the first weeks after you start taking this drug.

OVERDOSE
Symptoms: Nausea and abnormal vaginal bleeding.

What to Do: An overdose of ethinyl estradiol is unlikely to be life-threatening. However, if someone takes a much larger dose than prescribed, call your doctor, emergency medical services (EMS), or local poison control center.

▼ INTERACTIONS

DRUG INTERACTIONS
Consult your doctor for specific advice if you are taking acetaminophen, amiodarone, anabolic steroids, androgens, anti-infectives, antithyroid drugs, carbamazepine, carmustine, chloroquine, dantrolene, daunorubicin, disulfiram, divalproex, etretinate, gold salts, hydroxychloroquine, mercaptopurine, naltrexone, oral contraceptives, phenothiazines, phenytoin, valproic acid, bromocriptine, or cyclosporine.

FOOD INTERACTIONS
No known food interactions.

DISEASE INTERACTIONS
Caution is advised when taking ethinyl estradiol. Consult your doctor if you have any of the following: a history of blood clots while taking estrogens, breast cancer, endometriosis, fibroid tumors of the uterus, gallbladder disease or gallstones, jaundice, liver disease, or porphyria.

ETHOSUXIMIDE

Available in: Capsules, syrup
Available OTC? No   **As Generic?** Yes
Drug Class: Anticonvulsant/succinimide

▼ USAGE INFORMATION

WHY IT'S PRESCRIBED
To control seizures in patients with certain types of epilepsy.

HOW IT WORKS
Ethosuximide acts on the central nervous system to control the number and severity of seizures. It is thought to depress the activity of certain parts of the brain and suppress the abnormal transmission of nerve impulses that causes absence seizures.

▼ DOSAGE GUIDELINES

RANGE AND FREQUENCY
Adults: 750 to 1,500 mg a day, in 2 divided doses. A higher dose may be required. Children: 4 to 5 mg a day, in 2 divided doses. A low dose is used to start, and is gradually increased by your doctor.

ONSET OF EFFECT
Several hours.

DURATION OF ACTION
The drug is most effective for 24 hours or longer. After this time, effectiveness gradually decreases.

DIETARY ADVICE
Take it with food to minimize the risk of stomach upset.

STORAGE
Store in a tightly sealed container away from heat and direct light. Do not refrigerate or freeze the syrup.

MISSED DOSE
Take it as soon as you remember, unless your next scheduled dose is within the next 4 hours. If so, skip the missed dose. Take your next dose at the proper time, and resume your regular dosage schedule. Do not double the next dose, unless advised to do so by your doctor.

STOPPING THE DRUG
The decision to stop taking the drug should be made by your doctor. Ethosuximide should never be stopped abruptly, since this may cause seizures. The dose is typically tapered over a period of weeks to months.

PROLONGED USE
Ethosuximide can be taken on a long-term basis. Some side effects that are prominent in the first few weeks of therapy usually diminish over time.

▼ PRECAUTIONS

Over 60: Older patients may require lower doses to minimize side effects.

Driving and Hazardous Work: Ethosuximide may cause drowsiness and impair your ability to perform such tasks safely. Do not drive or engage in hazardous work until you determine how the medicine affects you.

Alcohol: May contribute to excessive drowsiness.

Pregnancy: Use of anticonvulsants is associated with an increased risk of birth defects, although studies with ethosuximide are incomplete. However, seizures during pregnancy can also increase risks to the fetus. Discuss with your doctor the potential risks and benefits of using this drug during pregnancy. Folate supplementation is recommended 1 to 2 months prior to conception, and continuing throughout pregnancy.

Breast Feeding: Ethosuximide passes into breast milk, although at low levels. Consult your doctor for advice if you are breast feeding.

Infants and Children: No special problems are expected.

Special Concerns: The generic form is not recommended. Your doctor may want you to wear a medical bracelet or carry an identification card saying that you are taking this drug.

OVERDOSE
Symptoms: Severe nausea and vomiting, difficulty breathing, severe drowsiness, coma.

What to Do: Call your doctor, emergency medical services (EMS), or the nearest poison control center immediately.

▼ INTERACTIONS

DRUG INTERACTIONS
Ethosuximide may be affected by other drugs or alter the blood levels of other medications, including other anticonvulsants (carbamazepine, phenacemide, phenobarbital, phenytoin, primidone, valproic acid) and certain psychiatric drugs (tricyclic antidepressants, MAO inhibitors, haloperidol).

FOOD INTERACTIONS
No known food interactions.

DISEASE INTERACTIONS
Special caution is advised if you have liver disease, kidney disease, a blood disorder, or intermittent porphyria.

≡ SIDE EFFECTS ≡

SERIOUS
Sore throat, fever, swollen glands, red or purple pointlike rash on the skin or mucous membranes, blistering or peeling skin lesions, mouth sores, easy bruising, paleness, weakness, confusion, lethargy, muscle pain, or seizures may be a sign of a potentially fatal blood reaction or other complication. Call your doctor immediately.

COMMON
Nausea and vomiting, loss of appetite, stomach upset, gastrointestinal cramps, weight loss, diarrhea, sedation, mild sensory nerve impairment.

LESS COMMON
Irritability, headache, dizziness, sleep disturbances. There are numerous additional side effects associated with the use of this drug; consult your physician if you are concerned about any adverse or unusual reactions.

ETIDRONATE DISODIUM

Available in: Tablets, injection
Available OTC? No   **As Generic?** No
Drug Class: Bisphosphonate inhibitor of bone resorption

▼ USAGE INFORMATION

WHY IT'S PRESCRIBED
To treat Paget's disease, a disorder characterized by rapid breakdown and reformation of bone, which can lead to fragility and malformation of bones. May also be used to treat elevated blood levels of calcium (hypercalcemia) caused by cancer; to treat and prevent calcium and bone deposits around artificial joint replacements (especially hip replacements) or around an area of spinal cord injury. Etidronate is also commonly used to treat postmenopausal osteoporosis.

HOW IT WORKS
Etidronate slows bone resorption (the speed at which bone is broken down before it is replaced), promoting the formation of healthy bone. It prevents the bone pain, deformity, and fractures associated with Paget's disease. In cancer-related hypercalcemia, this drug slows bone resorption and thus the flow of calcium from bone into the blood. It slows the progression of abnormal bone deposition after hip replacement and spinal cord injury. In osteoporosis, it helps to slow the breakdown of bone tissue.

▼ DOSAGE GUIDELINES

RANGE AND FREQUENCY
Usual adult oral dosage for Paget's disease: 2.3 mg per lb of body weight per day, or 2.7 to 4.6 mg per lb, in alternating 6 month courses of treatment and abstention. For hypercalcemia related to cancer: 9 mg per lb of body weight for 30 to 90 days. For prevention of calcium deposits, with hip replacement: 9 mg per lb for 1 month before and 3 months after surgery; for spinal cord injury: 9 mg per lb for 2 weeks, then 4.5 mg per lb for 10 weeks.

ONSET OF EFFECT
Within 1 to 3 months.

DURATION OF ACTION
Possibly up to a year or more after therapy is stopped.

DIETARY ADVICE
Take the tablets with water on an empty stomach at least 2 hours before or after eating. Eat a well-balanced diet with adequate calcium and vitamin D intake.

STORAGE
Store in a tightly sealed container away from heat, moisture, and direct light.

MISSED DOSE
Take it as soon as possible. However, if it is near the time for the next dose, skip the missed dose, and resume the normal dosage schedule. Do not double the next dose.

STOPPING THE DRUG
Do not stop taking the drug on your own.

PROLONGED USE
Regular visits to your doctor are necessary—even between treatments—to evaluate the drug's effect.

▼ PRECAUTIONS

Over 60: Elderly patients may be more prone to excess fluid retention when treated with injected etidronate in conjunction with hydration therapy. Careful monitoring of fluid and electrolyte levels is important.

Driving and Hazardous Work: No special warnings.

Alcohol: Alcohol should be restricted in high risk women because it is a risk factor for osteoporosis.

Pregnancy: Consult your doctor about whether the benefits of taking the medicine outweigh the potential risks to the unborn child.

Breast Feeding: It is not known if etidronate passes into breast milk.

Infants and Children: Safety and effectiveness have not been established.

OVERDOSE
Symptoms: Vomiting or diarrhea; palpitations; numbness or tingling in the hands, feet, lips, and tongue; facial pain.

What to Do: Call your doctor, emergency medical services (EMS), or the nearest poison control center immediately.

▼ INTERACTIONS

DRUG INTERACTIONS
Antacids or other medications containing calcium, magnesium, or aluminum may interfere with your body's absorption of oral etidronate. Warfarin may also interact with etidronate.

FOOD INTERACTIONS
Foods containing large amounts of calcium, and mineral supplements containing calcium, iron, magnesium, or aluminum should not be consumed within 2 hours of taking etidronate.

DISEASE INTERACTIONS
Consult your doctor for advice if you have a bone fracture, intestinal or bowel disease, kidney disease, or a heart condition.

 SIDE EFFECTS

SERIOUS
Bone fractures—especially in the long bones of the limbs—may occur, usually in patients on high doses or those taking the drug continuously for longer than 6 months.

COMMON
Bone pain or tenderness, often developing 4 to 6 weeks after treatment begins; it may persist, get worse, or sporadically ease and then return in patients with Paget's disease. Nausea and diarrhea may occur with higher doses. Headache, stomach upset, leg cramps, and joint pain may also occur.

LESS COMMON
Hives, skin rash, itching, swelling of the arms, legs, face, lips, tongue, or throat. The injectable form may cause loss of taste or metallic taste in the mouth.

ETODOLAC

Available in: Capsule, tablet, extended-release tablets
Available OTC? No   **As Generic?** Yes
Drug Class: Nonsteroidal anti-inflammatory drug (NSAID)

▼ USAGE INFORMATION

WHY IT'S PRESCRIBED
To treat mild to moderate pain and inflammation caused by tendinitis, arthritis, bursitis, gout, soft tissue injuries, migraine and other vascular headaches, menstrual cramps, and other conditions. When patients fail to respond to one NSAID, another may be tried. The greatest effectiveness often requires trial and error of several different NSAIDs.

HOW IT WORKS
NSAIDs work by interfering with the formation of prostaglandins, substances in the body that cause inflammation and make nerves more sensitive to pain impulses. NSAIDs have other modes of action that are less well understood.

▼ DOSAGE GUIDELINES

RANGE AND FREQUENCY
For osteoarthritis— Adults: To start, 400 mg, 2 or 3 times a day, or 300 mg, 3 or 4 times a day. For pain— Adults: To start, 400 mg. Then, 200 to 400 mg every 6 to 8 hours as needed. Consult your pediatrician for children's dose.

ONSET OF EFFECT
Within 30 minutes.

DURATION OF ACTION
4 to 6 hours.

DIETARY ADVICE
Take with food; maintain your usual food and fluid intake.

STORAGE
Store in a tightly sealed container away from heat, moisture, and direct light.

MISSED DOSE
Take it as soon as you remember. If it is near the time for the next dose, skip the missed dose and resume your regular dosage schedule. Do not double the next dose.

STOPPING THE DRUG
The decision to stop taking the drug should be made in consultation with your doctor.

PROLONGED USE
Prolonged use can cause gastrointestinal problems, including ulceration and bleeding, kidney dysfunction, and liver inflammation. See your doctor for regular evaluation.

▼ PRECAUTIONS

Over 60: Because of the potentially greater consequences of gastrointestinal side effects, the dose of NSAIDs for older patients, especially those over age 70, is often cut in half.

Driving and Hazardous Work: Do not drive or engage in hazardous work until you determine how the medicine affects you.

Alcohol: Avoid alcohol when using this medication because it increases the risk of stomach irritation.

Pregnancy: Avoid or discontinue this drug if you are pregnant or are planning to become pregnant.

Breast Feeding: Etodolac passes into breast milk; avoid use while nursing.

Infants and Children: Etodolac may be used in exceptional circumstances; consult your doctor.

Special Concerns: Because NSAIDs can interfere with blood coagulation, this drug should be stopped at least 3 days prior to any surgery.

OVERDOSE
Symptoms: Nausea, vomiting, severe headache, confusion, seizures.

What to Do: Call your doctor, emergency medical services (EMS), or the nearest poison control center immediately.

▼ INTERACTIONS

DRUG INTERACTIONS
Do not take this drug with aspirin or any other NSAIDs without your doctor's approval. In addition, consult your doctor if you are taking antihypertensives, steroids, anticoagulants, antibiotics, itraconazole or ketoconazole, plicamycin, penicillamine, valproic acid, phenytoin, cyclosporine, digitalis drugs, lithium, methotrexate, probenecid, triamterene, or zidovudine.

FOOD INTERACTIONS
No known food interactions.

DISEASE INTERACTIONS
Caution is advised when taking etodolac. Consult your doctor if you have any of the following: bleeding problems, inflammation or ulcers of the stomach and intestines, diabetes, lupus, anemia, asthma, epilepsy, Parkinson's disease, kidney stones, or a history of heart disease or alcohol abuse. Use of etodolac may cause complications in patients with liver or kidney disease, since these organs work together to remove the medication from the body.

SIDE EFFECTS

SERIOUS
Shortness of breath or wheezing, with or without swelling of legs or other signs of heart failure; chest pain; peptic ulcer disease with vomiting of blood; black, tarry stools; decreasing kidney function. Call your doctor immediately.

COMMON
Nausea, vomiting, heartburn, diarrhea, constipation, headache, dizziness, sleepiness.

LESS COMMON
Ulcers or sores in mouth, depression, rashes or blistering of skin, ringing sound in the ears, unusual tingling or numbness of the hands or feet, seizures, blurred vision. Also elevated potassium levels, decreased blood counts; such problems can be detected by your doctor.

ETOPOSIDE

Available in: Capsules, injection
Available OTC? No **As Generic?** Yes
Drug Class: Antineoplastic (anticancer) agent

▼ USAGE INFORMATION

WHY IT'S PRESCRIBED
To treat recurrent or persistent testicular cancer or lymphoma (cancer of the lymph nodes). It is also used to treat certain types of lung cancer.

HOW IT WORKS
Etoposide kills cancer cells by interfering with the activity of their genetic material, which prevents the cells from dividing normally and multiplying. The drug may also affect the growth and development of other kinds of cells in the body, which may cause unpleasant side effects.

▼ DOSAGE GUIDELINES

RANGE AND FREQUENCY
Usual adult dose by intravenous infusion for testicular carcinoma: 50 to 100 mg per square meter of body surface for 5 days to 100 mg per square meter on days 1, 3, and 5. Usual adult oral dose for small-cell lung cancer: 70 mg per square meter of body surface per day for 4 days to 100 mg per square meter per day for 5 days. Both regimens are repeated every 3 to 4 weeks, depending on the severity of any side effects.

ONSET OF EFFECT
Variable.

DURATION OF ACTION
Unknown.

DIETARY ADVICE
No special concerns.

STORAGE
Keep liquid forms of the drug refrigerated, but do not allow them to freeze.

MISSED DOSE
Skip the missed dose and continue your normal dosage schedule; do not double the next dose. Notify your doctor right away.

STOPPING THE DRUG
Continue to take the medicine exactly as prescribed by your doctor, even if you begin to feel ill. Certain side effects such as stomach upset and vomiting are common. Notify your doctor if vomiting occurs shortly after dosing.

PROLONGED USE
Follow the treatment schedule determined by your doctor. Periodic evaluation of the drug's effect and blood tests are an important part of treatment; blood cell counts need to be closely monitored.

▼ PRECAUTIONS

Over 60: Adverse reactions may be more likely and more severe in older patients.

Driving and Hazardous Work: Check with your doctor before engaging in activities where you are at risk for bruising or injury.

Alcohol: Limit alcohol to moderate intake.

Pregnancy: Birth defects may result if etoposide is used at the time of conception or during pregnancy. Sterility is another potential side effect. Tell your doctor before taking the drug if you are pregnant; use birth control while taking etoposide, and notify your doctor immediately if you think you have become pregnant while taking the drug.

Breast Feeding: Etoposide is distributed into breast milk and may cause serious side effects; consult your doctor for advice.

Infants and Children: Consult your pediatric oncologist.

Special Concerns: Advise your doctor if you or a family member plans to receive a vaccination; there is a danger you might get the infection the immunization is meant to prevent. Patients with low blood counts should avoid crowds and people with infections, and should be alert for signs of infection and bleeding. Exercise caution when cleaning your teeth, and check with your doctor before having any dental work done.

OVERDOSE
Symptoms: Increased severity of nausea or vomiting, rapid pulse, shortness of breath, fainting.

What to Do: Call your doctor, emergency medical services (EMS), or the nearest poison control center immediately.

▼ INTERACTIONS

DRUG INTERACTIONS
Any or all of the following drugs may cause undesirable effects when taken together with etoposide: bone marrow depressants, antivirals, antifungals, anticoagulants, cyclosporine, or aspirin.

FOOD INTERACTIONS
No known food interactions.

DISEASE INTERACTIONS
Advise your doctor if you have any of the following conditions: chickenpox, shingles, infection, or kidney or liver disease.

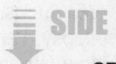

SIDE EFFECTS

SERIOUS
Bone marrow suppression (myelosuppression) causing fatigue, bleeding, bruising, fever, sore throat, chills. Severe gastrointestinal upset. Contact your doctor immediately if such symptoms appear.

COMMON
Loss of appetite, mild to moderate nausea, vomiting. Check with your doctor if these symptoms continue. Hair loss, sometimes progressing to total baldness, is generally temporary; hair will usually begin to grow back when the therapy is discontinued.

LESS COMMON
Allergic reactions, diarrhea, fatigue. Temporary drop in blood pressure (hypotension) causing dizziness and light-headedness may occur with intravenous infusion.

EXEMESTANE

Available in: Tablets
Available OTC? No **As Generic?** No
Drug Class: Antineoplastic (anticancer) agent

▼ USAGE INFORMATION

WHY IT'S PRESCRIBED
To treat advanced breast cancer in postmenopausal women whose tumors stop responding to tamoxifen therapy.

HOW IT WORKS
The growth of some breast cancers is stimulated by the hormone estrogen. The estrogen in postmenopausal women arises primarily from the conversion by the enzyme aromatase of male hormones (androgens) made in the adrenal and ovaries. Exemestane inactivates aromatase, thus preventing the natural synthesis of estrogen and inhibiting the growth of estrogen-dependent tumors.

▼ DOSAGE GUIDELINES

RANGE AND FREQUENCY
25 mg a day following a meal.

ONSET OF EFFECT
Unknown.

DURATION OF ACTION
Unknown.

DIETARY ADVICE
It is recommended that exemestane be taken after a meal.

STORAGE
Store in a tightly sealed container away from heat, moisture, and direct light.

MISSED DOSE
Exemestane is prescribed for once-daily use only. If you are unable to take the medication on a particular day, simply resume your regular dosage schedule the following day. Do not double the next dose.

STOPPING THE DRUG
The decision to stop taking the drug must be made in consultation with your doctor. Do not stop taking exemestane on your own.

PROLONGED USE
There is no standard duration of therapy with exemestane, although you can expect to remain on it for at least several weeks in order to determine if it is effective. Your doctor will determine whether your response to the drug is satisfactory or not, and will recommend continuation or discontinuation of therapy.

≡ SIDE EFFECTS ≡

SERIOUS
No serious side effects have been reported.

COMMON
Hot flashes, nausea, fatigue, pain, depression, insomnia, anxiety, shortness of breath.

LESS COMMON
Sweating, flulike symptoms, swelling, dizziness, headache, vomiting, abdominal pain, loss of appetite, constipation, diarrhea, increased appetite, weight gain, cough.

▼ PRECAUTIONS

Over 60: No special problems are expected.

Driving and Hazardous Work: Do not drive or engage in hazardous work until you determine how the medicine affects you.

Alcohol: No special problems are expected, but you should consult your doctor about drinking alcohol while taking exemestane.

Pregnancy: Exemestane must not be used in pregnant women. Although exemestane is only prescribed for postmenopausal women, it is important that patients be sure they are not pregnant before starting treatment with this drug.

Breast Feeding: Not applicable; this drug is prescribed only for postmenopausal women.

Infants and Children: Not applicable.

Special Concerns: Exemestane often lowers blood levels of lymphocytes (a type of infection-fighting white blood cell), but no increase in infections was seen in clinical trials.

OVERDOSE
Symptoms: No cases of overdose have been reported.

What to Do: An overdose is unlikely; however, if you have any reason to suspect that one has occurred, call emergency medical services (EMS) to receive evaluation and treatment at the closest emergency facility.

▼ INTERACTIONS

DRUG INTERACTIONS
None reported.

FOOD INTERACTIONS
None reported.

DISEASE INTERACTIONS
None reported.

FAMCICLOVIR

Available in: Tablets
Available OTC? No   **As Generic?** No
Drug Class: Antiviral

▼ USAGE INFORMATION

WHY IT'S PRESCRIBED
To treat shingles (herpes zoster) and recurrent genital herpes.

HOW IT WORKS
Famciclovir interferes with the activity of specific enzymes needed for the replication of DNA in viral cells, thus preventing the virus from multiplying.

▼ DOSAGE GUIDELINES

RANGE AND FREQUENCY
For shingles (herpes zoster): 500 mg every 8 hours for 7 days. The effectiveness of famciclovir in treating herpes zoster is usually determined after 2 days of regular use. The best effect is achieved if the medicine is prescribed immediately after the diagnosis is made. For recurrent genital herpes: 250 mg twice a day for up to 1 year. It should be taken at the first sign of recurrence.

ONSET OF EFFECT
Within 1 hour.

DURATION OF ACTION
Unknown.

DIETARY ADVICE
No special restrictions.

STORAGE
Store in a tightly sealed container away from heat, moisture, and direct light.

MISSED DOSE
Take it as soon as you remember. If it is near the time for the next dose, skip the missed dose and resume your regular dosage schedule. Do not double the next dose.

STOPPING THE DRUG
Take it as prescribed for the full treatment period, even if you feel better before the end of therapy. The decision to stop taking the drug should be made by your doctor.

PROLONGED USE
This drug is not intended for prolonged use, but under some circumstances it may be used for an extended period for the suppression of a chronic herpesvirus infection.

▼ PRECAUTIONS

Over 60: No special problems expected except for older persons with impaired kidney or liver function.

Driving and Hazardous Work: Famciclovir may cause dizziness and fatigue. Do not drive or engage in hazardous work until you determine how the medicine affects you.

Alcohol: No special precautions are necessary.

Pregnancy: Studies of the use of famciclovir in pregnant women have not been done. Consult your doctor about the risk of taking famciclovir during pregnancy.

Breast Feeding: Famciclovir may pass into breast milk; avoid or discontinue use while nursing.

Infants and Children: The safety and effectiveness of famciclovir for anyone under 18 have not been established. It should be used only under close medical supervision.

Special Concerns: This medicine is not recommended for use if you have had a bone marrow transplant or a kidney transplant. Before taking famciclovir, tell the doctor if your immune system is compromised. Do not take famciclovir if you have had an allergic response to it previously. Keep the affected area of skin clean and dry; wear loose-fitting clothing. Your doctor may periodically wish to take blood tests to evaluate your kidney function.

OVERDOSE
Symptoms: No cases of overdose have been reported.

What to Do: An overdose is unlikely to occur. However, if you have any reason to suspect an overdose, call your doctor, emergency medical services (EMS), or the nearest poison control immediately.

▼ INTERACTIONS

DRUG INTERACTIONS
Other drugs may interact with famciclovir. Consult your doctor for specific advice if you are taking probenecid or any other prescription or over-the-counter drug.

FOOD INTERACTIONS
No known food interactions.

DISEASE INTERACTIONS
Consult your doctor if you have any disorder or condition associated with a weakened immune system, such as HIV infection or AIDS. Use of famciclovir may cause complications in patients with impaired liver or kidney function, since these organs work together to remove the medication from the body.

≡ SIDE EFFECTS ≡

SERIOUS
Extreme drowsiness. Call your doctor immediately.

COMMON
Headache, nausea.

LESS COMMON
Fatigue, vomiting, diarrhea, itchiness, rash, hallucinations, confusion, sore throat, back or joint pain, sinus infection, fever, shivering.

FAMOTIDINE

Available in: Tablets, powder for suspension, orally disintegrating and chewable tablets
Available OTC? Yes   **As Generic?** No
Drug Class: Histamine (H2) blocker

▼ USAGE INFORMATION

WHY IT'S PRESCRIBED
To treat heartburn, ulcers of the stomach and duodenum, conditions that cause excess production of stomach acid (such as Zollinger-Ellison syndrome), and gastroesophageal reflux (backwash of stomach acid into the esophagus, resulting in heartburn). Chewable tablets are taken for prevention or treatment of heartburn.

HOW IT WORKS
Famotidine blocks the action of histamine (a compound produced in the body's cells), which in turn decreases the stomach's secretion of hydrochloric acid. Once the production of stomach acid is decreased, the body is better able to heal itself.

▼ DOSAGE GUIDELINES

RANGE AND FREQUENCY
To prevent heartburn: 10 mg, 1 hour before meals. For excess stomach acid: 20 to 160 mg every 6 hours. For acid reflux disease: 20 mg twice a day for up to 6 weeks. For stomach ulcers: 40 mg once a day for 8 weeks. For duodenal ulcers: To start, 40 mg once a day at bedtime or 20 mg twice a day; later, 20 mg once a day. Chewable tablets— For treatment of heartburn: Chew one tablet. For prevention of heartburn: Chew one tablet 15 to 60 minutes before eating.

ONSET OF EFFECT
Prescription form: Within 30 minutes. The lower dosage in the nonprescription form may take 45 minutes to relieve heartburn.

DURATION OF ACTION
Up to 12 hours.

DIETARY ADVICE
Take it after meals or with milk to minimize stomach irritation. Avoid foods that cause stomach irritation. Take chewable tablet with a glass of water.

STORAGE
Store tablets in a tightly sealed container away from heat, moisture, and direct light. After powder vials are reconstituted, store the medicine in the refrigerator, but keep it from freezing. Discard after 30 days.

MISSED DOSE
Take it as soon as you remember. If it is near the time for the next dose, skip the missed dose and resume your regular dosage schedule. Do not double the next dose.

STOPPING THE DRUG
The decision to stop taking the prescription drug should be made in consultation with your doctor.

PROLONGED USE
Do not take the prescription drug for more than 8 weeks unless your doctor orders it. Do not take the over-the-counter drug for more than 2 weeks unless otherwise instructed by your doctor.

▼ PRECAUTIONS

Over 60: Adverse reactions may be more likely and more severe in older patients.

Driving and Hazardous Work: Do not drive or engage in hazardous work until you determine how the medicine affects you.

Alcohol: Avoid alcohol while taking this drug; it may slow recovery. Also, this drug increases blood alcohol levels.

Pregnancy: Risks vary, depending on patient and dosage. Consult your physician for advice.

Breast Feeding: Famotidine passes into breast milk; you should avoid or discontinue use while breast feeding.

Infants and Children: Famotidine is not generally prescribed for infants and children.

Special Concerns: If necessary, famotidine may be given with antacids. Avoid cigarette smoking because it may increase secretion of stomach acid and thus worsen the disease.

OVERDOSE
Symptoms: Confusion, slurred speech, rapid heartbeat, difficulty breathing, delirium.

What to Do: Call your doctor, emergency medical services (EMS), or the nearest poison control center immediately.

▼ INTERACTIONS

DRUG INTERACTIONS
None reported.

FOOD INTERACTIONS
Carbonated drinks, citrus fruits and juices, caffeine-containing beverages, and other acidic foods or liquids may irritate the stomach or interfere with the therapeutic action of famotidine.

DISEASE INTERACTIONS
Patients with kidney disease should use famotidine in smaller, limited doses under careful supervision by a physician.

SIDE EFFECTS

SERIOUS
Irregular heart rhythm (palpitations), slowed heartbeat, severe blood problems resulting in unusual bleeding, bruising, fever, chills, and increased susceptibility to infection. Call your doctor immediately.

COMMON
Headache, fatigue, drowsiness, dizziness, nausea, vomiting, abdominal pain, diarrhea, constipation.

LESS COMMON
Blurred vision, decreased sexual desire or function, temporary hair loss, hallucinations, depression, insomnia, skin rash, hives, or redness.

FELBAMATE

BRAND NAME

Felbatol

Available in: Oral suspension, tablets
Available OTC? No   **As Generic?** No
Drug Class: Anticonvulsant

▼ USAGE INFORMATION

WHY IT'S PRESCRIBED
To control certain types of seizures due to epilepsy or other disorders. Because felbamate has a relatively high rate of potentially fatal side effects (including a serious blood disorder called aplastic anemia as well as liver disease), it is used only when other drugs have failed to control seizures. It may be used alone or combined with other anticonvulsants.

HOW IT WORKS
Felbamate is thought to depress the activity of certain parts of the brain and suppress the abnormal firing of neurons that causes seizures.

▼ DOSAGE GUIDELINES

RANGE AND FREQUENCY
Adults: 1,800 to 3,600 mg a day, in 3 or 4 divided doses. Children: 7 to 20 mg per lb

of body weight, in 3 or 4 divided doses. Some patients may require higher doses. Low doses are used to start; the dose is gradually increased by your doctor to achieve the maximum therapeutic benefit. When switching to felbamate from other anticonvulsants, doses of the other drugs should be reduced gradually.

ONSET OF EFFECT
1 to 4 hours.

DURATION OF ACTION
Maximum effect persists for 18 to 24 hours or longer; effectiveness then gradually decreases.

DIETARY ADVICE
Take with food to minimize stomach upset.

STORAGE
Store in a tightly sealed container away from heat, moisture, and direct light.

MISSED DOSE
Take it as soon as you remember. If it is near the time for the next dose, skip the missed dose and resume regular dosage schedule. Do not double the next dose, unless so advised by your doctor.

STOPPING THE DRUG
Never stop it abruptly; this may cause seizures. Your doctor will taper the dose over a period of weeks.

PROLONGED USE
Periodic examinations or laboratory tests to check blood counts and liver function may be needed.

▼ PRECAUTIONS

Over 60: Older patients may require lower doses to minimize side effects.

Driving and Hazardous Work: Felbamate may cause drowsiness or dizziness. Do not drive or engage in hazardous work until you determine how the medication affects you.

Alcohol: May contribute to excessive drowsiness.

Pregnancy: Adequate studies of felbamate use during pregnancy have not been done, but many anticonvulsants are associated with an increased rate of birth defects. However, seizures during pregnancy can also increase the risks to the fetus. Discuss with your doctor the potential risks and benefits of using this drug while pregnant. Folate supplementation is recommended beginning 1 to 2

months before conception and throughout pregnancy.

Breast Feeding: Felbamate passes into breast milk, although at low levels. Consult your doctor for advice.

Infants and Children: Close medical supervision is advised.

Special Concerns: Your doctor may want you to wear a medical bracelet or carry an identification card saying that you are taking this drug.

OVERDOSE
Symptoms: Unknown; reports of felbamate overdose are very rare.

What to Do: If an excessive dose is taken, call your doctor, emergency medical services (EMS), or poison control center immediately.

▼ INTERACTIONS

DRUG INTERACTIONS
Felbamate can increase blood levels of certain anticonvulsants (phenytoin, valproic acid) and decrease blood levels of others (carbamazepine). Phenytoin and carbamazepine can decrease blood levels of felbamate. Patients sensitive to chemically related drugs, such as meprobamate or carisoprodol, may also be sensitive to felbamate.

FOOD INTERACTIONS
No known food interactions.

DISEASE INTERACTIONS
Special caution is advised if you have a history of any blood disorder, bone marrow depression (causing anemia), or liver disease.

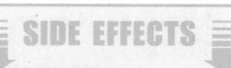
SIDE EFFECTS

SERIOUS
Fever, weakness, sore throat, swollen glands, purple or red pointlike spots on the skin, easy bruising, skin blistering, or yellowing of the eyes or skin may be signs of aplastic anemia, liver failure, or other potentially fatal complications. Call your doctor at once.

COMMON
Headache, nausea and vomiting, loss of appetite, stomach upset, constipation, sleepiness, insomnia, dizziness, anxiety, nervousness, tremor, muscle incoordination, runny nose and upper respiratory tract infection.

LESS COMMON
Blurred or double vision, coughing, diarrhea, abdominal pain, dry mouth. There are numerous additional side effects; consult your doctor if you are concerned about any adverse or unusual reactions.

FELODIPINE

Available in: Tablets, extended-release tablets
Available OTC? No **As Generic?** No
Drug Class: Calcium channel blocker

▼ USAGE INFORMATION

WHY IT'S PRESCRIBED
To control high blood pressure (hypertension).

HOW IT WORKS
Felodipine interferes with the movement of calcium into heart muscle cells and the smooth muscle cells in the walls of the arteries. This action relaxes blood vessels (causing them to widen), which lowers blood pressure, increases the blood supply to the heart, and decreases the heart's overall workload.

▼ DOSAGE GUIDELINES

RANGE AND FREQUENCY
To start, 5 to 10 mg once a day. The dose may be increased to a maximum of 20 mg once a day. For patients over 65, starting dose is 2.5 mg per day, to a maximum of 10 mg a day.

ONSET OF EFFECT
Within 2 to 5 hours.

DURATION OF ACTION
24 hours.

DIETARY ADVICE
Felodipine should be taken either on an empty stomach or with a light meal. Do not crush or chew tablets.

STORAGE
Store in a tightly sealed container away from heat, moisture, and direct light.

MISSED DOSE
Take it as soon as you remember. However, if it is near the time for the next dose, skip the missed dose and resume your regular dosage schedule. Do not double the next dose.

STOPPING THE DRUG
Do not stop taking felodipine suddenly, as this may cause potentially serious health problems. If therapy is to be discontinued, the dosage should be reduced gradually, according to your doctor's instructions.

PROLONGED USE
Consult your doctor about the need for medical examinations or laboratory studies to check liver function, kidney function, and heart function.

▼ PRECAUTIONS

Over 60: Older patients are prescribed lower starting doses, which may be gradually increased until the doctor determines the appropriate individual maintenance dose.

Driving and Hazardous Work: Do not drive or engage in hazardous work until you determine how felodipine affects you.

Alcohol: Avoid alcohol while taking this medication as it may cause an excessive drop in blood pressure.

Pregnancy: Consult your physician to determine whether the benefits of felodipine outweigh its possible risks while pregnant.

Breast Feeding: Felodipine may pass into breast milk; caution is advised. Consult your doctor for advice.

Infants and Children: Felodipine is generally not prescribed for children.

Special Concerns: Tell all your health care providers that you are taking felodipine and carry a note that says you take this medicine. Felodipine can cause erectile dysfunction in some men. Nicotine can reduce the effectiveness of the medicine. Hot environments can exaggerate the blood-pressure-lowering effect of felodipine.

OVERDOSE
Symptoms: Weakness, lightheadedness, rapid pulse, shortness of breath, tremors, flushed skin, fainting, slurred speech.

What to Do: Call your doctor, emergency medical services (EMS), or the nearest poison control center immediately.

▼ INTERACTIONS

DRUG INTERACTIONS
Consult your doctor for advice if you are taking anticonvulsants, beta-blockers, digitalis drugs, carbamazepine, cyclosporine, digoxin, disopyramide, magnesium, phenobarbital, phenytoin, quinidine, rifampin, cimetidine, or erythromycin.

FOOD INTERACTIONS
Grapefruit juice should be avoided because it can amplify the effect of the drug and cause a serious drop in blood pressure. Avoid excessive salt intake.

DISEASE INTERACTIONS
Caution is advised when taking felodipine. Consult your doctor if you have any of the following: congestive heart failure, a history of heart attack or stroke, heart rhythm disturbances, or impaired liver or kidney function.

SIDE EFFECTS

SERIOUS
Irregular or slow heartbeat, low blood pressure (causing dizziness or faintness).

COMMON
Flushing or skin rash, headache, swelling of the lower legs or feet.

LESS COMMON
Dizziness, numbness or tingling sensation, chest pain, palpitations, weakness, runny nose, rapid pulse, sore throat, abdominal discomfort, nausea, constipation or diarrhea, cough, muscle cramps, back pain, overgrowth of the gums.

FENOFIBRATE

Available in: Capsules
Available OTC? No   **As Generic?** No
Drug Class: Antilipidemic (triglyceride-lowering agent)

▼ USAGE INFORMATION

WHY IT'S PRESCRIBED
To treat high levels of blood triglyceride. Usually prescribed after other treatments—including diet, weight loss, exercise, and control of diabetes (when present)—fail to lower triglyceride levels adequately.

HOW IT WORKS
Fenofibrate speeds the removal of triglycerides from the lipoprotein known as "very low density lipoprotein (VLDL)," which is converted to low density lipoprotein (LDL). In some people total and LDL cholesterol levels may rise while triglycerides fall.

▼ DOSAGE GUIDELINES

RANGE AND FREQUENCY
Adults: 67 mg (1 capsule) once a day. The dose may be increased by your doctor to no more than 201 mg (3 capsules) a day.

ONSET OF EFFECT
Unknown.

DURATION OF ACTION
Unknown.

DIETARY ADVICE
Follow your doctor's dietary advice to improve control over high blood pressure and help prevent heart disease. The American Heart Association publishes a "Healthy Heart" diet; discuss this with your doctor. Limit intake of alcohol, which can raise triglyceride levels.

STORAGE
Store in a tightly sealed container away from heat, moisture, and direct light.

MISSED DOSE
If you miss a dose on one day, do not double the dose the next day.

STOPPING THE DRUG
Do not stop taking on your own; the level of triglycerides in your blood will increase.

PROLONGED USE
During therapy, your doctor will conduct periodic tests to measure triglyceride levels. Therapy should be discontinued if there is an inadequate response to the medication following two months of therapy at the maximum dose of 3 capsules per day.

▼ PRECAUTIONS

Over 60: No special warnings.

Driving and Hazardous Work: The use of fenofibrate should not impair your ability to perform such tasks safely.

Alcohol: Alcohol intake should be limited because it can raise triglyceride levels.

Pregnancy: Do not take fenofibrate while pregnant unless your doctor indicates that the risks of stopping the drug are too great. Triglycerides increase substantially during pregnancy and extremely high triglycerides can trigger an attack of acute pancreatitis.

Breast Feeding: Avoid or discontinue use while nursing.

Infants and Children: Safety and effectiveness have not been established for children under age 18.

Special Concerns: The most important treatment for high levels of blood triglycerides is a proper diet, weight loss, regular moderate exercise, the avoidance of certain medications, and control of diabetes. Because fenofibrate has potential side effects, it is important that you maintain a healthy diet and cooperate with other treatment strategies your physician may suggest. Fenofibrate may increase the chances of gallbladder, liver, and pancreas problems; your physician will order periodic blood tests.

OVERDOSE
Symptoms: No specific ones have been reported.

What to Do: If someone takes a much larger dose than prescribed, call your doctor, emergency medical services (EMS), or the nearest poison control immediately.

▼ INTERACTIONS

DRUG INTERACTIONS
Certain drugs may interact adversely with fenofibrate, particularly anticoagulants, such as warfarin, niacin, and any of the group of cholesterol-lowering drugs referred to as "statins." It is usually necessary to reduce the dose of warfarin to prevent bleeding. The combination of fenofibrate with either niacin or a statin drug can cause severe myositis (muscle inflammation), which can release a protein that damages the kidneys. Consult your doctor for advice.

FOOD INTERACTIONS
No known food interactions.

DISEASE INTERACTIONS
Inform your doctor if you have any of the following problems: gallstones, stomach or intestinal ulcer, kidney disease, muscle disease, or liver disease. The dose of fenofibrate must be reduced in those with significant kidney damage.

SIDE EFFECTS

SERIOUS
Fever, unusual or unexplained muscle aches and tenderness. Call your doctor right away.

COMMON
Skin rash, infection, flulike symptoms.

LESS COMMON
Fatigue, general feeling of pain, headache, belching, flatulence, nausea, vomiting, constipation, decreased libido, dizziness, nasal congestion, itching, visual disturbances, eye irritation.

FENOPROFEN CALCIUM

Available in: Capsules, tablets
Available OTC? No **As Generic?** Yes
Drug Class: Nonsteroidal anti-inflammatory drug (NSAID)

▼ USAGE INFORMATION

WHY IT'S PRESCRIBED
To treat mild to moderate pain and inflammation caused by tendinitis, arthritis, bursitis, gout, soft tissue injuries, migraine and other vascular headaches, menstrual cramps, and other conditions. When patients fail to respond to one NSAID, another may be tried. The greatest effectiveness often requires trial and error of several different NSAIDs.

HOW IT WORKS
NSAIDs work by interfering with the formation of prostaglandins, naturally occurring substances in the body that cause inflammation and make nerves more sensitive to pain impulses. NSAIDs also have other modes of action that are less well understood.

▼ DOSAGE GUIDELINES

RANGE AND FREQUENCY
Adults— For arthritis: 300 to 600 mg, 3 or 4 times a day, to a maximum of 3,200 mg a day. Full effect may take 2 to 4 weeks to begin. For mild to moderate pain: 200 mg every 4 to 6 hours.

ONSET OF EFFECT
15 to 30 minutes.

DURATION OF ACTION
4 to 6 hours.

DIETARY ADVICE
Take with food; maintain your usual food and fluid intake.

STORAGE
Store in a tightly sealed container away from heat, moisture, and direct light.

MISSED DOSE
Take it as soon as you remember. If it is near the time for the next dose, skip the missed dose and resume your regular dosage schedule. Do not double the next dose.

STOPPING THE DRUG
The decision to stop taking the drug should be made in consultation with your doctor.

PROLONGED USE
Prolonged use can cause gastrointestinal problems, including ulceration and bleeding, kidney dysfunction, and liver inflammation. See your doctor for regular evaluation.

▼ PRECAUTIONS

Over 60: Because of the potentially greater consequences of gastrointestinal side effects, the dose of NSAIDs for older patients, especially those over age 70, is often cut in half.

Driving and Hazardous Work: Do not drive or engage in hazardous work until you determine how the medicine affects you.

Alcohol: Avoid alcohol when using this medication because it increases the risk of stomach irritation.

Pregnancy: Avoid or discontinue this drug if you are pregnant or are planning to become pregnant.

Breast Feeding: Fenoprofen passes into breast milk; avoid or discontinue use while breast feeding.

Infants and Children: May be used in exceptional circumstances; consult your doctor.

Special Concerns: Because NSAIDs can interfere with blood coagulation, this drug should be stopped at least 3 days prior to any surgery.

OVERDOSE
Symptoms: Nausea, vomiting, severe headache, confusion, seizures.

What to Do: Call your doctor, emergency medical services (EMS), or the nearest poison control center immediately.

▼ INTERACTIONS

DRUG INTERACTIONS
Do not take this drug with aspirin or any other NSAIDs without your doctor's approval. In addition, consult your doctor if you are taking antihypertensives, steroids, anticoagulants, antibiotics, itraconazole or ketoconazole, plicamycin, penicillamine, valproic acid, phenytoin, cyclosporine, digitalis drugs, lithium, methotrexate, probenecid, triamterene, or zidovudine.

FOOD INTERACTIONS
No known food interactions.

DISEASE INTERACTIONS
Caution is advised when taking fenoprofen. Consult your doctor if you have any of the following: bleeding problems, inflammation or ulcers of the stomach and intestines, diabetes, lupus, anemia, asthma, epilepsy, Parkinson's disease, kidney stones, or a history of heart disease or alcohol abuse. Use of fenoprofen may cause complications in patients with liver or kidney disease, since these organs work together to remove the drug from the body.

SIDE EFFECTS

SERIOUS
Shortness of breath or wheezing, with or without swelling of legs or other signs of heart failure; chest pain; peptic ulcer disease with vomiting of blood; black, tarry stools; decreasing kidney function. Call your doctor immediately.

COMMON
Nausea, vomiting, heartburn, diarrhea, constipation, headache, dizziness, sleepiness.

LESS COMMON
Ulcers or sores in mouth, depression, rashes or blistering of skin, ringing sound in the ears, unusual tingling or numbness of the hands or feet, seizures, blurred vision. Also elevated potassium levels, decreased blood counts; such problems can be detected by your doctor.

FENTANYL TRANSDERMAL

Available in: Transdermal (skin) patch
Available OTC? No   **As Generic?** No
Drug Class: Opioid (narcotic) analgesic

▼ USAGE INFORMATION

WHY IT'S PRESCRIBED
To control severe chronic pain.

HOW IT WORKS
Fentanyl, a narcotic, relieves pain by acting on specific areas of the spinal cord and brain that process pain signals from nerves throughout the body.

▼ DOSAGE GUIDELINES

RANGE AND FREQUENCY
Attach the patch to the skin using the dose recommended by your doctor. Replace the patch every 72 hours or as your doctor directs. To apply, remove the patch from its protective pouch and remove the liner from the sticky side of the patch. Place the patch on a site that is hairless and dry, and hold it in place for 10 to 30 seconds to ensure adhesion. Wash the area with water if necessary, but do not use soap, lotion, alcohol, or other substances that may irritate the skin. Do not apply it in the same place more than once within a 3-day period. Avoid any area that is burned, irritated, or excessively oily. Wash your hands after applying a new patch. Remove an old patch after 72 hours (3 days), fold it onto itself and dispose of it in the toilet. Fentanyl transdermal patches are available in the following concentrations: 25 micrograms per hour (mcg/hr); 50 mcg/hr; 75 mcg/hr; 100 mcg/hr.

ONSET OF EFFECT
12 to 24 hours.

DURATION OF ACTION
Up to 72 hours.

DIETARY ADVICE
The patch can be applied without regard to diet.

STORAGE
Store the patch in its protective pouch away from heat, moisture, and direct light.

MISSED DOSE
Apply a new patch as soon as you remember. Do not apply more than one patch at a time, unless directed to do otherwise by your doctor. Remove the patch 3 days after applying it.

STOPPING THE DRUG
The decision to stop using the drug should be made by your doctor. It may be necessary to reduce the dose gradually if the medication is used for a long time, to decrease the risk of suffering withdrawal symptoms.

PROLONGED USE
Prolonged use may result in physical dependence.

▼ PRECAUTIONS

Over 60: Adverse reactions may be more likely and more severe in older patients. The smallest-dose patch is generally used at the beginning of therapy.

Driving and Hazardous Work: The use of fentanyl may impair your ability to perform such tasks safely.

Alcohol: Avoid alcohol.

Pregnancy: Adequate human studies have not been done. Before taking fentanyl, discuss with your doctor the relative risks and benefits of using this drug while pregnant.

Breast Feeding: This drug passes into breast milk; avoid or discontinue using it while nursing.

Infants and Children: This drug should not be used by patients under age 18 who weigh less than 110 pounds. Safety and effectiveness for children under the age of 12 have not been determined.

Special Concerns: Do not alter your dose or suddenly stop using this drug without consulting your doctor. Abruptly stopping its use may cause withdrawal symptoms. Heat can cause fentanyl to be absorbed more rapidly. Avoid heating pads, sunbathing, or long showers or baths in hot water. Not recommended for postoperative pain.

OVERDOSE
Symptoms: Seizures, severe drowsiness, hallucinations, slow heartbeat, very slow or weak breathing, cold, clammy skin, pinpoint pupils of eyes.

What to Do: Call your doctor, emergency medical services (EMS), or the nearest poison control center immediately.

▼ INTERACTIONS

DRUG INTERACTIONS
Consult your doctor for specific advice if you are taking benzodiazepines; central nervous system depressants such as opiates, barbiturates, and tranquilizers; or antidepressants, amiodarone, clonidine, or MAO inhibitors.

FOOD INTERACTIONS
No known food interactions.

DISEASE INTERACTIONS
Consult your doctor if you have any of the following: liver disease; kidney disease; prostate problems; gallbladder disease; intestinal problems, such as colitis; underactive thyroid; brain tumor; any heart disease; anemia; or a history of alcohol or drug abuse. Fever may increase the rate at which the drug is absorbed by the body, thus increasing risk of overdose.

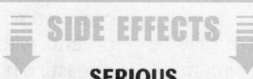
SIDE EFFECTS

SERIOUS
Seizures, severe drowsiness, hallucinations, slow heartbeat, very slow or weak breathing, cold, clammy skin, pinpoint pupils of eyes. Call your doctor immediately.

COMMON
Dizziness, nausea or vomiting, constipation, drowsiness, urine retention, itching.

LESS COMMON
Sweating, skin reaction at patch site, rigid muscles, fainting, jerking body movements (myoclonus).

FENTANYL TRANSMUCOSAL

Available in: Oral transmucosal (inside the mouth) lozenge
Available OTC? No   **As Generic?** No
Drug Class: Opioid (narcotic) analgesic

▼ USAGE INFORMATION

WHY IT'S PRESCRIBED
To manage flare-ups of cancer pain in people who are already receiving and who are tolerant to narcotic (opioid) therapy for underlying cancer pain. Fentanyl lozenges are not for short-term pain, including pain from injuries or surgery.

HOW IT WORKS
Fentanyl, a narcotic, relieves pain by acting on specific areas of the spinal cord and brain that process pain signals from nerves throughout the body.

▼ DOSAGE GUIDELINES

RANGE AND FREQUENCY
Your oncologist or physician will determine the appropriate dosage. Dosage will be individually adjusted to provide adequate pain relief with minimal side effects. Do not open the package until you are ready to use the medication. Place the lozenge in your mouth between your cheeks and gums. Move it around in your mouth, especially along the cheeks, twirling the han-

dle often. Finish the drug completely within 15 minutes for best results. If you finish too quickly, less drug will be absorbed through the cheeks and you will get less relief. Do not bite or chew the lozenge. Do not consume more than 4 lozenges per day (no more than 2 per flare-up); if you are not getting adequate pain relief, consult your doctor.

ONSET OF EFFECT
Within 15 to 45 minutes.

DURATION OF ACTION
Unknown.

DIETARY ADVICE
You may drink water before using the drug. Do not eat or drink anything while using it.

STORAGE
Store in its protective package away from heat, moisture, and direct light in a child-resistant locked storage space. Do not freeze or refrigerate.

MISSED DOSE
Not applicable. It is used as needed for breakthrough cancer pain that is not successfully controlled by regularly prescribed pain medication.

STOPPING THE DRUG
The lozenges are used on an as needed basis. However, because fentanyl can be addictive, it may be necessary to reduce the dose gradually if the medication is used for a long time, to decrease the risk of withdrawal symptoms.

PROLONGED USE
Prolonged use may result in physical dependence.

▼ PRECAUTIONS

Over 60: Adverse reactions may be more likely and more severe in older patients. The smallest-dose lozenge is generally used at the beginning of therapy.

Driving and Hazardous Work: The use of fentanyl may impair your ability to perform such tasks safely.

Alcohol: Avoid alcohol.

Pregnancy: Adequate human studies have not been done. Before taking fentanyl, discuss with your doctor the relative risks and benefits of using this drug while pregnant.

Breast Feeding: This drug passes into breast milk; avoid or discontinue using it while nursing.

Infants and Children: Safety and effectiveness for children under the age of 16 have not been determined. The lozenges contain a high concentration of fentanyl, which can be fatal to a child.

Special Concerns: You must be opioid tolerant to use this form of fentanyl. It contains a

high concentration of the drug and can cause serious, possibly fatal side effects in those not already taking narcotic pain relievers. If you do not finish the lozenge within 15 minutes, dispose of the remainder appropriately. Your doctor or health care provider will teach you how to do so.

OVERDOSE
Symptoms: Seizures, severe drowsiness, hallucinations, slow heartbeat, very slow or weak breathing, cold, clammy skin, pinpoint pupils of eyes.

What to Do: Call your doctor, emergency medical services (EMS), or the nearest poison control center immediately.

▼ INTERACTIONS

DRUG INTERACTIONS
Consult your doctor if you are taking benzodiazepines; central nervous system depressants, such as barbiturates, and tranquilizers; or antidepressants, amiodarone, clonidine, or MAO inhibitors.

FOOD INTERACTIONS
No known food interactions.

DISEASE INTERACTIONS
Consult your doctor if you have any of the following: liver disease; kidney disease; prostate problems; gallbladder disease; intestinal problems, such as colitis; underactive thyroid; brain tumor; any heart disease; anemia; chronic obstructive pulmonary disease or other respiratory illnesses; or a history of alcohol or drug abuse. Fever may increase the rate at which the drug is absorbed by the body, thus increasing risk of overdose.

 SIDE EFFECTS

SERIOUS
Seizures; severe drowsiness; hallucinations; slow heartbeat; very slow or weak breathing; cold, clammy skin; pinpoint pupils of eyes. Call your doctor immediately.

COMMON
Dizziness, nausea or vomiting, constipation, drowsiness, urine retention, itching.

LESS COMMON
Sweating, skin reaction at patch site, rigid muscles, fainting, jerking body movements (myoclonus).

FERROUS SALTS

Available in: Capsules, drops, elixir, solution, tablets
Available OTC? Yes   **As Generic?** Yes
Drug Class: Dietary supplement

▼ USAGE INFORMATION

WHY IT'S PRESCRIBED
To help increase the body's stores of iron, a mineral essential to the manufacture of red blood cells. An insufficient number of red blood cells results in anemia.

HOW IT WORKS
Ferrous salts are required for the production of hemoglobin in developing red blood cells. Hemoglobin is a complex iron-based protein in the red cell that carries oxygen to the body's tissues and carries carbon dioxide gas away from the tissues to be exhaled by the lungs.

▼ DOSAGE GUIDELINES

RANGE AND FREQUENCY
For iron deficiency, 325 mg, 3 times a day. Children: 5 to 10 mg for every 2.2 lbs (1 kg) of body weight 3 times a day.

ONSET OF EFFECT
From 5 to 7 days. Depending on the extent of the deficiency, more than 3 months of therapy may be needed for maximum benefit to be realized.

DURATION OF ACTION
Depends on the body's ability to utilize it.

DIETARY ADVICE
Take 1 hour before or 2 hours after eating.

STORAGE
Store in a tightly sealed container away from heat and direct light. Keep the liquid form from freezing.

MISSED DOSE
Take it as soon as you remember. If it is near the time for the next dose, skip the missed dose and resume your regular dosage schedule. Do not double the next dose.

STOPPING THE DRUG
If the medication was prescribed, the decision to stop taking this supplement should be made by your doctor.

PROLONGED USE
Prolonged use may result in the accumulation of iron in the tissues, the effects of which can include liver damage, heart problems, diabetes, erectile dysfunction, and unusually bronzed skin. Do not take iron supplements without consulting your doctor.

≣ SIDE EFFECTS ≣

SERIOUS
No serious side effects are associated with ferrous salts, except for iron overload due to prolonged, inappropriate use of the mineral.

COMMON
Nausea, constipation, black stools.

LESS COMMON
Stained teeth (with liquid forms), stomach pain, vomiting, diarrhea.

▼ PRECAUTIONS

Over 60: Problems in older adults have not been reported with intake of normal daily recommended amounts.

Driving and Hazardous Work: No problems expected.

Alcohol: Avoid alcohol while taking this medication because it may cause excess absorption of iron.

Pregnancy: This medication should be taken during pregnancy only if your doctor so advises.

Breast Feeding: No problems are expected during breast feeding; however, consult your doctor before taking ferrous salts.

Infants and Children: No unusual problems reported in infants and children. Close medical supervision is nonetheless recommended, and iron tablets should be stored out of reach of small children to avoid accidental ingestion, which can be severely toxic.

Special Concerns: The genetic disorder hemochromatosis, in which iron absorption is excessive, is very common. Iron deficiency may also be the first indication of a gastrointestinal malignancy. Therefore, iron should only be taken on the advice of a physician. Liquid forms of iron can stain the teeth. To prevent stains, mix each dose in water, fruit juice, or tomato juice and drink it through a straw. When using a dropper, place the dose on the back of the tongue and drink a glass of water or juice. Tooth stains can be removed by brushing with baking soda or 3% hydrogen peroxide.

OVERDOSE
Symptoms: Lethargy, nausea, vomiting, weak and rapid pulse, dehydration, loss of consciousness.

What to Do: Call your doctor, emergency medical services (EMS), or the nearest poison control center immediately.

▼ INTERACTIONS

DRUG INTERACTIONS
The following drugs may interact with ferrous salts and prevent their absorption: antacids, antibiotics, fluoroquinolones, levodopa, cholestyramine, or vitamin E. Consult your doctor for specific advice.

FOOD INTERACTIONS
Some foods can reduce the effect of this drug. The following foods should be avoided or taken in small amounts for at least 1 hour before and 2 hours after iron is taken: eggs, milk, spinach, cheese, yogurt, tea, coffee, whole-grain bread, cereal, and bran.

DISEASE INTERACTIONS
Consult your doctor if you have any of the following: a history of alcoholism; kidney disease; liver disease; porphyria; rheumatoid arthritis; asthma; allergies; heart disease; or a stomach ulcer, colitis, or another intestinal problem.

FEXOFENADINE

Available in: Capsules
Available OTC? No   **As Generic?** No
Drug Class: Antihistamine

▼ USAGE INFORMATION

WHY IT'S PRESCRIBED
To prevent or relieve symptoms of hay fever and other allergies, and to treat itchy skin and hives.

HOW IT WORKS
Fexofenadine blocks the effects of histamine, a naturally occurring substance within the body that causes swelling, itching, sneezing, watery eyes, hives, and other symptoms of allergic reaction.

▼ DOSAGE GUIDELINES

RANGE AND FREQUENCY
For adults and children age 12 and over: 60 mg, 2 times a day. For patients with decreased kidney function, a starting dose of 60 mg once a day is recommended. Children under age 12: Safety and effectiveness of fexofenadine in this age group have not been established.

ONSET OF EFFECT
Within 1 to 2 hours.

DURATION OF ACTION
12 hours or longer.

DIETARY ADVICE
This drug can be taken without regard to food or drink.

STORAGE
Store in a tightly sealed container in a dry place away from heat and direct light at room temperature.

MISSED DOSE
Take it as soon as you remember. If it is near the time for the next dose, skip the missed dose and resume your regular dosage schedule. Do not double the next dose.

STOPPING THE DRUG
You should take it as prescribed for the full treatment period, but you may stop if you are feeling better before the scheduled end of therapy. Fexofenadine can be used as needed to relieve symptoms of hay fever or other allergies.

PROLONGED USE
Tolerance, or decreased responsiveness to the drug, generally does not develop with prolonged use of fexofenadine; if it does, consult your physician. No special problems are expected with long-term use.

▼ SIDE EFFECTS

SERIOUS
No serious side effects are associated with the use of fexofenadine.

COMMON
No common side effects are associated with the use of fexofenadine.

LESS COMMON
Drowsiness, fatigue, stomach upset, painful menstrual bleeding.

▼ PRECAUTIONS

Over 60: No special problems are expected.

Driving and Hazardous Work: In rare cases fexofenadine may cause drowsiness and fatigue. Do not drive or engage in hazardous work until you determine how the medicine affects you.

Alcohol: No special precautions are necessary.

Pregnancy: Adequate and well-controlled studies in humans have not been done. Consult your doctor about taking fexofenadine if you are pregnant or are planning to become pregnant.

Breast Feeding: Fexofenadine may pass into breast milk; caution is advised. Consult your doctor for specific advice about the use of fexofenadine while nursing.

Infants and Children: Side effects are not expected to be any different in children ages 12 to 18 than those in patients 18 and older. The safety and effectiveness of fexofenadine for children up to 12 years of age have not been established.

OVERDOSE
Symptoms: Extreme drowsiness or fatigue.

What to Do: An overdose of fexofenadine is unlikely to be life-threatening. However, if someone takes a much larger dose than prescribed, call your doctor, emergency medical services (EMS), or local poison control right away.

▼ INTERACTIONS

DRUG INTERACTIONS
There are no known interactions between fexofenadine and other drugs.

FOOD INTERACTIONS
No known food interactions.

DISEASE INTERACTIONS
Consult your physician if you have impaired kidney function.

FEXOFENADINE/PSEUDOEPHEDRINE

Available in: Extended-release tablets
Available OTC? No   **As Generic?** No
Drug Class: Antihistamine/decongestant

▼ USAGE INFORMATION

WHY IT'S PRESCRIBED
To prevent or relieve symptoms of seasonal allergies, such as hay fever.

HOW IT WORKS
Fexofenadine blocks the effects of histamine, a naturally occurring substance within the body that causes swelling, itching, sneezing, watery eyes, hives, and other symptoms of allergic reaction. Pseudoephedrine narrows and constricts blood vessels to decrease the blood flow to swollen nasal passages and other tissues, which in turn reduces nasal secretions, shrinks swollen nasal mucous membranes, and improves airflow in nasal passages.

▼ DOSAGE GUIDELINES

RANGE AND FREQUENCY
Adults and teenagers: 1 tablet (60 mg fexofenadine/120 mg pseudoephedrine) twice a day.

ONSET OF EFFECT
Within 1 to 2 hours.

DURATION OF ACTION
12 hours or longer.

DIETARY ADVICE
This medication should be taken at least 1 hour before or 2 hours after a meal. Taking it with food delays the onset of the drug's effects. The tablet should be swallowed whole.

STORAGE
Store in a tightly sealed container away from heat, moisture, and direct light.

MISSED DOSE
Take it as soon as you remember. If it is near the time for the next dose, skip the missed dose and resume your regular dosage schedule. Do not double the next dose.

STOPPING THE DRUG
You may stop taking it before the scheduled end of therapy if you are feeling better.

PROLONGED USE
Consult your doctor about taking this drug for more than 5 to 7 days.

▼ PRECAUTIONS

Over 60: Adverse reactions may be more likely and more severe in older patients.

≡ SIDE EFFECTS ≡

SERIOUS
Palpitations, shortness of breath, breathing difficulty. Stop taking the medication and call your doctor right away.

COMMON
Headache, insomnia, nausea.

LESS COMMON
Dry mouth, indigestion, throat irritation, dizziness, agitation, back pain, anxiety, nervousness, stomach pain, upper respiratory infection.

Driving and Hazardous Work: Do not drive or engage in hazardous work until you determine how the medicine affects you.

Alcohol: No special warnings.

Pregnancy: Adequate human studies have not been done. Before taking this drug, tell your doctor if you are pregnant or are planning to become pregnant. Discuss with your doctor the relative risks and benefits of using this drug while pregnant.

Breast Feeding: The pseudoephedrine component of this drug passes into breast milk; avoid or discontinue taking this drug while breast feeding.

Infants and Children: Not recommended for use by children under age 12.

Special Concerns: If your symptoms do not improve within 7 days, check with your doctor. To help prevent insomnia, take the last dose at least 2 hours before your bedtime.

OVERDOSE
Symptoms: No cases of overdose have been reported.

What to Do: An overdose is unlikely; however, if you have reason to suspect an overdose has occurred, call emergency medical services (EMS) to receive evaluation and treatment.

▼ INTERACTIONS

DRUG INTERACTIONS
This drug and MAO inhibitors should not be used within 14 days of each other. Consult your doctor for advice if you are taking antihypertensives or digitalis drugs.

FOOD INTERACTIONS
No known food interactions.

DISEASE INTERACTIONS
You should not take this drug if you have a history of narrow-angle glaucoma, urinary retention, severe high blood pressure, or severe coronary artery disease. Caution is advised if you have mild to moderate high blood pressure, diabetes mellitus, a history of angina or heart attack, an overactive thyroid gland, impaired kidney function, or an enlarged prostate.

FINASTERIDE

Available in: Tablets
Available OTC? No   **As Generic?** No
Drug Class: 5-alpha reductase inhibitor

▼ USAGE INFORMATION

WHY IT'S PRESCRIBED
To treat benign prostatic hyperplasia (BPH)—that is, noncancerous enlargement of the prostate gland, which is extremely common among men over 50. Also used to treat male pattern hair loss.

HOW IT WORKS
Finasteride halts or reverses enlargement of the prostate by blocking the action of the enzyme 5-alpha reductase, which the body needs to produce dihydrotestosterone (DHT), a chemical involved in the mechanism that enlarges the prostate. DHT is also integral to the processs of male pattern hair loss; by decreasing DHT concentrations in the scalp, finasteride may slow or reverse this process.

▼ DOSAGE GUIDELINES

RANGE AND FREQUENCY
For BPH: 5 mg once a day. For male pattern hair loss: 1 mg once a day.

ONSET OF EFFECT
Unknown.

DURATION OF ACTION
For BPH: 24 hours for a single dose; up to 2 weeks after standard therapy is ended. For hair loss: New hair resulting from finasteride treatments will likely regress following discontinuation of the medication.

DIETARY ADVICE
Finasteride can be taken without regard to diet. If you have trouble swallowing the tablet whole, you can crush it and take it with liquid or food.

STORAGE
Store in a tightly sealed container away from heat, moisture, and direct light.

MISSED DOSE
If you miss a dose on one day, do not double the dose the next day.

STOPPING THE DRUG
The decision to stop taking the drug should be made by your doctor.

PROLONGED USE
If you take this drug for a prolonged period for BPH, see your doctor regularly so that changes in prostate size can be monitored. For hair loss, continued use is recommended to sustain the drug's benefits.

▼ PRECAUTIONS

Over 60: No special problems are expected.

Driving and Hazardous Work: The use of finasteride should not impair your ability to perform such tasks safely.

Alcohol: No special precautions are necessary.

Pregnancy: Although finasteride is not prescribed for women, those who are pregnant or planning to become pregnant should not handle the medication, especially if it is crushed or broken, because it can have an adverse effect on a male fetus. Men who take finasteride should use a barrier method of birth control (such as a condom), which prevents the female sexual partner from being exposed to small quantities of the drug present in semen.

Breast Feeding: Women who are nursing should avoid contact with finasteride or the sperm of a man who is taking the drug.

Infants and Children: Finasteride is not prescribed for children.

Special Concerns: Before taking this medicine for BPH, you should have a digital rectal examination and other tests for prostate cancer. Note that finasteride may affect the results of the prostate-specific antigen (PSA) test for prostate cancer; be sure any doctor you see for treatment, including your dentist, knows that you are taking this drug.

OVERDOSE
Symptoms: No specific ones have been reported.

What to Do: An overdose of finasteride is unlikely to be life-threatening. However, if someone takes a much larger dose than prescribed, call your doctor, emergency medical services (EMS), or the nearest poison control center.

▼ INTERACTIONS

DRUG INTERACTIONS
Consult your doctor for specific advice if you are taking amantadine, amphetamines, antihistamines, antidepressants, antidyskinetics (medications for Parkinson's disease or similar conditions), antipsychotics, appetite suppressants, anticholinergics (medications for stomach spasms or cramps), bronchodilators, decongestants, ephedrine, phenylpropanolamine, or pseudoephedrine.

FOOD INTERACTIONS
No known food interactions.

DISEASE INTERACTIONS
Caution is advised when taking finasteride. Before you start, consult your doctor if you have liver disease, which may magnify the effects of finasteride.

≡ SIDE EFFECTS ≡

SERIOUS
No serious side effects are associated with the use of finasteride.

COMMON
No common side effects are associated with the use of finasteride.

LESS COMMON
Reduced sex drive, erectile dysfunction (impotence), decreased quantity of ejaculate. It should be noted that this decrease is not a sign of reduced fertility.

379

FLAVOXATE

Available in: Tablets
Available OTC? No   **As Generic?** No
Drug Class: Urinary tract antispasmodic

▼ USAGE INFORMATION

WHY IT'S PRESCRIBED
To relieve the symptoms of urinary tract spasms, which may include chronic urinary urgency, frequent urination, pain, and incontinence.

HOW IT WORKS
Flavoxate blocks nerve impulses to the smooth muscles of the urinary tract, preventing muscle contraction in the bladder.

▼ DOSAGE GUIDELINES

RANGE AND FREQUENCY
Adults and teenagers: 100 to 200 mg, 3 or 4 times a day.

ONSET OF EFFECT
45 to 60 minutes.

DURATION OF ACTION
Unknown.

DIETARY ADVICE
Take flavoxate with water 30 minutes before meals unless your physician advises otherwise. If it causes stomach upset, ask your physician if you can take it with food or milk.

STORAGE
Store in a tightly sealed container away from heat, moisture, and direct light.

MISSED DOSE
Take it as soon as you remember. If it is near the time for the next dose, skip the missed dose and resume your regular dosage schedule. Do not double the next dose.

STOPPING THE DRUG
Take as prescribed for the full treatment period, even if you begin to feel better before the scheduled end of therapy.

PROLONGED USE
Tell your doctor if symptoms do not improve after prolonged use of this drug.

▼ PRECAUTIONS

Over 60:
Adverse reactions, especially confusion, may be more likely and more severe in older patients.

Driving and Hazardous Work:
Do not drive or engage in hazardous work until you determine how the medicine affects you.

SIDE EFFECTS

SERIOUS
Rash, fever, rapid pulse. Call your doctor right away.

COMMON
Confusion, dry mouth and throat, blurred vision, heightened sensitivity of the eyes to light (photophobia), decreased ability to sweat.

LESS COMMON
Dizziness, headache, nervousness, drowsiness, difficulty concentrating, abdominal pain, difficulty focusing the eyes, constipation, nausea, vomiting, hives, fever.

Alcohol: No special warnings.

Pregnancy: Flavoxate has not been shown to cause birth defects in animals. Adequate human studies have not been done. Before you take the medicine, tell your doctor if you are pregnant or plan to become pregnant; you must weigh the drug's benefits against the risks.

Breast Feeding: Flavoxate may pass into breast milk; caution is advised. Consult your doctor for advice.

Infants and Children: Not generally recommended for use by children under the age of 12. If flavoxate is prescribed for children, the dose should be determined by your pediatrician, and it should be given under close medical supervision.

Special Concerns: Limit exposure to sunlight and wear sunglasses in bright light. Avoid overexertion, since flavoxate interferes with the ability to sweat, which may lead to heatstroke. Use sugarless gum, candy, or ice chips to relieve dry mouth. Contact your doctor 2 months prior to having any surgery (including dental surgery) that will require general or spinal anesthesia. Tell your doctor if you experience abdominal bloating or difficulty emptying your bladder completely.

OVERDOSE

Symptoms: Rapid pulse and breathing, dilated pupils, dizziness, fever, hallucinations, slurred speech, confusion, agitation, unusual excitability, flushed face, convulsions, loss of consciousness.

What to Do: Call your doctor, emergency medical services (EMS), or the nearest poison control center immediately.

▼ INTERACTIONS

DRUG INTERACTIONS
Certain drugs may interact adversely with flavoxate or interfere with its action. Consult your doctor if you are taking cholinergic drugs. Also, tell your doctor if you are taking any other prescription or over-the-counter medicine before you take flavoxate.

FOOD INTERACTIONS
No known food interactions.

DISEASE INTERACTIONS
Caution is advised when taking flavoxate. Consult your doctor if you have any of the following: severe bleeding, narrow-angle glaucoma, angina, intestinal obstruction, urinary tract blockage, hiatal hernia, an enlarged prostate, myasthenia gravis, or a peptic ulcer.

FLECAINIDE ACETATE

Available in: Tablets
Available OTC? No   **As Generic?** No
Drug Class: Antiarrhythmic

▼ USAGE INFORMATION

WHY IT'S PRESCRIBED
To stabilize irregular heart-beats (cardiac arrhythmias).

HOW IT WORKS
Flecainide slows nerve impulses in the heart and makes heart tissue less sensitive to nerve impulses, thus stabilizing heartbeat.

▼ DOSAGE GUIDELINES

RANGE AND FREQUENCY
For paroxysmal supraventricular tachycardia or paroxysmal atrial fibrillation, or flutter, in persons without structural heart disease: Starting with 50 mg every 12 hours, increased by 50 mg every 4 days if necessary to a maximum of 150 mg every 12 hours. For life-threatening heart arrhythmias: Starting with 100 mg every 12 hours, increased by 50 mg every 4 days if necessary to a maximum of 200 mg every 12 hours. Initial dose should be lower in patients who have impaired heart or kidney function.

ONSET OF EFFECT
1 to 6 hours. May require daily doses for 3 to 5 days for full effect to occur.

DURATION OF ACTION
12 to 27 hours (longer in patients with impaired heart or kidney function).

DIETARY ADVICE
Take tablet with liquid. May be taken with or between meals.

STORAGE
Store in a tightly sealed container in a dry place away from heat and direct light.

MISSED DOSE
Take it as soon as you remember, up to 6 hours late. If more than 6 hours, skip the missed dose and resume your regular dosage schedule as prescribed. Do not double the next dose.

STOPPING THE DRUG
Take as prescribed for the full treatment period, even if you begin to feel better before the scheduled end of therapy. The decision to stop taking the drug should be made by your doctor.

PROLONGED USE
Lifelong therapy may be necessary. See your doctor regularly for examinations and diagnostic tests if you must take this medicine for a prolonged period.

▼ PRECAUTIONS

Over 60: Adverse reactions, especially heartbeat irregularities, may be more common and more severe in older patients.

Driving and Hazardous Work: Do not drive or engage in hazardous work until you determine how the medicine affects you.

Alcohol: Alcohol should be avoided while taking this medicine because it may further depress normal heart function.

Pregnancy: In animal studies large doses of flecainide have been shown to cause birth defects. Human studies have not been done. Before taking flecainide, tell your doctor if you are pregnant or plan to become pregnant.

Breast Feeding: Flecainide passes into breast milk and may cause harm to the infant; avoid or discontinue use while nursing.

Infants and Children: Not recommended for use by patients under age 18.

Special Concerns: Before you have any surgery (including dental surgery) or receive emergency medical care, be sure to tell the doctor or dentist that you are using flecainide. If you have a pacemaker, its function should be assessed shortly after starting therapy with flecainide.

OVERDOSE
Symptoms: Dizziness or faintness, rapid or irregular heartbeat, tremor, unusual or profuse sweating, drowsiness, loss of consciousness.

What to Do: Call your doctor, emergency medical services (EMS), or the nearest poison control center immediately.

▼ INTERACTIONS

DRUG INTERACTIONS
The following drugs may interact with flecainide. Consult your doctor if you are taking antacids, amiodarone or other antiarrhythmic drugs, beta-blockers, calcium channel blockers, bone marrow depressants, carbonic anhydrase inhibitors, carbamazepine, cimetidine, digitalis drugs, doxepin, nicotine, phenobarbital, or phenytoin.

FOOD INTERACTIONS
Caffeine-containing beverages can decrease flecainide activity. No other food interactions are expected.

DISEASE INTERACTIONS
Use of flecainide may cause complications in patients with heart disease, heart block, or slow heart rates, and may cause complications in patients with liver or kidney disease, since these organs work together to remove the medication from the body.

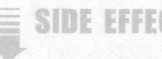
SIDE EFFECTS

SERIOUS
Shortness of breath, chest pain, irregular or rapid heartbeat, fainting, swollen feet or lower extremities, shaking or trembling. Call your doctor immediately.

COMMON
Headache; dizziness or lightheadedness; blurred vision or other visual disturbances, such as seeing spots.

LESS COMMON
Nausea, constipation, tremor, fatigue, abdominal pain, swollen hands, skin rash, anxiety, mental depression.

FLUCONAZOLE

Available in: Tablets, oral suspension, injection
Available OTC? No   **As Generic?** No
Drug Class: Antifungal

▼ USAGE INFORMATION

WHY IT'S PRESCRIBED
To treat fungal infections of the mouth and throat (thrush), of the vagina (yeast infection), or throughout the body, as well as meningitis (inflammation of the protective membranes surrounding the brain). Often used to treat AIDS-related fungal infections. May also be used to prevent recurring fungal infections in susceptible patients weakened by AIDS or by chemotherapy or radiation treatment.

HOW IT WORKS
Fluconazole prevents fungal organisms from manufacturing vital substances required for their growth and function. This drug is effective only for infections caused by fungal organisms. It will not work for bacterial or viral infections.

▼ DOSAGE GUIDELINES

RANGE AND FREQUENCY
Adults and teenagers— For fungal infections: 200 to 400 mg on the first day, then 100 to 400 mg once a day. For vaginal yeast infection: 1 dose of 150 mg, tablet or oral suspension.

ONSET OF EFFECT
Oral forms: Unknown. Injection: Immediate.

DURATION OF ACTION
Unknown.

DIETARY ADVICE
Swallow tablets with liquid. Oral suspension should be shaken and carefully measured out before you take it. This drug can be taken without regard to diet.

STORAGE
Store in a tightly sealed container away from heat, moisture, and direct light. Keep any liquid form refrigerated, but do not allow it to freeze.

MISSED DOSE
Take it as soon as you remember. This will help keep a constant level of medication in your system. If it is near the time for the next dose, skip the missed dose and resume your regular dosage schedule. Do not double the next dose.

STOPPING THE DRUG
Take it as prescribed for the full treatment period, even if you begin to feel better before the scheduled end of therapy. The decision to stop taking the drug should be made by your doctor. Gradual reduction of the dose may be necessary if you have been taking this medicine for a long time.

PROLONGED USE
Notify your doctor if your condition does not improve, or instead becomes worse, within a few weeks.

▼ PRECAUTIONS

Over 60: Dosage may need to be reduced in older patients with impaired kidney function.

Driving and Hazardous Work: The use of fluconazole should not impair your ability to perform such tasks safely.

Alcohol: No special precautions are necessary.

Pregnancy: Adequate studies of fluconazole use during pregnancy have not been done. Consult your doctor for specific advice if you are currently pregnant or plan to become pregnant.

Breast Feeding: Fluconazole may pass into breast milk; caution is advised. Consult your doctor for advice.

Infants and Children: Fluconazole is not generally prescribed for children under 14.

Special Concerns: Your doctor should monitor your kidney function while you take fluconazole. Tell any doctor or dentist whom you consult that you are taking this medicine. Be sure to shake the oral suspension well before taking it.

OVERDOSE
Symptoms: An overdose with fluconazole is unlikely.

What to Do: Emergency instructions not applicable.

▼ INTERACTIONS

DRUG INTERACTIONS
Do not take cisapride with fluconazole. Other drugs may interact with fluconazole. Consult your doctor for advice if you are taking oral antidiabetic drugs, cyclosporine, rifampin, phenytoin, rifabutin, tacrolimus, astemizole, or warfarin.

FOOD INTERACTIONS
No food interactions have been reported.

DISEASE INTERACTIONS
Caution is advised when taking fluconazole. Consult your doctor if you have a history of alcohol abuse (and associated liver problems), or any type of liver or kidney disease, since these organs work together to remove the medication from the body.

 SIDE EFFECTS

SERIOUS
Skin rash or itching, fever or chills. Call your doctor right away.

COMMON
No common side effects have been reported with the use of fluconazole.

LESS COMMON
Diarrhea, nausea, vomiting, constipation, dizziness, headache, redness or flushing of skin.

FLUCYTOSINE

Available in: Capsules
Available OTC? No   **As Generic?** No
Drug Class: Antifungal

▼ USAGE INFORMATION

WHY IT'S PRESCRIBED
To treat general fungal infections and severe fungal infections of the bone and bone marrow (osteomyelitis), the protective layers of tissue surrounding the brain (meningitis), the respiratory tract (pneumonia), the blood (septicemia), and the genitourinary tract (particularly those infections associated with AIDS).

HOW IT WORKS
Flucytosine kills infectious microorganisms by preventing them from synthesizing genetic material (RNA and DNA), thereby preventing the cells from reproducing.

▼ DOSAGE GUIDELINES

RANGE AND FREQUENCY
Adults and children: Usual dose is 12.5 to 37.5 mg per 2.2 lbs (1 kg) of body weight every 6 hours.

ONSET OF EFFECT
Unknown.

DURATION OF ACTION
Unknown.

DIETARY ADVICE
Flucytosine can be taken without regard to diet. You should take a few capsules at a time, over a 15-minute period, with food to reduce stomach distress.

STORAGE
Store in a tightly sealed container away from heat, moisture, and direct light.

MISSED DOSE
Take it as soon as you remember. If it is near the time for the next dose, skip the missed dose and resume your regular dosage schedule. Do not double the next dose.

STOPPING THE DRUG
Take it as prescribed for the full treatment period, even if you begin to feel better before the scheduled end of therapy. The decision to stop taking the drug should be made by your doctor.

PROLONGED USE
Prolonged use may cause or aggravate bone marrow depression (reduced bone marrow function), liver damage, or kidney damage. Consult your doctor about the need for periodic blood cell counts and liver and kidney function tests.

▼ PRECAUTIONS

Over 60: Dosage must be reduced in older patients who have impaired kidney function.

Driving and Hazardous Work: Do not drive or engage in hazardous work until you determine how the medicine affects you. Use of this drug may be a disqualification for piloting aircraft.

Alcohol: No special precautions are necessary.

Pregnancy: Adequate studies of flucytosine use during pregnancy have not been done. Consult your doctor for specific advice if you are pregnant or are planning to become pregnant.

Breast Feeding: Flucytosine may pass into breast milk; it is unclear if this poses any risks to the nursing infant. Consult your doctor for specific advice.

Infants and Children: No special problems are expected in young patients.

Special Concerns: Stay out of direct sunlight, especially between 10 am and 3 pm. Wear protective clothing, including a hat, and sunglasses. Apply a sun block with a sun protection factor (SPF) of at least 15. This medicine is generally given in conjunction with amphotericin B to avoid development of drug resistance. Flucytosine may cause infection of the gums. Be careful when using a toothbrush, toothpick, or dental floss. Avoid dental work while taking this drug.

OVERDOSE
Symptoms: Severe nausea, vomiting, abdominal pain, diarrhea, mental confusion.

What to Do: An overdose of flucytosine is unlikely to be life-threatening. However, if someone takes a much larger dose than prescribed, call your doctor, emergency medical services (EMS), or nearest poison control center immediately.

▼ INTERACTIONS

DRUG INTERACTIONS
Other drugs may interact with flucytosine. Consult your doctor for advice if you are taking amphotericin B injection, cytosine, or bone marrow depressants, or if you are undergoing radiation therapy.

FOOD INTERACTIONS
No known food interactions.

DISEASE INTERACTIONS
Caution is advised when taking flucytosine. Consult your doctor if you have bone marrow depression or liver or kidney disease. Use of flucytosine may cause complications in patients with liver or kidney disease, since these organs work together to remove the medication from the body.

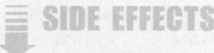 SIDE EFFECTS

SERIOUS
Unusual fatigue, yellow eyes or skin, unusual bleeding or bruising, skin rash, redness, or itching, sore throat, fever, increased sensitivity of eyes to sunlight, confusion, hallucinations. Call your doctor immediately.

COMMON
Loss of appetite, abdominal pain, stomach upset, nausea and vomiting, diarrhea.

LESS COMMON
Dizziness or lightheadedness, headache, unusual drowsiness.

FLUDROCORTISONE

Available in: Tablets
Available OTC? No   **As Generic?** No
Drug Class: Corticosteroid

▼ USAGE INFORMATION

WHY IT'S PRESCRIBED
To supplement inadequate production of a specific salt-retaining corticosteroid hormone in the body, which leads to conditions known as adrenocortical insufficiency and adrenogenital syndrome. Untreated, these disorders can cause premature puberty in boys, masculinization in females, and even death.

HOW IT WORKS
Fludrocortisone performs the same functions as one of the body's normal corticosteroid hormones called "aldosterone."

▼ DOSAGE GUIDELINES

RANGE AND FREQUENCY
For adrenocortical insufficiency— Adults: 50 to 200 micrograms (mcg) once a day. Children: 50 to 100 mcg once a day. For adrenogenital syndrome— Adults: 100 to 200 mcg once a day.

ONSET OF EFFECT
Variable.

DURATION OF ACTION
1 to 2 days.

DIETARY ADVICE
Can be taken with or between meals. Best taken with a full glass of water. Carefully monitor the amount of sodium in your diet. Excess sodium will increase potassium loss. Eat foods rich in potassium.

STORAGE
Store in a tightly sealed container in a dry place away from heat and direct light.

MISSED DOSE
Take it as soon as you remember. If it is near the time for the next dose, skip the missed dose and resume your regular dosage schedule. Do not double the next dose. Notify your physician if more than one dose is missed or a dose cannot be taken due to vomiting or nausea.

STOPPING THE DRUG
The decision to stop taking the drug should be made by your doctor.

PROLONGED USE
Your doctor may need to monitor your blood pressure, blood serum electrolyte (mineral salt) concentration, and other variables if you must take this medicine for a prolonged period.

▼ PRECAUTIONS

Over 60: Adverse reactions may be more likely and more severe in older patients.

Driving and Hazardous Work: Do not drive or engage in hazardous work until you determine how the medicine affects you.

Alcohol: No special warnings.

Pregnancy: Studies on birth defects in animals and humans have not been done. Before you take fludrocortisone, tell your doctor if you are pregnant or plan to become pregnant, to determine whether benefits outweigh potential risks.

Breast Feeding: Fludrocortisone passes into breast milk; consult your doctor.

Infants and Children: It can be used safely when needed; consult your pediatrician.

Special Concerns: Your doctor may ask you to follow a diet that is low in sodium and high in potassium and protein to avoid high blood pressure and excessive accumulation of water in the body. You should drink lots of water every day, unless your doctor directs otherwise.

OVERDOSE
Symptoms: Dizziness, weakness, swelling of hands and feet, excessive weight gain.

What to Do: Call your doctor, emergency medical services (EMS), or the nearest poison control center immediately.

▼ INTERACTIONS

DRUG INTERACTIONS
Consult your doctor for specific advice if you are taking acetazolamide, amphotericin B, capreomycin, carbenicillin, corticotropin (ACTH), dichlorphenamide, a diuretic, an antiglaucoma drug, insulin or oral antidiabetic agents, laxatives, methazolamide, mezlocillin, piperacillin, a salicylate, aspirin, sodium bicarbonate, ticarcillin, vitamin B, vitamin D, a barbiturate, carbamazepine, griseofulvin, phenylbutazone, phenytoin, primidone, rifampin, digitalis drugs, another steroid, or any medication that contains sodium.

FOOD INTERACTIONS
High-sodium foods should be avoided.

DISEASE INTERACTIONS
Caution is advised if you have any of the following: bone disease, edema (swelling due to fluid retention), heart disease, high blood pressure, kidney disease, liver disease, or thyroid disease. Use of fludrocortisone may cause complications in patients with liver or kidney disease, since these organs work together to remove the medication from the body.

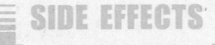

SIDE EFFECTS

SERIOUS
Headache and blurred vision caused by high blood pressure; low body potassium levels, causing cramps, weakness, and heart palpitations. Call your doctor immediately.

COMMON
Mild swelling of hands and feet.

LESS COMMON
Dizziness, difficulty swallowing, headache, hives, itchiness, rash, cough, vomiting, sudden weight gain, retention of sodium and water in the body.

FLUNISOLIDE

BRAND NAMES

AeroBid, AeroBid-M, Nasalide, Nasarel

Available in: Oral inhalation, nasal spray
Available OTC? No   **As Generic?** No
Drug Class: Respiratory corticosteroid

▼ USAGE INFORMATION

WHY IT'S PRESCRIBED
To treat bronchial asthma; to treat allergic rhinitis (seasonal allergies, such as hay fever); to prevent recurrence of nasal polyps after they have been removed surgically.

HOW IT WORKS
Respiratory corticosteroids such as flunisolide primarily reduce or prevent inflammation of the lining of the airways (the underlying cause of asthma), reduce the allergic response to inhaled allergens, and inhibit the secretion of mucus within the airways.

▼ DOSAGE GUIDELINES

RANGE AND FREQUENCY
Oral inhalation– Adults: 2 inhalations of 250 micrograms (mcg) each twice a day, morning and evening. Maximum dose is 4 inhalations twice a day. Children: Do not exceed 2 inhalations twice a day. Nasal spray– Adults and teenagers 15 and older: 2 sprays of 25 mcg in each nostril twice a day. Maximum dose is 8 sprays in each nostril a day. Children ages 6 to 14: One spray of 25 mcg in each nostril 3 times a day, or 2 sprays in each nostril twice a day. Maximum dose is 4 sprays in each nostril a day.

ONSET OF EFFECT
Usually within 1 week; it may take 3 weeks for the full effect to occur.

DURATION OF ACTION
Unknown.

DIETARY ADVICE
No special restrictions.

STORAGE
Store the inhaler in a dry place away from heat and direct light.

MISSED DOSE
Take it as soon as you remember. If it is near the time for the next dose, skip the missed dose and resume your regular dosage schedule. Do not double the next dose.

STOPPING THE DRUG
If you have been using flunisolide for a long period, do not stop taking it suddenly. Consult your doctor about how to stop.

PROLONGED USE
Consult your doctor about the need for continuing medical exams or laboratory tests.

▼ PRECAUTIONS

Over 60: No special problems are expected with older patients.

Driving and Hazardous Work: Do not drive or engage in hazardous work until you determine how the medicine affects you.

Alcohol: No special precautions are necessary.

Pregnancy: Flunisolide has not been reported to cause birth defects if taken during pregnancy. Before using this drug, tell your doctor if you are pregnant or plan to become pregnant.

Breast Feeding: Flunisolide may pass into breast milk; caution is advised. Consult your doctor for advice.

Infants and Children: Not recommended for children under the age of 6. The drug may inhibit growth and make children more susceptible to infection. If a younger person takes this medicine, be careful to avoid exposure to chicken pox and measles.

Special Concerns: Inhaled steroids will not help an asthma attack in progress. They can lower resistance to yeast infections of the mouth, throat, or voice box. To prevent yeast infections, gargle or rinse your mouth with water after each use; do not swallow the water. Know how to use the spray; read and follow the directions that come with the device. Before you have surgery, tell the doctor or dentist that you are using a steroid.

OVERDOSE
Symptoms: No specific ones have been reported.

What to Do: An overdose of flunisolide is unlikely to be life-threatening. However, if someone takes a much larger dose than prescribed, or if you have any reason to suspect an overdose, call your doctor, emergency medical services (EMS), or the nearest poison control center.

▼ INTERACTIONS

DRUG INTERACTIONS
Consult your doctor for specific advice if you are taking systemic corticosteroids, other inhaled corticosteroids, or drugs that suppress the immune system.

FOOD INTERACTIONS
No known food interactions.

DISEASE INTERACTIONS
Consult your doctor if you have a history of tuberculosis, herpes simplex infection of the eye, chickenpox, chronic bronchitis or bronchiectasis, osteoporosis, underactive thyroid, liver disease, glaucoma, measles, recent injury to the nose or nose surgery, or any active infection.

≣ SIDE EFFECTS ≣

SERIOUS
No serious side effects are associated with the use of flunisolide.

COMMON
Oral inhalation: Sore throat, white patches in mouth or throat, hoarseness. Nasal spray: Nosebleeds or bloody nasal secretions, nasal burning or irritation, sore throat.

LESS COMMON
Eye pain, watering eyes, gradual decrease of vision, stomach pain and digestive disturbances.

FLUOROMETHOLONE

Available in: Ophthalmic ointment, suspension
Available OTC? No   **As Generic?** No
Drug Class: Corticosteroid

▼ USAGE INFORMATION

WHY IT'S PRESCRIBED
To control inflammation and prevent potentially permanent damage that may result from various conditions involving inflammation in the tissues of the eye.

HOW IT WORKS
Fluorometholone inhibits the release of substances that stimulate an inflammatory reaction and pain in eye tissues.

▼ DOSAGE GUIDELINES

RANGE AND FREQUENCY
Ointment: Apply to eye 1 to 3 times a day, according to doctor's instructions. Suspension: 1 or 2 drops, 2 to 4 times a day. For severe conditions, more frequent application of either form may be recommended initially; the dosage will be decreased as inflammation subsides.

ONSET OF EFFECT
Unknown.

DURATION OF ACTION
Unknown.

≡ SIDE EFFECTS ≡

SERIOUS
Decreased or blurred vision (from cataract); eye pain, nausea, vomiting (from increased eye pressure); pain, redness, sensitivity to bright light, discharge (from eye infection). Call your doctor immediately if you experience any of these signs or symptoms.

COMMON
Increased eye pressure; this is usually reversed once the drug is stopped.

LESS COMMON
Burning, stinging, redness, or watering of eyes.

DIETARY ADVICE
No special restrictions.

STORAGE
Store in a tightly sealed container away from heat, moisture, and direct light. Do not allow it to freeze.

MISSED DOSE
Apply it as soon as you remember. If it is near the time for the next dose, skip the missed dose and resume your regular dosage schedule. Do not double the next dose.

STOPPING THE DRUG
It is very important to take this drug as prescribed for the full treatment period, even if symptoms improve before the scheduled end of therapy.

PROLONGED USE
See your doctor regularly for tests and examinations if you must take this drug for a prolonged period.

▼ PRECAUTIONS

Over 60: No special problems are expected.

Driving and Hazardous Work: Do not drive or engage in hazardous work until you determine how the medicine affects your vision.

Alcohol: No special precautions are necessary.

Pregnancy: Adequate human studies have not been done, although there have been no reports of birth defects. Before taking fluorometholone, tell your doctor if you are pregnant or are planning to become pregnant.

Breast Feeding: This medicine has not been reported to cause problems in nursing babies. Consult your doctor for specific advice.

Infants and Children: Safety and effectiveness have not been established for children under 2 years of age.

Special Concerns: To use the eye drops or the ointment, first wash your hands. Tilt your head back. Gently apply pressure to the inside corner of the eyelid and with the index finger of the same hand, pull downward on the lower eyelid to make a space. Drop the medicine or put a short strip of ointment (about 1/3 inch long) into this space and close your eye. Apply pressure for 1 or 2 minutes while keeping the eye closed without blinking. Then wash your hands again. Make sure the tip of the dropper or the applicator does not touch your eye, finger, or any other surface. If your symptoms do not improve in 5 to 7 days or if they become worse, check with your doctor. Wearing contact lenses while using this medication may increase the risk of infection. Your doctor may tell you not to wear contact lenses during treatment and for a day or two afterward.

OVERDOSE
Symptoms: When used topically, an overdose of fluorometholone is very unlikely. Inadvertent oral ingestion, however, may cause fever, muscle pain, loss of appetite, dizziness, fainting, and difficulty breathing.

What to Do: In case of accidental ingestion, call your doctor, emergency medical services (EMS), or the nearest poison control right away.

▼ INTERACTIONS

DRUG INTERACTIONS
Other medications may interact with fluorometholone. Consult your doctor for specific advice if you are taking any other prescription or over-the-counter medication, especially any preparation designed for use in the eyes.

FOOD INTERACTIONS
No known food interactions.

DISEASE INTERACTIONS
Consult your doctor if you have a history of cataracts, diabetes mellitus, glaucoma, herpes infection of the eye, fungal infection of the eye, or any other eye infection.

FLUOROURACIL (5-FLUOROURACIL; 5-FU)

Available in: Cream, topical solution
Available OTC? No   **As Generic?** No
Drug Class: Antimetabolite

▼ USAGE INFORMATION

WHY IT'S PRESCRIBED
To treat actinic keratosis (a type of precancerous skin lesion). It is prescribed generally for multiple lesions or when limited access to a lesion makes other methods of removal difficult.

HOW IT WORKS
Topical fluorouracil kills precancerous cells by interfering with the activity of their genetic material, thus preventing the cells from reproducing. The drug selectively destroys cells that multiply rapidly, as many malignant cells do.

▼ DOSAGE GUIDELINES

RANGE AND FREQUENCY
For precancerous skin lesions— Adults: Apply 1% cream or 5% solution to the affected area 1 or 2 times a day. The 5% cream is sometimes prescribed. Children: Consult your pediatrician.

ONSET OF EFFECT
From 2 to 7 days. The complete effect may require 2 to 6 weeks, or even 12 weeks for some patients. Complete healing may require 1 or 2 months after the drug has been stopped.

DURATION OF ACTION
Up to 24 hours.

DIETARY ADVICE
Fluorouracil may be applied without regard to diet.

STORAGE
Store in a tightly sealed container away from heat and direct light.

MISSED DOSE
Apply it as soon as you remember. If it is near the time for the next application, skip the missed dose and resume your regular dosage schedule. Do not double the next dose.

STOPPING THE DRUG
Apply fluorouracil for the entire duration of therapy, as prescribed. The decision to stop the drug should be made by your doctor.

PROLONGED USE
No problems are expected with prolonged use, but check regularly with your physician. Treatment usually lasts 2 to 8 weeks for precancerous lesions. Your physician may order a biopsy if the condition does not clear up.

▼ PRECAUTIONS

Over 60: No special problems are expected.

Driving and Hazardous Work: The use of fluorouracil should not impair your ability to perform such tasks safely.

Alcohol: No special precautions are necessary.

Pregnancy: Some fluorouracil is absorbed through the skin and may affect the unborn child. Before using, tell your doctor if you are pregnant or plan to become pregnant.

Breast Feeding: Fluorouracil passes into breast milk; avoid or discontinue usage while nursing.

Infants and Children: Fluorouracil is generally not prescribed for infants and children, but you should consult your doctor about its use for young patients.

Special Concerns: While you use fluorouracil, and for 1 or 2 months afterward, your skin may become much more sensitive to sunlight, and sunlight may increase the effect of the drug. During this period, stay out of direct sunlight, especially between 10 am and 3 pm. Wear protective clothing, including a hat and sunglasses. Apply a sun block that has a sun protection factor (SPF) of at least 15. When applying fluorouracil, wash the area with soap and water and use a cotton-tipped applicator or your fingertips to apply the drug. Wash your hands immediately to prevent any of the medicine from accidentally getting into your eyes or mouth.

OVERDOSE
Symptoms: No specific ones have been reported.

What to Do: An overdose is unlikely. However, if topical fluorouracil is accidentally swallowed, call your doctor, emergency medical services (EMS), or nearest poison control center.

▼ INTERACTIONS

DRUG INTERACTIONS
None known.

FOOD INTERACTIONS
No known food interactions.

DISEASE INTERACTIONS
Caution is advised when taking fluorouracil. Consult your doctor if you have any other skin problem.

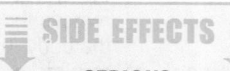
≣ SIDE EFFECTS ≣

SERIOUS
Severe redness, swelling, and tenderness of otherwise healthy regions of skin.

COMMON
Burning sensation where medicine is applied, increased sensitivity of skin to sunlight, redness, swelling, itching, rash, tenderness, pain, or oozing and crusting of the skin.

LESS COMMON
Hyperpigmentation (darkening) of skin, scaling, scarring, watery eyes.

FLUOXETINE HYDROCHLORIDE

Available in: Capsules, oral solution
Available OTC? No   **As Generic?** No
Drug Class: Selective serotonin reuptake inhibitor (SSRI) antidepressant

▼ USAGE INFORMATION

WHY IT'S PRESCRIBED
To treat major depression, obsessive-compulsive disorder, panic disorder, and chronic pain.

HOW IT WORKS
Fluoxetine affects levels of serotonin, a brain chemical that is thought to be linked to mood, emotions, and mental state.

▼ DOSAGE GUIDELINES

RANGE AND FREQUENCY
To start, 20 mg a day, taken in the morning. Your doctor may increase the dose gradually to a maximum of 80 mg a day. Older adults: To start, 10 to 20 mg a day. It may be increased gradually by your doctor to a maximum of 40 to 60 mg a day.

ONSET OF EFFECT
1 to 4 weeks.

DURATION OF ACTION
Unknown.

DIETARY ADVICE
Taking the drug with liquid or food can lessen stomach irritation. Capsules may be opened and mixed with food or juice if the patient has difficulty swallowing them.

STORAGE
Store in a tightly sealed container away from heat, moisture, and direct light. Keep the liquid form refrigerated, but do not allow it to freeze.

MISSED DOSE
Take it as soon as you remember. If it is near the time for the next dose, skip the missed dose and resume your regular dosage schedule. Do not double the next dose.

STOPPING THE DRUG
Take it as prescribed for the full treatment period, even if you begin to feel better. Discontinuing the drug abruptly may produce unpleasant withdrawal symptoms. Dosage should be reduced gradually according to your doctor's instructions.

PROLONGED USE
The usual course of therapy lasts 6 months to 1 year; some patients benefit from additional therapy. The usual course of therapy for obsessive-compulsive disorder lasts 1 year or more.

▼ PRECAUTIONS

Over 60: Adverse reactions may be more likely and more severe in older patients, since their metabolism is slower. A lower dose may be warranted.

Driving and Hazardous Work: Use caution when driving or engaging in hazardous work until you determine how the medicine affects you.

Alcohol: Avoid alcohol.

Pregnancy: Fluoxetine should be used during pregnancy only if the potential benefit justifies the potential risk to the fetus. Before you take this medicine, tell your doctor if you are pregnant or plan to become pregnant.

Breast Feeding: Fluoxetine may pass into breast milk; caution is advised. Consult your doctor for advice.

Infants and Children: Not recommended for use by children under age 12.

Special Concerns: Take it at least 6 hours before bedtime to prevent insomnia, unless the drug causes drowsiness.

OVERDOSE
Symptoms: Agitation, excitement, severe nausea and vomiting, seizures.

What to Do: Call your doctor, emergency medical services (EMS), or the nearest poison control center immediately.

▼ INTERACTIONS

DRUG INTERACTIONS
Fluoxetine and MAO inhibitors should not be used within 5 weeks of each other. The following drugs may interact with fluoxetine. Consult your doctor for specific advice if you are taking nortriptyline, caffeine, oral anticoagulants, central nervous system depressants, digitalis preparations, lithium, loratadine, dextromethorphan, ketorolac, buspirone, phenytoin, trazodone, tryptophan, sumatriptan, naratriptan, or zolmitriptan.

FOOD INTERACTIONS
No known food interactions.

DISEASE INTERACTIONS
Use of fluoxetine may cause complications in patients with liver or kidney disease, since these organs work together to remove the medication from the body. Use of the drug may make diabetes or seizures worse.

≡ SIDE EFFECTS ≡

SERIOUS
Agitation, shaking, difficulty breathing, rash, hives, itching, joint or muscle pain, chills or fever. If such symptoms occur, call your doctor immediately.

COMMON
Nervousness, drowsiness, anxiety, insomnia, headache, diarrhea, excessive sweating, nausea, decreased appetite, decreased initiative.

LESS COMMON
Nasal congestion, unusual or vivid dreams, cough, increased appetite, chest pain, constipation, vision disturbances, abdominal pain, stomach gas, constipation, vomiting, frequent urination, difficulty concentrating, sexual dysfunction, heartbeat irregularities, trembling, fatigue, dizziness, change in taste, flushing of the skin on the face and neck, dry mouth, menstrual pain.

FLUOXYMESTERONE

BRAND NAMES
Android-F, Halotestin

Available in: Tablets
Available OTC? No   **As Generic?** Yes
Drug Class: Hormone treatment (androgen); antineoplastic (anticancer) agent

▼ USAGE INFORMATION

WHY IT'S PRESCRIBED
For hormone replacement in men; to treat delayed sexual development in boys; to treat certain types of breast cancer in women.

HOW IT WORKS
Fluoxymesterone replaces natural testosterone in men deficient of the hormone. Fluoxymesterone also blocks the action of certain other hormones that promote the growth of some types of breast tumors.

▼ DOSAGE GUIDELINES

RANGE AND FREQUENCY
For hormone replacement in men: 5 to 20 mg daily, in single or divided doses. For treatment of delayed sexual development in boys: 2.5 to 10 mg a day for 4 to 6 months. For treatment of breast cancer in women: 10 to 40 mg daily, in divided doses.

ONSET OF EFFECT
1 month.

DURATION OF ACTION
Unknown.

DIETARY ADVICE
It can be taken with food to prevent stomach upset.

STORAGE
Store in a tightly sealed container away from heat and direct light.

MISSED DOSE
Take it as soon as you remember. If it is near the time for the next dose, skip the missed dose and resume your regular dosage schedule. Do not double the next dose.

STOPPING THE DRUG
The decision to stop taking the drug should be made by your doctor.

PROLONGED USE
You should see your doctor regularly for tests and examinations if you must take this drug for a prolonged period.

▼ PRECAUTIONS

Over 60: An increased risk of prostate enlargement or prostate cancer is found in older men.

Driving and Hazardous Work: Use of this drug should not impair your ability to perform such tasks safely.

Alcohol: No special precautions are necessary.

Pregnancy: Fluoxymesterone can affect both male and female fetuses; it should not be used during pregnancy.

Breast Feeding: Fluoxymesterone passes into breast milk; avoid or discontinue use while nursing.

Infants and Children: Fluoxymesterone can profoundly affect the growth and sexual development of infants and children. Risks must be weighed against benefits; consult your pediatrician.

Special Concerns: This drug contains the dye tartrazine, which may cause allergic reactions in some people. The risk of some cancers is increased with long-term, high-dose use. In some cases this drug can pass to a sexual partner and cause side effects. A nonhormonal (barrier) method of contraception is advised during therapy.

OVERDOSE
Symptoms: No specific ones have been reported.

What to Do: An overdose is unlikely to be life-threatening. However, if someone takes a much larger dose than prescribed, call your doctor, emergency medical services (EMS), or the nearest poison control center immediately.

▼ INTERACTIONS

DRUG INTERACTIONS
Consult your doctor for specific advice if you are taking acetaminophen, amiodarone, anabolic steroids, anticoagulants, anti-infective drugs, antithyroid agents, carbamazepine, carmustine, chloroquine, cyclosporine, dantrolene, daunorubicin, disulfiram, divalproex, estrogens, etretinate, gold salts, hydroxychloroquine, insulin, mercaptopurine, methotrexate, methyldopa, naltrexone, oral contraceptives, phenothiazines, phenytoin, plicamycin, or valproic acid.

FOOD INTERACTIONS
No known food interactions.

DISEASE INTERACTIONS
Consult your doctor if you have a history of prostate cancer, diabetes, edema (swelling owing to excess fluid retention), kidney disease, liver disease, enlarged prostate, heart disease, or blood vessel disease.

≡ SIDE EFFECTS ≡

SERIOUS
Itching of skin, yellowish tinge to eyes or skin. Call your doctor immediately.

COMMON
Women: Acne or oily skin, decreased breast size, hoarseness or deepening of voice, irregular menstrual periods, male-type baldness, excessive hair growth. Men: Enlarged or sore breasts, frequent or prolonged erections, frequent urination, temporary infertility. Notify your doctor if any of these symptoms occur.

LESS COMMON
Changes in skin coloration, confusion, constipation, dizziness, frequent headaches, increased thirst and urination, depression, nausea, vomiting, swelling of feet or lower legs, unusual bleeding, unusual fatigue, rapid weight gain, diarrhea, increased risk of infection, insomnia, increase or decrease in sexual desire. Men only: Testicular shrinkage, erectile dysfunction, skin irritation of the scrotum. Boys only: Acne, early growth of pubic hair, penis enlargement, increased frequency of erections.

FLUPHENAZINE

Available in: Tablets, oral concentrate, elixir, injection
Available OTC? No   **As Generic?** Yes
Drug Class: Antipsychotic; phenothiazine

▼ USAGE INFORMATION

WHY IT'S PRESCRIBED
To treat psychotic conditions such as schizophrenia.

HOW IT WORKS
Fluphenazine inhibits the activity of the brain chemical dopamine, thereby helping to prevent the overstimulation of specific nerve centers in the brain that are thought to be responsible for certain psychiatric disorders.

▼ DOSAGE GUIDELINES

RANGE AND FREQUENCY
Oral forms— Adults: To start, 2.5 to 10 mg a day, taken in divided doses every 6 to 8 hours; may be increased to a maximum of 20 mg a day. Maintenance dose is 1 to 20 mg a day. Children: 0.25 to 0.75 mg, 1 to 4 times a day. Older adults: 1 to 2.5 mg a day. Injection— 12.5 to 50 mg every 2 to 4 weeks.

ONSET OF EFFECT
Within 1 hour for oral forms; 24 to 72 hours for injection. Full therapeutic effect may take several weeks.

DURATION OF ACTION
From 6 to 8 hours with oral forms; 1 to 6 weeks with injection.

DIETARY ADVICE
It can be taken with liquid or food to minimize stomach upset. If your medicine comes with a dropper bottle, dilute your dose in half a glass of grapefruit or orange juice or water.

STORAGE
Store in a tightly sealed container in a dry place away from heat and direct light. Do not refrigerate, and keep liquid forms from freezing.

MISSED DOSE
Take it as soon as you remember. However, if it is more than 2 hours late, skip the missed dose and resume your regular dosage schedule. Do not double the next dose.

STOPPING THE DRUG
Do not stop taking the drug abruptly or without your doctor's approval. Dosage should be reduced gradually by your doctor to prevent withdrawal symptoms.

PROLONGED USE
Prolonged use may lead to tardive dyskinesia (involuntary movements of the jaw, lips, and tongue). Consult your doctor about the need for follow-up evaluations and tests.

▼ PRECAUTIONS

Over 60: Adverse reactions, especially shuffling gait, shaking, stiffness, and constipation, are more common in older patients.

Driving and Hazardous Work: Do not drive or engage in hazardous work until you determine how the medicine affects you.

Alcohol: Avoid alcohol.

Pregnancy: Discuss with your doctor the relative risks and benefits of taking this drug if you are, or plan to become, pregnant.

Breast Feeding: Either avoid taking the drug if possible or refrain from breast feeding.

Infants and Children: Not for use by children under age 12.

Special Concerns: Avoid getting overheated or chilled. Avoid getting the liquid form of the medicine on the skin, because it can cause irritation or a rash.

OVERDOSE
Symptoms: Extreme drowsiness, heartbeat irregularities, dry mouth, paradoxical restlessness or agitation, seizures, loss of consciousness.

What to Do: Call your doctor, emergency medical services (EMS), or the nearest poison control center immediately.

▼ INTERACTIONS

DRUG INTERACTIONS
The following drugs may interact with fluphenazine. Consult your doctor for specific advice if you are taking anticholinergics, antidepressants, antihistamines, antihypertensives, barbiturates, anesthetics, beta-blockers, diuretics, thyroid drugs, appetite suppressants, epinephrine, bupropion, cisapride, or calcium supplements.

FOOD INTERACTIONS
Avoid caffeinated beverages, apple juice, and tea.

DISEASE INTERACTIONS
Consult your doctor if you have a history of alcohol abuse, any blood disorder, breast cancer, enlarged prostate, epilepsy or a seizure disorder, glaucoma, lung disease, heart or blood vessel disease, liver disease, Parkinson's disease, peptic ulcer, or urinary difficulty.

SIDE EFFECTS

SERIOUS
Extreme and persistent restlessness; uncontrolled movements, including tics, twitching, twisting movements, and muscle spasms in the face, neck, and back; loss of coordination and balance; trembling, weakness, and stiffness in the extremities; difficulty swallowing or speaking; persistent, uncontrolled chewing, lip-smacking, or tongue movements; staring and absence of facial expression; fainting; increased skin sensitivity to the sun; skin rash; yellowish tinge to eyes or skin.

COMMON
Constipation, decreased sweating, dizziness or faintness, drowsiness, dry mouth, shaking, mild stiffness, shuffling gait, restlessness, blurred vision.

LESS COMMON
Menstrual irregularities, sexual dysfunction, unusual milk secretion, breast pain or swelling, unexpected weight gain, difficulty urinating.

FLURAZEPAM HYDROCHLORIDE

Available in: Capsules
Available OTC? No   **As Generic?** Yes
Drug Class: Benzodiazepine tranquilizer; sedative/hypnotic

▼ USAGE INFORMATION

WHY IT'S PRESCRIBED
For the short-term treatment of insomnia.

HOW IT WORKS
In general, flurazepam produces a mild sedative effect by depressing activity in the central nervous system (the brain and spinal cord). In particular, flurazepam appears to enhance the effect of gamma-aminobutyric acid (GABA), a natural chemical that inhibits the firing of neurons and dampens the transmission of nerve signals, thus decreasing nervous excitation.

▼ DOSAGE GUIDELINES

RANGE AND FREQUENCY
15 or 30 mg, taken in a single dose at bedtime.

ONSET OF EFFECT
From 30 to 60 minutes.

DURATION OF ACTION
Unknown.

DIETARY ADVICE
Limit your intake of caffeine-containing foods and beverages while taking this drug.

STORAGE
Store in a tightly sealed container away from heat, moisture, and direct light.

MISSED DOSE
Take it as soon as you remember, unless it is late at night. Do not take the medicine unless your schedule permits a full night's sleep.

STOPPING THE DRUG
Discontinuing the drug abruptly may produce withdrawal symptoms (sleep disruption, nervousness, irritability, diarrhea, abdominal cramps, muscle aches, memory impairment). The dosage should be reduced gradually according to your doctor's instructions.

PROLONGED USE
Do not use flurazepam for more than 8 weeks without consulting your doctor.

▼ PRECAUTIONS

Over 60: Adverse reactions are more likely and more severe. A lower dose may be warranted.

Driving and Hazardous Work: Flurazepam can impair mental alertness and physical coordination. Adjust your activities accordingly.

Alcohol: Avoid alcohol.

Pregnancy: Use during pregnancy should be avoided if possible. Be sure to tell your doctor if you are pregnant or plan to become pregnant.

Breast Feeding: Flurazepam passes into breast milk; do not take it while nursing.

Infants and Children: Flurazepam is not recommended for use by children under 6 months, and it is not generally prescribed for children under age 15. It should be used by older children only under close medical supervision.

Special Concerns: Use of this drug can lead to psychological or physical dependence.

OVERDOSE
Symptoms: Extreme drowsiness, confusion, slurred speech, slow reflexes, poor coordination, staggering gait, tremor, slowed breathing, loss of consciousness.

What to Do: Call your doctor, emergency medical services (EMS), or the nearest poison control center immediately.

▼ INTERACTIONS

DRUG INTERACTIONS
Other drugs may interact with flurazepam. Consult your doctor for specific advice if you are taking any drugs that depress the central nervous system; these include antihistamines, antidepressants or other psychiatric medications, barbiturates, sedatives, cough medicines, decongestants, and painkillers. Be sure your doctor knows about any over-the-counter medication you may take.

FOOD INTERACTIONS
None reported.

DISEASE INTERACTIONS
Caution is advised when taking flurazepam. Consult your doctor if you have a history of alcohol or drug abuse, stroke or other brain disease, any chronic lung disease, hyperactivity, depression or other mental illness, myasthenia gravis, sleep apnea, epilepsy, porphyria, kidney disease, or liver disease.

SIDE EFFECTS

SERIOUS
Difficulty concentrating, outbursts of anger, other behavior problems, depression, hallucinations, low blood pressure (causing faintness or confusion), memory impairment, muscle weakness, skin rash or itching, sore throat, fever and chills, sores or ulcers in throat or mouth, unusual bruising or bleeding, extreme fatigue, yellowish tinge to eyes or skin. Call your doctor immediately.

COMMON
Daytime drowsiness, dizziness, lightheadedness, loss of coordination, headaches, slurred speech.

LESS COMMON
Stomach cramps or pain, vision disturbances, change in sexual desire or ability, constipation, false sense of well-being, nausea and vomiting, urinary problems, unusual weakness or fatigue.

FLURBIPROFEN OPHTHALMIC

BRAND NAME

Ocufen

Available in: Ophthalmic solution
Available OTC? No   **As Generic?** No
Drug Class: Nonsteroidal anti-inflammatory drug (NSAID)

▼ USAGE INFORMATION

WHY IT'S PRESCRIBED
To treat some eye conditions and problems that occur during or after eye surgery.

HOW IT WORKS
Ophthalmic flurbiprofen inhibits the release of substances that stimulate inflammation and cause pain in eye tissues.

▼ DOSAGE GUIDELINES

RANGE AND FREQUENCY
Adults: 1 drop in each eye every 4 hours. Children: Consult your pediatrician.

ONSET OF EFFECT
Unknown.

DURATION OF ACTION
Unknown.

DIETARY ADVICE
No special restrictions.

STORAGE
Store in a tightly sealed container away from heat, moisture, and direct light. Do not allow it to freeze.

MISSED DOSE
Apply it as soon as you remember. If it is near the time for the next dose, skip the missed dose and resume your regular dosage schedule. Do not double the next dose.

STOPPING THE DRUG
Use it as prescribed for the full treatment period, even if you feel better before the scheduled end of therapy.

PROLONGED USE
See your doctor regularly for tests and examinations if you must use this drug for a prolonged period.

▼ PRECAUTIONS

Over 60: No special problems are expected.

Driving and Hazardous Work: The use of ophthalmic flurbiprofen should not impair your ability to perform such tasks safely.

Alcohol: No special warnings.

Pregnancy: Adequate human studies have not been completed. Before taking ophthalmic flurbiprofen, tell your doctor if you are pregnant or plan to become pregnant.

Breast Feeding: Ophthalmic flurbiprofen may pass into breast milk; caution is advised. Consult your doctor for specific advice.

Infants and Children: Use and dosage for infants and children must be determined by your doctor.

Special Concerns: To use the eye drops, first wash your hands. Tilt your head back. Gently apply pressure to the inside corner of the eyelid and with the index finger of the same hand, pull downward on the lower eyelid to make a space. Drop the medicine into this space and close your eye. Apply pressure for 1 or 2 minutes while keeping the eye closed without blinking. Then wash your hands again. Make sure the tip of the dropper does not touch your eye, finger, or any other surface. If your symptoms do not improve or if they become worse, check with your doctor. Ophthalmic flurbiprofen may cause problems in patients who wear soft contact lenses. Your doctor may want you to stop wearing the lenses while you take it.

OVERDOSE
Symptoms: No specific ones have been reported.

What to Do: An overdose of ophthalmic flurbiprofen is unlikely to be life-threatening. However, if someone takes a much larger dose of the drug than prescribed or accidentally ingests the medicine, call your doctor, emergency medical services (EMS), or the nearest poison control center.

▼ INTERACTIONS

DRUG INTERACTIONS
Consult your doctor for specific advice if you are taking aspirin or another salicylate, difunisal, etodolac, fenoprofen, floctafenine, oral flurbiprofen, ibuprofen, indomethacin, ketoprofen, ketorolac, meclofenamate, mefanamic acid, nabumetone, naproxen, oxyphenbutazone, phenylbutazone, piroxicam, sulindac, suprofen, tenoxicam, tiaprofenic acid, tolmetin, or zomepirac. Ophthalmic flurbiprofen reduces the effectivness of acetylcholine or carbachol, two drugs used to treat glaucoma. These drugs are rarely used today, but if you take them, be sure to let your doctor know.

FOOD INTERACTIONS
No known food interactions.

DISEASE INTERACTIONS
Caution is advised when taking ophthalmic flurbiprofen. Consult your doctor if you have hemophilia or any other bleeding problem.

≡ SIDE EFFECTS ≡

SERIOUS
Rarely, ophthalmic flurbiprofen will cause bleeding in the eye, redness or swelling of the eye or eyelid not present before the start of therapy, itching of the eye, or excessive tear production. Call your doctor immediately.

COMMON
Mild and temporary burning or stinging of eyes after application.

LESS COMMON
There are no less-common side effects associated with ophthalmic flurbiprofen.

FLURBIPROFEN ORAL

Available in: Tablets, extended-release capsules
Available OTC? No   **As Generic?** Yes
Drug Class: Nonsteroidal anti-inflammatory drug (NSAID)

▼ USAGE INFORMATION

WHY IT'S PRESCRIBED
To treat mild to moderate pain and inflammation caused by tendinitis, arthritis, bursitis, gout, soft tissue injuries, migraine and other vascular headaches, menstrual cramps, and other conditions. When patients fail to respond to one NSAID, another may be tried. The greatest effectiveness often requires trial and error of several different NSAIDs.

HOW IT WORKS
NSAIDs work by interfering with the formation of prostaglandins, substances that cause inflammation and make nerves more sensitive to pain impulses. NSAIDs also have other modes of action that are less well understood.

▼ DOSAGE GUIDELINES

RANGE AND FREQUENCY
Adults: Tablets: 50 mg, 4 times daily or 100 mg, 2 times daily. Extended-release capsules: 200 mg once a day. Maximum dose is 300 mg a day. For children's dose, consult your pediatrician.

ONSET OF EFFECT
Several hours.

DURATION OF ACTION
Varies; some patients require daily maintenance doses to control pain.

DIETARY ADVICE
Take flurbiprofen with food.

STORAGE
Store in a tightly sealed container away from heat, moisture, and direct light.

MISSED DOSE
Take it as soon as you remember. If it is near the time for the next dose, skip the missed dose and resume your regular dosage schedule. Do not double the next dose.

STOPPING THE DRUG
The decision to stop taking the drug should be made in consultation with your doctor.

PROLONGED USE
Prolonged use can cause gastrointestinal problems, including ulceration and bleeding, kidney dysfunction, and liver inflammation. Consult your doctor about the need for medical examinations and laboratory tests.

▼ PRECAUTIONS

Over 60: Because of the potentially greater consequences of gastrointestinal side effects, the dose of NSAIDs for older patients, especially those over age 70, is often cut in half.

Driving and Hazardous Work: Do not drive or engage in hazardous work until you determine how the medicine affects you.

Alcohol: Avoid alcohol when using this medication because it increases the risk of stomach irritation.

Pregnancy: Do not use this drug during pregnancy.

Breast Feeding: Flurbiprofen passes into breast milk; avoid use while breast feeding.

Infants and Children: Flurbiprofen may be used in exceptional circumstances; consult your doctor.

Special Concerns: Because NSAIDs can interfere with blood coagulation, this drug should be stopped at least 3 days prior to any surgery.

OVERDOSE
Symptoms: Severe nausea, vomiting, headache, confusion, seizures.

What to Do: Call your doctor, emergency medical services (EMS), or the nearest poison control center immediately.

▼ INTERACTIONS

DRUG INTERACTIONS
Do not take this drug with aspirin or any other NSAIDs without your doctor's approval. In addition, consult your doctor if you are taking antihypertensives, steroids, anticoagulants, antibiotics, itraconazole or ketoconazole, plicamycin, penicillamine, valproic acid, phenytoin, cyclosporine, digitalis drugs, lithium, methotrexate, probenecid, triamterene, or zidovudine.

FOOD INTERACTIONS
No known food interactions.

DISEASE INTERACTIONS
Caution is advised when taking flurbiprofen. Consult your doctor if you have any of the following: bleeding problems, inflammation or ulcers of the stomach and intestines, diabetes, lupus, anemia, asthma, epilepsy, Parkinson's disease, kidney stones, or a history of heart disease or alcohol abuse. Use of flurbiprofen may cause complications in patients with liver or kidney disease, since these organs work together to remove the drug from the body.

SIDE EFFECTS

SERIOUS
Shortness of breath or wheezing, with or without swelling of legs or other signs of heart failure; chest pain; peptic ulcer disease with vomiting of blood; black, tarry stools; decreasing kidney function. Call your doctor immediately.

COMMON
Nausea, vomiting, heartburn, diarrhea, constipation, headache, dizziness, sleepiness.

LESS COMMON
Ulcers or sores in mouth, depression, rashes or blistering of skin, ringing sound in the ears, unusual tingling or numbness of the hands or feet, seizures, blurred vision. Also elevated potassium levels, decreased blood counts; such problems can be detected by your doctor.

FLUTAMIDE

Available in: Capsules
Available OTC? No   **As Generic?** No
Drug Class: Antiandrogen

▼ USAGE INFORMATION

WHY IT'S PRESCRIBED
To treat cancer of the prostate gland.

HOW IT WORKS
The growth of some types of prostate tumors is stimulated by the hormone testosterone. Flutamide interferes with the activity of testosterone, thus slowing or halting the growth of such tumors.

▼ DOSAGE GUIDELINES

RANGE AND FREQUENCY
250 mg every 8 hours, in conjunction with leuprolide, a synthetic form of luteinizing hormone-releasing hormone (LHRH), a hormone that also blocks the release of testosterone.

ONSET OF EFFECT
Unknown.

DURATION OF ACTION
Unknown.

DIETARY ADVICE
Take with or without food. Be sure to drink plenty of fluids.

STORAGE
Store in a tightly sealed container away from heat and direct light.

MISSED DOSE
Take it as soon as you remember. If it is near the time for the next dose, skip the missed dose and resume your regular dosage schedule. Do not double the next dose.

STOPPING THE DRUG
The decision to stop taking the drug should be made in consultation with your doctor.

PROLONGED USE
You should see your doctor regularly for tests and examinations if you take this drug for a prolonged period.

▼ PRECAUTIONS

Over 60: The dosage may be reduced, because the medication takes longer to be eliminated from the body in older patients, but flutamide is not otherwise expected to cause different side effects or problems in older persons than it does in younger people.

Driving and Hazardous Work: Use of flutamide should not impair your ability to perform such tasks safely.

Alcohol: Limit alcohol to moderate intake only.

Pregnancy: Flutamide lowers sperm count, and the medication taken with it causes sterility that may be permanent. If you intend to have children, consult your doctor before you begin to take this medication to discuss utilizing a sperm bank.

Breast Feeding: Not applicable, since flutamide is not given to women.

Infants and Children: Flutamide is not recommended for children.

Special Concerns: If an anticoagulant is taken in combination with flutamide, close monitoring of blood clotting time is necessary, so that the dose of the anticoagulant can be adjusted if needed.

OVERDOSE
Symptoms: Dramatically slowed movement and activity, slow respiration, loss of muscle coordination, excessive tear production (weeping), loss of appetite, breast tenderness, gooseflesh, and vomiting.

What to Do: An overdose of flutamide is unlikely to be life-threatening. However, if someone takes a much larger dose than prescribed, call your doctor, emergency medical services (EMS), or the nearest poison control center immediately.

▼ INTERACTIONS

DRUG INTERACTIONS
The activity of an anticoagulant such as warfarin may be increased by flutamide. Consult your doctor for advice if you are taking an anticoagulant. Also consult your doctor if you are taking cholestyramine, cyclosporine, erythromycin, gemfibrozil, digoxin, cimetidine, ranitidine, omeprazole, or rifampin.

FOOD INTERACTIONS
No known food interactions.

DISEASE INTERACTIONS
You should not take flutamide if you have severe liver impairment. Consult your doctor if you have any other medical condition.

SIDE EFFECTS

SERIOUS
Bluish coloring of lips, fingernails, or palms of hands (a sign of inadequate blood and oxygen supply to body tissues), dark urine, extreme dizziness or fainting, feeling of extreme pressure in the head, itching, loss of appetite, nausea or vomiting, pain in the right flank, shortness of breath, weak and rapid heartbeat, yellow discoloration of the skin or eyes (jaundice). Call your doctor immediately.

COMMON
Diarrhea, erectile dysfunction (impotence) or loss of sexual desire, sudden sweating and feeling of warmth.

LESS COMMON
Loss of appetite, tingling or numbness of hands or feet, swollen and tender breasts, swelling of feet or lower legs.

FLUTICASONE

Available in: Oral inhalation, nasal spray
Available OTC? No **As Generic?** No
Drug Class: Respiratory corticosteroid

BRAND NAMES
Flonase, Flovent

▼ USAGE INFORMATION

WHY IT'S PRESCRIBED
To preventively treat bronchial asthma, and to treat allergic rhinitis (seasonal or perennial allergies such as hay fever).

HOW IT WORKS
Respiratory corticosteroids such as fluticasone primarily reduce or prevent inflammation of the lining of the airways (the underlying cause of asthma), reduce the allergic response to inhaled allergens, and inhibit the secretion of mucus within the airways.

▼ DOSAGE GUIDELINES

RANGE AND FREQUENCY
For asthma– Oral inhalation: 88 to 220 micrograms (mcg) a day, 2 times per day; not to exceed 440 mcg a day. For patients previously treated with oral corticosteroids: 880 mcg, 2 times a day. Dosage may gradually be reduced after 1 week of therapy. For allergic rhinitis– Nasal spray: Adults: 2 sprays (50 mcg each) in each nostril once per day, or 1 spray in each nostril twice a day (in the morning and at night). Children ages 4 to 17: One spray in each nostril once a day. Dose, if needed, may be increased to 2 sprays in each nostril once a day. Maximum daily dose should not exceed 200 mcg. After relief is achieved, the dose may be reduced to 1 spray per day.

ONSET OF EFFECT
Usually within 1 week; it may take 3 weeks for the full effect to occur.

DURATION OF ACTION
Unknown.

DIETARY ADVICE
No special restrictions.

STORAGE
Store the inhaler in a dry place away from heat and direct light.

MISSED DOSE
Take it as soon as you remember. If it is near the time for the next dose, skip the missed dose and resume your regular dosage schedule. Do not double the next dose.

STOPPING THE DRUG
If you have been using fluticasone for a long period, do not stop taking it suddenly. Consult your doctor about how to stop.

PROLONGED USE
Consult your doctor about the need for regular medical tests and examinations if you must take this drug for a prolonged period of time.

▼ PRECAUTIONS

Over 60: No special problems are expected.

Driving and Hazardous Work: The use of fluticasone should not impair your ability to perform such tasks safely.

Alcohol: No special precautions are necessary.

Pregnancy: Well-controlled studies of fluticasone use during pregnancy have not been done; it is generally not recommended unless the benefits clearly outweigh the risks. Consult your doctor.

Breast Feeding: Fluticasone may pass into breast milk; caution is advised. Consult your doctor for advice.

Infants and Children: Safety and effectiveness have not been established for children under age 4.

Special Concerns: Inhaled steroids will not help an asthma attack in progress. Inhaled steroids can lower resistance to yeast infections of the mouth, throat, or voice box. To prevent yeast infections, gargle or rinse your mouth with water after each use; do not swallow the water. Know how to use the spray properly; read and follow the directions that come with the device. Before you have surgery, tell the doctor or dentist that you are using a steroid.

OVERDOSE
Symptoms: No cases of overdose have been reported.

What to Do: An overdose of fluticasone is unlikely. If you have any reason to suspect an overdose, contact your doctor or seek medical assistance right away.

▼ INTERACTIONS

DRUG INTERACTIONS
Consult your doctor for specific advice if you are taking systemic corticosteroids, other inhaled corticosteroids, or drugs that suppress the immune system.

FOOD INTERACTIONS
No known food interactions.

DISEASE INTERACTIONS
Caution is advised when taking fluticasone. Consult your doctor if you have any of the following: a lung disease such as tuberculosis; a herpes infection of the eye; nasal ulcers or recent nose surgery or injury; or any bacterial, viral, or fungal infection. If you are exposed to chicken pox or measles, tell your doctor at once.

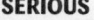
≡ SIDE EFFECTS ≡

SERIOUS
No serious side effects are associated with the use of fluticasone.

COMMON
Oral inhalation: Sore throat, white patches in mouth or throat, hoarseness. Nasal spray: Nosebleeds or bloody nasal secretions, nasal burning or irritation, sore throat.

LESS COMMON
Eye pain, watering eyes, gradual decrease of vision, stomach pain and digestive disturbances.

FLUVASTATIN

Available in: Capsules
Available OTC? No   **As Generic?** No
Drug Class: Antilipidemic (cholesterol-lowering agent)

▼ USAGE INFORMATION

WHY IT'S PRESCRIBED
To treat high cholesterol. Usually prescribed after first lines of treatment—including diet, weight loss, and exercise—fail to reduce total and low-density lipoprotein (LDL) cholesterol to acceptable levels.

HOW IT WORKS
Fluvastatin blocks the action of an enzyme required for the manufacture of cholesterol, thereby interfering with its formation. By lowering the amount of cholesterol in the liver cells, fluvastatin increases the formation of receptors for LDL, and thereby reduces blood levels of total and LDL cholesterol. In addition to lowering LDL cholesterol, fluvastatin also modestly reduces triglyceride levels and raises HDL (the so-called "good" cholesterol) levels.

▼ DOSAGE GUIDELINES

RANGE AND FREQUENCY
Initial dose is 20 mg, taken once a day in the evening.

Dose may be increased by your doctor to 40 mg, taken once a day in the evening.

ONSET OF EFFECT
Within 2 to 4 weeks after starting therapy.

DURATION OF ACTION
The effect persists for the duration of therapy.

DIETARY ADVICE
Cholesterol-lowering drugs are only one part of a total program that should include regular exercise and a healthy diet. The American Heart Association publishes a "Healthy Heart" diet, which is recommended.

STORAGE
Store in a tightly sealed container away from heat and direct light. Keep away from moisture and extremes in temperature.

MISSED DOSE
Take it as soon as you remember. Take your next dose at the proper time and resume your regular dosage schedule. Do not double the next dose.

STOPPING THE DRUG
The decision to stop taking the drug should be made in consultation with your doctor. Once the medication is discontinued, blood cholesterol is likely to return to original elevated levels.

PROLONGED USE
Side effects are more likely with prolonged use. As you continue with fluvastatin, your doctor will periodically order blood tests to evaluate liver function.

▼ PRECAUTIONS

Over 60: No special problems are expected in older patients.

Driving and Hazardous Work: The use of fluvastatin should not impair your ability to perform such tasks safely.

Alcohol: No special precautions are necessary.

Pregnancy: Should not be used during pregnancy or by women who plan to become pregnant in the near future.

Breast Feeding: Fluvastatin passes into breast milk and is not recommended while breast feeding.

Infants and Children: Rarely used in children.

Special Concerns: Important elements of treatment for high cholesterol include proper diet, weight loss, regular moderate exercise, and the avoidance of certain medications that may increase cholesterol levels. Because fluvastatin has potential side effects, it is important that you maintain a recommended healthy diet and cooperate with other treatments your physician may suggest.

OVERDOSE
Symptoms: An overdose of fluvastatin is unlikely.

What to Do: Emergency instructions not applicable.

▼ INTERACTIONS

DRUG INTERACTIONS
Consult your doctor if you are taking cyclosporine, gemfibrozil, niacin, antibiotics, especially erythromycin, or medications for fungus infections. All of these drugs may increase the risk of myositis (muscle inflammation) when taken with fluvastatin and may lead to kidney failure.

FOOD INTERACTIONS
No known food interactions.

DISEASE INTERACTIONS
Consult your doctor if you have any of the following problems: liver, kidney, or muscle disease, or a medical history involving organ transplant or recent surgery.

SIDE EFFECTS

SERIOUS
Fever, unusual or unexplained muscle aches and tenderness. Call your doctor right away.

COMMON
Side effects occur in only 1% to 2% of patients. These include constipation or diarrhea, dizziness or lightheadedness, bloating or gas, heartburn, nausea, skin rash, stomach pain, rise in liver enzymes.

LESS COMMON
Sleeping difficulty.

FLUVOXAMINE MALEATE

BRAND NAME

Luvox

Available in: Tablets
Available OTC? No   **As Generic?** Yes
Drug Class: SSRI antidepressant/anti-obsessive-compulsive agent

▼ USAGE INFORMATION

WHY IT'S PRESCRIBED
To treat obsessive-compulsive disorder.

HOW IT WORKS
Fluvoxamine affects levels of serotonin, a brain chemical that is thought to be linked to mood, emotions, and mental state.

▼ DOSAGE GUIDELINES

RANGE AND FREQUENCY
To start, 50 mg taken at bedtime; may be increased gradually by your doctor to 300 mg a day. Doses greater than 100 mg a day may be taken in 2 divided doses.

ONSET OF EFFECT
Unknown.

DURATION OF ACTION
Unknown.

DIETARY ADVICE
Fluvoxamine can be taken without regard to diet. Do not chew the tablet.

STORAGE
Store in a tightly sealed container away from heat, moisture, and direct light.

MISSED DOSE
Take it as soon as you remember. If it is near the time for the next dose, skip the missed dose and resume your regular dosage schedule. Do not double the next dose.

STOPPING THE DRUG
Take it as prescribed for the full treatment period, even if you begin to feel better before the scheduled end of therapy. Discontinuing the drug abruptly may produce unpleasant withdrawal symptoms. Dosage should be reduced gradually according to your doctor's instructions.

PROLONGED USE
Consult your doctor about the need for follow-up evaluation and tests if you must take this drug for an extended period.

▼ PRECAUTIONS

Over 60: Adverse reactions may be more likely and more severe in older patients. A lower dose may be warranted.

Driving and Hazardous Work: Use caution when driving or engaging in hazardous work until you determine how the medication affects you.

Alcohol: Avoid alcohol.

Pregnancy: Adequate human studies have not been done. Before taking fluvoxamine, tell your doctor if you are pregnant or plan to become pregnant. Discuss with your doctor the relative risks and benefits of using this drug while pregnant.

Breast Feeding: Fluvoxamine passes into breast milk; avoid or discontinue use while breast feeding.

Infants and Children: Not recommended for use by children under age 18.

OVERDOSE
Symptoms: Severe diarrhea; extreme dizziness, drowsiness, difficulty awakening, or coma; rapid or slow heartbeat; seizures; or severe vomiting.

What to Do: Call your doctor, emergency medical services (EMS), or the nearest poison control center immediately.

▼ INTERACTIONS

DRUG INTERACTIONS
You should not take fluvoxamine if you are taking terfenadine, astemizole, or cisapride. Fluvoxamine and MAO inhibitors should not be used within 14 days of each other.

Very serious side effects such as myoclonus (uncontrolled muscle jerking), hyperthermia (excessive rise in body temperature), and extreme stiffness may result. Consult your doctor for specific advice if you are taking or have recently taken alprazolam, diazepam, midazolam, triazolam, beta-blockers, tricyclic antidepressants, carbamazepine, clozapine, theophylline, tryptophan, lithium, warfarin, or methadone. Also consult your doctor if you smoke tobacco.

FOOD INTERACTIONS
No known food interactions.

DISEASE INTERACTIONS
Caution is advised when taking fluvoxamine. Consult your doctor if you have a history of alcohol or drug abuse, mania, or seizures.

≡ SIDE EFFECTS ≡

SERIOUS
Decreased libido, sexual dysfunction, diarrhea, dizziness, rapid heartbeat, difficulty breathing, seizures, trembling, vomiting, difficulty swallowing, fainting, psychotic reaction. Call your doctor immediately.

COMMON
Insomnia, decreased appetite, constipation, dry mouth, drowsiness, heartburn, runny nose, unexpected weight loss, headache, frequent urination, increased sweating, change in taste, yawning.

LESS COMMON
Swelling of the feet or lower legs, chills, gas, weight gain.

FOLIC ACID (FOLACIN; FOLATE)

Available in: Tablets, injectable form (for use in hospitals)
Available OTC? Yes   **As Generic?** Yes
Drug Class: Vitamin

▼ USAGE INFORMATION

WHY IT'S PRESCRIBED
The vitamin folic acid (also known as folacin and folate) is prescribed for treatment or prevention of certain types of anemia that result from folic acid deficiency. Such deficiencies may occur due to insufficient intake of folic acid (a result of poor diet or malnutrition), an inability to absorb the vitamin (as occurs in gastrointestinal disease), impaired ability to utilize the vitamin (due to excessive alcohol intake or phenytoin use), or as a result of conditions requiring increased amounts of folic acid (as occurs with pregnancy, breast feeding, hemodialysis, hemolytic anemia, and bone marrow failure).

HOW IT WORKS
Folic acid enhances chemical reactions that contribute to the production of red blood cells, the manufacture of DNA needed for cell replication, and the metabolism of amino acids (compounds necessary for the manufacture of proteins).

▼ DOSAGE GUIDELINES

RANGE AND FREQUENCY
For severe deficiency— Adults and children, regardless of age: 1 mg daily. For daily supplementation following correction of severe deficiency— Adults and adolescents: 1 mg, once daily. During pregnancy: 400 micrograms (mcg), once daily. While breast feeding: 260 to 280 mcg, once daily. Children, newborn to 3 years of age: 25 to 50 mcg, once daily; child 4 to 6 years of age: 75 mcg, once daily; child 7 to 10 years of age: 100 mcg, once daily.

ONSET OF EFFECT
Folic acid is used immediately by the body for a number of vital chemical functions.

DURATION OF ACTION
Folic acid is required by your body on a daily basis throughout a lifetime.

DIETARY ADVICE
Maintain your usual food and fluid intake. Increase fluids if you have a fever or diarrhea, in hot weather, or during exercise. Follow your doctor's dietary advice (such as low-fat, low-salt, or low-cholesterol restrictions) to improve control over high blood pressure and heart disease.

STORAGE
Store in a tightly sealed container away from heat and direct light. Keep away from moisture and extremes in temperature.

MISSED DOSE
Take it as soon as you remember. If it is near the time for the next dose, skip the missed dose and resume your regular dosage schedule. Do not double the next dose.

STOPPING THE DRUG
The decision to stop taking the drug should be made by your doctor.

PROLONGED USE
Therapy with folacin may require weeks or months.

▼ PRECAUTIONS

Over 60: No special problems are expected in older patients.

Driving and Hazardous Work: The use of folic acid should not impair your ability to perform such tasks safely.

Alcohol: Alcohol impairs the body's utilization of folic acid; avoid it completely if you are taking folic acid.

Pregnancy: Folic acid supplementation is recommended during pregnancy.

Breast Feeding: Folic acid supplementation is recommended while nursing.

Infants and Children: Folic acid may be used regardless of age.

Special Concerns: Folic acid ingestion can mask vitamin B12 deficiency and lead to irreversible neurological damage; therefore, folic acid should be taken only upon the recommendation of your doctor. Folic acid deficiency should not occur and supplementation is not necessary in healthy individuals who consume a normal balanced diet.

OVERDOSE
Symptoms: No specific ones have been reported.

What to Do: An overdose of folic acid is not life-threatening. No emergency procedures are warranted.

▼ INTERACTIONS

DRUG INTERACTIONS
Consult your doctor for advice if you are taking pain relievers, antibiotics, anticonvulsants, epoetin, estrogens, oral contraceptives, methotrexate, pyrimethamine, triamterene, sulfasalazine, or zinc supplements.

FOOD INTERACTIONS
No known food interactions.

DISEASE INTERACTIONS
Consult your doctor if you have pernicious anemia.

≡ SIDE EFFECTS ≡

SERIOUS
Wheezing, breathing difficulty, chest pain, swelling, tightness in throat or chest, dizziness, rash, itching. Such symptoms may indicate a serious allergic reaction, although this is extremely rare.

COMMON
The are no known common side effects associated with the use of folic acid.

LESS COMMON
Mild allergic reactions.

FOSCARNET SODIUM (PHOSPHONOFORMIC ACID)

Available in: Injection
Available OTC? No   **As Generic?** No
Drug Class: Antiviral

▼ USAGE INFORMATION

WHY IT'S PRESCRIBED
To treat the eye disorder cytomegalovirus (CMV) retinitis in patients with acquired immunodeficiency syndrome (AIDS). Sometimes prescribed for other viral infections.

HOW IT WORKS
Foscarnet interferes with the activity of enzymes needed for the replication of viral DNA in cells, thus preventing CMV from multiplying.

▼ DOSAGE GUIDELINES

RANGE AND FREQUENCY
60 mg for every 2.2 lbs (1 kg) of body weight, injected into a vein every 8 hours for 2 to 3 weeks, followed by a maintenance dose of 90 to 120 mg for every 2.2 lbs, injected daily.

ONSET OF EFFECT
Immediate.

DURATION OF ACTION
24 hours.

DIETARY ADVICE
No special restrictions.

STORAGE
Not applicable, since this drug is administered exclusively in a health care facility or by a home intravenous (I.V.) infusion team.

MISSED DOSE
Consult your doctor.

STOPPING THE DRUG
The decision to stop taking the drug should be made by your doctor.

PROLONGED USE
Your doctor should check your progress periodically.

▼ PRECAUTIONS

Over 60: Adverse reactions may be more likely and more severe in older patients.

Driving and Hazardous Work: Do not drive or engage in hazardous work until you determine how the medicine affects you.

Alcohol: Avoid alcohol.

Pregnancy: In animal studies, foscarnet has been shown to cause birth defects. Human studies have not been done. Before taking this drug, tell your doctor if you are pregnant or are planning to become pregnant.

Breast Feeding: Foscarnet may pass into breast milk; caution is advised. Consult your doctor for advice.

Infants and Children: There is no specific information about the use of foscarnet by infants and children. Consult your doctor about the possible risks and benefits.

Special Concerns: Drink several glasses of water every day unless your doctor advises otherwise. While taking foscarnet, your doctor may conduct periodic tests on the function of your kidneys. Anemia caused by foscarnet may be severe enough to require blood transfusions. If you are receiving the drug as therapy for CMV retinitis, you should periodically receive eye examinations by an ophthalmologist to check for signs of vision loss. Foscarnet may cause sores on the genital organs. Washing the genitals after urinating may decrease the likelihood of this problem.

OVERDOSE
Symptoms: Sudden or severe onset of serious side effects.

What to Do: Call your doctor, emergency medical services (EMS), or the nearest poison control center immediately.

▼ INTERACTIONS

DRUG INTERACTIONS
Other drugs may interact with foscarnet. Consult your doctor for specific advice if you are taking amphotericin B, carmustine, cisplatin, combination pain medicines containing acetaminophen or aspirin, cyclosporine, deferoxamine, gentamicin, gold salts, any pain medicine, lithium, methotrexate, pentamidine, penicillamine, plicamycin, streptozocin, or tiopronin.

FOOD INTERACTIONS
No known food interactions.

DISEASE INTERACTIONS
Caution is advised when taking foscarnet. Consult your doctor if you have anemia, kidney disease, or dehydration.

≡ SIDE EFFECTS ≡

SERIOUS
Kidney damage, causing symptoms such as increased or decreased urine output, increased or decreased urge to urinate, and increased thirst; toxicity of the nervous system, causing twitching or seizures, or numbness, tingling, or prickling in the extremities; fever and chills; pain at injection site; extreme fatigue. Call your doctor right away.

COMMON
Headache, abdominal pain or upset, nausea and vomiting, loss of weight or appetite, nervousness, anxiety, restlessness, mental confusion, lightheadedness, unusual fatigue.

LESS COMMON
Sores on the mouth, throat, penis, or vulva.

FOSFOMYCIN TROMETHAMINE

Available in: Powder for solution
Available OTC? No   **As Generic?** No
Drug Class: Antibiotic

▼ USAGE INFORMATION

WHY IT'S PRESCRIBED
To treat uncomplicated urinary tract infections (acute cystitis) in women.

HOW IT WORKS
Fosfomycin interferes with the formation of bacterial cell walls, rendering bacteria unable to multiply and spread.

▼ DOSAGE GUIDELINES

RANGE AND FREQUENCY
Adult and teenage females: 3 g in a single dose, given orally.

ONSET OF EFFECT
Within 3 hours.

DURATION OF ACTION
Unknown.

DIETARY ADVICE
No special dietary recommendations. Mix the powder with half a glass of water. (Do not use hot water.)

STORAGE
Store in a tightly sealed container away from heat, moisture, and direct light.

MISSED DOSE
Not applicable. Fosfomycin is intended for one-time use.

STOPPING THE DRUG
Not applicable.

PROLONGED USE
Fosfomycin is intended for one-time use only. Repeated doses increase the likelihood of adverse side effects. Call your doctor if the infection has not improved, or has worsened, within 2 to 3 days.

▼ PRECAUTIONS

Over 60: No special problems are expected.

Driving and Hazardous Work: Do not drive or engage in hazardous work until you determine how the medicine affects you.

Alcohol: No special precautions are necessary.

Pregnancy: Adequate studies of the use of this drug during pregnancy have not been done. Before taking fosfomycin, tell your doctor if you are pregnant or plan to become pregnant; discuss the relative risks and benefits of using the drug, and weigh them carefully.

Breast Feeding: It is not known whether fosfomycin passes into breast milk; caution is advised. Consult your doctor for specific advice.

Infants and Children: Not recommended for use by children under age 12.

Special Concerns: Urine tests to determine the type of bacteria causing the infection and its susceptibility to treatment should be done before and after the completion of therapy with fosfomycin.

OVERDOSE
Symptoms: An overdose with fosfomycin is unlikely to occur; no cases of overdose have been reported.

What to Do: Emergency instructions not applicable.

▼ INTERACTIONS

DRUG INTERACTIONS
Consult your doctor for specific advice if you are concurrently taking metoclopramide. Before taking fosfomycin, tell your doctor if you are taking any other drug.

FOOD INTERACTIONS
No known food interactions.

DISEASE INTERACTIONS
Caution is advised when taking fosfomycin. Consult your doctor if you have kidney disease or any other medical condition. Use of fosfomycin may cause complications in patients with kidney disease, since this organ works to remove the medication from the body.

≣ SIDE EFFECTS ≣

SERIOUS
No serious side effects are associated with the use of fosfomycin.

COMMON
Diarrhea, headache, vaginal itching, nausea, runny nose, back pain, painful menstruation, throat irritation, dizziness, abdominal pain, generalized pain, weakness, skin rash, indigestion or stomach upset. Call your doctor if such symptoms persist or interfere with daily activities.

LESS COMMON
Abnormal stools, loss of appetite, constipation, dry mouth, failure to urinate, ear disorders, fever, gas, flu-like symptoms, blood in urine, infection, insomnia, swollen lymph glands, nerve pain, nervousness, burning sensation, sleepiness, vomiting.

FOSINOPRIL SODIUM

Available in: Tablets
Available OTC? No **As Generic?** Yes
Drug Class: Angiotensin-converting enzyme (ACE) inhibitor

▼ USAGE INFORMATION

WHY IT'S PRESCRIBED
To control high blood pressure; to treat congestive heart failure; to treat patients with left ventricular dysfunction (damage to the pumping chamber of the heart); and to minimize further kidney damage in diabetics with mild kidney disease.

HOW IT WORKS
Angiotensin-converting enzyme (ACE) inhibitors block an enzyme that produces angiotensin, a naturally occurring substance that causes blood vessels to constrict and stimulates production of the adrenal hormone, aldosterone, which promotes sodium retention in the body. As a result, ACE inhibitors relax blood vessels (causing them to widen) and reduces sodium retention, which lowers blood pressure and so decreases the workload of the heart.

▼ DOSAGE GUIDELINES

RANGE AND FREQUENCY
Initial dose: 10 mg once a day. Maintenance dose: 20 to 80 mg a day, in 1 or 2 doses.

ONSET OF EFFECT
Within 1 hour.

DURATION OF ACTION
24 hours.

DIETARY ADVICE
Take fosinopril on an empty stomach, about 1 hour before mealtime. Follow your doctor's dietary advice (such as low-salt or low-cholesterol restrictions) to improve control over high blood pressure and heart disease. Avoid high-potassium foods like bananas and citrus fruits and juices, unless you are also taking drugs, such as diuretics, that lower potassium levels.

STORAGE
Store in a tightly sealed container away from heat, moisture, and direct light.

MISSED DOSE
Take it as soon as you remember. If it is near the time for the next dose, skip the missed dose and resume your regular dosage schedule. Do not double the next dose.

STOPPING THE DRUG
Do not stop taking this drug abruptly, as this may cause potentially serious health problems. Dosage should be reduced gradually, according to your doctor's instructions.

PROLONGED USE
Therapy with this medication may require months or years. Prolonged use may increase the risk of adverse effects.

▼ PRECAUTIONS

Over 60: Side effects may be more likely and more severe.

Driving and Hazardous Work: Avoid such activities until you determine how this medication affects you.

Alcohol: Alcohol may increase the effect of the drug and cause an excessive drop in blood pressure.

Pregnancy: Do not use fosinopril if you are pregnant or trying to become pregnant. Use of this drug during the last 6 months of pregnancy may cause severe defects, even death, in the fetus.

Breast Feeding: Fosinopril passes into breast milk and may be harmful to the infant; avoid using while nursing.

Infants and Children: Fosinopril is generally not recommended for children.

OVERDOSE
Symptoms: No specific ones have been reported.

What to Do: While overdose is unlikely, call your doctor, emergency medical services (EMS), or the nearest poison control center immediately if you suspect that someone has taken a much larger dose than prescribed.

▼ INTERACTIONS

DRUG INTERACTIONS
Consult your doctor if you are taking diuretics (especially potassium-sparing diuretics), potassium supplements or drugs containing potassium (check ingredient labels), lithium, anticoagulants (such as warfarin), indomethacin or other anti-inflammatory drugs, antacids, allopurinol, or any over-the-counter medications (especially cold remedies and diet pills).

FOOD INTERACTIONS
Avoid low-salt milk and salt substitutes. Many brands contain high amounts of potassium. Avoid high-potassium foods like bananas and citrus fruits and juices.

DISEASE INTERACTIONS
Consult your doctor if you have systemic lupus erythematosus or if you have had a prior allergic reaction to ACE inhibitors. This medication should be used with caution by patients with severe kidney disease or renal artery stenosis (narrowing of one or both of the arteries that supply blood to the kidneys).

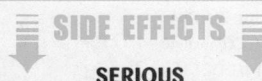

SIDE EFFECTS

SERIOUS
Fever and chills; sore throat and hoarseness; sudden difficulty breathing or swallowing; swelling of the face, mouth, or extremities; impaired kidney function (ankle swelling, decreased urination); confusion; yellow discoloration of the eyes or skin (indicating liver disorder); intense itching; chest pain or palpitations; abdominal pain. Serious side effects are very rare; contact your doctor immediately.

COMMON
Dry, persistent cough.

LESS COMMON
Dizziness or fainting; skin rash; numbness or tingling in the hands, feet, or lips; unusual fatigue or muscle weakness; nausea; drowsiness; loss of taste; headache.

FUROSEMIDE

Available in: Tablets, oral solution, injection
Available OTC? No   **As Generic?** Yes
Drug Class: Loop diuretic

▼ USAGE INFORMATION

WHY IT'S PRESCRIBED
To reduce fluid (salt and water) accumulation that leads to edema (swelling) and breathlessness in patients with heart disease, cirrhosis of the liver, and kidney disease. Furosemide is also sometimes used to help control high blood pressure.

HOW IT WORKS
Loop diuretics work on a specific portion of the kidney (the loop of Henle) to increase the excretion of water and sodium in urine.

▼ DOSAGE GUIDELINES

RANGE AND FREQUENCY
20 to 600 mg a day. Tablets and solution: dosage is given in 1, 2, or 3 divided doses daily. Injection (given in a hospital setting only): dosage given in divided doses every 2 to 3 hours or as a continuous infusion.

ONSET OF EFFECT
20 to 60 minutes.

DURATION OF ACTION
Tablets and solution: 6 to 8 hours. Injection: 2 hours.

DIETARY ADVICE
Take with food to reduce stomach irritation.

STORAGE
Keep in refrigerator, in a light-resistant container. Do not allow liquid forms to freeze.

MISSED DOSE
Take it as soon as you remember. If it is near the time for the next dose, skip the missed dose and resume your regular dosage schedule. Do not double the next dose.

STOPPING THE DRUG
The decision to stop taking the drug should be made by your doctor.

PROLONGED USE
No apparent problems. Regular examinations by your doctor are advised.

▼ PRECAUTIONS

Over 60: No special problems are expected.

Driving and Hazardous Work: No special precautions are required.

Alcohol: No special precautions are required.

Pregnancy: Diuretics are not useful for the normal fluid retention that occurs with pregnancy. In patients who do need diuretic therapy, furosemide is generally preferred, but should be taken only after careful consultation with your primary care doctor or OB/GYN specialist.

Breast Feeding: Furosemide passes into breast milk; avoid or discontinue use while breast feeding.

Infants and Children: Use furosemide only under careful supervision by a pediatrician.

Special Concerns: To prevent sleep disruption, avoid taking furosemide in the evening. You may have to take a potassium supplement or consume foods or fluids high in potassium while taking this drug. Diabetic patients should monitor their blood sugar levels carefully.

OVERDOSE
Symptoms: Weakness, lethargy, mental confusion, muscle cramps.

What to Do: Call your doctor, emergency medical services (EMS), or the nearest poison control center immediately.

▼ INTERACTIONS

DRUG INTERACTIONS
Consult your doctor about any other drugs you are taking, especially antibiotics, other blood pressure drugs, any ACE inhibitor, any pain reliever, lithium, cortisone-related drugs, digitalis-related drugs, or any nonsteroidal anti-inflammatory drug.

FOOD INTERACTIONS
None reported.

DISEASE INTERACTIONS
Caution is advised when taking this medication. Consult your doctor if you have diabetes, gout, or a hearing problem, or have had a recent heart attack.

▦ SIDE EFFECTS ▦

SERIOUS
Skin rash, hives, intense itching, swelling of the mouth and throat, breathing difficulty, mood or mental changes, nausea and vomiting, unusual fatigue, black or tarry stools. Call your doctor immediately.

COMMON
Muscle cramps or pain. Potassium depletion may lead to heart palpitations and weakness. Fluid depletion may lead to dizziness, especially upon arising from a sitting or lying position, as well as thirst, dry mouth, and constipation.

LESS COMMON
Buzzing or ringing in ears, loss of hearing (particularly after intravenous treatment), diarrhea, loss of appetite, gout, increased blood sugar (a problem for diabetic patients).

GABAPENTIN

Available in: Capsules, tablets
Available OTC? No   **As Generic?** No
Drug Class: Anticonvulsant

▼ USAGE INFORMATION

WHY IT'S PRESCRIBED
To control certain kinds of seizures in the treatment of epilepsy. Gabapentin is often prescribed in combination with another anticonvulsant medication.

HOW IT WORKS
The mechanism of action is not well understood. It is believed that gabapentin inhibits activity in certain parts of the brain and suppresses the abnormal firing of neurons that causes seizures.

▼ DOSAGE GUIDELINES

RANGE AND FREQUENCY
Adults: 900 to 6,000 mg a day, in 3 or 4 divided doses. Some patients require higher doses. The dose is started low and then gradually increased by your doctor to achieve maximum therapeutic benefit with a minimum of side effects. The dosage for children has not been clearly established.

ONSET OF EFFECT
Several hours.

DURATION OF ACTION
Maximum effectiveness lasts 5 to 8 hours or longer; effectiveness then gradually decreases.

DIETARY ADVICE
No special restrictions.

STORAGE
Store in a tightly sealed container away from heat, moisture, and direct light.

MISSED DOSE
Take it as soon as you remember. If your next dose is scheduled within the next 2 hours, take the missed dose, and take the next dose 1 to 2 hours later. Resume your regular dosage schedule. Do not double the next dose unless advised to do so by your doctor. Do not wait more than 12 hours between doses.

STOPPING THE DRUG
The decision to stop taking the drug should be made by your doctor. Never stop this drug abruptly because this may cause seizures. The dose is typically tapered over a period of weeks.

PROLONGED USE
Therapy with gabapentin may be required for months or years. Some side effects that are prominent during the first few weeks of therapy may subsequently diminish.

▼ PRECAUTIONS

Over 60: Older persons may require lower doses to minimize side effects.

Driving and Hazardous Work: Avoid such activities until you determine how the medication affects you.

Alcohol: May contribute to excessive drowsiness.

Pregnancy: Adequate human studies of gabapentin during pregnancy have not been done, but the use of other anticonvulsants is associated with an increased risk of birth defects. However, seizures during pregnancy can also increase the risks to the unborn child. Discuss with your doctor the potential risks and benefits of using gabapentin during pregnancy. Folate supplementation is recommended beginning 1 to 2 months before conception and throughout pregnancy.

Breast Feeding: Gabapentin may pass into breast milk, although at low levels. Consult your doctor for specific advice if you are nursing.

Infants and Children: There are few published studies regarding the use of gabapentin in children age 12 and younger, but effectiveness should be similar to that seen in older patients.

Special Concerns: Your doctor may want you to wear a medical bracelet or carry an identification card saying that you are taking this drug.

OVERDOSE
Symptoms: There have been few reports of gabapentin overdose. Symptoms include double vision, slurred speech, drowsiness, lethargy, and diarrhea.

What to Do: Call your doctor, emergency medical services (EMS), or the nearest poison control center immediately.

▼ INTERACTIONS

DRUG INTERACTIONS
Gabapentin has no significant drug interactions.

FOOD INTERACTIONS
No known food interactions.

DISEASE INTERACTIONS
The dose of gabapentin may need to be lower in patients with kidney disease.

SIDE EFFECTS

SERIOUS
Fever, sore throat, swollen glands, red or purple pointlike rash on the skin or mucous membranes, blistering or peeling skin lesions, mouth sores, easy bruising, paleness, weakness, confusion, lethargy, or seizures may be a sign of a potentially fatal blood disorder (aplastic anemia) or other complication. Call your physician immediately.

COMMON
Fatigue, dizziness, sedation, clumsiness or unsteadiness, unusual eye movements, blurred or altered vision, nausea, vomiting, tremor.

LESS COMMON
Diarrhea, muscle aches or weakness, dry mouth, headache, sleep disturbances, irritability, slurred speech. There are numerous additional side effects associated with the use of this drug; consult your doctor if you are concerned about any adverse or unusual reactions.

GANCICLOVIR SODIUM

Available in: Capsules, injection, intraocular implant
Available OTC? No   **As Generic?** Yes
Drug Class: Antiviral

▼ USAGE INFORMATION

WHY IT'S PRESCRIBED
To treat or prevent infections caused by cytomegalovirus (CMV). CMV infection of the eyes occurs in patients with weakened immune systems and is prevalent among people with AIDS. A more widespread infection with CMV may occur in patients who have received organ or bone marrow transplants and who are being treated with medications (immunosuppressants) to prevent rejection.

HOW IT WORKS
Ganciclovir interferes with the activity of enzymes needed for the replication of viral DNA in cells, thus preventing the virus from multiplying.

▼ DOSAGE GUIDELINES

RANGE AND FREQUENCY
Adults: Capsules (for maintenance and prevention therapy only; not for treatment of active infection): 1,000 mg, 3 times a day with food, or 500 mg every 3 hours while awake, for a total of 6 consecutive doses. Patients with kidney problems may require smaller doses. An injection form is available for hospitalized patients and those in special home care situations. The intraocular insert must be surgically implanted in the eye and replaced every 6 months.

ONSET OF EFFECT
Unknown.

DURATION OF ACTION
About 24 to 48 hours.

DIETARY ADVICE
Take the capsules with food. Increase fluids if you have a fever or diarrhea. Patients with AIDS are often weakened and may be unable to consume adequate amounts of nutritious food. Use special liquid supplements if necessary. Your doctor may refer you to a nutritionist.

STORAGE
Store in a tightly sealed container away from heat and direct light.

MISSED DOSE
Take it as soon as you remember. If it is near the time for the next dose, skip the missed dose and resume your regular dosage schedule. Do not double the next dose.

STOPPING THE DRUG
Take it as prescribed for the full treatment period, even if you feel better before the scheduled end of therapy.

PROLONGED USE
Your doctor should check your progress periodically during prolonged use.

▼ PRECAUTIONS

Over 60: Adverse reactions may be more likely and more severe in older patients.

Driving and Hazardous Work: Avoid such activities until you determine how the medicine affects you.

Alcohol: Avoid alcohol.

Pregnancy: Avoid use of this drug if you are pregnant or trying to become pregnant. If you must use the drug, use a reliable birth control method (both men and women) throughout therapy and for at least 3 months afterward.

Breast Feeding: Ganciclovir passes into breast milk and may be harmful to the nursing infant; do not breast feed when taking this drug.

Infants and Children: Not recommended for infants and children.

Special Concerns: Therapy with oral ganciclovir requires many weeks or months. Relapse of eye problems is common, once the drug is stopped. Remember that infection is a great threat to people with weakened immune systems. Do not receive any vaccinations without your doctor's approval, and try to avoid people with infections. Watch for unusual bleeding, bruising, or fevers.

OVERDOSE
Symptoms: Extreme weakness and dizziness, severe diarrhea and stomach upset, shortness of breath.

What to Do: Call your doctor, emergency medical services (EMS), or the nearest poison control center immediately.

▼ INTERACTIONS

DRUG INTERACTIONS
Consult your doctor for specific advice if you are taking amphotericin B, azathioprine, carmustine, chloramphenicol, cisplatin, cyclosporine, dapsone, deferoxamine, didanosine (ddI), flucytosine, gold salts, any pain medicine, lithium, methotrexate, pentamidine, penicillamine, plicamycin, probenecid, streptozocin, tiopronin, trimethoprim/ sulfamethoxazole, or zidovudine (AZT).

FOOD INTERACTIONS
No known food interactions.

DISEASE INTERACTIONS
Consult your doctor for advice if you have been diagnosed as having a low white blood cell count, low platelet count, clotting or bleeding problems, or kidney disease.

 SIDE EFFECTS

SERIOUS
Unusual or persistent fevers, chills, unusual fatigue, sore throat, bruising, or bleeding (these may be signs of serious anemia or problems with the cells of your immune system); skin rash, tremor, eye pain, or sudden change in vision (blurring or partial loss of sight), pain at the injection site. Call your doctor immediately.

COMMON
No common side effects are associated with the use of ganciclovir.

LESS COMMON
Abdominal discomfort, decreased appetite, nausea, vomiting, sweating.

GATIFLOXACIN

Available in: Tablets, injection
Available OTC? No   **As Generic?** No
Drug Class: Fluoroquinolone antibiotic

▼ USAGE INFORMATION

WHY IT'S PRESCRIBED
To treat mild to severe bacterial infections, including acute sinusitis, community-acquired pneumonia, urinary tract infections, kidney infections, acute bacterial complications due to chronic bronchitis, and gonorrhea.

HOW IT WORKS
Gatifloxacin inhibits the activity of bacterial enzymes (DNA gyrase and a topoisomerase) necessary for proper DNA formation and replication. This fights infection by preventing bacteria from reproducing.

▼ DOSAGE GUIDELINES

RANGE AND FREQUENCY
For most infections: 400 mg once a day for 7 to 10 days. For community-acquired pneumonia: 400 mg a day for 7 to 14 days. For uncomplicated urinary tract infections: 400 mg as a one-time dose or 200 mg once a day for 3 days. For gonorrhea: 400 mg as a one-time dose. For those with impaired kidney function: Your doctor will determine the appropriate dosage.

ONSET OF EFFECT
Varies depending on the infection being treated.

DURATION OF ACTION
Unknown.

DIETARY ADVICE
No special precautions.

STORAGE
Store in a tightly sealed container away from heat, moisture, and direct light.

MISSED DOSE
Take it as soon as you remember. If it is near the time for the next dose, skip the missed dose and resume your regular dosage schedule. Do not double the next dose.

STOPPING THE DRUG
It is very important to take this drug as prescribed for the full treatment period.

PROLONGED USE
If your symptoms do not improve or instead become worse after a few days, consult your doctor promptly.

▼ PRECAUTIONS

Over 60: No special problems are expected.

Driving and Hazardous Work: Do not drive or engage in hazardous work until you determine how the medicine affects you.

Alcohol: It is advisable to abstain from alcohol when fighting an infection.

Pregnancy: It should be used during pregnancy only if potential benefits clearly justify the risks. Before you take gatifloxacin, tell your doctor if you are pregnant or plan to become pregnant.

Breast Feeding: Gatifloxacin may pass into breast milk and cause serious side effects in the nursing infant; its use is discouraged when nursing.

Infants and Children: Not recommended for children.

Special Concerns: Do not take this medicine if you are allergic to any quinolone antibiotic.

OVERDOSE
Symptoms: An overdose is unlikely to occur. Possible symptoms after an excessive dose may include decreased activity and rate of breathing, vomiting, tremors, seizures.

What to Do: If you have any reason to suspect an overdose, call your doctor, emergency medical services (EMS), or the nearest poison control.

▼ INTERACTIONS

DRUG INTERACTIONS
Because gatifloxacin can affect the function of the heart, it should not be used if you are taking antiarrhythmic drugs, such as amiodarone. It should be used with caution in those taking cisapride, antipsychotics, tricylic antidepressants, erythromycin, warfarin, nonsteroidal anti-inflammatory drugs, or digoxin. Gatifloxacin should be taken at least 4 hours before using iron supplements, dietary supplements containing zinc, didanosine, or antacids containing aluminum or magnesium salts.

FOOD INTERACTIONS
No known food interactions.

DISEASE INTERACTIONS
Gatifloxacin should not be taken by people with prolongation of the QT interval on an electrocardiogram, known heart rhythm disturbances, uncorrected hypokalemia (low blood potassium levels), or those taking antiarrhythmic drugs. This drug should be used with caution in people with significant bradycardia (slow heart rate), recent myocardial ischemia, known or suspected nervous system disorders, or those who are predisposed to seizures. People with impaired kidney function may require a reduced dose depending on the severity of kidney dysfunction.

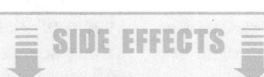

SIDE EFFECTS

SERIOUS
Serious reactions are rare and include seizures, rapid heartbeat, confusion, hallucinations, agitation, nightmares, depression, shortness of breath, unusual swelling in face or extremities, unconsciousness; redness, blisters, rash, or itching on exposure to sunlight; increased risk of tendinitis or tendon rupture. Call your doctor immediately.

COMMON
Nausea, vaginitis, diarrhea, headache, dizziness.

LESS COMMON
Chills, fever, back pain, abdominal pain, constipation, heartburn, inflammation of the tongue, mouth sores, vomiting, swelling, insomnia, numbness, shortness of breath, sore throat, sweating, abnormal vision, change in sense of taste, ringing in the ears, painful urination, blood in urine.

GEMFIBROZIL

Available in: Tablets
Available OTC? No   **As Generic?** Yes
Drug Class: Antilipidemic (triglyceride-lowering agent)

▼ USAGE INFORMATION

WHY IT'S PRESCRIBED
To treat high levels of blood triglyceride. Usually prescribed after other treatments—including diet, weight loss, exercise, and control of diabetes (when present)—fail to lower triglyceride levels adequately.

HOW IT WORKS
Gemfibrozil speeds the removal of triglycerides from the lipoprotein known as very-low-density lipoprotein (VLDL), which is converted to low-density lipoprotein (LDL). In some people total and LDL cholesterol levels may rise while triglycerides fall.

▼ DOSAGE GUIDELINES

RANGE AND FREQUENCY
Adults: 600 milligrams, 2 times per day. Usually taken 30 to 60 minutes before morning and evening meals.

ONSET OF EFFECT
Improvement begins in about 1 week and becomes most noticeable in about 4 weeks.

DURATION OF ACTION
Blood triglyceride levels increase within a few weeks of stopping gemfibrozil.

DIETARY ADVICE
Follow your doctor's dietary advice to improve control over high blood pressure and help prevent heart disease. The American Heart Association publishes a "Healthy Heart" diet; discuss this with your doctor. Limit intake of alcohol, which can raise triglyceride levels.

STORAGE
Store in a tightly sealed container away from heat and direct light.

MISSED DOSE
Take your missed dose as soon as you remember, unless the time for your next scheduled dose is within the next 2 hours. If so, do not take the missed dose. Take your next scheduled dose at the proper time, and resume your regular dosage schedule. Do not double the next dose.

STOPPING THE DRUG
Do not stop taking gemfibrozil on your own; the level of triglycerides in your blood will increase.

PROLONGED USE
Gemfibrozil is often taken for long periods of time. If your blood triglycerides do not diminish, your physician may stop the medication.

▼ PRECAUTIONS

Over 60: Adverse reactions may be more likely and more severe in older patients.

Driving and Hazardous Work: The use of gemfibrozil should not impair your ability to perform such tasks safely.

Alcohol: Alcohol intake should be limited because it can raise triglyceride levels.

Pregnancy: Do not take gemfibrozil while pregnant unless your doctor indicates that the risks of stopping the drug are too great. Triglycerides increase substantially during pregnancy and extremely high triglycerides can trigger an attack of acute pancreatitis.

Breast Feeding: Avoid or discontinue usage while nursing.

Infants and Children: Rarely used in infants and children.

Special Concerns: The most important treatment for high levels of blood triglycerides is a proper diet, weight loss, regular moderate exercise, the avoidance of certain medications, and control of diabetes. Because gemfibrozil has potential side effects, it is important that you maintain a healthy diet and cooperate with other treatment strategies your physician may suggest. Gemfibrozil may increase the chances of gallbladder, liver, and pancreas problems; your physician will order periodic blood tests.

OVERDOSE
Symptoms: No specific ones have been reported.

What to Do: Emergency instructions not applicable.

▼ INTERACTIONS

DRUG INTERACTIONS
Certain drugs may interact adversely with gemfibrozil, particularly anticoagulants, niacin, and any of the group of cholesterol-lowering drugs referred to as "-statins." It may be necessary to reduce the dose of warfarin to prevent bleeding. The combination of gemfibrozil with either niacin or a statin drug can cause severe myositis (muscle inflammation), which can release a protein that damages the kidneys.

FOOD INTERACTIONS
No known food interactions.

DISEASE INTERACTIONS
Inform your doctor if you have any of the following problems: gallstones, stomach or intestinal ulcer, kidney disease, muscle disease, or liver disease. The dose of gemfibrozil must be reduced in those with significant kidney damage.

  SIDE EFFECTS

SERIOUS
Muscle aches and tenderness; crampy abdominal pain, especially in the area under the ribs on the right side, with nausea and vomiting (this is an uncommon, serious side effect that may indicate gallbladder disease); decreased urine output.

COMMON
Diarrhea, nausea, gas.

LESS COMMON
Decreased sexual ability; headache; weight gain; feelings similar to the flu, with muscle aches or cramps, weakness, and unusual tiredness; inflammation of mouth and lips; heartburn.

GENTAMICIN TOPICAL

Available in: Cream, ointment
Available OTC? No   **As Generic?** Yes
Drug Class: Antibacterial (topical)

▼ USAGE INFORMATION

WHY IT'S PRESCRIBED
To treat minor bacterial infections of the skin, including infected bites, burns, abrasions, and other wounds; infected cysts, hair follicles, and other skin structures; and infections complicating rashes, eczema, dermatitis, and other inflammatory skin conditions. Gentamicin is not effective against fungal infections or viruses.

HOW IT WORKS
Gentamicin works by preventing bacterial organisms from manufacturing the vital proteins they require for growth and function.

▼ DOSAGE GUIDELINES

RANGE AND FREQUENCY
Adults and children over age 1: Apply it to the affected site 3 or 4 times a day.

ONSET OF EFFECT
Gentamicin begins killing susceptible bacteria shortly after contact. The drug's effects may not be noticeable for several days.

DURATION OF ACTION
The exact duration of action of gentamicin is not known, but replenishing the topical antibiotic 3 or 4 times a day is sufficient for treatment.

DIETARY ADVICE
No special restrictions.

STORAGE
Store in a tightly sealed container away from heat, moisture, and direct light.

MISSED DOSE
Apply it as soon as you remember. If it is near the time for the next dose, skip the missed dose and resume your regular dosage schedule. Do not double the next dose or apply excessive amounts of the drug to compensate for a missed application.

STOPPING THE DRUG
Apply the medicine as prescribed by your doctor for the full treatment period, even if you begin to feel better before the scheduled end of therapy.

PROLONGED USE
Therapy with gentamicin is usually completed within 7 to 14 days. Use of any antibiotic drug for longer than your doctor recommends increases your risk of infection by drug-resistant bacteria or other microorganisms (known as superinfection).

▼ PRECAUTIONS

Over 60: Adverse reactions may be more likely and more severe in older patients.

Driving and Hazardous Work: No special precautions are necessary.

Alcohol: No special precautions are necessary.

Pregnancy: Problems in pregnant women using gentamicin have not been reported. Consult your doctor for specific advice.

Breast Feeding: Gentamicin may pass into breast milk; caution is advised. Consult your doctor for advice.

Infants and Children: This drug is not recommended for use by children under 1 year of age.

Special Concerns: Make sure you tell your doctor about allergies that you might have before taking any antibiotic. There is varying opinion as to whether or not topical antibiotics are effective to treat infections. Tell your doctor if your condition has not improved within a few days of starting gentamicin. As with any other antibiotic, gentamicin is useful only against strains of bacteria that are susceptible to its effects.

OVERDOSE
Symptoms: No specific ones have been reported.

What to Do: An overdose of gentamicin is unlikely to be life-threatening. However, if someone takes a much larger dose than prescribed or accidentally ingests the cream or ointment, call your doctor, emergency medical services (EMS), or the nearest poison control center.

▼ INTERACTIONS

DRUG INTERACTIONS
No drug interactions have been reported. If you are concerned about whether a prescription or nonprescription medication you are taking may interact with topical gentamicin, consult your doctor or pharmacist for current information.

FOOD INTERACTIONS
No known food interactions.

DISEASE INTERACTIONS
Caution is advised when using gentamicin. Consult your doctor if you have hearing problems, kidney disease, any prior reactions to a skin cream or ointment, or any history of allergic reaction to antibiotics.

≡ SIDE EFFECTS ≡

SERIOUS
No serious side effects are associated with topical gentamicin when used as directed.

COMMON
No common side effects are associated with topical gentamicin when used as directed.

LESS COMMON
Itching, swelling, increased redness, or discomfort at the application site not present prior to therapy (as a result of allergic reaction).

GLATIRAMER ACETATE (COPOLYMER-1)

Available in: Powder that is used for injection
Available OTC? No   **As Generic?** No
Drug Class: Immunomodulator

▼ USAGE INFORMATION

WHY IT'S PRESCRIBED
To prevent or reduce the frequency of relapses in patients with relapsing-remitting multiple sclerosis (the most common form of MS, in which periods of active disease alternate with periods of remission or reduced severity of symptoms).

HOW IT WORKS
Nerves are insulated by a layer of fatty material known as myelin. MS is a frequently progressive, often debilitating, disorder that occurs when the protective myelin is damaged at various (multiple) sites throughout the central nervous system (brain and spinal cord) by the body's own immune system, with the subsequent development of scar-like tissue, a process referred to by doctors as sclerosis. Glatiramer acetate is believed to block the attack on the myelin sheath, slowing the progress of the disease.

▼ DOSAGE GUIDELINES

RANGE AND FREQUENCY
20 mg injected under the skin once a day.

ONSET OF EFFECT
Unknown.

DURATION OF ACTION
Unknown.

DIETARY ADVICE
No special restrictions.

STORAGE
The powder should be kept refrigerated; if refrigeration is not available, it may be stored at room temperature for up to one week. The vials of sterile water with which the powder is mixed should be stored at room temperature. The powder and water should be kept in tightly sealed containers away from direct light.

MISSED DOSE
Take it as soon as you remember. However, if it is near the time for the next dose, skip the missed dose and resume your regular dosage schedule. Do not double the next dose.

STOPPING THE DRUG
The decision to stop taking the drug should be made by your doctor.

PROLONGED USE
You should see your doctor regularly for tests and examinations if you must take this medicine for a prolonged period of time.

▼ PRECAUTIONS

Over 60: No special problems are expected.

Driving and Hazardous Work: Do not drive or engage in hazardous activities until you determine how the drug affects you.

Alcohol: No special warnings.

Pregnancy: Human studies have not been done. Before you take glatiramer acetate, tell your doctor if you are pregnant or plan to become pregnant.

Breast Feeding: Glatiramer acetate may pass into breast milk; caution is advised. Consult your doctor for specific information.

Infants and Children: The safety and effectiveness of glatiramer acetate in persons under age 18 have not been established.

Special Concerns: Glatiramer acetate should be injected at a different site every day during the week; 7 sites in all.

Sites for self-injection are the arms, stomach, thighs, and hips. The injection is best given at the same time every day. To prepare the medication for injection, use a sterile syringe and needle to transfer the sterile water into the glatiramer acetate vial. Swirl the vial gently and let it stand at room temperature until the solid material is completely dissolved. Discard the preparation if it contains visible sediment. Put the preparation into a sterile syringe fitted with a new 27-gauge needle and make the injection under the skin at the selected site of the day. After the injection, a cotton ball should be held against the injection site for a few seconds, but the site should not be rubbed.

OVERDOSE
Symptoms: No specific ones have been reported.

What to Do: If someone receives a much larger dose than prescribed or accidentally ingests glatiramer acetate, call the nearest poison control center immediately.

▼ INTERACTIONS

DRUG INTERACTIONS
Other drugs potentially may interact with glatiramer acetate. Consult your doctor for advice if you are taking any other medication.

FOOD INTERACTIONS
No known food interactions.

DISEASE INTERACTIONS
Caution is advised when taking glatiramer acetate. Consult your physician if you have any other medical condition.

▼ SIDE EFFECTS

SERIOUS
Severe pain or rash at injection site immediately after injection. Call your doctor immediately.

COMMON
Flushed skin, dizziness, depression, palpitations, anxiety, difficulty breathing, throat constriction, fast heartbeat, tremor, hives, transient chest pain, enlarged blood vessels, fever, chills, infection, migraine headache, loss of appetite, gastrointestinal disorders, nausea, vomiting, swelling of arms and legs, joint pains, anxiety, muscle tension, bronchitis, nasal inflammation, itching skin, ear pain, urge to urinate frequently.

LESS COMMON
There are no less-common side effects associated with glatiramer acetate.

GLIMEPIRIDE

Available in: Tablets
Available OTC? No   **As Generic?** Yes
Drug Class: Antidiabetic agent/sulfonylurea

▼ USAGE INFORMATION

WHY IT'S PRESCRIBED
To treat diabetes (high blood sugar) in patients who require little or no injectable insulin. It is used in conjunction with a special diet and exercise. Some patients may fail to respond initially or gradually lose their responsiveness to glimepiride. The antidiabetic agent metformin may be used with glimepiride to achieve the desired results.

HOW IT WORKS
Glimepiride stimulates the release of insulin from the pancreas and makes the tissues of your body more responsive to insulin.

▼ DOSAGE GUIDELINES

RANGE AND FREQUENCY
Adults: 1 to 4 mg once daily, 30 minutes before breakfast. Children: Not recommended for use by children.

ONSET OF EFFECT
2 to 3 hours.

DURATION OF ACTION
12 to 24 hours.

DIETARY ADVICE
Maintain special diets as recommended by your doctor. Restrict excessive intake of sugar-containing snacks.

STORAGE
Keep away from direct light, moisture, and extremes in temperature.

MISSED DOSE
Take it as soon as you remember. If it is near the time for the next dose, skip the missed dose and resume your regular dosage schedule. Do not double the next dose.

STOPPING THE DRUG
The decision to stop taking glimepiride should be made by your doctor.

PROLONGED USE
Therapy with glimepiride may require months or years. Its prolonged use may be associated with an increased risk of side effects.

▼ PRECAUTIONS

Over 60: Adverse reactions from this drug may be more likely and more severe.

Driving and Hazardous Work: Do not drive or engage in hazardous work until you determine how the medicine affects you.

Alcohol: Use only in a moderate, responsible fashion. Consult your doctor.

Pregnancy: Glimepiride should not be used during pregnancy.

Breast Feeding: It should not be used by nursing mothers.

Infants and Children: Not recommended for children.

Special Concerns: Understand the symptoms of low blood sugar. Always have easy access to sources of simple sugar—juice, candy bars, energy bars, hard candy, honey, sugar cubes, sugar dissolved in water—in the event you experience symptoms of hypoglycemia. Inform your doctor promptly about changes in the way you are feeling, changes in your lifestyle and level of activity, drugs that you may have been prescribed by other specialists, medications that you have stopped taking, unusually high or low results for any at-home tests you use to check your urine or blood, episodes of low blood sugar, and pregnancy. Wear a special medical ID bracelet. Do not miss meals. Use caution when exercising.

OVERDOSE
Symptoms: Symptoms are similar to serious side effects.

What to Do: Call emergency medical services (EMS), your doctor, or the nearest poison control center immediately.

▼ INTERACTIONS

DRUG INTERACTIONS
Consult your doctor for specific advice if you are taking steroids and nonsteroidal anti-inflammatory drugs (such as ibuprofen, aspirin, or aspirin-containing drugs), anticoagulants, certain antibiotics, especially for fungal infections, diuretics, lithium, beta-blockers, ulcer medications, ciprofloxacin, cyclosporine, guanethidine, MAO inhibitors, quinidine, quinine, chloramphenicol, estrogen, isoniazid, thyroid hormones, theophylline, pentamidine phenothiazines, or phenytoin.

FOOD INTERACTIONS
No known food interactions.

DISEASE INTERACTIONS
Consult your doctor if you have diarrhea, persistent vomiting, malabsorption disease, liver, thyroid, kidney, or adrenal gland disease, fever, or infection.

▼ SIDE EFFECTS

SERIOUS
Serious side effects are related to hypoglycemia, or low blood sugar, whose symptoms include perspiration or a cold sweat, restlessness, rapid pulse, anxious feeling, nausea, feelings of dizziness, weakness, or lightheadedness, poor coordination, slurred speech, confusion, sleepiness, seizures or convulsions, weakness of an arm, leg, or an entire side of the body, fainting. Seek emergency assistance. Administer sugar-containing substances only if the patient is conscious and alert. Other serious but less common side effects include low white blood cell count and elevation of liver-associated enzymes; these problems can be detected by your doctor.

COMMON
Dizziness, weakness, nausea, headache.

LESS COMMON
Skin reactions, such as itching, peeling, rashes, and hives; blurred vision; edema (swelling due to fluid retention) of face or extremities; severe tiredness; abdominal pain.

GLIPIZIDE

Available in: Tablets, extended-release tablets
Available OTC? No **As Generic?** Yes
Drug Class: Antidiabetic agent/sulfonylurea

▼ USAGE INFORMATION

WHY IT'S PRESCRIBED
To treat diabetes (high blood sugar) in patients who require little or no injectable insulin. It is used in conjunction with a special diet and exercise. Some patients may fail to respond initially or gradually lose their responsiveness to glipizide. Other antidiabetic agents may be used in conjunction with glipizide to achieve the desired results.

HOW IT WORKS
Glipizide stimulates the release of insulin from special cells in the pancreas and therefore helps to lower blood glucose.

▼ DOSAGE GUIDELINES

RANGE AND FREQUENCY
Usual starting dose: 5 mg a day, taken 30 minutes before breakfast. Dosage should be adjusted by 2.5 to 5 mg per day based on blood sugar response. When greater than 15 mg a day, dosages should be divided. In the elderly or patients with liver disease, the initial dose should be 2.5 mg a day. Extended-release tablets: 5 to 10 mg, once daily, usually with breakfast.

ONSET OF EFFECT
Within 30 minutes.

DURATION OF ACTION
12 to 24 hours.

DIETARY ADVICE
Maintain special diets as recommended by your doctor, nutritionist, or the American Diabetes Association. Restrict excessive intake of sugar-laden snacks. Read labels carefully when buying food.

STORAGE
Store away from direct light, moisture, and extremes in temperature.

MISSED DOSE
Take it as soon as you remember. If it is near the time for the next dose, skip the missed dose and resume your regular dosage schedule. Do not double the next dose.

STOPPING THE DRUG
The decision to stop taking it should be made by your doctor.

PROLONGED USE
Therapy may require months or years. Prolonged use may be associated with an increased risk of side effects.

▼ PRECAUTIONS

Over 60: Adverse reactions from this drug may be more likely and more severe.

Driving and Hazardous Work: Do not drive or engage in hazardous work until you determine how the medication affects you.

Alcohol: Drink in moderation.

Pregnancy: Insulin is the treatment of choice for pregnant diabetic women.

Breast Feeding: This drug passes into breast milk, although it is uncertain whether this is harmful to nursing infants.

Infants and Children: Not recommended for children.

Special Concerns: Keep simple sugars (juice, candy bars, hard candy) on hand in the event of hypoglycemia. Inform your doctor promptly of changes in how you feel, unusually high or low results for any at-home tests, episodes of low blood sugar, or pregnancy. Wear a medical ID bracelet. Do not miss meals. Use caution when exercising.

OVERDOSE
Symptoms: Symptoms similar to serious side effects.

What to Do: Call emergency medical services (EMS), your doctor, or the nearest poison control center immediately.

▼ INTERACTIONS

DRUG INTERACTIONS
Consult your doctor for specific advice if you are taking anticoagulants, antibiotics (especially sulfa-containing antibiotics or those used to treat fungal infections), steroids, diuretics, seizure medications, beta-blockers (which may include eye drops for glaucoma) or other blood pressure medications, lithium, ulcer drugs, guanethidine, MAO inhibitors, quinidine, quinine, salicylates, chloramphenicol, estrogens, isoniazid, thyroid hormones, theophylline, or pentamidine.

FOOD INTERACTIONS
Food delays the absorption of immediate-release tablets.

DISEASE INTERACTIONS
Consult your doctor if you have diarrhea, persistent vomiting, malabsorption disease, liver, thyroid, kidney, or adrenal gland disease, fever, infection, or impending or recent surgery.

 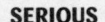

SIDE EFFECTS

SERIOUS
Serious side effects are related to hypoglycemia, or low blood sugar, whose symptoms include perspiration or a cold sweat, restlessness, rapid pulse, anxious feeling, nausea, feelings of dizziness, weakness, or lightheadedness, poor coordination, slurred speech, confusion, drowsiness, seizures, weakness of an arm, leg, or an entire side of the body, and fainting. Seek emergency assistance. Administer sugar-containing substances only if the patient is conscious and alert. Other serious but less common side effects include low white blood cell count and elevation of liver-associated enzymes; these can be detected by your doctor.

COMMON
Dizziness, constipation, nausea, heartburn, unusual or changed taste of food, or unusual taste in the mouth.

LESS COMMON
Peeling, red, bruised, or itching skin, pale skin, edema (swelling) of face or extremities, reduced ability to exercise, headache, fever.

GLUCAGON

Available in: Injection
Available OTC? No   **As Generic?** Yes
Drug Class: Hormone; antidote; antidiabetic agent

▼ USAGE INFORMATION

WHY IT'S PRESCRIBED
Glucagon is an injectable drug that is used for the emergency treatment of low blood sugar in diabetics who are unable to take any sugar-containing foods or liquids by mouth. These patients are usually unconscious or very confused and sleepy.

HOW IT WORKS
Glucagon stimulates the liver to release glucose (sugar) into the bloodstream.

▼ DOSAGE GUIDELINES

RANGE AND FREQUENCY
Adults and children weighing more than 45 pounds: 1 mg, by injection. Children less than 45 pounds: 0.5 mg. Doses may be repeated twice, at 15 minute intervals. Glucagon emergency kits usually contain two vials. One is glucagon. The other is a fluid that must be used to dilute glucagon before it can be drawn up in a syringe and injected.

ONSET OF EFFECT
Within 15 minutes.

DURATION OF ACTION
The effect persists for 1 to 2 hours.

DIETARY ADVICE
Solutions containing glucose (sugar) must be administered following glucagon injections for the drug to work properly.

STORAGE
Store in a tightly sealed container away from heat and direct light. If you prepared glucagon for injection but did not use it, it may be refrigerated and kept for no more than 48 hours.

MISSED DOSE
Not applicable; glucagon is used only in emergencies.

STOPPING THE DRUG
If the patient has not responded within 15 minutes of the first injection, do not stop glucagon treatments. You may administer 2 more injections at 15-minute intervals.

PROLONGED USE
Not applicable.

▼ PRECAUTIONS

Over 60: No unusual problems are expected.

Driving and Hazardous Work: Not applicable.

Alcohol: Not applicable.

Pregnancy: Glucagon may be administered.

Breast Feeding: It is unlikely that glucagon is hazardous to nursing infants, since the drug is used only occasionally, although no studies have been done to confirm this.

Infants and Children: Not applicable.

Special Concerns: Glucagon is effective only if given by injection. Therefore, it is very important that family members or caregivers know exactly how to prepare glucagon for injection. The best time to read and understand glucagon instructions is before an emergency occurs. Any diabetic patient who is confused, drowsy, sleepy, or unconscious should be assumed to have low blood sugar. Do not attempt to feed drowsy, disoriented, or unconscious individuals. Administer glucagon promptly. If not already notified, emergency personnel should be contacted immediately after the first glucagon dose has been injected. Do not wait for further doses to be given before calling for emergency assistance. Do not wait for additional 15-minute intervals. Glucagon is not a cure for low blood sugar. It is an emergency treatment that may be lifesaving, but it is only a temporary treatment that buys time. Even after glucagon injection, blood sugar may fall again to dangerously low levels. Do not assume that the danger has passed after successful treatment with glucagon. Any patient who was ill enough to receive glucagon needs to be evaluated fully by a physician.

OVERDOSE
Symptoms: Nausea, vomiting, severe weakness, irregular heartbeat, hoarseness, or cramps.

What to Do: An overdose of glucagon is unlikely to be life-threatening. However, if someone receives a much larger dose than prescribed, call your doctor, emergency medical services (EMS), or the nearest poison control center immediately.

▼ INTERACTIONS

DRUG INTERACTIONS
None known.

FOOD INTERACTIONS
No known food interactions.

DISEASE INTERACTIONS
Inform your doctor if you have insulinoma or pheochromocytoma. While these conditions may complicate the use of glucagon, they do not prohibit a patient from receiving the drug in an emergency.

▼ SIDE EFFECTS

SERIOUS
No serious side effects are associated with glucagon.

COMMON
Nausea may be associated with higher dosages.

LESS COMMON
Rare allergic reactions (wheezing, itching, weakness); redness and pain at site of injection. Consult your doctor if such side effects persist or recur.

GLYBURIDE

Available in: Tablets
Available OTC? No   **As Generic?** Yes
Drug Class: Antidiabetic agent/sulfonylurea

▼ USAGE INFORMATION

WHY IT'S PRESCRIBED
To help control adult-onset (non-insulin-dependent, or type 2) diabetes. Glyburide is sometimes used in conjunction with metformin (another oral antidiabetic).

HOW IT WORKS
Glyburide stimulates the release of insulin by the pancreas and decreases sugar production in the liver.

▼ DOSAGE GUIDELINES

RANGE AND FREQUENCY
Starting dose is 2.5 to 5 mg daily, 30 minutes before breakfast. It can be increased by your doctor in increments of 2.5 mg to a maximum of 20 mg per day, or decreased if needed. Elderly patients or those with kidney or liver dysfunction should receive an initial dose of 1.25 mg per day. If the daily maintenance dose is increased to 10 mg or more, the total dose should be divided equally between breakfast and dinner.

ONSET OF EFFECT
1 hour.

DURATION OF ACTION
24 hours.

DIETARY ADVICE
It is usually taken 30 minutes before breakfast.

STORAGE
Store in a tightly sealed container away from heat and direct light.

MISSED DOSE
Take it as soon as you remember. If it is near the time for the next dose, skip the missed dose and resume your regular dosage schedule. Do not double the next dose.

STOPPING THE DRUG
The decision to stop taking the drug should be made by your doctor. You may need to take glyburide for the rest of your life.

PROLONGED USE
Periodic blood tests should be done to determine how prolonged use affects blood sugar levels.

▼ PRECAUTIONS

Over 60: Treatment should start with lower doses, which should be increased slowly as determined by periodic tests. Adverse reactions may be more likely and more severe in older patients.

Driving and Hazardous Work: Do not drive or engage in hazardous work until you determine how the medication affects you.

Alcohol: Avoid alcohol.

Pregnancy: Uncontrolled blood sugar levels during pregnancy are associated with an increased risk of birth defects, so many experts recommend a switch to insulin during pregnancy.

Breast Feeding: Glyburide may pass into breast milk; caution is advised. Consult your doctor for advice.

Infants and Children: Glyburide does not work in juvenile-onset, insulin-dependent diabetes.

Special Concerns: Carry medical identification that says you have diabetes. If you are under stress due to an infection, fever, an injury, or surgery, you may need insulin therapy in addition to or instead of glyburide.

OVERDOSE
Symptoms: Symptoms are similar to serious side effects.

What to Do: An overdose of glyburide is unlikely to be life-threatening. However, if someone takes a much larger dose than prescribed, call your doctor, emergency medical services (EMS), or the nearest poison control center.

▼ INTERACTIONS

DRUG INTERACTIONS
Consult your doctor for specific advice if you are taking anabolic steroids, aspirin or other salicylates, cimetidine, gemfibrozil, fenfluramine, MAO inhibitors, phenylbutazone, ranitidine, sulfa drugs, beta-blockers, bumetanide, diazoxide, ethacrynic acid, furosemide, phenytoin, rifampin, thiazide diuretics, thyroid hormone, antacids, antifungal agents, enalapril, steroids, or warfarin.

FOOD INTERACTIONS
Glyburide is just part of the treatment for diabetes; be sure to follow the diet recommended by your doctor.

DISEASE INTERACTIONS
Use of this medication may cause complications in patients with liver or kidney disease, since these organs work together to remove the drug from the body.

 SIDE EFFECTS

SERIOUS
Serious side effects are related to hypoglycemia, or low blood sugar, whose symptoms include perspiration or a cold sweat, restlessness, rapid pulse, anxious feeling, nausea, feelings of dizziness, weakness, or lightheadedness, poor coordination, slurred speech, confusion, sleepiness, seizures, weakness of an arm, leg, or an entire side of the body, and fainting. Seek emergency assistance. Administer sugar-containing substances only if the patient is conscious and alert. Other serious but less common side effects include bone marrow suppression, hemolytic anemia, and elevation of liver-associated enzymes; these problems can be detected by your doctor.

COMMON
Bloating, heartburn, nausea, indigestion.

LESS COMMON
Blurred vision, changes in taste, itching, hives, joint or muscle pain.

GLYCERIN ORAL

Available in: Oral solution
Available OTC? No   **As Generic?** Yes
Drug Class: Diuretic, antiglaucoma agent

▼ USAGE INFORMATION

WHY IT'S PRESCRIBED
To treat glaucoma.

HOW IT WORKS
Glaucoma, a sight-threatening disorder, occurs when aqueous humor (the fluid inside the eye) cannot drain properly, causing an increase in pressure within the eyeball (intraocular pressure). This can damage the optic nerve and lead to a gradually progressive loss of vision. Oral glycerin promotes outflow of aqueous humor, thereby reducing intraocular pressure. It is used on a short-term basis to reduce eye pressure until further medical intervention, such as other medications or surgery, can be implemented for more long-term control of glaucoma.

▼ DOSAGE GUIDELINES

RANGE AND FREQUENCY
Adults: To start, 1 dose of 1 to 2 grams (g) per 2.2 lbs (1 kg) of body weight. Additional doses of 500 mg per 2.2 lbs may be given 4 times a day if needed. Children: To start, 1 dose of 1 to 1.5 g per 2.2 lbs. Dose may be repeated in 4 to 8 hours if needed.

ONSET OF EFFECT
Within 10 minutes.

DURATION OF ACTION
About 5 hours.

DIETARY ADVICE
No special restrictions.

STORAGE
Store in a tightly sealed container away from heat and direct light. Do not allow it to freeze.

MISSED DOSE
If this drug is prescribed beyond immediate short-term use, take the missed dose as soon as you remember. However, if it is near the time for the next dose, skip the missed dose and resume your regular dosage schedule. Do not double the next dose.

STOPPING THE DRUG
If this drug is prescribed beyond immediate short-term use, take it as prescribed for the full treatment period.

PROLONGED USE
In most cases oral glycerin is used exclusively on a short-term basis, either in a doctor's office or hospital, until other forms of treatment can be implemented.

▼ PRECAUTIONS

Over 60: Excessive dehydration may be more likely to occur in older patients.

Driving and Hazardous Work: Do not drive or engage in hazardous work until you determine how the medicine affects you.

Alcohol: No special warnings.

Pregnancy: Adequate studies have not been done. Before taking oral glycerin, tell your doctor if you are pregnant or plan to become pregnant.

Breast Feeding: Glycerin may pass into breast milk; caution is advised. Consult your doctor for specific advice.

Infants and Children: No special problems expected.

Special Concerns: To improve the taste of glycerin, it can be mixed with a small amount of unsweetened orange, lemon, or lime juice, poured over ice, and sipped through a straw. If you experience a headache while taking glycerin, you should lie down while you take it and for a short time afterward. If your headaches continue or become severe, consult your doctor. Diabetic patients must be sure their ophthalmologist and other doctors know they have diabetes and that it is under good control. This medication may interfere with blood sugar control.

OVERDOSE
Symptoms: Severe dehydration, heart rhythm abnormalities (cardiac arrhythmias), loss of consciousness, coma.

What to Do: Call your doctor, emergency medical services (EMS), or the nearest poison control center immediately.

▼ INTERACTIONS

DRUG INTERACTIONS
Consult your doctor for specific advice if you are taking a diuretic or any other prescription or over-the-counter medication.

FOOD INTERACTIONS
No known food interactions.

DISEASE INTERACTIONS
Caution is advised when taking glycerin. Consult your doctor if you have any of the following: diabetes mellitus, heart disease, hypovolemia (insufficient fluid volume in the body, due to dehydration or other causes), hypervolemia (excess fluid volume in the body, causing circulatory problems and swelling at various sites, due to fluid retention in the tissues), or a psychological condition associated with persistent confusion. Use of glycerin may cause complications in patients with kidney disease, since this organ works to remove the medication from the body.

SIDE EFFECTS

SERIOUS
Confusion, heart rhythm irregularities. Call your doctor immediately.

COMMON
Headache, nausea, and vomiting.

LESS COMMON
Dizziness, diarrhea, dry mouth, increased thirst.

GLYCERIN RECTAL

Available in: Rectal solution, rectal suppositories
Available OTC? Yes   **As Generic?** Yes
Drug Class: Hyperosmotic laxative

▼ USAGE INFORMATION

WHY IT'S PRESCRIBED
To treat constipation.

HOW IT WORKS
Glycerin attracts and retains water in the intestine, softening stools and inducing the urge to defecate.

▼ DOSAGE GUIDELINES

RANGE AND FREQUENCY
Adults and children age 6 and older: Insert one suppository or 5 to 15 ml of solution as rectal enema and retain for 15 minutes. Do not lubricate suppositories with anything other than water.

ONSET OF EFFECT
Within 15 to 60 minutes.

DURATION OF ACTION
Only while the solution or suppository is within the rectum.

DIETARY ADVICE
Maintain your usual food and fluid intake. Increase your intake of fluids if you have a fever or diarrhea, during hot weather, or during exercise.

STORAGE
Store away from heat, moisture, and direct light. Suppositories may be refrigerated, but do not allow them to freeze.

MISSED DOSE
Laxatives are usually prescribed for use only on an as-needed basis and are not meant to be taken regularly or for a prolonged period.

STOPPING THE DRUG
Take rectal glycerin only as needed. However, you may stop using it if you are feeling better before the scheduled end of therapy.

PROLONGED USE
Prolonged, excessive use of glycerin may be associated with an increased risk of side effects, including laxative dependence. Therefore, do not use glycerin for more than 3 to 5 days unless your doctor instructs you to do otherwise.

▼ PRECAUTIONS

Over 60:
Adverse reactions may be more likely and more severe in older patients.

Driving and Hazardous Work:
Do not drive or engage in hazardous work until you determine how the medicine affects you.

Alcohol:
No special precautions are required.

Pregnancy:
Adequate human studies have not been done. Before taking glycerin, tell your doctor if you are or are planning to become pregnant.

Breast Feeding:
Glycerin suppositories may be used safely by nursing mothers.

Infants and Children:
Not recommended for use by children under age 6.

Special Concerns:
A single missed bowel movement does not constitute constipation; do not use glycerin under such circumstances. Prolonged constipation or persistent rectal pain and discomfort should be evaluated by your doctor. Remember that chronic use of glycerin or any laxative can lead to laxative dependence. You should be sure to consume adequate amounts of bulk in your diet; good sources include bran or other cereals, fresh fruit, and vegetables.

OVERDOSE
Symptoms: No specific ones have been reported.

What to Do: An overdose of glycerin is unlikely to be life-threatening. However, if someone takes a much larger dose than prescribed, call your doctor.

▼ INTERACTIONS

DRUG INTERACTIONS
No significant drug interactions have been reported.

FOOD INTERACTIONS
No known food interactions.

DISEASE INTERACTIONS
Caution is advised when taking glycerin laxatives. Consult your doctor if you have any of the following: abdominal pain and fever, rectal bleeding, ostomy (an artificial surgical opening in the body to allow the release of urine or feces), diabetes mellitus, heart or kidney disease, or high blood pressure.

 SIDE EFFECTS

SERIOUS
There are no serious side effects associated with the use of rectal glycerin.

COMMON
Cramping.

LESS COMMON
Rectal pain, itching, or burning sensation. This is thought to be more common with dosage forms that require an applicator. If you notice increased pain or bleeding from the rectum after use of glycerin products, call your doctor. Weakness, sweating, and symptoms of dehydration (thirst, dizziness) also may occur.

GLYCOPYRROLATE

Available in: Tablets
Available OTC? No   **As Generic?** Yes
Drug Class: Anticholinergic, antispasmodic

▼ USAGE INFORMATION

WHY IT'S PRESCRIBED
To treat stomach ulcers and ease cramps and spasms of the stomach and intestines.

HOW IT WORKS
Glycopyrrolate inhibits gastrointestinal nerve receptor sites that stimulate both the secretion of stomach acid and smooth muscle activity in the digestive tract.

▼ DOSAGE GUIDELINES

RANGE AND FREQUENCY
Usually 1 to 2 mg, 2 to 3 times a day, with a maximum of 8 mg per day.

ONSET OF EFFECT
15 to 30 minutes.

DURATION OF ACTION
Up to 7 hours.

DIETARY ADVICE
Unless your doctor tells you otherwise, take glycopyrrolate 30 minutes to 1 hour before meals.

STORAGE
Store in a tightly sealed container away from heat and direct light.

MISSED DOSE
Take it as soon as you remember. If it is near the time for the next dose, skip the missed dose and resume your regular dosage schedule. Do not double the next dose.

STOPPING THE DRUG
Take it as prescribed for the full treatment period, or stop taking it if you are feeling better before the scheduled end of therapy. Do not stop the drug suddenly; consult your doctor about reducing the dose gradually.

PROLONGED USE
Prolonged use may cause chronic constipation and fecal impaction. Consult your doctor immediately.

▼ PRECAUTIONS

Over 60: Adverse reactions may be more likely and more severe in older patients.

Driving and Hazardous Work: Do not drive or engage in hazardous work until you determine how glycopyrrolate affects you. Use of this medicine disqualifies you from piloting aircraft.

Alcohol: No special warnings.

Pregnancy: Safety of using this drug during pregnancy has not been established. Before taking glycopyrrolate, tell your doctor if you are pregnant or plan to become pregnant and discuss whether the benefits clearly outweigh any potential risks.

Breast Feeding: Glycopyrrolate passes into breast milk; avoid or discontinue use while nursing.

Infants and Children: Smaller doses are recommended for infants and children. Glycopyrrolate should be given to young patients only under close medical supervision.

Special Concerns: Be sure that any doctor or dentist you go to knows that you are taking glycopyrrolate. To prevent heatstroke, avoid becoming overheated during exertion. Take this drug 2 to 3 hours before or after any antacids you are taking.

OVERDOSE
Symptoms: Blurred vision, dry mouth, low blood pressure, decreased breathing rate, rapid heartbeat, drowsiness, inability to urinate, flushed, hot, dry skin.

What to Do: Call your doctor, emergency medical services (EMS), or the nearest poison control center immediately.

▼ INTERACTIONS

DRUG INTERACTIONS
Consult your doctor for specific advice if you are taking antacids, other anticholinergics, tricyclic antidepressants, cyclopropane, cortisone drugs, digitalis drugs, haloperidol, ketoconazole, meperidine, methylphenidate, molindone, narcotic pain relievers, potassium chloride, quinidine, sedatives, or any central nervous system depressants.

FOOD INTERACTIONS
Avoid taking large amounts of vitamin C. No other food interactions are known.

DISEASE INTERACTIONS
Caution is advised while taking glycopyrrolate. Consult your doctor if you have any of the following: open-angle glaucoma, angina, chronic bronchitis, asthma, liver disease, hiatal hernia, enlarged prostate, myasthenia gravis, peptic ulcer, kidney disease, or thyroid disease.

SIDE EFFECTS

SERIOUS
Hives, rash, intense itching, faintness, or swelling soon after a dose. Call your doctor immediately.

COMMON
Enlarged pupils, blurred vision, constipation, dry mouth, difficulty urinating or inability to urinate, breathing difficulty.

LESS COMMON
Disorientation, irritability, incoherence, weakness, rapid or slow pulse, heart palpitations, unusual sensitivity of eyes to light, difficulty swallowing, nausea, vomiting, bloated abdomen, stomach upset, decreased sweating, skin problems, fever, loss of taste, impotence.

GOLD SODIUM THIOMALATE

Available in: Injection
Available OTC? No   **As Generic?** Yes
Drug Class: Antirheumatic

▼ USAGE INFORMATION

WHY IT'S PRESCRIBED
To treat rheumatoid arthritis. Gold sodium thiomalate is generally prescribed for patients who have not responded adequately to more conservative arthritis treatments, such as aspirin, nonsteroidal anti-inflammatory drugs (NSAIDs), and corticosteroids.

HOW IT WORKS
Gold sodium thiomalate contains gold. It is not precisely known how gold compounds work, but evidently they reduce some of the painful joint inflammation associated with arthritis. This drug can halt the progress of severe rheumatoid arthritis, preventing further joint damage, and in some cases it may bring about a remission from the disease.

▼ DOSAGE GUIDELINES

RANGE AND FREQUENCY
Adults: 10 mg given once by intramuscular injection during week 1. This is followed by 25 mg given once by injection during week 2, then 25 to 50 mg given once weekly until satisfactory relief is achieved or until 1,000 mg have been administered. If a satisfactory response is achieved, your doctor will begin a maintenance dose of 25 to 50 mg given once by injection every 2 to 4 weeks. Children: 10 mg given once by injection during week 1. This is followed by 1 mg per 2.2 lbs (1 kg) of body weight (but not more than 50 mg) given once by injection during week 2. Further doses are spaced similarly to the adult schedule, with the amount of drug determined by the weight of the child.

ONSET OF EFFECT
Within 6 to 8 weeks at the earliest.

DURATION OF ACTION
Unknown.

DIETARY ADVICE
Maintain your usual food and fluid intake.

STORAGE
Not applicable.

MISSED DOSE
Consult your physician.

STOPPING THE DRUG
Your doctor will stop this medication depending on whether you respond satisfactorily, develop side effects that make continuation impossible, or approach the maximum amount of drug that can be taken safely.

PROLONGED USE
Several months of therapy may be necessary to determine whether this medication is helping you. Prolonged use may be associated with an increased risk of side effects.

▼ PRECAUTIONS

Over 60: Adverse reactions may be more likely and severe.

Driving and Hazardous Work: Do not drive or engage in hazardous work until you determine how the medicine affects you.

Alcohol: Avoid alcohol.

Pregnancy: Do not use this drug during pregnancy.

Breast Feeding: This drug may pass into breast milk; caution is advised. Consult your doctor for advice.

Infants and Children: Consult your pediatrician.

Special Concerns: Gold compounds may have many adverse effects. Your doctor may order periodic blood tests to determine if you are having any undesirable reactions, such as anemia, low white blood cell count, or protein in the urine. This drug may increase your sensitivity to sunlight. Avoid direct sunlight during peak hours; wear protective clothing and use sunscreens.

OVERDOSE
Symptoms: No specific ones have been reported.

What to Do: Not applicable; an overdose of gold sodium thiomalate is unlikely to be administered by your doctor.

▼ INTERACTIONS

DRUG INTERACTIONS
Consult your doctor for advice if you are taking penicillamine or drugs that may depress bone marrow production, such as seizure medications or chemotherapy agents to treat cancer.

FOOD INTERACTIONS
No known food interactions.

DISEASE INTERACTIONS
Consult your doctor if you have anemia or any other blood disease, skin disease, colitis or any other intestinal disease, ulcers or heartburn, kidney disease, or systemic lupus erythematosus (SLE).

 SIDE EFFECTS

SERIOUS
Severe abdominal pain or bloody, black, or tarry stools; confusion; seizures.

COMMON
Temporary joint pain shortly after injection, itching, skin rash, indigestion, heartburn, constipation.

LESS COMMON
Hives, bloody or cloudy urine, sore tongue, bleeding, red, sore, swollen gums; painful sores in the mouth or throat.

GOSERELIN ACETATE

Available in: Implant
Available OTC? No   **As Generic?** No
Drug Class: Antineoplastic (anticancer) agent

▼ USAGE INFORMATION

WHY IT'S PRESCRIBED
To treat advanced forms of prostate cancer in men, and to treat advanced forms of breast cancer in women. It may also be used by women to relieve the pain and discomfort of endometriosis.

HOW IT WORKS
In men, goserelin decreases blood levels of testosterone. This slows the growth of cells in the prostate gland, which may lead to improvement of some of the pain and discomfort of advanced prostate cancer. In women, it decreases blood levels of estrogen and thereby may relieve some of the symptoms of advanced breast cancer. In women with endometriosis, reduced blood levels of estrogen lead to shrinking of endometrial tissue (uterine lining) and thus eases the painful cyclical flare-ups of endometriosis.

▼ DOSAGE GUIDELINES

RANGE AND FREQUENCY
Goserelin implants containing 3.6 mg of medication are placed just under the skin of the upper abdominal wall once every 28 days.

ONSET OF EFFECT
Within 2 to 4 weeks.

DURATION OF ACTION
Blood levels of the hormones testosterone and estrogen remain low for the duration of therapy with goserelin.

DIETARY ADVICE
Maintain your usual food and fluid intake. Increase fluids if you have a fever or diarrhea. Patients with cancer are often weakened by their illness, medications, or other treatments, and may be unable to consume adequate quantities of nutritious food. They should use liquid nutritional supplements if necessary.

STORAGE
Not applicable.

MISSED DOSE
Not applicable; the medication is delivered continuously in the form of an implant under the skin.

STOPPING THE DRUG
The decision to stop taking the drug should be made by your doctor.

PROLONGED USE
You should see your doctor regularly for tests and examinations while taking this medicine. Therapy with goserelin for prostate and breast cancer may be required for an indefinite period. Therapy with goserelin for endometriosis is usually completed within 6 months.

▼ PRECAUTIONS

Over 60: Adverse reactions may be more likely and more severe in older patients.

Driving and Hazardous Work: Do not drive or engage in hazardous work until you determine how the medication affects you.

Alcohol: Use alcohol only in moderation.

Pregnancy: Avoid or immediately discontinue taking the drug if you are pregnant or trying to become pregnant.

Breast Feeding: Avoid or discontinue use while nursing.

Infants and Children: This drug is not recommended for use by nonmenstruating females under the age of 18.

Special Concerns: Women of childbearing age must use effective non-hormonal contraception (that is, a form other than birth control pills) during treatment with goserelin and for 12 weeks following the end of therapy. In men, goserelin will cause sterility for at least the duration of therapy.

OVERDOSE
Symptoms: No specific ones have been reported.

What to Do: An overdose of goserelin is unlikely to be life-threatening.

▼ INTERACTIONS

DRUG INTERACTIONS
No specific ones known.

FOOD INTERACTIONS
No known food interactions.

DISEASE INTERACTIONS
No specific ones known.

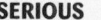

SIDE EFFECTS

SERIOUS
Bone pain; numbness or tingling of hands or feet; difficulty urinating; muscle weakness of the arms or legs. This may occur shortly after therapy begins. Call your doctor.

COMMON
Hot flashes, change in sex drive or decreased interest in sexual activity, erectile dysfunction (impotence), pelvic pain during sex, vaginal dryness and itching.

LESS COMMON
Edema (swelling in the extremities due to fluid retention); dizziness; headache; increased appetite; nausea or vomiting; abdominal pain; pain at application site; sore throat; change in voice; itching; leg cramps; breast pain or swelling; weight gain; chest pain; joint pain; acne or skin rash; increased anxiety or irritability, mood swings, or depression; fatigue; difficulty sleeping; nausea; increase in body or facial hair (in women); decrease in breast size.

GRISEOFULVIN

BRAND NAMES

Fulvicin P/G, Fulvicin U/F, Grifulvin V, Gris-PEG, Grisactin, Grisactin Ultra

Available in: Microsize capsules, oral suspension, tablets, ultramicrosize tablets
Available OTC? No   **As Generic?** Yes
Drug Class: Antifungal

▼ USAGE INFORMATION

WHY IT'S PRESCRIBED
To treat various forms of fungal infection, including ringworm (tinea barbae, tinea capitis, tinea corporis), jock itch (tinea cruris), athlete's foot (tinea pedis), and nail fungus (tinea unguium).

HOW IT WORKS
Griseofulvin prevents fungal organisms from manufacturing vital substances required for reproduction.

▼ DOSAGE GUIDELINES

RANGE AND FREQUENCY
Microsize capsules, oral suspension, tablets— Adults and teenagers: For feet and nails: 500 mg every 12 hours. For scalp, skin, and groin: 250 mg every 12 hours or 500 mg once a day. Children: 5 mg per 2.2 lbs (1 kg) of body weight every 12 hours, or 10 mg per 2.2 lbs once a day. Ultramicrosize tablets— Adults and teenagers: For feet and nails: 250 to 375 mg every 12 hours. For scalp, skin, and groin: 125 to 187.5 mg every 12 hours, or 250 to 375 mg once a day. Children age 2 and older: 2.75 to 3.65 mg per 2.2 lbs every 12 hours, or 5.5 to 7.3 mg per 2.2 lbs once a day.

ONSET OF EFFECT
Unknown.

DURATION OF ACTION
Unknown.

DIETARY ADVICE
Take griseofulvin with or after meals or milk. Milk, cheese, and other fatty foods increase the amount of medication absorbed from your stomach. Check with your physician if you are on a low-fat diet. Otherwise, maintain your usual food and fluid intake.

STORAGE
Store in a tightly sealed container away from heat, moisture, and direct light. Keep the liquid form refrigerated, but do not allow it to freeze.

MISSED DOSE
Take it as soon as you remember. However, if it is near the time for the next dose, skip the missed dose and resume your regular dosage schedule. Do not double the next dose.

STOPPING THE DRUG
Take it as prescribed for the full treatment period, even if you begin to feel better before the scheduled end of therapy. Recurrence of the infection is likely if you stop before the full treatment period is complete.

PROLONGED USE
Prolonged use may cause or aggravate bone marrow depression (reduced bone marrow function), liver damage, or kidney damage. Consult your doctor about the need for periodic blood cell counts and liver and kidney function tests.

▼ PRECAUTIONS

Over 60: Adverse reactions may be more likely and more severe in older patients.

Driving and Hazardous Work: Do not drive or engage in hazardous work until you determine how the medicine affects you.

Alcohol: Avoid alcohol.

Pregnancy: Do not use griseofulvin if you are pregnant or trying to become pregnant.

Breast Feeding: The drug may pass into breast milk; caution is advised. Consult your doctor for advice.

Infants and Children: Griseofulvin is not recommended for use by children under the age of 2.

Special Concerns: Stay out of direct sunlight, especially between 10 am and 3 pm. Wear protective clothing, including a hat, and sunglasses. Apply a sun block with a sun protection factor (SPF) of at least 15. Griseofulvin is usually used in conjunction with a topical antifungal to aid in the healing process and to reduce the likelihood of relapse.

OVERDOSE
Symptoms: An overdose with griseofulvin is unlikely.

What to Do: Emergency instructions not applicable.

▼ INTERACTIONS

DRUG INTERACTIONS
Other drugs may interact with griseofulvin. Consult your doctor for advice if you are taking anticoagulants or oral contraceptives.

FOOD INTERACTIONS
No known food interactions.

DISEASE INTERACTIONS
Caution is advised when taking griseofulvin. Consult your doctor if you have lupus, porphyria, or liver disease.

  SIDE EFFECTS

SERIOUS
Irritation or soreness of mouth or tongue; skin rash, hives, or itching; confusion; increased sensitivity of eyes to sunlight. Call your doctor immediately.

COMMON
Headache.

LESS COMMON
Insomnia, stomach pain, nausea or vomiting, unusual fatigue, dizziness, diarrhea.

GUAIFENESIN

Available in: Capsules, tablets, oral solution, syrup, extended-release forms
Available OTC? Yes **As Generic?** Yes
Drug Class: Expectorant

▼ USAGE INFORMATION

WHY IT'S PRESCRIBED
Guaifenesin is classified as an expectorant; that is, it is designed to reduce the thickness of mucus and phlegm, making it easier to cough up and out of the lungs and so improve breathing. It is used to treat minor upper respiratory infections and related conditions, such as bronchitis, colds, and sinus or throat infections. Guaifenesin is not a cough suppressant, and despite its popularity and its FDA approval as an expectorant, there is little scientific evidence that it is truly effective at reducing the thickness of mucus.

HOW IT WORKS
Guaifenesin supposedly increases the production of fluids in the respiratory tract and helps to liquefy and thin mucus secretions.

▼ DOSAGE GUIDELINES

RANGE AND FREQUENCY
Adults— Capsules, tablets, oral solution, syrup: 200 to 400 mg every 4 hours, to a maximum of 2,400 mg a day. Extended-release capsules and tablets: 600 to 1,200 mg every 12 hours, to a maximum of 2,400 mg a day. Children 2 to 12 years of age— Consult your doctor.

ONSET OF EFFECT
Usually within several hours.

DURATION OF ACTION
The exact duration of action is not known.

DIETARY ADVICE
Maintain your usual food and fluid intake. Increase fluids if you have a fever or diarrhea. Coughing also increases your daily fluid requirements.

STORAGE
Store in a tightly sealed container away from heat and direct light. Keep liquid forms of guaifenesin refrigerated, but do not allow it to freeze. Keep away from moisture and extremes in temperature.

MISSED DOSE
Take it as soon as you remember. If it is near the time for the next dose, skip the missed dose and resume your regular dosage schedule. Do not double the next dose.

STOPPING THE DRUG
You may stop taking guaifenesin before the scheduled end of therapy if you are feeling better; otherwise, take as prescribed for the full treatment period.

PROLONGED USE
Therapy with guaifenesin is usually completed within 7 to 10 days. Persistent cough may require special evaluation. Do not take nonprescription guaifenesin for more than 7 days without your doctor's approval.

▼ PRECAUTIONS

Over 60: Adverse reactions may be more likely and more severe.

Driving and Hazardous Work: Do not drive or engage in hazardous work until you determine how the medicine affects you.

Alcohol: No special warnings.

Pregnancy: Thorough studies have not been done, although no serious problems have been reported; consult your doctor for advice.

Breast Feeding: Guaifenesin may pass into breast milk, although no problems have been documented. Consult your doctor for advice.

Infants and Children: Generally, it should not be given to children under 2 unless directed otherwise by a pediatrician; children under 12 who have a persistent cough should be examined by a doctor before they are given guaifenesin.

Special Concerns: Guaifenesin is present in numerous nonprescription cough and cold remedies, so ask your pharmacist if you are unsure whether a product you are buying contains it. Do not treat a persistent cough on your own for more than a week or so without seeking medical advice. When treating young children, avoid capsules or tablets, since it is difficult to rely on children to swallow these dosage forms in one piece. Capsules and tablets should not be chewed.

OVERDOSE
Symptoms: No specific ones have been reported.

What to Do: An overdose of guaifenesin is unlikely to be life-threatening. However, if someone takes a much larger dose than prescribed, call your doctor, emergency medical services (EMS), or the nearest poison control center.

▼ INTERACTIONS

DRUG INTERACTIONS
None reported.

FOOD INTERACTIONS
None reported.

DISEASE INTERACTIONS
None reported.

≣ SIDE EFFECTS ≣

SERIOUS
No serious side effects are associated with guaifenesin.

COMMON
No common side effects are associated with guaifenesin.

LESS COMMON
Diarrhea; dizziness; headache; abdominal pain, nausea, or vomiting; skin rash; itching; hives.

GUANABENZ ACETATE

BRAND NAME
Wytensin

Available in: Tablets
Available OTC? No   **As Generic?** Yes
Drug Class: Centrally acting antihypertensive

▼ USAGE INFORMATION

WHY IT'S PRESCRIBED
To treat high blood pressure (hypertension).

HOW IT WORKS
Guanabenz acts upon certain areas of the central nervous system (the brain and spinal cord) that regulate the activity of the heart and the smooth muscle tissue surrounding the arteries. The drug causes the blood vessels to relax and widen, which in turn lowers blood pressure.

▼ DOSAGE GUIDELINES

RANGE AND FREQUENCY
Adults: Initially, 4 mg, 2 times a day. Your doctor will increase this dose gradually over a period of a few weeks until your blood pressure is acceptable. The usual maximum dose of guanabenz is 32 mg per day, given in divided doses.

ONSET OF EFFECT
Within 1 hour.

DURATION OF ACTION
12 hours.

DIETARY ADVICE
Follow a healthy diet (low-salt, low-fat, low-cholesterol) as advised by your doctor to help control blood pressure and prevent heart disease.

STORAGE
Store in a tightly sealed container away from heat, moisture, and direct light.

MISSED DOSE
Take it as soon as you remember. If it is near the time for the next dose, skip the missed dose and resume your regular dosage schedule. Do not double the next dose. Call your doctor if you have missed more than one day of medication.

STOPPING THE DRUG
Do not stop taking this drug suddenly, as this may cause potentially serious health problems. If therapy is to be discontinued, dosage should be reduced gradually, according to doctor's instructions.

PROLONGED USE
Extended therapy with guanabenz may be necessary. Side effects may be more likely with prolonged use.

▼ PRECAUTIONS

Over 60: Adverse reactions may be more likely and more severe.

Driving and Hazardous Work: The use of guanabenz may impair your ability to perform such tasks safely. Do not drive or engage in hazardous work until you determine how the medicine affects you.

Alcohol: Avoid alcohol.

Pregnancy: Avoid or discontinue the drug if you are pregnant or are planning to become pregnant.

Breast Feeding: Guanabenz may pass into breast milk; caution is advised. Consult your doctor for advice.

Infants and Children: Guanabenz is not recommended for use in children.

Special Concerns: If you miss several doses of guanabenz or upon completion of therapy, your blood pressure may return to dangerously high levels (known as rebound effect). Symptoms of rebound hypertension include: severe headache; nausea, vomiting, and abdominal pain; confusion; blurred vision; chest pain; sweating; nervousness, restlessness, anxiety, or trembling; heartbeat irregularities; trouble breathing. Call your doctor immediately. To avoid rebound hypertension, make every effort to follow your dosage schedule. Be sure to have adequate supplies of guanabenz available for vacations, travel, and holidays. Avoid nonprescription decongestants and cough, cold, and flu remedies. Drowsiness is common with guanabenz; take your last dose of the day around bedtime if possible. Remember that control of high blood pressure requires medication, diet, weight loss, and careful supervision by your physician.

OVERDOSE
Symptoms: Very low blood pressure causing faintness, extreme drowsiness, weakness, dizziness, or confusion; unusually slow heartbeat; irritability; tiny, constricted pupils.

What to Do: Call emergency medical services (EMS), your doctor, or the nearest poison control center immediately.

▼ INTERACTIONS

DRUG INTERACTIONS
Consult your doctor for specific advice if you are taking medicines that causes drowsiness, such as barbiturates, sedatives, cough medicines, or decongestants; alcohol; psychiatric medications; pain medications; anti-inflammatory drugs; beta-blockers or other medicines to lower blood pressure.

FOOD INTERACTIONS
No known food interactions.

DISEASE INTERACTIONS
Consult your doctor if you have any of the following: blood vessel disease of the brain, including a history of strokes or transient ischemic attacks (TIAs); angina or other heart disease; liver disease; or kidney disease.

≡ SIDE EFFECTS ≡

SERIOUS
There are no serious side effects associated with recommended doses of guanabenz. However, serious side effects may occur from missing several doses or upon completion of therapy (see Special Concerns).

COMMON
Dizziness or lightheadedness, faintness, drowsiness, dry mouth, general weakness.

LESS COMMON
Headache, decreased sexual ability, nausea.

GUANADREL SULFATE

BRAND NAME

Hylorel

Available in: Tablets
Available OTC? No **As Generic?** Yes
Drug Class: Peripherally acting antihypertensive

▼ USAGE INFORMATION

WHY IT'S PRESCRIBED
To treat high blood pressure. Guanadrel is used in conjunction with other established treatments, such as weight loss and sodium restriction.

HOW IT WORKS
Guanadrel acts on special nerve pathways that regulate the size of blood vessels by interfering with the release of a natural substance called norepinephrine, which constricts muscles surrounding the vessels. The drug relaxes these muscles, causing blood vessels to widen, which in turn lowers blood pressure.

▼ DOSAGE GUIDELINES

RANGE AND FREQUENCY
Adults: To start, 5 mg, 2 times a day. Your doctor will increase this dose as needed over a period of weeks until satisfactory blood pressure is achieved. This usually requires a dose of 20 to 75 mg per day, given in 2 to 4 equally divided doses.

ONSET OF EFFECT
Within 2 hours.

DURATION OF ACTION
About 9 hours.

DIETARY ADVICE
Follow a healthy diet (low-salt, low-fat, low-cholesterol) as advised by your doctor to help control blood pressure and prevent heart disease.

STORAGE
Store in a tightly sealed container away from heat and direct light. Keep it away from moisture and extremes in temperature.

MISSED DOSE
Take it as soon as you remember. However, if it is near the time for the next dose, skip the missed dose and resume your regular dosage schedule. Do not double the next dose.

STOPPING THE DRUG
Take the drug as prescribed for the full treatment period, even if you begin to feel better before the scheduled end of therapy.

PROLONGED USE
Lifelong therapy may be necessary. See your doctor regularly for examinations and tests if you must take this medicine for an extended period of time.

▼ PRECAUTIONS

Over 60: Adverse reactions may be more likely and more severe in older patients.

Driving and Hazardous Work: Do not drive or engage in hazardous work until you determine how the medicine affects you.

Alcohol: Avoid alcohol.

Pregnancy: Before taking guanadrel, tell your doctor if you are pregnant or plan to become pregnant.

Breast Feeding: Guanadrel may pass into breast milk; caution is advised. Consult your doctor for advice.

Infants and Children: Guanadrel is not recommended for use by children.

Special Concerns: Guanadrel frequently causes dizziness or lightheadedness, which is most noticeable when you change position, such as rising from a seated or lying position, or when getting out of bed or bending to pick up something. This may lead to fainting, falls, and injury. Sit or lie down immediately if you feel dizzy or lightheaded. This side effect may be worsened by alcohol, hot weather, dehydration, fever, prolonged standing, prolonged sitting, or exercise.

▼ OVERDOSE

Symptoms: Severe dizziness, confusion, weakness, fainting.

What to Do: Call emergency medical services (EMS), your doctor, or the nearest poison control center immediately.

▼ INTERACTIONS

DRUG INTERACTIONS
Consult your doctor for specific advice if you are taking antidepressants, appetite suppressants, cyclobenzaprine, haloperidol, loxapine, maprotiline, methylphenidate, phenothiazines, thioxanthenes, trimeprazine, MAO inhibitors, metaraminol, methoxamine, norepinephrine, phenylephrine, or phenylpropanolamine.

FOOD INTERACTIONS
No known food interactions.

DISEASE INTERACTIONS
Consult your doctor if you have any of the following: asthma; poor circulation to the brain, with any history of stroke, fainting, convulsions, or epilepsy; angina, recent heart attack, problems with pulse, unusual heart rhythms, pacemaker, or heart failure; conditions that lead to dehydration, such as fever, diarrhea, or colitis; diabetes; or pheochromocytoma.

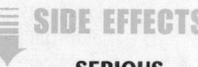
SIDE EFFECTS

SERIOUS
Excess fluid retention, which can cause swelling of lower legs and feet; chest pain; shortness of breath; fainting; repeated episodes of dizziness or falling, especially when changing position.

COMMON
Drowsiness, dizziness or lightheadedness, weight gain. In men, impotence and impaired ejaculation.

LESS COMMON
Diarrhea; dry mouth; headache; muscle aches; increased urination, especially at night.

GUANETHIDINE MONOSULFATE

Available in: Tablets
Available OTC? No **As Generic?** Yes
Drug Class: Peripherally acting antihypertensive

▼ USAGE INFORMATION

WHY IT'S PRESCRIBED
To help control moderate to severe high blood pressure, usually after other medications have failed to achieve satisfactory results.

HOW IT WORKS
Guanethidine interferes with the release of norepinephrine, a natural substance that constricts the muscles surrounding blood vessels. The drug relaxes these muscles, causing blood vessels to widen, thus lowering blood pressure.

▼ DOSAGE GUIDELINES

RANGE AND FREQUENCY
Adults: To start, 10 or 12.5 mg once a day. Your doctor may increase this gradually over weekly intervals until your blood pressure reaches an acceptable level. Your doctor will then prescribe a maintenance dose, usually 25 to 50 mg, taken once a day. Children: Dosage depends on age and weight of the child. Consult your pediatrician.

ONSET OF EFFECT
Blood pressure begins to drop shortly after ingestion; maximum benefits require 1 to 3 weeks.

DURATION OF ACTION
Blood pressure returns to previously high levels within 1 to 3 weeks after stopping.

DIETARY ADVICE
Increase fluids if you have a fever or diarrhea, in hot weather, or during exercise. Follow a healthy diet (low-salt, low-fat, low-cholesterol) as advised by your doctor to help control blood pressure and prevent heart disease.

STORAGE
Store in a tightly sealed container away from heat and direct light.

MISSED DOSE
Take it as soon as you remember. However, if it is near the time for the next dose, skip the missed dose and resume your regular dosage schedule. Do not double the next dose. Inform your doctor if you miss more than a full day of medication.

STOPPING THE DRUG
The decision to stop taking the drug should be made by your doctor. Do not stop this medication abruptly.

PROLONGED USE
Lifelong therapy may be necessary. See your doctor regularly for examinations and tests if you must take this drug for an extended period.

▼ PRECAUTIONS

Over 60: Adverse reactions may be more likely and more severe in older patients.

Driving and Hazardous Work: Do not drive or engage in hazardous work until you determine how the medicine affects you.

Alcohol: Avoid alcohol.

Pregnancy: Before taking guanethidine, tell your doctor if you are pregnant or plan to become pregnant.

Breast Feeding: Guanethidine may pass into breast milk; consult your doctor.

Infants and Children: May be used; consult your doctor.

Special Concerns: Guanethidine frequently causes dizziness or lightheadedness, especially when you change position. This may lead to fainting, falls, and injury. Sit or lie down immediately if you feel dizzy or lightheaded. This side effect may be worsened by alcohol, hot weather, dehydration, fever, prolonged standing or sitting or exercise.

OVERDOSE
Symptoms: Severe dizziness, confusion, weakness, or fainting; very slow pulse; severe diarrhea; severe nausea; cold, clammy skin; unresponsiveness, loss of consciousness.

What to Do: Call emergency medical services (EMS), your doctor, or the nearest poison control center immediately.

▼ INTERACTIONS

DRUG INTERACTIONS
Consult your doctor for specific advice if you are taking antidepressants, appetite suppressants, cyclobenzaprine, haloperidol, loxapine, maprotiline, methylphenidate, minoxidil, phenothiazines, thioxanthenes, trimeprazine, MAO inhibitors, metaraminol, methoxamine, norepinephrine, phenylephrine, phenylpropanolamine, insulin or oral medicines to control blood sugar, or anti-inflammatory drugs, especially NSAIDs.

FOOD INTERACTIONS
No known food interactions.

DISEASE INTERACTIONS
Consult your doctor if you have any of the following: asthma; poor circulation to the brain in association with history of stroke, fainting, epilepsy or other seizure disorders; angina, recent heart attack, heart rhythm irregularities, or heart failure; conditions that lead to dehydration, such as fever, diarrhea, or colitis; diabetes; pheochromocytoma; or impaired liver or kidney function.

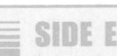

SIDE EFFECTS

SERIOUS
Excess fluid retention, which can cause swelling of lower legs and feet; chest pain; shortness of breath; fainting; dizziness or falling, especially when changing position.

COMMON
Dizziness or lightheadedness, drowsiness, weight gain, slow pulse, stuffy nose. In men, impotence and impaired ejaculation.

LESS COMMON
Diarrhea; dry mouth; headache; muscle aches; increased urination, especially at night; rash; vision problems.

GUANFACINE HYDROCHLORIDE

Available in: Tablets
Available OTC? No   **As Generic?** Yes
Drug Class: Centrally acting antihypertensive

▼ USAGE INFORMATION

WHY IT'S PRESCRIBED
To treat high blood pressure (hypertension).

HOW IT WORKS
Guanfacine acts upon certain areas of the central nervous system that regulate the activity of the heart and the smooth muscle tissue surrounding the arteries. The drug causes the blood vessels to relax and widen, which in turn lowers blood pressure.

▼ DOSAGE GUIDELINES

RANGE AND FREQUENCY
Adults: To start, 1 mg once daily, at bedtime. Your doctor will increase the dose as needed over a period of 4 to 8 weeks until satisfactory blood pressure is achieved. Maintenance dose is usually 2 to 3 mg per day, taken once daily at bedtime.

ONSET OF EFFECT
Peak effect within 7 days.

DURATION OF ACTION
24 hours.

DIETARY ADVICE
Increase fluid intake in hot weather, during exercise, or if you have a fever or diarrhea. Follow a healthy diet (low-salt, low-fat, low-cholesterol) as advised by your doctor to help control blood pressure and prevent heart disease.

STORAGE
Store in a tightly sealed container away from heat and direct light.

MISSED DOSE
Take it as soon as you remember. If it is near the time for the next dose, skip the missed dose and resume your regular dosage schedule. Do not double the next dose. Call your doctor if you have missed more than one day of medication.

STOPPING THE DRUG
Do not stop taking this drug suddenly, as this may cause potentially serious health problems. If therapy is to be discontinued, the dosage should be tapered, according to your physician's instructions.

PROLONGED USE
Extended therapy with this drug may be necessary. Side effects may be more likely with prolonged use.

▼ PRECAUTIONS

Over 60: Adverse reactions may be more likely and more severe.

Driving and Hazardous Work: Do not drive or engage in hazardous work until you determine how the medicine affects you.

Alcohol: Avoid alcohol.

Pregnancy: Avoid or discontinue use if you are pregnant or plan to become pregnant.

Breast Feeding: Guanfacine may pass into breast milk; caution is advised. Consult your doctor.

Infants and Children: Guanfacine is not recommended for use by children.

Special Concerns: If you miss several doses of guanfacine or upon completion of therapy, your blood pressure may return to dangerously high levels (known as rebound effect). Symptoms of rebound hypertension include: severe headache; nausea, vomiting, and abdominal pain; confusion; blurred vision; chest pain; sweating; nervousness, restlessness, anxiety, or trembling; heartbeat irregularities; trouble breathing. Call your doctor immediately. To avoid rebound hypertension, make every effort to follow your dosage schedule. Be sure to have adequate supplies of

guanfacine available for vacations, travel, and holidays. Drowsiness is common with guanfacine; take your last dose of the day around bedtime if possible. Remember that control of high blood pressure requires medication, diet, weight loss, and careful supervision by your doctor.

OVERDOSE
Symptoms: Extreme drowsiness, weakness, dizziness, or confusion; unusually slow heartbeat; irritability; tiny, constricted pupils.

What to Do: Call emergency medical services (EMS), your doctor, or the nearest poison control center immediately.

▼ INTERACTIONS

DRUG INTERACTIONS
Many patients taking guanfacine also require treatment with a diuretic to control their blood pressure. Consult your doctor for specific advice if you are taking medicines that cause drowsiness, such as barbiturates, sedatives, cough medicines, or decongestants; alcohol; psychiatric drugs; pain medications; anti-inflammatory drugs; beta-blockers or other medicines to lower blood pressure.

FOOD INTERACTIONS
No known food interactions.

DISEASE INTERACTIONS
Consult your doctor if you have any of the following: blood vessel disease of the brain, including a history of strokes or transient ischemic attacks (TIAs); angina or other heart disease; liver disease; or kidney disease.

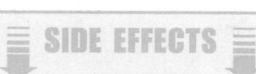

SIDE EFFECTS

SERIOUS
There are no serious side effects associated with recommended doses of guanfacine. However, serious side effects may occur from missing several doses or upon completion of therapy (see Special Concerns).

COMMON
Dry mouth, dizziness or lightheadedness, fatigue or drowsiness, weakness, constipation.

LESS COMMON
Headache, decreased sexual ability, depression, dry, burning eyes.

HALOPERIDOL

Available in: Tablets, liquid, injection
Available OTC? No **As Generic?** Yes
Drug Class: Neuroleptic; antipsychotic

▼ USAGE INFORMATION

WHY IT'S PRESCRIBED
To treat moderate to severe psychiatric conditions including schizophrenia, manic states, and drug-induced psychosis. It is also used to treat extreme behavior problems in children (including infantile autism), to ease the symptoms of Tourette's syndrome, and to reduce nausea and vomiting associated with chemotherapy for cancer.

HOW IT WORKS
Haloperidol blocks receptors of dopamine (a chemical that aids in the transmission of nerve impulses) in the central nervous system. Presumably, this produces a tranquilizing or antipsychotic effect.

▼ DOSAGE GUIDELINES

RANGE AND FREQUENCY
For psychotic disorders—
Adults: Initial dose is 0.5 to 5 mg, 2 or 3 times a day; maximum dose is 100 mg a day. Children ages 3 to 12: 0.05 to 0.15 mg for every 2.2 lbs (1 kg) of body weight. For Tourette's syndrome—Adults: 0.5 to 5 mg, 2 or 3 times a day. Children ages 3 to 12: 0.075 mg for every 2.2 lbs daily.

ONSET OF EFFECT
Sedation may occur within minutes, but onset of antipsychotic effect may take hours to occur or may not occur until days or weeks after the beginning of therapy.

DURATION OF ACTION
12 to 24 hours, but effects may persist for several days.

DIETARY ADVICE
Take haloperidol with food or a full glass of milk or water. To prevent stomach irritation, the oral solution can be diluted in beverages such as orange, apple, or tomato juice, or cola.

STORAGE
Store in a tightly sealed container away from heat and direct light.

MISSED DOSE
Take it as soon as you remember. Do not double the next dose. Space any remaining doses for that day at regular intervals. Return to your regular schedule the next day.

STOPPING THE DRUG
The decision to stop taking the drug should be made in consultation with your doctor. Gradual reduction of doses may be required if you have taken it for a long period.

PROLONGED USE
Prolonged use may lead to tardive dyskinesia (involuntary movements of the jaw, lips, tongue, and, in rare cases, the arms, legs, hands, or body). Consult your doctor about the need for periodic evaluation and lab tests.

▼ PRECAUTIONS

Over 60: Adverse reactions are more likely and more severe in older patients.

Driving and Hazardous Work: Exercise caution until you determine how the medication affects you.

Alcohol: Avoid alcohol.

Pregnancy: Before taking haloperidol, be sure to tell your doctor if you are, or plan to become, pregnant.

Breast Feeding: Haloperidol passes into breast milk and may be harmful to the child; do not use it while nursing.

Infants and Children: Not recommended for children under age 3 or those weighing less than 33 pounds.

Special Concerns: Avoid prolonged exposure to high temperatures or hot climates. Drink plenty of fluids and stay cool in the summertime. Avoid overexposure to sunlight until you determine if the drug heightens your skin's sensitivity to ultraviolet light.

OVERDOSE
Symptoms: Shallow, slow breathing, weak or rapid pulse, muscle weakness or tremor, dizziness, confusion, seizures, deep sleep, coma.

What to Do: Call your doctor, emergency medical services (EMS), or the nearest poison control center immediately.

▼ INTERACTIONS

DRUG INTERACTIONS
Consult your doctor for specific advice if you are taking anticholinergics, anticonvulsants, antidepressants, antihistamines, antihypertensives, bupropion, central nervous system depressants such as barbiturates, clozapine, dronabinol, ethinamate, fluoxetine, guanethidine, guanfacine, lithium, methyldopa, carbamazepine, rifampin, or trihexyphenidyl.

FOOD INTERACTIONS
No known food interactions.

DISEASE INTERACTIONS
Consult your doctor if you have Parkinson's disease or any movement disorder, glaucoma, epilepsy, or liver or kidney disease.

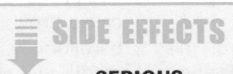
SIDE EFFECTS

SERIOUS
Rapid heartbeat, profuse sweating, seizures, difficulty breathing, neck stiffness, swelling of the tongue, difficulty swallowing. Also a rare condition can develop called neuroleptic malignant syndrome, characterized by stiffness or spasms of the muscles, high fever, and confusion or disorientation. Call your doctor immediately.

COMMON
Nausea, reduced sweating, dry mouth, blurred vision, drowsiness, shaking of hands, stiffness, stooped posture.

LESS COMMON
Difficult urination, menstrual irregularities, breast pain or swelling, unexpected weight gain, uncontrolled movements of the tongue, fever, chills, sore throat, unusual bruising or bleeding, heart palpitations, skin rash, itching, increased sensitivity of the skin to sunlight.

HALOPROGIN

Available in: Cream, solution
Available OTC? No   **As Generic?** No
Drug Class: Topical antifungal

▼ USAGE INFORMATION

WHY IT'S PRESCRIBED
To treat fungal infections of the skin, such as tinea corporis (ringworm), tinea cruris (jock itch), tinea pedis (athlete's foot), tinea manuum ("ringworm of the hand"), pityriasis versicolor ("sun fungus," a skin condition characterized by the formation of fine scaly patches of varying shapes, sizes, and colors).

HOW IT WORKS
Haloprogin prevents the growth and reproduction of fungus cells.

▼ DOSAGE GUIDELINES

RANGE AND FREQUENCY
For many conditions, rub the medicine gently into the affected area of skin 2 times a day for 2 to 4 weeks. (Note: This is simply the average dose of haloprogin. If the dose recommended by your physician is different, do not change it unless your physician advises you otherwise.)

ONSET OF EFFECT
Unknown.

DURATION OF ACTION
Unknown.

DIETARY ADVICE
Haloprogin can be used without regard to diet.

STORAGE
Store in a tightly sealed container away from heat and direct light. Do not allow the medicine to freeze.

MISSED DOSE
Apply it as soon as you remember. If it is near the time for the next dose, skip the missed dose and resume your regular dosage schedule. Do not apply a double dose.

STOPPING THE DRUG
Use the medication as prescribed for the full treatment period, even if you begin to feel better before the scheduled end of therapy. Discontinuing the drug prematurely may lead to an even worse fungal infection later (known as a rebound infection).

PROLONGED USE
If your skin problem does not improve within 4 weeks of starting therapy or if it becomes worse, notify your doctor.

▼ PRECAUTIONS

Over 60: Although there is no specific information comparing use of haloprogin in older patients with use in other age groups, the medicine is not expected to cause different side effects or problems in older people than in younger patients.

Driving and Hazardous Work: The use of haloprogin should not impair your ability to perform such tasks safely.

Alcohol: No special problems are expected with moderate use of alcohol.

Pregnancy: In animal studies, haloprogin has not been shown to cause birth defects or other problems. Human studies have not been done. Before you use haloprogin, be sure to tell your doctor if you are pregnant or plan to become pregnant.

Breast Feeding: It is not known whether haloprogin passes into breast milk; caution is advised. Consult your doctor for specific advice.

Infants and Children: Studies on the relationship of age to the effects of haloprogin have not been done in children. The safety and efficacy of the medicine on children have not been established. Use and dosage should be determined by your doctor.

Special Concerns: Avoid contact of the medicine with the eyes. Do not use haloprogin if you have had a prior allergic reaction to it or to any other topical antifungal drug.

OVERDOSE
Symptoms: No specific ones have been reported.

What to Do: An overdose of haloprogin is unlikely. However, if someone accidentally ingests the drug, call your doctor, emergency medical services (EMS), or the nearest poison control right away.

▼ INTERACTIONS

DRUG INTERACTIONS
Consult your doctor for specific advice if you are taking any other antifungal medication for the skin.

FOOD INTERACTIONS
No known food interactions.

DISEASE INTERACTIONS
Caution is advised when taking haloprogin. Consult your doctor if you have any other medical condition.

≡ SIDE EFFECTS ≡

SERIOUS
No serious side effects have been reported.

COMMON
A mild, temporary stinging when the solution form of haloprogin is applied.

LESS COMMON
Blistering, burning, itching, or other forms of skin irritation that were not present before the start of therapy. Call your doctor immediately.

HEPATITIS A VACCINE

Available in: Injection
Available OTC? No   **As Generic?** No
Drug Class: Vaccine

▼ USAGE INFORMATION

WHY IT'S PRESCRIBED
To protect against infection by the hepatitis A virus in people over the age of 2. The vaccine is recommended for people traveling to Africa, Asia (except Japan), parts of the Caribbean, Central and South America, eastern Europe, the Mediterranean basin, the Middle East, and Mexico. The vaccine is also recommended for people who live in or are moving to other areas that have frequent outbreaks of hepatitis A or those who may be at increased risk of infection. These people include military personnel, Alaskan Eskimos, Native Americans, persons engaging in high-risk sexual activity, such as homosexual males; people who use illegal injectable drugs, people working in facilities for the mentally retarded, employees of and children in day-care centers, people who work with hepatitis A virus in the laboratory, people who handle primate animals, food handlers, and people with chronic liver disease.

HOW IT WORKS
Hepatitis A vaccine stimulates the body's immune system to produce protective antibodies against the disease.

▼ DOSAGE GUIDELINES

RANGE AND FREQUENCY
All doses are administered by a health care professional. Adults: 1 dose injected into a muscle in the upper arm. A booster dose is given 6 months after the first dose. Children ages 2 to 18: 1 pediatric dose injected into a muscle in the upper arm. A similar booster is given 6 to 18 months later.

ONSET OF EFFECT
Within 4 weeks.

DURATION OF ACTION
Unknown.

DIETARY ADVICE
No special restrictions.

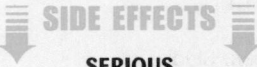

SIDE EFFECTS

SERIOUS
Serious allergic reaction involving difficulty swallowing or breathing; reddened skin, especially around the ears; itching, particularly of the hands or feet; hives; unusual and severe fatigue; and swollen face, eyes, or nasal passages. Call your doctor immediately.

COMMON
Soreness at the site of injection.

LESS COMMON
Fever, general feeling of illness or discomfort, lack of appetite, headache, nausea, tenderness or warmth at site of injection, aches or pain in joints or muscles, diarrhea or stomach cramps or pain, itching, swelling of the glands in armpits or neck, vomiting, welts.

STORAGE
Not applicable; the dose is administered only at a health care facility.

MISSED DOSE
If you miss a scheduled vaccination, contact your doctor.

STOPPING THE DRUG
The full schedule of injections should be followed unless a medical problem intervenes. A full course of injections must be completed to ensure adequate immunization.

PROLONGED USE
Not applicable.

▼ PRECAUTIONS

Over 60: Hepatitis A vaccine is not expected to cause different or more severe side effects in older patients than it does in younger persons. However, patients over age 50 may not develop as strong an immunity as their younger counterparts.

Driving and Hazardous Work: The vaccine should not impair your ability to perform such tasks safely.

Alcohol: No special precautions are necessary.

Pregnancy: Adequate human studies have not been done. Before taking hepatitis A vaccine, tell your physician if you are pregnant or planning to become pregnant.

Breast Feeding: No problems have been reported in nursing babies, but caution is advised. Consult your doctor.

Infants and Children: Not recommended for use by children under the age of 2. No special problems are expected in children over the age of 2.

OVERDOSE
Symptoms: Not applicable.

What to Do: No cases of overdose have been reported.

▼ INTERACTIONS

DRUG INTERACTIONS
There are no known drug interactions. Tell your doctor if you are taking any prescription or over-the-counter medication.

FOOD INTERACTIONS
No known food interactions.

DISEASE INTERACTIONS
Consult your doctor if you have a bleeding disorder, an immune deficiency condition, or any other medical condition. Vaccine injection may be postponed in persons with a fever or acute illness.

HEPATITIS B VACCINE

Available in: Injection
Available OTC? No **As Generic?** No
Drug Class: Vaccine

▼ USAGE INFORMATION

WHY IT'S PRESCRIBED
To protect against infection by the hepatitis B virus.

HOW IT WORKS
Hepatitis B vaccine stimulates the body's immune system to produce protective antibodies against the disease.

▼ DOSAGE GUIDELINES

RANGE AND FREQUENCY
Adults age 20 and older: A first injection of 10 micrograms (mcg) (Recombivax HB) or 20 mcg (Engerix-B) into upper arm, followed by an injection 1 month later and another 6 months after the first dose, for a total of 3 doses. Adults receiving dialysis: A first injection of 40 mcg (Recombivax HD Dialysis Formulation) followed by doses 1 month and 6 months after the first dose; some patients may receive a dose at 2 months. Dialysis patients receiving 4 doses will use Engerix-B. Children ages 11 to 20: A first injection of 5 mcg (Recombivax HB) or 20 mcg (Engerix-B) into upper arm, followed by an injection 1 month later and another 6 months after the first dose, for a total of 3 doses. Infants and children up to age 11: A first dose of 2.5 mcg (Recombivax HB) or 10 mcg (Engerix-B) into the thigh, with doses 1 month and 6 months after the first dose, for a total of 3 doses.

ONSET OF EFFECT
Unknown.

DURATION OF ACTION
Unknown.

DIETARY ADVICE
No special restrictions.

STORAGE
Not applicable; the dose is administered only at a health care facility.

MISSED DOSE
If you miss a scheduled vaccination, contact your doctor.

STOPPING THE DRUG
The full schedule of injections should be followed unless a medical problem intervenes. A full course of injections must be completed to ensure adequate immunization.

PROLONGED USE
No special problems are expected.

▼ PRECAUTIONS

Over 60: Hepatitis B vaccine is not expected to cause different or more severe side effects in older patients than it does in younger persons. However, patients over age 50 may not develop as strong an immunity as their younger counterparts.

Driving and Hazardous Work: Hepatitis B vaccine should not impair your ability to perform such tasks safely.

Alcohol: No special precautions are necessary.

Pregnancy: Adequate human studies have not been done. However, problems during pregnancy are not expected. Before you take hepatitis B vaccine, tell your doctor if you are pregnant or plan to become pregnant.

Breast Feeding: Hepatitis B vaccine may pass into breast milk; caution is advised. Consult your doctor for more information.

Infants and Children: Hepatitis B vaccine, with recommended doses, does not cause different or more severe side effects in infants and children than it does in older persons. Studies of the vaccine strength for use by dialysis patients have only been conducted on adult subjects. Consult your pediatrician for specific advice if your child is receiving dialysis.

OVERDOSE
Symptoms: Not applicable.

What to Do: No cases of overdose have been reported.

▼ INTERACTIONS

DRUG INTERACTIONS
Other drugs may interact with hepatitis B vaccine. Tell your doctor if you are taking any prescription or over-the-counter medication.

FOOD INTERACTIONS
No known food interactions.

DISEASE INTERACTIONS
Consult your doctor if you have any of the following: severe heart or lung disease, a moderate or severe illness with or without fever, or an immune deficiency condition.

 SIDE EFFECTS

SERIOUS
Serious allergic reaction involving difficulty swallowing or breathing; reddened skin, especially around the ears; itching, particularly of the hands or feet; hives; unusual and severe fatigue; and swollen face, eyes, or nasal passages. Call your doctor immediately.

COMMON
Soreness at the site of injection.

LESS COMMON
Dizziness, fever, unusual fatigue, headache. Also tenderness, warmth, hard lump, swelling, pain, itching, or purple spot at site of injection.

HOMATROPINE HYDROBROMIDE

Available in: Ophthalmic solution
Available OTC? No   **As Generic?** Yes
Drug Class: Eye muscle relaxant, pupil enlarger

▼ USAGE INFORMATION

WHY IT'S PRESCRIBED
To protect the eye before and after surgery, and to treat certain types of eye conditions, including iritis (inflammation of the iris, the colored or pigmented portion of the eye). It may also be used in eye examinations to help determine the proper prescription for eyeglasses.

HOW IT WORKS
Homatropine relaxes the ciliary muscle, which controls the shape of the eye's lens as it focuses, and another eye muscle called the sphincter, which controls the narrowing and widening of the pupil. Relaxation of these muscles prevents the lens from focusing and widens the pupil. This allows the doctor to view the interior of the eye during an ophthalmologic procedure. And, by immobilizing the tiny structures within the eye, the drug prevents scarring of eye tissue and may also alleviate pain somewhat.

▼ DOSAGE GUIDELINES

RANGE AND FREQUENCY
To aid in ophthalmic surgery or eye examinations: 1 drop (applied by doctor) every 5 to 10 minutes as needed. For treatment of iritis: 1 drop in affected eye(s), 2 or 3 times a day, or up to every 2 or 3 hours in more severe cases.

ONSET OF EFFECT
Within 1 hour.

DURATION OF ACTION
From 24 to 72 hours.

DIETARY ADVICE
It can be taken without regard to diet.

STORAGE
Store in a tightly sealed container away from heat, moisture, and direct light. Do not allow it to freeze.

MISSED DOSE
Apply it as soon as you remember. If it is near the time for the next dose, skip the missed dose and resume your regular dosage schedule. Do not double the next dose.

STOPPING THE DRUG
The decision to stop taking the drug should be made by your ophthalmologist.

PROLONGED USE
Not recommended.

▼ PRECAUTIONS

Over 60: Adverse reactions may be more likely and more severe.

Driving and Hazardous Work: Do not drive or engage in hazardous work until you determine how the medicine affects your vision. Extreme caution should be observed for activities requiring sharp vision for close objects (less than an arm's length away).

Alcohol: No special warnings.

Pregnancy: Adequate studies have not been done. Inform your doctor if you are pregnant or are planning to become pregnant.

Breast Feeding: Small amounts of homatropine pass into breast milk; either discontinue breast feeding or stop taking the drug. Consult your doctor for advice.

Infants and Children: Young children, especially those with blond hair or blue eyes, may be more sensitive to the drug and may have an increased risk of side effects. Use with extreme caution. This medication should not be used at all by infants younger than 3 months old.

Special Concerns: To use the eye drops, first wash your hands. Tilt your head back. Gently apply pressure to the inside corner of the eyelid and with the index finger of the same hand, pull downward on the lower eyelid to make a space. Drop the medicine into this space and close your eye. Apply pressure for 1 or 2 minutes while keeping the eye closed without blinking. Then wash your hands again. Make sure that the tip of the dropper does not touch your eye, finger, or any other surface.

OVERDOSE
Symptoms: Drowsiness, hallucinations, memory problems, dry mouth, dry skin, restlessness, palpitations, dizziness and disorientation, delirium.

What to Do: Call your doctor, emergency medical services (EMS), or the nearest poison control center immediately.

▼ INTERACTIONS

DRUG INTERACTIONS
Consult your doctor if you are taking any other prescription or over-the-counter drugs, especially those preparations designed for use in the eyes.

FOOD INTERACTIONS
No known food interactions.

DISEASE INTERACTIONS
Consult your doctor if you have a history of glaucoma, Down syndrome, or spastic paralysis.

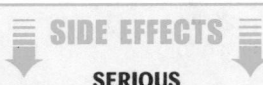

SIDE EFFECTS

SERIOUS
If absorbed into the bloodstream: Loss of coordination or unsteadiness, confusion or changes in behavior, hallucinations, slurred speech, rapid or irregular pulse, flushing, fever, unusual fatigue, dizziness, unusually dry skin, skin rash, dry mouth; in infants, abdominal swelling. Seek medical assistance immediately.

COMMON
Eye irritation and redness not present prior to treatment, swelling of the eyelids, blurred vision, increased sensitivity to bright light.

LESS COMMON
There are no less-common side effects associated with the use of homatropine.

HYDRALAZINE HYDROCHLORIDE

Available in: Tablets, injection
Available OTC? No   **As Generic?** Yes
Drug Class: Antihypertensive vasodilator

▼ USAGE INFORMATION

WHY IT'S PRESCRIBED
To treat moderate to severe high blood pressure and congestive heart failure.

HOW IT WORKS
Hydralazine hydrochloride acts upon the smooth muscle tissue surrounding the blood vessels, causing them to relax. The vessels widen and blood pressure decreases.

▼ DOSAGE GUIDELINES

RANGE AND FREQUENCY
To start, 10 mg, 4 times a day for 2 to 4 days. The dose is then increased to 25 mg, 4 times a day. The dose may be further increased to 50 mg, 4 times a day if needed. The total dose generally should not exceed 200 mg per day, but some patients may require 300 or 400 mg per day.

ONSET OF EFFECT
Within 20 to 30 minutes.

DURATION OF ACTION
3 to 8 hours.

DIETARY ADVICE
This medication should be taken with food. Follow a healthy diet (low-salt, low-fat, low-cholesterol) as advised by your doctor to help control blood pressure and prevent heart disease.

STORAGE
Store in a tightly sealed container away from heat and direct light.

MISSED DOSE
Take it as soon as you remember. If it is near the time for the next dose, skip the missed dose and resume your regular dosage schedule. Do not double the next dose.

STOPPING THE DRUG
Take the medicine as prescribed, even if you begin to feel better before the scheduled end of therapy.

PROLONGED USE
Prolonged use may cause an arthritis-like illness similar to lupus, numbness and tingling in hands or feet, and mental effects. Consult your doctor about the need for continuing medical examinations, including blood cell counts and other laboratory studies.

▼ PRECAUTIONS

Over 60: Adverse reactions may be more likely and more severe in older patients.

Driving and Hazardous Work: Do not drive or engage in hazardous work until you determine how the medicine affects you.

Alcohol: Alcohol should be avoided while taking this medication because it may trigger an excessive drop in blood pressure.

Pregnancy: In animal studies, hydralazine has caused birth defects. Human studies have not been done. Before taking hydralazine, tell your doctor if you are pregnant or plan to become pregnant.

Breast Feeding: Hydralazine passes into breast milk; you should avoid or discontinue its use while nursing.

Infants and Children: In children, this medicine is not expected to cause side effects different from those in adults. However, hydral-azine should be given to young patients only under close medical supervision.

Special Concerns: It may be necessary to take a diuretic along with hydralazine to reduce its side effects. Several weeks may be needed to determine the effectiveness of hydralazine in reducing blood pressure.

OVERDOSE

Symptoms: Rapid and weak heartbeat, extreme weakness, loss of consciousness, cold and sweaty skin, flushing.

What to Do: Call your doctor, emergency medical services (EMS), or the nearest poison control center immediately.

▼ INTERACTIONS

DRUG INTERACTIONS
Consult your doctor for specific advice if you are taking diazoxide, MAO inhibitors, loop diuretics, beta-blockers, nitrates, or nonsteroidal anti-inflammatory agents such as indomethacin.

FOOD INTERACTIONS
No known food interactions.

DISEASE INTERACTIONS
Caution is advised when taking hydralazine. Consult your doctor if you have any of the following: rheumatic heart disease, mitral valve heart disease, lupus erythematosus, or impaired brain circulation. Use of hydralazine may cause complications in patients with liver or kidney disease, since these organs work together to remove the medication from the body.

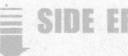 SIDE EFFECTS

SERIOUS
Lupus-like syndrome causing fast pulse and palpitations; rapid or irregular heartbeat; hives, itching, or rash; swollen lymph glands; weakness and fainting when standing up; swelling of the feet or legs; and joint pain. Call your doctor immediately.

COMMON
Headache, chest pain, nausea, vomiting, diarrhea, loss of appetite, stomach pain, blood in urine or stools, fatigue.

LESS COMMON
Dizziness; numbness, tingling, and weakness in hands or feet; chills; fever; skin rash.

HYDROCHLOROTHIAZIDE/TRIAMTERENE

Available in: Capsules, tablets
Available OTC? No   **As Generic?** Yes
Drug Class: Thiazide diuretic

▼ USAGE INFORMATION

WHY IT'S PRESCRIBED
To treat high blood pressure (hypertension); to treat conditions that cause edema (swelling of body tissues resulting from excess salt and water retention).

HOW IT WORKS
This drug combines a thiazide diuretic (hydrochlorothiazide) and a potassium-sparing diuretic (triamterene). Diuretics increase the excretion of salt and water in the urine. By reducing the overall fluid volume in the body, these drugs reduce blood volume and so reduce pressure within the blood vessels.

▼ DOSAGE GUIDELINES

RANGE AND FREQUENCY
Adults: 1 or 2 capsules or tablets once a day. Children: The dose must be determined by your doctor.

ONSET OF EFFECT
Within 2 hours.

DURATION OF ACTION
6 to 12 hours.

DIETARY ADVICE
This medication should be taken in the morning after breakfast.

STORAGE
Store in a tightly sealed container away from heat and direct light.

MISSED DOSE
Take it as soon as you remember. If it is near the time for the next dose, skip the missed dose and resume your regular dosage schedule. Do not double the next dose.

STOPPING THE DRUG
The decision to stop taking the drug should be made by your doctor.

PROLONGED USE
See your doctor regularly for examinations and tests if you must take this medicine for an extended period.

▼ PRECAUTIONS

Over 60: Adverse reactions may be more likely and more severe.

Driving and Hazardous Work: No special precautions are necessary.

Alcohol: No special precautions are necessary.

Pregnancy: This drug should not be taken during pregnancy unless recommended by your doctor. Other diuretics are generally preferred.

Breast Feeding: This drug passes into breast milk; avoid or discontinue use while breast feeding.

Infants and Children: No unusual side effects are expected in children. The dose must be determined by a pediatrician.

Special Concerns: To prevent hydrochlorothiazide from interfering with sleep, take it in the morning. If you are taking it for high blood pressure, follow the diet and weight control measures recommended by your doctor. Avoid exposure to sunlight, use a sunblock, or wear protective clothing. This medicine may cause your body to lose potassium. Follow your doctor's instructions about eating potassium-rich foods or taking a potassium supplement.

OVERDOSE
Symptoms: Dehydration, muscle weakness, cramps, heart arrhythmias.

What to Do: Call your doctor, emergency medical services (EMS), or the nearest poison control center immediately.

▼ INTERACTIONS

DRUG INTERACTIONS
Consult your doctor for specific advice if you are taking ACE inhibitors, cyclosporine, medications or dietary supplements that contain potassium, cholestyramine, colestipol, digitalis drugs, lithium, or any over-the-counter medication.

FOOD INTERACTIONS
Avoid consuming large servings of high-potassium foods, which include bananas, citrus fruits and juices, melons, prunes, (and most fruits in general), avocados, potatoes, nuts, baked beans, brussels sprouts, and skim milk.

DISEASE INTERACTIONS
Caution is advised when taking this medicine. Consult your doctor if you have diabetes, gout, kidney stones, lupus erythematosus, pancreatitis, heart disease, blood vessel disease, menstrual problems, liver disease, or kidney disease.

▼ SIDE EFFECTS

SERIOUS
Skin rash, hives, intense itching, swelling of the mouth and throat, breathing difficulty, heart rhythm irregularities or palpitations, lightheadedness or dizziness, unusual bleeding or bruising. Call your doctor immediately.

COMMON
Fluid depletion may lead to dizziness, especially upon arising from a sitting or lying position, as well as thirst, dry mouth, and constipation.

LESS COMMON
Decreased sexual ability, increased sensitivity to sunlight, loss of appetite, gout, increased blood sugar (a problem for diabetic patients).

HYDROCHLOROTHIAZIDE (HCTZ)

Available in: Tablets, oral suspension
Available OTC? No   **As Generic?** Yes
Drug Class: Thiazide diuretic

▼ USAGE INFORMATION

WHY IT'S PRESCRIBED
To treat high blood pressure (hypertension); to treat conditions that cause edema (swelling of body tissues resulting from excess salt and water retention).

HOW IT WORKS
Diuretics increase the excretion of salt and water in the urine. By reducing the overall fluid volume in the body, these drugs reduce pressure within the blood vessels.

▼ DOSAGE GUIDELINES

RANGE AND FREQUENCY
Adults– To reduce excess body water: 25 to 100 mg, 1 or 2 times a day. Your doctor may change the frequency to every other day or 3 to 5 days a week. For high blood pressure: 25 to 100 mg a day. Children, to reduce body water– Ages 2 to 12: 37.5 to 100 mg a day in 2 doses. Ages 6 months to 2 years:
12.5 to 37.5 mg a day in 2 doses. Infants under 6 months: Up to 3.3 mg per 2.2 lbs (1 kg) of body weight in 2 doses.

ONSET OF EFFECT
Within 2 hours.

DURATION OF ACTION
6 to 12 hours.

DIETARY ADVICE
It can be be taken with food to avoid stomach upset.

STORAGE
Store in a tightly sealed container away from heat and direct light. Keep the liquid form from freezing.

MISSED DOSE
Take it as soon as you remember. If it is near the time for the next dose, skip the missed dose and resume your regular dosage schedule. Do not double the next dose.

STOPPING THE DRUG
The decision to stop taking the drug should be made by your doctor.

PROLONGED USE
See your doctor regularly for examinations and tests if you must take this medicine for an extended period.

▼ PRECAUTIONS

Over 60: Adverse reactions may be more likely and more severe in older patients.

Driving and Hazardous Work: No special precautions are necessary.

Alcohol: No special precautions are necessary.

Pregnancy: Hydrochlorothiazide has caused birth defects in animals. Human studies have not been done. This medicine should not be taken during pregnancy unless recommended by your doctor; other diuretics are generally preferred for pregnant women.

Breast Feeding: Hydrochlorothiazide passes into breast milk; avoid or discontinue use during the first month of nursing.

Infants and Children: No unusual side effects are expected in children. The dose must be determined by a pediatrician.

Special Concerns: Hydrochlorothiazide is usually prescribed once a day. To prevent it from interfering with sleep, take it in the morning. If you are taking this drug for high blood pressure, follow the diet and weight control measures recommended by your doctor. Avoid exposure to sunlight,
use a sunblock, or wear protective clothing. This medicine may cause your body to lose potassium. Follow your doctor's instructions about eating potassium-rich foods or taking a potassium supplement.

OVERDOSE
Symptoms: Fainting, lethargy, dizziness, drowsiness, confusion, gastrointestinal irritation.

What to Do: Call your doctor, emergency medical services (EMS), or the nearest poison control center immediately.

▼ INTERACTIONS

DRUG INTERACTIONS
Consult your doctor for specific advice if you are taking anticoagulants, cholestyramine, colestipol, drugs for diabetes, nonsteroidal anti-inflammatory drugs, digitalis drugs, or lithium.

FOOD INTERACTIONS
No known food interactions.

DISEASE INTERACTIONS
Caution is advised when taking hydrochlorothiazide. Consult your doctor if you have any of the following: diabetes, gout, lupus erythematosus, pancreatitis, heart disease, blood vessel disease, liver disease, or kidney disease.

▤ SIDE EFFECTS ▤

SERIOUS
Skin rash, hives, intense itching, swelling of the mouth and throat, breathing difficulty, heart rhythm irregularities, lightheadedness, unusual bleeding or bruising. Call your doctor immediately.

COMMON
Muscle cramps or pain. Potassium depletion may lead to heart palpitations and weakness. Fluid depletion may lead to dizziness, especially upon arising from a sitting or lying position, as well as thirst, dry mouth, and constipation.

LESS COMMON
Decreased sexual ability, increased sensitivity to sunlight, loss of appetite, gout, increased blood sugar (a problem for diabetic patients), pancreatitis (rare).

HYDROCODONE BITARTRATE/ACETAMINOPHEN

Available in: Capsules, oral solution, tablets
Available OTC? No   **As Generic?** Yes
Drug Class: Opioid (narcotic) analgesic

▼ USAGE INFORMATION

WHY IT'S PRESCRIBED
To relieve moderate to severe pain, when nonprescription pain relievers prove inadequate. Hydrocodone, in combination with acetaminophen, may provide better pain relief at lower doses than either medication used alone at higher doses.

HOW IT WORKS
Hydrocodone, a narcotic, is believed to relieve pain by acting on specific areas in the spinal cord and brain that process pain signals from nerves throughout the body. Acetaminophen appears to interfere with the action of prostaglandins, substances in the body that cause inflammation and make nerves more sensitive to pain impulses.

▼ DOSAGE GUIDELINES

RANGE AND FREQUENCY
Adults– Capsules: 1 every 4 to 6 hours. Oral solution: 1 to 3 teaspoons every 4 to 6 hours. Tablets: 1 or 2 containing 2.5 mg of hydrocodone, or 1 containing 5, 7.5, or 10 mg of hydrocodone, every 4 to 6 hours.

ONSET OF EFFECT
30 to 60 minutes.

DURATION OF ACTION
4 to 6 hours.

DIETARY ADVICE
This drug can be taken without regard to diet.

STORAGE
Store in a tightly sealed container away from heat, moisture, and direct light.

MISSED DOSE
If you are taking this medicine on a fixed schedule, take it as soon as you remember. If it is near the time for the next dose, skip the missed dose and resume your regular dosage schedule. Do not double the next dose.

STOPPING THE DRUG
The decision to stop taking the drug should be made by your doctor.

PROLONGED USE
See your doctor regularly for tests and examinations. Prolonged use can lead to mental or physical dependence.

▼ PRECAUTIONS

Over 60: Adverse reactions may be more likely and more severe in older patients.

Driving and Hazardous Work: Do not drive or engage in hazardous work until you determine how the medicine affects you.

Alcohol: Avoid alcohol.

Pregnancy: Overuse during pregnancy can cause drug dependence in the fetus.

Breast Feeding: It is not known whether this drug passes into breast milk; caution is advised. Consult your doctor for specific advice.

Infants and Children: Adverse reactions may be more likely and more severe in children.

Special Concerns: If you feel the drug is not working properly after a few weeks, do not increase the dose.

OVERDOSE
Symptoms: Severe dizziness or drowsiness; cold, clammy skin; slow breathing or shortness of breath; severe confusion; seizures; stomach cramps or pain; diarrhea; sweating; constricted pupils; nausea or vomiting; irregular heartbeat; severe weakness.

What to Do: Call your doctor, emergency medical services (EMS), or the nearest poison control center immediately.

▼ INTERACTIONS

DRUG INTERACTIONS
Consult your doctor for specific advice if you are taking any prescription or over-the-counter medications, especially drugs with acetaminophen or central nervous system depressants such as barbiturates, seizure medicine, muscle relaxants, anesthetics, tranquilizers, or sedatives.

FOOD INTERACTIONS
No known food interactions.

DISEASE INTERACTIONS
Consult your doctor if you have a head injury or brain disease, hypothyroidism, an enlarged prostate, seizures, kidney or liver disease, gall bladder problems, a blood disorder, or a history of alcohol or drug abuse.

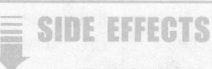
SIDE EFFECTS

SERIOUS
Bloody, dark, or cloudy urine; severe pain in lower back or side; pale or black, tarry stools; yellow-tinged eyes or skin; hallucinations; frequent urge to urinate; painful or difficult urination; sudden decrease in amount of urine; increased sweating; unusual bleeding or bruising; irregular heartbeat; skin rash, hives, or itching; unusual excitement; irregular breathing or wheezing; ringing or buzzing in ears; pinpoint red spots on skin; sore throat and fever; confusion; trembling or uncontrolled muscle movements; flushing or swelling of face. Call your doctor immediately.

COMMON
Dizziness, lightheadedness, nausea or vomiting, drowsiness, constipation, itching.

LESS COMMON
Stomach pain, allergic reaction, false sense of well-being, depression, loss of appetite, blurring or change in vision, feeling of illness, headache, nervousness, insomnia.

HYDROCODONE BITARTRATE/IBUPROFEN

BRAND NAME

Vicoprofen

Available in: Tablets
Available OTC? No   **As Generic?** No
Drug Class: Opioid (narcotic) analgesic

▼ USAGE INFORMATION

WHY IT'S PRESCRIBED
For short-term (generally less than 10 days) relief of acute pain, when nonprescription pain relievers prove inadequate. Hydrocodone, in combination with ibuprofen, may provide better pain relief at lower doses than either medicine used alone.

HOW IT WORKS
Hydrocodone, a narcotic, is believed to relieve pain by acting on specific areas in the spinal cord and brain that process pain signals from nerves throughout the body. Ibuprofen, a nonsteroidal anti-inflammatory drug (NSAID), works by interfering with the formation of prostaglandins, substances that cause inflammation and make nerves more sensitive to pain impulses. NSAIDs also have other modes of action that are less well understood.

▼ DOSAGE GUIDELINES

RANGE AND FREQUENCY
Adults and teenagers age 16 and over: 1 tablet every 4 to 6 hours, as needed. Do not take more than 5 tablets in a 24-hour period.

ONSET OF EFFECT
Unknown.

DURATION OF ACTION
Less than 10 hours.

DIETARY ADVICE
Take this drug with food.

STORAGE
Store in a tightly sealed container away from heat, moisture, and direct light.

MISSED DOSE
If you are taking this medicine on a fixed schedule, take it as soon as you remember. If it is near the time for the next dose, skip the missed dose and resume your regular dosage schedule. Do not double the next dose.

STOPPING THE DRUG
You may stop taking this drug whenever you choose.

PROLONGED USE
Opioids may be habit-forming, and prolonged use may increase the risk of dependency. Hydrocodone is used only for short-term (10 days or less) treatment of pain.

▼ PRECAUTIONS

Over 60: Adverse reactions may be more likely and more severe in older patients.

Driving and Hazardous Work: The use of this drug may impair your ability to perform such tasks safely.

Alcohol: Avoid alcohol. The combination of alcohol and this drug may increase the depressant effects of the medicine. Drinking alcoholic beverages while taking ibuprofen may increase the risk of stomach irritation.

Pregnancy: Avoid or discontinue this drug if you are pregnant or planning to become pregnant. Overuse during pregnancy can cause drug dependence in the fetus.

Breast Feeding: Ibuprofen passes into breast milk; avoid use while nursing.

Infants and Children: Not recommended for use by children under age 16.

Special Concerns: If you feel the drug is not working properly, do not increase your dose. Call your doctor. Because NSAIDs can interfere with blood coagulation, this drug should be stopped at least 3 days prior to any surgery.

OVERDOSE
Symptoms: Severe nausea; vomiting; difficult or slow breathing or shortness of breath; severe dizziness or drowsiness; cold, clammy or bluish skin; irregular or slow heartbeat; severe weakness; headache; confusion; loss of consciousness.

What to Do: Call your doctor, emergency medical services (EMS), or the nearest poison control center immediately.

▼ INTERACTIONS

DRUG INTERACTIONS
Consult your doctor for advice if you are taking: ACE inhibitors; anticholinergics; MAO inhibitors; tricyclic antidepressants; aspirin; central nervous system depressants, such as barbiturates, seizure medicines, muscle relaxants, anesthetics, tranquilizers, or sedatives; diuretics; lithium; methotrexate; or warfarin.

FOOD INTERACTIONS
No known food interactions.

DISEASE INTERACTIONS
Consult your doctor if you have an underactive thyroid, Addison's disease, an enlarged prostate, urinary difficulty, asthma, any lung disease, bleeding problems, inflammation or ulcers of the stomach and intestine, lupus, anemia, high blood pressure, or a history of heart disease. Use of this drug may cause complications in patients with severely impaired liver or kidney function.

▒ SIDE EFFECTS ▒

SERIOUS
Shallow or labored breathing; bloody, dark, or cloudy urine; severe pain in lower back or side; frequent urge to urinate; painful or difficult urination; sudden decrease in urine output; unusual bleeding or bruising; irregular heartbeat; skin rash, hives, or itching; confusion; trembling or uncontrolled muscle movements. Call your doctor immediately.

COMMON
Headache, dizziness, lightheadedness, nausea, stomach upset, drowsiness, constipation.

LESS COMMON
Abdominal pain, weakness, insomnia, nervousness, diarrhea, flatulence, dry mouth, swelling of the limbs or other areas, unusual sweating.

HYDROCORTISONE OPHTHALMIC

Available in: Ointment
Available OTC? No   **As Generic?** No
Drug Class: Corticosteroid

▼ USAGE INFORMATION

WHY IT'S PRESCRIBED
To control inflammation and prevent potentially permanent damage that may result from conditions that involve inflammation in the eye tissues.

HOW IT WORKS
Hydrocortisone inhibits the release of natural substances that stimulate an inflammatory reaction.

▼ DOSAGE GUIDELINES

RANGE AND FREQUENCY
Adults and children: Ointment is applied to eye 3 or 4 times a day to start; doses are spaced further apart as therapeutic effect is achieved.

ONSET OF EFFECT
Unknown.

DURATION OF ACTION
Unknown.

DIETARY ADVICE
This medication can be used without regard to diet.

SIDE EFFECTS

SERIOUS
Decreased vision or blurring of vision (from cataract); eye pain, nausea, vomiting (from increased eye pressure); pain, redness, sensitivity to bright light, discharge (from eye infection). Call your doctor immediately if you experience any of these signs or symptoms. This drug may trigger a recurrence of herpes infection of the eye; mention any previous herpes infection to your doctor.

COMMON
Mild and temporary blurred vision.

LESS COMMON
Burning, stinging, redness, or watering of eyes.

STORAGE
Store in a tightly sealed container away from heat and direct light.

MISSED DOSE
Apply it as soon as you remember. If it is near the time for the next dose, skip the missed dose and resume your regular dosage schedule. Do not double the next dose.

STOPPING THE DRUG
It is very important to use this drug as prescribed for the full treatment period, even if symptoms improve before the scheduled end of therapy.

PROLONGED USE
You should see your doctor regularly for tests and examinations if you must use this drug for a prolonged period.

▼ PRECAUTIONS

Over 60:
While there is no information comparing use of this drug in older patients with use in younger persons, no different side effects or problems are expected.

Driving and Hazardous Work:
Do not drive or engage in hazardous work until you determine how the medicine affects you.

Alcohol:
No special precautions are necessary.

Pregnancy:
This drug has caused birth defects in animals. Reliable human studies have not been done, but no human birth defects have been reported. Before you take ophthalmic hydrocortisone, tell your doctor if you are pregnant or plan to become pregnant.

Breast Feeding:
Ophthalmic hydrocortisone has not been reported to cause problems in nursing babies. Consult your doctor for advice.

Infants and Children:
Children under 2 years of age may be especially sensitive to the effects of ophthalmic hydrocortisone.

Special Concerns:
To use the ointment, first wash your hands. Tilt your head back. Gently apply pressure to the inside corner of the eyelid and with the index finger of the same hand, pull downward on the lower eyelid to make a space. Put a short strip of ointment (about ⅓ inch long) into this space and close your eye. Apply pressure for 1 or 2 minutes while keeping the eye closed without blinking. Then wash your hands again. Make sure the tip of the applicator does not touch your eye, finger, or any other surface. If your symptoms do not improve in a few days or if they become worse, check with your doctor.

OVERDOSE

Symptoms: When used topically, an overdose of ophthalmic hydrocortisone is extremely unlikely. Inadvertent oral ingestion, however, may cause fever, muscle aches, general feeling of weakness and illness, loss of appetite, dizziness, fainting, trouble breathing.

What to Do: An overdose of ophthalmic hydrocortisone is unlikely to be life-threatening. However, if someone applies a much larger dose of the drug than prescribed or accidentally ingests the medicine, call your doctor, emergency medical services (EMS), or the nearest poison control center right away.

▼ INTERACTIONS

DRUG INTERACTIONS
Other drugs may interact with ophthalmic hydrocortisone. Consult your doctor for specific advice if you are taking any other prescription or over-the-counter medication.

FOOD INTERACTIONS
No known food interactions.

DISEASE INTERACTIONS
Caution is advised when taking ophthalmic hydrocortisone. Consult your doctor if you have any of the following: cataracts, diabetes, glaucoma, herpes infection of the eye, tuberculosis of the eye, or any other eye infection.

HYDROCORTISONE SYSTEMIC

Available in: Oral suspension, tablets, injection, enema, rectal aerosol foam
Available OTC? No   **As Generic?** No
Drug Class: Corticosteroid

▼ USAGE INFORMATION

WHY IT'S PRESCRIBED
To treat numerous conditions that involve inflammation (a response by body tissues, producing redness, warmth, swelling, and pain). Such conditions include arthritis, allergic reactions, asthma, some skin diseases, multiple sclerosis flare-ups, and other autoimmune diseases. Also prescribed to treat deficiency of natural steroid hormones.

HOW IT WORKS
This hormone mimics the effects of the body's natural corticosteroids. It depresses the synthesis, release, and activity of inflammation-producing body chemicals. It also suppresses the activity of the immune system.

▼ DOSAGE GUIDELINES

RANGE AND FREQUENCY
Oral dose: 20 to 240 mg a day, depending on condition, in 1 or several doses. Injection: 15 to 240 mg a day, injected into a muscle, or 5 to 75 mg every 2 or 3 weeks, injected into a joint or lesion, or 100 to 500 mg every 2 to 6 hours, into muscle or vein or under skin, depending on condition. Enema: 100 mg taken nightly. Rectal aerosol foam: 90 mg, 1 or 2 times a day. Consult pediatrician for children's dosage.

ONSET OF EFFECT
Varies widely depending on the form of the drug used.

DURATION OF ACTION
Variable.

DIETARY ADVICE
Can be taken with food or milk to minimize stomach upset. Your doctor may recommend a special diet.

STORAGE
Store in a tightly sealed container away from heat, moisture, and direct light. Do not allow liquid form to freeze.

MISSED DOSE
If you take several doses a day and it is close to the next dose, double the next dose. If you take 1 dose a day and you do not remember until the next day, skip the missed dose and do not double the next dose.

STOPPING THE DRUG
With long-term therapy, do not stop taking the drug abruptly; the dosage should be decreased gradually.

PROLONGED USE
See your doctor regularly for tests and examinations. Long-term use may lead to cataracts, diabetes, hypertension, or osteoporosis.

▼ PRECAUTIONS

Over 60: Adverse reactions may be more likely and more severe in older patients.

Driving and Hazardous Work: Do not drive or engage in hazardous work until you determine how the medicine affects you.

Alcohol: May cause stomach problems; avoid it unless your physician approves occasional moderate drinking.

Pregnancy: Overuse during pregnancy can retard the child's growth and cause other developmental problems. Consult your doctor.

Breast Feeding: Do not use this drug while nursing.

Infants and Children: Hydrocortisone may retard the normal growth and development of bone and other tissues.

Special Concerns: This drug can lower your resistance to infection. Avoid immunizations with live vaccines. Patients undergoing long-term therapy should wear a medical-alert bracelet. Call your doctor if you develop a fever.

OVERDOSE
Symptoms: Fever, muscle or joint pain, nausea, dizziness, fainting, difficulty breathing. Prolonged overuse: Moonface, obesity, unusual hair growth, acne, loss of sexual function, muscle wasting.

What to Do: Seek medical assistance immediately.

▼ INTERACTIONS

DRUG INTERACTIONS
Consult your doctor for specific advice if you are taking aminoglutethimide, antacids, barbiturates, carbamazepine, griseofulvin, mitotane, phenylbutazone, phenytoin, primidone, rifampin, injectable amphotericin B, oral antidiabetes agents, insulin, digitalis drugs, diuretics, or medications containing potassium or sodium.

FOOD INTERACTIONS
Avoid excess sodium.

DISEASE INTERACTIONS
Consult your doctor if you have a history of bone disease, chickenpox, measles, gastrointestinal disorders, diabetes, recent serious infection, tuberculosis, glaucoma, heart disease, hypertension, liver or kidney disorders, high blood cholesterol, overactive or underactive thyroid, myasthenia gravis, or lupus.

SIDE EFFECTS

SERIOUS
Vision problems, frequent urination, increased thirst, rectal bleeding, blistering skin, confusion, hallucinations, paranoia, euphoria, depression, mood swings, redness and swelling at injection site. Call your doctor immediately.

COMMON
Increased appetite, indigestion, nervousness, insomnia, greater susceptibility to infections, increased blood pressure, slowed healing of wounds, rapid weight gain, easy bruising, fluid retention.

LESS COMMON
Change in skin color, dizziness, headache, increased sweating, unusual growth of body or facial hair, increased blood sugar, peptic ulcers, adrenal insufficiency, muscle weakness, cataracts, glaucoma, osteoporosis.

HYDROCORTISONE TOPICAL

Available in: Cream, lotion, ointment, topical solution, dental paste
Available OTC? Yes   **As Generic?** Yes
Drug Class: Topical corticosteroid

▼ USAGE INFORMATION

WHY IT'S PRESCRIBED
To treat certain skin conditions that are associated with itching, redness, scaling and peeling, pain, and other signs of inflammation. It is also used to treat inflammatory conditions within the mouth.

HOW IT WORKS
Topical hydrocortisone appears to interfere with the formation of natural substances within the body that are directly responsible for the process of inflammation, which produces swelling, redness, and pain.

▼ DOSAGE GUIDELINES

RANGE AND FREQUENCY
Adults using dental paste: Apply at bedtime to affected areas of the mouth. Adults using cream, lotion, ointment, solution: Apply sparingly to affected areas of the skin 1 to 2 (sometimes 3) times daily. Children: Consult your pediatrician for specific dosage and other advice.

ONSET OF EFFECT
Steroids begin to exert their effect soon after application. However, recognizable changes in your condition may take several days or more to develop.

DURATION OF ACTION
Unknown.

DIETARY ADVICE
Maintain your usual food and fluid intake.

STORAGE
Store in a tightly sealed container away from heat and direct light. Keep away from moisture and extremes in temperature.

MISSED DOSE
Apply it as soon as you remember. If it is near the time for the next dose, skip the missed dose and resume your regular dosage schedule. Do not double the next dose.

STOPPING THE DRUG
Take as prescribed for the full treatment period, even if you begin to feel better before the scheduled end of therapy.

PROLONGED USE
Therapy with this medication may require weeks or months; long-term therapy requires monitoring by your physician even with a low-potency product.

▼ PRECAUTIONS

Over 60: Adverse reactions may be more likely and more severe; therapy with topical corticosteroids should therefore be brief and infrequent.

Driving and Hazardous Work: The use of hydrocortisone topical preparation should not impair your ability to perform such tasks safely.

Alcohol: No special precautions are necessary.

Pregnancy: It should not be used for prolonged periods in pregnant women or in those trying to become pregnant.

Breast Feeding: Although problems have not been documented, caution is advised. Do not apply to breasts prior to nursing. Consult your doctor for specific advice.

Infants and Children: Not recommended for prolonged use. Consult your doctor.

Special Concerns: Avoid use of this medication around the eye. Hydrocortisone is not a treatment for acne, burns, infections, or disorders of pigmentation. Do not bandage or wrap the medicated area of skin with any special dressings or coverings unless specifically told to do so by your doctor.

OVERDOSE
Symptoms: No specific ones have been reported.

What to Do: An overdose is unlikely to be life-threatening. However, in the event of accidental ingestion or an apparent overdose, call your doctor, emergency medical services (EMS), or the nearest poison control immediately.

▼ INTERACTIONS

DRUG INTERACTIONS
None reported.

FOOD INTERACTIONS
None reported.

DISEASE INTERACTIONS
Consult your doctor if you have any of the following: diabetes; skin infection, or skin sores and ulcers; infection at another site in your body; tuberculosis; unusual bleeding or bruising; glaucoma; or cataracts.

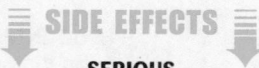

SIDE EFFECTS

SERIOUS
Serious side effects from the use of topical hydrocortisone are very rare.

COMMON
Burning, itching, irritation, redness, dryness, acne, stinging and cracking of skin, numbness or tingling in the extremities (in 0.5% to 1% of patients).

LESS COMMON
Blistering and pus near hair follicles, unusual bleeding or easy bruising, darkening or prominence of small surface veins, increased susceptibility to infection.

HYDROMORPHONE HYDROCHLORIDE

BRAND NAMES

Dilaudid, Dilaudid-5, Dilaudid-HP, Hydrostat IR

Available in: Oral solution, tablets, injection, rectal suppositories
Available OTC? No   **As Generic?** Yes
Drug Class: Opioid (narcotic) analgesic

▼ USAGE INFORMATION

WHY IT'S PRESCRIBED
To treat severe pain.

HOW IT WORKS
Opioids such as hydromorphone relieve pain by acting on specific areas of the spinal cord and brain that process pain signals from nerves throughout the body.

▼ DOSAGE GUIDELINES

RANGE AND FREQUENCY
Adults: Oral solution or tablets: 2 or 2.5 mg every 3 to 6 hours as needed. Injection: 1 to 2 mg into a muscle or under the skin every 3 to 6 hours as needed. Suppositories: 3 mg every 4 to 8 hours as needed. All doses may be increased by your physician, depending on the severity of your pain.

ONSET OF EFFECT
Oral forms and suppositories: Within 30 minutes. Injection: Within 10 to 15 minutes.

DURATION OF ACTION
Oral forms and suppositories: 4 hours. Injection: 2 to 5 hours. These times may decrease as a tolerance to hydromorphone develops.

DIETARY ADVICE
Take hydromorphone with food. Maintain your usual food and fluid intake. Narcotics cause constipation, so make sure your diet contains adequate amounts of fiber and vegetables.

STORAGE
Store in a tightly sealed container away from heat, moisture, and direct light. Keep the liquid form refrigerated, but do not allow it to freeze.

MISSED DOSE
If you are taking it on a fixed schedule, take it as soon as you remember. If it is near time for the next dose, skip the missed dose and resume your regular dosage schedule. Do not double the next dose.

STOPPING THE DRUG
You should take it as prescribed for the full treatment period, but you may stop taking the drug if you are feeling better before the scheduled end of therapy.

PROLONGED USE
Therapy with hydromorphone varies, depending on the cause of your pain. Some patients require long-term narcotic therapy. Side effects may be more likely with prolonged use.

▼ PRECAUTIONS

Over 60:
Adverse reactions may be more likely and more severe in older patients.

Driving and Hazardous Work:
The use of hydromorphone may impair your ability to perform such tasks safely.

Alcohol:
Avoid alcohol.

Pregnancy:
Adequate human studies have not been done. Before taking hydromorphone, tell your doctor if you are pregnant or are planning to become pregnant.

Breast Feeding:
Hydromorphone passes into breast milk; caution is advised. Consult your doctor for advice.

Infants and Children:
This drug may be used by young patients. Side effects may be more likely in children under the age of 2. Consult your pediatrician for advice.

Special Concerns:
This medication may be habit-forming. Do not exceed recommended doses or increase the dose on your own. This drug is more effective if taken before pain becomes too severe.

OVERDOSE
Symptoms: Confusion; sleepiness; slurred speech; unconsciousness; small, pinpoint pupils; cold, clammy skin; slow breathing; seizures; severe drowsiness, weakness, or dizziness.

What to Do: Call your doctor, emergency medical services (EMS), or the nearest poison control center immediately.

▼ INTERACTIONS

DRUG INTERACTIONS
Consult your doctor for specific advice if you are taking carbamazepine or other medicine for seizures, barbiturates, sedatives, cough medicines, decongestants, antidepressants, other prescription pain medications, MAO inhibitors, naltrexone, rifampin, or zidovudine.

FOOD INTERACTIONS
No known food interactions.

DISEASE INTERACTIONS
Consult your doctor if you have any of the following: history of alcohol or drug abuse; emotional illness; brain disorders or head injury; seizures; lung disease; prostate problems or other problems with urination; gallstones; colitis; or heart, kidney, liver, or thyroid disease.

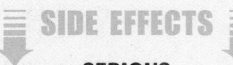

SIDE EFFECTS

SERIOUS
Serious side effects of hydromorphone are indistinguishable from those of overdose: confusion; sleepiness; slurred speech; unconsciousness; small, pinpoint pupils; cold, clammy skin; slow breathing; seizures; severe drowsiness, weakness, or dizziness.

COMMON
Dizziness or lightheadedness, nausea or vomiting, constipation, itching.

LESS COMMON
Dry mouth, mood swings or false sense of well-being and euphoria, hallucinations, nightmares.

HYDROXYCHLOROQUINE SULFATE

Available in: Tablets
Available OTC? No   **As Generic?** Yes
Drug Class: Anti-infective/antimalarial; antirheumatic

▼ USAGE INFORMATION

WHY IT'S PRESCRIBED
To prevent and treat malaria caused by specific strains of plasmodia (the parasite that causes malaria) that are chloroquine-sensitive, but when chloroquine is not available. It is also used to treat rheumatoid arthritis and lupus.

HOW IT WORKS
Hydroxychloroquine is poisonous to the malarial parasite. For rheumatoid arthritis and lupus, it may suppress the release of certain chemicals that cause inflammation.

▼ DOSAGE GUIDELINES

RANGE AND FREQUENCY
All dosages are for adults and adolescents. Consult your pediatrician for children's doses, which are based on body weight and should not exceed adult doses. To prevent malaria: 400 mg (310 mg base) once a week. To treat malaria: 800 mg (620 mg base) taken once; or 800 mg, followed by 400 mg (310 mg base), 6 to 8 hours after the first dose, then 400 mg once a day for 2 more days. For rheumatoid arthritis or lupus : 6.5 mg (5 mg base) per 2.2 lbs (1 kg) of body weight daily.

ONSET OF EFFECT
Unknown. When taking this drug for arthritis, it may take up to 6 months for the effect to occur. Consult your physician if your condition has not improved within this time.

DURATION OF ACTION
Unknown.

DIETARY ADVICE
Take it with food or milk to reduce stomach upset.

STORAGE
Store in a tightly sealed container away from heat, moisture, and direct light.

MISSED DOSE
Take it as soon as you remember. However, if it is near the time for the next dose, skip the missed dose and resume your regular dosage schedule. Do not double the next dose.

STOPPING THE DRUG
Take it as prescribed for the full treatment period.

PROLONGED USE
You may need to take this medication for an extended period of time. If you are taking it to prevent malaria, your doctor will want you to begin 1 to 2 weeks before you travel to an area where malaria is prevalent. Keep taking this medication while you are in the area and for 4 weeks after you leave.

▼ PRECAUTIONS

Over 60: Adverse reactions may be more likely and more severe in older patients.

Driving and Hazardous Work: The use of this drug may impair your ability to perform such tasks safely. Exercise caution.

Alcohol: No special precautions are necessary.

Pregnancy: The use of hydroxychloroquine is generally discouraged during pregnancy because of the risks it poses to the unborn child. However, in some cases it may be prescribed to prevent or treat malaria, since the risks of malaria are potentially more serious than those posed by the drug. Discuss with your doctor the relative risks and benefits of using this drug while pregnant.

Breast Feeding: Hydroxychloroquine passes into breast milk; extreme caution is advised. Consult your doctor for specific advice.

Infants and Children: Children are extremely sensitive to toxic effects of this drug. Use by children is considered risky, although it may be prescribed if benefits outweigh the potential risks. Consult your pediatrician for advice.

Special Concerns: Malaria is spread by mosquitoes. Take appropriate precautions to guard against being bitten by malaria-carrying mosquitoes. Note that hydroxychloroquine is not effective against all types of malaria.

OVERDOSE
Symptoms: Excitability, headache, drowsiness.

What to Do: Call your doctor, emergency medical services (EMS), or the nearest poison control center immediately.

▼ INTERACTIONS

DRUG INTERACTIONS
Consult your doctor for specific advice if you are taking magnesium or aluminum salts, cimetidine, or digoxin.

FOOD INTERACTIONS
No known food interactions.

DISEASE INTERACTIONS
Consult your doctor if you have any blood disorders, including anemia, unexplained bleeding or bruising, porphyria, or low white blood cells; liver, neurological, or vision disorders; or psoriasis.

SIDE EFFECTS

SERIOUS
Blurred or altered vision; blood problems, including low white blood cell count (sore throat, fever); anemia (fatigue, weakness); and low platelet count (easy bleeding and bruising). Such side effects are extremely rare; call your doctor immediately if they occur.

COMMON
No common side effects have been reported.

LESS COMMON
Diarrhea, loss of appetite, headache, stomach cramps or pain, nausea or vomiting, itching, dizziness, fatigue, confusion, loss or bleaching of hair, skin rash. Also blue-black discoloration of the skin, the inside of the mouth, or the fingernails.

HYDROXYUREA

Available in: Capsules
Available OTC? No   **As Generic?** Yes
Drug Class: Antimetabolite

▼ USAGE INFORMATION

WHY IT'S PRESCRIBED
To treat various types of cancer, including malignant melanoma, certain kinds of leukemia, inoperable ovarian tumors, and cancers of the head and neck.

HOW IT WORKS
Hydroxyurea prevents cancer cell growth by interfering with the synthesis of DNA in cancer cells and inhibits cell repair, thus decreasing the cell survival rate. The drug may also affect the growth and development of other kinds of cells in the body, resulting in unpleasant side effects.

▼ DOSAGE GUIDELINES

RANGE AND FREQUENCY
For intermittent therapy of solid tumors, with radiation therapy: 60 to 80 mg per 2.2 lbs (1 kg) of body weight every 3 days. For continuous therapy of solid tumors and chronic myelocytic leukemia: 500 to 2,000 mg per day, in 1 or 2 doses.

ONSET OF EFFECT
Unknown.

DURATION OF ACTION
Up to 24 hours.

DIETARY ADVICE
If you cannot swallow the capsule, empty the contents into a glass of water and consume immediately.

STORAGE
Store in a tightly sealed container away from heat and direct light.

MISSED DOSE
Take it as soon as you remember. If it is close to the next dose, skip the missed dose and resume your regular dosage schedule. Do not double the next dose.

STOPPING THE DRUG
The decision to stop taking the drug should be made in consultation with your physician.

PROLONGED USE
Hydroxyurea should be discontinued if there is no clinical response as determined by your doctor. If there is a response, the drug may be continued indefinitely.

▼ PRECAUTIONS

Over 60: Adverse reactions may be more likely and more severe in older patients.

Driving and Hazardous Work: Do not drive or engage in hazardous work until you determine how the medicine affects you.

Alcohol: Avoid alcohol.

Pregnancy: Hydroxyurea may cause birth defects if it is taken at the time of conception. Before taking it, tell your doctor if you are pregnant or plan a pregnancy.

Breast Feeding: Not recommended during therapy.

Infants and Children: Adverse reactions may be more likely and more severe in children.

Special Concerns: Be careful when you use a toothbrush, toothpick, or dental floss. Check with your doctor before having any dental work done. Avoid people with infections. Be careful not to cut yourself when you are using sharp objects such as a nail cutter or razor. Wash your hands regularly to decrease the likelihood of spreading bacteria or viruses. Avoid contact sports or other situations where an injury could occur. Watch closely for signs of infection, and take your temperature if you feel ill. Do not receive any immunizations without your doctor's approval. After you stop taking hydroxyurea, check with your doctor if you notice black, tarry stools; blood in urine or stools; cough or hoarseness; fever or chills; pain in lower back or side; painful or difficult urination; red spots on skin; or unusual bleeding or bruising.

OVERDOSE
Symptoms: Excessive side effects.

What to Do: Call your doctor, emergency medical services (EMS), or the nearest poison control center immediately.

▼ INTERACTIONS

DRUG INTERACTIONS
Consult your doctor for specific advice if you are taking amphotericin B, antithyroid agents, azathioprine, chloramphenicol, colchicine, flucytosine, ganciclovir, interferon, plicamycin, zidovudine, probenecid, or sulfinpyrazone.

FOOD INTERACTIONS
No known food interactions.

DISEASE INTERACTIONS
Caution is advised when taking hydroxyurea. Consult your doctor if you have a history of any of the following: anemia, chickenpox, shingles, gout, kidney stones, any infection, or kidney disease.

SIDE EFFECTS

SERIOUS
Cough or hoarseness; fever or chills; pain in lower back or side; painful or difficult urination; black, tarry stools; blood in urine or stools; red spots on skin; unusual bleeding or bruising; sores in mouth or on lips; confusion; seizures; dizziness; hallucinations; headache; joint pain; swelling of feet or lower legs. Call your doctor immediately.

COMMON
Diarrhea, loss of appetite, nausea or vomiting.

LESS COMMON
Constipation, reddened skin, skin rash, itching, drowsiness.

HYDROXYZINE

Available in: Tablets, syrup, injection
Available OTC? No **As Generic?** Yes
Drug Class: Antihistamine/mild sedative

▼ USAGE INFORMATION

WHY IT'S PRESCRIBED
Hydroxyzine is used for several conditions. Its mild sedative effect is useful in treating insomnia and agitation in some patients. It is also used to treat itching, hives, and other allergy symptoms; to control nausea and vomiting; to ease the symptoms of alcohol withdrawal; and to provide mild sedation prior to a dental procedure or to the administration of general anesthesia before surgery.

HOW IT WORKS
Hydroxyzine is an antihistamine; that is, it blocks the effects of histamine, a naturally occurring substance in the body that causes swelling, itching, sneezing, watery eyes, hives, and other symptoms of allergic reactions. In addition to its antihistamine effect, hydroxyzine also has a sedative effect and appears to suppress activity in some regions of the central nervous system (the brain and spinal cord) associated with nausea and psychological distress.

▼ DOSAGE GUIDELINES

RANGE AND FREQUENCY
For sedation— Adults: 50 to 100 mg a day. For allergy symptoms— Adults: 25 to 100 mg, 3 or 4 times a day, as needed. Children age 6 and older: 12.5 to 25 mg, every 6 hours as needed. Children up to age 6: 12.5 mg every 6 hours as needed. For nausea and vomiting— Adults: 25 to 100 mg, 3 or 4 times a day. Children: 0.6 mg per 2.2 lbs of body weight per day.

ONSET OF EFFECT
15 to 30 minutes.

DURATION OF ACTION
Approximately 6 to 8 hours.

DIETARY ADVICE
Drink plenty of fluids.

STORAGE
Store in a tightly sealed container away from heat and direct light. Keep tablets away from moisture and extremes in temperature. Keep liquid forms refrigerated, but do not allow to freeze.

MISSED DOSE
Take it as soon as you remember. If it is near the time for the next dose, skip the missed dose and resume your regular dosage schedule. Do not double the next dose.

STOPPING THE DRUG
The decision to stop taking the drug should be made in consultation with your doctor.

PROLONGED USE
Therapy with hydroxyzine may require days or weeks, depending on the condition. Side effects may be more likely with prolonged use.

▼ PRECAUTIONS

Over 60: Adverse reactions may be more likely and more severe in older patients.

Driving and Hazardous Work: Hydroxyzine may impair mental alertness; caution is advised.

Alcohol: Avoid alcohol.

Pregnancy: Adequate studies of hydroxyzine use during pregnancy have not been done; consult your doctor for specific advice.

Breast Feeding: Hydroxyzine may pass into breast milk and cause side effects in the nursing infant; do not use.

Infants and Children: Use this drug only under close supervision by your pediatrician.

Special Concerns: Antihistamines are widely available without prescription; if you are taking a prescription anti-histamine, avoid other cough, cold, flu, sinus, or allergy preparations.

OVERDOSE
Symptoms: Severe dryness in mouth, nose, and throat; extreme drowsiness; loss of coordination; faintness; flushing; tremor; hallucinations; breathing difficulty.

What to Do: Call emergency medical services (EMS), your doctor, or the nearest poison control center immediately.

▼ INTERACTIONS

DRUG INTERACTIONS
Consult your doctor for specific advice if you are taking any drugs that depress the central nervous system; these include antidepressants or other psychiatric medications, other antihistamines, barbiturates, sedatives, cough medicines, decongestants, and painkillers. Be sure your doctor knows about any over-the-counter drug you may take.

FOOD INTERACTIONS
None are known.

DISEASE INTERACTIONS
Consult your doctor if you have any of the following: asthma, glaucoma or another eye disorder, thyroid disease, heart or blood vessel disease, high blood pressure, enlarged prostate, or urinary difficulty.

SIDE EFFECTS

SERIOUS
Loss of coordination, seizures, extreme drowsiness, breathing difficulty, inability to urinate.

COMMON
Drowsiness; dryness in the mouth, nasal passages, and other mucous membranes.

LESS COMMON
Difficult urination, dizziness, rash, sore throat, fever, nightmares, restlessness, sleep disruption, irritability, increased skin sensitivity to sunlight, loss of appetite, stomach upset, decreased sexual ability in men.

IBUPROFEN

Available in: Tablets, oral solution, chewable tablets
Available OTC? Yes **As Generic?** Yes
Drug Class: Nonsteroidal anti-inflammatory drug (NSAID)

▼ USAGE INFORMATION

WHY IT'S PRESCRIBED
To treat mild to moderate pain and inflammation caused by tendinitis, arthritis, bursitis, gout, soft tissue injuries, migraine and other vascular headaches, menstrual cramps, and other conditions. It is also used to reduce fever.

HOW IT WORKS
NSAIDs work by interfering with the formation of prostaglandins, substances that cause inflammation and make nerves more sensitive to pain impulses. NSAIDs also have other modes of action that are less well understood.

▼ DOSAGE GUIDELINES

RANGE AND FREQUENCY
Adults— For mild to moderate pain, arthritis, and menstrual pain: 200 to 400 mg every 4 to 6 hours. For fever: 200 to 400 mg every 4 to 6 hours, but not more than 1,200 mg a day. Children ages 6 months to 12 years— For fevers below 102.5°F, 5 mg for every 2.2 lbs (1 kg) of body weight every 6 to 8 hours. For higher fevers, 10 mg per 2.2 lbs every 6 to 8 hours, but not more than 40 mg per 2.2 lbs a day.

ONSET OF EFFECT
For pain and fever, 30 minutes. For arthritis, up to 3 weeks.

DURATION OF ACTION
4 hours or more.

DIETARY ADVICE
Take ibuprofen with food.

STORAGE
Store in a tightly sealed container away from heat, moisture, and direct light.

MISSED DOSE
Take it as soon as you remember. However, if it is near the time for the next dose, skip the missed dose and resume your regular dosage schedule. Do not double the next dose.

STOPPING THE DRUG
If taking this drug by prescription, do not stop without consulting your doctor.

PROLONGED USE
Prolonged use can cause gastrointestinal problems, including ulceration and bleeding, kidney dysfunction, and liver inflammation. See your doctor regularly for laboratory tests and examinations.

▼ PRECAUTIONS

Over 60: Because of the potentially greater consequences of gastrointestinal side effects, the dose of NSAIDs for older patients, especially those over age 70, is often cut in half.

Driving and Hazardous Work: Do not drive or engage in hazardous work until you determine how the medicine affects you.

Alcohol: Avoid alcohol, as it may increase the risk of stomach irritation.

Pregnancy: Avoid or discontinue this drug if you are pregnant or are planning to become pregnant.

Breast Feeding: Ibuprofen passes into breast milk; avoid use while nursing.

Infants and Children: May be used in exceptional circumstances; consult your doctor.

Special Concerns: Because NSAIDs can interfere with blood coagulation, this drug should be stopped at least 3 days prior to any surgery.

OVERDOSE
Symptoms: Severe nausea, vomiting, headache, confusion, seizures.

What to Do: Call your doctor, emergency medical services (EMS), or the nearest poison control center immediately.

▼ INTERACTIONS

DRUG INTERACTIONS
Do not take this drug with aspirin or any other NSAIDs without your doctor's approval. In addition, consult your doctor if you are taking antihypertensives, steroids, anticoagulants, antibiotics, itraconazole or ketoconazole, plicamycin, penicillamine, valproic acid, phenytoin, cyclosporine, digitalis drugs, lithium, methotrexate, probenecid, triamterene, or zidovudine.

FOOD INTERACTIONS
No known food interactions.

DISEASE INTERACTIONS
Consult your doctor if you have any of the following: bleeding problems, inflammation or ulcers of the stomach and intestines, diabetes mellitus, systemic lupus erythematosus (SLE, lupus), anemia, asthma, epilepsy, Parkinson's disease, kidney stones, or a history of heart disease or alcohol abuse. Use of ibuprofen may cause complications in patients with liver or kidney disease, since these organs work together to remove the medication from the body.

SIDE EFFECTS

SERIOUS
Shortness of breath or wheezing, with or without swelling of legs or other signs of heart failure; chest pain; peptic ulcer disease with vomiting of blood; black, tarry stools; decreasing kidney function. Call your doctor immediately.

COMMON
Nausea, vomiting, heartburn, diarrhea, constipation, headache, dizziness, sleepiness.

LESS COMMON
Ulcers or sores in mouth, depression, rashes or blistering of skin, ringing sound in the ears, unusual tingling or numbness of the hands or feet, seizures, blurred vision. Also: elevated potassium levels, decreased blood counts; such problems can be detected by your doctor.

IDOXURIDINE (IDU)

Available in: Drops, ointment
Available OTC? No   **As Generic?** No
Drug Class: Ophthalmic antiviral drug

▼ USAGE INFORMATION

WHY IT'S PRESCRIBED
To treat viral infections of the eye, especially those caused by the herpes simplex virus.

HOW IT WORKS
Idoxuridine interferes with the activity of enzymes necessary for the replication of viral DNA in cells, thus preventing the virus from multiplying.

▼ DOSAGE GUIDELINES

RANGE AND FREQUENCY
The dosage may vary considerably from patient to patient, depending on a number of factors. The following guidelines represent typical doses; follow your doctor's specific dosing instruction. Eye drops: Apply 1 drop in the eye every hour during the day and every 2 hours at night. When the condition improves, apply it every 2 hours during the day and every 4 hours at night. Ointment: Apply a ⅜-inch strip of ointment every 4 hours (5 times a day), making the last application at bedtime.

ONSET OF EFFECT
Within 1 hour.

DURATION OF ACTION
Up to 6 hours.

DIETARY ADVICE
No special restrictions.

STORAGE
Keep the liquid form of idoxuridine refrigerated, but do not allow it to freeze.

MISSED DOSE
Apply the missed dose as soon as you remember. If it is near time for the next dose, skip the missed dose and resume your regular dosage schedule. Do not double the next dose.

STOPPING THE DRUG
Take the drug as prescribed for the full treatment period, even if you begin to feel better before the scheduled end of therapy.

PROLONGED USE
Idoxuridine is not intended for prolonged use. If your symptoms do not improve in 7 days, consult your doctor.

▼ PRECAUTIONS

Over 60: No special problems are expected.

Driving and Hazardous Work: The use of idoxuridine should not impair your ability to perform such tasks safely.

Alcohol: No special precautions are necessary.

Pregnancy: Before taking idoxuridine, tell your doctor if you are pregnant or plan to become pregnant.

Breast Feeding: Idoxuridine may pass into breast milk; caution is advised. Consult your doctor for advice.

Infants and Children: Studies of the use of idoxuridine specifically in children have not been done; this drug should be used by young patients only under close medical supervision.

Special Concerns: Be sure you know how to apply idoxuridine. For the eye drops, first wash your hands. Then apply pressure to the inside corner of the eye with your middle finger. Tilt your head backward and pull the lower lid away from the eye with the index finger of the same hand. Drop the eye drops into the pouch you have created and close your eyes without blinking. Keep your eyes closed for 1 to 2 minutes. Then wash your hands. For the ointment, first wash your hands. Pull the lower lid down from the eye to form a pouch. Squeeze the tube to apply a thin strip of the ointment into the pouch. Close your eyes for 1 to 2 minutes.

Then wash your hands. Do not let the applicator touch any surface, including the eye. If you accidentally touch its tip, clean it with warm water and soap. Family members should use separate washcloths and towels to prevent the spread of infection.

OVERDOSE
Symptoms: No specific ones have been reported.

What to Do: An overdose of idoxuridine is unlikely to occur. Emergency instructions are not applicable.

▼ INTERACTIONS

DRUG INTERACTIONS
Consult your doctor if you are using any eye product containing boric acid.

FOOD INTERACTIONS
No known food interactions.

DISEASE INTERACTIONS
Caution is advised when taking idoxuridine; consult your doctor if you have a history of any other eye problems.

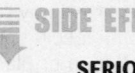

SIDE EFFECTS

SERIOUS
Allergic reaction causing itching, swelling, redness, pain, and constant burning; corneal ulcer causing painful sensation of having something lodged in the eye. In either case, call your doctor or ophthalmologist immediately.

COMMON
Heightened sensitivity of the eyes to bright light, stinging or burning in the eyes.

LESS COMMON
Blurred vision, excessive tear production.

IMIPRAMINE

Available in: Tablets, capsules
Available OTC? No   **As Generic?** Yes
Drug Class: Tricyclic antidepressant

▼ USAGE INFORMATION

WHY IT'S PRESCRIBED
To relieve symptoms of major depression. Also used to treat bed-wetting in children age 6 and older and incontinence in older women.

HOW IT WORKS
Imipramine affects levels of specific brain chemicals (serotonin and norepinephrine) that are thought to be linked to mood, emotions, and mental state.

▼ DOSAGE GUIDELINES

RANGE AND FREQUENCY
For depression— Tablets: Adults: To start, 25 to 50 mg, 3 to 4 times a day; may be increased to 200 mg a day. Teenagers: 25 to 50 mg a day; may be increased to 100 mg a day. Older adults: To start, 25 mg a day at bedtime; may be increased to 100 mg a day. Children ages 6 to 12: 10 to 30 mg a day.

Capsules: Adults: To start, 75 mg a day at bedtime; may be increased to 200 mg a day. For bed-wetting— Tablets: Children age 6 and older: 25 mg a day, 1 hour before bedtime. Dose may be increased based on the child's age.

ONSET OF EFFECT
1 to 6 weeks.

DURATION OF ACTION
Unknown.

DIETARY ADVICE
To lessen stomach upset, take with food, unless your doctor instructs otherwise. Increase intake of fiber and fluids.

STORAGE
Store in a tightly sealed container away from heat, moisture, and direct light.

MISSED DOSE
If you take a one-time daily bedtime dose, do not take a missed dose in the morning because it may cause drowsiness. Call your doctor. If you take more than 1 dose a day, take it as soon as you remember. If it is near the time for the next dose, skip the missed dose and resume your regular dosage schedule. Do not double the next dose.

STOPPING THE DRUG
Take as prescribed for the full treatment period, even if you begin to feel better before the scheduled end of therapy. The decision to stop taking the drug should be made in consultation with your doctor.

PROLONGED USE
The usual course of therapy lasts 6 months to 1 year; some patients benefit from additional therapy.

▼ PRECAUTIONS

Over 60: Adverse reactions may be more likely and more severe in older patients. A lower dose may be warranted.

Driving and Hazardous Work: Use caution until you determine how the medicine affects you. Drowsiness and lightheadedness can occur.

Alcohol: Avoid alcohol.

Pregnancy: Adequate studies have not been done. Consult your doctor for advice.

Breast Feeding: Do not use this drug while nursing.

Infants and Children: Not prescribed for children under the age of 6.

Special Concerns: This is a potentially dangerous drug, especially if taken in excess. Tricyclic antidepressants should not be within easy reach of suicidal patients.

OVERDOSE
Symptoms: Difficulty breathing, severe fatigue, seizures, confusion, hallucinations, distractibility, dilated pupils, irregular heartbeat, fever.

What to Do: Call your doctor, emergency medical services (EMS), or the nearest poison control center immediately.

▼ INTERACTIONS

DRUG INTERACTIONS
Consult your doctor for specific advice if you are taking antithyroid agents, cimetidine, cisapride, clonidine, guanadrel, guanethidine, metrizamide, appetite suppressants, isoproterenol, ephedrine, epinephrine, amphetamines, phenylephrine, antipsychotic drugs, pimozide, methyldopa, metyrosine, metoclopramide, pemoline, promethazine, trimeprazine, rauwolfia alkaloids, MAO inhibitors, or any drugs that depress the central nervous system.

FOOD INTERACTIONS
No known food interactions.

DISEASE INTERACTIONS
Consult your physician if you have any of the following: a history of alcohol abuse, difficulty urinating, asthma, bipolar disorder, high blood pressure, stomach or intestinal problems, glaucoma, overactive thyroid, enlarged prostate, schizophrenia, seizures a blood disorder, or kidney, heart, or liver disease.

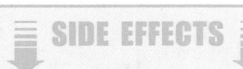

SIDE EFFECTS

SERIOUS
Confusion, heartbeat irregularities, hallucinations, seizures, extreme fatigue or drowsiness, blurred or altered vision, breathing difficulty, constipation, impaired concentration, difficult urination, fever, extreme and persistent restlessness, loss of coordination and balance, difficulty swallowing or speaking, dilated pupils, eye pain, fainting. Also trembling, shaking, weakness, and stiffness in the extremities; shuffling gait. Call your doctor immediately.

COMMON
Drowsiness, dizziness, or lightheadedness, headache, dry mouth or unpleasant taste, fatigue, heightened sensitivity of skin to sunlight, weight gain, increased appetite, nausea.

LESS COMMON
Heartburn, insomnia, diarrhea, increased sweating, vomiting.

IMIQUIMOD

Available in: Cream
Available OTC? No   **As Generic?** No
Drug Class: Immunomodulator

▼ USAGE INFORMATION

WHY IT'S PRESCRIBED
To treat external condylomata acuminata (genital and perianal warts) in adults.

HOW IT WORKS
Imiquimod's mechanism of action is unknown.

▼ DOSAGE GUIDELINES

RANGE AND FREQUENCY
Apply a thin layer to the affected area 3 times a week at bedtime. Leave it on the skin for 6 to 10 hours. The cream should then be removed by washing with mild soap and water.

ONSET OF EFFECT
Unknown.

DURATION OF ACTION
Unknown.

DIETARY ADVICE
No special restrictions.

STORAGE
Store in a tightly sealed container away from heat, moisture, and direct light. Do not allow it to freeze.

MISSED DOSE
If you miss a scheduled dose, skip it and resume your regular dosage schedule on the appointed day; do not apply the cream 2 days in a row.

STOPPING THE DRUG
Treatment should continue until there is total clearance of the warts or for no more than 16 weeks. If the warts do not clear up within this time, do not continue to apply imiquimod to the area; consult your doctor.

PROLONGED USE
Imiquimod is prescribed for no more than 16 weeks.

▼ PRECAUTIONS

Over 60: No special problems are expected.

Driving and Hazardous Work: The use of imiquimod should not impair your ability to perform such tasks safely.

Alcohol: No special precautions are necessary.

Pregnancy: Adequate human studies have not been done.

Before taking imiquimod, tell your physician if you are pregnant or plan to become pregnant.

Breast Feeding: Imiquimod may pass into breast milk; caution is advised. Consult your doctor for advice.

Infants and Children: Not recommended for use by children under age 18.

Special Concerns: The treated area should not be covered by tight bandages or clothing. Wash your hands before and after applying imiquimod to the skin. Avoid getting the drug in your eyes. Sexual relations should be avoided while the cream is on the skin. Imiquimod cream may weaken condoms and diaphragms, compromising the protection they provide. If serious irritation of the treated area occurs, discontinue the medication for several days to allow the reaction to subside. You may then resume therapy.

OVERDOSE
Symptoms: No cases of overdose have been reported.

What to Do: An overdose with imiquimod is unlikely. If someone accidentally ingests imiquimod, call your doctor, emergency medical services (EMS), or the nearest poison control center immediately.

▼ INTERACTIONS

DRUG INTERACTIONS
None known.

FOOD INTERACTIONS
No known food interactions.

DISEASE INTERACTIONS
Imiquimod should be used with caution by anyone with a history of inflammatory skin conditions. If you have had any recent medical or surgical treatment in the genital or perianal area, therapy with imiquimod should be delayed until the affected tissue has healed.

≡ SIDE EFFECTS ≡

SERIOUS
Swollen eyelids, face, or lips, wheezing, or rash may be signs of a drug allergy. Call your doctor immediately.

COMMON
Common side effects are limited to the treated area of the skin. The following have been observed: redness, thinning of the skin, flaking, swelling of the treated area.

LESS COMMON
Hardening or stiffening of the treated area, sores, scabbing, blisters.

INDAPAMIDE

Available in: Tablets
Available OTC? No   **As Generic?** Yes
Drug Class: Thiazide diuretic

▼ USAGE INFORMATION

WHY IT'S PRESCRIBED
To help control high blood pressure and to treat conditions that cause edema (swelling of body tissues resulting from excess salt and water retention).

HOW IT WORKS
Diuretics increase the excretion of salt and water in the urine. By reducing the overall fluid volume in the body, these drugs reduce blood volume and so reduce pressure within the blood vessels.

▼ DOSAGE GUIDELINES

RANGE AND FREQUENCY
For high blood pressure: Initial dose is 1.5 mg once a day. It can be increased to 5 mg a day. To reduce edema: 2.5 mg once a day; it can be increased to 5 mg a day.

ONSET OF EFFECT
From 2 to 3 hours.

DURATION OF ACTION
24 hours.

DIETARY ADVICE
A single daily dose should be taken in the morning after breakfast.

STORAGE
Store in a tightly sealed container away from heat and direct light.

MISSED DOSE
Take it as soon as you remember. If it is near the time for the next dose, skip the missed dose and resume your regular dosage schedule. Do not double the next dose.

STOPPING THE DRUG
The decision to stop taking the drug should be made by your doctor.

PROLONGED USE
See your doctor regularly for examinations and tests if you must take this medicine for an extended period.

▼ PRECAUTIONS

Over 60: Adverse reactions may be more likely and more severe in older patients.

Driving and Hazardous Work: No special warnings.

Alcohol: No special precautions are necessary.

Pregnancy: Indapamide should not be used during pregnancy unless recommended by your doctor.

Breast Feeding: Indapamide may pass into breast milk; caution is advised. Consult your doctor for advice.

Infants and Children: The safety and effectiveness of indapamide for children under 12 have not been determined. Consult your doctor for specific advice.

Special Concerns: Follow your doctor's instructions about consuming potassium-rich foods or taking a potassium supplement. It may be necessary to discontinue indapamide 5 to 7 days before undergoing major surgery. If you are taking more than 1 dose a day, the last dose should be taken no later than 6 pm unless your doctor advises otherwise.

OVERDOSE
Symptoms: Stomach irritation, thirst, muscle cramps, nausea, vomiting, increased urination, lethargy, loss of consciousness.

What to Do: Call your doctor, emergency medical services (EMS), or the nearest poison control center immediately.

▼ INTERACTIONS

DRUG INTERACTIONS
Consult your doctor for advice if you are taking other drugs for high blood pressure, lithium, oral antidiabetic drugs, digitalis preparations, nonsteroidal anti-inflammatory drugs, cholestyramine, or colestipol.

FOOD INTERACTIONS
Follow your doctor's advice about salt use and potassium-rich foods.

DISEASE INTERACTIONS
Caution is advised when taking indapamide. Consult your doctor if you have diabetes, gout, or lupus. Use of indapamide may cause complications in patients with liver or kidney disease, since these organs work together to remove the medication from the body.

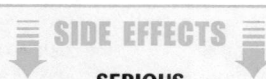

SIDE EFFECTS

SERIOUS
Skin rash, hives, intense itching, swelling of the mouth and throat, breathing difficulty, heart rhythm irregularities, light-headedness, unusual bleeding or bruising. Call your doctor immediately.

COMMON
Muscle cramps or pain. Potassium depletion may lead to heart palpitations and weakness. Fluid depletion may lead to dizziness, especially upon arising from a sitting or lying position, as well as thirst, dry mouth, and constipation.

LESS COMMON
Decreased sexual ability, increased sensitivity to sunlight, loss of appetite, gout, increased blood sugar (a problem for diabetic patients).

INDINAVIR

Available in: Capsules
Available OTC? No   **As Generic?** No
Drug Class: Antiviral/protease inhibitor

▼ USAGE INFORMATION

WHY IT'S PRESCRIBED
To treat advanced HIV (human immunodeficiency virus) infection and AIDS (acquired immunodeficiency syndrome), usually in combination with other drugs. While not a cure for HIV infection, this drug may suppress the replication of the virus and delay the progression of the disease.

HOW IT WORKS
Indinavir blocks the activity of a viral protease, an enzyme that is needed by HIV to reproduce. Blocking the protease causes HIV to make copies that cannot infect new cells.

▼ DOSAGE GUIDELINES

RANGE AND FREQUENCY
800 mg every 8 hours, alone or in combination with other antiviral agents. Higher or lower doses are sometimes prescribed when indinavir is being combined with medications such as nevirapine and delavirdine, which alter indinavir blood levels.

ONSET OF EFFECT
Unknown. With most anti-retroviral drugs, an early response can be seen within the first few days of therapy, but the maximum effect may take 12 to 16 weeks.

DURATION OF ACTION
Unknown. Effects of the drug may be prolonged if indinavir is used in combination with other effective drugs and the virus is maximally suppressed.

DIETARY ADVICE
Indinavir should be taken with plenty of water or other liquid, preferably at least 1 hour before or 2 hours after a meal. It may also be taken with a light, nonfat snack.

STORAGE
Store in a tightly sealed container away from heat, moisture, and direct light.

MISSED DOSE
Take it as soon as you remember. However, if it is near the time for the next dose, skip the missed dose and resume your regular dosage schedule. Do not double the next dose.

STOPPING THE DRUG
The decision to stop taking the drug should be made by your doctor.

PROLONGED USE
See your doctor regularly for tests and examinations.

▼ PRECAUTIONS

Over 60: No special studies have been done on older patients.

Driving and Hazardous Work: Do not drive or engage in hazardous work until you determine how the medicine affects you.

Alcohol: Avoid alcohol if liver function is impaired.

Pregnancy: Indinavir has been shown to cause birth defects in animals. Human studies have not been done. Nevertheless, indinavir is increasingly being used in combination with other anti-retroviral drugs to treat pregnant HIV-infected women.

Breast Feeding: Women infected with HIV should not breast-feed, so as to avoid transmitting the virus to an uninfected child.

Infants and Children: Safety and effectiveness of indinavir for children under the age of 16 have not been established.

Special Concerns: It is important to drink at least 48 ounces of water or other liquids every 24 hours to help prevent kidney stones. Therapy may be interrupted for patients who develop kidney stones. Be sure to tell any doctor or dentist treating you that you are taking indinavir. Remember that taking indinavir does not eliminate the chance of passing the AIDS virus to other persons.

OVERDOSE
Symptoms: Pain in the lower back, blood in the urine, nausea, vomiting, diarrhea.

What to Do: An overdose of indinavir is unlikely to be life-threatening. However, if someone takes a much larger dose than prescribed, call your doctor, emergency medical services (EMS), or the nearest poison control center immediately.

▼ INTERACTIONS

DRUG INTERACTIONS
Consult your doctor for specific advice if you are taking any other drug, especially astemizole, cisapride, didanosine, delavirdine, efavirenz, itraconazole, ketoconazole, midazolam, triazolam, didanosine, rifabutin, rifampin, phenobarbital, phenytoin, carbamazepine, cholesterol-lowering drugs, or dexamethasone.

FOOD INTERACTIONS
Food, especially fatty foods, will decrease absorption of the drug.

DISEASE INTERACTIONS
Use of indinavir may cause complications in patients with liver disease.

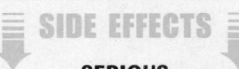

SIDE EFFECTS

SERIOUS
Blood in urine and sharp back pain caused by kidney stones. High blood sugar (diabetes) has occurred in patients taking drugs of this class, although a cause-and-effect relationship has not been established. Call your doctor if you develop increased thirst or excessive urination.

COMMON
Generalized weakness, abdominal pains, diarrhea, nausea, vomiting, headache, insomnia, changes in taste, dry skin, chapped lips.

LESS COMMON
Dizziness, drowsiness, depression, memory changes, abdominal bloating, muscle wasting.

INDOMETHACIN

Available in: Capsules, suspension, rectal suppositories
Available OTC? No **As Generic?** Yes
Drug Class: Nonsteroidal anti-inflammatory drug (NSAID)

▼ USAGE INFORMATION

WHY IT'S PRESCRIBED
To treat mild to moderate pain and inflammation occurring in association with tendinitis, arthritis, bursitis, gout, soft tissue injuries, migraine and other types of vascular headache, menstrual cramps, and other conditions. Because of its greater risk of toxicity, indomethacin should be taken only when other NSAIDs prove ineffective.

HOW IT WORKS
NSAIDs such as indomethacin work by interfering with the formation of prostaglandins. These are naturally occurring substances in the body that cause inflammation and make nerves more sensitive to pain impulses. NSAIDs also have other modes of action that are less well understood.

▼ DOSAGE GUIDELINES

RANGE AND FREQUENCY
Adults— Capsules: For arthritis: 25 to 50 mg, 2 to 4 times daily, up to a usual maximum of 200 mg a day at first. For gout: 100 mg immediately, then 50 mg taken 3 times a day. This may be decreased gradually by your doctor. For bursitis or tendinitis: 25 mg, 3 to 4 times a day, or 50 mg, 3 times a day. Extended-release capsules: For arthritis: 75 mg, 1 to 2 times a day. Rectal suppositories: For arthritis, gout, bursitis, and tendinitis: 50 mg suppository, inserted 1 to 4 times a day. Children— Consult a pediatrician for dosage for all forms.

ONSET OF EFFECT
30 minutes to several hours.

DURATION OF ACTION
4 hours or more.

DIETARY ADVICE
Take with food; maintain your usual food and fluid intake.

STORAGE
Store in a tightly sealed container away from heat, moisture, and direct light.

MISSED DOSE
Take it as soon as you remember. If it is near the time for the next dose, skip the missed dose and resume your regular dosage schedule. Do not double the next dose.

STOPPING THE DRUG
Take it as prescribed for the full treatment period. Ask your doctor about stopping the drug if you are feeling better before the scheduled end of therapy.

PROLONGED USE
Therapy may require weeks or months.

▼ PRECAUTIONS

Over 60: Because of the potentially greater consequences of gastrointestinal side effects, the dose in older patients, especially those over age 70, is often cut in half.

Driving and Hazardous Work: Avoid such activities until you determine how the medicine affects you.

Alcohol: Avoid alcohol.

Pregnancy: Do not use this drug while pregnant.

Breast Feeding: Do not use indomethacin while nursing.

Infants and Children: May be used in exceptional circumstances only when other NSAIDs prove ineffective; consult a pediatrician.

Special Concerns: Because NSAIDs can interfere with blood coagulation, this drug should be stopped at least 3 days prior to any surgery.

OVERDOSE
Symptoms: Severe nausea, vomiting, headache, confusion, seizures.

What to Do: Call your doctor, emergency medical services (EMS), or the nearest poison control center immediately.

▼ INTERACTIONS

DRUG INTERACTIONS
Do not take with aspirin or other NSAIDs. Consult your doctor if you are taking anticoagulants, antibiotics, itraconazole or ketoconazole, plicamycin, penicillamine, valproic acid, phenytoin, cyclosporine, digitalis drugs, lithium, medication for high blood pressure, methotrexate, probenecid, steroids, triamterene, or zidovudine.

FOOD INTERACTIONS
No known food interactions.

DISEASE INTERACTIONS
Consult your doctor if you have a history of alcohol abuse, bleeding problems, inflammation or ulcers of the stomach and intestines, diabetes mellitus, heart, liver, or kidney disease (including kidney stones), systemic lupus erythematosus (SLE, lupus), anemia, asthma, epilepsy, or Parkinson's disease.

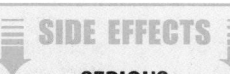

SIDE EFFECTS

SERIOUS
Wheezing or breathing difficulty, with or without swelling of the legs or other signs of heart failure; chest pain; peptic ulcers with vomiting of blood; black, tarry stools; decreased kidney function causing blood in the urine, decreased urine output, and shortness of breath. NSAIDs may cause constriction of the airways or severe allergic reactions in patients who are sensitive to aspirin, especially those with aspirin-induced nasal polyps or asthma.

COMMON
Nausea, vomiting, heartburn, diarrhea, constipation, headache, dizziness, drowsiness.

LESS COMMON
Ulcers or sores in mouth, rashes or blistering, unusual tingling or numbness of the hands and feet, depression, ringing in the ears, seizures, blurred vision. Also high blood potassium levels and decreased blood counts; such problems can be detected by your doctor.

INFLUENZA VIRUS VACCINE

Available in: Injection
Available OTC? No **As Generic?** No
Drug Class: Vaccine

▼ USAGE INFORMATION

WHY IT'S PRESCRIBED
To help prevent infection by the influenza (flu) virus.

HOW IT WORKS
The influenza vaccine is an injection that works by introducing a dead (inactive) flu virus into the body, which stimulates the immune system to produce protective antibodies against the disease. The virus used for the vaccine at any given time is similar to the one that the World Health Organization and the U.S. Public Health Service believe is likely to appear during the upcoming flu season, since the strains of influenza change from season to season and year to year.

▼ DOSAGE GUIDELINES

RANGE AND FREQUENCY
Adults and children age 9 and older: 1 injection into the upper arm annually, usually in early November. Children ages 6 months to 9 years: 1 or 2 injections into the thigh annually, usually in early November.

ONSET OF EFFECT
Most patients develop immunity within 2 to 4 weeks.

DURATION OF ACTION
Unknown. The antibodies may be available for protection against a particular strain of flu for many years following the injection, but the antibodies will only protect against a flu virus that is identical or very similar to the one that was used in the vaccine. A different strain of the flu may not be affected by the antibodies, leading to infection.

DIETARY ADVICE
No special restrictions.

STORAGE
Not applicable; the dose is administered only at a health care facility.

MISSED DOSE
Not applicable.

STOPPING THE DRUG
Not applicable.

PROLONGED USE
Not applicable.

▼ PRECAUTIONS

Over 60: Influenza vaccine is not expected to cause different or more severe side effects in older patients than it does in younger persons. However, older adults may not develop as strong an immunity as younger persons.

Driving and Hazardous Work: The vaccine should not impair your ability to perform such tasks safely.

Alcohol: No special precautions are necessary.

Pregnancy: The vaccine has not been shown to cause problems in pregnant women. Consult your doctor for more information.

Breast Feeding: The vaccine has not been shown to cause any problems in nursing babies. Consult your doctor for advice.

Infants and Children: Not recommended for use by children under the age of 6 months. Only the "split-virus" vaccine should be administered to children under the age of 13.

Special Concerns: If you want to decrease your chances of coming down with the flu, discuss appropriate health care measures with your doctor. Remember that the vaccine is not effective against all strains of the flu. The ability of the vaccine to stimulate your immune system is affected by your age, by the presence of other diseases, and by the use of other medications. Protection from flu infection during the flu season may be less in these circumstances. Make sure to tell your doctor if you or your child are ill on the day the injection is scheduled. Your doctor may decide to reschedule your vaccination.

OVERDOSE
Symptoms: An overdose with the influenza vaccine is unlikely.

What to Do: No cases of overdose have been reported.

▼ INTERACTIONS

DRUG INTERACTIONS
Other drugs may interact with influenza vaccine. Tell your doctor if you are taking any prescription or over-the-counter medication.

FOOD INTERACTIONS
No known food interactions.

DISEASE INTERACTIONS
Consult your doctor if you have any of the following: bronchitis, pneumonia, or other respiratory problems, seizures, allergies to eggs, or allergies to antibiotics, especially gentamicin.

≡ SIDE EFFECTS ≡

SERIOUS
Serious allergic reaction involving difficulty swallowing or breathing; reddened skin, especially around the ears; itching, particularly of the hands or feet; hives; unusual and severe fatigue; and swollen face, eyes, or nasal passages. Call your doctor immediately.

COMMON
Pain, redness, or hard lump at site of injection.

LESS COMMON
Fever, muscle aches, general feeling of illness.

INSULIN GLARGINE (RDNA ORIGIN)

Available in: Injection
Available OTC? No   **As Generic?** No
Drug Class: Antidiabetic agent

▼ USAGE INFORMATION

WHY IT'S PRESCRIBED
For long-term treatment of diabetes mellitus. All patients with type 1 diabetes require lifelong insulin treatment. Patients with type 2 diabetes may require insulin if they are unable to control their blood glucose (sugar) levels with diet and oral medications. Insulin glargine is a slightly modified form of human insulin that maintains a relatively constant glucose-lowering effect over a 24-hour period and thus permits dosing once a day.

HOW IT WORKS
Insulin, a hormone secreted by the beta cells of the pancreas, plays an essential role in controlling the metabolism and storage of carbohydrates, fat, and protein. Insulin is secreted in response to a rise in blood sugar (glucose). Insulin lowers blood glucose by increasing its uptake by body cells, especially muscle, and by reducing the release of glucose from the liver between meals.

▼ DOSAGE GUIDELINES

RANGE AND FREQUENCY
Injected under the skin (stomach, thigh, or upper arm) once a day at bedtime. Doses are determined by your doctor. The solution should be clear and colorless, without any visible particles. Insulin glargine must not be diluted or mixed with any other insulin or solution.

ONSET OF EFFECT
About 1 to 2 hours.

DURATION OF ACTION
At least 24 hours.

≣ SIDE EFFECTS ≣

SERIOUS
Symptoms of hypoglycemia can be caused by the release of adrenaline or by an inadequate supply of glucose to the brain. With severe hypoglycemia, lack of sufficient glucose to the brain may cause slurred speech, impaired concentration, confusion, seizures, coma, irreversible brain damage, and death. Mild hypoglycemia may cause restless sleep, nightmares, or a cold sweat that awakens patients at night.

COMMON
Symptoms resulting from release of adrenaline are common manifestations of mild to moderate hypoglycemia. They include cold sweats, anxiety, shakiness, hunger, rapid heartbeat, headache, and nervousness. Weight gain is common when taking insulin.

LESS COMMON
Allergic reactions, lipoatrophy (depressions in the skin due to loss of fat tissue), and lipohypertrophy (excessive accumulation of fat tissue).

DIETARY ADVICE
All patients with diabetes should follow the general dietary recommendations of the American Diabetes Association. Though intake of simple sugars is not forbidden, consuming a large amount of sugary foods at one time may trigger a rapid rise in blood glucose that can increase urination and thirst. In addition, patients who take insulin must remain consistent from day to day in the timing and caloric content of their meals. Depending on the timing, dose, and types of insulin prescribed, snacks may be recommended in the late afternoon, before bedtime, or prior to unusual physical activity. Diabetic patients must always have available a juice, food, or tablets that can raise blood glucose levels rapidly to counter an episode of hypoglycemia.

STORAGE
Refrigerate insulin but do not allow it to freeze. If refrigeration is not possible, the 10-milliliter (mL) vial or 3-mL cartridge in use can be kept unrefrigerated for up to 28 days away from direct heat and light, as long as the temperature is not greater than 86°F. Unrefrigerated 10-mL vials and 3-mL cartridges must be used within the 28-day period or they must be discarded. If refrigeration is not possible, the 5-mL vial in use can be kept unrefrigerated for up to 14 days away from direct heat and light, as long as the temperature is not greater than 86°F. Unrefrigerated 5-mL vials must be used within the 14-day period or they must be discarded. If refrigerated, the 5-mL vial in use can be kept for up to 28 days. Once the 3-mL cartridge is placed in an OptiPen One, it should not be put in the refrigerator.

MISSED DOSE
Timing of insulin doses is extremely important. The best approach is to measure blood glucose and add a dose of regular insulin if glucose levels are too high. Otherwise, wait for the next scheduled dose.

STOPPING THE DRUG
Do not stop taking insulin injections unless ordered by your doctor. Patients with diabetes are often given general instructions for modifying their insulin doses based on home blood glucose measurements.

PROLONGED USE
After many years with diabetes, some patients become insensitive to the symptoms of hypoglycemia and are at risk for serious brain complications of prolonged, unrecognized hypoglycemia.

▼ PRECAUTIONS

Over 60: No special warnings. Some older people may, however, have vision problems that may make it difficult to draw up the correct dose of insulin.

Driving and Hazardous Work: Patients taking insulin must be very careful to avoid hypoglycemia when driving or engaging in hazardous work.

Alcohol: Moderate alcohol intake, especially when taken with large meals, does not

(continued) **449**

adversely affect control of diabetes or alter the dose of insulin. However, large amounts of alcohol increase the risk of hypoglycemia.

Pregnancy: Strict metabolic control—using insulin injections in most women—must be maintained during pregnancy to reduce the risk of birth defects, fetal complications, or death at the time of delivery. In women who had diabetes before the onset of pregnancy, the dose of insulin is often smaller during the first third (trimester) of pregnancy and then higher during the final two trimesters. When women first develop diabetes during pregnancy (gestational diabetes), insulin requirements drop rapidly after delivery and most do not need to continue with insulin treatment.

Breast Feeding: Insulin requirements tend to be lower during breast feeding. Home glucose monitoring is important to avoid hypoglycemia. Insulin glargine may pass into breast milk; consult your doctor for advice.

Infants and Children: Treatment with insulin in young patients age 6 and older is the same as that in older people with diabetes. The safety and effectiveness of insulin glargine in children under the age of 6 have not been established.

Special Concerns: Inadequate amounts of insulin in type 1 diabetes may lead to the serious complication of diabetic ketoacidosis, characterized by loss of appetite, excessive thirst and urination, nausea, vomiting, deep breathing, fruity breath odor, drowsiness, confusion, and loss of consciousness. Insulin glargine is not the insulin of choice for treatment of diabetic ketoacidosis. An intravenous short-acting insulin is the preferred treatment.

OVERDOSE

Symptoms: Insulin overdose results in hypoglycemia (see Side Effects for symptoms).

What to Do: For mild to moderate hypoglycemia, ingest drinks or food containing sugar. For more severe hypoglycemia, administer injections of glucagon or call emergency medical services (EMS) immediately.

▼ INTERACTIONS

DRUG INTERACTIONS
A large number of drugs can promote either elevated blood glucose levels or hypoglycemia. Be sure that your doctor knows about all of the medications you take and is informed before you start taking any new drugs, either by prescription or over the counter. Corticosteroids in particular are likely to raise blood glucose levels and insulin requirements. Beta-blockers (commonly pre-scribed for hypertension) may cause either high blood glucose levels or hypoglycemia; in addition, because these medications may dampen the symptoms of hypoglycemia that are caused by adrenaline release, mild degrees of hypoglycemia may progress unnoticed to more serious hypoglycemia affecting the brain.

FOOD INTERACTIONS
Insulin requirements are increased by the ingestion of large amounts of calories, especially simple sugars and other carbohydrates.

DISEASE INTERACTIONS
Insulin requirements are increased by infections, psychological stress, or an uncontrolled overactive thyroid, and often at a time of surgery. Requirements may diminish with kidney disease or an underactive adrenal or pituitary gland.

INSULIN (INTERMEDIATE-ACTING, NPH, LENTE)

Available in: Injection
Available OTC? Yes **As Generic?** No
Drug Class: Antidiabetic agent

▼ USAGE INFORMATION

WHY IT'S PRESCRIBED
For long-term treatment of diabetes mellitus. All patients with type 1 diabetes require lifelong insulin treatment. Patients with type 2 diabetes may require insulin if they are unable to control their blood glucose (sugar) levels with diet and oral medications.

HOW IT WORKS
Insulin, a hormone secreted by the beta cells of the pancreas, plays an essential role in controlling the metabolism and storage of carbohydrates, fat, and protein. Insulin is secreted in response to a rise in blood sugar (glucose). Insulin lowers blood glucose by increasing its uptake by body cells, especially muscle, and by reducing the release of glucose from the liver between meals.

▼ DOSAGE GUIDELINES

RANGE AND FREQUENCY
Injected 1 or 2 times a day. Doses and frequency are determined by your doctor. Intermediate-acting (NPH or Lente) insulin can be mixed in the same syringe with rapid-acting insulin; draw up the rapid-acting insulin first. Intermediate-acting insulin solutions are cloudy (insulin settles to the bottom of the bottle) and must be rolled or gently shaken to distribute the insulin evenly in the solution before drawing it up into the syringe.

ONSET OF EFFECT
Within 1 hour; peak effect occurs within 8 to 12 hours.

DURATION OF ACTION
From 12 to 18 hours.

DIETARY ADVICE
All patients with diabetes should follow the general dietary recommendations of the American Diabetes Association. Though intake of simple sugars is not forbidden, consuming a large amount of sugary foods at one time may trigger a rapid rise in blood glucose that can increase urination and thirst. In addition, patients who take insulin must remain consistent from day to day in the timing and caloric content of their meals. Depending on the timing, dose, and types of insulin prescribed, snacks may be recommended in the late afternoon, before bedtime, or prior to unusual physical activity. Diabetic patients must always have available a juice, food, or tablets that can raise blood glucose levels rapidly to counter an episode of hypoglycemia.

STORAGE
Refrigerate insulin but do not allow it to freeze. Insulin does not have to be kept refrigerated when you're traveling for short periods, but exposure to high temperatures must be avoided.

MISSED DOSE
Timing of insulin doses is extremely important. The best approach is to measure blood glucose and add a dose of regular insulin if your glucose levels are too high. Otherwise, wait for the next scheduled dose.

STOPPING THE DRUG
Do not stop taking insulin injections unless ordered by your doctor. Patients with diabetes are often given general instructions for modifying

their insulin doses based on home blood glucose measurements.

PROLONGED USE
After many years with diabetes, some patients become insensitive to the symptoms of hypoglycemia and are at risk for serious brain complications of prolonged, unrecognized hypoglycemia.

▼ PRECAUTIONS

Over 60: No special warnings. Some older people may, however, have vision problems that may make it difficult to draw up the correct dose of insulin.

Driving and Hazardous Work: Patients taking insulin must be very careful to avoid hypoglycemia when driving or engaging in hazardous work.

Alcohol: Moderate alcohol intake, especially when taken with large meals, does not adversely affect control of diabetes or alter the dose of insulin. However, large amounts of alcohol increase the risk of hypoglycemia.

Pregnancy: Strict metabolic control—using insulin injections in most women—must

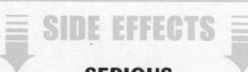

SIDE EFFECTS

SERIOUS
Symptoms of hypoglycemia can be caused by the release of adrenaline or by an inadequate supply of glucose to the brain. With severe hypoglycemia, lack of sufficient glucose to the brain may cause slurred speech, impaired concentration, confusion, seizures, coma, irreversible brain damage, and death. Mild hypoglycemia may cause restless sleep, nightmares, or a cold sweat that awakens patients at night.

COMMON
Symptoms resulting from the release of adrenaline are common with mild to moderate hypoglycemia. They include cold sweats, anxiety, shakiness, hunger, rapid heartbeat, and headache. Weight gain is also common when taking insulin.

LESS COMMON
Allergic reactions, lipoatrophy (depressions in the skin due to loss of fat tissue), and lipohypertrophy (excessive accumulation of fat tissue).

be maintained during pregnancy to reduce the risk of birth defects, fetal complications, or death at the time of delivery. In women who had diabetes before the onset of pregnancy, the dose of insulin is often smaller during the first third (trimester) of pregnancy and then higher during the final two trimesters. When women first develop diabetes during pregnancy (gestational diabetes), insulin requirements drop rapidly after delivery and most do not need to continue with insulin treatment.

Breast Feeding: Insulin requirements tend to be lower during breast feeding. Home glucose monitoring is important to avoid hypoglycemia. Insulin is not present in breast milk.

Infants and Children: Treatment with insulin in children is the same as in older people with diabetes.

Special Concerns: Inadequate amounts of insulin in type 1 diabetes may lead to the serious complication of diabetic ketoacidosis, characterized by loss of appetite, excessive thirst and urination, nausea, vomiting, deep breathing, fruity breath odor, drowsiness, confusion, and loss of consciousness.

OVERDOSE

Symptoms: Insulin overdose results in hypoglycemia (see Side Effects for symptoms).

What to Do: For mild to moderate hypoglycemia, ingest drinks or food containing sugar. For more severe hypoglycemia, administer injections of glucagon or call emergency medical services (EMS) immediately.

▼ INTERACTIONS

DRUG INTERACTIONS

A large number of drugs can promote either elevated blood glucose levels or hypoglycemia. Be sure that your doctor knows about all of the medications you take and is informed before you start taking any new drugs, either by prescription or over the counter. Corticosteroids in particular are likely to raise blood glucose levels and insulin requirements. Betablockers (commonly prescribed for hypertension) may cause either high blood glucose levels or hypoglycemia; in addition, because these medications may dampen the symptoms of hypoglycemia that are caused by adrenaline release, mild degrees of hypoglycemia may progress unnoticed to more serious hypoglycemia affecting the brain.

FOOD INTERACTIONS

Insulin requirements are increased when larger amounts of calories are ingested, especially simple sugars and carbohydrates.

DISEASE INTERACTIONS

Insulin requirements are increased by infections, psychological stress, or an uncontrolled overactive thyroid, and often at a time of surgery. Requirements may diminish with kidney disease or an underactive adrenal or pituitary gland.

INSULIN (LISPRO RDNA ORIGIN)

Available in: Injection
Available OTC? Yes   **As Generic?** No
Drug Class: Antidiabetic agent

▼ USAGE INFORMATION

WHY IT'S PRESCRIBED
For long-term treatment of
diabetes mellitus. All patients
with type 1 diabetes require
lifelong insulin treatment.
Patients with type 2 diabetes
may require insulin if they are
unable to control their blood
glucose (sugar) levels with
diet and oral medications.

HOW IT WORKS
Insulin, a hormone secreted
by the beta cells of the pancreas, plays an essential role
in controlling the metabolism
and storage of carbohydrates,
fat, and protein. Insulin is
secreted in response to a rise
in blood sugar (glucose).
Insulin lowers blood glucose
by increasing its uptake by
body cells, especially muscle,
and by reducing the release
of glucose from the liver
between meals.

▼ DOSAGE GUIDELINES

RANGE AND FREQUENCY
It may be taken 1 to 4 times
daily, before meals and possibly at bedtime. Doses and
frequency are determined by
your doctor. Rapid-acting
(lispro rDNA origin) insulin
should be administered 15
minutes before a meal.

ONSET OF EFFECT
Within 30 to 45 minutes; the
peak effect occurs within 1
hour.

DURATION OF ACTION
From 3 to 4 hours.

DIETARY ADVICE
All patients with diabetes
should follow the general
dietary recommendations of
the American Diabetes Association. Though intake of simple sugars is not forbidden,
consuming a large amount of

sugary foods at one time may
trigger a rapid rise in blood
glucose that can increase urination and thirst. In addition,
patients who take insulin must
remain consistent from day to
day in the timing and caloric
content of their meals.
Depending on the timing,
dose, and types of insulin
prescribed, snacks may be
recommended in the late
afternoon, before bedtime,
or prior to unusual physical
activity. Diabetic patients must
always have available a juice,
food, or tablets that can raise
blood glucose levels rapidly
to counter an episode of
hypoglycemia.

STORAGE
Refrigerate insulin but do not
allow it to freeze. Insulin does
not have to be kept refrigerated when you're traveling for
short periods, but exposure
to high temperatures must be
avoided.

MISSED DOSE
Timing of insulin doses is
extremely important. The best
approach is to measure blood
glucose and add a dose of
regular insulin if your glucose
levels are too high. Otherwise, wait for the next scheduled dose.

STOPPING THE DRUG
Do not stop taking insulin
injections unless ordered by
your doctor. Patients with diabetes are often given general
instructions for modifying
their insulin doses based on
home blood glucose mea-
surements.

PROLONGED USE
After many years with diabetes, some patients become
insensitive to the symptoms

of hypoglycemia and are at
risk for serious brain complications of prolonged, unrecognized hypoglycemia.

▼ PRECAUTIONS

Over 60: No special warnings. Some older people may,
however, have vision problems that may make it difficult
to draw up the correct dose
of insulin.

**Driving and Hazardous
Work:** Patients taking insulin
must be extremely careful to
avoid hypoglycemia when
driving or engaging in hazardous work.

Alcohol: Moderate alcohol
intake, especially when taken
with large meals, does not
adversely affect control of
diabetes or alter the dose of
insulin. However, large
amounts of alcohol increase
the risk of hypoglycemia.

Pregnancy: Strict metabolic
control—using insulin injections in most women—must
be maintained during pregnancy to reduce the risk of
birth defects, fetal complications, or death at the time
of delivery. In women who
had diabetes before the
onset of pregnancy, the
dose of insulin is often
smaller during the first third
(trimester) of pregnancy
and then higher during the
final two trimesters. When
women first develop diabetes during pregnancy (gestational diabetes), insulin
requirements drop rapidly
after delivery and most do
not need to continue with
insulin treatment.

SIDE EFFECTS

SERIOUS
Symptoms of hypoglycemia can be caused by the release
of adrenaline or by an inadequate supply of glucose to the
brain. With severe hypoglycemia, lack of sufficient glucose
to the brain may cause slurred speech, impaired concentration, confusion, seizures, coma, irreversible brain damage, and death. Mild hypoglycemia may cause restless
sleep, nightmares, or a cold sweat that awakens patients at
night.

COMMON
Symptoms resulting from release of adrenaline are common manifestations of mild to moderate hypoglycemia.
They include cold sweats, anxiety, shakiness, hunger, rapid
heartbeat, headache, and nervousness. Weight gain is
common when taking insulin.

LESS COMMON
Allergic reactions, lipoatrophy (depressions in the skin due
to loss of fat tissue), and lipohypertrophy (excessive accumulation of fat tissue).

Breast Feeding: Insulin requirements tend to be lower during breast feeding. Home glucose monitoring is important to avoid hypoglycemia. Insulin is not present in breast milk.

Infants and Children: Treatment with insulin in young patients is the same as that in older people with diabetes.

Special Concerns: Inadequate amounts of insulin in type 1 diabetes may lead to the serious complication of diabetic ketoacidosis, characterized by loss of appetite, excessive thirst and urination, nausea, vomiting, deep breathing, fruity breath odor, drowsiness, confusion, and loss of consciousness.

OVERDOSE

Symptoms: Insulin overdose results in hypoglycemia (see Side Effects for symptoms).

What to Do: For mild to moderate hypoglycemia, ingest drinks or food containing sugar. For more severe hypoglycemia, administer injections of glucagon or call emergency medical services (EMS) immediately.

▼ INTERACTIONS

DRUG INTERACTIONS

A large number of drugs can promote either elevated blood glucose levels or hypoglycemia. Be sure that your doctor knows about all of the medications you take and is informed before you start taking any new drugs, either by prescription or over the counter. Corticosteroids in particular are likely to raise blood glucose levels and insulin requirements. Beta-blockers (commonly prescribed for hypertension) may cause either high blood glucose levels or hypoglycemia; in addition, because these medications may dampen the symptoms of hypoglycemia that are caused by adrenaline release, mild degrees of hypoglycemia may progress unnoticed to more serious hypoglycemia affecting the brain.

FOOD INTERACTIONS

Insulin requirements are increased when larger amounts of calories are ingested, especially simple sugars and carbohydrates.

DISEASE INTERACTIONS

Insulin requirements are increased by infections, psychological stress, or an uncontrolled overactive thyroid, and often at a time of surgery. Requirements may diminish with kidney disease or an underactive adrenal or pituitary gland.

INSULIN (LONG-ACTING, ULTRALENTE)

Available in: Injection
Available OTC? Yes   **As Generic?** No
Drug Class: Antidiabetic agent

▼ USAGE INFORMATION

WHY IT'S PRESCRIBED
For long-term treatment of diabetes mellitus. All patients with type 1 diabetes require lifelong insulin treatment. Patients with type 2 diabetes may require insulin if they are unable to control their blood glucose (sugar) levels with diet and oral medications.

HOW IT WORKS
Insulin, a hormone secreted by the beta cells of the pancreas, plays an essential role in controlling the metabolism and storage of carbohydrates, fat, and protein. Insulin is secreted in response to a rise in blood sugar (glucose). Insulin lowers blood glucose by increasing its uptake by body cells, especially muscle, and by reducing the release of glucose from the liver between meals.

▼ DOSAGE GUIDELINES

RANGE AND FREQUENCY
Injected 1 or 2 times a day. Doses and frequency are determined by your doctor. Long-acting (Ultralente) insulin can be mixed in the same syringe with rapid-acting insulin; draw up the rapid-acting insulin first. Long-acting insulin solutions are cloudy (insulin settles to the bottom of the bottle) and must be rolled or gently shaken to distribute the insulin evenly in the solution before drawing it up into the syringe.

ONSET OF EFFECT
Within 6 to 8 hours; the peak effect occurs within 10 to 20 hours.

DURATION OF ACTION
From 24 to 36 hours.

SIDE EFFECTS

SERIOUS
Symptoms of hypoglycemia can be caused by the release of adrenaline or by an inadequate supply of glucose to the brain. With severe hypoglycemia, lack of sufficient glucose to the brain may cause slurred speech, impaired concentration, confusion, seizures, coma, irreversible brain damage, and death. Mild hypoglycemia may cause restless sleep, nightmares, or a cold sweat that awakens patients at night.

COMMON
Symptoms resulting from release of adrenaline are common manifestations of mild to moderate hypoglycemia. They include cold sweats, anxiety, shakiness, hunger, rapid heartbeat, headache, and nervousness. Weight gain is common when taking insulin.

LESS COMMON
Allergic reactions, lipoatrophy (depressions in the skin due to loss of fat tissue), and lipohypertrophy (excessive accumulation of fat tissue).

DIETARY ADVICE
All patients with diabetes should follow the general dietary recommendations of the American Diabetes Association. Though intake of simple sugars is not forbidden, consuming a large amount of sugary foods at one time may trigger a rapid rise in blood glucose that can increase urination and thirst. In addition, patients who take insulin must remain consistent from day to day in the timing and caloric content of their meals. Depending on the timing, dose, and types of insulin prescribed, snacks may be recommended in the late afternoon, before bedtime, or prior to unusual physical activity. Diabetic patients must always have available a juice, food, or tablets that can raise blood glucose levels rapidly to counter an episode of hypoglycemia.

STORAGE
Refrigerate insulin but do not allow it to freeze. Insulin does not have to be kept refrigerated when you're traveling for short periods, but exposure to high temperatures must be avoided.

MISSED DOSE
Timing of insulin doses is extremely important. The best approach is to measure blood glucose and add a dose of regular insulin if your glucose levels are too high. Otherwise, wait for the next scheduled dose.

STOPPING THE DRUG
Do not stop taking insulin injections unless ordered by your doctor. Patients with diabetes are often given general instructions for modifying their insulin doses based on home blood glucose measurements.

PROLONGED USE
After many years with diabetes, some patients become insensitive to the symptoms of hypoglycemia and are at risk for serious brain complications of prolonged, unrecognized hypoglycemia.

▼ PRECAUTIONS

Over 60: No special warnings. Some older people may, however, have vision problems that may make it difficult to draw up the correct dose of insulin.

Driving and Hazardous Work: Patients taking insulin must be very careful to avoid hypoglycemia when driving or engaging in hazardous work.

Alcohol: Moderate alcohol intake, especially when taken with large meals, does not adversely affect control of diabetes or alter the dose of insulin. However, large amounts of alcohol increase the risk of hypoglycemia.

Pregnancy: Strict metabolic control—using insulin injections in most women—must be maintained during pregnancy to reduce the risk of birth defects, fetal complications, or death at the time of delivery. In women who had diabetes before the onset of pregnancy, the dose of insulin is often smaller during the first third (trimester) of pregnancy and then higher during the final two trimesters. When women first develop diabetes during pregnancy

(continued)   **455**

(gestational diabetes), insulin requirements drop rapidly after delivery and most do not need to continue with insulin treatment.

Breast Feeding: Insulin requirements tend to be lower during breast feeding. Home glucose monitoring is important to avoid hypoglycemia. Insulin is not present in breast milk.

Infants and Children: Treatment with insulin in young patients is the same as that in older people with diabetes.

Special Concerns: Inadequate amounts of insulin in type 1 diabetes may lead to the serious complication of diabetic ketoacidosis, characterized by loss of appetite, excessive thirst and urination, nausea, vomiting, deep breathing, fruity breath odor, drowsiness, confusion, and loss of consciousness.

OVERDOSE

Symptoms: Insulin overdose results in hypoglycemia (see Side Effects for symptoms).

What to Do: For mild to moderate hypoglycemia, ingest drinks or food containing sugar. For more severe hypoglycemia, administer injections of glucagon or call emergency medical services (EMS) immediately.

▼ INTERACTIONS

DRUG INTERACTIONS

A large number of drugs can promote either elevated blood glucose levels or hypoglycemia. Be sure that your doctor knows about all of the medications you take and is informed before you start taking any new drugs, either by prescription or over the counter. Corticosteroids in particular are likely to raise blood glucose levels and insulin requirements. Beta-blockers (commonly prescribed for hypertension) may cause either high blood glucose levels or hypoglycemia; in addition, because these medications may dampen the symptoms of hypoglycemia that are caused by adrenaline release, mild degrees of hypoglycemia may progress unnoticed to more serious hypoglycemia affecting the brain.

FOOD INTERACTIONS

Insulin requirements are increased when larger amounts of calories are ingested, especially simple sugars and carbohydrates.

DISEASE INTERACTIONS

Insulin requirements are increased by infections, psychological stress, or an uncontrolled overactive thyroid, and often at a time of surgery. Requirements may diminish with kidney disease or an underactive adrenal or pituitary gland.

INSULIN (REGULAR, RAPID-ACTING, OR SEMILENTE)

Available in: Injection
Available OTC? Yes **As Generic?** No
Drug Class: Antidiabetic agent

▼ USAGE INFORMATION

WHY IT'S PRESCRIBED
For long-term treatment of diabetes mellitus. All patients with type 1 diabetes require lifelong insulin treatment. Patients with type 2 diabetes may require insulin if they are unable to control their blood glucose (sugar) levels with diet and oral medications.

HOW IT WORKS
Insulin, a hormone secreted by the beta cells of the pancreas, plays an essential role in controlling the metabolism and storage of carbohydrates, fat, and protein. Insulin is secreted in response to a rise in blood sugar (glucose). Insulin lowers blood glucose by increasing its uptake by body cells, especially muscle, and by reducing the release of glucose from the liver between meals.

▼ DOSAGE GUIDELINES

RANGE AND FREQUENCY
It may be taken 1 to 4 times daily, before meals and possibly at bedtime. Doses and frequency are determined by your doctor. Regular (or rapid-acting or semilente) insulin should be administered 30 to 45 minutes before a meal. It can be mixed in the same syringe with intermediate-acting insulins. Draw up the regular insulin first.

ONSET OF EFFECT
Within 45 minutes; peak effect occurs within 2 to 4 hours.

DURATION OF ACTION
From 4 to 6 hours.

DIETARY ADVICE
All patients with diabetes should follow the general dietary recommendations of the American Diabetes Association. Though intake of simple sugars is not forbidden, consuming a large amount of sugary foods at one time may trigger a rapid rise in blood glucose that can increase urination and thirst. In addition, patients who take insulin must remain consistent from day to day in the timing and caloric content of their meals. Depending on the timing, dose, and types of insulin prescribed, snacks may be recommended in the late afternoon, before bedtime, or prior to unusual physical activity. Diabetic patients must always have available a juice, food, or tablets that can raise blood glucose levels rapidly to counter an episode of hypoglycemia.

STORAGE
Refrigerate insulin but do not allow it to freeze. Insulin does not have to be kept refrigerated when you're traveling for short periods, but exposure to high temperatures must be avoided.

MISSED DOSE
Timing of insulin doses is extremely important. The best approach is to measure blood glucose and add a dose of regular insulin if glucose levels are too high. Otherwise, wait for the next scheduled dose.

STOPPING THE DRUG
Do not stop taking insulin injections unless ordered by your doctor. Patients with diabetes are often given general instructions for modifying their insulin doses based on home blood glucose measurements.

PROLONGED USE
After many years with diabetes, some patients become insensitive to the symptoms of hypoglycemia and are at risk for serious brain complications of prolonged, unrecognized hypoglycemia.

▼ PRECAUTIONS

Over 60: No special warnings. Some older people may, however, have vision problems that may make it difficult to draw up the correct dose of insulin.

Driving and Hazardous Work: Patients taking insulin must be very careful to avoid hypoglycemia when driving or engaging in hazardous work.

Alcohol: Moderate alcohol intake, especially when taken with large meals, does not adversely affect control of diabetes or alter the dose of insulin. However, large amounts of alcohol increase the risk of hypoglycemia.

Pregnancy: Strict metabolic control—using insulin injections in most women—must be maintained during pregnancy to reduce the risk of birth defects, fetal complications, or death at the time of delivery. In women who had diabetes before the onset of

▤ SIDE EFFECTS ▤

SERIOUS
Symptoms of hypoglycemia can be caused by the release of adrenaline or by an inadequate supply of glucose to the brain. With severe hypoglycemia, lack of sufficient glucose to the brain may cause slurred speech, impaired concentration, confusion, seizures, coma, irreversible brain damage, and death. Mild hypoglycemia may cause restless sleep, nightmares, or a cold sweat that awakens patients at night.

COMMON
Symptoms resulting from release of adrenaline are common manifestations of mild to moderate hypoglycemia. They include cold sweats, anxiety, shakiness, hunger, rapid heartbeat, headache, and nervousness. Weight gain is common when taking insulin.

LESS COMMON
Allergic reactions, lipoatrophy (depressions in the skin due to loss of fat tissue), and lipohypertrophy (excessive accumulation of fat tissue).

(continued) 457

INSULIN (REGULAR, RAPID-ACTING, OR SEMILENTE) (continued)

pregnancy, the dose of insulin is often smaller during the first third (trimester) of pregnancy and then higher during the final two trimesters. When women first develop diabetes during pregnancy (gestational diabetes), insulin requirements drop rapidly after delivery and most do not need to continue with insulin treatment.

Breast Feeding: Insulin requirements tend to be lower during breast feeding. Home glucose monitoring is important to avoid hypoglycemia. Insulin is not present in breast milk.

Infants and Children: Treatment with insulin in young patients is the same as that in older people with diabetes.

Special Concerns: Inadequate amounts of insulin in type 1 diabetes may lead to the serious complication of diabetic ketoacidosis, characterized by loss of appetite, excessive thirst and urination, nausea, vomiting, deep breathing, fruity breath odor, drowsiness, confusion, and loss of consciousness.

OVERDOSE
Symptoms: Insulin overdose results in hypoglycemia (see Side Effects for symptoms).

What to Do: For mild to moderate hypoglycemia, ingest drinks or food containing sugar. For more severe hypoglycemia, administer injections of glucagon or call emergency medical services (EMS) immediately.

▼ INTERACTIONS

DRUG INTERACTIONS
A large number of drugs can promote either elevated blood glucose levels or hypoglycemia. Be sure that your doctor knows about all of the medications you take and is informed before you start taking any new drugs, either by prescription or over the counter. Corticosteroids in particular are likely to raise blood glucose levels and insulin requirements. Beta-blockers (commonly prescribed for hypertension) may cause either high blood glucose levels or hypoglycemia; in addition, because these medications may dampen the symptoms of hypoglycemia that are caused by adrenaline release, mild degrees of hypoglycemia may progress unnoticed to more serious hypoglycemia affecting the brain.

FOOD INTERACTIONS
Insulin requirements are increased when larger amounts of calories are ingested, especially simple sugars and carbohydrates.

DISEASE INTERACTIONS
Insulin requirements are increased by infections, psychological stress, or an uncontrolled overactive thyroid, and often at a time of surgery. Requirements may diminish with kidney disease or an underactive adrenal or pituitary gland.

INTERFERON ALFA-2A

Available in: Injection
Available OTC? No   **As Generic?** No
Drug Class: Immunomodulator

▼ USAGE INFORMATION

WHY IT'S PRESCRIBED
To treat hairy-cell leukemia, AIDS-associated Kaposi's sarcoma, or chronic myelogenous leukemia.

HOW IT WORKS
Interferon alfa-2a acts in the same way as the body's natural interferons, which are proteins released by cells of the immune system to fight viruses and cancer cells.

▼ DOSAGE GUIDELINES

RANGE AND FREQUENCY
For hairy-cell leukemia: 3 million units daily by injection for 16 to 24 weeks. Then 3 million units 3 times a week for maintenance. For AIDS-related Kaposi's sarcoma: 36 million units daily for 10 to 12 weeks, then 36 million units 3 times a week. For Philadelphia chromosome-positive (Ph+) chronic myelogenous leukemia: 9 million units daily for the duration of treatment or as determined by your doctor.

ONSET OF EFFECT
Unknown.

DURATION OF ACTION
Unknown.

DIETARY ADVICE
Drink plenty of fluids to reduce the risk of excessively low blood pressure.

STORAGE
Keep interferon alfa-2a refrigerated but do not allow it to freeze.

MISSED DOSE
If you miss a dose, do not take the missed dose and do not double the next dose. Check with your doctor on what to do.

STOPPING THE DRUG
The decision to stop taking the drug should be made by your doctor.

PROLONGED USE
See your doctor regularly for tests and examinations if you must take this drug for a prolonged period.

▼ PRECAUTIONS

Over 60: Adverse reactions may be more likely and more severe in older patients.

Driving and Hazardous Work: Avoid such activities until you determine how the medicine affects you. Administering interferon at bedtime may help to minimize daytime sleepiness.

Alcohol: Avoid alcohol.

Pregnancy: Adequate studies have not been done. Consult your doctor for advice.

Breast Feeding: Interferon alfa-2a may pass into breast milk; caution is advised. Consult your doctor for advice.

Infants and Children: Severe adverse effects have been noted in some children treated with high doses of interferon. Consult your pediatrician for advice.

Special Concerns: Do not change to another brand of alfa interferon without consulting your doctor. They have different dosage schedules. Try to avoid people with infections, because this drug can lower white blood cell levels temporarily and increase susceptibility to disease. Be careful when cleaning your teeth, and avoid cutting yourself when using sharp objects such as a razor. Avoid contact sports or other situations where bruising could occur.

OVERDOSE
Symptoms: No specific ones have been reported.

What to Do: Call your doctor or emergency medical services (EMS) immediately if you suspect an overdose.

▼ INTERACTIONS

DRUG INTERACTIONS
Consult your doctor for specific advice if you are taking any prescription or over-the-counter medication, especially theophylline, or central nervous system depressants including antihistamines, alcohol, tranquilizers, or psychiatric medications.

FOOD INTERACTIONS
None are known.

DISEASE INTERACTIONS
Consult your doctor if you have a history of bleeding or clotting disorders, chickenpox, shingles, psychological or neurological disorders, seizures, diabetes, heart attack, heart disease, kidney disease, liver disease, lung disease, autoimmune disorders, or thyroid disease.

SIDE EFFECTS

SERIOUS
Confusion, depression, nervousness, distractibility, impaired thinking, or thoughts of suicide; numbness or tingling of fingers, toes, and face; black, tarry, or bloody stools; blood in urine; chest pain; hoarseness; fever or chills after 3 weeks of treatment; irregular heartbeat; pain in lower back or side; difficult or painful urination; red spots on skin; unusual bleeding or bruising; increased incidence of infections. Call your doctor immediately.

COMMON
Flulike symptoms, fatigue, muscle aches, fever, or chills in first weeks of treatment; general discomfort or ill feeling; headache; loss of appetite; nausea and vomiting; odd, metallic, or altered taste; skin rash; temporary hair loss. Side effects are more common with higher doses. Tolerance to high doses may be improved by gradually increasing the doses over the first weeks of treatment.

LESS COMMON
Back pain, blurred vision, dizziness, dry mouth, dry or itching skin, profuse or unusual sweating, joint pain, leg cramps, lip or mouth sores, weight loss.

INTERFERON ALFA-2B

Available in: Injection
Available OTC? No **As Generic?** No
Drug Class: Immunomodulator

▼ USAGE INFORMATION

WHY IT'S PRESCRIBED
To treat hairy-cell leukemia, AIDS-associated Kaposi's sarcoma, condylomata acuminata (genital warts), and types of chronic hepatitis; also used as an adjuvant (supplemental) treatment to surgery for malignant melanoma.

HOW IT WORKS
It acts in the same way as the body's natural interferons, which are proteins released by the cells of the immune system to fight viruses and cancer cells.

▼ DOSAGE GUIDELINES

RANGE AND FREQUENCY
For hairy-cell leukemia: 2 million units per square meter of body surface 3 times a week. For AIDS-related Kaposi's sarcoma: 30 million units 3 times a week. For condylomata acuminata: 1 million units per lesion 3 times a week for 3 weeks. For chronic hepatitis: 3 million units 3 times a week for 6 months (in patients with evidence of response). For malignant melanoma: 20 million units per square meter of body surface for 5 consecutive days per week for 4 weeks, followed by maintenance with 10 million units per square meter 3 times a week for 48 weeks.

ONSET OF EFFECT
Unknown.

DURATION OF ACTION
Unknown.

SIDE EFFECTS

SERIOUS
Confusion, depression, nervousness, distractibility, or impaired thinking; numbness or tingling of fingers, toes, and face; sleeping difficulty; black, tarry, or bloody stools; blood in urine; chest pain, cough, or hoarseness; fever or chills after 3 weeks of treatment; irregular heartbeat; pain in lower back or side; difficult or painful urination; red spots on skin; unusual bleeding or bruising; increased incidence of infections. Call your doctor immediately.

COMMON
Flulike symptoms, fatigue, muscle aches, fever, or chills in first weeks of treatment; general discomfort or ill feeling; headache; loss of appetite; nausea and vomiting; odd, metallic, or altered taste; skin rash; temporary hair loss. Side effects are more common with higher doses. Tolerance to high doses may be improved by gradually increasing the doses over the first weeks of treatment.

LESS COMMON
Back pain, blurred vision, dizziness, dry mouth, dry or itching skin, profuse or unusual sweating, joint pain, leg cramps, lip or mouth sores, weight loss.

DIETARY ADVICE
Drink plenty of fluids to reduce the risk of excessively low blood pressure.

STORAGE
Keep interferon alfa-2b refrigerated but do not allow it to freeze.

MISSED DOSE
If you miss a dose, do not take the missed dose and do not double the next dose. Check with your doctor on what to do.

STOPPING THE DRUG
The decision to stop taking the drug should be made by your doctor.

PROLONGED USE
See your doctor regularly for tests and examinations if you must take this drug for a prolonged period.

▼ PRECAUTIONS

Over 60: Adverse reactions may be more likely and more severe in older patients.

Driving and Hazardous Work: Do not drive or engage in hazardous work until you determine how the medicine affects you. Administering interferon at bedtime may help to minimize daytime sleepiness.

Alcohol: Avoid alcohol.

Pregnancy: Adequate studies have not been done. Consult your doctor for advice.

Breast Feeding: This drug may pass into breast milk; caution is advised. Consult your doctor for advice.

Infants and Children: May be used to treat chronic hepatitis B in children aged 1 and older; consult a pediatrician.

Special Concerns: Do not change to another brand without consulting your doctor. They have different dosage schedules. Try to avoid people with infections, because this drug can lower white blood cell levels temporarily and increase susceptibility to disease. Be careful when cleaning your teeth, and avoid cutting yourself when using sharp objects such as a razor. Avoid contact sports or other situations where bruising could occur.

OVERDOSE
Symptoms: No specific ones.

What to Do: Call your doctor or emergency medical services (EMS) immediately if you suspect an overdose.

▼ INTERACTIONS

DRUG INTERACTIONS
Consult your doctor for specific advice if you are taking any medication, especially central nervous system depressants including antihistamines, alcohol, tranquilizers, or psychiatric medications.

FOOD INTERACTIONS
None are known.

DISEASE INTERACTIONS
Consult your doctor if you have a history of bleeding or clotting disorders, chickenpox, shingles, psychological or neurological disorders, diabetes, autoimmune disorders, or heart, kidney, liver, lung, or thyroid disease.

INTERFERON ALFA-N1

Available in: Injection
Available OTC? No   **As Generic?** No
Drug Class: Immunomodulator

▼ USAGE INFORMATION

WHY IT'S PRESCRIBED
To treat hairy-cell leukemia, condylomata acuminata (genital warts), or juvenile laryngeal papillomatosis (abnormal growths in the voice box, occurring in children).

HOW IT WORKS
It acts in the same way as the body's natural interferons, which are proteins released by the cells of the immune system to fight viruses and cancer cells.

▼ DOSAGE GUIDELINES

RANGE AND FREQUENCY
For hairy-cell leukemia: 3 million units a day by injection for 16 to 24 weeks, then 3 million units 3 times a week.

For condylomata acuminata: 1 million units per square meter of body surface 5 times a week, then the same dose 5 times a week for 2 weeks, then 3 times a week for 4 weeks, then 3 times a week for 1 month. For juvenile laryngeal papillomatosis: The dose is based on area of body surface and is given daily for 26 days, followed by maintenance dosage 3 times a week for at least 6 months.

ONSET OF EFFECT
Unknown.

DURATION OF ACTION
Unknown.

DIETARY ADVICE
Drink plenty of fluids to reduce the risk of excessively low blood pressure.

▼ SIDE EFFECTS

SERIOUS
Confusion, depression, nervousness, distractibility, impaired thinking, or thoughts of suicide; numbness or tingling of fingers, toes, and face; black, tarry, or bloody stools; blood in urine; chest pain; hoarseness; fever or chills after 3 weeks of treatment; irregular heartbeat; pain in lower back or side; difficult or painful urination; red spots on skin; unusual bleeding or bruising; increased incidence of infections. Call your doctor immediately.

COMMON
Flulike symptoms, fatigue, muscle aches, fever, or chills in first weeks of treatment; general discomfort or ill feeling; headache; loss of appetite; nausea and vomiting; odd, metallic, or altered taste; skin rash; temporary hair loss. Side effects are more common with higher doses. Tolerance to high doses may be improved by gradually increasing the doses over the first weeks of treatment.

LESS COMMON
Back pain, blurred vision, dizziness, dry mouth, dry or itching skin, profuse or unusual sweating, joint pain, leg cramps, lip or mouth sores, weight loss.

STORAGE
Keep interferon alfa-n1 refrigerated but do not allow it to freeze.

MISSED DOSE
If you miss a dose, do not take the missed dose and do not double the next dose. Check with your doctor on what to do.

STOPPING THE DRUG
The decision to stop taking the drug should be made by your doctor.

PROLONGED USE
See your doctor regularly for tests and examinations if you must take this drug for a prolonged period.

▼ PRECAUTIONS

Over 60: Adverse reactions may be more likely and more severe in older patients.

Driving and Hazardous Work: Do not drive or engage in hazardous work until you determine how the medicine affects you. Administering interferon at bedtime may help to minimize daytime sleepiness.

Alcohol: Avoid alcohol.

Pregnancy: Adequate studies have not been done. Consult your doctor for advice.

Breast Feeding: Interferon alfa-n1 may pass into breast milk; caution is advised. Consult your doctor for advice.

Infants and Children: No special studies have been done; consult a pediatrician.

Special Concerns: Do not change to another brand of alfa interferon without consulting your doctor. They have different dosage schedules. Try to avoid people with infections, because this drug can lower white blood cell levels temporarily and increase susceptibility to disease. Be careful when cleaning your teeth, and avoid cutting yourself when using sharp objects, such as a razor. Avoid contact sports or other situations where bruising could occur.

OVERDOSE
Symptoms: No specific ones have been reported.

What to Do: Call your doctor or emergency medical services (EMS) immediately if you suspect an overdose.

▼ INTERACTIONS

DRUG INTERACTIONS
Consult your doctor for specific advice if you are taking any prescription or over-the-counter medication, especially central nervous system depressants including antihistamines, alcohol, tranquilizers, or psychiatric medications.

FOOD INTERACTIONS
None are known.

DISEASE INTERACTIONS
Consult your doctor if you have a history of bleeding or clotting disorders, chickenpox, shingles, psychological or neurological disorders, diabetes, autoimmune disorders, heart disease, kidney disease, liver disease, lung disease, or thyroid disease.

461

INTERFERON ALFA-N3

Available in: Injection
Available OTC? No   **As Generic?** No
Drug Class: Immunomodulator

▼ USAGE INFORMATION

WHY IT'S PRESCRIBED
To treat condylomata acuminata (genital or venereal warts) in patients 18 years of age or older.

HOW IT WORKS
It acts in the same way as the body's natural interferons, which are proteins released by the immune system to fight viruses, cancer cells, and other types of disease. Interferon alfa-n3 is derived from human white blood cells and has an antiviral effect.

▼ DOSAGE GUIDELINES

RANGE AND FREQUENCY
0.05 ml injected into each wart 2 times a week for up to 8 weeks. Total dose for each session should not exceed 0.5 ml (2.5 million units).

ONSET OF EFFECT
Unknown.

DURATION OF ACTION
Unknown; however, warts will continue to disappear after completion of 8 weeks of therapy and discontinuation of the drug.

DIETARY ADVICE
Drink plenty of fluids to reduce risk of excessively low blood pressure.

STORAGE
Keep interferon alfa-n3 refrigerated but do not allow it to freeze.

MISSED DOSE
If you miss a dose, do not take the missed dose and do not double the next dose. Check with your doctor on what to do.

STOPPING THE DRUG
The decision to stop taking the drug should be made by your doctor.

PROLONGED USE
See your doctor regularly for tests and examinations if you must take this drug for a prolonged period.

▼ PRECAUTIONS

Over 60: Adverse reactions may be more likely and more severe in older patients.

Driving and Hazardous Work: Do not drive or engage in hazardous work until you determine how the medicine affects you. Administering interferon at bedtime may help to minimize daytime sleepiness.

Alcohol: Avoid alcohol.

Pregnancy: Adequate studies have not been done. Consult your doctor for advice.

Breast Feeding: Interferon alfa-n3 may pass into breast milk; caution is advised. Consult your doctor for advice.

Infants and Children: No special studies have been done; consult a pediatrician.

Special Concerns: Do not change to another brand of alfa interferon without consulting your doctor. They have different dosage schedules. Try to avoid people with infections, because this drug can lower white blood cell levels temporarily and increase susceptibility to disease. Be careful when cleaning your teeth, and avoid cutting yourself when using sharp objects such as a razor. Avoid contact sports or other situations where bruising could occur.

OVERDOSE
Symptoms: No specific ones have been reported.

What to Do: Call your doctor or emergency medical services (EMS) immediately if you suspect an overdose.

▼ INTERACTIONS

DRUG INTERACTIONS
Consult your doctor for specific advice if you are taking any prescription or over-the-counter medication, especially central nervous system depressants including antihistamines, alcohol, tranquilizers, or psychiatric medications.

FOOD INTERACTIONS
None are known.

DISEASE INTERACTIONS
Caution is advised when taking interferon alfa-n3. Consult your doctor if you have a history of bleeding or clotting disorders, chickenpox, shingles, psychological or neurological disorders, diabetes, autoimmune disorders, heart disease, kidney disease, liver disease, lung disease, or thyroid disease.

 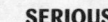 **SIDE EFFECTS**

SERIOUS
Confusion, depression, nervousness, distractibility, impaired thinking, or thoughts of suicide; numbness or tingling of fingers, toes, and face; black, tarry, or bloody stools; blood in urine; chest pain; hoarseness; fever or chills after 3 weeks of treatment; irregular heartbeat; pain in lower back or side; difficult or painful urination; red spots on skin; unusual bleeding or bruising; increased incidence of infections. Call your doctor immediately.

COMMON
Flulike symptoms, fatigue, muscle aches, fever, or chills in first weeks of treatment; general discomfort or ill feeling; headache; loss of appetite; nausea and vomiting; odd, metallic, or altered taste; skin rash; temporary hair loss. Side effects are more common with higher doses. Tolerance to high doses may be improved by gradually increasing the doses over the first weeks of treatment.

LESS COMMON
Back pain, blurred vision, dizziness, dry mouth, dry or itching skin, profuse or unusual sweating, joint pain, leg cramps, lip or mouth sores, weight loss.

INTERFERON ALFACON-1

BRAND NAME

Infergen

Available in: Injection
Available OTC? No **As Generic?** No
Drug Class: Immunomodulator

▼ USAGE INFORMATION

WHY IT'S PRESCRIBED
To treat chronic hepatitis C infection in adults who have developed liver disease.

HOW IT WORKS
It acts in the same way as the body's natural interferons, which are proteins released by the cells of the immune system to fight viruses.

▼ DOSAGE GUIDELINES

RANGE AND FREQUENCY
For people who have never been treated with interferons: 9 micrograms (mcg) injected under the skin 3 times a week for 24 weeks, with at least 48 hours between doses. For people who have undergone previous interferon therapy and either did not respond to it or relapsed following discontinuation of therapy: 15 mcg under the skin 3 times a week for 6 months.

ONSET OF EFFECT
Unknown.

DURATION OF ACTION
Unknown.

DIETARY ADVICE
Drink plenty of fluids to reduce the risk of excessively low blood pressure.

STORAGE
Refrigerate, but do not allow it to freeze. Do not expose it to high temperatures or direct sunlight. Store away from food. Just prior to administration, interferon alfacon-1 may be allowed to reach room temperature.

MISSED DOSE
If you miss a dose, do not take the missed dose and do not double the next dose. Check with your doctor on what to do.

STOPPING THE DRUG
The decision to stop taking the drug should be made by your doctor.

PROLONGED USE
See your doctor regularly for tests and exams if you take it for a prolonged period.

▼ PRECAUTIONS

Over 60: Adverse reactions may be more likely and more severe in older patients.

Driving and Hazardous Work: Do not drive or engage in hazardous work until you determine how the medicine affects you.

Alcohol: No special precautions are necessary.

Pregnancy: Adequate human studies have not been done. Interferon alfacon-1 should not be used when pregnant.

Breast Feeding: Interferon alfacon-1 may pass into breast milk; caution is advised. Consult your doctor.

Infants and Children: Not recommended for patients under age 18.

Special Concerns: Do not shake the vial prior to administration. If the liquid in the vial is cloudy or discolored, do not use it. Discard any unused portion. Do not change to another brand of interferon without consulting your doctor. They have different dosage schedules.

OVERDOSE

Symptoms: An overdose is unlikely. However, with a very high dose, you may experience some side effects more acutely, particularly loss of appetite, chills, fever, and muscle pain.

What to Do: If you take a much larger dose than prescribed, call your doctor or get emergency medical attention immediately.

▼ INTERACTIONS

DRUG INTERACTIONS
Consult your doctor if you are taking any prescription or other drug, especially central nervous system depressants, including antihistamines, alcohol, tranquilizers, or psychiatric medications.

FOOD INTERACTIONS
No known food interactions.

DISEASE INTERACTIONS
Interferon alfacon-1 should not be taken by patients with severe depression, suicidal feelings, or a history of other severe psychiatric disorders. Those with preexisting heart disease must use this drug with special caution. Consult your doctor for specific advice if you have a history of bleeding or clotting disorders, chickenpox, shingles, psychological or neurological disorders, diabetes, autoimmune disorders, kidney disease, liver disease, lung disease, or thyroid disease.

 SIDE EFFECTS

SERIOUS
Confusion, depression, nervousness, distractibility, or impaired thinking; numbness or tingling of fingers, toes, and face; sleeping difficulty; black, tarry, or bloody stools; blood in urine; chest pain, cough, or hoarseness; fever or chills after 3 weeks of treatment; irregular heartbeat; pain in lower back or side; difficult or painful urination; red spots on skin; unusual bleeding or bruising; increased incidence of infections. Call your doctor immediately.

COMMON
Flulike symptoms, fatigue, muscle aches, fever, or chills in first weeks of treatment; general discomfort or ill feeling; headache; loss of appetite; nausea and vomiting; odd, metallic, or altered taste; skin rash; temporary hair loss. Side effects are more common with higher doses. Tolerance to high doses may be improved by gradually increasing the doses over the first weeks of treatment.

LESS COMMON
Back pain, blurred vision, dizziness, dry mouth, dry or itching skin, profuse or unusual sweating, joint pain, leg cramps, lip or mouth sores, weight loss.

INTERFERON BETA-1A

BRAND NAME

Avonex

Available in: Powder for injection
Available OTC? No **As Generic?** No
Drug Class: Immunomodulator

▼ USAGE INFORMATION

WHY IT'S PRESCRIBED
To treat relapsing-remitting multiple sclerosis (the most common form of MS, in which periods of active disease alternate with periods of remission or reduced severity of symptoms).

HOW IT WORKS
It acts in the same way as the body's natural interferons, which are proteins released by the immune system to fight viruses, cancer cells, and other types of disease. The exact way in which the drug fights MS is unknown, but it appears to interfere with the immune system's attack on healthy tissue (the apparent cause of MS).

▼ DOSAGE GUIDELINES

RANGE AND FREQUENCY
6 million units once a week by injection.

ONSET OF EFFECT
Unknown.

DURATION OF ACTION
Unknown.

DIETARY ADVICE
Drink plenty of fluids to reduce the risk of excessively low blood pressure.

STORAGE
Keep liquid form of interferon beta-1a refrigerated but do not allow it to freeze.

MISSED DOSE
If you miss a dose, do not take the missed dose and do not double the next dose. Check with your doctor on what to do.

STOPPING THE DRUG
The decision to stop taking the drug should be made by your doctor.

PROLONGED USE
See your doctor regularly for tests and examinations if you must take this drug for a prolonged period.

▼ PRECAUTIONS

Over 60: Adverse reactions may be more likely and more severe in older patients.

Driving and Hazardous Work: Do not drive or engage in hazardous work until you determine how the medicine affects you.

Alcohol: Avoid alcohol.

Pregnancy: Adequate studies have not been done. Consult your doctor for advice.

Breast Feeding: Interferon beta-1a may pass into breast milk; caution is advised. Consult your doctor for advice.

Infants and Children: No special studies have been done on the effects of beta interferon in children.

Special Concerns: Interferon beta-1a should be used with caution in patients with a history of depression, since it has been linked to an increase in suicidal impulses. Try to avoid people with infections, because this drug can lower white blood cell levels temporarily and increase susceptibility to disease. Be careful when using a toothbrush, dental floss, or toothpick. Your doctor or dentist may recommend other ways to clean your teeth. Check with your doctor before having any dental work done. Be careful not to cut yourself when using sharp objects such as a razor. Avoid contact sports or other situa-tions where bruising could occur. Do not touch your eyes or the inside of your mouth unless you have just washed your hands.

OVERDOSE
Symptoms: No specific ones have been reported.

What to Do: Call your doctor or emergency medical services (EMS) immediately if you suspect an overdose.

▼ INTERACTIONS

DRUG INTERACTIONS
Consult your doctor for specific advice if you are taking any prescription or over-the-counter medication.

FOOD INTERACTIONS
None are known.

DISEASE INTERACTIONS
Caution is advised when taking interferon beta-1a. Consult your doctor if you have a history of bleeding or clotting disorders, chickenpox, shingles, psychological or neurological disorders, diabetes, autoimmune disorders, heart disease, kidney disease, liver disease, lung disease, or thyroid disease.

 SIDE EFFECTS

SERIOUS
Seizures, swelling and fluid retention, pelvic pain, pounding in the chest, breast pain, frequent urination, sweating, anxiety, confusion, joint pain, breathing difficulty, depression, suicidal thoughts or impulses. Call your doctor right away.

COMMON
Pain, inflammation, or allergic reaction at injection site (most common side effect); flulike symptoms, including headache, fever, muscle aches, general weakness, and fatigue (these symptoms tend to diminish as the body adjusts to therapy); insomnia; increased susceptibility to infection; nausea and vomiting; diarrhea; abdominal pain; temporary hair loss.

LESS COMMON
Dizziness, dry mouth, dry or itching skin, increased sweating, joint pain, changes in vision, hearing problems.

INTERFERON BETA-1B (RIFN-B)

Available in: Powder for injection
Available OTC? No   **As Generic?** No
Drug Class: Immunomodulator

▼ USAGE INFORMATION

WHY IT'S PRESCRIBED
To treat relapsing-remitting multiple sclerosis (the most common form of MS, in which periods of active disease alternate with periods of remission or reduced severity of symptoms).

HOW IT WORKS
It acts in the same way as the body's natural interferons, which are proteins released by the immune system to fight viruses, cancer cells, and other types of disease. The exact way in which this drug fights MS is unknown, but it appears to interfere with the immune system's attack on healthy tissue.

▼ DOSAGE GUIDELINES

RANGE AND FREQUENCY
8 million units (0.25 mg) by injection every other day.

ONSET OF EFFECT
Unknown.

DURATION OF ACTION
Unknown.

DIETARY ADVICE
Drink plenty of fluids to reduce the risk of excessively low blood pressure.

STORAGE
Keep the liquid form refrigerated but do not allow it to freeze.

MISSED DOSE
If you miss a dose, do not take the missed dose and do not double the next dose. Notify your doctor.

STOPPING THE DRUG
The decision to stop taking the drug should be made by your doctor.

PROLONGED USE
See your doctor regularly for tests and examinations if you must take this drug for a prolonged period.

▼ PRECAUTIONS

Over 60: Adverse reactions may be more likely and more severe in older patients.

Driving and Hazardous Work: Do not drive or engage in hazardous work until you determine how the medicine affects you.

Alcohol: Avoid alcohol.

Pregnancy: Adequate studies have not been done. Consult your doctor for advice.

Breast Feeding: Interferon beta-1b may pass into breast milk; caution is advised. Consult your doctor for advice.

Infants and Children: No special studies have been done on the effects of beta interferon in children.

Special Concerns: Interferon beta-1b should be used with caution in patients with a history of depression, since it has been linked to an increase in suicidal impulses. Try to avoid people with infections, because this drug can lower white blood cell levels temporarily and increase susceptibility to disease. Be careful when using a toothbrush, dental floss, or toothpick. Your doctor or dentist may recommend other ways to clean your teeth. Check with your doctor before having any dental work done. Be careful not to cut yourself when using sharp objects such as a razor. Avoid contact sports or other situations where bruising could occur. Do not touch your eyes or the inside of your mouth unless you have just washed your hands.

OVERDOSE
Symptoms: No specific ones have been reported.

What to Do: Call your doctor or emergency medical services (EMS) immediately if you suspect an overdose.

▼ INTERACTIONS

DRUG INTERACTIONS
Consult your doctor for specific advice if you are taking any prescription or over-the-counter medication.

FOOD INTERACTIONS
None are known.

DISEASE INTERACTIONS
Caution is advised when taking interferon beta-1b. Consult your doctor if you have a history of bleeding or clotting disorders, chickenpox, shingles, psychological or neurological disorders, diabetes, autoimmune disorders, heart disease, kidney disease, liver disease, lung disease, or thyroid disease.

SIDE EFFECTS

SERIOUS
Seizures, swelling and fluid retention, pelvic pain, pounding in the chest, breast pain, frequent urination, sweating, anxiety, confusion, joint pain, breathing difficulty, depression, suicidal thoughts or impulses. Call your doctor right away.

COMMON
Pain, inflammation, or allergic reaction at injection site (most common side effect); flulike symptoms, including headache, fever, muscle aches, general weakness, and fatigue (these symptoms tend to diminish as the body adjusts to therapy); insomnia; increased susceptibility to infection; nausea and vomiting; diarrhea; abdominal pain; temporary hair loss.

LESS COMMON
Dizziness, dry mouth, dry or itching skin, increased sweating, joint pain, vision or hearing problems. Tissue death at the site of injection has occurred in a few patients.

INTERFERON GAMMA-1B

Available in: Injection
Available OTC? No **As Generic?** No
Drug Class: Immunomodulator

▼ USAGE INFORMATION

WHY IT'S PRESCRIBED
To treat chronic granulomatous disease (an inherited disorder characterized by recurring infections and the widespread growth of lesions or tumors in the skin, lungs, and lymphatic system).

HOW IT WORKS
It acts in the same way as the body's natural interferons, which are proteins released by the immune system to fight viruses, cancer cells, and other types of disease. Of all the interferons, interferon gamma has the greatest immunomodulator properties (ability to alter the efficacy of the immune system).

▼ DOSAGE GUIDELINES

RANGE AND FREQUENCY
For adults with body surface area greater than 0.5 square meters: 1.5 million units (50 micrograms) per square meter by injection 3 times a week. For adults with body surface area less than 0.5 square meters: 1.5 micrograms per 2.2 lbs (1 kg) of body weight 3 times a week. The preferred injection sites are the deltoid (shoulder) muscle or the front thigh muscle.

ONSET OF EFFECT
Unknown.

DURATION OF ACTION
Unknown.

DIETARY ADVICE
Drink plenty of fluids to reduce the risk of excessively low blood pressure.

STORAGE
Keep interferon gamma-1b refrigerated but do not allow it to freeze.

MISSED DOSE
If you miss a dose, do not take the missed dose and do not double the next dose. Check with your doctor on what to do.

STOPPING THE DRUG
The decision to stop taking the drug should be made by your doctor.

PROLONGED USE
See your doctor regularly for tests and examinations if you must take this drug for a prolonged period.

▼ PRECAUTIONS

Over 60: No special problems are expected.

Driving and Hazardous Work: Do not drive or engage in hazardous work until you determine how the medicine affects you.

Alcohol: Avoid alcohol.

Pregnancy: Very large doses of interferon gamma-1b have increased fetal deaths and uterine bleeding in animals. Before you take interferon gamma-1b, tell your doctor if you are pregnant or plan to become pregnant.

Breast Feeding: Interferon gamma-1b may pass into breast milk; caution is advised. Consult your doctor for specific advice.

Infants and Children: Interferon gamma-1b is not expected to cause different side effects or problems in infants and children than it does in other age groups.

Special Concerns: Taking interferon gamma-1b at bedtime can help to minimize its flulike side effects. Your doctor may want you to take acetaminophen before each injection to avoid such side effects. Your doctor may tell you to drink extra fluids to prevent low blood pressure caused by loss of too much water. Interferon gamma-1b may make you more sensitive to sunlight. Use sunscreen or wear protective clothing.

OVERDOSE
Symptoms: No specific ones have been reported.

What to Do: Call your doctor or emergency medical services (EMS) immediately if you have any reason to suspect an overdose.

▼ INTERACTIONS

DRUG INTERACTIONS
Consult your doctor for specific advice if you are taking any prescription or over-the-counter medication.

FOOD INTERACTIONS
No known food interactions.

DISEASE INTERACTIONS
Caution is advised when taking interferon gamma-1b. Consult your doctor if you have a history of seizures, mental or psychiatric illness, heart disease, multiple sclerosis, or lupus (which may be worsened by gamma interferon).

▼ SIDE EFFECTS

SERIOUS
Black, tarry, or bloody stools; blood in the urine; painful or difficult urination; pain in the lower back or side; loss of balance or coordination; mental confusion and impaired thinking; masklike facial expression; trouble walking or shuffling gait; red spots on the skin; stiffness of arms or legs; trembling and shaking of hands and fingers; trouble speaking or swallowing. Call your doctor right away.

COMMON
Muscle aches, diarrhea, fever and chills, general discomfort or feelings of illness, headache, nausea or vomiting, skin rash, unusual fatigue, increased incidence of infections, unusual bleeding or bruising.

LESS COMMON
Dizziness, joint pain, loss of appetite, weight loss, cough or hoarseness.

IODINE, STRONG

Available in: Oral solution
Available OTC? No   **As Generic?** Yes
Drug Class: Thyroid agent

▼ USAGE INFORMATION

WHY IT'S PRESCRIBED
To treat an overactive thyroid gland (hyperthyroidism); to treat iodine deficiency; to prepare for thyroid surgery.

HOW IT WORKS
Strong iodine blocks production and release of thyroid hormone by the thyroid gland.

▼ DOSAGE GUIDELINES

RANGE AND FREQUENCY
For overactive thyroid gland, adults and children over age 10: 1 ml, 3 times a day. To prepare for thyroid surgery: 0.1 ml, 3 times a day for 10 to 14 days.

ONSET OF EFFECT
Unknown.

DURATION OF ACTION
Unknown.

DIETARY ADVICE
Take with a glass of fruit juice, milk, or broth to minimize stomach upset. Drink all of the liquid to get the full dose of the medicine.

STORAGE
Keep the solution refrigerated, but do not allow it to freeze.

MISSED DOSE
Take it as soon as you remember. If it is near the time for the next dose, skip the missed dose and resume your regular dosage schedule. Do not double the next dose.

STOPPING THE DRUG
The decision to stop taking the drug should be made by your doctor.

PROLONGED USE
It is necessary to see your physician regularly to check the progress of treatment when taking strong iodine for a prolonged period.

▼ PRECAUTIONS

Over 60: No special problems or side effects are expected in older patients.

Driving and Hazardous Work: Use of strong iodine should not impair your ability to perform such tasks safely.

Alcohol: No special warnings.

Pregnancy: Iodine can cross the placenta and cause thyroid problems or goiter in the fetus. Before you take strong iodine, tell your doctor if you are pregnant or plan to become pregnant.

Breast Feeding: Strong iodine passes into breast milk; avoid or discontinue use while nursing.

Infants and Children: The use and dose of strong iodine in an infant or a child must be determined by your doctor.

Special Concerns: Take the oral solution by mouth even if it comes in a dropper bottle. Do not use the medicine if the solution turns reddish brown. If crystals form in the solution, they can be dissolved by warming the closed container in warm water and then shaking the container gently. Take the liquid through a straw to lessen tooth discoloration. If stomach upset continues, consult your doctor.

OVERDOSE
Symptoms: Gastrointestinal pain and diarrhea, sometimes bloody; loss of consciousness.

What to Do: Call your doctor, emergency medical services (EMS), or the nearest poison control center immediately.

▼ INTERACTIONS

DRUG INTERACTIONS
Consult your doctor for specific advice if you are taking amiloride, spironolactone, triamterene, other thyroid agents, or lithium.

FOOD INTERACTIONS
This drug contains potassium. Consult your doctor if you are on a low-potassium diet.

DISEASE INTERACTIONS
Caution is advised when taking strong iodine. Consult your doctor if you have any of the following: bronchitis or another lung condition, kidney disease, or hyperkalemia (excess potassium in the blood).

≣ SIDE EFFECTS ≣

SERIOUS
Fever, swollen glands, rash, joint pain. Call your doctor immediately.

COMMON
Nausea, metallic taste.

LESS COMMON
Fever, headache, inflamed salivary glands, runny nose, stained teeth, swelling around eyes, warm and reddened skin, pinkeye, stomach upset, vomiting, diarrhea, sores on mucous membranes.

IODINE TOPICAL

Available in: Topical solution
Available OTC? Yes   **As Generic?** Yes
Drug Class: Antibacterial (topical); antiseptic

▼ USAGE INFORMATION

WHY IT'S PRESCRIBED
Iodine is a very effective disinfectant used for prevention and treatment of minor skin infections caused by bacteria. It is also used to disinfect the skin prior to needle procedures and minor surgeries (such as blood drawing, dialysis, and injections).

HOW IT WORKS
Iodine poisons bacteria on contact, by causing the proteins comprising the organism to congeal.

▼ DOSAGE GUIDELINES

RANGE AND FREQUENCY
Adults: Apply to affected site as directed by a physician or according to manufacturer's instructions on the label. Children 1 month of age and over: Consult a pediatrician.

ONSET OF EFFECT
Immediate.

DURATION OF ACTION
Unknown.

DIETARY ADVICE
Maintain your usual food and fluid intake. Increase fluids if you have a fever or diarrhea, in hot weather, or during exercise.

STORAGE
Store in a tightly sealed container away from heat and direct light. Keep away from moisture and extremes in temperature.

MISSED DOSE
Apply as soon as you remember. If it is near the time for the next dose, skip the missed dose and resume your regular dosage schedule.

STOPPING THE DRUG
Use as prescribed for the full treatment period, even if you begin to feel better before the scheduled end of therapy.

PROLONGED USE
Therapy with this medication should be concluded within 7 to 10 days. Consult your physician if your condition has not improved—or especially if it has worsened—anytime after starting therapy with iodine.

▼ PRECAUTIONS

Over 60: No special problems are expected.

Driving and Hazardous Work: The use of iodine should not impair your ability to perform such tasks safely.

Alcohol: No special precautions are necessary.

Pregnancy: Avoid or discontinue using iodine if you are pregnant or trying to become pregnant.

Breast Feeding: Iodine passes into breast milk; avoid or discontinue usage while nursing.

Infants and Children: Iodine is not recommended for use on children under 1 month of age.

Special Concerns: Iodine has serious side effects if it is absorbed in large amounts into your blood. Therefore, do not apply excessive amounts to affected skin. Do not swallow iodine solutions. Above all, never apply this medication to open wounds, to deep cuts, or to bleeding or ulcerated skin. Do not use this medication near your eyes; therefore, use caution when applying iodine to the skin of your forehead or cheeks, and be sure to use small quantities applied carefully, rather than large volumes of liquid. If iodine gets into your eyes, wash with water immediately.

OVERDOSE
Symptoms: Overdose with topical iodine is unlikely when used as directed. If this medication is swallowed, symptoms include abdominal pain, diarrhea, nausea, vomiting, fever, excessive thirst, decreased passage of urine.

What to Do: Call your doctor, emergency medical services (EMS), or the nearest poison control center immediately.

▼ INTERACTIONS

DRUG INTERACTIONS
No specific drug interactions have yet been documented. If you are concerned about whether a prescription or nonprescription medication you are taking may interact with topical iodine, consult your doctor or pharmacist for current information.

FOOD INTERACTIONS
No known food interactions.

DISEASE INTERACTIONS
Consult your doctor if you have any of the following: animal bites; large sores, blisters, ulcerations, or broken skin at the application site; severe injury at the application site; puncture wounds or other deep wounds; serious burns; or allergies to shellfish.

SIDE EFFECTS

SERIOUS
Used as directed, topical iodine is not expected to produce any serious side effects.

COMMON
Momentary burning or tingling at the site of application.

LESS COMMON
Irritation or skin allergy, with blistering, crusting, itching, or reddening of skin at site of application.

IPECAC SYRUP

BRAND NAME

Ipecac syrup is available in generic form only.

Available in: Syrup
Available OTC? Yes **As Generic?** Yes
Drug Class: Emetic

▼ USAGE INFORMATION

WHY IT'S PRESCRIBED
To cause vomiting in persons who have ingested certain toxic substances or have taken an overdose of a drug.

HOW IT WORKS
Ipecac induces vomiting by chemically irritating the stomach lining, triggering the vomiting reflex.

▼ DOSAGE GUIDELINES

RANGE AND FREQUENCY
Adults and teenagers: 15 to 30 ml, followed by 1 full glass of water. Children ages 1 to 12: 15 ml followed by ½ to 1 full glass of water. Children ages 6 months to 1 year: 5 to 10 ml, followed by ½ to 1 full glass of water. If vomiting does not occur, the first dose may be repeated one time after 20 minutes.

ONSET OF EFFECT
Within 20 to 30 minutes.

DURATION OF ACTION
From 20 to 25 minutes.

DIETARY ADVICE
Drink water immediately after taking ipecac syrup.

STORAGE
Store in a tightly sealed container away from heat, moisture, and direct light.

MISSED DOSE
Not applicable. It should be used more than 1 time only if clearly necessary.

STOPPING THE DRUG
Do not give more than 2 doses. If not effective, consult your doctor, emergency medical services (EMS), or local poison control center.

PROLONGED USE
Ipecac is not intended for prolonged use.

▼ PRECAUTIONS

Over 60:
No special problems are expected.

Driving and Hazardous Work:
Do not drive or engage in hazardous work until you determine how the drug affects you.

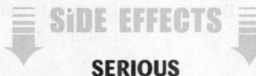

≡ SIDE EFFECTS ≡

SERIOUS
Heartbeat irregularities; nausea or vomiting lasting for more than 30 minutes; excessive diarrhea; weakness or stiffness of the muscles in the neck, arms, and legs; stomach pain or cramps; unusual fatigue; difficulty breathing. Call your doctor right away.

COMMON
Drowsiness and mild diarrhea.

LESS COMMON
There are no less-common side effects associated with the use of ipecac syrup.

Alcohol:
Avoid alcohol.

Pregnancy:
No studies of the use of ipecac syrup during pregnancy have been done. Discuss with your doctor the relative risks and benefits of using it while pregnant.

Breast Feeding:
Ipecac syrup may pass into breast milk; caution is advised. Consult your doctor for advice.

Infants and Children:
Use by children should be under strict supervision. There is an increased risk of swallowing the vomited substance in children under 1 year of age. Consult your doctor before using ipecac syrup.

Special Concerns:
Before giving ipecac syrup, consult your doctor, emergency medical services (EMS), or the nearest poison control center. Ipecac syrup should not be given to anyone who has ingested gasoline, paint thinner, kerosene, or a caustic substance such as lye. Do not give ipecac syrup to anyone who is unconscious or very drowsy, because of an increased risk that the vomited substance can enter the lung. If you have a child over 1 year of age in the house, keep 30 ml (1 oz) of ipecac syrup on hand for emergencies. Ipecac syrup should not be used to induce vomiting as a means of losing weight. It can be toxic to the heart.

OVERDOSE

Symptoms: Breathing difficulty, muscle stiffness, diarrhea.

What to Do: Call your doctor, emergency medical services (EMS), or the nearest poison control center immediately.

▼ INTERACTIONS

DRUG INTERACTIONS
Do not give any other medicines, including over-the-counter drugs, with ipecac unless you first consult your doctor. Antiemetics can decrease the syrup's effect and increase its toxicity. If using activated charcoal, wait until vomiting (induced by ipecac) has stopped before administering it.

FOOD INTERACTIONS
Ipecac syrup should not be taken with milk, milk products, or carbonated beverages. Milk and milk products prevent ipecac syrup from working properly. Carbonated beverages can cause the stomach to swell.

DISEASE INTERACTIONS
You should not take ipecac syrup if you suffer from or have heart disease, a history of seizures, shock, reduced gag reflex, drowsiness, or unconsciousness.

IPRATROPIUM BROMIDE

BRAND NAME

Atrovent

Available in: Inhalation aerosol, inhalation solution
Available OTC? No **As Generic?** Yes
Drug Class: Respiratory inhalant

▼ USAGE INFORMATION

WHY IT'S PRESCRIBED
To control the symptoms of lung diseases, such as asthma, chronic bronchitis, and emphysema.

HOW IT WORKS
It inhibits the cough reflex by blocking the activity of acetylcholine, a chemical that, in the lungs, causes the smooth muscles surrounding the airways to constrict. Therefore, when inhaled, ipratropium bromide causes the airways to widen (bronchodilation).

▼ DOSAGE GUIDELINES

RANGE AND FREQUENCY
The drug may be used as needed to relieve respiratory symptoms. For chronic obstructive lung disease such as bronchitis or emphysema—Inhalation aerosol: Adults and children 6 and over: 2 to 4 inhalations 3 or 4 times a day at regularly spaced intervals. Some patients may need 6 to 8 inhalations a day. Inhalation solution, adults and children 12 and over: 250 to 500 micrograms in a nebulizer 3 or 4 times a day, every 6 to 8 hours.

ONSET OF EFFECT
5 to 15 minutes.

DURATION OF ACTION
3 to 4 hours.

DIETARY ADVICE
Sugarless hard candy or gum can be taken to relieve dry mouth.

STORAGE
Store in a tightly sealed container away from heat and direct light. Open bottles of the solution should be refrigerated, but do not allow the solution to freeze.

MISSED DOSE
Take it as soon as you remember. If it is near the time for the next dose, skip the missed dose and resume your regular dosage schedule. Do not double the next dose.

STOPPING THE DRUG
It may not be necessary to continue using the medication for as long as originally prescribed; consult your doctor.

PROLONGED USE
You should see your doctor regularly if you must take this drug for a prolonged period.

▼ PRECAUTIONS

Over 60: Ipratropium is not expected to cause different problems in older patients than in younger persons.

Driving and Hazardous Work: Do not drive or engage in hazardous work until you determine how the medicine affects you.

Alcohol: No special precautions are necessary.

Pregnancy: Ipratropium has not caused birth defects in animals. Human studies have not been done. Before you take ipratropium, tell your doctor if you are pregnant or plan to become pregnant.

Breast Feeding: It is not known whether ipratropium passes into breast milk; caution is advised. Consult your doctor for specific advice.

Infants and Children: Ipratropium has been tested in children and has not been shown to cause different effects than in adults.

Special Concerns: To test the inhaler, insert the canister into the mouthpiece, take the cap off the mouthpiece, shake the inhaler 3 or 4 times, and spray once into the air. To use the inhaler, hold it upright, with the mouthpiece end down, shake it 3 or 4 times, then breathe out. Spray into open mouth or with mouth closed over inhaler, as recommended by your doctor. Clean the inhaler, mouthpiece, and spacer at least twice a week. To take the inhalation solution, use a power-operated nebulizer with a face mask or mouthpiece. Get instructions for using the nebulizer from your doctor.

OVERDOSE
Symptoms: No specific ones have been reported.

What to Do: An overdose of ipratropium is unlikely to be life-threatening. However, if someone takes a much larger dose than prescribed, call your doctor, emergency medical services (EMS), or the nearest poison control center.

▼ INTERACTIONS

DRUG INTERACTIONS
Before you use ipratropium, tell your doctor if you are using any other prescription or over-the-counter drug.

FOOD INTERACTIONS
No known food interactions.

DISEASE INTERACTIONS
Consult your doctor if you have glaucoma or difficulty urinating.

SIDE EFFECTS

SERIOUS
Persistent constipation; lower abdominal pain or bloating; wheezing or difficulty breathing; tightness in chest; severe eye pain; skin rash or hives; swelling of face, lips, or eyelids. Call your doctor immediately.

COMMON
Dry mouth, cough, unpleasant taste.

LESS COMMON
Blurred vision, other changes in vision, burning eyes, difficult urination, dizziness, headache, nausea, pounding heartbeat, nervousness, sweating, trembling.

IRBESARTAN

Available in: Tablets
Available OTC? No   **As Generic?** No
Drug Class: Antihypertensive/angiotensin II antagonist

▼ USAGE INFORMATION

WHY IT'S PRESCRIBED
To control high blood pressure. This drug appears to have the same benefits as the class of antihypertensive drugs known as "ACE inhibitors," without producing the common side effect (experienced by as many as 30% of patients) of a dry cough. Irbesartan may be used by itself or in conjunction with other antihypertensive medications.

HOW IT WORKS
Irbesartan blocks the effects of angiotensin II, a naturally occurring substance that causes blood vessels to narrow. Irbesartan causes the blood vessels to dilate, thereby lowering blood pressure and decreasing the workload of the heart.

▼ DOSAGE GUIDELINES

RANGE AND FREQUENCY
To start, 150 mg once a day. It may be increased by your doctor to a maximum dose of 300 mg per day.

ONSET OF EFFECT
Within 2 to 4 hours.

DURATION OF ACTION
More than 24 hours.

DIETARY ADVICE
No special restrictions, unless your doctor has advised a low-sodium diet or other dietary modifications to help control your blood pressure.

STORAGE
Store in a tightly sealed container away from heat, moisture, and direct light.

MISSED DOSE
If you miss a dose on one day, do not double the dose the next day. Resume your regular dosage schedule.

STOPPING THE DRUG
Take it as prescribed for the full treatment period. The decision to stop taking the drug should be made in consultation with your physician.

PROLONGED USE
Lifelong therapy may be necessary. However, if you do change certain health habits (for example, increasing exercise or losing weight), a reduced dose may be possible under a doctor's supervision.

▼ PRECAUTIONS

Over 60: Adverse reactions may be more likely and more severe in older patients.

Driving and Hazardous Work: Do not drive or engage in hazardous work until you determine how the medicine affects you.

Alcohol: No special precautions are necessary.

Pregnancy: Irbesartan should not be used by pregnant women. Discontinue taking the drug as soon as possible when pregnancy is detected and discuss treatment alternatives with your doctor.

Breast Feeding: Irbesartan may pass into breast milk; caution is advised. Consult your doctor for advice.

Infants and Children: The safety and effectiveness of use in children have not been established.

Special Concerns: Irbesartan may cause excessively low blood pressure with dizziness or lightheadedness, which is most noticeable when you change position. This may lead to fainting, falls, and injury. Sit or lie down immediately if you feel dizzy or lightheaded. This side effect may be worsened by alcohol, hot weather, dehydration, salt depletion from diuretic use, fever, prolonged standing, prolonged sitting, or exercise.

OVERDOSE

Symptoms: No cases of overdose have been reported. However, if you take a much larger dose than prescribed, you may experience extremely low blood pressure or heartbeat irregularities.

What to Do: If you take a much larger dose than prescribed, contact your doctor.

▼ INTERACTIONS

DRUG INTERACTIONS
No drug interactions have yet been observed with irbesartan. Consult your doctor for specific advice if you are taking any other medication, including other drugs for high blood pressure. Irbesartan can be taken together with diuretics or other medications for high blood pressure, if your doctor approves.

FOOD INTERACTIONS
No known food interactions.

DISEASE INTERACTIONS
Patients with liver or kidney disease are advised to exercise caution when taking irbesartan.

▼ SIDE EFFECTS

SERIOUS
No serious side effects are associated with the use of irbesartan. (In clinical trials, the incidence of adverse effects was not significantly greater with the medication than with a placebo.)

COMMON
No common side effects are associated with the use of irbesartan.

LESS COMMON
Diarrhea, indigestion, heartburn, fatigue, muscle pain, edema, sexual dysfunction, low blood pressure.

ISOETHARINE

Available in: Inhalation solution, inhalation aerosol
Available OTC? No **As Generic?** Yes
Drug Class: Bronchodilator/sympathomimetic

▼ USAGE INFORMATION

WHY IT'S PRESCRIBED
Isoetharine is used to dilate air passages in the lungs that have become narrowed as a result of disease or inflammation. It is used in the treatment of asthma and chronic obstructive pulmonary disease (COPD).

HOW IT WORKS
Isoetharine widens constricted airways in the lungs by relaxing the smooth muscles that surround the bronchial passages.

▼ DOSAGE GUIDELINES

RANGE AND FREQUENCY
May be used when needed to relieve breathing difficulty. Adults, using inhalation solution for nebulizers: Usual dose is 4 inhalations, not to be taken more frequently than every 4 hours, for a usual maximum of 3 to 4 times a day. Note that isoetharine for nebulizers may or may not require dilution with saline. Check with your doctor to determine whether your medication requires dilution; if so, follow directions accordingly. Children: Consult your pediatrician. Adults using inhalation aerosol: A treatment consists of 340 micrograms (1 puff), repeated after 1 to 2 minutes if necessary. Treatments may be repeated every 4 hours if necessary. Children: Not recommended in children younger than 12 years of age.

ONSET OF EFFECT
Within 5 minutes.

DURATION OF ACTION
1 to 4 hours.

DIETARY ADVICE
Maintain your usual food and fluid intake.

STORAGE
Store in a tightly sealed container away from heat and direct light. Do not refrigerate inhalation solutions.

MISSED DOSE
Skip the missed dose and resume your regular dosage schedule. Do not double the next dose.

STOPPING THE DRUG
It may not be necessary to finish the recommended course of therapy. Consult your doctor.

PROLONGED USE
Therapy may require months or years. Excessive use may result in temporary loss of effectiveness.

▼ PRECAUTIONS

Over 60: Adverse reactions may be more likely and more severe in older patients.

Driving and Hazardous Work: Do not drive or engage in hazardous work until you determine how the medicine affects you.

Alcohol: No special precautions are necessary.

Pregnancy: Adequate studies have not been done; benefits must be weighed against potential risks. Consult your doctor for specific advice.

Breast Feeding: It is not known if isoetharine passes into breast milk. Mothers who wish to breast-feed while taking this drug should discuss the matter with their doctor.

Infants and Children: Nebulized solutions may be used to treat breathing difficulties in infants and children. Consult your pediatrician. Use of the inhalation aerosol is not recommended in children younger than 12 years old.

Special Concerns: Pay heed to any asthma attack or other breathing problem that does not improve after your usual nebulizer treatment or usual number of puffs. Seek help immediately if you feel your lungs are persistently constricted, if you are using more than the recommended number of treatments or puffs per day, or if you feel a recent attack is somehow different from others.

OVERDOSE
Symptoms: See Serious Side Effects.

What to Do: Call your doctor, emergency medical services (EMS), or the nearest poison control center immediately.

▼ INTERACTIONS

DRUG INTERACTIONS
Consult your doctor for specific advice if you are taking a beta-blocker, ergotamine or ergotaminelike medications, antidepressants, digitalis drugs, or an MAO inhibitor.

FOOD INTERACTIONS
No known food interactions.

DISEASE INTERACTIONS
Consult your doctor if you have a history of substance abuse (especially cocaine), seizures, brain damage, heart disease, heartbeat irregularities, high blood pressure, anxiety disorders, or a thyroid condition.

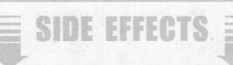

SIDE EFFECTS

SERIOUS
Isoetharine may become ineffective if used too often, resulting in more-severe breathing difficulty that does not improve. Signs include persistent wheezing, coughing, or shortness of breath; confusion; bluish color to lips or fingernails; inability to speak. Other side effects include chest pain or heaviness; irregular, racing, fluttering, or pounding heartbeat; lightheadedness; fainting; severe weakness; severe headache.

COMMON
Trouble sleeping, dry mouth, sore throat, nervousness, restlessness.

LESS COMMON
Trembling, sweating, headache, nausea or vomiting, flushing or redness to cheeks or other skin, muscle aches, unpleasant or unusual taste in mouth.

ISONIAZID

Available in: Syrup, tablets, injection
Available OTC? No   **As Generic?** Yes
Drug Class: Anti-infective/antitubercular agent

▼ USAGE INFORMATION

WHY IT'S PRESCRIBED
To prevent and treat tuberculosis (TB). It may be taken alone to prevent TB, but must be used with other antitubercular agents to treat an active case of TB.

HOW IT WORKS
Isoniazid interferes with the formation of DNA and lipids, needed to manufacture the TB bacteria's cell walls.

▼ DOSAGE GUIDELINES

RANGE AND FREQUENCY
For prevention— Adults and teenagers: 300 mg once a day. Children: 10 mg per 2.2 lbs (1 kg) of body weight once a day (not more than 300 mg a day). For treatment— Adults and teenagers: 300 mg once a day, or 15 mg per 2.2 lbs 2 or 3 times a week (not more than 900 mg per dose). Children: 10 to 20 mg per 2.2 lbs (not more than 300 mg a day) once a day, or 20 to 40 mg per 2.2 lbs 2 or 3 times a week (not more than 900 mg per dose). Ten to 25 mg a day of vitamin B6 may be given to prevent nerve damage.

ONSET OF EFFECT
Unknown.

DURATION OF ACTION
Unknown.

DIETARY ADVICE
Take this medicine 1 hour before or 2 hours after meals. Taking it with food or an antacid will prevent stomach irritation but decrease the absorption of the drug. Do not take an antacid containing aluminum within 1 hour of taking isoniazid.

STORAGE
Store in a tightly sealed container away from heat, moisture, and direct light. Do not freeze the liquid forms.

MISSED DOSE
Take it as soon as you remember, to help keep a constant level of medication in your system. If it is near the time for the next dose, skip the missed dose and resume your regular dosage schedule. Do not double the next dose.

STOPPING THE DRUG
Take it as prescribed for the full treatment period, even if you feel better before the scheduled end of therapy. Treatment may continue for months or years. The decision to stop the drug should be made by your doctor.

PROLONGED USE
See your doctor regularly for tests and examinations if you must take this medicine for a prolonged period. If your symptoms do not improve or instead become worse after 3 weeks, consult your doctor.

▼ PRECAUTIONS

Over 60: Adverse reactions may be more likely and more severe in older patients.

Driving and Hazardous Work: Do not drive or engage in hazardous work until you determine how the medicine affects you.

Alcohol: Avoid alcohol; it may diminish isoniazid's effectiveness and may interact with the drug, increasing the risk of hepatitis (liver inflammation).

Pregnancy: In human studies, isoniazid has not caused birth defects. Tell your doctor if you are pregnant or are planning to become pregnant and discuss the relative risks and benefits of using this drug.

Breast Feeding: Isoniazid passes into breast milk; caution is advised. Consult your doctor for specific advice.

Infants and Children: No special problems are expected. Discuss with your pediatrician the relative risks and benefits of your child's using this drug.

Special Concerns: Isoniazid can cause false results on urine sugar tests for people with diabetes.

OVERDOSE
Symptoms: Severe seizures, nausea, vomiting, difficulty breathing, slurred speech, blurred vision, hallucinations, dizziness, loss of consciousness, stupor.

What to Do: Call your doctor, emergency medical services (EMS), or the nearest poison control center immediately.

▼ INTERACTIONS

DRUG INTERACTIONS
Consult your doctor for specific advice if you are taking narcotic pain relievers, antacids, acetaminophen, carbamazepine, disulfiram, phenytoin, rifampin, ketoconazole, itraconazole, warfarin, or diazepam. Ask your doctor if any of the medications you take are toxic to the liver; such drugs should be avoided.

FOOD INTERACTIONS
Swiss cheese, fish, chocolate, and beer can react with this medication. Consult your doctor for advice.

DISEASE INTERACTIONS
Consult your doctor if you have epilepsy or another seizure disorder, or a history of alcohol abuse. Use of isoniazid may cause complications in patients with liver or kidney disease, since these organs work together to remove the medication from the body.

▼ SIDE EFFECTS

SERIOUS
Numbness, pain, burning, or tingling in hands and feet; loss of appetite; stomach pain; clumsiness; yellowish tinge to the eyes or skin; nausea; vomiting; darkened urine; unusual fatigue. Call your doctor immediately.

COMMON
Diarrhea, rash, fever.

LESS COMMON
Irritability, seizures.

ISOPROTERENOL

BRAND NAMES

Isuprel,
Isuprel Mistometer,
Medihaler-Iso

Available in: Inhalation solution or aerosol
Available OTC? No   **As Generic?** Yes
Drug Class: Bronchodilator/sympathomimetic

▼ USAGE INFORMATION

WHY IT'S PRESCRIBED
To dilate air passages in the lungs that have become narrowed as a result of disease or inflammation. It is used in the treatment of asthma and chronic obstructive pulmonary disease (COPD).

HOW IT WORKS
Isoproterenol widens constricted airways in the lungs by relaxing smooth muscles that surround the bronchial passages.

▼ DOSAGE GUIDELINES

RANGE AND FREQUENCY
For use when needed to relieve wheezing or difficulty breathing— By nebulizer: Adults: 6 to 12 inhalations of 0.25% solution. May be repeated if necessary every 15 minutes for a maximum of 3 doses. Take no more than 8 treatments every 24 hours. Or: 5 to 10 inhalations of 0.5% solution, or 3 to 7 inhalations of 1.0% solution, repeated once after 5 to 10 minutes if necessary. Take no more than 5 treatments per day. If you are on a program of scheduled, daily isoproterenol treatments, do not take a treatment more often than every 3 to 4 hours. Children: Follow directions above for 0.25% and 0.5% solutions. A 1.0% solution is not used in children. By inhalation aerosol, adults and children: 1 puff. Wait 1 minute to assess effect. May be repeated after 1 to 5 minutes if needed. This treatment may be repeated 4 to 6 times per day. For scheduled, daily use— 1 puff every 3 to 4 hours.

ONSET OF EFFECT
Within 5 minutes.

DURATION OF ACTION
From 30 to 120 minutes.

DIETARY ADVICE
Maintain your usual food and fluid intake.

STORAGE
Store at room temperature in a tightly sealed container away from heat and direct light.

MISSED DOSE
Skip the missed dose and resume your regular dosage schedule. Do not double the next dose.

STOPPING THE DRUG
It may not be necessary to finish the recommended course of therapy. Consult your doctor.

PROLONGED USE
Therapy may require months or years. Excessive use may result in temporary loss of effectiveness.

▼ PRECAUTIONS

Over 60: Adverse reactions may be more likely and more severe in older patients.

Driving and Hazardous Work: Do not drive or engage in hazardous work until you determine how the medicine affects you.

Alcohol: No special precautions are necessary.

Pregnancy: Benefits must be weighed against potential risks; consult your doctor.

Breast Feeding: Mothers who wish to breast feed while taking this drug should discuss the matter with their doctor.

Infants and Children: May be used to treat breathing difficulties in infants and children.

Special Concerns: Pay heed to any breathing problem that does not improve after your usual nebulizer treatment or usual number of puffs. Seek help immediately if you feel your lungs are persistently constricted, if you are using more than the recommended number of treatments per day, or if you feel a recent attack is somehow different from others.

OVERDOSE
Symptoms: Chest pain or heaviness; irregular, racing, fluttering, or pounding heartbeat; dizziness; lightheadedness; fainting; severe weakness; severe headache.

What to Do: Call your doctor, emergency medical services (EMS), or the nearest poison control center immediately.

▼ INTERACTIONS

DRUG INTERACTIONS
Consult your doctor for specific advice if you are taking a beta-blocker, ergotamine or ergotamine-like medications, antidepressants, digitalis drugs, or an MAO inhibitor.

FOOD INTERACTIONS
No known food interactions.

DISEASE INTERACTIONS
Consult your doctor if you have a history of substance abuse (especially cocaine), seizures, brain damage, heart disease, heartbeat irregularities, high blood pressure, anxiety disorders, or a thyroid condition.

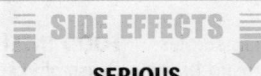

SIDE EFFECTS

SERIOUS
Isoproterenol may become ineffective if used too often, resulting in more-severe breathing difficulty that does not improve. Signs include persistent wheezing, coughing, or shortness of breath; confusion; bluish color to lips or fingernails; inability to speak. Other side effects include chest pain or heaviness; irregular, racing, fluttering, or pounding heartbeat; lightheadedness; fainting; severe weakness; severe headache.

COMMON
Trouble sleeping, dry mouth, sore throat, pinkish color to saliva, nervousness, restlessness.

LESS COMMON
Trembling, sweating, headache, nausea or vomiting, flushing or redness to cheeks or other skin surfaces.

ISOSORBIDE DINITRATE

Available in: Capsules, tablets, chewable tablets, sublingual and buccal forms
Available OTC? No   **As Generic?** Yes
Drug Class: Nitrate

▼ USAGE INFORMATION

WHY IT'S PRESCRIBED
To prevent or relieve attacks of angina (chest pain associated with heart disease).

HOW IT WORKS
Isosorbide dinitrate relaxes the smooth muscle of the blood vessels and increases the supply of blood and oxygen to the heart. It also reduces the heart's workload and demand for oxygen.

▼ DOSAGE GUIDELINES

RANGE AND FREQUENCY
To prevent angina attacks: Extended-release capsules or tablets, 20 to 80 mg every 8 to 12 hours. For short-acting capsules or tablets, 5 to 40 mg, 4 times a day. To treat angina attack: When you feel an attack of angina starting, place a sublingual (under tongue) or buccal (inside the cheek) tablet in your mouth or chew a chewable tablet. If pain is not relieved in 5 minutes with a sublingual tablet, take a second tablet. A third tablet may be used after another 5 minutes. If pain continues to persist, call your doctor or go to the nearest hospital emergency room.

ONSET OF EFFECT
Chewable and sublingual (under the tongue) tablets: 2 to 5 minutes; tablets: 15 to 40 minutes; extended-release capsules and tablets: 30 minutes.

DURATION OF ACTION
1 to 2 hours for chewable tablets, 4 to 6 hours for tablets and capsules, 12 hours for extended-release forms.

DIETARY ADVICE
Take capsules or tablets 30 minutes before or 1 to 2 hours after meals.

STORAGE
Store in a tightly sealed container away from heat and direct light.

MISSED DOSE
Take it as soon as you remember. If it is near the time for the next dose, skip the missed dose and resume your regular dosage schedule as prescribed. Do not double the next dose.

STOPPING THE DRUG
The decision to stop taking the drug should be made by your doctor. Do not stop taking this medicine suddenly. Consult your doctor about reducing the dose gradually.

PROLONGED USE
You should see your doctor regularly if you must take this medicine for an extended period.

▼ PRECAUTIONS

Over 60: Adverse reactions may be more likely and more severe in older patients.

Driving and Hazardous Work: Do not drive or engage in hazardous work until you determine how the medicine affects you.

Alcohol: Avoid alcohol.

Pregnancy: Animal tests have shown adverse effects on the fetus. Human tests have not been done. Before taking isosorbide dinitrate, tell your doctor if you are pregnant or plan to become pregnant.

Breast Feeding: Isosorbide dinitrate may pass into breast milk; caution is advised. Consult your doctor for advice.

Infants and Children: No studies on the use of this medicine in children have been done. Use and dose should be determined by your doctor.

Special Concerns: Use extra care in hot weather or during exercise, or when standing for long periods of time.

OVERDOSE

Symptoms: Bluish fingernails, lips, or palms; extreme dizziness or fainting; unusual weakness, fever, weak and rapid heartbeat; seizures.

What to Do: Call your doctor, emergency medical services (EMS), or the nearest poison control center immediately.

▼ INTERACTIONS

DRUG INTERACTIONS
Do not take isosorbide dinitrate within 24 hours of taking sildenafil citrate. Sildenafil can enhance the action of nitrates (such as isosorbide), causing potentially dangerous decreases in blood pressure. Consult your doctor for specific advice if you are taking other heart medicines, or antihypertensives.

FOOD INTERACTIONS
No known food interactions.

DISEASE INTERACTIONS
Caution is advised when taking isosorbide dinitrate. Consult your doctor if you have any of the following: anemia, glaucoma, a recent head injury or stroke, hyperthyroidism, or a recent heart attack. Use of isosorbide dinitrate may cause complications in patients with severe liver or kidney disease, since these organs work together to remove the medication from the body.

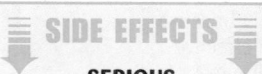

SIDE EFFECTS

SERIOUS
Blurred vision, dry mouth, severe or prolonged headache. Call your doctor immediately.

COMMON
Dizziness or lightheadedness, especially when getting up from a seated or lying position; flushing of the face and neck; unusually rapid pulse or heartbeat; nausea and vomiting; restlessness.

LESS COMMON
Skin rash.

ISOSORBIDE MONONITRATE

Available in: Tablets, extended-release tablets
Available OTC? No   **As Generic?** Yes
Drug Class: Nitrate

▼ USAGE INFORMATION

WHY IT'S PRESCRIBED
To prevent or relieve attacks of angina (chest pain associated with heart disease).

HOW IT WORKS
Isosorbide relaxes the smooth muscle of the blood vessels and increases the supply of blood and oxygen to the heart. It also reduces the heart's workload and demand for oxygen.

▼ DOSAGE GUIDELINES

RANGE AND FREQUENCY
To prevent angina attacks—Tablets: 20 mg, 2 times a day, with doses 7 hours apart. Extended-release tablets: 30 to 240 mg once a day.

ONSET OF EFFECT
60 minutes.

DURATION OF ACTION
Unknown.

DIETARY ADVICE
Take tablets on an empty stomach, at least 30 minutes before or 1 to 2 hours after mealtime.

STORAGE
Store in a tightly sealed container away from heat and direct light.

MISSED DOSE
Take it as soon as you remember. If it is near the time for the next dose, skip the missed dose and resume your regular dosage schedule as prescribed. Do not double the next dose.

STOPPING THE DRUG
The decision to stop taking the drug should be made by your doctor.

PROLONGED USE
You should see your doctor regularly if you take this medicine for an extended period.

▼ PRECAUTIONS

Over 60: Adverse reactions may be more likely and more severe in older patients.

Driving and Hazardous Work: Avoid such activities until you determine how the medicine affects you.

Alcohol: Avoid alcohol.

Pregnancy: Animal tests have shown adverse effects on the fetus. Human tests have not been done. Before taking this drug, tell your doctor if you are pregnant or plan to become pregnant.

Breast Feeding: Isosorbide mononitrate may pass into breast milk; caution is advised. Consult your doctor for specific advice.

Infants and Children: No studies on the use of this medicine in children have been done. Use and dose should be determined by your doctor.

Special Concerns: Do not stop taking this medicine suddenly because it can cause a spasm of the blood vessels in the heart. Consult your doctor about reducing the dose gradually. Use extra care in hot weather or during exercise, or when you must stand for long periods of time. This medicine may cause headaches at the beginning of therapy. Headaches can be treated with aspirin or acetaminophen and usually stop after your body becomes accustomed to the medication. The dose may be reduced temporarily because of headaches. The effectiveness of the medicine may decrease over time; notify your doctor if this occurs.

OVERDOSE
Symptoms: Bluish fingernails, lips or palms; extreme dizziness or fainting; unusual weakness, fever, weak and fast heartbeat, seizures.

What to Do: Call your doctor, emergency medical services (EMS), or the nearest poison control center immediately.

▼ INTERACTIONS

DRUG INTERACTIONS
Do not take isosorbide mononitrate within 24 hours of taking sildenafil citrate. Sildenafil can enhance the action of nitrates (such as isosorbide), causing potentially dangerous decreases in blood pressure. Consult your doctor for specific advice if you are taking other heart medicines, or antihypertensives.

FOOD INTERACTIONS
No known food interactions.

DISEASE INTERACTIONS
Consult your doctor if you have any of the following: anemia, glaucoma, a recent head injury or stroke, an overactive thyroid, or a recent heart attack. Use of isosorbide mononitrate may cause complications in patients with severe liver or kidney disease, since these organs work together to remove the medication from the body.

▤ SIDE EFFECTS ▤

SERIOUS
Blurred vision, dry mouth, severe or prolonged headache. Call your doctor immediately.

COMMON
Dizziness or lightheadedness, especially when rising suddenly to a standing position; flushing of the face and neck; rapid pulse or heartbeat; nausea or vomiting; restlessness.

LESS COMMON
Skin rash.

ISOTRETINOIN

Available in: Capsules
Available OTC? No   **As Generic?** No
Drug Class: Acne drug

▼ USAGE INFORMATION

WHY IT'S PRESCRIBED
Isotretinoin is used to treat severe acne that has not responded adequately to other treatments, such as oral antibiotics. Because of the risk for potentially serious side effects, isotretinoin is prescribed only as a last resort.

HOW IT WORKS
Isotretinoin decreases the size of and interferes with the functioning of structures in the skin called sebaceous glands. These tiny glands, located along hair shafts all over the body's surface, produce sebum—a thick, oily substance that serves as the skin's natural lubricant. Hormonal activity (during pregnancy, puberty, or menstruation, for example) can stimulate overproduction of sebum by the sebaceous glands so that it is secreted faster than it can exit the pores. This may lead to blockage of the hair follicle and result in the sort of skin lesion that characterizes acne. By thinning the composition of sebum and reducing sebum production (as well as causing other, only partly-understood changes), isotretinoin improves acne.

▼ DOSAGE GUIDELINES

RANGE AND FREQUENCY
Adults and teenagers: 0.5 to 1 mg per 2.2 lbs (1 kg) of body weight, in 1 or 2 doses per day, taken for a total period of 20 weeks (average) for complete treatment. Children: Not recommended. Capsules should be swallowed whole; do not open, crush, or chew them.

ONSET OF EFFECT
Variable, usually within several weeks after starting therapy.

DURATION OF ACTION
Most patients have complete and prolonged improvement of acne following therapy with isotretinoin, while others do not. Good results are usually achieved only with the appropriate dose and duration of treatment.

DIETARY ADVICE
Isotretinoin should be taken with food. Maintain your usual food and fluid intake. Do not take vitamin supplements containing vitamin A while taking isotretinoin.

STORAGE
Store in a tightly sealed container away from heat and direct light. Keep away from moisture and extremes in temperature.

MISSED DOSE
Take it as soon as you remember. If it is near the time for the next dose, skip the missed dose and resume your regular dosage schedule. Do not double the next dose.

STOPPING THE DRUG
Take it as prescribed for the full treatment period, even if your acne clears before the scheduled end of therapy. Special exception: Stop taking the medication immediately if you become pregnant or believe that there is a possibility that you might be pregnant.

PROLONGED USE
Therapy with isotretinoin usually lasts 15 to 20 weeks. A second course of therapy may be initiated if the first yields less-than-satisfactory results; a period of two months without using the drug is required between the first and second course of therapy.

▼ PRECAUTIONS

Over 60: It is possible that adverse reactions may be more likely or more severe in older patients.

Driving and Hazardous Work: The use of isotretinoin should not impair your ability to perform such tasks safely during daytime. Exercise caution at night, since the drug may impair night vision.

Alcohol: Simultaneous use of alcohol and isotretinoin may cause an unhealthy rise in triglyceride levels.

Pregnancy: Do not use this medication under any circumstances during pregnancy or within one month of intended pregnancy.

Breast Feeding: Do not use this medication while nursing.

Infants and Children: Not recommended for use by children under age 13.

Special Concerns: Isotretinoin can lead to a severely deformed infant if used during pregnancy, even if only for a very short time. Therefore, this medication should not be used by any woman of childbearing age

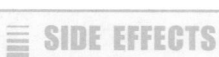

SIDE EFFECTS

SERIOUS
Severe headache that may occur in conjunction with blurred vision, nausea, and vomiting. Discontinue isotretinoin and contact your doctor immediately as this may be an indication of a very serious condition known as "pseudotumor cerebri," marked by increased pressure within the skull, which may damage the brain. Severe central abdominal pain, penetrating through to the back, may indicate acute pancreatitis (inflammation of the pancreas); call your doctor or get to an emergency room immediately.

COMMON
Dry, itching, or cracked skin or lips; easy bruising; nosebleeds; dry, red, or inflamed eyes, difficulty wearing contact lenses; increased susceptibility to sunburn; muscle or joint pain. Consult your doctor if such symptoms persist or interfere with daily activities.

LESS COMMON
Rashes, peeling of skin on palms and soles, nausea, dizziness, poor night vision (night blindness), cataracts, appearance of small spots or shadows passing slowly across the line of vision ("floaters"), thinning hair, weight loss, swelling in the feet and ankles (known as "edema") due to excess fluid retention in the body tissues, mental depression.

who is not using established methods of contraception. If you are a woman starting on isotretinoin, you should first be using two reliable forms of contraception and have a pregnancy test done to exclude the possibility of pregnancy. Then, begin isotretinoin on the third day of the subsequent menstrual cycle to further ensure that you are not pregnant. You must also avoid pregnancy for 1 full month after discontinuing therapy. Your doctor may require you to sign a consent form before prescribing this medication. Once you have started isotretinoin, expect some drying, cracking, peeling, or itching of your skin, as well as dry nasal passages and mouth. About 9 out of every 10 people taking isotretinoin experience these problems. Avoid prolonged exposure to the sun and be sure to use sunblock when spending time outdoors, since isotretinoin may increase your skin's sensitivity to ultraviolet light and thus your risk of sunburn.

OVERDOSE

Symptoms: Headache, vomiting, facial flushing, dry or cracked lips, abdominal pain, dizziness. Such symptoms usually resolve on their own in a short period of time.

What to Do: An overdose is unlikely to be life-threatening. However, if overdose symptoms occur and persist, or if someone accidentally ingests isotretinoin, call your doctor, emergency medical services (EMS), or the nearest poison control center immediately.

▼ INTERACTIONS

DRUG INTERACTIONS

Consult your doctor for specific advice if you are taking etretinate, tretinoin, vitamin A supplements, multivitamins, tetracycline, topical sulfur, or topical benzoyl peroxide.

FOOD INTERACTIONS

No known food interactions. (Isotretinoin should be taken with food.)

DISEASE INTERACTIONS

Consult your doctor if you have any of the following: a history of alcohol abuse, diabetes mellitus, pancreatitis, high blood levels of cholesterol or triglycerides, severe weight problems, vision problems, or severe headaches.

ISOXSUPRINE HYDROCHLORIDE

Available in: Tablets
Available OTC? No   **As Generic?** No
Drug Class: Vasodilator

▼ USAGE INFORMATION

WHY IT'S PRESCRIBED
To treat problems resulting from poor blood circulation to the brain (cerebrovascular insufficiency) or the body (arteriosclerosis obliterans, thromboangiitis obliterans, and Raynaud's disease).

HOW IT WORKS
Isoxsuprine acts upon the smooth muscle tissue surrounding the arteries, causing it to relax, which widens the blood vessels and lowers blood pressure, as well as increasing heart output and improving blood circulation.

▼ DOSAGE GUIDELINES

RANGE AND FREQUENCY
10 to 20 mg, 3 or 4 times a day.

ONSET OF EFFECT
1 hour.

DURATION OF ACTION
Unknown.

DIETARY ADVICE
Isoxsuprine can be taken with meals or milk.

STORAGE
Store in a tightly sealed container in a dry place away from heat and direct light.

MISSED DOSE
Take a missed dose as soon as you remember. If it is near the time for the next dose, skip the missed dose and resume your regular dosage schedule. Do not double the next dose.

STOPPING THE DRUG
Take as prescribed for the full treatment period, even if you begin to feel better before the scheduled end of therapy. The decision to stop taking the drug should be made by your doctor.

PROLONGED USE
You should see your doctor regularly for tests and examinations if you take this drug for a prolonged period.

▼ PRECAUTIONS

Over 60: There is no specific information comparing use of isoxsuprine in older patients with use in other age groups. However, older patients may be more likely to experience an increased sensitivity to cold temperatures.

Driving and Hazardous Work: Do not drive or engage in hazardous work until you determine how the medicine affects you.

Alcohol: Alcohol should be avoided while taking this medication.

Pregnancy: Isoxsuprine has not been shown to cause birth defects. Given prior to delivery, it may cause low blood sugar, bowel problems, low blood pressure, and other problems in a newborn baby.

Breast Feeding: Isoxsuprine has not been shown to cause problems in nursing babies.

Infants and Children: Isoxsuprine is generally not prescribed for infants and children.

Special Concerns: You should avoid sudden changes in position to reduce the possibility of dizziness, lightheadedness, and falling. You should not smoke cigarettes if you take isoxsuprine. Taking blood pressure measurements in sitting, lying, and standing positions is recommended to detect the likelihood of episodes of low blood pressure in patients receiving isoxsuprine. Be sure to tell your doctor if you have had any unusual or allergic reaction to isoxsuprine in the past. Also tell your doctor if you are allergic to any other substances, such as foods, dyes, and preservatives.

OVERDOSE
Symptoms: Headache, vomiting, flushed face, abdominal pain, dizziness, loss of muscle coordination.

What to Do: Call your doctor, emergency medical services (EMS), or the nearest poison control center immediately.

▼ INTERACTIONS

DRUG INTERACTIONS
Consult your doctor for specific advice if you are taking any prescription or over-the-counter medicine. In some cases your doctor may want to change the dose or have you take other precautions.

FOOD INTERACTIONS
No known food interactions.

DISEASE INTERACTIONS
Caution is advised when taking isoxsuprine. Consult your doctor if you have any of the following: angina, bleeding problems, glaucoma, hardening of the arteries, pulmonary hypertension, low blood pressure, a recent heart attack, or a recent stroke.

≡ SIDE EFFECTS ≡

SERIOUS
Chest pain, dizziness, or faintness; rapid heartbeat; skin rash; shortness of breath; continuing nausea and repeated vomiting. Such side effects are rare but potentially serious; if they do occur, call your doctor immediately.

COMMON
There are no common side effects associated with the use of isoxsuprine.

LESS COMMON
Nausea, vomiting.

ISRADIPINE

Available in: Capsules
Available OTC? No   **As Generic?** No
Drug Class: Calcium channel blocker

▼ USAGE INFORMATION

WHY IT'S PRESCRIBED
To treat high blood pressure.

HOW IT WORKS
Isradipine interferes with the movement of calcium into heart muscle cells and the smooth muscle cells in the walls of the arteries. This action relaxes blood vessels (causing them to widen), which lowers blood pressure, increases the blood supply to the heart, and decreases the heart's overall workload.

▼ DOSAGE GUIDELINES

RANGE AND FREQUENCY
2.5 mg twice a day to start. The dose may be increased.

ONSET OF EFFECT
Within 20 minutes.

DURATION OF ACTION
More than 12 hours.

DIETARY ADVICE
No special restrictions.

STORAGE
Store in a tightly sealed container away from heat and direct light. Keep away from moisture and extremes in temperature.

MISSED DOSE
Take it as soon as you remember. If it is near the time for the next dose, skip the missed dose and resume your regular dosage schedule. Do not double the next dose.

STOPPING THE DRUG
Do not stop taking this drug suddenly, as this may cause potentially serious health problems. If therapy is to be discontinued, dosage should be reduced gradually, according to doctor's instructions.

PROLONGED USE
See your doctor regularly for examinations and tests if you take this medicine for a prolonged period. Remember that isradipine controls high blood pressure but does not cure it. Lifelong therapy may be necessary.

▼ PRECAUTIONS

Over 60: Adverse reactions may be more likely and more severe in older patients.

Driving and Hazardous Work: Do not drive or engage in hazardous work until you determine how the medicine affects you.

Alcohol: Avoid alcohol.

Pregnancy: In animal studies, large doses of isradipine have caused birth defects. Human studies have not been done. Before you take isradipine, tell your doctor if you are currently pregnant or plan to become pregnant.

Breast Feeding: Isradipine may pass into breast milk; caution is advised. Consult your doctor for advice.

Infants and Children: Safety and effectiveness of isradipine have not been determined for young patients.

Special Concerns: In addition to taking isradipine, be sure to follow all special instructions on weight control and diet. Your doctor will tell you which specific factors are most important for you. Check with your doctor before changing your diet.

OVERDOSE
Symptoms: Dizziness, slurred speech, nausea, weakness, drowsiness, and confusion.

What to Do: Call your doctor, emergency medical services (EMS), or the nearest poison control center immediately.

▼ INTERACTIONS

DRUG INTERACTIONS
Consult your physician for specific advice if you are taking acetazolamide, ampho-tericin B, corticosteroids, dichlorphenamide, diuretics, methazolamide, beta-blockers, carbamazepine, cyclosporine, procainamide, quinidine, digitalis, disopyramide or the following eye medicines: betaxolol, levobunolol, metipranolol, or timolol.

FOOD INTERACTIONS
Avoid foods high in sodium.

DISEASE INTERACTIONS
Caution is advised when taking isradipine. Consult your doctor if you have any of the following: abnormal heart rhythm (cardiac arrhythmia), or other disorders of the heart and blood vessels, mental depression, or Parkinson's disease. Use of isradipine may cause complications in patients with liver or kidney disease, since these organs work together to remove the medication from the body.

≡ SIDE EFFECTS ≡

SERIOUS
Breathing difficulty, coughing, or wheezing; irregular or pounding heartbeat; chest pain; fainting. Call your doctor immediately.

COMMON
Headache; dizziness; skin flushing and feeling of warmth; swelling in the feet, ankles, or calves; palpitations.

LESS COMMON
Constipation or diarrhea, nausea, unusual fatigue and weakness, skin rash, increased urination.

ITRACONAZOLE

Available in: Capsules, oral solution
Available OTC? No　**As Generic?** Yes
Drug Class: Antifungal

▼ USAGE INFORMATION

WHY IT'S PRESCRIBED
To treat serious fungal infections occurring in the lungs and other parts of the body. These infections may occur in patients who do not have other illnesses, although they frequently occur in patients with weakened immune systems. Itraconazole is sometimes prescribed for fungal infections that are limited only to the nails.

HOW IT WORKS
Itraconazole prevents fungal organisms from producing vital substances required for growth and function. This drug is effective only for infections caused by fungal organisms. It will not work against bacterial or viral infections.

▼ DOSAGE GUIDELINES

RANGE AND FREQUENCY
Capsules— Adults and teenagers 16 and older: 200 to 400 mg, taken once daily. Children under age 16: Consult your pediatrician for proper dosage. Oral solution— Adults and teenagers: 100 to 200 mg once a day for days or weeks, depending on the condition being treated. Children: Consult your pediatrician. Swish the solution vigorously in your mouth for several seconds before swallowing.

ONSET OF EFFECT
Unknown.

DURATION OF ACTION
Unknown.

DIETARY ADVICE
Take capsules with food, but do not take the oral solution with food. Maintain your usual food and fluid intake. Patients with compromised immune systems are often weakened by their illness, by medications, or by other treatments, and may be unable to consume adequate amounts of nutritious food. Use liquid supplements if necessary.

STORAGE
Store in a tightly sealed container away from heat, moisture, and direct light.

MISSED DOSE
Take it as soon as you remember. This will help keep a constant level of medication in your system. If it is near the time for the next dose, skip the missed dose and resume your regular dosage schedule. Do not double the next dose.

STOPPING THE DRUG
Take it as prescribed for the full treatment period, even if you begin to feel better before the scheduled end of therapy. The decision to stop taking the drug should be made by your doctor. Gradual reduction of the dose may be necessary if you have been taking this medicine for a long time.

PROLONGED USE
Therapy with this medication may require months. Prolonged use may increase the risk of adverse effects.

▼ PRECAUTIONS

Over 60: Adverse reactions may be more likely and more severe in older patients.

Driving and Hazardous Work: Do not drive or engage in hazardous work until you determine how the medicine affects you.

Alcohol: Avoid alcohol throughout therapy and for two days afterwards.

Pregnancy: Adequate studies of itraconazole use during pregnancy have not been done. Consult your doctor for specific advice if you are or plan to become pregnant.

Breast Feeding: This drug passes into breast milk; avoid use while nursing.

Infants and Children: Itraconazole is not recommended for use by children under the age of 16.

Special Concerns: Women should use effective contraception to prevent pregnancy while taking this medication. Continue these measures for at least 2 months following the end of therapy. The capsules and the oral solution should not be used interchangeably.

OVERDOSE
Symptoms: An overdose with itraconazole is unlikely.

What to Do: Emergency instructions not applicable.

▼ INTERACTIONS

DRUG INTERACTIONS
While taking itraconazole, do not take astemizole, cisapride, or terfenadine. Serious side effects involving the heart may result. You should not take medications containing alcohol, such as cough syrups, elixirs, and tonics. Consult your doctor for specific advice if you are taking antacids, anticholinergics, histamine H2-blockers, omeprazole, oral antidiabetics, sucralfate, carbamazepine, cyclosporine, isoniazid, didanosine, digoxin, phenytoin, rifampin, or warfarin. If you are taking an antacid, take it at least 2 hours after taking itraconazole.

FOOD INTERACTIONS
No known food interactions.

DISEASE INTERACTIONS
Consult your doctor if you have any of the following conditions: liver or kidney disease, low levels or absence of stomach acid, or a history of alcohol abuse.

≡ SIDE EFFECTS ≡

SERIOUS
Skin rash or itching, fever or chills. Call your doctor right away.

COMMON
No common side effects have been reported.

LESS COMMON
Diarrhea, nausea, vomiting, constipation, dizziness, headache, redness or flushing of skin.

KAOLIN WITH PECTIN

Available in: Oral suspension
Available OTC? Yes   **As Generic?** Yes
Drug Class: Antidiarrheal

▼ USAGE INFORMATION

WHY IT'S PRESCRIBED
To treat diarrhea.

HOW IT WORKS
Kaolin with pectin absorbs fluids and binds to and removes bacteria and toxins from the digestive tract.

▼ DOSAGE GUIDELINES

RANGE AND FREQUENCY
Adults: 4 to 8 tablespoons (60 to 120 ml) after each loose bowel movement. Children age 12 and older: 3 to 4 tbsp (45 to 60 ml) after each loose bowel movement. Children ages 6 to 12: 2 to 4 tbsp (30 to 60 ml) after each loose bowel movement. Children ages 3 to 6: 1 to 2 tbsp (15 to 30 ml) after each loose bowel movement.

ONSET OF EFFECT
Unknown.

DURATION OF ACTION
Unknown.

DIETARY ADVICE
A mild diet is recommended when recovering from diarrhea. Bananas, rice, applesauce, and plain toast are good choices. Be sure to get plenty of fluids.

SIDE EFFECTS

SERIOUS
No serious side effects have been reported.

COMMON
No common side effects have been reported.

LESS COMMON
Constipation.

STORAGE
Store in a tightly sealed container away from heat, moisture, and direct light.

MISSED DOSE
Take it as soon as you remember. If it is nearly time for another dose, skip the missed dose. Do not double the next dose.

STOPPING THE DRUG
Do not use this drug for more than 2 days without consulting your doctor.

PROLONGED USE
This drug is not intended for prolonged use. Consult your doctor if diarrhea continues for more than 2 days.

▼ PRECAUTIONS

Over 60: Adverse reactions associated with diarrhea may be more severe in older patients. They should be sure to consume enough liquids to replace body fluids lost because of diarrhea.

Driving and Hazardous Work: The use of kaolin with pectin should not impair your ability to perform such tasks safely.

Alcohol: Avoid alcohol.

Pregnancy: It is not absorbed into the body and is not expected to cause problems during pregnancy.

Breast Feeding: It is not absorbed into the body and is not expected to cause problems during breast feeding.

Infants and Children: Kaolin with pectin should be used in children under the age of 3 only under the supervision of a doctor.

Special Concerns: In addition to taking medicine for diarrhea, it is important to replace the fluid lost by your body and to eat a proper diet. During the first 24 hours, drink plenty of caffeine-free clear liquids like water, broth, ginger ale, and decaffeinated tea. During the second 24 hours you may eat bland foods such as applesauce, bread, crackers, and oatmeal. Avoid caffeine, fried or spicy foods, bran, candy, fruits, and vegetables. They can make your condition worse.

OVERDOSE
Symptoms: Constipation.

What to Do: An overdose of kaolin with pectin is unlikely to be life-threatening. However, if someone takes a much larger dose than prescribed, call your doctor, emergency medical services (EMS), or the nearest poison control center immediately.

▼ INTERACTIONS

DRUG INTERACTIONS
Consult your doctor for specific advice if you are taking anticholinergics, antidyskinet-ics, digitalis drugs, lincomycins, loxapine, phenothiazines, thioxanthenes, or any other oral medication. Do not take any medication within 2 to 3 hours of taking kaolin with pectin.

FOOD INTERACTIONS
Fruits, fried or spicy foods, bran, candy, and caffeine-containing beverages can make diarrhea worse.

DISEASE INTERACTIONS
Caution is advised when taking kaolin with pectin. Consult your doctor if the diarrhea is suspected to be caused by parasites or dysentery.

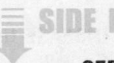

KETOCONAZOLE ORAL

Available in: Tablets
Available OTC? No   **As Generic?** No
Drug Class: Antifungal

▼ USAGE INFORMATION

WHY IT'S PRESCRIBED
To treat serious fungal infections occurring in the lungs and other parts of the body. Ketoconazole is used to treat fungal infections of the skin, such as tinea corporis (ringworm), tinea cruris (jock itch), tinea pedis (athlete's foot), and pityriasis versicolor ("sun fungus," a condition characterized by fine scaly patches of varying shapes, sizes, and colors), that are severe or are unresponsive to griseofulvin.

HOW IT WORKS
Ketoconazole prevents fungal organisms from producing vital substances required for growth and function. This drug is effective only for infections caused by fungal organisms. It will not work for bacterial or viral infections.

▼ DOSAGE GUIDELINES

RANGE AND FREQUENCY
Adults and teenagers: 200 to 400 mg once a day. Children over age 2: 3.3 to 6.6 mg per 2.2 lbs of body weight once a day. Treatment may last from 1 week to 6 months, depending on the type of infection being treated.

ONSET OF EFFECT
Unknown.

DURATION OF ACTION
Unknown.

DIETARY ADVICE
Take it with food to reduce stomach upset. Tablets may be crushed and mixed with a beverage or food to reduce the bitter taste.

STORAGE
Store in a tightly sealed container away from heat, moisture, and direct light.

MISSED DOSE
Take it as soon as you remember. This will help keep a constant level of medication in your system. If it is near the time for the next dose, skip the missed dose and resume your regular dosage schedule. Do not double the next dose.

STOPPING THE DRUG
Take it as prescribed for the full treatment period, even if you begin to feel better before the scheduled end of therapy. The decision to stop taking the drug should be made by your doctor. Dose should be reduced gradually if you have used the drug for a long time.

PROLONGED USE
Months of therapy may be necessary. Prolonged use increases the risk of adverse effects and may interfere with the body's synthesis of steroid hormones, which may cause erectile dysfunction in men and cessation of menstrual periods in women.

▼ PRECAUTIONS

Over 60: Adverse reactions may be more likely and more severe.

Driving and Hazardous Work: Avoid such activities until you determine how the medication affects you.

Alcohol: Avoid alcohol.

Pregnancy: Adequate studies of ketoconazole use during pregnancy have not been done. Consult your doctor for advice if you are pregnant or planning to become pregnant.

Breast Feeding: Ketoconazole passes into breast milk; caution is advised. Consult your doctor for specific advice.

Infants and Children: Not recommended for use by children under 2 years.

Special Concerns: Ketoconazole may make your eyes more sensitive to sunlight. If this occurs, avoid exposure to bright light and wear sunglasses. For full effectiveness, ketoconazole should be taken at the same time every day.

OVERDOSE
Symptoms: An overdose is unlikely to occur.

What to Do: Emergency instructions not applicable.

▼ INTERACTIONS

DRUG INTERACTIONS
While taking ketoconazole, do not take astemizole, cisapride, or terfenadine. Serious side effects involving the heart may result. Do not take medications containing alcohol, such as cough syrups, elixirs, and tonics. Consult your doctor for advice if you are taking cyclosporine, isoniazid, didanosine, phenytoin, rifampin, or warfarin. If you are taking antacids, anticholinergics, histamine H2-blockers, omeprazole, or sucralfate, take them at least 2 hours after taking ketoconazole.

FOOD INTERACTIONS
No known food interactions.

DISEASE INTERACTIONS
Caution is advised when taking ketoconazole. Consult your doctor if you have any of the following: history of alcohol abuse, decreased amount of stomach acid, liver disease, or kidney disease. Use of ketoconazole can cause complications in patients with liver or kidney disease, since these organs work together to remove the medication from the body. If you have no stomach acid or a decreased amount of stomach acid, your doctor may prescribe a special solution.

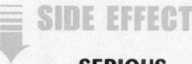 **SIDE EFFECTS**

SERIOUS
Skin rash, itching, fever, chills. Call your doctor right away.

COMMON
No common side effects have been reported.

LESS COMMON
Diarrhea, nausea, vomiting, constipation, dizziness, headache, redness or flushing of skin.

KETOCONAZOLE TOPICAL

Available in: Cream, shampoo
Available OTC? Yes   **As Generic?** Yes
Drug Class: Topical antifungal

▼ USAGE INFORMATION

WHY IT'S PRESCRIBED
Ketoconazole is used to treat fungal infections of the skin. These infections include tinea pedis (athlete's foot), tinea corporis (ringworm), tinea cruris (jock itch), yeast infections of the skin, seborrheic dermatitis, and others.

HOW IT WORKS
Ketoconazole prevents fungal organisms from manufacturing vital substances required for growth and function.

▼ DOSAGE GUIDELINES

RANGE AND FREQUENCY
Adults, for tinea and yeast: Apply once daily to affected skin. Treatment generally requires 2 to 6 weeks. Adults, for seborrheic dermatitis: Apply two times a day to affected skin. Treatment generally requires 4 weeks. Children: Consult your pediatrician.

ONSET OF EFFECT
Ketoconazole begins killing susceptible fungi shortly after contact. The effects may not be noticeable for several days or weeks.

DURATION OF ACTION
Unknown.

DIETARY ADVICE
Maintain your usual food and fluid intake. Increase fluid intake in hot weather, during exercise, or if you have a fever or diarrhea.

STORAGE
Store in a tightly sealed container away from heat and direct light.

MISSED DOSE
Apply it as soon as you remember. If it is near the time for the next dose, skip the missed dose and resume your regular dosage schedule. Do not double the next dose or apply an excessively thick film of topical medication to compensate for a missed application.

STOPPING THE DRUG
Apply ketoconazole as prescribed for the full treatment period, even if you notice marked improvement before the scheduled end of therapy.

PROLONGED USE
Therapy with this medication should not exceed 4 weeks.

▼ PRECAUTIONS

Over 60: Adverse reactions may be more likely and more severe in older patients.

Driving and Hazardous Work: The use of ketoconazole cream should not impair your ability to perform such tasks safely.

Alcohol: No special precautions are necessary.

Pregnancy: Avoid or discontinue use of ketoconazole if you are pregnant or trying to become pregnant.

Breast Feeding: Ketoconazole may pass into breast milk; avoid or discontinue usage while nursing. Consult your doctor for specific advice.

Infants and Children: Not recommended for use by young children.

Special Concerns: Avoid contact with eyes. Wash hands thoroughly after application. Tell your doctor if your condition has not improved within a few days of starting ketoconazole. As with any other antifungal, ketoconazole is useful only against organisms that are vulnerable to its effects. Therefore, it is important to tell your doctor if your condition has not improved— or has worsened—within a few days of starting ketoconazole. The particular organism causing your illness may be resistant to this medication.

OVERDOSE
Symptoms: No specific ones have been reported.

What to Do: An overdose of ketoconazole is unlikely to be life-threatening. However, if someone applies a much larger dose than prescribed or ingests the medication, call your doctor, emergency medical services (EMS), or the nearest poison control center.

▼ INTERACTIONS

DRUG INTERACTIONS
No specific drug interactions are known as of this writing. If you are concerned whether a prescription or over-the-counter medication you are taking may interact with ketoconazole, consult your physician or pharmacist for current information.

FOOD INTERACTIONS
No known food interactions.

DISEASE INTERACTIONS
Consult your physician if you have had previous allergies or an undesirable reaction to any other topical medication.

 SIDE EFFECTS

SERIOUS
Blistering or ulceration of the skin; blistering of the lips, nose, and mouth.

COMMON
Brief burning, itching, or irritation after application of cream; peeling.

LESS COMMON
Severe burning, itching, swelling, increased redness, or any discomfort at the application site not present prior to therapy (as a result of allergic reaction).

KETOPROFEN

Available in: Tablets and capsules (also extended-release forms), rectal suppositories
Available OTC? Yes   **As Generic?** Yes
Drug Class: Nonsteroidal anti-inflammatory drug (NSAID)

▼ USAGE INFORMATION

WHY IT'S PRESCRIBED
To treat mild to moderate pain and inflammation caused by tendinitis, arthritis, bursitis, gout, soft tissue injuries, migraine and other vascular headaches, menstrual cramps, and other conditions. When patients fail to respond to one NSAID, another may be tried. The greatest effectiveness often requires trial and error of several different NSAIDs.

HOW IT WORKS
NSAIDs work by interfering with the formation of prostaglandins, naturally occurring substances in the body that cause inflammation and make nerves more sensitive to pain impulses. NSAIDs also have other modes of action that are less well understood.

▼ DOSAGE GUIDELINES

RANGE AND FREQUENCY
Adults— Tablets or capsules: 50 mg, 4 times a day, or 75 mg, 3 times a day. Extended-release tablets or capsules: 200 mg once a day. Suppositories: 50 to 100 mg inserted twice a day (morning and evening). Sometimes, suppositories may be used only at night by people who take an oral dose during the day. Maximum dosage for all forms is 300 mg per day.

ONSET OF EFFECT
1 to 2 hours.

DURATION OF ACTION
3 to 4 hours.

DIETARY ADVICE
Take oral forms with food.

STORAGE
Store in a tightly sealed container away from heat, moisture, and direct light.

MISSED DOSE
Take it as soon as you remember. If it is near the time for the next dose, skip the missed dose and resume your regular dosage schedule. Do not double the next dose.

STOPPING THE DRUG
If taking this drug by prescription, do not stop without consulting your doctor.

PROLONGED USE
Prolonged use can cause gastrointestinal problems, including ulceration and bleeding, kidney dysfunction, and liver inflammation. Consult your doctor about the need for medical examinations and laboratory studies.

▼ PRECAUTIONS

Over 60: Because of the potentially greater consequences of gastrointestinal side effects, the dose of NSAIDs for older patients, especially those over age 70, is often cut in half.

Driving and Hazardous Work: Do not drive or engage in hazardous work until you determine how the medicine affects you.

Alcohol: Avoid alcohol when using this medication because it increases the risk of stomach irritation.

Pregnancy: Do not use ketoprofen while pregnant.

Breast Feeding: Ketoprofen passes into breast milk; avoid use while nursing.

Infants and Children: Ketoprofen may be used in exceptional circumstances; consult your doctor.

Special Concerns: Because NSAIDs can interfere with blood coagulation, this drug should be stopped at least 3 days prior to any surgery.

OVERDOSE
Symptoms: Severe nausea, vomiting, headache, confusion, seizures.

What to Do: Call your doctor, emergency medical services (EMS), or the nearest poison control center immediately.

▼ INTERACTIONS

DRUG INTERACTIONS
Do not take this drug with aspirin or any other NSAIDs without your doctor's approval. In addition, consult your doctor if you are taking antihypertensives, steroids, anticoagulants, antibiotics, itraconazole or ketoconazole, plicamycin, penicillamine, valproic acid, phenytoin, cyclosporine, digitalis drugs, lithium, methotrexate, probenecid, triamterene, or zidovudine.

FOOD INTERACTIONS
No known food interactions.

DISEASE INTERACTIONS
Consult your doctor if you have any of the following: bleeding problems, inflammation or ulcers of the stomach and intestines, diabetes mellitus, systemic lupus erythematosus (SLE, lupus), anemia, asthma, epilepsy, Parkinson's disease, kidney stones, or a history of heart disease or alcohol abuse. Use of ketoprofen may cause complications in patients with liver or kidney disease, since these organs work together to remove the medication from the body.

SIDE EFFECTS

SERIOUS
Shortness of breath or wheezing, with or without swelling of legs or other signs of heart failure; chest pain; peptic ulcer disease with vomiting of blood; black, tarry stools; decreasing kidney function. Call your doctor immediately.

COMMON
Nausea, vomiting, heartburn, diarrhea, constipation, headache, dizziness, sleepiness.

LESS COMMON
Ulcers or sores in mouth, depression, rashes or blistering of skin, ringing sound in the ears, unusual tingling or numbness of the hands or feet, seizures, blurred vision. Also elevated potassium levels, decreased blood counts; such problems can be detected by your doctor.

KETOROLAC TROMETHAMINE OPHTHALMIC

Available in: Ophthalmic solution
Available OTC? No   **As Generic?** No
Drug Class: Nonsteroidal anti-inflammatory drug (NSAID)

▼ USAGE INFORMATION

WHY IT'S PRESCRIBED
For short-term therapy of eye itching caused by seasonal allergic conjunctivitis. It is also used to treat inflammation and eye problems that may occur after cataract surgery.

HOW IT WORKS
Ophthalmic ketorolac inhibits the release of substances that stimulate inflammation and cause pain in eye tissues.

▼ DOSAGE GUIDELINES

RANGE AND FREQUENCY
Adults: 1 drop in each eye 4 times a day. Children: Consult your pediatrician.

ONSET OF EFFECT
Unknown.

DURATION OF ACTION
Unknown.

DIETARY ADVICE
No special restrictions.

STORAGE
Store this medication in a tightly sealed container away from heat, moisture, and direct light. Do not refrigerate or allow it to freeze.

MISSED DOSE
Apply it as soon as you remember. If it is near the time for the next dose, skip the missed dose and resume your regular dosage schedule. Do not double the next dose.

STOPPING THE DRUG
Use it as prescribed for the full treatment period, even if you feel better before the scheduled end of therapy.

PROLONGED USE
See your doctor regularly for tests and examinations if you must use this drug for a prolonged period.

▼ PRECAUTIONS

Over 60: Adverse reactions may be more likely and more severe in older patients.

Driving and Hazardous Work: Do not drive or engage in hazardous work until you determine how the medicine affects your vision.

Alcohol: Avoid alcohol.

Pregnancy: Adequate human studies have not been completed. Before taking ophthalmic ketorolac, tell your doctor if you are pregnant or plan to become pregnant.

Breast Feeding: Ophthalmic ketorolac may pass into breast milk; caution is advised. Consult your doctor for specific advice.

Infants and Children: Use and dosage for infants and children must be determined by your doctor.

Special Concerns: To use the eye drops, first wash your hands. Tilt your head back. Gently apply pressure to the inside corner of the eyelid and with the index finger of the same hand, pull downward on the lower eyelid to make a space. Drop the medicine into this space and close your eye. Apply pressure for 1 or 2 minutes while keeping the eye closed without blinking. Then wash your hands again. Make sure the tip of the dropper does not touch your eye, finger, or any other surface. If your symptoms do not improve or if they become worse, check with your doctor. Ophthalmic ketorolac may cause problems in patients who wear soft contact lenses. Your physician may want you to stop wearing the lenses while you take the medicine.

OVERDOSE
Symptoms: No specific ones have been reported.

What to Do: An overdose of ophthalmic ketorolac is unlikely to be life-threatening. However, if someone applies a much larger dose of the drug than prescribed or accidentally ingests the medicine, call your doctor, emergency medical services (EMS), or the nearest poison control center.

▼ INTERACTIONS

DRUG INTERACTIONS
Consult your doctor for specific advice if you are taking aspirin or another salicylate, diflunisal, etodolac, fenoprofen, floctafenine, flurbiprofen, ibuprofen, indomethacin, ketoprofen, oral ketorolac, meclofenamate, mefenamic acid, nabumetone, naproxen, oxyphenbutazone, phenylbutazone, piroxicam, sulindac, suprofen, tenoxicam, tiaprofenic acid, tolmetin, or zomepirac.

FOOD INTERACTIONS
No known food interactions.

DISEASE INTERACTIONS
Caution is advised when taking ophthalmic ketorolac. Consult your doctor if you have hemophilia or any other bleeding problem.

≣ SIDE EFFECTS ≣

SERIOUS
Rarely, ophthalmic ketorolac tromethamine will cause bleeding in the eye, redness or swelling of the eye or eyelid not present before the start of therapy, or tearing or itching of the eye. Call your doctor immediately.

COMMON
Mild and temporary burning or stinging of eyes after application, eye infection.

LESS COMMON
There are no less-common side effects associated with ophthalmic ketorolac.

KETOROLAC TROMETHAMINE SYSTEMIC

Available in: Tablets, injection
Available OTC? No   **As Generic?** Yes
Drug Class: Nonsteroidal anti-inflammatory drug (NSAID)

▼ USAGE INFORMATION

WHY IT'S PRESCRIBED
To treat moderate to severe pain and inflammation, usually following surgery.

HOW IT WORKS
NSAIDs work by interfering with the action of prostaglandins, naturally occurring substances that cause inflammation and make nerves more sensitive to pain impulses. NSAIDs also have other modes of action that are less well understood.

▼ DOSAGE GUIDELINES

RANGE AND FREQUENCY
For acute pain— Initial adult dose is usually by injection, which may be followed (if necessary) by injections or tablets. Injection: 30 mg into a vein every 6 hours. Some people may receive one 60 mg dose into a muscle. The dose should not exceed 120 mg per 24-hour period. Tablets: 10 mg, 4 times a day, taken every 4 to 6 hours.

Your doctor may recommend a different dose, though it should not exceed 40 mg per day. For pain in children— Consult your pediatrician.

ONSET OF EFFECT
Into a vein: Immediate. Into a muscle: Within 10 minutes. Tablets: 30 to 60 minutes.

DURATION OF ACTION
6 to 8 hours.

DIETARY ADVICE
Tablets should be taken with food; maintain your usual food and fluid intake.

STORAGE
Not applicable for injection form; it is administered only at a health care facility. Store tablets in a tightly sealed container away from heat and direct light.

MISSED DOSE
Take tablets as soon as you remember. If it is near the time for the next dose, skip the missed dose and resume your regular dosage schedule. Do not double the next dose.

STOPPING THE DRUG
Take it as prescribed for the full treatment period. Ask your doctor about stopping the drug if you are feeling better before the scheduled end of therapy.

PROLONGED USE
Therapy generally does not last more than 5 days. Use beyond that period may cause serious side effects.

▼ PRECAUTIONS

Over 60: Because of the potentially greater consequences of gastrointestinal side effects, the dose of NSAIDs for older patients, especially those over age 70, is often cut in half.

Driving and Hazardous Work: Avoid such activities until you determine how the medicine affects you.

Alcohol: Avoid alcohol.

Pregnancy: Avoid or discontinue ketorolac if you are pregnant or are planning to become pregnant.

Breast Feeding: Ketorolac passes into breast milk; avoid use while nursing.

Infants and Children: May be used in exceptional circumstances; consult your doctor.

OVERDOSE
Symptoms: Nausea, vomiting, severe headache, confusion, seizures.

What to Do: Call your doctor, emergency medical services (EMS), or the nearest poison control center immediately.

▼ INTERACTIONS

DRUG INTERACTIONS
Do not take this drug with aspirin or any other NSAIDs. In addition, consult your doctor if you are taking acetaminophen, anticoagulants, enoxaparin, lithium, methotrexate, diuretics, beta-blockers, sulfinpyrazone, valproic acid, or warfarin.

FOOD INTERACTIONS
No known food interactions.

DISEASE INTERACTIONS
Caution is advised when taking ketorolac. Consult your doctor if you have any of the following: nasal polyps, severe hives, any stomach or intestinal disorder, high blood pressure, a blood coagulation defect, or a history of heart disease. Use of ketorolac may cause complications in patients with liver or kidney disease, since these organs work together to remove the medication from the body.

 SIDE EFFECTS

SERIOUS
Gastrointestinal bleeding, causing dark or bloody stools or vomiting; severe high blood pressure, causing headache and blurred vision; prolonged bleeding from a cut; burnlike rash. Call your doctor immediately. This drug may cause breathing difficulty or a severe allergic reaction in persons who are sensitive to aspirin, especially those with aspirin-induced nasal polyps or asthma.

COMMON
Stomach distress.

LESS COMMON
Drowsiness, diarrhea, confusion, ringing in ears, sensitivity to sunlight, water retention, hives, headache.

KETOTIFEN FUMARATE

Available in: Ophthalmic solution
Available OTC? No   **As Generic?** No
Drug Class: Histamine (H1) blocker

▼ USAGE INFORMATION

WHY IT'S PRESCRIBED
For short-term therapy of eye itching caused by seasonal allergic conjunctivitis (inflammation of the mucous membranes that line the inner surface of the eyelids and whites of the eyes).

HOW IT WORKS
Ketotifen blocks the effects of histamine, a naturally occurring substance within the body that causes swelling, itching, sneezing, watery eyes, hives, and other symptoms associated with allergic reactions.

▼ DOSAGE GUIDELINES

RANGE AND FREQUENCY
Instill 1 drop in the affected eye(s) every 8 to 12 hours.

ONSET OF EFFECT
Unknown.

DURATION OF ACTION
Unknown.

DIETARY ADVICE
Ketotifen can be used without regard to diet.

STORAGE
Store in a tightly sealed container away from heat, moisture, and direct light. Do not allow it to freeze.

MISSED DOSE
Apply it as soon as you remember. If it is near the time for the next dose, skip the missed dose and resume your regular dosage schedule. Do not double the next dose.

STOPPING THE DRUG
You may stop using ketotifen whenever you choose.

PROLONGED USE
Ketotifen is prescribed for short-term use only.

▼ PRECAUTIONS

Over 60: No special problems are expected.

Driving and Hazardous Work: Avoid such activities until you determine how the medicine affects you.

Alcohol: No special precautions are necessary.

Pregnancy: No adequate human studies have been done. Before taking ketotifen, tell your doctor if you are pregnant or plan to become pregnant.

Breast Feeding: Ketotifen may pass into breast milk; caution is advised. Consult your doctor for specific advice.

Infants and Children: Not recommended for use by children under 3 years of age.

Special Concerns: To use the eye drops, first wash your hands. Tilt your head back. Gently apply pressure to the inside corner of the eyelid and with the index finger of the same hand, pull downward on the lower eyelid to make a space. Drop the medicine into this space and close your eye. Apply pressure for 1 or 2 minutes while keeping the eye closed without blinking. Then wash your hands again. Make sure the tip of the dropper does not touch your eye, finger, or any other surface. You should not wear a contact lens if your eye is red. Ketotifen should not be used to treat contact-lens-related irritation. If you wear soft contact lenses and your eyes are not red, wait at least 10 minutes after instilling the drops before inserting your contact lenses.

OVERDOSE
Symptoms: No specific ones have been reported.

What to Do: An overdose with ketotifen is unlikely to be life-threatening. However, if someone accidentally ingests the medicine, seek emergency medical attention immediately.

▼ INTERACTIONS

DRUG INTERACTIONS
None reported.

FOOD INTERACTIONS
None reported.

DISEASE INTERACTIONS
None reported.

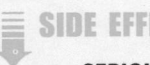

▼ SIDE EFFECTS

SERIOUS
No serious side effects are associated with ketotifen.

COMMON
Headache, runny nose.

LESS COMMON
Allergic reaction, burning or stinging of the eye, tearing, eye dryness, eye pain, itching, corneal inflammation, pupil dilation, light sensitivity, rash, flulike symptoms, sore throat.

LABETALOL HYDROCHLORIDE

Available in: Tablets (Injection is for hospital use only.)
Available OTC? No **As Generic?** Yes
Drug Class: Beta-blocker

▼ USAGE INFORMATION

WHY IT'S PRESCRIBED
To treat severe high blood pressure (hypertension).

HOW IT WORKS
Labetalol hydrochloride is a beta-blocker with alpha-blocker activity. Such drugs work by preventing—or blocking—nerve impulses from exerting an accelerating or intensifying effect on specific parts of the body, especially the blood vessels and heart. Unlike other beta-blockers, this drug does not significantly slow the heart rate.

▼ DOSAGE GUIDELINES

RANGE AND FREQUENCY
Usual adult dose: 100 mg twice daily, 6 to 12 hours apart, increased to a maintenance dose of 200 to 400 mg twice daily. Maximum dose: 800 mg, 3 times daily.

ONSET OF EFFECT
Within 20 minutes.

DURATION OF ACTION
12 to 24 hours.

DIETARY ADVICE
Follow your doctor's dietary restrictions, such as a low-salt or low-fat diet, to improve control over high blood pressure and heart disease. Take the tablets with food.

STORAGE
Store in a tightly sealed container away from heat and direct light.

MISSED DOSE
Take it as soon as you remember. If it is within 8 hours of your next dose, skip the missed dose, and go back to your regular schedule. Do not double the next dose.

STOPPING THE DRUG
Do not stop this drug suddenly, as this may lead to angina or a heart attack in patients with advanced heart disease. Slow reduction of the dose over a period of 2 to 3 weeks is advised. Do not stop taking the drug or make any changes in dosage without consulting your doctor.

PROLONGED USE
Lifelong therapy may be necessary. See your doctor regularly for examinations and tests if you must take this medication for a prolonged period.

▼ PRECAUTIONS

Over 60: Adverse reactions may be more likely and more severe in older patients.

Driving and Hazardous Work: Do not drive or engage in hazardous work until you determine how the medicine affects you.

Alcohol: Drink in careful moderation if at all. Alcohol may interact with the drug and cause a dangerous drop in blood pressure.

Pregnancy: Discuss with your doctor the relative risks and benefits of using this drug while pregnant.

Breast Feeding: Adverse effects in infants have not been reported. Consult your doctor for specific advice.

Infants and Children: No special problems.

Special Concerns: Get up slowly from a sitting or lying position to avoid dizziness or lightheadedness, especially when you first start taking the drug or if the dosage has been increased.

OVERDOSE
Symptoms: Unusually slow or rapid heartbeat, severe dizziness or fainting, poor circulation in the hands (bluish skin), breathing difficulty, seizures.

What to Do: Call your doctor, emergency medical services (EMS), or the nearest poison control center immediately.

▼ INTERACTIONS

DRUG INTERACTIONS
Consult your physician for specific advice if you are taking amphetamines, oral antidiabetic agents, asthma medication (such as aminophylline or theophylline), calcium channel blockers, clonidine, guanabenz, halothane, allergy shots, insulin, MAO inhibitors, reserpine, other beta-blockers, any over-the-counter medicine, sodium bicarbonate injection.

FOOD INTERACTIONS
None reported.

DISEASE INTERACTIONS
Labetalol hydrochloride should be used with caution in people with diabetes, especially insulin-dependent diabetes, since the drug may mask symptoms of hypoglycemia. Consult your doctor if you have allergies or asthma; heart or blood vessel disease (including congestive heart failure and peripheral vascular disease); hyperthyroidism; irregular (slow) heartbeat; myasthenia gravis; psoriasis; respiratory problems, such as bronchitis or emphysema; kidney or liver disease; or a history of depression.

SIDE EFFECTS

SERIOUS
Shortness of breath, wheezing; chest pain or tightness; swelling of the ankles, feet, and lower legs; mental depression. If you experience such symptoms, stop taking the drug and call your doctor immediately.

COMMON
Dizziness or lightheadedness, especially when rising suddenly to a standing position; decreased sexual ability; unusual fatigue, weakness, or drowsiness; insomnia; scalp tingling, especially at the beginning of treatment.

LESS COMMON
Changes in taste; itching, numbness, or tingling; vivid dreams or nightmares; nausea or vomiting; irregular or slow heartbeat (50 beats per minute or less).

LACTULOSE

BRAND NAMES

Cholac, Chronulac, Constilac, Constulose, Duphalac, Enulose, Evalose, Heptalac, Portalac

Available in: Syrup
Available OTC? No   **As Generic?** Yes
Drug Class: Hyperosmotic laxative

▼ USAGE INFORMATION

WHY IT'S PRESCRIBED
For long-term treatment of chronic constipation. It is also sometimes used for treatment of severe liver disease.

HOW IT WORKS
Lactulose draws water into the bowel to help loosen and soften the stool and stimulate bowel activity.

▼ DOSAGE GUIDELINES

RANGE AND FREQUENCY
For constipation: 15 to 30 ml once a day. The dose may be increased to 60 ml once a day, if needed. For severe liver disease: 30 to 45 ml, 3 or 4 times a day until 2 or 3 soft stools are produced daily.

ONSET OF EFFECT
24 to 48 hours.

DURATION OF ACTION
Up to 24 hours.

DIETARY ADVICE
Take it with a full glass (8 oz) of water or fruit juice, or 2 glasses of water if your doctor directs. You should not use lactulose if you are on a low-galactose diet.

STORAGE
Store in a tightly sealed container away from heat, moisture, and direct light. Do not allow to freeze.

MISSED DOSE
Take it as soon as you remember. If it is near the time for the next dose, skip the missed dose and resume your regular dosage schedule. Do not double the next dose.

STOPPING THE DRUG
Take it as prescribed for the full treatment period. However, you may stop taking the drug if you are feeling better before the scheduled end of therapy.

PROLONGED USE
Do not take lactulose for more than 1 week unless you are under a doctor's supervision. Prolonged use may cause laxative dependence.

▼ PRECAUTIONS

Over 60: No special problems are expected in older patients.

Driving and Hazardous Work:
The use of lactulose should not impair your ability to perform such tasks safely.

Alcohol: No special precautions are necessary.

Pregnancy: Caution is advised. Discuss with your doctor the relative risks and benefits of using this drug while pregnant.

Breast Feeding: Lactulose may pass into breast milk; caution is advised. Consult your doctor for advice.

Infants and Children: Lactulose is not recommended for use by children under the age of 6 unless prescribed by your doctor.

Special Concerns: Excessive use of lactulose or any laxative in teenagers may indicate an eating disorder such as anorexia nervosa or bulimia nervosa. Consult your doctor if you observe such behavior. If you have a sudden change in bowel function or habits that lasts more than 2 weeks, consult your doctor.

OVERDOSE
Symptoms: Diarrhea, severe abdominal cramps.

What to Do: An overdose of lactulose is unlikely to be life-threatening. However, if someone takes a much larger dose than prescribed, call your doctor, emergency medical services (EMS), or the nearest poison control center.

▼ INTERACTIONS

DRUG INTERACTIONS
Consult your doctor for specific advice if you are taking other laxatives, antacids, antibiotics, anticoagulants, digitalis drugs, oral tetracyclines, sodium polystyrene sulfonate, ciprofloxacin, or potassium supplements.

FOOD INTERACTIONS
If you are on a low-calorie, low-salt, or low-sugar diet, check with your doctor before taking lactulose.

DISEASE INTERACTIONS
Caution is advised when taking lactulose. Consult your doctor if you have symptoms of appendicitis or an inflamed bowel (abdominal pain, cramps, soreness, bloating, nausea, and vomiting), diabetes mellitus, difficulty swallowing, heart disease or blood pressure disorder, intestinal problems, or kidney disease.

SIDE EFFECTS

SERIOUS
Unusual weakness, confusion, muscle cramps, dizziness or lightheadedness, irregular heartbeat.

COMMON
Diarrhea, gas, intestinal cramps, increased thirst.

LESS COMMON
No less-common side effects are associated with lactulose.

LAMIVUDINE (3TC)

Available in: Solution, tablets
Available OTC? No **As Generic?** No
Drug Class: Antiviral

▼ USAGE INFORMATION

WHY IT'S PRESCRIBED
To treat HIV (human immun-odeficiency virus) infection in combination with zidovudine (AZT) or other antiretroviral agents. While not a cure for HIV infection, these drugs may suppress the replication of the virus and delay the progression of the disease.

HOW IT WORKS
Lamivudine interferes with the activity of enzymes needed for the replication of DNA in viral cells, thus preventing HIV from reproducing. HIV that has become resistant to lamivudine may be less likely to become resistant to zidovudine.

▼ DOSAGE GUIDELINES

RANGE AND FREQUENCY
Adults and teenagers weigh-ing 110 lbs or more: 150 mg, 2 times a day. Adults weighing less than 110 lbs: 2 mg per 2.2 lbs (1 kg) of body weight 2 times a day.

Children 3 months to 12 years: 4 mg per 2.2 lbs of body weight 2 times a day, up to 150 mg per dose. In all cases lamivudine should be taken with other anti-retroviral agents.

ONSET OF EFFECT
Unknown. With most anti-retroviral drugs, an early response can be seen within the first few days of therapy, but the maximum effect may take 12 to 16 weeks.

DURATION OF ACTION
Unknown. Effects of the drug may be prolonged if lamivudine is used in combi-nation with other effective drugs and the virus is maxi-mally suppressed.

DIETARY ADVICE
Can be taken with or without food. Be sure to drink plenty of fluids.

STORAGE
Store in a tightly sealed con-tainer away from heat and direct light.

MISSED DOSE
Take it as soon as you remember. If it is near the time for the next dose, skip the missed dose and resume your regular dosage schedule. Do not double the next dose. It is especially important to take lamivudine on schedule, to assure constant, proper blood levels of the drug.

STOPPING THE DRUG
Take it as prescribed for the full treatment period, even if you begin to feel better.

PROLONGED USE
See your doctor regularly for tests and examinations if you must take this medicine for a prolonged period.

▼ PRECAUTIONS

Over 60: No special studies have been done on older patients. A lower dose may be warranted, especially if liver or kidney function is impaired.

Driving and Hazardous Work: Avoid such activities until you determine how the medicine affects you.

Alcohol: Avoid alcohol if liver function is impaired.

Pregnancy: In animal studies, lamivudine has been shown to cause birth defects. Neverthe-less, lamivudine is increasingly used in combination with other antiretroviral drugs to treat pregnant HIV-infected women.

Breast Feeding: Women infected with HIV should not breast feed, so as to avoid transmitting the virus to an uninfected child.

Infants and Children: Adverse reactions may be more likely and more severe in young patients.

Special Concerns: If you are taking the solution, use a spe-cial measuring spoon or other precisely marked scoop to dispense the proper dose. The risk of transmitting the HIV to other persons is not reduced by lamivudine. Be sure to take precautionary measures.

OVERDOSE
Symptoms: No cases of over-dose have been reported. The symptoms would likely include diarrhea or abdominal cramps.

What to Do: An overdose of lamivudine is unlikely to occur. Nonetheless, if you have any reason to suspect an overdose, call your doctor, emergency medical services (EMS), or the nearest poison control center as soon as possible.

▼ INTERACTIONS

DRUG INTERACTIONS
Consult your doctor for spe-cific advice if you are taking any other prescription or over-the-counter medication.

FOOD INTERACTIONS
No known food interactions.

DISEASE INTERACTIONS
Consult your doctor if you have any other medical con-dition. Use of lamivudine may cause complications in patients with impaired liver or kidney function, since these organs work together to remove the medication from the body.

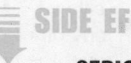
SIDE EFFECTS

SERIOUS
Severe stomach or abdominal pain; nausea; vomiting; unusual fatigue; fever; chills; sore throat; numbness, burn-ing, tingling, or pain in hands, arms, legs or feet; breathing difficulty; itching; hives; skin rash; swelling of face, mouth, lips, throat, or tongue. Call your doctor immediately if any of these side effects arise.

COMMON
No common side effects are associated with lamivudine.

LESS COMMON
Mild to moderate abdominal pain, diarrhea, dizziness, cough, headache, mild nausea or vomiting, insomnia, loss of hair.

LAMIVUDINE/ZIDOVUDINE

Available in: Tablets
Available OTC? No   **As Generic?** No
Drug Class: Antiviral

▼ USAGE INFORMATION

WHY IT'S PRESCRIBED
To treat HIV (human immu-nodeficiency virus) infection. While not a cure for HIV, this combination of lamivudine (3TC) and zidovudine (AZT) may suppress the replication of the virus and delay the progression of the disease.

HOW IT WORKS
This drug combination inter-feres with the activity of enzymes needed for the repli-cation of DNA in viral cells, thus preventing HIV from reproducing.

▼ DOSAGE GUIDELINES

RANGE AND FREQUENCY
Adults and teenagers: 1 tablet (containing 150 mg of lamivu-dine and 300 mg of zidovu-dine) twice a day. Children: Should not be taken by chil-dren because it is a fixed-dose combination that cannot be adjusted.

ONSET OF EFFECT
Unknown. With most anti-retroviral drugs, an early response can be seen within the first few days of therapy, but the maximum effect may take 12 to 16 weeks.

DURATION OF ACTION
Unknown. Effects of the drug combination may be pro-longed if the virus is maxi-mally suppressed.

DIETARY ADVICE
Can be taken with or without food. Be sure to drink plenty of fluids.

STORAGE
Store in a tightly sealed con-tainer away from heat, mois-ture, and direct light.

MISSED DOSE
Take it as soon as you remem-ber. If it is near the time for the next dose, skip the missed dose and resume your regular dosage schedule. Do not dou-ble the next dose. It is espe-cially important to take this medication on schedule, to assure constant, proper blood levels of the drug.

STOPPING THE DRUG
The decision to stop taking the drug should be made in consultation with your doctor.

PROLONGED USE
See your doctor regularly for tests and examinations as long as you take this medication.

▼ PRECAUTIONS

Over 60: No special studies have been done on older patients. A lower dose may be warranted, especially if liver or kidney function is impaired.

Driving and Hazardous Work: Use of this drug com-bination should not diminish your ability to perform such tasks safely.

Alcohol: Avoid alcohol if liver function is impaired.

Pregnancy: Adequate human studies have not been done. Discuss with your doctor the relative risks and benefits of using this drug while pregnant.

Breast Feeding: Women infected with HIV should not breast-feed, so as to avoid transmitting the virus to an uninfected child.

Infants and Children: Not recommended for children under the age of 12.

Special Concerns: Use of this drug combination does not eliminate the risk of passing the AIDS virus (HIV) to other persons. Be sure to take all appropriate preventive mea-sures. This medication should not be used in patients with low body weight.

OVERDOSE
Symptoms: No cases of over-dose with this combination have been reported. How-ever, cases of overdose have been reported for zidovudine taken alone (see Zidovudine).

What to Do: If you suspect an overdose or if someone takes a much larger dose than prescribed, call your doctor, emergency medical services (EMS), or the nearest poison control center immediately.

▼ INTERACTIONS

DRUG INTERACTIONS
Consult your doctor for spe-cific advice if you are taking amphotericin B (by injection), anticancer agents, thyroid drugs, azathioprine, chloram-phenicol, colchicine, cyclophosphamide, flucyto-sine, ganciclovir, interferon, mercaptopurine, methotrex-ate, plicamycin, clarithro-mycin, or probenecid. Also consult your doctor for spe-cific advice if you are taking any other prescription or over-the-counter medication.

FOOD INTERACTIONS
No known food interactions.

DISEASE INTERACTIONS
Caution is advised when tak-ing this drug combination. Consult your doctor if you have anemia or another blood problem. Use of this drug is not recommended in patients with impaired kidney function or risk factors for liver disease.

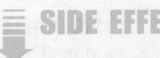
SIDE EFFECTS

SERIOUS
Severe stomach or abdominal pain; anemia (low red blood cell count) causing paleness, fatigue, or shortness of breath; fever; chills; sore throat. Also numbness, burning, tingling, or pain in the hands, arms, legs or feet; breathing difficulty; itching; hives; skin rash; swelling of the face, mouth, lips, throat, or tongue. Call your doctor immediately.

COMMON
Headaches, nausea and vomiting, insomnia, stomach upset, loss of appetite, diarrhea, dizziness, cough.

LESS COMMON
Mild to moderate abdominal pain or cramping, muscle aches and pain, hepatitis (liver inflammation, which may cause yellowish discoloration of skin and eyes), joint pain, loss of hair.

LAMOTRIGINE

BRAND NAME

Lamictal

Available in: Tablets, chewable tablets
Available OTC? No   **As Generic?** No
Drug Class: Anticonvulsant

▼ USAGE INFORMATION

WHY IT'S PRESCRIBED
To control certain kinds of seizures in the treatment of epilepsy. Lamotrigine is generally taken in conjunction with other anticonvulsants.

HOW IT WORKS
Lamotrigine acts on the central nervous system to control the number and severity of seizures. It is thought to depress the activity of certain parts of the brain and suppress the abnormal firing of neurons that causes seizures.

▼ DOSAGE GUIDELINES

RANGE AND FREQUENCY
Adults: 200 to 900 mg a day, in 2 divided doses. Some patients may require higher doses. A low dose is used to start; the dose is gradually increased by your doctor. The increase in dose is very slow if you are also taking valproic acid (Depakene, Depakote).

Lamotrigine is generally not recommended for use in children younger than age 16.

ONSET OF EFFECT
Several hours.

DURATION OF ACTION
Maximum effectiveness lasts 24 hours or longer; effectiveness then gradually decreases.

DIETARY ADVICE
Take it with food to minimize the likelihood of stomach upset. Chewable tablets can be taken with a small amount of water or diluted fruit juice.

STORAGE
Store in a tightly sealed container away from heat, moisture, and direct light.

MISSED DOSE
Take it as soon as you remember. If it is near the time for the next dose, skip the missed dose and resume your regular dosage schedule. Do not double the next dose,

unless advised to do so by your doctor.

STOPPING THE DRUG
Never stop taking this drug abruptly because seizures may ensue. The dose is typically tapered over a period of weeks under your doctor's supervision.

PROLONGED USE
See your doctor regularly for tests if you must take this drug for an extended period.

▼ PRECAUTIONS

Over 60: Adverse reactions may be more likely in older patients. Lower dosages may be warranted.

Driving and Hazardous Work: This drug may cause drowsiness or dizziness. Do not drive or engage in hazardous work until you determine how it affects you.

Alcohol: May contribute to excessive drowsiness.

Pregnancy: Anticonvulsants have been associated with an increased risk of birth defects, though adequate studies of lamotrigine have not been done. However, seizures during pregnancy can also increase the risks to the fetus. Discuss with your doctor the potential risks and benefits of using this drug during pregnancy. Folate supplementation is advised beginning 1 to 2 months before conception, continuing throughout pregnancy.

Breast Feeding: Lamotrigine passes into breast milk, although at low levels. Cau-

tion is advised; consult your doctor for specific advice.

Infants and Children: Because side effects are more common and may be more severe in young patients, lamotrigine is generally not recommended.

Special Concerns: Your doctor may want you to wear a medical bracelet or carry an identification card saying that you are taking this drug.

OVERDOSE
Symptoms: Severe clumsiness and unsteadiness; severe dizziness or drowsiness; extremely slurred speech; severe, unusual, rapid, side-to-side, or rolling eye movements; rapid heartbeat; loss of consciousness; dry mouth.

What to Do: Call your doctor, emergency medical services (EMS), or the nearest poison control center immediately.

▼ INTERACTIONS

DRUG INTERACTIONS
Lamotrigine can interact with many other drugs, including other anticonvulsants (carbamazepine, phenobarbital, phenytoin, primidone, valproic acid), as well as acetaminophen, methotrexate, pyrimethamine, and trimethoprim.

FOOD INTERACTIONS
No known food interactions.

DISEASE INTERACTIONS
Special caution is advised in those with kidney or liver disease or folate deficiency.

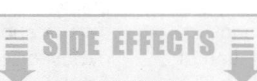

SIDE EFFECTS

SERIOUS
Fever, sore throat, swollen glands, red or purple pointlike rash on the skin or mucous membranes, blistering or peeling skin lesion, weakness, confusion, lethargy, or seizures may be a sign of a potentially fatal blood reaction or other complication. Call your doctor immediately.

COMMON
Dizziness, blurred or double vision, clumsiness or incoordination, drowsiness, nausea, vomiting, headache.

LESS COMMON
Indigestion, runny nose, loss of strength, insomnia, depression, mood changes, trembling or shaking, slurred speech. Numerous additional side effects are associated with the use of this drug; consult your doctor if you are concerned about any adverse or unusual reactions.

LANSOPRAZOLE

Available in: Delayed-release capsules
Available OTC? No   **As Generic?** No
Drug Class: Antacid/proton pump inhibitor

▼ USAGE INFORMATION

WHY IT'S PRESCRIBED
To treat stomach and duodenal (intestinal) ulcers, gastroesophageal reflux disease (chronic heartburn caused by the backwash of stomach acid into the esophagus), and conditions that cause increased stomach acid secretion, such as Zollinger-Ellison syndrome. Lansoprazole is also prescribed in conjunction with the antibiotics amoxicillin and clarithromycin to eradicate the bacterium H. pylori and thus prevent the recurrence of duodenal ulcers caused by this bacterium.

HOW IT WORKS
Lansoprazole blocks the action of a specific enzyme in the cells that line the stomach, thus decreasing the production of stomach acid. Reduction of stomach acid creates a more favorable environment for the eradication of H. pylori and promotes the healing of ulcers.

▼ DOSAGE GUIDELINES

RANGE AND FREQUENCY
Prevacid– To treat duodenal ulcers: Initial dose is 15 mg once a day; it may later be increased. To treat gastroesophageal reflux disease: 15 mg once a day for up to 8 weeks. To treat other conditions: Initial dose is 60 mg once a day; it may be increased. Treatment usually runs 4 to 8 weeks. A second course of treatment may be necessary. For Zollinger-Ellison syndrome: Initial dose is 60 mg once a day; it may be increased. Prevpac– To prevent duodenal ulcers: 30 mg lansoprazole, 1 gram amoxicillin, and 500 mg clarithromycin every 12 hours for 14 days.

ONSET OF EFFECT
1 to 3 hours.

DURATION OF ACTION
More than 24 hours.

DIETARY ADVICE
The drug is best taken 30 minutes or more before a meal, preferably breakfast.

STORAGE
Store in a tightly sealed container away from heat, moisture, and direct light.

MISSED DOSE
Take it as soon as you remember. However, if it is near the time for the next dose, skip the missed dose and resume your regular dosage schedule. Do not double the next dose.

STOPPING THE DRUG
Take as prescribed for the full treatment period, even if your symptoms improve before the scheduled end of therapy.

PROLONGED USE
See your doctor regularly for tests and examinations if you must take this drug for a prolonged period. Lansoprazole should not be used indefinitely as maintenance therapy for duodenal ulcer or esophagitis; other treatments are recommended.

▼ PRECAUTIONS

Over 60: No special problems are expected.

Driving and Hazardous Work: Avoid such activities until you determine how the drug affects you. Taking lansoprazole may be a disqualification for piloting aircraft.

Alcohol: Avoid alcohol throughout the duration of therapy with this drug.

Pregnancy: Adequate human studies have not been done. Before taking lansoprazole, tell your doctor if you are pregnant or plan to become pregnant.

Breast Feeding: Lansoprazole may pass into breast milk; caution is advised. Consult your doctor for advice.

Infants and Children: Use and dose for anyone under 18 should be determined by your doctor or pediatrician.

Special Concerns: Tell any doctor or dentist whom you see for treatment that you are taking lansoprazole. Do not chew the capsules. If you have trouble swallowing them, you may open them and sprinkle the contents on one tablespoon of applesauce, cottage cheese, yogurt, or similar food. If your doctor directs, you may take an antacid along with lansoprazole.

OVERDOSE
Symptoms: No cases of overdose have been reported.

What to Do: An overdose is unlikely to be life-threatening. However, if someone takes a much larger dose than prescribed, call your doctor, emergency medical services (EMS), or the nearest poison control center immediately.

▼ INTERACTIONS

DRUG INTERACTIONS
Consult your doctor for specific advice if you are taking ampicillin, sucralfate, iron salts or supplements, cyclosporine, diazepam, disulfiram, ketoconazole, phenytoin, or theophylline.

FOOD INTERACTIONS
No significant food interactions have been reported.

DISEASE INTERACTIONS
Caution is advised when taking lansoprazole. Consult your doctor if you have liver disease, since it may increase the risk of side effects.

SIDE EFFECTS

SERIOUS
No serious side effects have been reported.

COMMON
Diarrhea, itching or rash, headache, dizziness.

LESS COMMON
Abdominal or stomach pain, nausea, increase or decrease in appetite, anxiety, flulike symptoms, constipation, coughing, mental depression, muscle pain.

LATANOPROST

Available in: Ophthalmic solution
Available OTC? No **As Generic?** No
Drug Class: Antiglaucoma agent

▼ USAGE INFORMATION

WHY IT'S PRESCRIBED
To treat glaucoma.

HOW IT WORKS
Glaucoma, a sight-threatening disorder, occurs when the aqueous humor (fluid inside the eye) cannot drain properly, causing increased pressure within the eyeball (intraocular pressure). Increased eye pressure can damage the optic nerve and lead to a gradually progressive loss of vision. Latanoprost promotes outflow of aqueous humor, thereby reducing intraocular pressure.

▼ DOSAGE GUIDELINES

RANGE AND FREQUENCY
1 drop of latanoprost in each eye once daily in the evening.

ONSET OF EFFECT
3 to 4 hours.

DURATION OF ACTION
24 hours or more.

DIETARY ADVICE
This medication can be used without regard to diet.

STORAGE
Store in a tightly sealed container away from heat, moisture, and direct light. Do not allow the medicine to freeze.

MISSED DOSE
Apply it as soon as you remember. If it is near the time for the next dose, skip the missed dose and resume your regular dosage schedule. Do not double the next dose.

STOPPING THE DRUG
The decision to stop using the drug should be made by your doctor.

PROLONGED USE
See your doctor regularly for tests and examinations if you must take this drug for a prolonged period.

▼ PRECAUTIONS

Over 60: No special problems are expected.

Driving and Hazardous Work: Do not drive or engage in hazardous work until you determine how the medicine affects your vision.

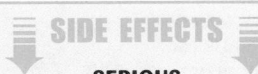

≣ SIDE EFFECTS ≣

SERIOUS
Chest pain, difficulty breathing. Call your doctor right away.

COMMON
Blurred vision, burning and stinging of the eye, sensation of something in the eye, increased brown pigmentation of the iris, eye redness.

LESS COMMON
Dry eye, excessive tearing, eye pain, lid crusting, swollen eyelid, eyelid pain or discomfort, sensitivity to light, upper respiratory tract infection, double vision, pain in the chest and back.

Alcohol: No special precautions are necessary.

Pregnancy: Latanoprost has not caused birth defects in animals. Human studies have not been done. Before you take latanoprost, tell your doctor if you are pregnant or plan to become pregnant.

Breast Feeding: Latanoprost may pass into breast milk; caution is advised. Consult your doctor for advice.

Infants and Children: The safety and effectiveness of latanoprost in infants and children have not been established.

Special Concerns: To use the eye drops, first wash your hands. Tilt your head back. Gently apply pressure to the inside corner of the eyelid and with the index finger of the same hand, pull downward on the lower eyelid to make a space. Drop the medicine into this space and close your eye. Apply pressure for 1 or 2 minutes while keeping the eye closed without blinking. Then wash your hands again. Make sure the tip of the dropper does not touch your eye, finger, or any other surface. Latanoprost may make your eyes more sensitive to sunlight. If this occurs, wear sunglasses or avoid exposure to bright light as necessary. Latanoprost may change eye color, increasing the brown pigment in the iris over a period of months or years. The color change may be permanent. Latanoprost contains ingredients that may damage contact lenses. Contact lenses should be removed 15 minutes before applying the medication and reinserted 15 minutes or more afterward.

OVERDOSE
Symptoms: No specific ones have been reported.

What to Do: An overdose of latanoprost is unlikely to be life-threatening. If a large volume enters the eyes, flush with water. If someone accidentally ingests the medication, call your doctor, emergency medical services (EMS), or the nearest poison control center.

▼ INTERACTIONS

DRUG INTERACTIONS
Other drugs may interact with latanoprost. Consult your doctor for specific advice if you are taking any other prescription or over-the-counter medication. If you are using other ophthalmic medications to reduce fluid pressure in the eye, administer them at least 5 minutes apart.

FOOD INTERACTIONS
No known food interactions.

DISEASE INTERACTIONS
Use of latanoprost may cause complications in patients with liver or kidney disease, since these organs work together to remove the drug from the body.

LEFLUNOMIDE

Available in: Tablets
Available OTC? No   **As Generic?** No
Drug Class: Antirheumatic

▼ USAGE INFORMATION

WHY IT'S PRESCRIBED
To reduce the signs and symptoms of moderate to severe active rheumatoid arthritis. Leflunomide is prescribed for patients who have not responded adequately to one or more antirheumatic medications.

HOW IT WORKS
Leflunomide appears to suppress overactivity of the immune system, which is believed to cause rheumatoid arthritis. It also appears to reduce inflammation.

▼ DOSAGE GUIDELINES

RANGE AND FREQUENCY
Adults: To start, 100 mg a day for 3 days. Maintenance dose: 20 mg a day. Dose may be lowered by your doctor to 10 mg a day, if necessary.

ONSET OF EFFECT
Unknown.

DURATION OF ACTION
Unknown.

DIETARY ADVICE
Maintain your usual food and fluid intake.

STORAGE
Store in a tightly sealed container away from heat, moisture, and direct light.

MISSED DOSE
If you miss a dose on one day, do not double the dose the next day.

STOPPING THE DRUG
Take it as prescribed for the full treatment period, even if you begin to feel better.

PROLONGED USE
See your doctor regularly for liver function tests while taking this medication.

▼ PRECAUTIONS

Over 60: No special problems are expected.

Driving and Hazardous Work: The use of leflunomide should not impair your ability to perform such tasks safely.

Alcohol: Drink only in moderation, if at all.

Pregnancy: Leflunomide can cause serious birth defects. Do not take the drug if you are pregnant. Before you start taking leflunomide, you must have had a negative pregnancy test within the previous 2 weeks. An effective method of birth control should be used while you are taking leflunomide. If you suspect you are pregnant, stop taking the drug immediately and consult your doctor.

Breast Feeding: It is unknown whether leflunomide passes into breast milk. However, do not take the drug while nursing. Consult your doctor for advice.

Infants and Children: Safety and effectiveness have not been established for children under age 18.

Special Concerns: Upon completion of treatment, it is recommended that you follow a specific procedure to lower the levels of leflunomide in the blood. Take 8 grams cholestyramine 3 times a day for 11 days (does not have to be 11 consecutive days, unless there is a need to reduce levels rapidly). Your doctor will conduct two tests (each at least 2 weeks apart) to monitor blood levels of the medication. Without following this procedure, it may take up to 2 years to reach undetectable blood levels of the drug.

OVERDOSE
Symptoms: No cases of overdose have been reported.

What to Do: If someone takes a much larger dose than prescribed, call your doctor, emergency medical services (EMS), or the nearest poison control center immediately.

▼ INTERACTIONS

DRUG INTERACTIONS
The following drugs may interact with leflunomide. Consult your doctor for specific advice if you are taking: methotrexate, rifampin, cholestyramine, charcoal, or tolbutamide.

FOOD INTERACTIONS
No known food interactions.

DISEASE INTERACTIONS
Do not take leflunomide if you have liver disease. Caution is advised in patients with kidney disease. Consult your doctor for advice.

 SIDE EFFECTS

SERIOUS
Liver toxicity may occur; it can be detected by your doctor with blood tests; it may be discerned by the patient if it causes jaundice, characterized by yellowish discoloration of the skin and eyes. Call your doctor immediately.

COMMON
Diarrhea, hair loss, rash.

LESS COMMON
Allergic reaction, back pain, bronchitis, pneumonia, nasal congestion, itching.

LETROZOLE

Available in: Tablets
Available OTC? No **As Generic?** No
Drug Class: Antiestrogen; antineoplastic (anticancer) agent

▼ USAGE INFORMATION

WHY IT'S PRESCRIBED
Letrozole is used for the treatment of advanced breast cancer. It is usually prescribed for postmenopausal women whose breast cancer has progressed following treatment with other antiestrogens, such as tamoxifen.

HOW IT WORKS
The growth of some breast tumors is stimulated by estrogens. After the menopause, women's ovaries produce little estrogen, but androgens formed in the adrenals can be converted to estrogen. Letrozole blocks the enzyme that carries out this conversion. Thus, letrozole is not directly toxic to cancer cells but rather inhibits the growth of some breast tumors by reducing blood levels of estrogen.

▼ DOSAGE GUIDELINES

RANGE AND FREQUENCY
2.5 mg once a day.

ONSET OF EFFECT
Unknown.

DURATION OF ACTION
Unknown.

DIETARY ADVICE
Letrozole can be taken without regard to meals. Maintain adequate food and fluid intake, since calorie, protein, and vitamin needs increase in patients with cancer.

STORAGE
Store in a tightly sealed container away from heat, moisture, and direct light.

MISSED DOSE
Letrozole is prescribed for once-daily use only. If you are unable to take this medication on a particular day, resume your regularly scheduled dose the following day. Do not double the next dose.

STOPPING THE DRUG
This drug is used to treat a chronic condition. You may need to use it for an extended period, and you should take it exactly as prescribed throughout the course of treatment. The decision to stop the drug must be made in consultation with your doctor. Do not stop taking letrozole on your own.

PROLONGED USE
There is no standard duration of therapy with letrozole, although you can expect to remain on it for several weeks in order to determine if it is effective. Your doctor will decide whether your response to the drug is satisfactory or not, and will recommend continuation or discontinuation of therapy.

▼ PRECAUTIONS

Over 60: No special problems are expected.

Driving and Hazardous Work: Use of this medication should not impair your ability to engage in such tasks safely.

Alcohol: No special precautions are necessary.

Pregnancy: Letrozole must not be used in pregnant women. Although letrozole is not generally prescribed for premenopausal women, it is important that patients be sure they are not pregnant before starting treatment with this drug.

Breast Feeding: Use of this drug is not recommended while nursing; the benefits must clearly outweigh potential risks. Consult your doctor for specific advice.

Infants and Children: Use of letrozole is not approved for infants and children.

Special Concerns: Patients with cancer are very often weakened by their illness, by poor nutrition, and by the effects of chemotherapy, radiation, and surgery. Such

patients are more likely to experience undesirable side effects of a medication. In addition, these side effects may be more pronounced. Follow all medication directions carefully.

OVERDOSE
Symptoms: No cases of overdose have been reported.

What to Do: An overdose is unlikely; however, if you have any reason to suspect that one has occurred, call emergency medical services (EMS) to receive evaluation and treatment in the closest emergency facility.

▼ INTERACTIONS

DRUG INTERACTIONS
No significant drug interactions are associated with the use of letrozole.

FOOD INTERACTIONS
No known food interactions.

DISEASE INTERACTIONS
No significant interactions.

 SIDE EFFECTS

SERIOUS
No serious side effects have been reported.

COMMON
Fatigue, nausea and vomiting, muscle and joint pain, headache, shortness of breath.

LESS COMMON
Chest pain, edema (swelling around the feet and ankles), weakness, increase in weight, high blood pressure, constipation, diarrhea, abdominal pain, loss of appetite, indigestion, viral infection, drowsiness or dizziness, cough, hot flashes, rash, itching.

LEUCOVORIN CALCIUM

Available in: Tablets, injection
Available OTC? No   **As Generic?** Yes
Drug Class: Folic acid derivative

▼ USAGE INFORMATION

WHY IT'S PRESCRIBED
To serve as an antidote to the toxic effects of high doses of methotrexate (a cancer drug) and other drugs that antagonize (block the action of) the essential nutrient folic acid. Leucovorin is also used in conjunction with another drug, fluorouracil, to treat some kinds of colon cancer. It may also be used to treat some forms of anemia.

HOW IT WORKS
Folic acid is needed by healthy cells in the body to grow, survive, and multiply. Leucovorin is a derivative of folic acid and thus prevents some of the damage done to healthy cells by therapy with methotrexate and other drugs that deplete folic acid in the body. Because leucovorin acts in the body the same way as folic acid, it is useful against anemia due to folic acid deficiency.

▼ DOSAGE GUIDELINES

RANGE AND FREQUENCY
To prevent drug side effects: 10 mg per square meter of body surface every 6 hours for 10 doses. For colon cancer, there are 3 accepted regimens: (a) 200 mg per square meter of body surface daily for 5 days; (b) 20 mg per square meter of body surface daily for 5 days; or (c) 500 mg per square meter of body surface in a single dose. In each regimen leucovorin is followed by appropriate doses of fluorouracil. The drug combination is cycled depending on the regimen. To treat megaloblastic anemia caused by congenital enzyme deficiency: 3 to 6 mg to start, then 1 mg per day. To treat folate-deficient megaloblastic anemia: Up to 1 mg of leucovorin daily; duration of treatment depends upon the response of the individual.

ONSET OF EFFECT
From 5 to 20 minutes after injection; 20 to 30 minutes after oral ingestion.

DURATION OF ACTION
From 3 to 6 hours.

DIETARY ADVICE
Leucovorin can be given between meals. The doses must be evenly spaced, day and night.

STORAGE
Store in a tightly sealed container away from heat and direct light.

MISSED DOSE
As soon as you remember, check with your doctor to learn if you should take an extra dose. Do not take more medicine without consulting your doctor. Resume your regular dosage schedule as soon as possible.

STOPPING THE DRUG
The decision to stop taking the drug should be made by your doctor.

PROLONGED USE
See your doctor regularly for tests and examinations if you take this medication for a prolonged period.

▼ PRECAUTIONS

Over 60: There is no specific information comparing use of leucovorin in older patients with use in younger persons.

Driving and Hazardous Work: The use of leucovorin should not impair your ability to perform such tasks safely.

Alcohol: Avoid alcohol while taking this medication, since alcohol only further depletes folic acid.

Pregnancy: Neither animal nor human studies on the effects of using leucovorin during pregnancy have been done. Before taking leucovorin, tell your doctor if you are pregnant or plan to become pregnant. It should be used during pregnancy only under the close supervision of a doctor who is experienced in anti-metabolite cancer therapy.

Breast Feeding: It is not known whether leucovorin passes into breast milk. It has not been reported to cause problems in nursing infants. Consult your doctor for specific advice.

Infants and Children: In children who suffer from seizure disorders, treatment with leucovorin may increase the frequency of seizures.

Special Concerns: Inform your doctor if you cannot tolerate the oral dose and it causes vomiting. Injection therapy may be warranted.

OVERDOSE
Symptoms: No specific ones have been reported.

What to Do: An overdose of leucovorin is unlikely to be life-threatening. However, if someone takes a much larger dose than prescribed, seek medical assistance right away.

▼ INTERACTIONS

DRUG INTERACTIONS
Consult your doctor for specific advice if you are taking any other prescription or over-the-counter drugs.

FOOD INTERACTIONS
No known food interactions.

DISEASE INTERACTIONS
Caution is advised when taking leucovorin. Consult your doctor if you have kidney disease or vitamin B12 deficiency.

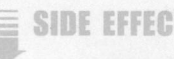

SIDE EFFECTS

SERIOUS
Skin rash, hives, itching, seizures. These may be signs of a serious allergic reaction; call your doctor right away.

COMMON
No common side effects have been reported.

LESS COMMON
There are no less-common side effects associated with the use of leucovorin.

LEUPROLIDE ACETATE

Available in: Injection, implanted capsule
Available OTC? No   **As Generic?** No
Drug Class: Synthetic hormone

▼ USAGE INFORMATION

WHY IT'S PRESCRIBED
To ease symptoms of advanced forms of prostate cancer in men (implanted capsule), and to relieve the pain and discomfort of endometriosis in women. It is also used by children with precocious (early onset) puberty and in certain patients with anemia owing to bleeding from fibroids.

HOW IT WORKS
In men, leuprolide decreases blood levels of testosterone. This slows the growth of cells in the prostate, which may ease the pain and discomfort of advanced prostate cancer. In women, leuprolide decreases blood levels of estrogen, which shrinks endometrial tissue (uterine lining) and thus eases flare-ups of endometriosis. It will suppress menstrual periods and thus help to correct the anemia associated with bleeding from fibroids.

▼ DOSAGE GUIDELINES

RANGE AND FREQUENCY
Injection— Men: 1 mg injected under the skin once a day or 7.5 mg of the Depot form injected into muscle once a month. Women: 3.75 mg injected into muscle once a month for up to 6 months. Children: Consult your pediatrician. Implanted capsule— Men: 1 capsule is implanted under the skin of the upper arm. The implant contains 65 mg of leuprolide that is continuously released for 12 months. After 12 months the implant must be removed. Another implant may be inserted to continue therapy.

≡ SIDE EFFECTS ≡

SERIOUS
In men: Pain in groin or leg, chest pain. In women: Increased hair growth, deepening of voice. In men and women: Rapid or irregular heartbeat. Call your doctor immediately.

COMMON
Injection— In women: Light, irregular vaginal bleeding, cessation of menstrual periods (amenorrhea), vaginal dryness. In both men and women: Sudden sweating and feelings of warmth (hot flashes). Implanted capsule— Hot flashes, lack of energy, depression, sweating, headache, bruising, and breast enlargement.

LESS COMMON
In men: Bone pain, constipation, decreased testicle size, impotence, loss of appetite, swollen and tender breasts. In women: Burning, itching, or dryness of vagina, decreased interest in sex, breast tenderness, pelvic pain, mood changes. In men and women: Blurred vision, burning or itching at injection or implant site, headache, nausea or vomiting, swollen feet or lower legs, insomnia, weight gain, numbness or tingling of the hands or feet.

ONSET OF EFFECT
Men: 2 to 4 weeks. Women: 1 to 2 months.

DURATION OF ACTION
Injection— Men: 4 to 12 weeks. Women: 60 to 90 days. Implanted capsule— 12 months.

DIETARY ADVICE
No special recommendations.

STORAGE
Keep liquid form refrigerated until the first dose, but do not allow it to freeze. Then store it in a tightly sealed container at room temperature away from heat and direct light. Implanted capsule: Not applicable.

MISSED DOSE
If you take the drug every day, take the missed dose as soon as you remember. If you do not remember until the next day, skip the missed dose and resume your regular dosage schedule. Do not double the next dose. Implanted capsule: Not applicable.

STOPPING THE DRUG
The decision to stop taking the drug should be made by your doctor.

PROLONGED USE
See your doctor for periodic examinations and lab tests.

▼ PRECAUTIONS

Over 60: No special advice.

Driving and Hazardous Work: Avoid such activities until you determine how the medicine affects you.

Alcohol: No special warnings.

Pregnancy: Leuprolide may cause birth defects if taken during pregnancy. Notify your doctor immediately if you think you are pregnant.

Breast Feeding: Leuprolide may pass into breast milk; caution is advised. Consult your doctor for advice.

Infants and Children: Leuprolide should be given to children only under close medical supervision.

Special Concerns: Use only the syringes provided in the kit. Other types may not deliver the same dose. When taking leuprolide, women should use nonhormonal contraception (that is, methods other than birth control pills).

OVERDOSE
Symptoms: None reported.

What to Do: An overdose is unlikely to be life-threatening. However, if someone takes a much larger dose than prescribed, call your doctor, emergency medical services (EMS), or the nearest poison control center.

▼ INTERACTIONS

DRUG INTERACTIONS
Consult your doctor for specific advice if you are taking any other medications or herbal remedies.

FOOD INTERACTIONS
No known food interactions.

DISEASE INTERACTIONS
Consult your doctor if you experience vaginal bleeding of unknown cause or, in men, difficulty urinating.

LEVAMISOLE HYDROCHLORIDE

BRAND NAME

Ergamisol

Available in: Tablets
Available OTC? No **As Generic?** No
Drug Class: Immunomodulator; antineoplastic (anticancer) agent

▼ USAGE INFORMATION

WHY IT'S PRESCRIBED
Levamisole enhances the effectiveness of fluorouracil, a drug used to treat cancer of the colon.

HOW IT WORKS
It is unknown precisely how levamisole works. It appears that it improves the responsiveness of the immune system, which is suppressed by other chemotherapy agents such as fluorouracil. Therefore it improves the patient's overall ability to fight disease. Unlike many other cancer drugs, levamisole does not directly attack malignant cells.

▼ DOSAGE GUIDELINES

RANGE AND FREQUENCY
50 mg every 8 hours for 3 days, beginning no later than 30 days after surgery. Usual maintenance dose is 50 mg for 3 days every 2 weeks for 1 year.

ONSET OF EFFECT
Unknown.

DURATION OF ACTION
Unknown.

DIETARY ADVICE
Maintain adequate food and fluid intake. Calorie, protein, and vitamin needs increase in patients with cancer. Good nutrition is essential to cope with the demands of chemotherapy.

STORAGE
Store in a tightly sealed container away from heat and direct light.

MISSED DOSE
Take it as soon as you remember. If it is near the time for the next dose, skip the missed dose and resume your regular dosage schedule. Do not double the next dose.

STOPPING THE DRUG
The decision to stop taking the drug should be made by your doctor.

PROLONGED USE
You should see your doctor regularly for tests and examinations if you take levamisole for a prolonged period.

▼ PRECAUTIONS

Over 60: Levamisole is not expected to cause different side effects or problems in older persons than it does in younger patients.

Driving and Hazardous Work: Do not drive or engage in hazardous work until you determine how the medicine affects you.

Alcohol: Avoid alcohol completely while taking this medication. When alcohol is consumed with the combination of levamisole and fluorouracil, severe nausea and vomiting may result.

Pregnancy: Levamisole has not been shown to cause birth defects in animals. Human studies have not been done. Consult your doctor for advice if you are pregnant or plan to become pregnant.

Breast Feeding: It is not known whether levamisole passes into breast milk; caution is advised. Consult your doctor for specific advice.

Infants and Children: There is no information comparing the use of levamisole in infants and children with use in older persons.

Special Concerns: If you vomit after taking a dose of levamisole, ask your doctor whether you should take the dose again or wait for the next dose. Avoid contact with persons who have infections. Do not receive any immunizations while you take this medication. Before you have dental work done, tell the dentist that you are taking levamisole. Rinse your mouth after eating and drinking and use a soft toothbrush and an electric razor.

OVERDOSE
Symptoms: Nausea, vomiting, infection, inflammation of the mouth.

What to Do: Call your doctor, emergency medical services (EMS), or the nearest poison control center immediately.

▼ INTERACTIONS

DRUG INTERACTIONS
Consult your doctor for specific advice if you are taking phenytoin or the anticoagulant warfarin. Side effects of levamisole may be more frequent when taken with fluorouracil.

FOOD INTERACTIONS
No known food interactions.

DISEASE INTERACTIONS
Caution is advised when taking levamisole. Consult your doctor if you have any other medical condition.

SIDE EFFECTS

SERIOUS
Flulike symptoms (such as fever or chills, body aches, general feeling of discomfort, weakness, and cough), unusual bleeding or bruising, blurred vision, trouble walking, uncontrolled movements of the arms or legs. Although such side effects are rare, they are serious; call your physician immediately if you experience such symptoms.

COMMON
Nausea, vomiting, and diarrhea.

LESS COMMON
Anxiety or nervousness, dizziness, headache, depression, nightmares, pain in joints or muscles, skin rash or itching, insomnia, unusual sleepiness or tiredness, metallic taste, sores in the mouth or on the lips.

LEVETIRACETAM

Available in: Tablets
Available OTC? No   **As Generic?** No
Drug Class: Anticonvulsant

▼ USAGE INFORMATION

WHY IT'S PRESCRIBED
Used in combination with one or more other anticonvulsant drugs to control partial seizures (those which begin with an abnormal burst of electrical activity in a small portion of the brain, often resulting in twitching or numbness in a localized part of the body).

HOW IT WORKS
The precise mechanism of action is unknown.

▼ DOSAGE GUIDELINES

RANGE AND FREQUENCY
To start, 500 mg twice a day. Dosage may be gradually increased by your doctor (1,000 mg a day every 2 weeks) to a maximum of 3,000 mg a day. People with impaired kidney function may require an adjustment in dose.

ONSET OF EFFECT
Within 48 hours.

DURATION OF ACTION
Unknown.

DIETARY ADVICE
Can be taken without regard to meals.

STORAGE
Store in a tightly sealed container away from heat, moisture, and direct light.

MISSED DOSE
Take it as soon as you remember. If it is near the time for the next dose, skip the missed dose and resume your regular dosage schedule. Do not double the next dose.

STOPPING THE DRUG
The decision to stop taking the drug should be made by your doctor. Never stop this drug abruptly because this may cause seizures. The dose is typically tapered over a period of weeks.

PROLONGED USE
This drug is often taken for prolonged periods. See your physician for periodic check-ups throughout treatment.

▼ PRECAUTIONS

Over 60: Decreased kidney function is more common in older persons. Because levetiracetam is eliminated from the body through the kidney, the risk of side effects is increased. Kidney function should be carefully monitored. A dosage adjustment may be warranted.

Driving and Hazardous Work: This drug may cause drowsiness or dizziness, particularly in the first few weeks it is used. Do not drive or engage in hazardous work until you determine how the medicine affects you.

Alcohol: Avoid alcohol; it may contribute to excessive drowsiness.

Pregnancy: Levetiracetam has caused birth defects in animal studies. Human studies with this drug have not been done, but other anticonvulsants are known to increase the risk of birth defects. However, seizures during pregnancy can also increase the risks to the fetus. Discuss with your doctor the potential risks and benefits of using this drug during pregnancy.

Breast Feeding: Levetiracetam may pass into breast milk; caution is advised. Consult your doctor for specific advice.

Infants and Children: Not recommended for use by children under age 16.

Special Concerns: See your doctor for regular check-ups to detect the onset of any serious side effects. Your doctor may advise you to carry an ID card or bracelet that says you are taking this drug.

OVERDOSE
Symptoms: Few cases of overdose have been reported. In clinical trials, the most common symptom following overdose was drowsiness.

What to Do: If an excessive dose is taken, call your doctor, emergency medical services (EMS), or poison control center immediately.

▼ INTERACTIONS

DRUG INTERACTIONS
No known drug interactions.

FOOD INTERACTIONS
No known food interactions.

DISEASE INTERACTIONS
A lower dose may be needed in patients with decreased kidney function.

SIDE EFFECTS

SERIOUS
Extreme drowsiness, psychotic symptoms. Call your physician immediately.

COMMON
Drowsiness, fatigue, increased susceptibility to infection, dizziness, lightheadedness.

LESS COMMON
Coordination difficulties, agitation, hostility, anxiety, nervousness, depression, hallucinations, attempted suicide, loss of appetite, amnesia, emotional instability, numbness, prickling or tingling sensations, cough, sore throat, runny nose, sinusitis, double vision.

LEVOBUNOLOL

Available in: Ophthalmic solution
Available OTC? No   **As Generic?** No
Drug Class: Antiglaucoma drug; ophthalmic beta-blocker

▼ USAGE INFORMATION

WHY IT'S PRESCRIBED
To treat glaucoma.

HOW IT WORKS
Glaucoma, a sight-threatening disorder, occurs when aqueous humor (fluid inside the eye) cannot drain properly, causing an increase in pressure within the eyeball (intraocular pressure). The increased eye pressure can damage the optic nerve and lead to a gradually progressive loss of vision. Levobunolol decreases the production of aqueous humor and promotes its outflow, thereby reducing intraocular pressure.

▼ DOSAGE GUIDELINES

RANGE AND FREQUENCY
Adults and older children: 1 drop in each affected eye, 1 or 2 times a day. Children: The dose must be determined by your doctor.

ONSET OF EFFECT
Within 60 minutes.

DURATION OF ACTION
Up to 24 hours.

SIDE EFFECTS

SERIOUS
Palpitations, trouble breathing, dizziness, and weakness caused by low blood pressure. Call your doctor right away.

COMMON
Burning, stinging, tearing, and irritation of the eye when medication is taken.

LESS COMMON
Eyebrow pain, itching, decreased night vision, crusted eyelashes, increased sensitivity of eye to light, dry eye.

DIETARY ADVICE
No special restrictions.

STORAGE
Store in a tightly sealed container away from heat, moisture, and direct light. Do not allow it to freeze.

MISSED DOSE
Apply it as soon as you remember. If it is near the time for the next dose, skip the missed dose and resume your regular dosage schedule.

STOPPING THE DRUG
The decision to stop using the drug should be made by your doctor.

PROLONGED USE
See your doctor regularly for tests and examinations if you must take this drug for a prolonged period.

▼ PRECAUTIONS

Over 60:
Adverse reactions may be more likely and more severe in older patients.

Driving and Hazardous Work:
Avoid such activities until you determine how the medication affects your vision.

Alcohol: Consume alcohol in moderation only.

Pregnancy: Levobunolol has not been shown to cause birth defects in animals. Human studies have not been done. Before you take levobunolol, tell your doctor if you are pregnant or plan to become pregnant.

Breast Feeding: Levobunolol may pass into breast milk; caution is advised. Consult your doctor for advice.

Infants and Children: Adverse reactions may be more likely and more severe in young patients.

Special Concerns: To use the eye drops, first wash your hands. Tilt your head back. Gently apply pressure to the inside corner of the eyelid and with the index finger of the same hand, pull downward on the lower eyelid to make a space. Drop the medicine into this space and close your eye. Apply pressure for 1 or 2 minutes while keeping the eye closed without blinking. Then wash your hands again. Make sure the tip of the dropper does not touch your eye, finger, or any other surface. If you are taking the medicine with the compliance cap (C Cap), make sure the number 1 or the correct day of the week appears in the window of the cap before using the eye drops for the first time. After every dose, rotate the bottle until the cap clicks to the position that tells you the next dose. Before you have any kind of surgery, dental treatment, or emergency treatment, tell the person in charge that you are taking levobunolol. This drug may make you more sensitive to sunlight. If this occurs, wear sunglasses or avoid bright light as comfort dictates.

OVERDOSE
Symptoms: Nervousness, chest pain, confusion, hallucinations, coughing, wheezing, drowsiness, dizziness, nausea or vomiting, irregular or pounding heartbeat, insomnia, unusual fatigue.

What to Do: If a large volume enters the eye, flush with water. If someone accidentally ingests the drug, call your doctor, emergency medical services (EMS), or the nearest poison control center immediately.

▼ INTERACTIONS

DRUG INTERACTIONS
It is not recommended to use two ophthalmic beta-blockers at the same time. Special caution is warranted in people taking antidiabetic drugs, since levobunolol may mask symptoms of low blood sugar. Other drugs may interact with levobunolol. Tell your doctor about any other prescription or over-the-counter medication that you take.

FOOD INTERACTIONS
No known food interactions.

DISEASE INTERACTIONS
Consult your doctor if you have asthma, emphysema or other lung disease, heart disease, hyperthyroidism, or diabetes mellitus.

LEVOCABASTINE

Available in: Ophthalmic suspension
Available OTC? No   **As Generic?** No
Drug Class: Histamine (H1) blocker

▼ USAGE INFORMATION

WHY IT'S PRESCRIBED
For temporary symptomatic relief of itching and irritation of the eyes associated with seasonal allergies.

HOW IT WORKS
Levocabastine blocks the effects of histamine, a naturally occurring substance within the body that causes swelling, itching, sneezing, watery eyes, hives, and other symptoms associated with allergic reactions.

▼ DOSAGE GUIDELINES

RANGE AND FREQUENCY
Instill 1 drop in affected eye(s), 4 times a day, for up to 2 weeks. Shake well before using the drug.

ONSET OF EFFECT
Within 10 to 15 minutes.

DURATION OF ACTION
From 2 to 4 hours.

DIETARY ADVICE
This drug can be used without regard to diet.

STORAGE
Store in a tightly sealed container away from heat, moisture, and direct light. Do not allow it to freeze.

MISSED DOSE
Apply it as soon as you remember. If it is near the time for the next dose, skip the missed dose and resume your regular dosage schedule. Do not double the next dose.

STOPPING THE DRUG
Take it as prescribed for the full treatment period, even if you feel better before the scheduled end of therapy.

PROLONGED USE
This medication is for short-term symptomatic relief only; treatment should not exceed 2 weeks. Check with your doctor if symptoms do not improve, or if your condition becomes worse, after 3 days.

▼ PRECAUTIONS

Over 60: No special problems are expected.

Driving and Hazardous Work: No problems are expected, but it is advisable not to engage in such activities until you determine how this drug affects your vision.

Alcohol: No special precautions are necessary.

Pregnancy: Adequate studies have not been done, although no problems have been reported. Before taking levocabastine, tell your doctor if you are pregnant or plan to become pregnant.

Breast Feeding: Levocabastine passes into breast milk; do not use it when nursing.

Infants and Children: The safety and effectiveness of levocabastine have not been established in children under the age of 12. This drug should not be used by patients in this age group.

Special Concerns: To use the eye drops, first wash your hands. Tilt your head back. Gently apply pressure to the inside corner of the eyelid and with the index finger of the same hand, pull downward on the lower eyelid to make a space. Drop the medicine into this space and close your eye. Apply pressure for 1 or 2 minutes while keeping the eye closed without blinking. Then wash your hands again. Make sure the tip of the dropper does not touch your eye, finger, or any other surface. The manufacturer of this drug recommends that soft contact lenses not be worn while undergoing treatment with levocabastine.

OVERDOSE
Symptoms: No cases of overdose have been reported.

What to Do: An overdose of levocabastine is unlikely to occur. In case of accidental ingestion, call your doctor, emergency medical services (EMS), or the nearest poison control center immediately.

▼ INTERACTIONS

DRUG INTERACTIONS
No drug interactions have been reported. Nonetheless, it is wise to consult your doctor before taking any other prescription or over-the-counter eye medication.

FOOD INTERACTIONS
No food interactions have been reported.

DISEASE INTERACTIONS
No disease interactions have been reported.

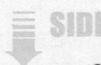

SIDE EFFECTS

SERIOUS
Cough, breathing difficulty, swelling around the eyes, eye pain or discharge, excessive tear production, unusual fatigue, nausea, sore throat, redness or irritation not present prior to treatment, visual disturbances. Such side effects are very rare, but if they occur, stop using the drug and call your doctor immediately.

COMMON
Temporary burning or stinging in the eyes upon application of the drops.

LESS COMMON
Headache, dry eyes, dry mouth, and drowsiness. Call your doctor if such symptoms persist or begin to interfere with daily activities.

LEVODOPA

Available in: Tablets, capsules
Available OTC? No **As Generic?** Yes
Drug Class: Antiparkinsonism drug

▼ USAGE INFORMATION

WHY IT'S PRESCRIBED
To treat Parkinson's disease and Parkinson-like syndromes. Such syndromes can occur following injury to or infection of the central nervous system, damage to the blood vessels in the brain (for example, after a stroke), or exposure to certain toxins.

HOW IT WORKS
Levodopa replenishes the supply of dopamine in the brain. Dopamine is a chemical in the central nervous system that plays an essential role in the initiation and smooth control of voluntary muscle movement.

▼ DOSAGE GUIDELINES

RANGE AND FREQUENCY
Adults: To start, 0.5 g per day in 2 or more divided doses. The dose is increased gradually (by 0.5 to 0.75 g per day) over the course of 4 to 7 days, until the desired therapeutic response is achieved. The onset of adverse side effects may preclude the use of higher doses. The maximum beneficial dose is usually 5 to 6 g per day. Children: Smaller doses are

used; consult your pediatrician for specific information.

ONSET OF EFFECT
Within 1 to 2 hours.

DURATION OF ACTION
From 4 to 5 hours.

DIETARY ADVICE
Eating food shortly after taking this medication may minimize the chance of stomach upset. Eating food before taking the medicine or at the same time may blunt levodopa's effects.

STORAGE
Store in a tightly sealed container away from heat, moisture, and direct light.

MISSED DOSE
Take it as soon as you remember. However, if it is near the time for the next dose, skip the missed dose and resume your regular dosage schedule. Do not double the next dose.

STOPPING THE DRUG
Consult your doctor for the best approach to stopping the drug. The dose should be decreased very gradually. Abruptly stopping the drug can cause an acute (sudden-onset) adverse reaction.

PROLONGED USE
Prolonged use of levodopa can result in a less predictable therapeutic response and bothersome involuntary muscle movements.

▼ PRECAUTIONS

Over 60: Adverse reactions to levodopa may be more likely and more severe in older patients. The dose should be increased very gradually in this age group.

Driving and Hazardous Work: Do not drive or engage in hazardous work until the full dose has been attained and you determine how the drug affects you.

Alcohol: Do not consume alcohol. Alcohol can cause pronounced confusion or delirium in patients taking this medication.

Pregnancy: Adequate human studies have not been done, and the effects of levodopa during pregnancy have not been determined. Pregnant women should therefore avoid taking levodopa.

Breast Feeding: Levodopa passes into breast milk; levodopa should not be used by nursing mothers.

Infants and Children: Levodopa should be used with caution by infants and children. The dose should be smaller than that for adults and should be determined by your pediatrician.

Special Concerns: Patients taking levodopa should not eat a high-protein diet,

because it can reduce the medication's effectiveness.

OVERDOSE
Symptoms: The symptoms of levodopa overdose are unknown.

What to Do: If you have any reason to suspect an overdose, call your doctor, emergency medical services (EMS), or the nearest poison control center.

▼ INTERACTIONS

DRUG INTERACTIONS
Consult your doctor for specific advice if you are taking any of the following drugs that may interact with levodopa: MAO inhibitor antidepressants (such as phenelzine sulfate or tranylcypromine sulfate) or antihypertensives.

FOOD INTERACTIONS
A high-protein diet can reduce the effectiveness of levodopa. Persons taking levodopa should therefore decrease their protein intake if it is high.

DISEASE INTERACTIONS
Caution is advised when taking levodopa. Consult your doctor if you have any of the following: heart disease or heart rhythm abnormalities, bronchial asthma, glaucoma, malignant melanoma, or changes in mental state.

 SIDE EFFECTS

SERIOUS
Irregular heartbeat, heart rhythm abnormalities, low blood pressure, fainting or near fainting, hallucinations.

COMMON
Nausea, confusion.

LESS COMMON
Breathing difficulty.

LEVODOPA/CARBIDOPA

Available in: Tablets, sustained-release tablets
Available OTC? No   **As Generic?** Yes
Drug Class: Antiparkinsonism drug

▼ USAGE INFORMATION

WHY IT'S PRESCRIBED
To treat Parkinson's disease and Parkinson-like syndromes, which can occur following injury to or infection of the central nervous system, damage to the blood vessels in the brain, or exposure to certain toxins. Levodopa/carbidopa improves or alleviates such symptoms as rigidity, slowness, loss of smoothness of movement, and tremor.

HOW IT WORKS
Levodopa/carbidopa increases brain levels of dopamine, a chemical that plays an essential role in the smooth movement of muscles.

▼ DOSAGE GUIDELINES

RANGE AND FREQUENCY
Adults: To start, 1 tablet of 100/10 levodopa/carbidopa (100 mg of levodopa and 10 mg of carbidopa), 3 or 4 times a day; or 1 tablet of 100/25 levodopa/carbidopa, 3 times a day. Dose is gradually increased every 5 to 7 days until the maximum therapeutic benefit is achieved without the onset of serious side effects. The maximum dose is variable, ranging from the equivalent of 4 to 10 tablets per day. Children: Smaller doses can be used; consult your pediatrician.

ONSET OF EFFECT
Within 90 to 120 minutes.

DURATION OF ACTION
From 3 to 4 hours.

DIETARY ADVICE
Eating food shortly after taking the medication may minimize the chance of stomach upset. Eating food before taking the medicine or at the same time may blunt levodopa's effects.

STORAGE
Store in a tightly sealed container away from heat, moisture, and direct light.

MISSED DOSE
Take it as soon as you remember, unless the time for your next scheduled dose is within the next 2 hours. If so, skip the missed dose and resume your regular dosage schedule. Do not double the next dose.

STOPPING THE DRUG
Consult your doctor before stopping the drug. The dosage should be decreased very gradually. Abruptly stopping the medication can result in an acute (sudden-onset) adverse reaction.

PROLONGED USE
Prolonged use of this drug may result in a less predictable therapeutic response as well as the onset of involuntary muscle movements.

▼ PRECAUTIONS

Over 60: Adverse reactions may be more likely and more severe in older patients.

Driving and Hazardous Work: Avoid such activities until you determine how the medicine affects you.

Alcohol: Avoid alcohol.

Pregnancy: This combination drug should not be used by pregnant women.

Breast Feeding: Levodopa passes into breast milk. This combination drug should not be used by nursing mothers.

Infants and Children: Levodopa/carbidopa can be used by children, with caution. The appropriate dosage will be determined by your pediatrician. Use of the sustained-release tablets in children under the age of 18 is not recommended.

Special Concerns: Levodopa/carbidopa should be used with special caution if you are also taking other antiparkinsonism drugs. Do not crush or chew the sustained-release tablets. Swallow them whole.

OVERDOSE
Symptoms: Sudden or severe confusion, delirium, hallucinations.

What to Do: Call your doctor, emergency medical services (EMS), or the nearest poison control center immediately.

▼ INTERACTIONS

DRUG INTERACTIONS
Do not take levodopa/carbidopa if you are taking, or took within the past 14 days, an MAO inhibitor (such as phenelzine sulfate or tranylcypromine sulfate). Consult your doctor for specific advice if you are taking selegiline, tricyclic antidepressants, risperidone, fluphenazine, phenytoin, papaverine, iron salts, metoclopramide, or any antihypertensive drugs.

FOOD INTERACTIONS
The effectiveness of levodopa/carbidopa may be impaired by a high-protein diet. Persons taking the drug should take care to limit their protein intake.

DISEASE INTERACTIONS
You should not take levodopa/carbidopa if you have malignant melanoma, ischemic heart disease, heart rhythm abnormalities, bronchial asthma, narrow-angle glaucoma, or any changes in mental state. Levodopa/carbidopa should be used with caution in people who have kidney, liver, or endocrine disease, a history of heart attack, peptic ulcer, or chronic wide-angle glaucoma.

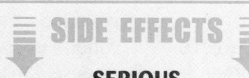
SIDE EFFECTS

SERIOUS
Nausea, fatigue, depression, dizziness or lightheadedness when standing or sitting up suddenly (orthostatic hypotension), fainting or near fainting.

COMMON
With long-term use, quirky involuntary muscle movements, an unpredictable therapeutic response.

LESS COMMON
Confusion, delirium; dark saliva, urine, or sweat.

LEVOFLOXACIN

Available in: Tablets, injection
Available OTC? No   **As Generic?** No
Drug Class: Fluoroquinolone antibiotic

▼ USAGE INFORMATION

WHY IT'S PRESCRIBED
To treat pneumonia, chronic bronchitis, and other infections caused by bacteria.

HOW IT WORKS
Levofloxacin inhibits the activity of a bacterial enzyme (gyrase) that is necessary for proper DNA formation and replication. This fights infection by preventing bacteria cells from reproducing.

▼ DOSAGE GUIDELINES

RANGE AND FREQUENCY
Adults: 250 to 500 mg once a day for 7 to 14 days. After an initial dose of 250 to 500 mg, patients with kidney problems receive 250 mg every day for 7 to 14 days.

ONSET OF EFFECT
Varies depending on the infection being treated.

DURATION OF ACTION
Unknown.

DIETARY ADVICE
Drink plenty of fluids.

STORAGE
Store in a tightly sealed container away from heat and direct light. Do not allow the injection form to freeze.

MISSED DOSE
Take it as soon as you remember. If it is near the time for the next dose, skip the missed dose and resume your regular dosage schedule. Do not double the next dose.

STOPPING THE DRUG
It is very important to take this drug as prescribed for the full treatment period, even if you begin to feel better before the scheduled end of therapy (unless you experience intolerable side effects, including increased sensitivity to sunlight).

PROLONGED USE
See your doctor regularly for tests and examinations if you must take this medicine for a prolonged period.

▼ PRECAUTIONS

Over 60: No special problems are expected.

Driving and Hazardous Work: Do not drive or engage in hazardous work until you determine how the medicine affects you.

Alcohol: It is advisable to abstain from alcohol when fighting an infection.

Pregnancy: In some animal tests, levofloxacin has caused birth defects. Adequate studies in humans have not been done. It should be used during pregnancy only if potential benefits clearly justify the risks. Before you take levofloxacin, tell your doctor if you are pregnant or plan to become pregnant.

Breast Feeding: Levofloxacin passes into breast milk and may cause serious side effects in the nursing infant; use of the drug is discouraged when nursing.

Infants and Children: Levofloxacin is not recommended for use by persons under the age of 18, as it has been shown to interfere with bone development.

Special Concerns: If levofloxacin causes sensitivity to sunlight, stop taking the drug and try to avoid exposure to sunlight for the next 5 days; also wear protective clothing and use a sunblock. Levofloxacin should not be taken by patients whose work makes it impossible to avoid exposure to sunlight. It is important to drink plenty of fluids while taking this drug.

OVERDOSE
Symptoms: No specific ones have been reported.

What to Do: If you have any reason to suspect an overdose, call your doctor, emergency medical services (EMS), or the nearest poison control center.

▼ INTERACTIONS

DRUG INTERACTIONS
Consult your doctor for specific advice if you are taking aminophylline, antacids, didanosine, iron supplements, sucralfate, or zinc salts. Also tell your doctor if you are taking any other prescription or over-the-counter drug.

FOOD INTERACTIONS
No known food interactions.

DISEASE INTERACTIONS
Caution is advised when taking levofloxacin. Consult your doctor if you have any other medical condition. Use of levofloxacin can cause complications in patients with kidney disease, since this organ works to remove the medication from the body.

≡ SIDE EFFECTS ≡

SERIOUS
Serious reactions to levofloxacin are rare and include seizures, mental confusion, hallucinations, agitation, nightmares, depression, shortness of breath, unusual swelling in the face or extremities, and loss of consciousness. Also skin burning, redness, blisters, rash, or itching on exposure to sunlight; increased risk of tendinitis or tendon rupture. Call your doctor immediately.

COMMON
Increased sensitivity to sunlight (and increased risk of sunburn) for days following therapy.

LESS COMMON
Diarrhea, nausea and vomiting, stomach pain and upset, gas, headache, dizziness, restlessness, insomnia, changes in taste perception, drowsiness, itching, dry mouth, unusual body aches or pains.

LEVOMETHADYL ACETATE HYDROCHLORIDE

Available in: Oral solution
Available OTC? No   **As Generic?** No
Drug Class: Narcotic

▼ USAGE INFORMATION

WHY IT'S PRESCRIBED
To prevent or ease withdrawal symptoms during detoxification from illegal narcotics, and to serve as maintenance therapy during narcotic addiction treatment programs.

HOW IT WORKS
Levomethadyl serves as a substitute for other narcotics that tend to produce more-pronounced effects.

▼ DOSAGE GUIDELINES

RANGE AND FREQUENCY
Addicts who have not begun treatment with methadone: To start, between 20 and 40 mg per day, 3 times a week. Addicts who have been receiving methadone: To start, the dose will be a little higher than the amount of methadone per day, but not more than 120 mg, 3 times a week. The dose will be reduced in detoxification programs, continued as long as needed in maintenance programs. Levomethadyl should not be taken daily due to risk of overdose.

ONSET OF EFFECT
Levomethadyl may not be fully effective for several days. Thus methadone may be the first drug used in a detoxification program, since its effect is more immediate; levomethadyl may then be used since, unlike methadone, it does not need to be taken every day.

DURATION OF ACTION
48 to 72 hours.

DIETARY ADVICE
No special restrictions.

STORAGE
Not applicable; dose may be taken only at approved treatment facilities.

MISSED DOSE
Not applicable; the dose is administered by a health care professional specializing in addiction treatment.

STOPPING THE DRUG
The decision to stop taking levomethadyl should be made by the addiction treatment specialist.

PROLONGED USE
See your health care professional regularly for tests and examinations.

▼ PRECAUTIONS

Over 60: Studies on older patients have not been conducted.

Driving and Hazardous Work: Do not drive or engage in hazardous work until you determine how the medicine affects you.

Alcohol: Avoid alcohol.

Pregnancy: Using this drug during pregnancy may cause withdrawal symptoms in the newborn baby. Federal law requires pregnancy tests before starting treatment and once-a-month exams during treatment.

Breast Feeding: Levomethadyl may pass into breast milk; caution is advised. Consult your doctor for advice.

Infants and Children: Federal law prohibits use of levomethadyl by persons under 18 years of age.

Special Concerns: Tell any doctor or dentist you see for treatment that you are taking levomethadyl. To prevent constipation, you may be advised to increase the fiber in your diet, drink a lot of fluids, or take laxatives.

OVERDOSE
Symptoms: See Serious Side Effects.

What to Do: Call your doctor, emergency medical services (EMS), or the nearest poison control center immediately.

▼ INTERACTIONS

DRUG INTERACTIONS
Consult your doctor for specific advice if you are taking barbiturates, buprenorphine, butorphanol, carbamazepine, central nervous system depressants, chloramphenicol, cimetidine, corticosteroids, dezocine, diltiazem, disulfiram, divalproex, erythromycin, griseofulvin, isoniazid, oral contraceptives, nalbuphine, naltrexone, pentazocine, phenylbutazone, phenytoin, primidone, quinine, rifampin, ranitidine, tricyclic antidepressants, valproic acid, or verapamil.

FOOD INTERACTIONS
No known food interactions.

DISEASE INTERACTIONS
Consult your doctor if you have any of the following: chronic lung disease, brain disease, head injury, colitis, Crohn's disease, enlarged prostate, gallbladder disease, heart disease, high blood pressure, kidney or liver disease, or an underactive thyroid.

⇒ SIDE EFFECTS ⇐

SERIOUS
Some serious side effects of levomethadyl are indistinguishable from those of overdose: Confusion; slurred speech; severe drowsiness; small, pinpoint pupils; cold, clammy skin; slow breathing; seizures; unconsciousness. Other serious side effects are depression; enlarged pupils; swelling of fingers, feet, face, and lower legs; skin rash; diarrhea; insomnia; rapid heartbeat; nervousness; runny nose; trembling; stomach cramps; fever. Call your doctor immediately.

COMMON
Abdominal or stomach pains, nausea, and constipation.

LESS COMMON
Back pain, watering eyes, anxiety, blurred vision, flu symptoms, chills, decreased sexual desire, dizziness when getting up, headache, cough, hot flashes, muscle pain, unusual dreams.

LEVONORGESTREL IMPLANTS

Available in: Implanted capsule
Available OTC? No   **As Generic?** No
Drug Class: Progestin (hormone)

▼ USAGE INFORMATION

WHY IT'S PRESCRIBED
As a birth control method.

HOW IT WORKS
The implant slowly releases levonorgestrel, a synthetic hormone, into the bloodstream. It prevents a woman's egg from developing fully and causes changes in the uterine lining that make it difficult for sperm to reach the egg. It may prevent ovulation in some patients.

▼ DOSAGE GUIDELINES

RANGE AND FREQUENCY
6 capsules are implanted under the skin of the upper arm. The capsules are placed in a fanlike position, 15 degrees apart. They are removed after 5 years.

ONSET OF EFFECT
Within 24 hours if implanted within 7 days of the menstrual period.

DURATION OF ACTION
Up to 5 years.

DIETARY ADVICE
No special restrictions.

STORAGE
Not applicable.

MISSED DOSE
Not applicable; the drug is delivered continuously from the implant under the skin.

STOPPING THE DRUG
The decision to stop using the implant can be made whenever you choose, but the implants should be removed by your doctor.

PROLONGED USE
See your doctor at least once a year for periodic examinations and lab tests.

▼ PRECAUTIONS

Over 60: Not normally prescribed for postmenopausal women.

Driving and Hazardous Work: No special precautions are necessary.

Alcohol: No special precautions are necessary.

Pregnancy: Extensive studies have shown that no special risks to mother or child are associated with pregnancies occurring prior to or shortly after implantation of levonorgestrel capsules. Nonetheless, it is advisable to have the implants removed if pregnancy occurs.

Breast Feeding: Levonorgestrel passes into breast milk but has not been shown to cause problems. It can be used by nursing mothers who desire contraception.

Infants and Children: Levonorgestrel implants have not been shown to cause problems in teenagers. However, birth control methods that protect against sexually transmitted diseases (for example, condoms) are preferred for those in this age group.

Special Concerns: Do not have this implant inserted until you are sure you are not pregnant. Call your doctor immediately if one of the capsules falls out before the skin heals over the implant. No contraceptive method is perfect: If you suspect a pregnancy, you should call your doctor immediately. If you have any laboratory test, tell the health professional that you are using these contraceptives. Cigarette smoking or alcohol abuse can increase the risk of osteoporosis and blood clot formation. Implants should be removed if you develop active thrombophlebitis (pain caused by a blot clot lodged in a blood vessel), thromboembolic disease, or jaundice (yellowish tinge to the eyes or skin), or if you will be immobilized for a significant period of time because of illness or some other factor. If you have sudden unexplained vision problems, including changes in tolerance for contact lenses, you should be evaluated by an ophthalmologist.

OVERDOSE
Symptoms: Not applicable.

What to Do: Emergency instructions not applicable.

▼ INTERACTIONS

DRUG INTERACTIONS
Consult your doctor for specific advice if you are taking aminoglutethimide, carbamazepine, phenytoin, rifabutin, or rifampin.

FOOD INTERACTIONS
No known food interactions.

DISEASE INTERACTIONS
Caution is advised when using this contraceptive. Consult your doctor if you have any of the following: asthma, epilepsy, heart or circulation problems, kidney disease, liver disease, migraine headaches, breast disease, bleeding disorders, central nervous system disorders (including depression), diabetes, or high blood cholesterol.

≣ SIDE EFFECTS ≣

SERIOUS
Changes in or cessation of menstrual bleeding, unexpected or increased flow of breast milk, mental depression, skin rash, loss of or change in speech, impaired coordination or vision, severe and sudden shortness of breath. Call your doctor immediately.

COMMON
Stomach pain; swelling of face, ankles, or feet; mild headache; mood changes; unusual fatigue; weight gain; pain or irritation at site of implant.

LESS COMMON
Acne, breast pain or tenderness, hot flashes, insomnia, loss of sexual desire, loss or gain of scalp hair or body hair, brown spots on skin.

LEVOTHYROXINE SODIUM

Available in: Tablets, injection
Available OTC? No **As Generic?** Yes
Drug Class: Hypothyroid agent

▼ USAGE INFORMATION

WHY IT'S PRESCRIBED
To treat patients with an underactive thyroid gland, goiter (enlarged thyroid gland), and benign and malignant (noncancerous and cancerous) thyroid nodules.

HOW IT WORKS
Levothyroxine acts in the body as a substitute for natural thyroid hormone.

▼ DOSAGE GUIDELINES

RANGE AND FREQUENCY
Tablets– Adults and teenagers: 0.016 mg per 2.2 lbs (1 kg) a day. Children less than 6 months old: 0.025 to 0.05 mg once a day. Children 6 to 12 months old: 0.05 to 0.075 mg once a day. Children ages 1 to 5: 0.075 to 0.1 mg once a day. Children ages 6 to 12: 0.1 to 0.15 mg a day. Injection– Adults and teenagers: 0.05 to 0.1 mg into a vein or muscle once a day. Children

less than 6 months old: 0.019 to 0.038 mg once a day. Children 6 to 12 months old: 0.038 to 0.056 mg once a day. Children ages 1 to 5: 0.056 to 0.075 mg once a day. Children ages 6 to 10: 0.075 to 0.113 mg once a day. Children ages 10 to 12: 0.113 to 0.15 mg once a day.

ONSET OF EFFECT
24 hours.

DURATION OF ACTION
1 to 3 weeks.

DIETARY ADVICE
Take it before breakfast on an empty stomach.

STORAGE
Store in a tightly sealed container away from heat, moisture, and direct light.

MISSED DOSE
If you miss your dose on one day, you may double the dose on the next day. If you miss two or more doses in a row, call your doctor.

STOPPING THE DRUG
The decision to stop taking the drug should be made in consultation with your doctor.

PROLONGED USE
If you must take this drug, it is very likely that lifelong therapy will be necessary. See your doctor regularly for routine tests and examinations to evaluate your condition.

▼ PRECAUTIONS

Over 60: Modificaton of the dosage may be required.

Driving and Hazardous Work: Avoid such activities until you determine how the medicine affects you.

Alcohol: Avoid alcohol.

Pregnancy: Using the recommended dose of levothyroxine has not been shown to cause birth defects. The dose may need to be changed during pregnancy. Consult your doctor for specific advice.

Breast Feeding: Using the recommended dose of levothyroxine has not been shown to cause problems while nursing. Consult your doctor for specific advice.

Infants and Children: No special problems expected.

Special Concerns: You should wear a medical bracelet or carry an identification card saying that you are taking this medication.

**OVERDOSE
Symptoms:** Rapid heartbeat, chest pain, shortness of breath.

What to Do: Call your doctor, emergency medical services (EMS), or the nearest poison control center immediately.

▼ INTERACTIONS

DRUG INTERACTIONS
Consult your doctor for advice if you are taking anticoagulants; cholestyramine; colestipol; amphetamines; appetite suppressants; asthma medication; or cold, sinus, or allergy medications.

FOOD INTERACTIONS
No known food interactions.

DISEASE INTERACTIONS
Caution is advised when taking levothyroxine. Consult your doctor if you have any of the following: diabetes mellitus, diabetes insipidus, myxedema, an overactive thyroid gland, atherosclerosis (so-called hardening of the arteries), heart disease, high blood pressure, an underactive adrenal gland, or an underactive pituitary gland.

 SIDE EFFECTS

SERIOUS
In rare instances, levothyroxine may cause severe headaches, skin rash, hives, rapid or irregular heartbeat, chest pain, or shortness of breath. These symptoms may signal an overdose or an allergic reaction. Seek emergency medical assistance immediately.

COMMON
No common side effects are associated with the use of levothyroxine.

LESS COMMON
Leg cramps, diarrhea, changes in menstrual cycle, changes in appetite, sweating, sensitivity to heat, shaking of the hands, fever, headache, insomnia, irritability, weight loss, vomiting, nervousness. These symptoms may indicate your dose needs adjustment by your doctor.

LIDOCAINE HYDROCHLORIDE TOPICAL

Available in: Gel, ointment, aerosol spray, transdermal patch
Available OTC? No   **As Generic?** Yes
Drug Class: Topical analgesic

▼ USAGE INFORMATION

WHY IT'S PRESCRIBED
For topical therapy of certain skin conditions associated with itching or pain, such as minor burns, insect bites, skin rashes (such as poison ivy), and minor cuts and scratches. The transdermal patch is used to relieve pain associated with post-herpetic neuralgia. Topical lidocaine is not meant to be used to relieve the pain of severe injuries, nor should it be prescribed for large or actively bleeding wounds.

HOW IT WORKS
Lidocaine interferes with the ability of certain nerves to conduct electrical signals, which blocks the transmission of nerve impulses that carry pain messages.

▼ DOSAGE GUIDELINES

RANGE AND FREQUENCY
Gel, ointment, and spray— Adults: Apply to affected area 3 to 4 times a day as needed. Children: Consult a pediatrician for advice. Transdermal patch— Adults: Apply a patch to intact skin to cover the most painful area. Up to 3 patches may be applied simultaneously, for no more than 12 hours at a time per 24-hour period.

ONSET OF EFFECT
Within minutes.

DURATION OF ACTION
Gel, ointment, and spray: About 45 minutes. Transdermal patch: Up to 12 hours.

DIETARY ADVICE
Maintain usual food and fluid intake. Increase fluids if you have a fever or diarrhea, in hot weather, or during exercise.

STORAGE
Store in a tightly sealed container away from heat and direct light. Keep away from moisture and extremes in temperature.

MISSED DOSE
Apply it as soon as you remember. If it is near the time for the next dose, skip the missed dose and resume your regular dosage schedule. Do not double the next dose or apply an excessively thick film of topical lidocaine to compensate for a missed application.

STOPPING THE DRUG
Apply as prescribed for the full treatment period. However, you may stop using the drug if you feel better before the scheduled end of therapy.

PROLONGED USE
Therapy with this medication is generally finished within several days. Prolonged use may increase the risk of undesirable side effects.

▼ PRECAUTIONS

Over 60: Adverse reactions may be more likely and more severe in older patients.

Driving and Hazardous Work: No special warnings.

Alcohol: No special warnings.

Pregnancy: Lidocaine may be used during pregnancy, but first consult your physician.

Breast Feeding: Lidocaine may pass into breast milk; caution is advised. Consult your doctor for advice.

Infants and Children: Not recommended for use by children under age 2. The transdermal patch is not recommended for children under the age of 18.

Special Concerns: Lidocaine has serious side effects if it is absorbed in large amounts into the blood. Therefore, do not apply excessive amounts of gel or ointment to the affected skin or wear a patch longer than 12 hours. Use only enough medication to make a thin film. Above all, never apply this medication to open wounds, deep cuts, or bleeding or ulcerated skin. Dispose of the patch to prevent access by children or pets because a significant amount of lidocaine remains in the patch following use.

OVERDOSE
Symptoms: Dizziness, slow or irregular heartbeat, confusion, seizures, shivering, unusual restlessness or agitation, hallucinations, difficulty breathing, bluish color to skin, lips, or fingertips.

What to Do: Call your doctor, emergency medical services (EMS), or the nearest poison control center immediately.

▼ INTERACTIONS

DRUG INTERACTIONS
The following drugs may interact with topical lidocaine, especially if excessive amounts of lidocaine are applied to the skin: medications to control heart rhythms, such as mexiletine or tocainide; beta-blockers; and cimetidine.

FOOD INTERACTIONS
No known food interactions.

DISEASE INTERACTIONS
Consult your doctor if you have any of the following: skin infection at or close to the application site; large sores, blisters, ulcerations, or broken skin at the application site; or severe injury at the application site.

 SIDE EFFECTS

SERIOUS
Hives, itching, rash, swelling of face, mouth, lips, throat, or tongue; burning, swelling, worsening redness, or pain at site of application. These may be signs of a potentially serious allergic reaction, which is rare.

COMMON
There are no significant common side effects of topical lidocaine when used in recommended amounts.

LESS COMMON
Mild redness, blanching (whitening), or swelling of skin at application sites. If irritation or a burning sensation occurs during application of the transdermal patch, remove the patch and do not reapply until the irritation recedes.

LINDANE

Available in: Cream, lotion, shampoo
Available OTC? No   **As Generic?** Yes
Drug Class: Insecticide

▼ USAGE INFORMATION

WHY IT'S PRESCRIBED
Lindane cream and lotion are used to treat scabies infestation. The shampoo form is used to treat lice infestation.

HOW IT WORKS
Lindane is absorbed directly into the bodies of scabies and lice, where it overstimulates nerve activity, ultimately causing convulsions and death of the insect.

▼ DOSAGE GUIDELINES

RANGE AND FREQUENCY
Cream and lotion: Wash, rinse, and dry your skin thoroughly before applying. Apply enough lindane to cover the entire surface of your body from the neck down, including the soles of the feet. Rub in well. Leave it on for no more than 8 hours, then remove it by washing thoroughly. Shampoo: Rinse and dry your hair and scalp. Apply enough lindane to thoroughly wet the scalp and affected areas. Allow it to remain in place for 4 minutes, then lather. Rinse thoroughly and dry with a clean towel. Then use a fine-tooth comb to remove nits. Treatment may be repeated after 7 days if necessary.

ONSET OF EFFECT
Unknown.

DURATION OF ACTION
Unknown.

DIETARY ADVICE
Lindane can be used without regard to diet. After applying the medication, be sure to wash your hands thoroughly before eating.

STORAGE
Store in a tightly sealed container away from heat and direct light.

MISSED DOSE
If you require a second dose of the shampoo (usually applied 7 days after the first dose) and forget it, administer it as soon as you remember.

STOPPING THE DRUG
In most cases lindane is needed only once; a second application may be necessary if living nits are found after initial treatment.

PROLONGED USE
Not applicable, since lindane is generally used only once or twice.

▼ PRECAUTIONS

Over 60: Adverse reactions may be more likely in older patients.

Driving and Hazardous Work: Do not drive or engage in hazardous work until you determine how the medicine affects you.

Alcohol: No special precautions are necessary.

Pregnancy: Lindane is absorbed through the skin and could reach the fetus. Before you use lindane, tell your doctor if you are currently pregnant or plan to become pregnant. Do not use lindane more than twice during pregnancy.

Breast Feeding: Lindane passes into breast milk; caution is advised. You should not breast feed for 2 days after using lindane. Consult your doctor for advice.

Infants and Children: Adverse reactions may be more likely and more severe in infants and children. Do not use on premature infants.

Special Concerns: Lindane is a poison that can depress the activity of the central nervous system (brain and spinal cord). Keep it away from the eyes and mouth. It may be fatal if swallowed. If you accidentally get some lindane in your eyes, wash them thoroughly with water and call your doctor. Do not use lindane on open wounds, such as cuts and sores. When applying lindane to another person, wear disposable plastic or rubber gloves, especially if you are breast feeding or pregnant. Do not keep lindane in your home any longer than needed. Be sure that any discarded lindane is out of the reach of children and pets.

OVERDOSE

Symptoms: Seizures, dizziness, vomiting.

What to Do: Call your doctor, emergency medical services (EMS), or the nearest poison control center immediately.

▼ INTERACTIONS

DRUG INTERACTIONS
Consult your doctor for specific advice if you are taking any prescription or over-the-counter medication.

FOOD INTERACTIONS
No known food interactions.

DISEASE INTERACTIONS
Caution is advised when using lindane. Consult your doctor if you have a seizure disorder, a skin rash, or any raw and broken skin.

≡ SIDE EFFECTS ≡

SERIOUS
Seizures; dizziness, clumsiness, or unsteady gait; rapid heartbeat; muscle cramps; nervousness, restlessness, or irritability; vomiting. Call your doctor immediately.

COMMON
There are no common side effects associated with lindane. However, when you stop using lindane, itching may occur and persist for 1 or more weeks; notify your doctor if this continues for more than a few weeks or interferes with daily activity.

LESS COMMON
Skin rash, redness or skin irritation that was not present prior to therapy.

LINEZOLID

Available in: Injection, tablets, oral suspension
Available OTC? No   **As Generic?** No
Drug Class: Oxazolidinone antibiotic

▼ USAGE INFORMATION

WHY IT'S PRESCRIBED
To treat certain hospital- or community-acquired pneumonias and some bacterial infections of the skin and blood.

HOW IT WORKS
Linezolid inhibits the growth of bacteria by interfering with the process of translating DNA messages into proteins. Because this drug works differently from other antibiotics, the development of cross-resistance between linezolid and other classes of antibiotics is unlikely.

▼ DOSAGE GUIDELINES

RANGE AND FREQUENCY
For vancomycin-resistant Enterococcus faecium infections: 600 mg every 12 hours for 14 to 28 days. For pneumonia and complicated skin infections: 600 mg every 12 hours for 10 to 14 days. For uncomplicated skin infections: 400 mg every 12 hours for 10 to 14 days. Length of therapy to be determined by your doctor.

ONSET OF EFFECT
Unknown.

DURATION OF ACTION
Unknown.

DIETARY ADVICE
No special recommendations.

STORAGE
Injection: Not applicable; injections are administered only at a health care facility. Tablets and oral solution: Store in a tightly sealed container away from heat, moisture, and direct light.

MISSED DOSE
Take it as soon as you remember. If it is near the time for the next dose, skip the missed dose and resume your regular dosage schedule. Do not double the next dose.

STOPPING THE DRUG
Take as prescribed for the full treatment period, even if your symptoms improve before the scheduled end of therapy.

PROLONGED USE
Prolonged use of any antibiotic increases the risk of superinfection (a more severe and drug-resistant infection). Use is generally limited to 10 to 28 days. People at risk for bleeding disorders or who have low platelets should have their blood platelet counts monitored by their doctor while taking linezolid.

▼ PRECAUTIONS

Over 60: No special advice.

Driving and Hazardous Work: Avoid such activities until you determine how the medicine affects you.

Alcohol: It is advisable to abstain from alcohol when treating a serious infection.

Pregnancy: Adequate human studies have not been done. Discuss with your doctor the relative risks and benefits of using this drug while pregnant.

Breast Feeding: Linezolid may pass into breast milk; caution is advised. Consult your doctor for advice.

Infants and Children: Safety and effectiveness have not been established for children under the age of 18.

Special Concerns: The oral suspension is supplied as a powder form. Tap the bottle gently to loosen the powder. Add a total of 123 milliliters (mL) distilled water in two portions. After adding the first half, shake the bottle well to wet all of the powder. Add the second portion of water and shake vigorously to mix the suspension. After constitution, each 5 mL of suspension contains 100 mg linezolid. Before using, gently mix by inverting the bottle 3 to 5 times. Do not shake. Store at room temperature and use the suspension within 21 days of reconstitution.

OVERDOSE

Symptoms: No cases of overdose have been reported. Symptoms may include lethargy, impaired coordination, vomiting, and tremor.

What to Do: If you suspect an overdose or if someone takes a much larger dose than prescribed, call your doctor, emergency medical services (EMS), or the nearest poison control center immediately.

▼ INTERACTIONS

DRUG INTERACTIONS
Consult your doctor for specific advice if you are taking an MAO inhibitor antidepressant (such as phenelzine or tranylcypromine), pseudoephedrine, phenylpropanolamine, dopamine, epinephrine, or SSRI antidepressants.

FOOD INTERACTIONS
Avoid tyramine-rich foods, which include aged cheeses, avocados, banana skins, bean curd, bologna and other processed lunch meats, chicken livers, chocolate, figs, canned or dried fish, pickled herring, meat extracts, pepperoni, raisins, raspberries, soy sauce, unpasteurized beer, Chianti, sherry, vermouth, and red wines in general.

DISEASE INTERACTIONS
Consult your doctor if you have a history of high blood pressure, hyperthyroidism, pheochromocytoma, carcinoid syndrome, thrombocytopenia or other bleeding disorders, diarrhea, or decreased kidney function.

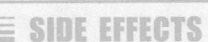

SIDE EFFECTS

SERIOUS
Serious side effects are rare, but may include: thrombocytopenia (reduced blood platelet numbers, resulting in uncontrolled bleeding) and pseudomembranous colitis. Consult your doctor immediately.

COMMON
Diarrhea, headache, nausea.

LESS COMMON
Insomnia, vomiting, constipation, dizziness.

LIOTHYRONINE SODIUM

Available in: Tablets
Available OTC? No **As Generic?** Yes
Drug Class: Thyroid hormone

▼ USAGE INFORMATION

WHY IT'S PRESCRIBED
Liothyronine is prescribed when the thyroid gland does not naturally produce enough thyroid hormone.

HOW IT WORKS
Liothyronine is a synthetic form of thyroid hormone. It functions in the same manner as (and so serves as a substitute for) the natural hormone when the body does not produce enough on its own.

▼ DOSAGE GUIDELINES

RANGE AND FREQUENCY
25 micrograms (mcg) per day to start. It can be increased to 50 mcg per day, taken in 2 or more daily doses.

ONSET OF EFFECT
Within 48 to 72 hours.

DURATION OF ACTION
Up to 72 hours after the drug is discontinued.

DIETARY ADVICE
Best if taken before breakfast, to minimize risk of insomnia.

STORAGE
Store in a tightly sealed container away from heat and direct light.

MISSED DOSE
Take it as soon as you remember. If it is near the time for the next dose, skip the missed dose and resume your regular dosage schedule. Do not double the next dose.

STOPPING THE DRUG
The decision to stop taking the drug should be made by your doctor.

PROLONGED USE
No special problems are expected.

▼ PRECAUTIONS

Over 60: A different dose may be needed for older patients. Consult your doctor about the proper dose.

Driving and Hazardous Work: The use of liothyronine should not impair your ability to perform such tasks safely.

Alcohol: Avoid alcohol.

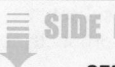

SIDE EFFECTS

SERIOUS
Severe headache in children; skin rash or hives. Call your physician immediately.

COMMON
Changes in appetite, changes in menstrual period, headache, hand tremors, increased sensitivity to heat, irritability, leg cramps, nervousness, sweating, insomnia, vomiting, weight loss, clumsiness, coldness, constipation, dry skin, muscle aches, weakness, weight gain.

LESS COMMON
Diarrhea or other forms of gastrointestinal upset.

Pregnancy: Use of proper amounts of liothyronine during pregnancy has not been shown to cause problems. Your doctor may want you to change the dose while you are pregnant. Regular visits to the doctor during pregnancy are advised.

Breast Feeding: Use of proper amounts of liothyronine in nursing women has not been shown to cause problems in their babies.

Infants and Children: The dose for infants and children must be carefully adjusted by the doctor.

Special Concerns: Before undergoing any kind of medical or dental procedure, be sure to tell the doctor or dentist in charge that you are taking liothyronine.

OVERDOSE
Symptoms: Headache, irritability, nervousness, sweating, rapid heartbeat, fever, palpitations or other heartbeat irregularities, increased bowel movements, menstrual irregularities, vomiting, seizures.

What to Do: An overdose of liothyronine is unlikely to be life-threatening. However, if someone takes a much larger dose than prescribed, call your doctor, emergency medical services (EMS), or nearest poison control center immediately.

▼ INTERACTIONS

DRUG INTERACTIONS
Consult your doctor for specific advice if you are taking amphetamines, anticoagulants, appetite suppressants, cholestyramine, colestipol, medicine for asthma or other breathing problems, or medicine for colds, sinus problems or hay fever.

FOOD INTERACTIONS
No known food interactions.

DISEASE INTERACTIONS
Caution is advised when taking liothyronine. Consult your doctor if you have any of the following: diabetes mellitus, hardening of the arteries, heart disease, high blood pressure, history of overactive thyroid, or underactive adrenal gland, underactive pituitary gland. If you have certain kinds of heart disease, this medicine may cause chest pains or shortness of breath during exertion. If these symptoms occur, consult your doctor.

LISINOPRIL

Available in: Tablets
Available OTC? No **As Generic?** No
Drug Class: Angiotensin-converting enzyme (ACE) inhibitor

▼ USAGE INFORMATION

WHY IT'S PRESCRIBED
To control high blood pressure (hypertension). Also used to treat congestive heart failure (CHF) and left ventricular dysfunction (damage to the primary pumping chamber of the heart), and to minimize further kidney damage in diabetic patients with mild kidney disease.

HOW IT WORKS
Angiotensin-converting enzyme (ACE) inhibitors block an enzyme that produces angiotensin, a naturally occurring substance that causes blood vessels to constrict and stimulates production of the adrenal hormone, aldosterone, which promotes sodium retention in the body. As a result, ACE inhibitors relax blood vessels (causing them to widen) and reduces sodium retention, which lowers blood pressure and so decreases the workload of the heart.

▼ DOSAGE GUIDELINES

RANGE AND FREQUENCY
For high blood pressure: 5 to 40 mg once a day. For congestive heart failure: 2.5 to 20 mg once a day.

ONSET OF EFFECT
Within 1 hour.

DURATION OF ACTION
24 hours.

DIETARY ADVICE
Take lisinopril on an empty stomach, about 1 hour before mealtime. Follow your doctor's dietary advice (such as low-salt or low-cholesterol restrictions) to improve control over high blood pressure and heart disease. Avoid high-potassium foods like bananas and citrus fruits and juices, unless you are also taking medications, such as diuretics, that lower potassium levels.

STORAGE
Store in a tightly sealed container away from heat and direct light.

MISSED DOSE
Take it as soon as you remember. If it is near the time for the next dose, skip the missed dose and resume your regular dosage schedule. Do not double the next dose.

STOPPING THE DRUG
Do not stop taking this drug abruptly, as this may cause potentially serious health problems. Dosage should be reduced gradually, according to your doctor's instructions.

PROLONGED USE
Lifelong therapy with lisinopril may be necessary. See your doctor regularly for examinations and tests if you must take this medicine for a prolonged period.

▼ PRECAUTIONS

Over 60: No unusual problems are expected in older patients.

Driving and Hazardous Work: Do not drive or engage in hazardous work until you determine how the medicine affects you.

Alcohol: Consume alcohol only in moderation since it may increase the effect of the drug and cause an excessive drop in blood pressure. Consult your doctor for advice.

Pregnancy: Use of lisinopril during the last 6 months of pregnancy may cause severe defects, even death, in the fetus. The drug should be discontinued if you are pregnant or plan to become pregnant.

Breast Feeding: Lisinopril may pass into breast milk; caution is advised. Consult your doctor for advice.

Infants and Children: Children may be especially sensitive to the effects of lisinopril. Benefits must be weighed against potential risks; consult your pediatrician for advice.

OVERDOSE
Symptoms: Dizziness, confusion, faintness.

What to Do: Call your doctor, emergency medical services (EMS), or the nearest poison control center immediately.

▼ INTERACTIONS

DRUG INTERACTIONS
Consult your doctor if you are taking diuretics (especially potassium-sparing diuretics), potassium supplements or drugs containing potassium (check ingredient labels), lithium, anticoagulants (such as warfarin), indomethacin or other anti-inflammatory drugs, or any over-the-counter medications (especially cold remedies and diet pills).

FOOD INTERACTIONS
Avoid low-salt milk and salt substitutes. Many of these products contain potassium.

DISEASE INTERACTIONS
Consult your doctor if you have systemic lupus erythematosus (SLE) or if you have had a prior allergic reaction to ACE inhibitors. Lisinopril should be used with caution by patients with severe kidney disease or renal artery stenosis (narrowing of one or both of the arteries that supply blood to the kidneys).

≡ SIDE EFFECTS ≡

SERIOUS
Fever and chills; sore throat and hoarseness; sudden difficulty breathing or swallowing; swelling of the face, mouth, or extremities; impaired kidney function (ankle swelling, decreased urination); confusion; yellow discoloration of the eyes or skin (indicating liver disorder); intense itching; chest pain or palpitations; abdominal pain. Serious side effects are very rare; contact your doctor immediately.

COMMON
Dry, persistent cough.

LESS COMMON
Dizziness or fainting; skin rash; numbness or tingling in the hands, feet, or lips; unusual fatigue or muscle weakness; nausea; drowsiness; loss of taste; headache.

LISINOPRIL/HYDROCHLOROTHIAZIDE

Available in: Tablets
Available OTC? No   **As Generic?** No
Drug Class: Angiotensin-converting enzyme (ACE) inhibitor/diuretic

▼ USAGE INFORMATION

WHY IT'S PRESCRIBED
To treat high blood pressure.

HOW IT WORKS
Angiotensin-converting enzyme (ACE) inhibitors, such as lisinopril, block an enzyme that produces angiotensin, a naturally occurring substance that causes blood vessels to constrict and stimulates production of the adrenal hormone, aldosterone, which promotes sodium retention in the body. As a result, ACE inhibitors relax blood vessels (causing them to widen) and reduce sodium retention, which lowers blood pressure and so decreases the workload of the heart. Hydrochlorothiazide (HCTZ), a diuretic, increases sodium and water in the urine output. By reducing the overall fluid volume in the body, diuretics reduce blood volume and so reduce blood pressure.

▼ DOSAGE GUIDELINES

RANGE AND FREQUENCY
This combination medication comes in three strengths: lisinopril/HCTZ 10/12.5, 20/12.5, and 20/25. The dose ranges from 10 to 40 mg lisinopril and 12.5 to 50 mg HCTZ per day. 1 or 2 tablets are taken once a day in the morning after breakfast.

ONSET OF EFFECT
Within 1 hour.

DURATION OF ACTION
Unknown.

DIETARY ADVICE
Follow your doctor's dietary advice (such as low-salt or low-fat restrictions) to improve control over high blood pressure and heart disease.

STORAGE
Store in a tightly sealed container away from heat, moisture, and direct light.

MISSED DOSE
Take it as soon as you remember. If it is near the time for the next dose, skip the missed dose and resume your regular dosage schedule. Do not double the next dose.

STOPPING THE DRUG
Discontinuing this drug abruptly may cause potentially serious problems. The dosage should be reduced gradually, according to your doctor's instructions.

PROLONGED USE
Lifelong therapy may be required; see your doctor regularly for evaluation.

▼ PRECAUTIONS

Over 60: Adverse reactions may be more likely and more severe in older patients.

Driving and Hazardous Work: Do not drive or engage in hazardous work until you determine how the medicine affects you.

Alcohol: Consume alcohol only in moderation since it may increase the effect of the drug and cause an excessive drop in blood pressure. Consult your doctor for advice.

Pregnancy: Before taking this medication, tell your doctor if you are pregnant or plan to become pregnant. Use of this drug during the last 6 months of pregnancy may cause severe defects, even death, in the fetus.

Breast Feeding: Lisinopril may pass into breast milk; caution is advised. Consult your doctor for advice.

Infants and Children: Children may be especially sensitive to the effects of lisinopril. Consult your pediatrician about the relative risks and benefits.

OVERDOSE
Symptoms: Overdose has not been reported; symptoms might include dizziness, faintness, or confusion.

What to Do: While overdose is unlikely, call your doctor, emergency medical services (EMS), or the nearest poison control center immediately if you suspect that someone has taken a much larger dose than prescribed.

▼ INTERACTIONS

DRUG INTERACTIONS
Consult your doctor for specific advice if you are taking cholestyramine, colestipol, digitalis drugs, lithium, potassium-containing medicines or supplements, or any over-the-counter drug (especially cold remedies and diet pills).

FOOD INTERACTIONS
Avoid low-salt milk and salt substitutes. Many of these products contain potassium.

DISEASE INTERACTIONS
Consult your doctor if you have systemic lupus erythematosus or if you have had a prior allergic reaction to ACE inhibitors. This medication should be used with caution by patients with severe kidney disease or renal artery stenosis (narrowing of one or both of the arteries that supply blood to the kidneys).

SIDE EFFECTS

SERIOUS
Fever and chills; sore throat and hoarseness; sudden difficulty breathing or swallowing; swelling of the face, mouth, or extremities; impaired kidney function (ankle swelling, decreased urination); confusion; yellow discoloration of the eyes or skin (indicating liver disorder); intense itching; chest pain or heartbeat irregularities; abdominal pain. Serious side effects are very rare; contact your doctor immediately.

COMMON
Dry, persistent cough.

LESS COMMON
Dizziness or fainting; skin rash; numbness or tingling in the hands, feet, or lips; change in color of the hands from white to blue to red (Raynaud's phenomenon) in cold weather; unusual fatigue or muscle weakness; nausea; drowsiness; loss of taste; headache; unusual dreams.

LITHIUM

Available in: Capsules, syrup, tablets, extended-release tablets
Available OTC? No   **As Generic?** Yes
Drug Class: Antimanic agent

▼ USAGE INFORMATION

WHY IT'S PRESCRIBED
To treat the manic phase of bipolar disorder (also known as manic-depression) and to enhance the effect of other antidepressant medications in patients with recurrent depression.

HOW IT WORKS
The exact mechanism of action of lithium is unknown.

▼ DOSAGE GUIDELINES

RANGE AND FREQUENCY
The dose is determined by measuring blood levels of lithium 12 hours after the drug is administered. The average adult dose is 900 to 1,800 mg a day. For older adults, the average dose is 150 to 900 mg a day.

ONSET OF EFFECT
1 to 2 weeks for mania. When used in conjunction with an antidepressant, symptoms may improve within a few days.

DURATION OF ACTION
24 hours.

DIETARY ADVICE
Can be taken with meals to lessen stomach upset. You should drink 8 to 10 glasses of water or caffeine-free beverages every day.

STORAGE
Store in a tightly sealed container away from heat and direct light.

MISSED DOSE
Take it as soon as you remember. If it is near the time for the next dose, skip the missed dose and resume your regular dosage schedule. Do not double the next dose.

STOPPING THE DRUG
The decision to stop taking the drug should be made in consultation with your doctor.

PROLONGED USE
See your doctor regularly for tests and examinations. Blood levels of lithium must be measured carefully to prevent lithium toxicity.

▼ PRECAUTIONS

Over 60: Adverse reactions may be more likely and more severe in older patients. A lower dose may be warranted.

Driving and Hazardous Work: Avoid such activities until you determine how the medicine affects you.

Alcohol: No special precautions are necessary.

Pregnancy: Lithium can cause problems in the unborn child, especially during the first 3 months of pregnancy. Before you take lithium, tell your doctor if you are pregnant or plan to become pregnant.

Breast Feeding: Lithium passes into breast milk; caution is advised. Consult your doctor for specific advice.

Infants and Children: Lithium can weaken the bones of infants and children. Use and dosage for children under the age of 12 must be determined by your pediatrician.

Special Concerns: Take care to avoid dehydration in hot weather and while engaging in vigorous activities. Be sure to drink plenty of fluids when using lithium. If you cannot consume enough fluids or you develop severe diarrhea while taking lithium, stop taking the drug and contact your doctor. Nonsteroidal anti-inflammatory drugs (NSAIDs) such as ibuprofen increase blood levels of lithium.

OVERDOSE
Symptoms: Twitching, tremor, slurred speech, extreme drowsiness, disorientation, confusion, seizures, muscle weakness, loss of consciousness, diarrhea, nausea, vomiting.

What to Do: Call your doctor, emergency medical services (EMS), or the nearest poison control center immediately.

▼ INTERACTIONS

DRUG INTERACTIONS
Other drugs may increase blood levels of lithium; consult your doctor for specific advice if you are taking another medicine for mental illness, a diuretic, medicine for pain or inflammation (especially NSAIDs), tetracycline, metronidazole, or ACE inhibitors. Some drugs lower blood levels of lithium; consult your doctor for advice if you are taking theophylline, caffeine, or acetazolamide.

FOOD INTERACTIONS
Avoid drinks and foods that contain caffeine.

DISEASE INTERACTIONS
You should not take lithium if you have seriously impaired kidney function, cardiovascular disease, or a history of leukemia. Before taking lithium, consult your doctor for specific advice if you have a history of brain disease, schizophrenia, diabetes, difficulty urinating, any infection, epilepsy, thyroid disease, Parkinson's disease, psoriasis, or leukemia.

SIDE EFFECTS

SERIOUS
Sedation, pronounced muscle weakness, confusion or disorientation, muscle twitching, vomiting, increased urination, slow heartbeat, fatigue, weight gain, dizziness, cold arms and legs, dry and rough skin, hoarseness, sensitivity to cold, swollen feet or legs, swollen neck. Call your physician immediately.

COMMON
Increased thirst, increased urination, nausea, loss of appetite, diarrhea, a slight tremor in the hands, fatigue, unexpected weight gain, metallic taste in mouth.

LESS COMMON
Skin rash, acne, hair loss.

LOMEFLOXACIN HYDROCHLORIDE

Available in: Tablets
Available OTC? No **As Generic?** No
Drug Class: Fluoroquinolone antibiotic

BRAND NAME
Maxaquin

▼ USAGE INFORMATION

WHY IT'S PRESCRIBED
To treat bacterial infections of the lower respiratory tract and urinary tract; to prevent urinary tract infections in patients preparing to undergo transurethral surgery (such as that performed to treat an enlarged prostate).

HOW IT WORKS
Lomefloxacin inhibits the activity of a bacterial enzyme (gyrase) that is necessary for proper DNA formation and replication. This prevents bacteria cells from reproducing.

▼ DOSAGE GUIDELINES

RANGE AND FREQUENCY
To treat infection— Adults age 18 and over: 400 mg, once a day for 10 to 14 days, depending on the type of infection being treated. To prevent infections presurgically— 400 mg, 2 to 6 hours before surgery.

ONSET OF EFFECT
Varies depending on the infection being treated.

DURATION OF ACTION
Unknown.

DIETARY ADVICE
Take it without regard to meals, although the drug is absorbed faster when taken on an empty stomach. Take it with a full glass of water, and drink lots of fluids, particularly citrus or cranberry juices.

STORAGE
Store in a tightly sealed container away from heat and direct light.

MISSED DOSE
Take it as soon as you remember. If it is near the time for the next dose, skip the missed dose and resume your regular dosage schedule. Do not double the next dose.

STOPPING THE DRUG
Take lomefloxacin as prescribed for the full treatment period, even if you begin to feel better before the scheduled end of therapy.

PROLONGED USE
See your doctor regularly for tests and examinations if you must take this medicine for a prolonged period.

▼ PRECAUTIONS

Over 60: No special problems are expected.

Driving and Hazardous Work: Avoid such activities until you determine how the medicine affects you.

Alcohol: It is advisable to abstain from alcohol when fighting an infection.

Pregnancy: In some animal tests, lomefloxacin has caused birth defects. Adequate studies in humans have not been done. It should be used during pregnancy only if potential benefits clearly justify the risks. Before you take lomefloxacin, tell your doctor if you are pregnant or plan to become pregnant.

Breast Feeding: Lomefloxacin passes into breast milk and may cause serious side effects in the nursing infant; use of the drug is discouraged when nursing.

Infants and Children: Lomefloxacin is not recommended for use by persons under the age of 18, as it has been shown to interfere with bone development.

Special Concerns: If lomefloxacin makes you unusually sensitive to sunlight, wear protective clothing, apply a sunblock, and try to stay out of direct sunlight, particularly between 10 am and 3 pm. Do not take any antacid or vitamin 4 hours before or 2 hours after taking this drug.

OVERDOSE
Symptoms: Severely reduced urination, weight gain, confusion, dryness and flakiness of skin, trembling, seizures.

What to Do: Call your doctor, emergency medical services (EMS), or the nearest poison control center immediately.

▼ INTERACTIONS

DRUG INTERACTIONS
Other drugs may interact with lomefloxacin. Consult your doctor for specific advice if you are taking aminophylline, antacids, didanosine, iron supplements, oxtriphylline, sucralfate, theophylline, warfarin, or zinc salts.

FOOD INTERACTIONS
No known food interactions.

DISEASE INTERACTIONS
Consult your doctor if you have a brain or spinal cord condition, epilepsy, or any other condition causing seizures. Use of lomefloxacin may cause complications in patients with liver or kidney disease, since these organs work together to remove the medication from the body.

SIDE EFFECTS

SERIOUS
Serious reactions to lomefloxacin are rare and include seizures, mental confusion, hallucinations, agitation, nightmares, depression, shortness of breath, unusual swelling in the face or extremities, and loss of consciousness. Also severe skin burning, redness, blisters, rash, or itching on exposure to sunlight. Call your doctor immediately.

COMMON
Increased sensitivity to sunlight (and increased risk of sunburn) for days following therapy.

LESS COMMON
Diarrhea, nausea and vomiting, stomach pain and upset, gas, headache, dizziness, restlessness, insomnia, changes in taste perception, drowsiness, itching, dry mouth, unusual body aches or pains.

LOMUSTINE

Available in: Capsules
Available OTC? No   **As Generic?** No
Drug Class: Alkylating agent

▼ USAGE INFORMATION

WHY IT'S PRESCRIBED
To treat brain tumors and Hodgkin's disease (a type of cancer affecting the lymph nodes and spleen).

HOW IT WORKS
Lomustine kills cancer cells by interfering with the activity of their genetic material, thus preventing the cells from reproducing. The drug may also affect the growth and development of normal cells in the body, resulting in unpleasant side effects.

▼ DOSAGE GUIDELINES

RANGE AND FREQUENCY
130 mg per square meter of body surface once every 6 weeks. The dose may need to be lowered, based on red blood cell counts.

ONSET OF EFFECT
Unknown.

DURATION OF ACTION
Unknown.

DIETARY ADVICE
Lomustine is best taken on an empty stomach at bedtime to minimize stomach upset.

STORAGE
Store in a tightly sealed container away from heat and direct light.

MISSED DOSE
Take it as soon as you remember. Do not double the next dose.

STOPPING THE DRUG
The decision to stop taking the drug should be made by your doctor.

PROLONGED USE
See your doctor regularly for tests and examinations if you take this medication for a prolonged period.

▼ PRECAUTIONS

Over 60: No special precautions are necessary.

Driving and Hazardous Work: Do not drive or engage in hazardous work until you determine how the medicine affects you.

Alcohol: Avoid alcohol.

Pregnancy: Lomustine can cause birth defects if taken by either the father or the mother. Persons of childbearing years should take steps to prevent pregnancy while being treated with this drug.

Breast Feeding: Not recommended while undergoing therapy with this drug.

Infants and Children: Lomustine is expected to have the same therapeutic effect and cause the same side effects in infants and children as it does in adults.

Special Concerns: Do not receive any immunizations without your doctor's approval. Avoid persons who have recently had oral polio vaccine and those with any infection. Consult your doctor or dentist about appropriate ways to clean your teeth to avoid injury. Be careful not to cut yourself when using sharp objects such as a safety razor or nail cutters. Avoid activities and contact sports where bruising or injury could occur. If you vomit shortly after taking a dose of lomustine, check with your doctor. You may be told to take the dose again. Lomustine may have cumulative effects on bone marrow, causing low blood counts. This drug has been reported to have an effect on the lungs, causing shortness of breath up to 15 years after taking it.

OVERDOSE
Symptoms: Swelling of the abdomen or glands, weakness, nosebleed.

What to Do: Call your doctor, emergency medical services (EMS), or the nearest poison control center immediately.

▼ INTERACTIONS

DRUG INTERACTIONS
Consult your doctor for specific advice if you are taking amphotericin B, antithyroid agents, aspirin, azathioprine, chloramphenicol, colchicine, coumadin, flucytosine, ganciclovir, interferon, plicamycin, or zidovudine (AZT). Also consult your doctor if you are taking any over-the-counter medications.

FOOD INTERACTIONS
No known food interactions.

DISEASE INTERACTIONS
Consult your doctor if you have any of the following: shingles, chickenpox, any infection, kidney disease, or lung disease.

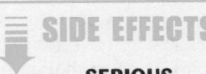
≡ SIDE EFFECTS ≡

SERIOUS
Black, tarry, or bloody stools; blood in urine; fever and chills, cough or hoarseness; pain in lower back or side; difficult, decreased, or painful urination; red spots on skin; unusual bleeding or bruising; confusion; loss of coordination; slurred speech; sores on lips or in mouth; swollen feet or lower legs; unusual fatigue; cough; shortness of breath. Call your doctor immediately.

COMMON
Loss of appetite, nausea and vomiting (for periods of less than 24 hours), temporary hair loss.

LESS COMMON
Darkened skin, diarrhea, itching or skin rash.

LOPERAMIDE HYDROCHLORIDE

BRAND NAMES

Imodium, Imodium A-D, Imodium A-D Caplets, Kaopectate II, Maalox Anti-Diarrheal, Pepto Diarrhea Control

Available in: Capsules, oral solution, tablets
Available OTC? Yes   **As Generic?** Yes
Drug Class: Antidiarrheal

▼ USAGE INFORMATION

WHY IT'S PRESCRIBED
To treat diarrhea.

HOW IT WORKS
Loperamide eases diarrhea by slowing the activity of the intestines.

▼ DOSAGE GUIDELINES

RANGE AND FREQUENCY
Capsules— Adults and teenagers: 4 mg after the first loose bowel movement, 2 mg after each subsequent loose bowel movement. Take no more than 16 mg every 24 hours. Children ages 8 to 12: 2 mg, 3 times a day. Children ages 6 to 8: 2 mg, 2 times a day. Oral solution— Adults and teenagers: 4 mg (4 tea-spoons) after the first loose bowel movement, 2 mg after each subsequent loose bowel movement. No more than 8 mg every 24 hours. Children ages 9 to 11: 2 mg after the first loose bowel movement, 1 mg after each subsequent loose bowel movement. No more than 6 mg every 24 hours. Children ages 6 to 8: 2 mg after the first loose bowel movement, 1 mg after each subsequent loose bowel movement. No more than 4 mg every 24 hours. Tablets— Adults and teen-agers: 4 mg after the first loose bowel movement, 1 mg after each subsequent loose bowel movement. No more than 8 mg every 24 hours. Children ages 9 to 11: 2 mg after the first loose bowel movement, 1 mg after each subsequent loose bowel movement. No more than 6 mg every 24 hours. Children ages 6 to 8: 2 mg after the first loose bowel movement, 1 mg after each subsequent loose bowel movement. No more than 4 mg every 24 hours.

ONSET OF EFFECT
Unknown.

DURATION OF ACTION
Up to 24 hours.

DIETARY ADVICE
Take it on an empty stomach (1 hour before or 2 hours after eating). A mild diet is recommended when recovering from diarrhea. Bananas, rice, applesauce, and plain toast are good choices. Be sure to drink plenty of fluids.

STORAGE
Store in a tightly sealed container away from heat, moisture, and direct light.

MISSED DOSE
Skip the missed dose and resume your regular dosage schedule. Do not double the next dose.

STOPPING THE DRUG
You may stop taking the drug whenever you choose.

PROLONGED USE
Loperamide should not be used for more than 2 days unless directed otherwise by your doctor.

▼ PRECAUTIONS

Over 60: Diarrhea may easily lead to dehydration, especially in older patients, and loperamide may mask the effects of dehydration. When using loperamide, older persons should be sure to get plenty of fluids.

Driving and Hazardous Work: Avoid such activities until you determine how the medicine affects you.

Alcohol: Avoid alcohol.

Pregnancy: Discuss with your doctor the relative risks and benefits of using loperamide while pregnant.

Breast Feeding: It is not known whether loperamide passes into breast milk; caution is advised. Consult your doctor for specific advice.

Infants and Children: Do not give to children under 6 years of age unless otherwise directed by your doctor.

Special Concerns: During the first 24 hours, drink plenty of caffeine-free clear liquids like water, broth, ginger ale, and decaffeinated tea. During the second 24 hours you may eat bland foods such as applesauce, bread, crackers, and oatmeal.

OVERDOSE
Symptoms: Constipation, central nervous system depression, gastrointestinal irritation.

What to Do: An overdose of loperamide is unlikely to be life-threatening. However, if someone takes a much larger dose than prescribed, call your doctor, emergency medical services (EMS), or the nearest poison control center.

▼ INTERACTIONS

DRUG INTERACTIONS
Consult your doctor for specific advice if you are taking antibiotics, such as cephalosporin, erythromycin, and tetracycline; or any narcotic pain medication.

FOOD INTERACTIONS
Fruits, fried or spicy foods, bran, candy, and caffeine-containing beverages can make diarrhea worse.

DISEASE INTERACTIONS
Consult your doctor if you have any of the following: dysentery, severe colitis, or liver disease.

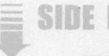

SIDE EFFECTS

SERIOUS
Bloating, skin rash, constipation, loss of appetite, stomach pains, nausea, vomiting. Call your doctor immediately.

COMMON
No common side effects are associated with loperamide.

LESS COMMON
Dizziness or drowsiness, dry mouth.

LOPERAMIDE/SIMETHICONE

Available in: Chewable tablet
Available OTC? Yes   **As Generic?** No
Drug Class: Antidiarrheal/antigas combination

▼ USAGE INFORMATION

WHY IT'S PRESCRIBED
To treat diarrhea and to relieve bloating, pain, pressure, and cramps caused by excess gas in the stomach and intestines.

HOW IT WORKS
Loperamide eases diarrhea by slowing the activity of the intestines. Simethicone disperses and prevents the formation of gas bubbles in the gastrointestinal tract.

▼ DOSAGE GUIDELINES

RANGE AND FREQUENCY
Adults and teenagers: Chew 2 tablets and drink a full glass of water after the first loose stool. If needed, chew 1 tablet and drink more water after the next loose stool. Take no more than 4 tablets per day. Children ages 6 to 11: Chew 1 tablet after the first loose stool. If needed, chew half a tablet after the next loose stool. Children ages 9 to 11 (or weighing 60 to 95 lbs) should take no more than 3 tablets per day. Children ages 6 to 8 (or weighing 48 to 59 lbs) should take no more than 2 tablets per day. Follow each dose with plenty of clear liquids.

ONSET OF EFFECT
Unknown.

DURATION OF ACTION
Unknown.

DIETARY ADVICE
A mild diet is recommended when recovering from diarrhea. Bananas, rice, applesauce, and plain toast are good choices. Be sure to drink plenty of fluids.

STORAGE
Store in a tightly sealed container away from heat, moisture, and direct light.

MISSED DOSE
Not applicable, since the drug is taken only when necessary.

STOPPING THE DRUG
You may stop taking the drug whenever you choose.

PROLONGED USE
This drug should not be used for more than 2 days unless directed otherwise by your physician.

▼ PRECAUTIONS

Over 60: Diarrhea may easily lead to dehydration, especially in older patients, and this drug may mask the symptoms of dehydration. When using this drug, older persons should be sure to get plenty of fluids.

Driving and Hazardous Work: No special precautions are necessary.

Alcohol: Avoid alcohol, as it may irritate the lining of the gastrointestinal tract and promote dehydration.

Pregnancy: Discuss with your doctor the relative risks and benefits of using this drug while pregnant.

Breast Feeding: This drug may pass into breast milk; caution is advised. Consult your doctor for advice.

Infants and Children: Not recommended for use by children under the age of 6 or who weigh less than 48 lbs.

Special Concerns: Chew the tablets thoroughly before swallowing for quicker and more complete relief. You should change position frequently and walk about to help eliminate gas. During the first 24 hours, drink plenty of caffeine-free clear liquids like water, broth, ginger ale, and decaffeinated tea. During the second 24 hours you may eat bland foods, such as applesauce, bread, crackers, and oatmeal. Tell your doctor if you are on a low-sodium, low-sugar, or other special diet. Do not smoke before meals.

OVERDOSE
Symptoms: Constipation, gastrointestinal irritation, drowsiness, confusion.

What to Do: An overdose of this drug is unlikely to be life-threatening. However, if someone takes a much larger dose than prescribed, call your doctor.

▼ INTERACTIONS

DRUG INTERACTIONS
Consult your doctor for specific advice if you are taking antibiotics, such as cephalosporin, erythromycin, and tetracycline; or any narcotic pain medication.

FOOD INTERACTIONS
Fruits, fried or spicy foods, bran, candy, and caffeine-containing beverages can make diarrhea worse. Avoid any foods that increase gas formation. Chew your food slowly and thoroughly.

DISEASE INTERACTIONS
Do not use this drug if you have a high fever (over 101°F) or stools containing blood or mucus. Consult your physician if you have dysentery, severe colitis, or liver disease.

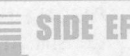
SIDE EFFECTS

SERIOUS
Skin rash, bloating, constipation, loss of appetite, stomach pain, nausea, vomiting. Call your doctor immediately.

COMMON
Expulsion of excess gas, causing belching and flatulence.

LESS COMMON
Dizziness or drowsiness, dry mouth.

LORACARBEF

BRAND NAME

Lorabid

Available in: Capsules, oral suspension
Available OTC? No **As Generic?** No
Drug Class: Antibiotic

▼ USAGE INFORMATION

WHY IT'S PRESCRIBED
To treat bacterial infections including urinary tract infections, bronchitis, pneumonia, and strep throat (streptococcal pharyngitis).

HOW IT WORKS
Loracarbef, an antibiotic similar to those in the cephalosporin family, kills bacteria or inhibits their growth and multiplication.

▼ DOSAGE GUIDELINES

RANGE AND FREQUENCY
For infections of the urinary tract— Adults and teenagers: 200 to 400 mg, 1 or 2 times a day for 7 to 14 days. For bronchitis— Adults and teenagers: 200 to 400 mg, 2 times a day for 7 days. For pneumonia— Adults and teenagers: 400 mg, 2 times a day for 14 days. For infections of skin and soft tissue— Adults and teenagers: 200 mg, 2 times a day for 7 days. For strep throat— Adults and teenagers: 200 mg, 2 times a day for 10 days. For all conditions, use and dosage of loracarbef for children ages 6 months to 12 years must be determined by your doctor.

ONSET OF EFFECT
Unknown.

DURATION OF ACTION
Unknown.

DIETARY ADVICE
Loracarbef should be taken on an empty stomach at least 1 hour before or 2 hours after meals. Drink plenty of fluids.

STORAGE
Store in a tightly sealed container away from heat and direct light.

MISSED DOSE
Take it as soon as you remember. If it is near the time for the next dose, skip the missed dose and resume your regular dosage schedule. Do not double the next dose.

STOPPING THE DRUG
It is very important to take antibiotics as prescribed for the full treatment period, even if you begin to feel better before the scheduled end of therapy. This is especially important when being treated for streptococcal infections.

PROLONGED USE
You should see your doctor regularly for tests and examinations if you must take this medicine for a prolonged period.

▼ PRECAUTIONS

Over 60: In older patients, loracarbef is not expected to cause side effects different from or more severe than those in younger persons.

Driving and Hazardous Work: Do not drive or engage in hazardous work until you determine how the medicine affects you.

Alcohol: No special problems are expected, although it is generally advisable to abstain from alcohol when fighting an infection.

Pregnancy: Loracarbef has not been shown to cause birth defects in animals. Human studies have not been done. Before you take loracarbef, tell your doctor if you are pregnant or plan to become pregnant.

Breast Feeding: Loracarbef may pass into breast milk; caution is advised. Consult your doctor for advice.

Infants and Children: Consult your doctor about use of loracarbef by children 12 years or younger.

Special Concerns: It is important to maintain consistent blood levels of loracarbef. You should be very careful not to miss a dose. If you have difficulty maintaining a proper dosage schedule, consult your physician.

OVERDOSE
Symptoms: Unusually rapid or slow heartbeat, unusual drop in blood pressure (causing dizziness, lightheadedness, confusion, or fainting).

What to Do: An overdose is unlikely to be life-threatening. However, if someone takes a larger dose than prescribed, call your doctor, emergency medical services (EMS), or the nearest poison control center right away.

▼ INTERACTIONS

DRUG INTERACTIONS
Other drugs may interact with loracarbef. Consult your doctor for specific advice if you are taking diuretics (water pills) or probenecid. Also tell your doctor if you are taking any other prescription or over-the-counter medication.

FOOD INTERACTIONS
No known food interactions.

DISEASE INTERACTIONS
Use of loracarbef may cause complications in patients with liver or kidney disease, since these organs work together to remove the medication from the body.

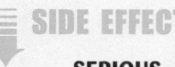
SIDE EFFECTS

SERIOUS
Severe diarrhea, skin rash, hives, intense itching. Call your doctor right away.

COMMON
Loss of appetite, mild diarrhea, stomach pain, nausea, vomiting. Consult your doctor.

LESS COMMON
Dizziness, drowsiness, headache, discharge from or itching of the vagina, insomnia, general nervousness. Consult your doctor if such symptoms persist.

LORATADINE

Available in: Tablets, syrup
Available OTC? No **As Generic?** No
Drug Class: Antihistamine

▼ USAGE INFORMATION

WHY IT'S PRESCRIBED
To prevent or relieve symptoms of hay fever and other allergies, such as watery or itchy eyes, runny nose, sneezing, or itchy skin. Loratadine is also used sometimes to treat chronic (persistent) hives.

HOW IT WORKS
Loratadine blocks the effects of histamine, a naturally occurring substance that causes swelling, itching, sneezing, watery eyes, hives, and other symptoms of allergic reaction.

▼ DOSAGE GUIDELINES

RANGE AND FREQUENCY
Tablets and syrup— Adults and children age 10 and older: 10 mg once a day. Children ages 2 to 9: 5 mg once a day. Do not increase the dose in an attempt to achieve quicker relief of symptoms.

ONSET OF EFFECT
Within 1 hour.

DURATION OF ACTION
24 hours or more.

DIETARY ADVICE
Loratadine can be taken without regard to diet, but taking this medicine with food may be beneficial because it may increase absorption of the drug from the gastrointestinal tract by up to 40%.

STORAGE
Store in a tightly sealed container at room temperature, away from heat, moisture, and direct light.

MISSED DOSE
Take it as soon as you remember. However, if it is near the time for the next dose, skip the missed dose and resume your regular dosage schedule. Do not double the next dose.

STOPPING THE DRUG
The decision to stop taking the drug should be made in consultation with your doctor.

PROLONGED USE
Loratadine can be taken safely for prolonged periods. Long-term use is not associated with decreased effectiveness of the drug (a problem with certain allergy medications and other drugs).

▼ PRECAUTIONS

Over 60: Adverse reactions may be more likely and more severe in older patients.

Driving and Hazardous Work: The use of loratadine, at recommended doses, should not impair your ability to perform such tasks safely.

Alcohol: No special precautions are necessary.

Pregnancy: Before you take loratadine, tell your doctor if you are pregnant or plan to become pregnant.

Breast Feeding: Loratadine passes into breast milk; avoid or discontinue use while breast feeding.

Infants and Children: Adverse reactions may be more likely and more severe in children.

Special Concerns: Stop taking loratadine 4 to 7 days before you have an allergy skin test.

OVERDOSE
Symptoms: Rapid heartbeat, headache, drowsiness.

What to Do: An overdose of loratadine is unlikely to be life-threatening. However, if someone takes a much larger dose than prescribed, call your doctor, emergency medical services (EMS), or the nearest poison control center.

▼ INTERACTIONS

DRUG INTERACTIONS
Consult your doctor for advice if you are taking clarithromycin, erythromycin, troleandomycin, itraconazole, or ketoconazole.

FOOD INTERACTIONS
There are no known interactions between loratadine and specific foods.

DISEASE INTERACTIONS
There are no known disease interactions.

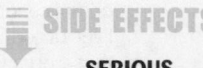

SIDE EFFECTS

SERIOUS
No serious side effects are associated with the use of loratadine.

COMMON
No common side effects are associated with the use of loratadine.

LESS COMMON
In rare cases adverse reactions have been reported in persons taking loratadine, but none of these reactions is clearly linked to use of the drug.

LORATADINE/PSEUDOEPHEDRINE

BRAND NAME

Claritin-D

Available in: Extended-release tablets
Available OTC? No **As Generic?** No
Drug Class: Antihistamine/decongestant

▼ USAGE INFORMATION

WHY IT'S PRESCRIBED
To relieve the symptoms of seasonal allergic rhinitis (hay fever), which include runny nose, nasal congestion, and sneezing.

HOW IT WORKS
Loratadine blocks the effects of histamine, a naturally occurring substance that causes swelling, itching, sneezing, nasal discharge and congestion, and other symptoms of an allergic reaction. Pseudoephedrine narrows and constricts blood vessels to reduce the blood flow to swollen nasal passages, which reduces nasal secretions, shrinks swollen nasal mucous membranes, and improves airflow through the nasal passages.

▼ DOSAGE GUIDELINES

RANGE AND FREQUENCY
The 12-hour formulation may be taken twice a day (every 12 hours). The 24-hour formulation should only be taken once a day. Tablets should be taken with a full glass of water.

ONSET OF EFFECT
Within 1 to 3 hours.

DURATION OF ACTION
12 to 24 hours or more.

DIETARY ADVICE
This drug can be taken without regard to meals. Take it with a full glass of water.

STORAGE
Store in a tightly sealed container away from heat, moisture, and direct light.

MISSED DOSE
Not applicable. This drug is taken as needed.

STOPPING THE DRUG
Not applicable. This drug is taken as needed.

PROLONGED USE
This drug is prescribed for short-term (seasonal) use only.

▼ PRECAUTIONS

Over 60: Adequate studies have not been done. However, older patients are more susceptible to the effects of the pseudoephedrine component (see Pseudoephedrine).

Driving and Hazardous Work: The use of this drug should not impair your ability to perform such tasks safely. However, exercise caution if the medication makes you drowsy.

Alcohol: No special precautions are necessary.

Pregnancy: Adequate human studies have not been done. Discuss with your doctor the relative risks and benefits of using this drug while pregnant.

Breast Feeding: Both drugs pass into breast milk. Discuss with your doctor the relative risks and benefits of using this drug while nursing.

Infants and Children: Not recommended for use by children under age 12.

Special Concerns: Do not break or chew the tablet. Patients with a history of esophageal narrowing or swallowing difficulty should not take this drug.

OVERDOSE
Symptoms: Drowsiness, heartbeat irregularities, headache, giddiness, nausea, vomiting, sweating, increased thirst, chest pain, urination difficulties, muscle weakness and tenseness, anxiety, restlessness, insomnia, hallucinations, delusions, seizures, difficulty breathing.

What to Do: Call your doctor, emergency medical services (EMS), or the nearest poison control center immediately.

▼ INTERACTIONS

DRUG INTERACTIONS
This drug and MAO inhibitors should not be used within 14 days of each other. Consult your doctor for specific advice if you are taking beta-blockers, digitalis drugs, or over-the-counter antihistamines or decongestants.

FOOD INTERACTIONS
No known food interactions.

DISEASE INTERACTIONS
You should not take this drug if you have narrow-angle glaucoma, severe hypertension, urinary retention, or severe coronary artery disease. Caution is advised when taking this drug if you have any of the following: high blood pressure, diabetes mellitus, heart disease, increased eye pressure, hyperthyroidism, or enlarged prostate. Use of this drug may cause complications in patients with liver or kidney disease, since these organs work together to remove the medication from the body.

 SIDE EFFECTS

SERIOUS
No serious side effects are associated with the use of loratadine/pseudoephedrine.

COMMON
Insomnia, dry mouth, drowsiness.

LESS COMMON
Nervousness, dizziness, indigestion.

LORAZEPAM

Available in: Oral solution, tablets, injection
Available OTC? No   **As Generic?** Yes
Drug Class: Benzodiazepine tranquilizer; antianxiety agent

▼ USAGE INFORMATION

WHY IT'S PRESCRIBED
To treat anxiety and insomnia. The injection form of lorazepam, administered in a hospital setting, is used to treat a type of seizure disorder (status epilepticus) and is used before surgery to sedate patients prior to the administration of anesthesia.

HOW IT WORKS
In general, lorazepam produces mild sedation by depressing activity in the central nervous system. In particular, lorazepam appears to enhance the effect of gamma-aminobutyric acid (GABA), a natural chemical that inhibits the firing of neurons and dampens the transmission of nerve signals, thus decreasing nervous excitation.

▼ DOSAGE GUIDELINES

RANGE AND FREQUENCY
For anxiety— Adults and teenagers: 1 to 2 mg every 8 or 12 hours, up to 6 mg a day. Older adults: 0.5 mg, 2 times a day to start; the dose may be increased. For insomnia— Adults and teenagers: 1 to 2 mg taken at bedtime. Note: In all cases, use and dosage for children under 12 years of age must be determined by your doctor.

ONSET OF EFFECT
30 minutes to 2 hours for oral forms.

DURATION OF ACTION
12 to 24 hours.

DIETARY ADVICE
Can be taken with food to prevent gastrointestinal upset.

STORAGE
Store in a tightly sealed container away from heat, moisture, and direct light.

MISSED DOSE
Take it as soon as you remember. However, if it is near the time for the next dose, skip the missed dose and resume your regular dosage schedule. Do not double the next dose. For insomnia, do not take it unless your schedule allows a full night's sleep.

STOPPING THE DRUG
Never stop taking the drug abruptly, as this can cause withdrawal symptoms. Dosage should be reduced gradually as directed by your doctor.

PROLONGED USE
Lorazepam may slowly lose its effectiveness with prolonged use. See your doctor for periodic evaluation if you must take this drug for an extended length of time.

▼ PRECAUTIONS

Over 60: Adverse reactions may be more likely and more severe in older patients. A lower dose may be warranted.

Driving and Hazardous Work: Lorazepam can impair mental alertness and physical coordination. Adjust your activities accordingly.

Alcohol: Avoid alcohol.

Pregnancy: Use during pregnancy should be avoided if possible. Tell your doctor if you are pregnant or plan to become pregnant.

Breast Feeding: Lorazepam passes into breast milk; do not take it while nursing.

Infants and Children: Lorazepam should be used by children only under close medical supervision.

Special Concerns: Lorazepam use can lead to psychological or physical dependence. Short-term therapy (8 weeks or less) is typical; do not take the drug for a longer period unless so advised by your doctor. Never take more than the prescribed daily dose.

OVERDOSE
Symptoms: Extreme drowsiness, confusion, slurred speech, slow reflexes, poor coordination, staggering gait, tremor, slowed breathing, loss of consciousness.

What to Do: Call your doctor, emergency medical services (EMS), or the nearest poison control center immediately.

▼ INTERACTIONS

DRUG INTERACTIONS
Consult your doctor for specific advice if you are taking any drugs that depress the central nervous system (such as antihistamines, antidepressants or other psychiatric medications, barbiturates, sedatives, cough medicines, decongestants, and painkillers). Be sure your doctor knows about any over-the-counter drug you may take.

FOOD INTERACTIONS
None reported.

DISEASE INTERACTIONS
Consult your doctor if you have a history of alcohol or drug abuse, stroke or other brain disease, any chronic lung disease, hyperactivity, depression or other mental illness, myasthenia gravis, sleep apnea, epilepsy, porphyria, kidney disease, or liver disease.

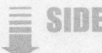 SIDE EFFECTS

SERIOUS
Difficulty concentrating, outbursts of anger, other behavior problems, depression, hallucinations, low blood pressure (causing faintness or confusion), memory impairment, muscle weakness, skin rash or itching, sore throat, fever and chills, sores or ulcers in throat or mouth, unusual bruising or bleeding, extreme fatigue, yellowish tinge to eyes or skin. Call your doctor immediately.

COMMON
Drowsiness, loss of coordination, unsteady gait, dizziness, lightheadedness, slurred speech.

LESS COMMON
Change in sexual desire or ability, constipation, false sense of well-being, nausea and vomiting, urinary problems, unusual fatigue.

LOSARTAN POTASSIUM

Available in: Tablets
Available OTC? No **As Generic?** No
Drug Class: Antihypertensive/angiotensin II antagonist

BRAND NAME
Cozaar

▼ USAGE INFORMATION

WHY IT'S PRESCRIBED
To control high blood pressure. This drug appears to have the same benefits as the class of antihypertensive drugs known as ACE inhibitors, without producing the common side effect (experienced by as many as 30% of patients) of a dry cough. Losartan may be used alone or in conjunction with other antihypertensive medications.

HOW IT WORKS
Losartan blocks the effects of angiotensin II, a naturally occurring substance that causes blood vessels to narrow. Losartan causes the blood vessels to dilate, thereby lowering blood pressure and decreasing the workload of the heart.

▼ DOSAGE GUIDELINES

RANGE AND FREQUENCY
Adults: To start, 25 to 50 mg once a day. Usual maintenance dose is 25 to 100 mg, taken once a day or divided into 2 doses. Children: Not recommended.

ONSET OF EFFECT
Within 1 hour.

DURATION OF ACTION
24 hours.

DIETARY ADVICE
Follow a healthy diet (low-salt, low-fat, low-cholesterol) as advised by your doctor to help control blood pressure and prevent heart disease.

STORAGE
Store in a tightly sealed container away from heat, moisture, and direct light.

MISSED DOSE
Take it as soon as you remember. If it is near the time for the next dose, skip the missed dose and resume your regular dosage schedule. Do not double the next dose.

STOPPING THE DRUG
Take it as prescribed for the full treatment period. The decision to stop taking the drug should be made in consultation with your physician.

PROLONGED USE
Lifelong therapy may be necessary. However, if you do change certain health habits (for example, increasing exercise or losing weight), it may

be possible, under your doctor's supervision, to reduce the dose.

▼ PRECAUTIONS

Over 60: Adverse reactions may be more likely and more severe in older patients.

Driving and Hazardous Work: Do not drive or engage in hazardous work until you determine how the medicine affects you.

Alcohol: Drink only in careful moderation. (See Special Concerns.)

Pregnancy: In certain ways losartan is similar to a class of drugs that have caused damage to the unborn child when taken in the second or third trimester of pregnancy. Because safer, more effective medications can lower blood pressure during pregnancy, and because adequate studies on the use of losartan during pregnancy have not been done, women who are pregnant or planning to become pregnant should not take this drug.

Breast Feeding: Losartan passes into breast milk; avoid use while nursing.

Infants and Children: The safety and effectiveness of this drug have not been established for children.

Special Concerns: Losartan may cause dizziness or lightheadedness, which is most noticeable when you change position. This may lead to fainting, falls, and injury. Sit or lie down immediately if

you feel dizzy or lightheaded. This side effect may be worsened by alcohol, hot weather, dehydration, fever, prolonged standing, prolonged sitting, or exercise.

OVERDOSE
Symptoms: Fainting, dizziness, weak pulse that might be very slow or very fast, nausea and vomiting, chest pain.

What to Do: Call your doctor, emergency medical services (EMS), or the nearest poison control center immediately.

▼ INTERACTIONS

DRUG INTERACTIONS
Consult your doctor for specific advice if you are taking diuretics, potassium-containing medicines or supplements, salt substitutes, low-salt milk, NSAIDs, allopurinol, over-the-counter drugs for colds, coughs, hay fever, asthma, sinus problems, or appetite control, or other prescription medications.

FOOD INTERACTIONS
No known food interactions.

DISEASE INTERACTIONS
Use of losartan may cause complications in patients with liver or kidney disease, since these organs work together to remove the medication from the body.

≡ SIDE EFFECTS ≡

SERIOUS
Sudden difficulty breathing or swallowing; hoarseness; swelling of the face, mouth, hands, or throat; dizziness; cough; fever or sore throat. Call your doctor immediately.

COMMON
Headache.

LESS COMMON
Back pain, fatigue, diarrhea, nasal congestion.

LOTEPREDNOL ETABONATE

Available in: Ophthalmic suspension
Available OTC? No   **As Generic?** No
Drug Class: Corticosteroid

▼ USAGE INFORMATION

WHY IT'S PRESCRIBED
Alrex is prescribed for temporary relief of eye symptoms due to seasonal allergic inflammation of the conjunctiva. Lotemax is used to control inflammation and prevent potentially permanent damage that may result from eye problems, such as conjunctivitis, herpes of the eye, and corneal injuries. It is also used to help relieve redness, irritation, and discomfort in the eye, and may be used after eye surgery to control any inflammatory response. Loteprednol is less potent than prednisolone but also less likely to cause adverse effects.

HOW IT WORKS
Ophthalmic loteprednol inhibits the release of natural substances that cause inflammation and pain in eye tissues.

▼ DOSAGE GUIDELINES

RANGE AND FREQUENCY
Alrex (0.2%)– To treat seasonal allergic conjunctivitis: 1 drop into the affected eye 4 times a day. Lotemax (0.5%)– 1 to 2 drops into the affected eye 4 times a day. Within the first week of treatment, dose may be increased, up to 1 drop per hour, if needed. For postoperative inflammation: 1 to 2 drops into the operated eye 4 times a day beginning 24 hours following surgery and for the next 2 weeks.

ONSET OF EFFECT
Unknown.

DURATION OF ACTION
Unknown.

DIETARY ADVICE
No special restrictions.

STORAGE
Store in a tightly sealed container away from heat, moisture, and direct light. Do not allow it to freeze.

MISSED DOSE
Apply it as soon as you remember. If it is near the time for the next dose, skip the missed dose and resume your regular dosage schedule. Do not double the next dose.

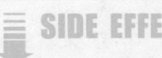

SIDE EFFECTS

SERIOUS
Decreased vision or blurring of vision (from cataract); eye pain, nausea, vomiting (from increased intraocular pressure); pain, redness, sensitivity to bright light, discharge (from eye infection). Call your doctor immediately if you experience any of these signs or symptoms. The drug may trigger a recurrence of herpes infection of the eye; mention any previous herpes infection to your doctor.

COMMON
Burning, stinging, redness, or watering of eyes.

LESS COMMON
Headache, runny nose, sore throat.

STOPPING THE DRUG
It is very important to use this drug as prescribed for the full treatment period, even if symptoms improve before the scheduled end of therapy.

PROLONGED USE
You should see your ophthalmologist to have your eye pressure monitored if you use this drug for 10 days or longer.

▼ PRECAUTIONS

Over 60: No special advice.

Driving and Hazardous Work: Do not drive or engage in hazardous work until you determine how the medicine affects your vision.

Alcohol: No special warnings.

Pregnancy: Adequate human studies have not been done, though no birth defects have been reported. Tell your doctor if you are pregnant or plan to become pregnant.

Breast Feeding: Ophthalmic loteprednol has not been reported to cause problems in nursing babies. Consult your doctor.

Infants and Children: Safety and effectiveness have not been established.

Special Concerns: Shake the bottle vigorously before administering. Wash your hands and tilt your head back. Gently apply pressure to the inside corner of the eyelid and with the index finger of the same hand, pull downward on the lower eyelid to make a space. Drop the medicine into this space and close your eye. Apply pressure for 1 or 2 minutes while keeping the eye closed without blinking. Then wash your hands again. Make sure the tip of the dropper does not touch your eye, finger, or any other surface. If your symptoms do not improve in 2 days or if they become worse, check with your doctor. Wearing contact lenses while using this medication may increase the risk of infection. Your doctor may tell you not to wear contact lenses during and for a day or two after treatment.

OVERDOSE
Symptoms: When used topically, an overdose is very unlikely. Inadvertent oral ingestion, however, may cause fever, muscle pain, loss of appetite, dizziness, fainting, and trouble breathing.

What to Do: An overdose is unlikely to be life-threatening. However, if someone accidentally ingests the medicine, call your doctor, emergency medical services (EMS), or the nearest poison control center.

▼ INTERACTIONS

DRUG INTERACTIONS
Consult your doctor for specific advice if you are taking any other medication.

FOOD INTERACTIONS
No known food interactions.

DISEASE INTERACTIONS
Consult your doctor if you have any of the following: cataracts, diabetes, glaucoma, herpes infection or tuberculosis of the eye, or any other eye infection.

LOVASTATIN

BRAND NAME

Mevacor

Available in: Tablets
Available OTC? No   **As Generic?** No
Drug Class: Antilipidemic (cholesterol-lowering agent)

▼ USAGE INFORMATION

WHY IT'S PRESCRIBED
To treat high cholesterol. Usually prescribed after first lines of treatment—including diet, weight loss, and exercise—fail to reduce total and low-density lipoprotein (LDL) cholesterol to acceptable levels. Lovastatin has also been approved for the primary prevention of coronary artery disease (CAD) in persons with no symptoms of CAD, but who have average to modestly elevated levels of total and LDL cholesterol and below average HDL.

HOW IT WORKS
Lovastatin blocks the action of an enzyme required for the manufacture of cholesterol, thereby interfering with its formation. By lowering the amount of cholesterol in the liver cells, lovastatin increases the formation of receptors for LDL, and thereby reduces blood levels of total and LDL cholesterol. In addition to lowering LDL cholesterol, lovastatin also modestly reduces triglyceride levels and raises HDL (the so-called good) cholesterol.

▼ DOSAGE GUIDELINES

RANGE AND FREQUENCY
20 to 80 mg per day, taken with meals. The 20 mg dose is taken with the evening meal; doses greater than 20 mg per day are taken in the morning and evening.

ONSET OF EFFECT
2 to 4 weeks.

DURATION OF ACTION
The effect persists for the duration of therapy.

DIETARY ADVICE
Cholesterol-lowering drugs are only one part of a total program that should include regular exercise and a healthy diet. The American Heart Association publishes a "Healthy Heart" diet, which is recommended.

STORAGE
Store in a tightly sealed container away from heat, moisture, and direct light.

MISSED DOSE
Take your missed dose as soon as you remember. Take your next scheduled dose at the proper time, and resume your regular dosage schedule. Do not take a double dose.

STOPPING THE DRUG
The decision to stop taking the drug should be made in consultation with your doctor. Once the medication is discontinued, blood cholesterol is likely to return to original elevated levels.

PROLONGED USE
Side effects are more likely with prolonged use. As you continue with lovastatin, your doctor will periodically order blood tests to evaluate liver function.

▼ PRECAUTIONS

Over 60: No special problems are expected.

Driving and Hazardous Work: The use of lovastatin should not impair your ability to perform such tasks safely.

Alcohol: No special precautions are necessary.

Pregnancy: Lovastatin should not be used during pregnancy nor by women who are trying to become pregnant.

Breast Feeding: This drug is not recommended for women who are nursing.

Infants and Children: The drug can be effective, but safety is not known; rarely used in children. Consult your pediatrician.

Special Concerns: Important elements of treatment for high cholesterol include proper diet, weight loss, regular moderate exercise, and the avoidance of certain medications that may increase cholesterol levels. Because lovastatin has potential side effects, it is important that you maintain a recommended healthy diet and cooperate with other treatments your physician may suggest.

OVERDOSE
Symptoms: An overdose of lovastatin is unlikely.

What to Do: Emergency instructions not applicable.

▼ INTERACTIONS

DRUG INTERACTIONS
Consult your doctor if you are taking cyclosporine, gemfibrozil, niacin, antibiotics, especially erythromycin, or medications for fungus infections. All of these drugs may increase the risk of myositis (muscle inflammation) when taken with lovastatin and may lead to kidney failure.

FOOD INTERACTIONS
None reported.

DISEASE INTERACTIONS
Consult your doctor if you have any of the following problems: liver, kidney, or muscle disease, or a medical history involving organ transplant or recent surgery.

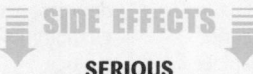
SIDE EFFECTS

SERIOUS
Fever, unusual or unexplained muscle aches and tenderness. Call your doctor right away.

COMMON
Side effects occur in only 1% to 2% of patients. These include constipation or diarrhea, dizziness or lightheadedness, bloating or gas, heartburn, nausea, skin rash, stomach pain, rise in liver enzymes.

LESS COMMON
Sleeping difficulty.

LOXAPINE

Available in: Tablets, oral solution, capsules, injection
Available OTC? No   **As Generic?** Yes
Drug Class: Neuroleptic; antipsychotic

▼ USAGE INFORMATION

WHY IT'S PRESCRIBED
To treat moderate to severe psychiatric conditions, such as schizophrenia.

HOW IT WORKS
Loxapine appears to block receptors of dopamine (a chemical that aids in the transmission of nerve impulses) in the central nervous system. Presumably, this produces a tranquilizing or antipsychotic effect.

▼ DOSAGE GUIDELINES

RANGE AND FREQUENCY
Oral forms: To start, 10 mg, 2 times a day. The dose may be gradually increased by your physician to a maximum of 250 mg a day. Injection: 12.5 to 50 mg, 4 to 6 times per day, injected into a muscle.

ONSET OF EFFECT
Sedation may occur within minutes, but onset of antipsychotic effect may take hours to occur or may not occur until days or weeks after the beginning of therapy.

DURATION OF ACTION
12 to 24 hours.

DIETARY ADVICE
Oral solution should be mixed with orange juice or grapefruit juice.

STORAGE
Store in a tightly sealed container away from heat, moisture, and direct light. Do not allow the solution or injection forms to freeze.

MISSED DOSE
Take it as soon as you remember. However, if it is near the time for the next dose, skip the missed dose and resume your regular dosage schedule. Do not double the next dose.

STOPPING THE DRUG
The decision to stop taking the drug should be made in consultation with your doctor.

PROLONGED USE
Prolonged use may lead to tardive dyskinesia (involuntary movements of the jaw, lips, tongue, and, in rare cases, the arms, legs, hands, or body). Consult your doctor about the need for follow-up evaluations and tests if you must take this drug for an extended period.

▼ PRECAUTIONS

Over 60: Adverse reactions may be more likely and more severe in older patients.

Driving and Hazardous Work: Do not drive or engage in hazardous work until you determine how the medicine affects you.

Alcohol: Avoid alcohol.

Pregnancy: Adequate studies have not been completed; consult your doctor for more information.

Breast Feeding: It is not known whether loxapine passes into breast milk, although no problems have been reported.

Infants and Children: The safety and effectiveness of loxapine in children have not been established. Use and dose for children up to age 16 should be determined by your doctor.

Special Concerns: Avoid prolonged exposure to high temperatures in hot climates. Drink plenty of fluids and stay cool in the summertime. Avoid overexposure to sunlight until you determine if the drug heightens your skin's sensitivity to ultraviolet light.

▼ OVERDOSE

Symptoms: Severe drowsiness, severe dizziness, muscle jerking, trembling, or stiffness, trouble breathing, unusual fatigue.

What to Do: Call your doctor, emergency medical services (EMS), or the nearest poison control center immediately.

▼ INTERACTIONS

DRUG INTERACTIONS
Do not take loxapine within 2 hours of taking an antacid or an antidiarrheal medication. Consult your doctor for specific advice if you are taking amoxapine, methyldopa, metoclopramide, metyrosine, other drugs for mental illness, pemoline, pimozide, promethazine, rauwolfia alkaloids, trimeprazine, any medication that depresses the central nervous system, tricyclic antidepressants, guanadrel, or guanethidine.

FOOD INTERACTIONS
None are known.

DISEASE INTERACTIONS
Consult your doctor if you have a history of alcohol or drug abuse, difficulty urinating, benign prostatic hyperplasia (BPH), glaucoma, Parkinson's disease, heart or blood vessel disease, liver disease, or a seizure disorder.

SIDE EFFECTS

SERIOUS
Seizures, breathing difficulty, heartbeat irregularities, high fever, unusual sweating, loss of bladder control, lip puckering or smacking, uncontrolled chewing and tongue movements, uncontrolled limb or body movements, difficulty speaking or swallowing, loss of balance, trembling, muscle spasms, severe constipation, difficulty urinating, rash, sore throat and fever, unusual bleeding or bruising, jaundice. Call your doctor immediately.

COMMON
Blurred vision, dizziness, confusion, fainting, drowsiness, shuffling gait, slow movements, staring and absence of facial expression, dry mouth.

LESS COMMON
Mild constipation, sexual dysfunction, headache, increased sensitivity of skin to sun, nausea or vomiting, insomnia, menstrual irregularities, breast swelling, unusual milk secretion, unexpected weight gain.

LYME DISEASE VACCINE (RECOMBINANT OSPA)

Available in: Injection
Available OTC? No **As Generic?** No
Drug Class: Vaccine

▼ USAGE INFORMATION

WHY IT'S PRESCRIBED
To protect against, but not treat, Lyme disease in people ages 15 to 70. The vaccine is recommended for people who live or work in grassy or wooded areas infested with ticks infected with Borrelia burgdorferi (the bacteria that causes Lyme disease) as well as for people planning to travel to those areas.

HOW IT WORKS
Lyme disease vaccine stimulates the body's immune system to produce antibodies against a protein on the outer surface of the tick. When infected ticks bite vaccinated humans, the vaccine-induced antibodies enter the tick and attack the B. burgdorferi inside the gut of the tick, thereby preventing transmission of the disease.

▼ DOSAGE GUIDELINES

RANGE AND FREQUENCY
All doses are administered by a health care professional. Adults and teenagers: 1 dose injected into a muscle in the upper arm. Booster doses are given 1 month and 12 months

after the first dose. All three doses are required to confer optimal protection.

ONSET OF EFFECT
Unknown.

DURATION OF ACTION
Unknown.

DIETARY ADVICE
No special restrictions.

STORAGE
Not applicable; the dose is administered only at a health care facility.

MISSED DOSE
If you miss a scheduled vaccination, contact your doctor. According to the Centers for Disease Control and Prevention (CDC), if you miss the one-month booster, you may take it as soon as possible within the first year. All 3 injections should be completed within 1 year.

STOPPING THE DRUG
The full schedule of injections should be followed unless a medical problem intervenes. A full course of injections must be completed to ensure adequate immunization.

PROLONGED USE
Periodic booster shots may be recommended.

▼ PRECAUTIONS

Over 60: Lyme disease vaccine is not expected to cause different or more severe side effects in older patients than in younger persons.

Driving and Hazardous Work: The vaccine should not impair your ability to perform such tasks safely.

Alcohol: No special precautions are necessary.

Pregnancy: Adequate human studies have not been done. Before taking Lyme disease vaccine, tell your physician if you are pregnant or planning to become pregnant.

Breast Feeding: Lyme disease vaccine may pass into breast milk; caution is advised. Consult your doctor for advice.

Infants and Children: Not recommended for use by children under the age of 15. No special problems are expected in persons over the age of 15.

Special Concerns: Previous infection with B. burgdorferi does not mean that you are immune to future infections of Lyme disease. As with any vaccine, Lyme disease vaccine may not protect all individuals. In clinical studies, the vaccine was effective in approximately 78% of cases after receiving all three doses. In addition to vaccination, people can decrease their chances of acquiring tick-borne infections by wearing pants and long-sleeved shirts, tucking pants into socks, spraying tick repellent on clothing, checking for ticks in

a tick-infested area, and removing attached ticks.

OVERDOSE
Symptoms: Not applicable.

What to Do: No cases of overdose have been reported.

▼ INTERACTIONS

DRUG INTERACTIONS
No drug interactions have been reported. However, as with other intramuscular injections, Lyme disease vaccine should not be administered to people taking anticoagulant drugs, such as warfarin, unless the potential benefit outweighs the risks.

FOOD INTERACTIONS
No known food interactions.

DISEASE INTERACTIONS
No known disease interactions. However, as with other intramuscular injections, Lyme disease vaccine should not be administered to people with blood clotting disorders. The safety of the vaccine has not been tested in people with joint or neurological complications of Lyme disease, disorders associated with chronic joint swelling, and in those with a pacemaker.

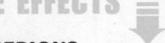 **SIDE EFFECTS**

SERIOUS
No serious side effects have been reported.

COMMON
Soreness or redness at the site of injection.

LESS COMMON
Muscle pain, chills, fever, flulike symptoms.

MAGALDRATE

Available in: Oral suspension
Available OTC? Yes   **As Generic?** Yes
Drug Class: Antacid

▼ USAGE INFORMATION

WHY IT'S PRESCRIBED
To relieve symptoms of heartburn, acid indigestion, sour stomach, and gastro-esophageal reflux. Also prescribed to treat hyperacidity associated with peptic ulcers, gastritis, and esophagitis.

HOW IT WORKS
Magaldrate neutralizes stomach acid and reduces the action of pepsin, a digestive enzyme. This provides symptomatic relief from excess stomach acid.

▼ DOSAGE GUIDELINES

RANGE AND FREQUENCY
Adults: 540 to 1,080 mg (5 to 10 ml). Children: 5 to 10 mg. Take it between meals and at bedtime.

ONSET OF EFFECT
Within 20 minutes.

DURATION OF ACTION
20 to 60 minutes in fasting patients; 3 hours when taken after meals.

DIETARY ADVICE
Eat a balanced diet.

STORAGE
Store in a tightly sealed container away from heat, moisture, and direct light.

MISSED DOSE
Take it as soon as you remember. If it is near the time for the next dose, skip the missed dose and resume your regular dosage schedule. Do not double the next dose.

STOPPING THE DRUG
Take as directed for the full treatment period.

PROLONGED USE
Do not take magaldrate for more than 2 weeks unless your doctor advises you to do otherwise.

SIDE EFFECTS

SERIOUS
Severe and continuing constipation, dizziness, lightheadedness, and heartbeat irregularities. Bone loss (osteomalacia) may occur, especially with prolonged use in dialysis patients. Hypophosphatemia (too little phosphate in the blood) may occur with prolonged use and a low-phosphate diet; symptoms include bone pain, fractures (due to bone loss), muscle weakness, loss of appetite, mood changes, a general feeling of discomfort, swelling of the wrists and ankles, unusual weight loss, and anemia (decreased number of red blood cells; symptoms include weakness and fatigue). Call your doctor immediately.

COMMON
Chalky taste in mouth.

LESS COMMON
Increased thirst, speckling or whitish color of stools, stomach cramps, diarrhea, mild constipation.

▼ PRECAUTIONS

Over 60: Constipation and intestinal trouble are more common in older persons. Older patients who have or who are at high risk for osteoporosis or other bone disorders should avoid frequent use of magaldrate.

Driving and Hazardous Work: No special precautions.

Alcohol: Avoid alcohol.

Pregnancy: Adequate studies have not been done. Before taking magaldrate, tell your doctor if you are pregnant or plan to become pregnant.

Breast Feeding: Magaldrate may pass into breast milk but has not been reported to cause problems in nursing babies. Consult your doctor for advice.

Infants and Children: Do not give antacids and other magnesium-containing medicines to young children unless prescribed by a physician.

Special Concerns: Use over-the-counter antacids only occasionally unless otherwise directed by your doctor. Persistent heartburn not readily relieved by antacids may be signaling a heart attack or other serious disorder. Seek medical help promptly.

OVERDOSE
Symptoms: Diarrhea, nausea, vomiting, constipation, confusion, palpitations, weakness, fatigue, bone pain, stupor.

What to Do: An overdose of magaldrate is unlikely to be life-threatening. However, if someone takes a much larger dose than prescribed, call your doctor, emergency medical services (EMS), or the nearest poison control center.

▼ INTERACTIONS

DRUG INTERACTIONS
Magaldrate and other magnesium-containing antacids may interact with vitamin D (including calcitediol and calcitriol), and may decrease the effectiveness of pancrelipase. Note that other medications may lose their effectiveness when taken within 1 hour of antacids. Consult your doctor for specific advice if you are taking amphetamines, bisacodyl, cellulose sodium phosphate, citrates, chenodiol, digoxin, enteric-coated medications, fluoroquinolones, isoniazid, ketoconazole, mecamylamine, methenamine, nitrofurantoin, penicillamine, phosphates, sodium polystyrene sulfonate resin, quinidine, or tetracyclines.

FOOD INTERACTIONS
No known food interactions.

DISEASE INTERACTIONS
Do not take magaldrate if you have any symptoms of appendicitis or an inflamed bowel (abdominal pain, cramps, soreness, bloating, nausea, and vomiting). Magaldrate is not recommended for Alzheimer's patients. Consult your doctor if you have any of the following: broken bones, colitis, diarrhea, intestinal blockage or bleeding, colostomy or ileostomy, edema, hypophosphatemia, heart disease, liver disease, toxemia of pregnancy, or kidney disease.

MAGNESIUM CITRATE

Available in: Oral solution
Available OTC? Yes   **As Generic?** Yes
Drug Class: Hyperosmotic laxative

▼ USAGE INFORMATION

WHY IT'S PRESCRIBED
To treat short-term constipation and for rapid emptying of the colon for rectal and bowel examinations.

HOW IT WORKS
Magnesium citrate attracts and retains water in the intestine, softening stools and inducing the urge to defecate.

▼ DOSAGE GUIDELINES

RANGE AND FREQUENCY
Adults and teenagers: 11 to 25 g daily in 1 or more doses. Children ages 6 to 12: 5.5 to 12.5 g daily in 1 or more doses.

ONSET OF EFFECT
30 minutes to 3 hours.

DURATION OF ACTION
Variable.

DIETARY ADVICE
Take it on an empty stomach with a full glass of cold water or juice.

STORAGE
Store in a tightly sealed container away from heat, moisture, and direct light.

MISSED DOSE
If you are taking this drug on a fixed schedule, take the missed dose as soon as you remember. If it is near the time for the next dose, skip the missed dose and resume your regular dosage schedule. Do not double the next dose.

STOPPING THE DRUG
Take it as prescribed for the full treatment period. However, you may stop taking the drug if you are feeling better before the scheduled end of the therapy.

PROLONGED USE
Magnesium citrate is intended for short-term therapy only.

▼ PRECAUTIONS

Over 60: No special problems are expected.

Driving and Hazardous Work: This medication should not impair your ability to perform such tasks safely.

Alcohol: Avoid alcohol.

Pregnancy: Pregnant women with impaired kidney function should avoid taking magnesium citrate.

≣ SIDE EFFECTS ≣

SERIOUS
Confusion, dizziness or lightheadedness, intestinal blockage, skin rash or itching, difficulty swallowing. Call your doctor immediately.

COMMON
Cramping, diarrhea, gas, increased thirst.

LESS COMMON
Sweating, weakness.

Breast Feeding: Magnesium citrate may pass into breast milk; caution is advised. Consult your doctor for advice.

Infants and Children: Do not give magnesium citrate and other laxatives to children under 6 years of age unless prescribed by a doctor.

Special Concerns: Chilling the medication or taking it with ice or following it with citrus fruit juice or citrus-flavored carbonated beverages may make it more palatable. Remember that chronic use of magnesium citrate or any laxative can lead to laxative dependence. You should consume adequate amounts of fiber in your diet, like bran, whole-grain cereals, fruit, and vegetables. Magnesium citrate should be taken on a schedule that doesn't interfere with activities or sleep, as it produces watery stools in 3 to 6 hours. It should not be taken within 2 hours of taking other medications.

OVERDOSE
Symptoms: Severe or protracted diarrhea.

What to Do: An overdose of magnesium citrate is unlikely to be life-threatening. However, if someone takes a much larger dose than prescribed, call your doctor, emergency medical services (EMS), or the nearest poison control center right away.

▼ INTERACTIONS

DRUG INTERACTIONS
Consult your doctor for specific advice if you are taking cellulose sodium phosphate; other magnesium-containing medications, such as antacids; other laxatives; sodium polystyrene sulfonate; and oral tetracycline antibiotics.

FOOD INTERACTIONS
No known food interactions.

DISEASE INTERACTIONS
Caution is advised when taking magnesium citrate. Consult your doctor if you have kidney problems, symptoms of appendicitis (abdominal pain, nausea, vomiting), heart damage, intestinal obstruction or perforation, heart block, or rectal fissures.

MAGNESIUM OXIDE

Mag-Ox 400, Maox 420, Uro-Mag

Available in: Capsules, tablets
Available OTC? Yes   **As Generic?** Yes
Drug Class: Antacid

▼ USAGE INFORMATION

WHY IT'S PRESCRIBED
To treat low magnesium in the blood (hypomagnesemia). Also used to replace or prevent magnesium loss due to other medications or conditions. It is used as an antacid to relieve heartburn, sour stomach, and acid indigestion.

HOW IT WORKS
Magnesium oxide neutralizes stomach acid and reduces the action of pepsin, a digestive enzyme. This provides symptomatic relief from excess stomach acid and heartburn.

▼ DOSAGE GUIDELINES

RANGE AND FREQUENCY
Capsules: 140 mg, 3 to 4 times a day. Tablets: 400 to 800 mg a day in evenly divided doses.

ONSET OF EFFECT
Within 20 minutes.

DURATION OF ACTION
For 20 minutes in fasting patients; 3 hours when taken after meals.

DIETARY ADVICE
Take this medication at least 1 hour after meals.

STORAGE
Store in a tightly sealed container away from heat, moisture, and direct light.

MISSED DOSE
Take it as soon as you remember. If it is near the time for the next dose, skip the missed dose and resume your regular dosage schedule. Do not double the next dose.

STOPPING THE DRUG
Take it as prescribed for the full treatment period. However, when magnesium oxide is used as an antacid, it may be taken as needed.

PROLONGED USE
You should see your doctor regularly for tests and examinations if you must take this drug for a prolonged period.

▼ PRECAUTIONS

Over 60: Adverse reactions may be more likely and more severe.

Driving and Hazardous Work: Do not drive or engage in hazardous work until you determine how the medicine affects you.

Alcohol: Avoid alcohol.

Pregnancy: Adequate studies have not been done. Be sure to tell your doctor if you are pregnant or planning to become pregnant.

Breast Feeding: Magnesium oxide may pass into breast milk; consult your doctor for advice.

Infants and Children: Not recommended for use by children under 6 unless prescribed by a doctor.

Special Concerns: Using magnesium oxide in large amounts or for prolonged periods may have a laxative effect; the drug should not be used regularly for this purpose. In general, do not take other medicines within 2 hours of taking magnesium-containing antacids. Heartburn or upper abdominal pain not readily relieved by antacids may be signaling a heart attack or other serious disorder. In such cases, seek medical help promptly.

OVERDOSE
Symptoms: Diarrhea, bloating, change in mental state, muscle pain or twitching, slowed or shallow breathing, coma.

What to Do: An overdose of magnesium oxide is unlikely to be life-threatening. However, if someone takes a much larger dose than prescribed, call your doctor,

emergency medical services (EMS), or the nearest poison control center immediately.

▼ INTERACTIONS

DRUG INTERACTIONS
Consult your doctor if you are taking fluoroquinolones, ketoconazole, methenamine, mecamylamine, sodium polystyrene sulfonate, tetracyclines, urinary acidifiers, digitalis drugs, misoprostol, pancrelipase, iron salts, phosphates, salicylates, or vitamin D (including calcifediol and calcitriol). Also, certain medications may lose their effectiveness or cause unexpected side effects when taken within 2 hours of magnesium oxide. These include enteric-coated medicines, folic acid, penicillamine, phenothiazines, and phenytoin. Take at least 2 hours apart (3 hours with phenytoin).

FOOD INTERACTIONS
No known food interactions.

DISEASE INTERACTIONS
Do not take magnesium oxide if you have any symptoms of appendicitis or an inflamed bowel (abdominal pain, cramps, soreness, bloating, nausea, and vomiting). Magnesium-containing antacids should not be taken by patients with kidney disease. Consult your doctor if you have any of the following: bone fractures, colitis, severe and continuing constipation, hemorrhoids, intestinal or rectal bleeding, a colostomy or ileostomy, persistent diarrhea, edema, heart disease, liver disease, toxemia of pregnancy, sarcoidosis, or underactive parathyroid glands.

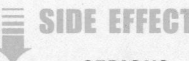
SIDE EFFECTS

SERIOUS
Dizziness, lightheadedness, continuing feeling of discomfort, irregular heartbeat, loss of appetite, mental or mood changes, muscle weakness, unusual fatigue or weakness, unusual weight loss. Call your doctor immediately.

COMMON
Chalky taste, laxative effect.

LESS COMMON
Diarrhea, increased thirst, speckling or discoloration of stools, stomach cramps, nausea or vomiting, elevated magnesium in the blood (detectable by your doctor).

532

MAGNESIUM SULFATE

Available in: Crystals, tablets
Available OTC? Yes **As Generic?** Yes
Drug Class: Laxative/dietary supplement

▼ USAGE INFORMATION

WHY IT'S PRESCRIBED
Magnesium sulfate is used to evacuate the bowel before surgery, and as a dietary supplement for people with a magnesium deficiency due to illness or as a result of the use of certain medications.

HOW IT WORKS
As a laxative, magnesium sulfate attracts and retains water in the intestine, softening stools and inducing the urge to defecate.

▼ DOSAGE GUIDELINES

RANGE AND FREQUENCY
As a laxative— Adults and teenagers: 10 to 30 g daily in 1 or more doses. Children ages 6 to 12: 5 to 10 g daily in 1 or more doses. To treat magnesium deficiency— The dose is determined by your doctor according to the severity of the deficiency.

ONSET OF EFFECT
Within 30 minutes to 3 hours.

DURATION OF ACTION
Variable.

DIETARY ADVICE
Take it on an empty stomach with a full glass of cold water or juice.

STORAGE
Store in a tightly sealed container away from heat, moisture, and direct light.

MISSED DOSE
If you are taking this drug on a fixed schedule, take the missed dose as soon as you remember. If it is near the time for the next dose, skip the missed dose and resume your regular dosage schedule. Do not double the next dose.

STOPPING THE DRUG
You should not take magnesium sulfate for more than 1 week unless your physician prescribes its continued use.

PROLONGED USE
You should see your doctor regularly for tests and examinations if you must take this drug for a prolonged period.

▼ PRECAUTIONS

Over 60: No special problems are expected.

Driving and Hazardous Work: The use of magnesium sulfate should not impair your ability to perform such tasks safely.

Alcohol: Avoid alcohol.

Pregnancy: Magnesium sulfate is used as a treatment, in the hospital only, for certain symptoms of toxemia of pregnancy. In proper amounts it can be used if necessary as a dietary supplement during pregnancy.

Breast Feeding: Magnesium sulfate passes into breast milk; caution is advised. Consult your doctor for advice.

Infants and Children: Magnesium sulfate and other laxatives should not be given to children under 6 years of age unless prescribed by your pediatrician.

Special Concerns: Taking it with ice or following it with citrus fruit juice or citrus-flavored carbonated beverages may make it more palatable. Remember that chronic use of magnesium sulfate or any laxative can lead to laxative dependence. Consume adequate amounts of fiber in your diet, such as bran, whole-grain cereals, fruit, and vegetables. Magnesium sulfate should be taken on a schedule that does not interfere with activities or sleep, as it produces watery stools within 3 to 6 hours. It should not be taken within 2 hours of taking other medications.

OVERDOSE
Symptoms: Blurred or double vision, dizziness or fainting, severe drowsiness, increased or decreased urination, slow heartbeat, trouble breathing.

What to Do: Call your doctor, emergency medical services (EMS), or the nearest poison control center immediately.

▼ INTERACTIONS

DRUG INTERACTIONS
Consult your doctor for specific advice if you are taking oral tetracycline, other magnesium-containing preparations, cellulose sodium phosphate, sodium polystyrene sulfonate, or digitalis drugs.

FOOD INTERACTIONS
No known food interactions.

DISEASE INTERACTIONS
Caution is advised when taking magnesium sulfate. Consult your doctor if you have any of the following: myasthenia gravis, severe kidney disease, heart blockage, intestinal obstruction or perforation, or any respiratory disease.

≡ SIDE EFFECTS ≡

SERIOUS
Abdominal cramps, nausea, diarrhea. Call your doctor immediately.

COMMON
There are no common side effects associated with the use of magnesium sulfate.

LESS COMMON
There are no less-common side effects associated with the use of magnesium sulfate.

MAPROTILINE HYDROCHLORIDE

Available in: Tablets
Available OTC? No   **As Generic?** Yes
Drug Class: Tetracyclic antidepressant

▼ USAGE INFORMATION

WHY IT'S PRESCRIBED
To relieve symptoms of major depression.

HOW IT WORKS
Maprotiline affects levels of norepinephrine, a brain chemical that is thought to be linked to mood, emotions, and mental state.

▼ DOSAGE GUIDELINES

RANGE AND FREQUENCY
Adults: To start, 25 mg, 1 to 3 times a day. The dose may be increased gradually by your doctor to 150 mg a day. Children: Dosage is determined by your doctor.

ONSET OF EFFECT
1 to 3 weeks.

DURATION OF ACTION
Unknown.

DIETARY ADVICE
No special restrictions.

STORAGE
Store in a tightly sealed container away from heat, moisture, and direct light.

MISSED DOSE
If you take a one-time daily bedtime dose, do not take a missed dose in the morning because it may cause drowsiness. Call your doctor. If you take more than 1 dose a day, take it as soon as you remember. If it is near the time for the next dose, skip the missed dose and resume your regular dosage schedule. Do not double the next dose.

STOPPING THE DRUG
Take it as prescribed for the full treatment period, even if you feel better before the scheduled end of therapy. The decision to stop taking the drug should be made by your doctor.

PROLONGED USE
See your doctor regularly for tests and examinations if you take it for a prolonged period.

▼ PRECAUTIONS

Over 60: Adverse reactions may be more likely and more severe in older patients.

Driving and Hazardous Work: Use caution while driving or engaging in hazardous work until you determine how the medicine affects you. Drowsiness or lightheadedness can occur.

Alcohol: Avoid alcohol.

Pregnancy: In animal studies, maprotiline has not caused problems. Human studies have not been done. Before you take maprotiline, tell your doctor if you are pregnant or plan to become pregnant.

Breast Feeding: Maprotiline passes into breast milk; caution is advised. Consult your doctor for specific advice.

Infants and Children: Use and dosage for infants and children must be determined by your doctor. It is not known whether maprotiline causes different or more severe side effects in infants and children than it does in older persons.

Special Concerns: Risk of seizures is increased if more than 150 mg is taken within a 24-hour period. If maprotiline causes dry mouth, use sugarless candy, gum, or ice chips for relief.

OVERDOSE
Symptoms: Severe dizziness or drowsiness, seizures, nausea or vomiting, heartbeat irregularities, difficulty breathing, fever, restlessness, muscle stiffness or fatigue.

What to Do: Call your doctor, emergency medical services (EMS), or the nearest poison control center immediately.

▼ INTERACTIONS

DRUG INTERACTIONS
Maprotiline and MAO inhibitors should not be used within 14 days of each other. Consult your doctor for specific advice if you are taking asthma medicine, amphetamines, cisapride, cold medicine, medicines that depress the central nervous system, or appetite suppressants.

FOOD INTERACTIONS
No known food interactions.

DISEASE INTERACTIONS
Caution is advised when taking maprotiline. Consult your doctor if you have any of the following: epilepsy or another seizure disorder, gastrointestinal problems, asthma, urinary problems, glaucoma, a history of alcohol abuse, an enlarged prostate, heart disease, blood vessel disease, liver disease, or an overactive thyroid.

 SIDE EFFECTS

SERIOUS
Severe constipation, trembling, weight loss, unusual excitability, severe dizziness or drowsiness, seizures, nausea or vomiting, palpitations or heartbeat irregularities, difficulty breathing, fever, restlessness, severe muscle stiffness or fatigue. Also skin redness, swelling, itching, or rash. Call your doctor right away.

COMMON
Dizziness, lightheadedness, drowsiness, visual disturbances, dry mouth, headache, sexual dysfunction, fatigue.

LESS COMMON
Diarrhea, constipation, heartburn, increased sensitivity to sunlight, increased sweating, weight loss, insomnia, increased appetite with weight gain.

MASOPROCOL

BRAND NAME

Actinex

Available in: Cream
Available OTC? No   **As Generic?** No
Drug Class: Topical antineoplastic (anticancer) agent

▼ USAGE INFORMATION

WHY IT'S PRESCRIBED
Masoprocol is used for therapy of actinic keratoses (precancerous skin growths that can become malignant if left untreated).

HOW IT WORKS
It is not known exactly how masoprocol works. Laboratory experiments have shown that masoprocol prevents cells similar to the ones found in actinic keratoses from multiplying.

▼ DOSAGE GUIDELINES

RANGE AND FREQUENCY
Adults: Apply cream to lesions 2 times a day. Use sufficient cream to cover lesions entirely. Do not apply a covering bandage or dressing to the site. Children: Consult a pediatrician.

ONSET OF EFFECT
The anticancer effect of masoprocol begins as soon as the medication comes in contact with diseased skin.

Significant improvement, however, may not be visible to the patient or physician until after therapy has continued for a period of time.

DURATION OF ACTION
Unknown.

DIETARY ADVICE
Maintain your usual food and fluid intake. Increase intake of fluids if you have a fever or diarrhea, in hot weather, or during exercise.

STORAGE
Store in a tightly sealed container away from heat and direct light. Keep away from moisture and extremes in temperature.

MISSED DOSE
Apply it as soon as you remember. If it is near the time for the next dose, skip the missed dose and resume your regular dosage schedule. Do not double the next dose.

STOPPING THE DRUG
Take it as prescribed for the full treatment period, even if you begin to feel better

before the scheduled end of the therapy.

PROLONGED USE
Therapy with this medication may require many weeks. The risk of an undesirable side effect increases with prolonged use.

▼ PRECAUTIONS

Over 60: Adverse reactions may be more likely and more severe in older patients.

Driving and Hazardous Work: Masoprocol may cause dizziness and allergic reactions. Therefore, do not drive or engage in hazardous work until you determine how the medicine affects you.

Alcohol: No special precautions are necessary.

Pregnancy: The effects are unknown. Consult your physician if you are pregnant or trying to become pregnant.

Breast Feeding: Masoprocol may pass into breast milk; caution is advised. Consult your doctor for advice.

Infants and Children: Safety and effectiveness of masoprocol are unknown in young patients. Your pediatrician will weigh the risks of using it.

Special Concerns: Masoprocol contains sulfites; be sure to inform your physician if you are allergic to sulfites or sulfur-containing compounds. This medication should be kept away from your eyes and mouth. Wash your hands thoroughly immediately after applying masoprocol to pre-

vent accidental contact with these sensitive areas. Your skin may appear reddened and blotchy wherever masoprocol has been in contact with it. These reactions usually disappear completely within 2 weeks of stopping the medication.

OVERDOSE
Symptoms: No specific ones have been reported.

What to Do: An overdose is unlikely to be life-threatening. However, if someone applies a much larger dose than prescribed, call your doctor, emergency medical services (EMS), or the nearest poison control center.

▼ INTERACTIONS

DRUG INTERACTIONS
No specific interactions are known at this time. Consult your doctor or pharmacist if you are concerned whether a prescription or nonprescription medication you are using may interact with masoprocol.

FOOD INTERACTIONS
No known food interactions.

DISEASE INTERACTIONS
Caution is advised when taking masoprocol. Consult your doctor if you have allergies to sulfites or had previous allergic reactions to masoprocol.

SIDE EFFECTS

SERIOUS
Shortness of breath, wheezing, difficulty breathing, confusion, hives, itching, rash, abdominal pain, facial swelling, sweating, weakness, and lightheadedness (allergic reaction to sulfites or other components of the preparation).

COMMON
Redness, pain, swelling, and dry, flaking skin at the site of application.

LESS COMMON
Blistering or wet discharge at the site of application; burning or other discomfort following application; rough, wrinkled skin.

MEASLES, MUMPS, AND RUBELLA VACCINE, LIVE

Available in: Injection
Available OTC? No   **As Generic?** No
Drug Class: Vaccine

▼ USAGE INFORMATION

WHY IT'S PRESCRIBED
To prevent infection by the measles, mumps, and rubella (German measles) viruses.

HOW IT WORKS
The measles, mumps, and rubella vaccine is an injection that works by introducing small amounts of live strains of the viruses into the body, which stimulate the immune system to produce its own protective antibodies against these viruses.

▼ DOSAGE GUIDELINES

RANGE AND FREQUENCY
The first dose, injected under the skin, should be given at 12 to 15 months of age. A second dose should be given between either ages 4 and 6 or ages 11 and 12. Adults born before 1957 are generally considered to be immune to measles and mumps.

ONSET OF EFFECT
Most patients develop immunity within 2 to 6 weeks.

DURATION OF ACTION
Up to 11 years or more.

DIETARY ADVICE
No special restrictions.

STORAGE
Not applicable; the dose is administered only at a health care facility.

MISSED DOSE
If your child misses a scheduled vaccination, contact your pediatrician.

STOPPING THE DRUG
The full schedule of injections should be followed unless a medical problem intervenes.

PROLONGED USE
No special problems are expected.

▼ PRECAUTIONS

Over 60: Measles, mumps, and rubella vaccine is not expected to cause different or more severe side effects in older patients than it does in younger persons.

Driving and Hazardous Work: The vaccine should not impair your ability to perform such tasks safely.

Alcohol: No special warnings.

Pregnancy: Generally, its use during pregnancy should be avoided. Before you have a measles, mumps, and rubella vaccination, tell your doctor if you are pregnant or plan to become pregnant. A pregnancy test should be done before the vaccine is given. Women should avoid pregnancy for 3 months following vaccination.

Breast Feeding: Components of the vaccine may pass into breast milk; caution is advised. Consult your doctor for specific advice.

Infants and Children: Measles, mumps, and rubella vaccine is not recommended for children younger than 12 months. The presence of the mother's antibodies in children under 12 months may prevent the vaccine from working. If a child is vaccinated before 12 months, another dose is recommended at 12 to 15 months of age.

Special Concerns: Applying a warm compress to the injection site can reduce redness and swelling. Do not use the vaccine within 3 months of an infusion of immunoglobulin. Immunosuppressive drugs and corticosteroids may decrease the vaccine's effect.

OVERDOSE
Symptoms: An overdose with measles, mumps, and rubella vaccine is unlikely.

What to Do: No cases of overdose have been reported.

▼ INTERACTIONS

DRUG INTERACTIONS
Other drugs may interact with measles, mumps, and rubella vaccine. Consult your doctor for specific advice if you are taking any prescription or over-the-counter medication.

FOOD INTERACTIONS
No known food interactions.

DISEASE INTERACTIONS
Consult your doctor if you have any of the following: a history of immune system deficiency, cancer, a blood disease, active tuberculosis, an allergic reaction to eggs or egg products, or an allergic reaction to neomycin.

 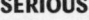

SIDE EFFECTS

SERIOUS
Serious allergic reaction involving difficulty swallowing or breathing; reddened skin, especially around the ears; itching, particularly of the hands or feet; hives; severe fatigue; swelling of face, eyes, or nasal passages; eye pain or tenderness; or high fever. Call your doctor immediately.

COMMON
Burning or stinging at site of injection, fever, skin rash.

LESS COMMON
Mild headache, sore throat, nausea, vomiting, diarrhea. Also redness, itching, swelling, or hard lump at site of injection; general feeling of illness; aches or pain in joints.

MEBENDAZOLE

Available in: Chewable tablets
Available OTC? No **As Generic?** Yes
Drug Class: Anthelmintic

▼ USAGE INFORMATION

WHY IT'S PRESCRIBED
To treat various intestinal roundworm infections, including ascariasis (common roundworm), hookworm infection, trichuriasis (whipworm), and enterobiasis or oxyuriasis (pinworm). It may be used to treat nonintestinal roundworm infections or more than one worm infection at a time.

HOW IT WORKS
Mebendazole interferes with the worm's energy-producing processes, including preventing the worm from absorbing glucose (sugar).

▼ DOSAGE GUIDELINES

RANGE AND FREQUENCY
For roundworms, hookworms, and whipworms— Adults and children age 2 and over: 100 mg, 2 times a day, in the morning and evening, for 3 days. Treatment may be repeated in 2 to 3 weeks. For pinworms— Adults and children age 2 and over: 100 mg for 1 day, repeated in 2 to 3 weeks. For multiple worm infections— Adults and children age 2 and over: 100 mg, 2 times a day, in the morning and evening, for 3 days. Treatment may be repeated in 2 to 3 weeks.

ONSET OF EFFECT
Unknown.

DURATION OF ACTION
Unknown.

DIETARY ADVICE
Take it with meals high in fat content to help the body better absorb the medication. If you are on a low-fat diet, consult your doctor for specific advice.

STORAGE
Store in a tightly sealed container away from heat, moisture, and direct light.

MISSED DOSE
Take it as soon as you remember. If it is near the time for the next dose, skip the missed dose and resume your regular dosage schedule. Do not double the next dose.

STOPPING THE DRUG
Take as prescribed for the full treatment period, even if you begin to feel better before the scheduled end of therapy.

PROLONGED USE
You should see your doctor regularly for tests and examinations if you take this medicine for a prolonged period.

▼ PRECAUTIONS

Over 60: No studies have been done specifically on older patients; adverse reactions may be more likely or more severe.

Driving and Hazardous Work: The use of mebendazole should not impair your ability to perform such tasks safely.

Alcohol: No special precautions are necessary.

Pregnancy: The use of mebendazole while pregnant is not recommended. Consult your doctor for advice.

Breast Feeding: Mebendazole may pass into breast milk; caution is advised. Consult your doctor for advice.

Infants and Children: Use and dose for children up to 2 years of age must be determined by your doctor.

Special Concerns: For pinworm infection, clothing, bedding, and towels should be washed daily. All members of the family may have to be treated to eradicate the infestation. A second treatment for all household members may be necessary after 2 or 3 weeks. All bedding and nightclothes should be washed after treatment. To prevent reinfection, you should wash the anal region daily, change your underwear and bedding every day, and wash your hands and fingernails before each meal and after bowel movements. Hookworm infection can cause anemia, and your doctor may tell you to take iron supplements during and after treatment.

OVERDOSE
Symptoms: Gastrointestinal upset lasting several hours; possible respiratory arrest or seizures.

What to Do: Call your doctor, emergency medical services (EMS), or the nearest poison control center immediately.

▼ INTERACTIONS

DRUG INTERACTIONS
Other drugs may interact with mebendazole. Consult your doctor for specific advice if you are taking carbamazepine or any other prescription or over-the-counter medication.

FOOD INTERACTIONS
No known food interactions.

DISEASE INTERACTIONS
Consult your doctor if you have liver disease, Crohn's disease, or ulcerative colitis.

SIDE EFFECTS

SERIOUS
Fever, sore throat, skin rash or itching, unusual fatigue. Call your doctor immediately.

COMMON
There are no common side effects associated with the use of this drug.

LESS COMMON
Nausea, vomiting, stomach pain or upset, diarrhea. Such symptoms tend to be short-lived and resolve on their own.

MECLIZINE

Available in: Capsules, tablets, chewable tablets
Available OTC? Yes   **As Generic?** Yes
Drug Class: Antiemetic; antivertigo agent

▼ USAGE INFORMATION

WHY IT'S PRESCRIBED
To treat and prevent nausea, vomiting, and dizziness caused by motion sickness and vertigo (dizziness) associated with other medical problems.

HOW IT WORKS
Meclizine acts on brain centers that control nausea, vomiting, and dizziness.

▼ DOSAGE GUIDELINES

RANGE AND FREQUENCY
To prevent and treat motion sickness— Adults and teenagers: 25 to 50 mg, 1 hour before travel; the dose may be repeated every 24 hours. To prevent and treat vertigo— Adults and teenagers: 25 to 100 mg a day as needed, in divided doses.

ONSET OF EFFECT
Within 1 hour.

DURATION OF ACTION
Up to 24 hours.

DIETARY ADVICE
Can be taken with food.

STORAGE
Store in a tightly sealed container away from heat, moisture, and direct light.

MISSED DOSE
Take it as soon as you remember. If it is near the time for the next dose, skip the missed dose and resume your regular dosage schedule. Do not double the next dose.

STOPPING THE DRUG
Take it as prescribed for the full treatment period. However, you may stop taking the medication if you are feeling better before the scheduled end of therapy.

PROLONGED USE
See your doctor regularly for tests and examinations if you must use this drug for a prolonged period.

▼ PRECAUTIONS

Over 60: Adverse reactions may be more likely and more severe in older patients.

Driving and Hazardous Work: Do not drive or engage in hazardous work until you determine how the medicine affects you.

Alcohol: Avoid alcohol when using this medication.

Pregnancy: Adequate human studies have not been completed. Before taking meclizine, tell your doctor if you are pregnant or plan to become pregnant.

Breast Feeding: Meclizine may pass into breast milk but has not been reported to cause problems in nursing babies. It may reduce the flow of breast milk. Consult your doctor for advice.

Infants and Children: Meclizine is not recommended for use by children under the age of 12.

Special Concerns: If dry mouth occurs, use sugarless candy or gum or bits of ice for temporary relief. If constipation occurs, a high-fiber diet and drinking plenty of fluids can help relieve the problem. Meclizine can cause false-negative results in allergy skin testing.

OVERDOSE
Symptoms: Extreme excitability, seizures, drowsiness, hallucinations.

What to Do: Call your doctor, emergency medical services (EMS), or the nearest poison control center immediately.

▼ INTERACTIONS

DRUG INTERACTIONS
Consult your doctor for specific advice if you are taking medications that can depress the central nervous system, such as antihistamines, medicines for hay fever, tranquilizers, sleep medications, prescription pain medicines, or muscle relaxants, or if you are taking any over-the-counter medication.

FOOD INTERACTIONS
No known food interactions.

DISEASE INTERACTIONS
Caution is advised when taking meclizine. Consult your doctor if you have any of the following: urinary tract blockage, glaucoma, asthma, bronchitis, emphysema, any other chronic lung disease, enlarged prostate, heart failure, or intestinal blockage.

SIDE EFFECTS

SERIOUS
No serious side effects have been reported with the use of meclizine.

COMMON
Drowsiness.

LESS COMMON
Blurred or double vision; upset stomach; constipation or diarrhea; insomnia; painful or difficult urination; dizziness; dry mouth, nose, and throat; headache; loss of appetite; fast heartbeat; nervousness; restlessness; skin rash.

MECLOFENAMATE SODIUM

Available in: Capsules
Available OTC? No   **As Generic?** Yes
Drug Class: Nonsteroidal anti-inflammatory drug (NSAID)

▼ USAGE INFORMATION

WHY IT'S PRESCRIBED
To treat mild to moderate pain and inflammation caused by tendinitis, arthritis, bursitis, gout, soft tissue injuries, migraine and other vascular headaches, menstrual cramps, and other conditions. When patients fail to respond to one NSAID, another may be tried. The greatest effectiveness often requires trial and error of several different NSAIDs.

HOW IT WORKS
NSAIDs work by interfering with prostaglandins, naturally occurring substances in the body that cause inflammation and make nerves more sensitive to pain impulses. NSAIDs also have other modes of action that are less well understood.

▼ DOSAGE GUIDELINES

RANGE AND FREQUENCY
Adults: 50 mg, 4 to 6 times a day. Maximum dose is 400 mg a day. Children: Consult your pediatrician.

ONSET OF EFFECT
From 30 minutes to several hours or longer.

DURATION OF ACTION
4 hours or more.

DIETARY ADVICE
Take with food; maintain your usual food and fluid intake.

STORAGE
Store in a tightly sealed container away from heat, moisture, and direct light. Keep away from extremes in temperature.

MISSED DOSE
Take it as soon as you remember. If it is near the time for the next dose, skip the missed dose and resume your regular dosage schedule. Do not double the next dose.

STOPPING THE DRUG
The decision to stop taking the drug should be made in consultation with your doctor.

PROLONGED USE
Prolonged use can cause gastrointestinal problems, including ulceration and bleeding, kidney dysfunction, and liver inflammation. See your doctor regularly for evaluation.

▼ PRECAUTIONS

Over 60: Because of the potentially greater consequences of gastrointestinal side effects, the dose of NSAIDs for older patients, especially those over age 70, is often cut in half.

Driving and Hazardous Work: Do not drive or engage in hazardous work until you determine how the medicine affects you.

Alcohol: Avoid alcohol when using this medication because it increases the risk of stomach irritation.

Pregnancy: Avoid or discontinue this drug if you are pregnant or plan to become pregnant.

Breast Feeding: Meclofenamate passes into breast milk; avoid or discontinue use while nursing.

Infants and Children: May be used in exceptional circumstances; consult your doctor.

Special Concerns: Because NSAIDs can interfere with blood coagulation, this drug should be stopped at least 3 days prior to any surgery.

OVERDOSE
Symptoms: Severe nausea, vomiting, headache, confusion, seizures.

What to Do: Call your doctor, emergency medical services (EMS), or the nearest poison control center immediately.

▼ INTERACTIONS

DRUG INTERACTIONS
Do not take this drug with aspirin or any other NSAIDs without your doctor's approval. In addition, consult your doctor if you are taking antihypertensives, steroids, anticoagulants, antibiotics, itraconazole or ketoconazole, plicamycin, penicillamine, valproic acid, phenytoin, cyclosporine, digitalis drugs, lithium, methotrexate, probenecid, triamterene, or zidovudine.

FOOD INTERACTIONS
No known food interactions.

DISEASE INTERACTIONS
Consult your doctor if you have any of the following: bleeding problems, inflammation or ulcers of the stomach and intestines, diabetes mellitus, systemic lupus erythematosus (SLE, lupus), anemia, asthma, epilepsy, Parkinson's disease, kidney stones, or a history of heart disease or alcohol abuse. Use of meclofenamate may cause complications in patients with liver or kidney disease, since these organs work together to remove the medication from the body.

▼ SIDE EFFECTS

SERIOUS
Shortness of breath or wheezing, with or without swelling of legs or other signs of heart failure; chest pain; peptic ulcer disease with vomiting of blood; black, tarry stools; decreasing kidney function. Call your doctor immediately.

COMMON
Nausea, vomiting, heartburn, diarrhea, constipation, headache, dizziness, sleepiness.

LESS COMMON
Ulcers or sores in mouth, depression, rashes or blistering of skin, ringing sound in the ears, unusual tingling or numbness of the hands or feet, seizures, blurred vision. Also elevated potassium levels, decreased blood counts; such problems can be detected by your doctor.

MEDROXYPROGESTERONE ACETATE

Available in: Tablets, injection
Available OTC? No   **As Generic?** Yes
Drug Class: Progestin (hormone)

▼ USAGE INFORMATION

WHY IT'S PRESCRIBED
To treat amenorrhea (cessation of menstrual periods) and abnormal uterine bleeding. It also may be used as a contraceptive.

HOW IT WORKS
Medroxyprogesterone inhibits secretion of pituitary hormones that in turn regulate menstrual and reproductive cycles. It also alters activity of uterine cells, resulting in, among other changes, thickening of the cervical mucus. These changes make it less likely for a partner's sperm to reach and fertilize an egg.

▼ DOSAGE GUIDELINES

RANGE AND FREQUENCY
For amenorrhea: Tablets, 5 to 10 mg a day for 5 to 10 days. For abnormal uterine bleeding: Tablets, 5 to 10 mg a day for 5 to 10 days beginning on the 16th or 21st day of the menstrual cycle. For contraception: 1 depo (Depo-Provera) injection (150 mg) every 3 months. For use in treating menopause: Tablets, 10 mg a day for 10 to 14 days, together with estrogen in each 25-day cycle.

ONSET OF EFFECT
Varies with mode of delivery. Protection against pregnancy can begin immediately if injection is given within 5 days of the menstrual period.

DURATION OF ACTION
Tablets: 24 hours or more. Injection: More than 3 months.

DIETARY ADVICE
Take it with meals to prevent gastrointestinal upset.

STORAGE
Store in a tightly sealed container away from heat and direct light.

MISSED DOSE
Take a missed dose of the tablet as soon as you remember. If it is near the time for the next dose, skip the missed dose and resume your regular dosage schedule. Do not double the next dose.

STOPPING THE DRUG
The decision to stop taking the drug should be made by your doctor.

PROLONGED USE
Consult your doctor about the need for periodic examinations and laboratory tests if you use this drug for a prolonged period.

▼ PRECAUTIONS

Over 60: No special problems are expected in older patients.

Driving and Hazardous Work: Do not drive or engage in hazardous work until you determine how the medicine affects you.

Alcohol: No special precautions are necessary.

Pregnancy: Before you use medroxyprogesterone, tell your doctor if you are pregnant or plan to become pregnant. This medicine must not be used during pregnancy.

Breast Feeding: Medroxyprogesterone passes into breast milk; avoid or discontinue use while nursing.

Infants and Children: This medication is not recommended for young patients.

Special Concerns: Remember that no contraceptive method is perfect; 1% of women using the medroxyprogesterone injections have become pregnant.

OVERDOSE
Symptoms: No specific ones have been reported.

What to Do: An overdose of medroxyprogesterone is unlikely to be life-threatening. However, if someone takes a much larger dose than prescribed, call your doctor, emergency medical services (EMS), or the nearest poison control center immediately.

▼ INTERACTIONS

DRUG INTERACTIONS
Consult your doctor for specific advice if you are taking aminoglutethimide, carbamazepine, phenytoin, rifabutin, or rifampin.

FOOD INTERACTIONS
No known food interactions.

DISEASE INTERACTIONS
Do not take medroxyprogesterone if you have known or suspected breast malignancies or tumors, acute liver disease or liver tumors, or active thrombophlebitis or thromboembolic disease. Consult your doctor if you have any of the following: asthma; epilepsy; migraine headaches; heart or circulation problems; bleeding problems; a history of thrombophlebitis or thromboembolic disease; diabetes mellitus; high blood cholesterol; kidney disease; risk factors for osteoporosis; or central nervous system disorders, such as depression.

⇊ SIDE EFFECTS ⇊

SERIOUS
Abnormal menstrual bleeding; unexpected or increased flow of breast milk; mental depression; skin rash; loss of or change in speech, coordination, or vision; severe and sudden shortness of breath. Call your doctor immediately.

COMMON
Stomach pain, swelling of face, ankles, or feet, mild headache, mood changes, unusual fatigue, weight gain.

LESS COMMON
Acne, breast pain or tenderness, hot flashes, insomnia, loss of sexual desire, loss or gain of scalp hair or body hair, brown spots on skin.

MEDRYSONE

Available in: Ophthalmic suspension
Available OTC? No   **As Generic?** No
Drug Class: Corticosteroid

▼ USAGE INFORMATION

WHY IT'S PRESCRIBED
To control inflammation and prevent potentially permanent damage that may result from conditions that involve inflammation in the tissues of the eye. Also used to help relieve redness, irritation, and discomfort in the eye. Medrysone is less effective than ophthalmic dexamethasone, hydrocortisone, or prednisolone but also less likely to cause adverse effects.

HOW IT WORKS
Medrysone inhibits the release of natural substances that stimulate inflammation and pain in eye tissues.

▼ DOSAGE GUIDELINES

RANGE AND FREQUENCY
1 drop in each eye up to every 4 hours.

ONSET OF EFFECT
Unknown.

DURATION OF ACTION
Unknown.

DIETARY ADVICE
This medication can be used without regard to diet.

STORAGE
Store in a tightly sealed container away from heat, moisture, and direct light. Do not allow it to freeze.

MISSED DOSE
Apply it as soon as you remember. If it is near the time for the next dose, skip the missed dose and resume your regular dosage schedule. Do not double the next dose.

STOPPING THE DRUG
Use as prescribed for the full treatment period, even if your symptoms improve before the scheduled end of therapy.

PROLONGED USE
You should see your doctor regularly for tests and examinations if you take this drug for a prolonged period.

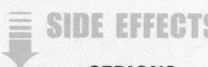

SIDE EFFECTS

SERIOUS
Serious side effects are less likely than with ophthalmic dexamethasone, hydrocortisone, or prednisolone but may include decreased vision or blurring of vision (from cataract); eye pain, nausea, vomiting (from increased eye pressure); and pain, redness, sensitivity to bright light, and discharge (from eye infection). Call your doctor immediately if you experience any of these signs or symptoms. This drug may trigger a recurrence of herpes infection of the eye; mention any previous herpes infection to your doctor.

COMMON
No common side effects are associated with medrysone.

LESS COMMON
Burning, stinging, redness, or watering of eyes.

▼ PRECAUTIONS

Over 60: No special problems are expected.

Driving and Hazardous Work: Do not drive or engage in hazardous work until you determine how the medicine affects your vision.

Alcohol: No special precautions are necessary.

Pregnancy: In animal studies, medrysone has caused problems during pregnancy. Reliable human studies have not been done, but no human birth defects have been reported. Before you take medrysone, tell your doctor if you are pregnant or plan to become pregnant.

Breast Feeding: Medrysone has not been reported to cause problems in nursing babies. Consult your doctor for specific advice.

Infants and Children: Children under 2 years of age may be especially sensitive to the effects of medrysone.

Special Concerns: To use the eye drops, first wash your hands. Tilt your head back. Gently apply pressure to the inside corner of the eyelid and with the index finger of the same hand, pull downward on the lower eyelid to make a space. Drop the medicine into this space and close your eye. Apply pressure for 1 or 2 minutes while keeping the eye closed without blinking. Then wash your hands again. Make sure the tip of the dropper does not touch your eye, finger, or any other surface. If your symptoms do not improve in 5 to 7 days or if they become worse, check with your doctor. Wearing contact lenses while using this medication may increase the risk of infection. Your doctor may tell you not to wear contact lenses during and for a day or two after treatment.

OVERDOSE
Symptoms: When used topically, an overdose of medrysone is very unlikely. Inadvertent oral ingestion, however, may cause fever, muscle pain, malaise, loss of appetite, dizziness, fainting, and breathing trouble.

What to Do: An overdose of medrysone is unlikely to be life-threatening. However, if someone applies a much larger dose than prescribed or accidentally ingests the medicine, call your doctor, emergency medical services (EMS), or the nearest poison control center immediately.

▼ INTERACTIONS

DRUG INTERACTIONS
Consult your doctor for specific advice if you are taking any other prescription or over-the-counter medication.

FOOD INTERACTIONS
No known food interactions.

DISEASE INTERACTIONS
Caution is advised when taking medrysone. Consult your doctor if you have any of the following: diabetes, tuberculosis of the eye, glaucoma, cataracts, herpes infection of the eye, or any other eye infection.

MEFENAMIC ACID

Available in: Capsules
Available OTC? No **As Generic?** No
Drug Class: Nonsteroidal anti-inflammatory drug (NSAID)

▼ USAGE INFORMATION

WHY IT'S PRESCRIBED
To treat mild to moderate pain and inflammation caused by tendinitis, arthritis, bursitis, gout, soft tissue injuries, migraine and other vascular headaches, menstrual cramps, and other conditions. When patients fail to respond to one NSAID, another may be tried. The greatest effectiveness often requires trial and error of several different NSAIDs.

HOW IT WORKS
NSAIDs work by interfering with prostaglandins, naturally occurring substances in the body that cause inflammation and make nerves more sensitive to pain impulses. NSAIDs also have other modes of action that are less well understood.

▼ DOSAGE GUIDELINES

RANGE AND FREQUENCY
Adults: 250 mg every 6 hours. The drug should not be used for more than 7 days. For children's dose, consult your pediatrician.

ONSET OF EFFECT
Several hours to several days.

DURATION OF ACTION
4 hours or more.

DIETARY ADVICE
Take with food; maintain your usual food and fluid intake.

STORAGE
Store in a tightly sealed container away from heat, moisture, and direct light. Keep away from extremes in temperature.

MISSED DOSE
Take it as soon as you remember. If it is near the time for the next dose, skip the missed dose and resume your regular dosage schedule. Do not double the next dose.

STOPPING THE DRUG
The decision to stop taking the drug should be made in consultation with your doctor.

PROLONGED USE
Mefenamic acid is not recommended for use longer than 7 days in a course of therapy.

▼ PRECAUTIONS

Over 60: Because of the potentially greater consequences of gastrointestinal side effects, the dose of NSAIDs for older patients, especially those over age 70, is often cut in half.

Driving and Hazardous Work: Avoid such activities until you determine how the medicine affects you.

Alcohol: Avoid alcohol when using this medication because it increases the risk of stomach irritation.

Pregnancy: Avoid or discontinue this drug if you are pregnant or plan to become pregnant.

Breast Feeding: Mefenamic acid passes into breast milk; avoid use while nursing.

Infants and Children: May be used in exceptional circumstances; consult your doctor.

Special Concerns: Because NSAIDs can interfere with blood coagulation, this drug should be stopped at least 3 days prior to any surgery.

OVERDOSE
Symptoms: Severe nausea, vomiting, headache, confusion, seizures.

What to Do: Call your doctor, emergency medical services (EMS), or the nearest poison control center immediately.

▼ INTERACTIONS

DRUG INTERACTIONS
Do not take this drug with aspirin or any other NSAIDs without your doctor's approval. In addition, consult your doctor if you are taking antihypertensives, steroids, anticoagulants, antibiotics, itraconazole or ketoconazole, plicamycin, penicillamine, valproic acid, phenytoin, cyclosporine, digitalis drugs, lithium, methotrexate, probenecid, triamterene, or zidovudine.

FOOD INTERACTIONS
No known food interactions.

DISEASE INTERACTIONS
Consult your doctor if you have any of the following: bleeding problems, inflammation or ulcers of the stomach and intestines, diabetes mellitus, systemic lupus erythematosus (SLE, lupus), anemia, asthma, epilepsy, Parkinson's disease, kidney stones, or a history of heart disease or alcohol abuse. Use of mefenamic acid may cause complications in patients with liver or kidney disease, since these organs work together to remove the medication from the body.

≡ SIDE EFFECTS ≡

SERIOUS
Shortness of breath or wheezing, with or without swelling of legs or other signs of heart failure; chest pain; peptic ulcer disease with vomiting of blood; black, tarry stools; decreasing kidney function. Call your doctor immediately.

COMMON
Nausea, vomiting, heartburn, diarrhea, constipation, headache, dizziness, sleepiness.

LESS COMMON
Ulcers or sores in mouth, depression, rashes or blistering of skin, ringing sound in the ears, unusual tingling or numbness of the hands or feet, seizures, blurred vision. Also elevated potassium levels, decreased blood counts; such problems can be detected by your doctor.

MEFLOQUINE HYDROCHLORIDE

Available in: Tablets
Available OTC? No   **As Generic?** No
Drug Class: Anti-infective/antimalarial

▼ USAGE INFORMATION

WHY IT'S PRESCRIBED
To treat mild to moderate acute malaria caused by strains of plasmodia (the parasite that causes malaria) that are susceptible to mefloquine—specifically, Plasmodium falciparum and Plasmodium vivax. Also used to prevent malaria caused by these strains.

HOW IT WORKS
Mefloquine is poisonous to the malarial parasite.

▼ DOSAGE GUIDELINES

RANGE AND FREQUENCY
Adults— To treat: 5 tablets (1,250 mg each) taken as a single dose. Patients with acute P. vivax malaria, treated with mefloquine, are at high risk of relapse. To avoid relapse after the initial treatment, patients should be treated with another antimalarial, such as primaquine. To prevent: 250 mg once a week. Begin taking mefloquine one week prior to departure and continue taking the drug for 4 weeks upon return. Children 6 months of age and older— To treat, 20 to 25 mg per 2.2 lbs (1 kg) of body weight. Split the total dose into 2 doses 6 to 8 hours apart in order to reduce the risk and severity of side effects. To prevent: Your pediatrician will determine the appropriate dose.

ONSET OF EFFECT
Unknown.

DURATION OF ACTION
Up to 3 weeks.

DIETARY ADVICE
Do not take on an empty stomach. Take with at least 8 oz of water.

STORAGE
Store in a tightly sealed container away from heat, moisture, and direct light.

MISSED DOSE
If taking 1 or more doses a day, take it as soon as you remember. If it is near the time for the next dose, skip the missed dose and resume your regular dosage schedule. Do not double the next dose. If taking 1 weekly dose, take it as soon as possible, then resume regular schedule.

STOPPING THE DRUG
Take it as prescribed for the full treatment period.

PROLONGED USE
Periodic liver function tests and eye exams are recommended.

▼ PRECAUTIONS

Over 60: Adverse reactions may be more likely and more severe in older patients.

Driving and Hazardous Work: Avoid such activities until you determine how the medicine affects you. Dizziness and coordination difficulties may occur after the drug is discontinued.

Alcohol: No special warnings.

Pregnancy: The use of mefloquine is discouraged during pregnancy because of the risks it poses to the unborn child. Women of childbearing age should practice contraception during preventive therapy.

Breast Feeding: Mefloquine passes into breast milk; extreme caution is advised. Consult your physician for specific advice.

Infants and Children: Safety and effectiveness have not been established for children under the age of 6 months. Early vomiting has been associated with mefloquine use in children and with treatment failure. If a second dose is not tolerated, alternative antimalarial measures should be considered.

Special Concerns: If you take mefloquine once a week, take it on the same day every week. Malaria is spread by mosquitoes. Take appropriate precautions, such as using mosquito netting, to guard against being bitten by malaria-carrying mosquitoes.

OVERDOSE
Symptoms: Side effects may be more pronounced.

What to Do: If you have reason to suspect overdose, call your doctor, emergency medical services (EMS), or the nearest poison control center immediately.

▼ INTERACTIONS

DRUG INTERACTIONS
Consult your doctor for more advice if you are taking a beta-blocker, quinidine, quinine, chloroquine, antiarrhythmic drugs, calcium channel blockers, halofantrine, antihistamines, histamine (H1) blockers, tricyclic antidepressants, phenothiazines, anticonvulsants. Also, tell your physician if you are taking any other prescription or over-the-counter drug.

FOOD INTERACTIONS
No known food interactions.

DISEASE INTERACTIONS
Consult your doctor for specific advice if you have a seizure or psychiatric disorder, impaired liver function, any eye condition, or heart disease.

≡ SIDE EFFECTS ≡

SERIOUS
Slowed heartbeat, seizures. Severe anxiety, depression, restlessness, or confusion during preventive therapy may be signs of more serious psychiatric problems. Call your doctor immediately.

COMMON
Treatment-related: dizziness, muscle pain, nausea, fever, headache, vomiting, chills, diarrhea, skin rash, abdominal pain, fatigue, loss of appetite, ringing in the ears. Prevention-related: vomiting, nausea.

LESS COMMON
Treatment-related: hair loss, emotional problems, itching, fatigue. Prevention-related: dizziness, lightheadedness.

MEGESTROL ACETATE

Available in: Oral suspension, tablets
Available OTC? No   **As Generic?** Yes
Drug Class: Progestin (hormone treatment); antineoplastic (anticancer) agent

▼ USAGE INFORMATION

WHY IT'S PRESCRIBED
To treat cancer of the breast or uterus, and to treat loss of appetite and loss of weight (wasting) caused by AIDS (acquired immunodeficiency syndrome).

HOW IT WORKS
Megestrol, a synthetic form of the hormone progestin, interferes with the activity of certain other hormones and proteins needed for some types of cancer cells to grow. The mechanism by which megestrol increases weight is unclear. It appears to stimulate the appetite and affect metabolism, resulting in weight gain.

▼ DOSAGE GUIDELINES

RANGE AND FREQUENCY
For breast cancer: 160 mg per day in 1 or several doses for 2 or more months. For uterine cancer: 40 to 320 mg per day for 2 or more months. For loss of weight and appetite associated with AIDS: 800 mg a day for the first month; the dose may be adjusted later.

ONSET OF EFFECT
Unknown.

DURATION OF ACTION
Unknown.

DIETARY ADVICE
No special restrictions.

STORAGE
Store in a tightly sealed container away from heat and direct light.

MISSED DOSE
Take it as soon as you remember. If it is near the time for the next dose, skip the missed dose and resume your regular dosage schedule. Do not double the next dose.

STOPPING THE DRUG
The decision to stop taking the drug should be made by your doctor.

PROLONGED USE
You should see your doctor regularly for tests and examinations if you take this drug for a prolonged period.

▼ PRECAUTIONS

Over 60: No special problems are expected in older patients.

Driving and Hazardous Work: Do not drive or engage in hazardous work until you determine how the medicine affects you.

Alcohol: Avoid alcohol while taking this drug.

Pregnancy: Megestrol should never be taken during pregnancy. Consult your doctor immediately if you believe you have become pregnant.

Breast Feeding: Megestrol passes into breast milk; caution is advised. Consult your doctor for specific advice.

Infants and Children: Safety and effectiveness have not been established; consult your pediatrician to weigh risks against benefits.

Special Concerns: If you take any laboratory or diagnostic test, tell the clinician that you are taking megestrol. Megestrol may cause tenderness, swelling, or bleeding of the gums. Brush and floss your teeth carefully and see your dentist regularly.

OVERDOSE

Symptoms: No specific ones have been reported.

What to Do: An overdose of megestrol is unlikely to be life-threatening. However, if someone takes a much larger dose than prescribed, call your doctor, emergency medical services (EMS), or the nearest poison control center.

▼ INTERACTIONS

DRUG INTERACTIONS
Consult your doctor for specific advice if you are taking aminogluthimide, carbamazepine, phenobarbital, phenytoin, rifabutin, or rifampin.

FOOD INTERACTIONS
No known food interactions.

DISEASE INTERACTIONS
Caution is advised when taking megestrol. Consult your doctor if you have a history of asthma, epilepsy, heart or circulation problems, kidney disease, migraine headaches, bleeding disorders, blood clots, stroke, varicose veins, breast disease, mental depression, high blood cholesterol, diabetes mellitus, or liver disease.

 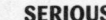 **SIDE EFFECTS**

SERIOUS
Abnormal vaginal discharge or bleeding, changes in menstrual cycle. Less frequently: High blood pressure; palpitations; heart failure; headache; loss of or change in speech, coordination, or vision; numbness or pain in chest, arm, or leg; shortness of breath; high blood sugar causing dry mouth, frequent urination, loss of appetite, and unusual thirst; depression; skin rash. Call your doctor promptly.

COMMON
Diarrhea; nausea; vomiting; impotence; diminished sex drive; abdominal cramps or pain; swollen face, ankles, or feet; mild increase in blood pressure; headache; mood changes; nervousness; fatigue; weight gain.

LESS COMMON
Acne, constipation, breast pain or tenderness, brown spots on skin, hot flashes, loss or gain of hair, insomnia, unusual or excessive sweating.

MELOXICAM

Available in: Tablets
Available OTC? No   **As Generic?** No
Drug Class: Nonsteroidal anti-inflammatory drug (NSAID)

▼ USAGE INFORMATION

WHY IT'S PRESCRIBED
To relieve the pain, inflammation, and stiffness of osteoarthritis.

HOW IT WORKS
NSAIDs work by interfering with the formation of prostaglandins, naturally occurring substances in the body that cause inflammation and make nerves more sensitive to pain impulses. NSAIDs also have other modes of action that are less well understood.

▼ DOSAGE GUIDELINES

RANGE AND FREQUENCY
Adults: To start, 7.5 mg a day. The dose may be adjusted later to no more than 15 mg a day.

ONSET OF EFFECT
Unknown.

DURATION OF ACTION
Unknown.

DIETARY ADVICE
Meloxicam may be taken with or without food.

STORAGE
Store in a tightly sealed container away from heat, moisture, and direct light.

MISSED DOSE
If you do not remember until the next day, skip the missed dose and resume your regular dosage schedule. Do not double the next dose.

STOPPING THE DRUG
The decision to stop taking the drug should be made in consultation with your physician.

PROLONGED USE
The risk of gastrointestinal side effects may be increased with extended use.

▼ PRECAUTIONS

Over 60: Caution should be exercised, as with any NSAID, in using meloxicam. Therapy should be started with the lowest recommended dose.

Driving and Hazardous Work: No special problems are expected.

Alcohol: Avoid alcohol when using this medication because it increases the risk of stomach irritation.

Pregnancy: Discuss with your doctor the relative risks and benefits of using this drug while pregnant. Do not use meloxicam during the last trimester.

Breast Feeding: Meloxicam may pass into breast milk; caution is advised. Consult your doctor for advice on whether to discontinue nursing or discontinue the drug.

Infants and Children: The safety and effectiveness of this drug have not been established for children under the age of 18.

OVERDOSE
Symptoms: Few cases of overdose have been reported. Symptoms may include lethargy; drowsiness; nausea; vomiting; abdominal pain; black, tarry stools; breathing difficulty; and coma.

What to Do: If you suspect an overdose or if someone takes a much larger dose than prescribed, call your doctor, emergency medical services (EMS), or the nearest poison control center immediately.

▼ INTERACTIONS

DRUG INTERACTIONS
Do not take this drug with aspirin or any other NSAIDs without your doctor's approval. In addition, consult your doctor if you are taking furosemide, ACE inhibitors, lithium, cholestyramine, or warfarin.

FOOD INTERACTIONS
No known food interactions.

DISEASE INTERACTIONS
Meloxicam should not be taken by people who have experienced asthma, hives, or allergic-type reactions after taking aspirin or other NSAIDs. People with a history of ulcer disease or gastrointestinal bleeding (especially if elderly or debilitated) should only take meloxicam with extreme caution. Consult your doctor if you have high blood pressure or heart failure. In patients with advanced liver or kidney disease meloxicam is not recommended, since these organs both work to remove the medication from the body.

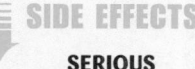

SIDE EFFECTS

SERIOUS
Shortness of breath or wheezing, with or without swelling of legs or other signs of congestive heart failure; chest pain; peptic ulcer disease with vomiting of blood; black, tarry stools; decreasing kidney function. Call your doctor immediately.

COMMON
Diarrhea.

LESS COMMON
Nausea, upper respiratory tract infection, sore throat, dizziness, swelling of the legs.

MELPHALAN

BRAND NAMES
Alkeran, L-PAM, Phenylalanine Mustard

Available in: Tablets, injection
Available OTC? No   **As Generic?** No
Drug Class: Alkylating agent

▼ USAGE INFORMATION

WHY IT'S PRESCRIBED
To treat multiple myeloma (a cancer of the bone marrow) and ovarian cancer.

HOW IT WORKS
Melphalan kills cancer cells by interfering with the activity of their genetic material, thus preventing the cells from reproducing. The drug may also affect the growth and development of normal cells in the body, resulting in unpleasant side effects.

▼ DOSAGE GUIDELINES

RANGE AND FREQUENCY
For multiple myeloma: 6 mg (3 tablets) per day for 2 to 3 weeks; the drug is discontinued for up to 4 weeks, then resumed at a dose of 2 mg a day, depending on blood counts. For ovarian cancer: Initial dose is 0.2 mg per 2.2 lbs (1 kg) of body weight once a day for 5 days. Dosage and duration of treatment may be altered to meet the needs of each patient.

ONSET OF EFFECT
Unknown.

DURATION OF ACTION
Unknown.

DIETARY ADVICE
Melphalan is best taken with food to minimize stomach upset.

STORAGE
Store in a tightly sealed container away from heat and direct light.

MISSED DOSE
Take it as soon as you remember. If it is near the time for the next dose, skip the missed dose and resume your regular dosage schedule. Do not double the next dose.

STOPPING THE DRUG
The decision to stop taking the drug should be made by your doctor.

PROLONGED USE
See your doctor regularly for tests and examinations if you must take this medication for a prolonged period.

▼ PRECAUTIONS

Over 60: No special problems are expected.

Driving and Hazardous Work: The use of melphalan should not impair your ability to perform such tasks safely.

Alcohol: Avoid alcohol.

Pregnancy: Melphalan can cause birth defects if taken by either the father or the mother. Before you take it, tell your doctor if you are pregnant or plan to become pregnant.

Breast Feeding: Melphalan passes into breast milk; avoid or discontinue use while nursing. Consult you doctor for specific advice.

Infants and Children: There is no specific information about the use of melphalan in children.

Special Concerns: While taking melphalan, do not receive any immunizations without your doctor's approval. Avoid persons who have recently had oral polio vaccine and those with any infection. Check with your doctor before having any dental work done. Consult your doctor or dentist about appropriate ways to clean your teeth to avoid injury. Be careful not to cut yourself when using sharp objects such as a safety razor or nail cutters. Avoid activities and contact sports where bruising or injury could occur. If you vomit shortly after taking a dose of melphalan, check with your doctor. You may be instructed to take the dose again.

OVERDOSE

Symptoms: Vomiting, mouth ulcerations, diarrhea, gastrointestinal hemorrhage (causing blood in the stool).

What to Do: Call your doctor, emergency medical services (EMS), or the nearest poison control center immediately.

▼ INTERACTIONS

DRUG INTERACTIONS
Consult your doctor for specific advice if you are taking amphotericin B, antithyroid agents, azathioprine, chloramphenicol, colchicine, flucytosine, interferon, plicamycin, probenecid, or sulfinpyrazone. Also consult your doctor if you are taking any over-the-counter medications.

FOOD INTERACTIONS
No known food interactions.

DISEASE INTERACTIONS
Consult your doctor if you have any of the following: shingles, chicken pox, any infection, kidney disease, or lung disease.

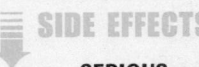

SIDE EFFECTS

SERIOUS
Black, tarry, or bloody stools; blood in the urine; fever and chills; cough or hoarseness; pain in lower back or side; difficult, decreased, or painful urination; red spots on skin; unusual bleeding or bruising; swollen feet or lower legs. Call your doctor immediately. Some of these side effects may recur after you stop taking melphalan. If so, consult your doctor.

COMMON
No common side effects are associated with melphalan.

LESS COMMON
Nausea and vomiting, mouth sores, allergic reaction.

MEPERIDINE HYDROCHLORIDE

BRAND NAME

Demerol

Available in: Syrup, tablets, injection
Available OTC? No   **As Generic?** Yes
Drug Class: Opioid (narcotic) analgesic

▼ USAGE INFORMATION

WHY IT'S PRESCRIBED
To treat moderate to severe pain.

HOW IT WORKS
Narcotics such as meperidine relieve pain by acting on specific areas of the spinal cord and brain that process pain signals from nerves throughout the body.

▼ DOSAGE GUIDELINES

RANGE AND FREQUENCY
Adults— Syrup or tablets: 50 to 150 mg every 3 or 4 hours as needed. Injection: 50 to 150 mg into a muscle or under the skin every 3 or 4 hours as needed. Children— Syrup, tablet, or injection into a muscle or under the skin: 1.1 to 1.76 mg per 2.2 lbs (1 kg) of body weight every 3 or 4 hours as needed.

ONSET OF EFFECT
Oral forms: 15 minutes. Injection: 10 to 15 minutes.

DURATION OF ACTION
2 to 4 hours.

DIETARY ADVICE
Tablets can be taken with food to lessen stomach upset. Syrup should be taken with a half glass of water.

STORAGE
Store the drug in a tightly sealed container away from heat, moisture, and direct light. Do not allow the liquid form to freeze.

MISSED DOSE
If you are taking meperidine on a fixed schedule, take it as soon as you remember. If it is near the time for the next dose, skip the missed dose and resume your regular dosage schedule. Do not double the next dose.

STOPPING THE DRUG
The decision to stop taking the drug should be made by your doctor.

PROLONGED USE
Meperidine should not be taken for a prolonged period. Prolonged use can cause nerve damage and physical dependence. Do not abruptly stop taking meperidine without consulting your doctor.

▼ PRECAUTIONS

Over 60:
Adverse reactions may be more likely and more severe in older patients.

Driving and Hazardous Work:
Do not drive or engage in hazardous work until you determine how the medicine affects you.

Alcohol:
Avoid alcohol.

Pregnancy:
Before you use this medication, tell your doctor if you are pregnant or plan to become pregnant. Overuse during pregnancy can cause physical dependence in the unborn baby. Meperidine use just before delivery can cause breathing problems in the newborn.

Breast Feeding:
Meperidine passes into breast milk; caution is advised. Consult your doctor for specific advice.

Infants and Children:
Adverse reactions may be more likely and more severe in infants and children. Consult your pediatrician for specific advice.

Special Concerns:
If you feel the medication is not working properly after a few weeks, do not increase the dose. Consult your doctor. Before having any surgery, tell the doctor or dentist in charge that you are taking meperidine.

OVERDOSE
Symptoms: Confusion; slurred speech; extreme sedation, weakness, or dizziness; small, pinpoint pupils; cold, clammy skin; slow breathing; seizures; loss of consciousness.

What to Do: Call your doctor, emergency medical services (EMS), or the nearest poison control center immediately.

▼ INTERACTIONS

DRUG INTERACTIONS
Consult your doctor for specific advice if you are taking carbamazepine or other medicine for seizures, barbiturates, sedatives, cough medicines, decongestants, antidepressants, other prescription pain medications, MAO inhibitors, naltrexone, rifampin, or zidovudine.

FOOD INTERACTIONS
No known food interactions.

DISEASE INTERACTIONS
Consult your doctor if you have any of the following: history of alcohol or drug abuse; emotional illness; brain disorders or head injury; seizures; lung disease; prostate problems or other problems with urination; gallstones; colitis; heart, kidney, liver, or thyroid disease.

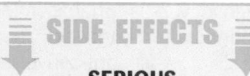 SIDE EFFECTS

SERIOUS
Serious side effects are indistinguishable from those of overdose and include confusion; slurred speech; extreme sedation, weakness, or dizziness; small, pinpoint pupils; cold, clammy skin; slow breathing; seizures; loss of consciousness.

COMMON
Dizziness or lightheadedness, nausea or vomiting, constipation, mild drowsiness, itching.

LESS COMMON
Mood swings or false sense of well-being (euphoria), redness or flushing of face.

MEPHENYTOIN

Available in: Tablets
Available OTC? No   **As Generic?** No
Drug Class: Hydantoin anticonvulsant

▼ USAGE INFORMATION

WHY IT'S PRESCRIBED
To control certain kinds of seizures due to epilepsy. It is often given along with another anticonvulsant, such as phenytoin, phenobarbital, or primidone.

HOW IT WORKS
Mephenytoin is thought to depress the activity of certain parts of the brain and suppress the abnormal firing of neurons that causes seizures.

▼ DOSAGE GUIDELINES

RANGE AND FREQUENCY
Adults: 200 to 800 mg a day, in 3 divided doses. Children: 100 to 400 mg a day, in 3 divided doses. Some patients require higher doses. A low dose is used to start; it may then be gradually increased by your physician.

ONSET OF EFFECT
30 minutes.

SIDE EFFECTS

SERIOUS
Fever, sore throat, swollen glands, red or purple pointlike rash on the skin or mucous membranes, blistering or peeling skin lesions, mouth sores or bleeding, easy bruising, paleness, weakness, confusion, lethargy, or seizures may be a sign of a potentially fatal blood disorder or other complication. Call your doctor immediately.

COMMON
Dizziness, drowsiness, fatigue, clumsiness or unsteadiness, double vision, nervousness, nausea, vomiting, insomnia.

LESS COMMON
Hair loss, weight gain, swelling, depression, disorientation. Numerous additional side effects are associated with the use of this drug; consult your doctor if you are concerned about any unusual reactions.

DURATION OF ACTION
Maximum effectiveness lasts 24 to 48 hours; effectiveness then gradually decreases.

DIETARY ADVICE
Take with food to minimize stomach upset.

STORAGE
Store in a tightly sealed container away from heat, moisture, and direct light.

MISSED DOSE
Take it as soon as you remember. However, if it is near the time for the next dose, skip the missed dose and resume you regular dosage schedule. Do not double the next dose unless advised to do so by your doctor.

STOPPING THE DRUG
Never stop taking this drug abruptly; seizures may ensue. The dose should be tapered gradually over a period of weeks under the supervision of your doctor.

PROLONGED USE
This drug is typically used on a long-term basis. If so, see your doctor regularly for tests and examinations.

▼ PRECAUTIONS

Over 60: Adverse reactions may be more likely and more severe in older patients. A lower dose may be used.

Driving and Hazardous Work: This drug may cause drowsiness or dizziness, particularly in the first few weeks it is used. Do not drive or engage in hazardous work until you determine how the medicine affects you.

Alcohol: Avoid alcohol; it may contribute to excessive drowsiness.

Pregnancy: Anticonvulsants are associated with an increased risk of birth defects, although studies with this drug are incomplete. However, seizures during pregnancy can also increase the risks to the fetus. Discuss with your doctor the potential risks and benefits of using this drug during pregnancy. Folate supplementation is advised starting 1 to 2 months before conception and throughout pregnancy.

Breast Feeding: Mephenytoin may pass into breast milk, although at low levels. Consult your doctor for advice.

Infants and Children: Adverse reactions may be more frequent and more severe in infants and children. Not generally recommended in those younger than age 16.

Special Concerns: See your doctor for regular check-ups to detect the onset of any serious side effects. Your doctor may advise you to carry an ID card or bracelet that says you are taking this drug.

OVERDOSE
Symptoms: Blurred or double vision, difficulty walking, extreme clumsiness or unsteadiness, severe confusion, dizziness or drowsiness.

What to Do: Call your doctor, emergency medical services (EMS), or the nearest poison control center immediately.

▼ INTERACTIONS

DRUG INTERACTIONS
Mephenytoin can interact with many other drugs, including central nervous system depressants, xanthines, amiodarone, antacids, medicines containing calcium, anticoagulants, chloramphenicol, cimetidine, disulfiram, isoniazid, fluconazole, phenylbutazone, sulfonamides, corticosteroids, estrogens or oral contraceptives, corticotropin, oral diazoxide, lidocaine, methadone, phenacemide, rifampin, streptozocin, sucralfate, or other anticonvulsants (such as valproic acid).

FOOD INTERACTIONS
No known food interactions.

DISEASE INTERACTIONS
Special caution is advised in those with a blood disease, porphyria, lupus, coronary artery disease, kidney disease, or liver disease.

MEPROBAMATE

Available in: Tablets, extended-release capsules
Available OTC? No   **As Generic?** Yes
Drug Class: Antianxiety drug

▼ USAGE INFORMATION

WHY IT'S PRESCRIBED
To treat anxiety. This drug is now rarely prescribed; other drugs are more commonly prescribed for this purpose.

HOW IT WORKS
The mechanism by which meprobamate works is unknown.

▼ DOSAGE GUIDELINES

RANGE AND FREQUENCY
Adults and teenagers—Tablets: 400 mg, 3 or 4 times a day, or 600 mg, 2 times a day. Extended-release capsules: 400 to 800 mg, 2 times a day.

ONSET OF EFFECT
Unknown.

DURATION OF ACTION
Unknown.

DIETARY ADVICE
Meprobamate can be taken with food to prevent gastrointestinal upset.

STORAGE
Store in a tightly sealed container away from heat, moisture, and direct light.

MISSED DOSE
Take it as soon as you remember. However, if it is near the time for the next dose, skip the missed dose and resume your regular dosage schedule. Do not double the next dose.

STOPPING THE DRUG
Do not stop taking meprobamate abruptly, as this may produce withdrawal symptoms. The dosage should be reduced gradually according to your doctor's instructions.

PROLONGED USE
See your doctor for periodic evaluation if you must take this drug for an extended length of time.

▼ PRECAUTIONS

Over 60: Adverse reactions may be more likely and more severe in older patients.

Driving and Hazardous Work: Meprobamate can impair mental alertness and physical coordination. If you experience such problems, consult your doctor about adjusting your dosage.

Alcohol: Alcohol intake should be extremely moderate or stopped altogether while taking this drug.

Pregnancy: Meprobamate may increase the risk of birth defects if taken early in pregnancy. Before you take it, be sure to tell your doctor if you are pregnant or plan to become pregnant.

Breast Feeding: Meprobamate passes into breast milk; do not take it while nursing.

Infants and Children: Meprobamate is not recommended for use by children under the age of 6.

Special Concerns: Meprobamate use can lead to psychological or physical dependence. Short-term therapy (8 weeks or less) is typical; do not take the drug for a longer period unless advised otherwise by your physician. Never take more than the prescribed daily dose.

OVERDOSE
Symptoms: Severe confusion, lightheadedness, dizziness, or drowsiness, lethargy, shortness of breath, loss of consciousness.

What to Do: Call your doctor, emergency medical services (EMS), or the nearest poison control center immediately.

▼ INTERACTIONS

DRUG INTERACTIONS
Consult your doctor for specific advice if you are taking any drugs that depress the central nervous system; these include antihistamines, antidepressants or other psychiatric medications, barbiturates, sedatives, cough medicines, decongestants, and painkillers. Be sure your doctor knows about any over-the-counter drug you may take.

FOOD INTERACTIONS
None reported.

DISEASE INTERACTIONS
Caution is advised when taking meprobamate. Consult your doctor if you have a history of alcohol or drug abuse, epilepsy, or porphyria. Use of meprobamate may cause complications in patients with impaired liver or kidney function, since these organs work together to remove the medication from the body.

SIDE EFFECTS

SERIOUS
Skin rash, itching, or hives, confusion, heartbeat irregularities, sore throat and fever, unusual bruising or bleeding, unusual excitability, wheezing, shortness of breath, slowed or labored breathing. Call your doctor immediately.

COMMON
Drowsiness, loss of coordination, poor balance, unsteadiness when walking or standing.

LESS COMMON
Blurred vision or other vision disturbances, diarrhea, dizziness, lightheadedness, euphoria (false sense of well-being), nausea, vomiting, headache, unusual fatigue.

MERCAPTOPURINE

Available in: Tablets
Available OTC? No   **As Generic?** No
Drug Class: Antimetabolite

▼ USAGE INFORMATION

WHY IT'S PRESCRIBED
To treat certain types of leukemia.

HOW IT WORKS
Mercaptopurine kills cancer cells by interfering with the synthesis of their genetic material, which prevents the cells from reproducing. The drug may also affect the growth and development of other kinds of cells in the body, resulting in unpleasant side effects.

▼ DOSAGE GUIDELINES

RANGE AND FREQUENCY
A variety of dosage schedules and regimens for mercaptopurine, with and without other antitumor drugs, is used. For acute myeloblastic leukemia, acute lymphocytic leukemia, and chronic myelocytic leukemia, the initial dose is 80 to 100 mg per square meter of body surface, once a day. Maintenance dose is 50 to 100 mg per square meter of body surface a day.

ONSET OF EFFECT
2 hours.

DURATION OF ACTION
Variable.

DIETARY ADVICE
Drink plenty of fluids.

STORAGE
Store in a tightly sealed container away from heat and direct light.

MISSED DOSE
Take it as soon as you remember. However, if it is near the time for the next dose, skip the missed dose and resume your regular dosage schedule. Do not double the next dose.

STOPPING THE DRUG
The decision to stop taking the drug should be made by your doctor.

PROLONGED USE
See your doctor regularly for tests and examinations if you must take this drug for a prolonged period.

▼ PRECAUTIONS

Over 60: No special problems are expected.

Driving and Hazardous Work: Do not drive or engage in hazardous work until you determine how the medicine affects you.

Alcohol: Avoid alcohol.

Pregnancy: Mercaptopurine may cause birth defects if either the father or the mother is taking it at the time of conception. Persons of childbearing years should take steps to prevent pregnancy when taking this medication.

Breast Feeding: Not recommended during therapy.

Infants and Children: No special warnings.

Special Concerns: Your doctor will want to check blood work (liver, kidney, and blood cell function) weekly or monthly while you are taking this medicine. If you vomit after taking a dose, call your doctor to learn if you should take the dose again or wait for the next dose. Do not receive any immunizations while you are taking mercaptopurine, and avoid people with infections. Be careful when brushing your teeth and check with your doctor before having dental work done. Take care not to cut yourself when using sharp objects such as a safety razor. Avoid contact sports.

OVERDOSE
Symptoms: Loss of appetite, nausea, vomiting, diarrhea, gastrointestinal upset.

What to Do: Call your doctor, emergency medical services (EMS), or the nearest poison control center immediately.

▼ INTERACTIONS

DRUG INTERACTIONS
Consult your doctor for specific advice if you are taking acetaminophen, amiodarone, anabolic steroids, androgens, antibiotics, carbamazepine, chloroquine, dantrolene, disulfiram, divalproex, estrogens, etretinate, gold salts, hydroxychloroquine, methyldopa, naltrexone, oral contraceptives, phenothiazines, phenytoin, plicamycin, valproic acid, azathioprine, corticosteroids, cyclosporine, monoclonal antibodies, allopurinol, amphotericin B, antithyroid agents, chloramphenicol, colchicine, flucytosine, ganciclovir, interferon, zidovudine, probenecid, or sulfinpyrazone.

FOOD INTERACTIONS
No known food interactions.

DISEASE INTERACTIONS
Consult your doctor if you have a history of chickenpox, shingles, gout, kidney stones, any infection, kidney disease, or liver disease.

≡ SIDE EFFECTS ≡

SERIOUS
Black or tarry stools; blood-tinged urine or stools; cough or hoarseness; fever; chills; lower back pain or pain in flanks; painful, difficult urination; small, red spots on the skin; bleeding from gums, nose, or other unusual places; easy bruising; shortness of breath. See your doctor right away if any of these occur. Other serious side effects include low white blood cell and platelet counts, anemia, and liver damage. Such problems can be detected by your doctor.

COMMON
Unusual fatigue, yellowish tinge to skin and eyes (jaundice). Notify your doctor.

LESS COMMON
Nausea, vomiting, abdominal pain or bloating, mouth sores, darkening of skin, diarrhea, headaches, skin rash and itching, weakness.

MESALAMINE

Available in: Extended-release capsules, delayed-release tablets, enema
Available OTC? No   **As Generic?** No
Drug Class: Gastrointestinal anti-inflammatory

▼ USAGE INFORMATION

WHY IT'S PRESCRIBED
To treat inflammatory bowel diseases such as ulcerative colitis.

HOW IT WORKS
The exact mechanism of action is uncertain, although it appears that mesalamine inhibits the production of substances known as metabolites of arachidonic acid (specifically, leukotrienes and prostaglandins), which produce inflammation in the digestive tract.

▼ DOSAGE GUIDELINES

RANGE AND FREQUENCY
Dosage can differ for different brands. Extended-release capsules— Adults: 1 g, 4 times a day for up to 8 weeks. Delayed-release tablets— Adults: Asacol: 800 mg, 3 times a day for 6 weeks. Enema— 4 g (1 unit) used every night for 3 to 6 weeks.

ONSET OF EFFECT
Unknown.

DURATION OF ACTION
Unknown.

DIETARY ADVICE
Take the oral forms before meals and at bedtime with a full glass of water unless you are directed otherwise by your doctor.

STORAGE
Store in a tightly sealed container away from heat and direct light.

MISSED DOSE
Take the oral forms as soon as you remember. If it is near the time for the next dose, skip the missed dose and resume your regular dosage schedule. If you miss a dose of mesalamine enema, take it if you remember the same night. Otherwise, skip the missed dose and resume your regular dosage schedule. In all cases, do not double the next dose.

STOPPING THE DRUG
Take as prescribed for the full treatment period, even if you begin to feel better before the scheduled end of therapy.

PROLONGED USE
You should see your doctor regularly for tests and examinations if you take this drug for a prolonged period.

▼ PRECAUTIONS

Over 60: There is no information comparing the use of mesalamine by older patients with use by other age groups.

Driving and Hazardous Work: Avoid such activities until you determine how the medicine affects you.

Alcohol: Avoid alcohol.

Pregnancy: Mesalamine has not caused birth defects in animals. Human studies have not been done. Before you take mesalamine, tell your doctor if you are pregnant or plan to become pregnant.

Breast Feeding: Mesalamine may pass into breast milk; caution is advised. Consult your doctor for advice.

Infants and Children: There is no specific information comparing use of mesalamine in infants and children with use in other age groups. Use and dose must be determined by your doctor.

Special Concerns: Do not change to another brand without consulting your doctor. The enema may stain clothing, fabrics, or any surface that it touches.

OVERDOSE

Symptoms: Confusion, severe diarrhea, dizziness or light-headedness, drowsiness, severe headache, hearing loss, buzzing or ringing in ear, continuing nausea or vomiting.

What to Do: An overdose of mesalamine is unlikely to be life-threatening. However, if someone takes a much larger dose than prescribed, call your doctor, emergency medical services (EMS), or the nearest poison control center.

▼ INTERACTIONS

DRUG INTERACTIONS
Be sure to consult your doctor if you are taking any other prescription or over-the-counter medication.

FOOD INTERACTIONS
No known food interactions.

DISEASE INTERACTIONS
Those with kidney disease should not take mesalamine, as it may make the condition worse. Patients with hypertension should be monitored closely.

SIDE EFFECTS

SERIOUS
Severe abdominal pains or cramps; bloody diarrhea; fever; severe headache; skin rash and itching; blue or pale skin; severe back or stomach pain, possibly moving to the left arm, neck, or shoulder; chills; rapid heartbeat; nausea or vomiting; shortness of breath; swollen stomach; unusual fatigue; yellow eyes or skin; rectal irritation (with enema). Call your doctor immediately.

COMMON
Mild abdominal cramping, mild diarrhea, dizziness, headache, runny or stuffy nose, sneezing.

LESS COMMON
Acne, back or joint pain, gas or flatulence, loss of appetite, loss of hair.

METAPROTERENOL

Available in: Inhalation aerosol or solution, syrup, tablets
Available OTC? No   **As Generic?** Yes
Drug Class: Bronchodilator/sympathomimetic

▼ USAGE INFORMATION

WHY IT'S PRESCRIBED
To dilate air passages in the lungs that have become narrowed as a result of disease or inflammation. It is used in the treatment of asthma and chronic obstructive pulmonary disease (COPD).

HOW IT WORKS
Metaproterenol widens constricted airways by relaxing the smooth muscles that surround the bronchial passages.

▼ DOSAGE GUIDELINES

RANGE AND FREQUENCY
Use when needed to relieve breathing difficulty. Inhalation solution for nebulizers—Adults and children over 12 years of age: Usual dose is 10 inhalations, not to be taken more frequently than every 3 to 4 hours, for a usual maximum of 3 to 4 times a day. Infants and children under 12 years of age: Consult a pediatrician. Inhalation aerosol—Adults and children 12 years and older: 2 to 3 puffs every 3 to 4 hours. Do not exceed more than 12 puffs per day. Infants and children under 12 years of age: Not recommended. Syrup and tablets—Adults and children 9 years of age and older: 20 mg, 3 or 4 times a day. Infants and children under 9 years of age: Consult a pediatrician.

ONSET OF EFFECT
Inhalation: Within 5 minutes. Oral: 15 to 30 minutes.

DURATION OF ACTION
Inhalation: 1 to 5 hours. Oral: Up to 4 hours.

DIETARY ADVICE
No special recommendations.

STORAGE
Store in a tightly sealed container away from heat and direct light. Do not refrigerate inhalation solutions.

MISSED DOSE
Skip the missed dose and resume your regular dosage schedule. Do not double the next dose.

STOPPING THE DRUG
It may not be necessary to finish the recommended course of therapy. Consult your doctor.

PROLONGED USE
Therapy may require months or years. Excessive use may result in temporary loss of effectiveness.

▼ PRECAUTIONS

Over 60: Adverse reactions may be more likely and more severe in older patients.

Driving and Hazardous Work: Avoid such activities until you determine how the medicine affects you.

Alcohol: No special precautions are necessary.

Pregnancy: Adequate studies have not been done; the benefits must be weighed against potential risks. Consult your doctor for specific advice.

Breast Feeding: Mothers who wish to breast feed while taking this drug should discuss the matter with their doctor.

Infants and Children: Use of the inhalation aerosol is not recommended in children younger than 12.

Special Concerns: Pay heed to any breathing problem that does not improve after your usual nebulizer treatment or usual number of puffs. Seek help immediately if you feel your lungs are persistently constricted, if you are using more than the recommended number of treatments per day, or if you feel a recent attack is somehow different from others.

OVERDOSE
Symptoms: Chest pain or heaviness; irregular, racing, fluttering, or pounding heartbeat; dizziness; lightheadedness; fainting; severe weakness; severe headache.

What to Do: Call your doctor, emergency medical services (EMS), or the nearest poison control center immediately.

▼ INTERACTIONS

DRUG INTERACTIONS
Consult your doctor for specific advice if you are taking a beta-blocker, ergotamine or ergotamine-like medications, antidepressants, digitalis drugs, or an MAO inhibitor.

FOOD INTERACTIONS
No known food interactions.

DISEASE INTERACTIONS
Consult your doctor if you have a history of substance abuse (especially cocaine), seizures, brain damage, heart disease, heartbeat irregularities, high blood pressure, anxiety disorders, or a thyroid condition.

≡ SIDE EFFECTS ≡

SERIOUS
Inhaled form: May become ineffective if used too often, resulting in more-severe breathing difficulty that does not improve. Signs include persistent wheezing, coughing, or shortness of breath; confusion; bluish color to lips or fingernails; inability to speak. Ingested form: Chest pain or heaviness; irregular, racing, fluttering, or pounding heartbeat; lightheadedness; fainting; severe weakness; severe headache.

COMMON
Trouble sleeping, dry mouth, sore throat, nervousness, restlessness.

LESS COMMON
Trembling, sweating, headache, nausea or vomiting, flushing or redness to cheeks or other skin, muscle aches, unpleasant or unusual taste in mouth.

METFORMIN

BRAND NAME
Glucophage

Available in: Tablets
Available OTC? No **As Generic?** No
Drug Class: Antidiabetic agent/biguanide

▼ USAGE INFORMATION

WHY IT'S PRESCRIBED
Used to lower abnormally high blood glucose (sugar) levels in patients with non-insulin-dependent (type 2) diabetes whose blood sugar levels cannot be adequately controlled by diet or exercise alone. The drug may be used alone or in conjunction with sulfonylurea drugs or insulin.

HOW IT WORKS
Metformin decreases the liver's production of glucose, inhibits the breakdown of fatty acids used to produce glucose, and increases the removal of glucose from muscle, the liver, and other body tissues where it is stored.

▼ DOSAGE GUIDELINES

RANGE AND FREQUENCY
Available in 500 mg or 850 mg tablets. Initial dose: 500 mg a day, taken with dinner. If tolerated, a second dose can be added, taken with breakfast. The dose may be slowly increased (1 tablet every 1 or 2 weeks) to a maximum of 2,500 mg a day. Alternatively, 850 mg daily, increased by 850 mg every other week to a maximum of 2,550 mg per day.

ONSET OF EFFECT
Within 2 hours.

DURATION OF ACTION
From 12 to 15 hours.

DIETARY ADVICE
Take with meals to reduce risk of stomach upset.

STORAGE
Store in a sealed container at room temperature away from heat and direct light.

MISSED DOSE
Take it with food as soon as you remember. However, if it is almost time for the next dose, skip the missed dose and resume your regular dosage schedule. Do not double the next dose.

STOPPING THE DRUG
Stop taking metformin only when your doctor advises.

PROLONGED USE
Because metformin helps to manage diabetes but does not cure the disease, its use will be ongoing as long as your blood glucose levels are being adequately controlled. If not, the metformin dosage may be adjusted or a different treatment prescribed.

▼ PRECAUTIONS

Over 60: Because metformin is metabolized in the kidneys, extra caution is warranted in thin, elderly patients with mild adrenal insufficiency (not often detected by the usual tests for kidney impairment).

Driving and Hazardous Work: No special precautions are necessary.

Alcohol: Excessive amounts of alcohol can increase the effect of metformin, possibly resulting in abnormally low blood glucose levels.

Pregnancy: Taking metformin is not advised during pregnancy. Consult your doctor if you become pregnant or plan to become pregnant; insulin is usually the treatment of choice for pregnant diabetic women.

Breast Feeding: Metformin passes into breast milk, although it has not been shown to cause harm to nursing infants. Consult your doctor for specific advice.

Infants and Children: Not recommended for children.

Special Concerns: Do not take metformin if you have previously had an allergic reaction to it.

OVERDOSE
Symptoms: Symptoms of lactic acidosis or hypoglycemia (see Serious Side Effects).

What to Do: Seek emergency medical assistance right away.

▼ INTERACTIONS

DRUG INTERACTIONS
Consult your doctor if you are taking any of the following: amiloride, calcium channel blockers, cimetidine, digoxin, furosemide, morphine, procainamide, quinidine, quinine, ranitidine, trimethoprim, triamterene, or vancomycin.

FOOD INTERACTIONS
The amount and type of food you eat affect your blood glucose levels and must be taken into account while you receive metformin therapy.

DISEASE INTERACTIONS
Do not take metformin if you have any condition that requires careful control of blood glucose levels, such as severe infection; any condition contributing to abnormally low blood oxygen levels, such as congestive heart failure or emphysema; metabolic acidosis (buildup of acid in the blood); a history of alcohol abuse; or kidney or liver disease.

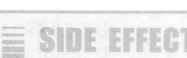

SIDE EFFECTS

SERIOUS
In rare cases, metformin may lead to lactic acidosis, an abnormal and potentially life-threatening buildup of lactic acid in the blood. Symptoms include rapid, shallow breathing; unusual sleepiness or weakness; muscle pain; and abdominal distress. Metformin also occasionally causes abnormally low blood glucose levels (hypoglycemia); symptoms include blurred vision, cold sweats, confusion, anxiousness, rapid heartbeat, shakiness, and nausea. Seek medical assistance immediately.

COMMON
Diarrhea, nausea, vomiting, abdominal bloating, gas, diminished appetite. Usually such symptoms are mild and transient. Consult your doctor if the symptoms persist or increase in severity.

LESS COMMON
Unpleasant or metallic taste in mouth.

METHADONE HYDROCHLORIDE

Available in: Oral concentrate, oral solution, tablets, injection
Available OTC? No   **As Generic?** Yes
Drug Class: Opioid (narcotic) analgesic

▼ USAGE INFORMATION

WHY IT'S PRESCRIBED
To relieve severe pain. It is also used to prevent or ease withdrawal symptoms during detoxification from illegal narcotics, and to serve as maintenance therapy during narcotic addiction treatment programs.

HOW IT WORKS
Methadone is a long-acting opioid. It binds with natural opiate receptors throughout the central nervous system, thereby altering the perception of and emotional response to pain.

▼ DOSAGE GUIDELINES

RANGE AND FREQUENCY
For pain— Oral solution: 5 to 20 mg every 6 to 8 hours. Tablets: 5 to 10 mg every 6 to 8 hours. For narcotic addiction maintenance therapy— Oral solution or tablets: Up to 120 mg a day, depending on individual needs. Children: Dosages must be determined by your doctor. The injectable form is administered only when patients are unable to take methadone orally.

ONSET OF EFFECT
Oral forms: 30 minutes to 1 hour.

DURATION OF ACTION
Oral forms: 4 to 8 hours.

DIETARY ADVICE
Oral forms can be taken with food to lessen stomach upset. Dispersible tablets should be stirred into water or juice before taking.

STORAGE
Store the medication in a tightly sealed container away from heat, moisture, and direct light. Do not freeze the liquid forms.

MISSED DOSE
If you are taking methadone on a fixed schedule, take as soon as you remember. If it is near the time for the next dose, skip the missed dose and resume your regular dosage schedule. Do not double the next dose.

STOPPING THE DRUG
The decision to stop taking the drug should be made by your doctor.

PROLONGED USE
Prolonged use can cause physical dependence.

▼ PRECAUTIONS

Over 60: Adverse reactions may be more likely and more severe in older patients.

Driving and Hazardous Work: Avoid such activities until you determine how the medicine affects you.

Alcohol: Avoid alcohol.

Pregnancy: Adequate studies have not been done. Discuss with your doctor the relative risks and benefits of methadone use during pregnancy.

Breast Feeding: Methadone passes into breast milk; caution is advised. Taking large doses in a maintenance program can cause physical dependence in the baby. Consult your doctor for specific advice.

Infants and Children: Adverse reactions may be more likely and more severe in children. Consult your doctor for advice.

Special Concerns: If you feel the medication is not working properly after a few weeks, do not increase the dose. Consult your doctor. Before having any surgery, tell the doctor or dentist in charge that you are taking methadone.

OVERDOSE

Symptoms: Confusion; slurred speech; extreme sedation, weakness, or dizziness; small, pinpoint pupils; cold, clammy skin; slow breathing; seizures; loss of consciousness.

What to Do: Call your doctor, emergency medical services (EMS), or the nearest poison control center immediately.

▼ INTERACTIONS

DRUG INTERACTIONS
Consult your doctor for specific advice if you are taking carbamazepine or other medicine for seizures, barbiturates, sedatives, cough medicines, decongestants, antidepressants, other prescription pain medications, MAO inhibitors, naltrexone, rifampin, or zidovudine.

FOOD INTERACTIONS
None are known.

DISEASE INTERACTIONS
Consult your doctor if you have any of the following: history of alcohol or drug abuse; emotional illness; brain disorders or head injury; seizures; lung disease; prostate problems or other problems with urination; gallstones; colitis; heart, kidney, liver, or thyroid disease.

≡ SIDE EFFECTS ≡

SERIOUS
Serious side effects of methadone are indistinguishable from those of overdose: confusion; severe drowsiness, weakness, or dizziness; slurred speech; small, pinpoint pupils; cold, clammy skin; slow breathing; seizures; loss of consciousness.

COMMON
Dizziness or lightheadedness, nausea or vomiting, constipation, drowsiness, itching.

LESS COMMON
Sweating, swelling of the feet and ankles, redness or flushing of face.

METHAMPHETAMINE HYDROCHLORIDE

Available in: Tablets, extended-release tablets
Available OTC? No   **As Generic?** No
Drug Class: Central nervous system stimulant/amphetamine

▼ USAGE INFORMATION

WHY IT'S PRESCRIBED
To treat narcolepsy and attention-deficit hyperactivity disorder (ADHD) in children and adults.

HOW IT WORKS
Methamphetamine activates nerve cells in the brain and spinal cord to increase motor activity and alertness, and lessen drowsiness and fatigue. In hyperactivity disorders and narcolepsy, amphetamines improve the ability to pay attention.

▼ DOSAGE GUIDELINES

RANGE AND FREQUENCY
Children age 6 and older– To start, regular tablets are used, 5 mg, 1 or 2 times a day. The dose is gradually increased to 20 to 25 mg a day, either as regular tablets (in 2 or 3 divided doses) or extended-release tablets (once a day). Adults– Tablets: To start, 5 mg, 2 or 3 times a day. Extended-release tablets: To start, 10 mg, 1 or 2 times a day. The dosage may be increased to a total of 60 mg a day, in 2 or 3 divided doses.

ONSET OF EFFECT
Variable.

DURATION OF ACTION
Variable.

DIETARY ADVICE
This drug can be taken without regard to food. Avoid caffeine-containing beverages like tea, coffee, and some carbonated colas. Avoid acidic foods that are rich in vitamin C, such as fruit juices and other citrus products. Avoid vitamin C tablets.

STORAGE
Store in a tightly sealed container away from heat, moisture, and direct light.

MISSED DOSE
Take the missed dose as soon as you remember. If it is close to the next dose or within 6 hours of bedtime, skip the missed dose and resume your regular dosage schedule. Do not double the next dose.

STOPPING THE DRUG
Take it as prescribed for the full treatment period, even if you begin to feel better before the scheduled end of therapy. The decision to stop taking the drug should be made in consultation with your doctor. The doctor may decrease your dosage gradually to reduce the possibility of withdrawal symptoms.

PROLONGED USE
Amphetamines can be habit-forming, and prolonged use may increase the risk of drug dependency.

▼ PRECAUTIONS

Over 60: There is no specific information comparing use of methamphetamine in older patients with use in younger persons.

Driving and Hazardous Work: Do not drive or engage in hazardous work until you determine how the medicine affects you.

Alcohol: Avoid alcohol.

Pregnancy: Adequate human studies have not been completed. Before taking methamphetamine, tell your doctor if you are pregnant or plan to become pregnant.

Breast Feeding: Methamphetamine passes into breast milk; do not use it while nursing.

Infants and Children: This drug is not recommended for use by children under age 6.

Special Concerns: Take methamphetamine only as directed and do not increase the dose on your own. Remember that fatigue, excessive drowsiness, or depression while taking stimulants may mean an emergency situation is developing. Difficulty sleeping may be improved by taking the last scheduled dose several hours before bedtime.

OVERDOSE
Symptoms: Extreme degrees of restlessness, agitation, bizarre behavior; panic; rapid breathing; confusion; high fever; hallucinations; seizures; coma.

What to Do: Call your doctor, emergency medical services (EMS), or the nearest poison control center immediately.

▼ INTERACTIONS

DRUG INTERACTIONS
Consult your doctor for specific advice if you are taking tricyclic antidepressants, caffeine, beta-blockers, digitalis drugs, central nervous system stimulants, meperidine, MAO inhibitors, sympathomimetic agents, or thyroid hormones.

FOOD INTERACTIONS
Citrus juices and caffeinated beverages and foods may interact with this drug.

DISEASE INTERACTIONS
Consult your doctor if you have any of the following: advanced blood vessel disease, heart disease, hyperthyroidism, hypertension, severe anxiety, Tourette's syndrome, glaucoma, or a history of drug abuse.

 SIDE EFFECTS

SERIOUS
Irregular heartbeat, chest pain, increased blood pressure, skin rash, uncontrollable movements of arms and legs, mental changes, unusual weakness, very high fever. Call your doctor immediately.

COMMON
Mood changes, insomnia, drowsiness, restlessness.

LESS COMMON
Blurred vision, constipation, diarrhea, loss of appetite, headache, increased sweating, stomach cramps or abdominal pain, nausea or vomiting, changes in sexual desire or decreased sexual ability.

METHENAMINE AND METHENAMINE SALTS

Available in: Tablets, enteric-coated tablets, oral suspension, granules for solution
Available OTC? No   **As Generic?** Yes
Drug Class: Anti-infective

▼ USAGE INFORMATION

WHY IT'S PRESCRIBED
To prevent and treat urinary tract infections.

HOW IT WORKS
Methenamine and methenamine salts kill bacteria in the urinary tract by forming ammonia and formaldehyde, chemicals that are toxic to the microorganisms that cause infection.

▼ DOSAGE GUIDELINES

RANGE AND FREQUENCY
For prevention of infection— Adults and teenagers: 1,000 mg, 2 times a day. Children ages 6 to 12: 500 mg to 1,000 mg, 2 times a day. For treatment of infection— Adults and teenagers: 1,000 mg, 4 times a day. Children ages 6 to 12: 500 mg, 4 times a day. Children up to age 6: 8.3 mg per lb of body weight, 4 times a day.

ONSET OF EFFECT
Within 1 hour.

DURATION OF ACTION
Up to 8 hours.

DIETARY ADVICE
Take it after meals and at bedtime. Drink plenty of liquids, ensuring that your fluid intake is at least 2 quarts a day. This drug works best in highly acidic urine. Maintain a protein-rich diet and consume liberal amounts of cranberries or cranberry juice, plums, or prunes to ensure sufficiently acidic urine. If this cannot be achieved through diet alone, take vitamin C supplements. Avoid citrus fruits and juices.

STORAGE
Store in a tightly sealed container away from heat and direct light.

MISSED DOSE
Take it as soon as you remember. However, if it is near the time for the next dose, skip the missed dose and resume your regular dosage schedule. Do not double the next dose.

STOPPING THE DRUG
Take as prescribed for the full treatment period, even if you begin to feel better before the scheduled end of therapy.

PROLONGED USE
Consult your doctor about the need for liver function tests and other tests during prolonged therapy.

▼ PRECAUTIONS

Over 60: Adverse reactions may be more likely and more severe in older patients.

Driving and Hazardous Work: Avoid such activities until you determine how the medication affects you.

Alcohol: No special precautions are necessary.

Pregnancy: It is not known whether methenamine is harmful during pregnancy. Discuss with your physician the relative risks and benefits.

Breast Feeding: Methenamine passes into breast milk but has not been reported to cause problems in nursing babies. Consult your doctor about its use during nursing.

Infants and Children: No special problems expected.

Special Concerns: If you take the dry granule form of methenamine, dissolve the contents of each packet in 2 to 4 ounces of water and stir well before drinking it. Avoid use of antacids while taking this medicine. Urine pH should be monitored before starting and throughout therapy.

OVERDOSE
Symptoms: No specific ones have been reported.

What to Do: An overdose of methenamine is unlikely to be life-threatening. However, if someone takes a much larger dose than prescribed, call your doctor, emergency medical services (EMS), or the nearest poison control center.

▼ INTERACTIONS

DRUG INTERACTIONS
Consult your doctor for advice if you are taking thiazide diuretics; sodium bicarbonate; methazolamide; sulfamethoxazole; or urinary alkalizers, such as acetazolamide.

FOOD INTERACTIONS
While taking methenamine, avoid milk products, citrus fruits and juices, and alkaline foods like vegetables and peanuts.

DISEASE INTERACTIONS
Use of methenamine may cause complications in patients with liver or kidney disease, since these organs work together to remove the medication from the body. Before you take methenamine, tell your doctor if you have ever experienced severe dehydration.

⬇ SIDE EFFECTS ⬇

SERIOUS
Skin rash, blood in urine, lower back pain, burning or pain while urinating. Call your physician immediately.

COMMON
No common side effects are associated with the use of methenamine.

LESS COMMON
Nausea or vomiting may occur. Contact your doctor if such symptoms persist.

METHIMAZOLE

Available in: Tablets
Available OTC? No   **As Generic?** No
Drug Class: Antithyroid agent

▼ USAGE INFORMATION

WHY IT'S PRESCRIBED
To treat conditions in which the thyroid gland produces too much thyroid hormone.

HOW IT WORKS
Methimazole interferes with the body's ability to use iodine in the manufacture of thyroid hormone.

▼ DOSAGE GUIDELINES

RANGE AND FREQUENCY
Adults: 15 to 60 mg a day in 1 daily dose or in 2 divided daily doses. Usual maintenance dose is 5 to 15 mg a day. Children: 0.2 mg per 2.2 lbs (1 kg) of body weight a day in 1 daily dose or in 2 divided daily doses. To treat a thyroid crisis: 12 to 20 mg every 4 hours.

ONSET OF EFFECT
5 days or more.

DURATION OF ACTION
Unknown.

DIETARY ADVICE
Methimazole can be taken with or without food. It should be taken consistently in the same way, either with or between meals.

STORAGE
Store in a tightly sealed container away from heat and direct light.

MISSED DOSE
Take it as soon as you remember. However, if it is near the time for the next dose, skip the missed dose and resume your regular dosage schedule. Do not double the next dose.

STOPPING THE DRUG
Take it as prescribed for the full treatment period, even if you begin to feel better before the scheduled end of therapy.

PROLONGED USE
No special problems are expected. It may be necessary to take this medication for several years.

▼ PRECAUTIONS

Over 60:
Adverse reactions may be more common and more severe in older patients.

Driving and Hazardous Work:
The use of this medication should not impair your ability to perform such tasks safely.

Alcohol:
Consult your doctor about using alcohol while taking methimazole.

Pregnancy:
Too large a dose during pregnancy may cause problems in the fetus. Use of the prescribed dose, with careful monitoring, is not likely to cause problems.

Breast Feeding:
Methimazole passes into breast milk, but your doctor may allow you to continue to nurse if the dose is low and the infant is checked regularly.

Infants and Children:
No special problems expected.

Special Concerns:
Before undergoing any kind of medical or dental procedure, tell the doctor or dentist in charge that you are taking methimazole. During and after treatment with methimazole, do not receive any immunizations without your doctor's approval, and avoid persons who have taken oral polio vaccine recently.

OVERDOSE
Symptoms: Nausea, vomiting, coldness, constipation, changes in menstrual period, dry and puffy skin, headache, listlessness, swollen neck, sleepiness, muscle aches, unusual weight gain.

What to Do: An overdose of methimazole is unlikely to be life-threatening. However, if someone takes a much larger dose than prescribed, call your doctor, emergency medical services (EMS), or the local poison control center right away.

▼ INTERACTIONS

DRUG INTERACTIONS
Consult your doctor for specific advice if you are taking amiodarone, iodinated glycerol, potassium iodide, anticoagulants, or digitalis drugs.

FOOD INTERACTIONS
Consult your doctor about a special low-iodine diet.

DISEASE INTERACTIONS
Use of methimazole may cause complications in patients with liver disease, since this organ works to remove the medication from the body.

≡ SIDE EFFECTS ≡

SERIOUS
Cough; continuing or severe fever or chills; hoarseness; mouth sores; pain, swelling, or redness in joints; throat infection; yellow discoloration of the skin or eyes; general feeling of illness. Call your doctor immediately.

COMMON
Mild and temporary fever; rash or itching.

LESS COMMON
Backache; black and tarry stools; blood in urine or stools; shortness of breath; increased or decreased urination; swelling of feet or lower legs; swollen lymph or salivary glands; numbness or tingling of face, fingers, or toes; dizziness; nausea; stomach pain; vomiting.

METHOCARBAMOL

Available in: Tablets, injection
Available OTC? No   **As Generic?** Yes
Drug Class: Muscle relaxant

▼ USAGE INFORMATION

WHY IT'S PRESCRIBED
Muscle relaxants are used to relieve stiffness and discomfort caused by severe sprains and strains, muscle spasms, or other muscle problems. They may be prescribed in conjunction with other treatment methods, such as physical therapy.

HOW IT WORKS
Muscle relaxants such as methocarbamol depress activity in the central nervous system (brain and spinal cord), which in turn interferes with the transmission of nerve impulses from the spinal cord to the skeletal muscles.

▼ DOSAGE GUIDELINES

RANGE AND FREQUENCY
Adults and teenagers—
Tablets: 1,500 mg, 4 times a day to start, then the dose may be reduced. Injection: 1 to 3 g a day, in 1 or several doses. Children— Consult your pediatrician.

ONSET OF EFFECT
Immediate after injection; within 30 minutes after oral administration.

DURATION OF ACTION
Unknown.

DIETARY ADVICE
Take the tablets with food to reduce stomach irritation.

STORAGE
Store in a tightly sealed container away from heat and direct light.

MISSED DOSE
Take it as soon as you remember. However, if it is near the time for the next dose, skip the missed dose and resume your regular dosage schedule. Do not double the next dose.

STOPPING THE DRUG
The decision to stop taking the drug should be made by your doctor.

PROLONGED USE
You should see your doctor regularly for tests and examinations if you take this drug for a prolonged period.

▼ PRECAUTIONS

Over 60: No special problems are expected.

Driving and Hazardous Work: Do not drive or engage in hazardous work until you determine how the medicine affects you.

Alcohol: Avoid alcohol while taking this drug because it may compound the sedative effect and may cause liver damage.

Pregnancy: Adequate studies of methocarbamol during pregnancy have not been done; discuss relative risks and benefits with your doctor.

Breast Feeding: Methocarbamol may pass into breast milk; caution is advised. Consult your doctor for advice.

Infants and Children: No special problems have been documented; consult your pediatrician for advice.

Special Concerns: Methocarbamol can cause false results in tests of sugar levels for diabetic patients. This drug will intensify the effect that alcohol, sedatives, and other central nervous system depressants have on the brain. Do not take methocarbamol if you are allergic to any skeletal muscle relaxant. Use of this drug should be accompanied by bed rest, physical therapy, and other measures to relieve discomfort.

OVERDOSE
Symptoms: Nausea, vomiting, diarrhea, loss of appetite, headache, severe weakness, fainting, breathing difficulties, irritability, seizures, feeling of paralysis, profuse sweating, loss of consciousness.

What to Do: Call your doctor, emergency medical services (EMS), or the nearest poison control center immediately.

▼ INTERACTIONS

DRUG INTERACTIONS
Consult your doctor for specific advice if you are taking any drug that depresses the central nervous system or any tricyclic antidepressant.

FOOD INTERACTIONS
No known food interactions.

DISEASE INTERACTIONS
Caution is advised when taking methocarbamol. Consult your doctor if you have a history of any of the following: alcohol or drug abuse, allergies, a blood disease caused by an allergy or another medication, kidney disease, liver disease, porphyria, or epilepsy.

 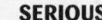
SIDE EFFECTS

SERIOUS
Fainting; palpitations or rapid heartbeat; fever; hives or severe swelling of face, lips, or tongue along with shortness of breath, chest tightness, or wheezing (indicating a potentially life-threatening allergic reaction); seizures; mental depression. Seek medical help immediately.

COMMON
Blurred, double, or altered vision, dizziness or lightheadedness, drowsiness, dry mouth.

LESS COMMON
Inability to pass urine; sores on lips, ulcers in mouth; abdominal cramps or pain; clumsiness; unsteady gait; confusion; constipation; diarrhea; excitability, nervousness, restlessness, or irritability; flushing or redness of face; headache; heartburn; hiccups; muscle weakness; nausea and vomiting; trembling; insomnia or fitful sleep; burning, red eyes; stuffy nose.

METHOTREXATE

BRAND NAMES

Folex, Folex PFS,
Mexate, Mexate-AQ,
Rheumatrex

Available in: Tablets, injection
Available OTC? No   **As Generic?** Yes
Drug Class: Antineoplastic agent/antimetabolite; antipsoriatic; antirheumatic

▼ USAGE INFORMATION

WHY IT'S PRESCRIBED
To treat certain kinds of cancer, psoriasis, and rheumatoid arthritis.

HOW IT WORKS
Methotrexate interferes with the activity of an enzyme needed for the maintenance and replication of cells, especially those that divide and proliferate rapidly. Such cells include many types of cancer cells, as well as those that compose the bone marrow and the cells that line the mouth, intestine, and bladder. Consequently, in addition to its cancer-fighting effects, methotrexate may also harm healthy tissues in the body, causing unpleasant or serious side effects. It is unknown how methotrexate works to ease rheumatoid arthritis, but it appears to modify the function of the immune system, whose activity is believed to play a role in the progression of the disease.

▼ DOSAGE GUIDELINES

RANGE AND FREQUENCY
For psoriasis or rheumatoid arthritis— Tablets: 2.5 to 5 mg every 12 hours for 3 doses in 1 week; or 10 mg once a week. Injection: 10 mg, once a week. For cancer— Use and dose depends on type and stage of disease. Your doctor may alter dosage as needed. Consult pediatrician for children's dose.

ONSET OF EFFECT
Unknown.

DURATION OF ACTION
Unknown.

DIETARY ADVICE
This drug is best taken 1 to 2 hours before meals.

STORAGE
Store in a tightly sealed container away from heat, moisture, and direct light.

MISSED DOSE
If you miss a dose, do not take the missed dose and do not double the next dose. Resume your regular schedule and check with your doctor.

STOPPING THE DRUG
The decision to stop taking the drug should be made by your doctor.

PROLONGED USE
See your doctor regularly for tests and examinations.

▼ PRECAUTIONS

Over 60: Adverse reactions may be more likely and more severe in older patients.

Driving and Hazardous Work: Avoid such activities until you determine how the medicine affects you.

Alcohol: Avoid alcohol.

Pregnancy: Methotrexate can cause birth defects and other problems; avoid use during pregnancy.

Breast Feeding: Methotrexate passes into breast milk and may cause serious side effects in the nursing infant; do not use while breast feeding.

Infants and Children: Infants are more sensitive to the effects of methotrexate. No special problems are expected in older children.

Special Concerns: Methotrexate may lower your resistance to infection by reducing the number of white blood cells in the blood. Do not have any immunizations without your doctor's approval. Avoid people with infections. Use care when shaving, trimming nails, or using sharp objects. Inform your doctor immediately if you have fever, chills, unusual bleeding or bruising, diarrhea, or a cough. Methotrexate may increase skin sensitivity to sunlight. Limit sun exposure until you see how the medicine affects you. After you stop taking methotrexate, you may experience back pain, blurred vision, confusion, seizures, dizziness, fever, or unusual fatigue; consult your doctor immediately.

OVERDOSE
Symptoms: Severe damage to the liver, kidneys, stomach, intestines, bone marrow, and lungs, causing a wide array of symptoms.

What to Do: If you suspect an overdose, seek medical assistance immediately.

▼ INTERACTIONS

DRUG INTERACTIONS
A number of drugs may interact with methotrexate. Consult your doctor for specific advice if you are taking any drugs that may affect the liver, such as azathioprine, retinoids, and sulfasalazine; or any other prescription or over-the-counter medication.

FOOD INTERACTIONS
No known food interactions.

DISEASE INTERACTIONS
Consult your doctor if you have any of the following: a history of alcohol abuse, chickenpox, shingles, colitis, any disease of the immune system, kidney stones, any infection, intestinal blockage, kidney disease, liver disease, mouth sores or inflammation, or stomach ulcers.

≡ SIDE EFFECTS ≡

SERIOUS
Black, tarry stools; bloody vomit; diarrhea; flushing or redness of skin; sores in mouth and on lips; stomach pain; blood in urine or stools; confusion; seizures; cough or hoarseness; fever or chills; pain in lower back or side; painful or difficult urination; red spots on skin; shortness of breath; swollen feet or lower legs; unusual bleeding or bruising; back pain; dark urine; drowsiness; dizziness; headache; joint pain; unusual fatigue; yellow-tinged eyes or skin. Call your doctor immediately.

COMMON
Loss of appetite, nausea and vomiting, minor mouth ulcers.

LESS COMMON
Acne, boils, pale skin, skin rash, or itching.

METHYLDOPA

Available in: Oral suspension, tablets, injection
Available OTC? No   **As Generic?** Yes
Drug Class: Centrally acting antihypertensive

▼ USAGE INFORMATION

WHY IT'S PRESCRIBED
To treat high blood pressure (hypertension).

HOW IT WORKS
Methyldopa acts upon certain areas of the central nervous system (the brain and spinal cord) that regulate the activity of the heart and the smooth muscle tissue surrounding the arteries. The drug causes blood vessels to relax and widen, which in turn lowers blood pressure.

▼ DOSAGE GUIDELINES

RANGE AND FREQUENCY
Suspension or tablets—Adults: 250 mg to 2 g a day in 2 to 4 doses. Children: 10 mg per 2.2 lbs (1 kg) of body weight in 2 to 4 doses. Injection— Adults: 250 to 500 mg injected into a vein every 6 hours. Children: 20 to 40 mg per 2.2 lbs injected every 6 hours.

ONSET OF EFFECT
Unknown.

DURATION OF ACTION
12 to 24 hours after single oral dose, 24 to 48 hours after multiple oral doses; 10 to 16 hours after injection.

DIETARY ADVICE
Methyldopa can be taken without regard to the timing of meals. Follow a healthy diet (low-salt, low-fat, low-cholesterol) as advised by your doctor to help control blood pressure and prevent heart disease.

STORAGE
Store tablets and injection in a tightly sealed container away from heat, moisture, and direct light. Keep oral suspension refrigerated, but do not allow it to freeze.

MISSED DOSE
Take it as soon as you remember. However, if it is near the time for the next dose, skip the missed dose and resume your regular dosage schedule. Do not double the next dose.

STOPPING THE DRUG
Do not stop taking this drug suddenly, as this may cause potentially serious health problems. If therapy is to be discontinued, dosage should be reduced gradually, according to a doctor's instructions.

PROLONGED USE
Lifelong therapy may be required. See your doctor regularly for tests and examinations if you take this medicine for a prolonged period.

▼ PRECAUTIONS

Over 60: Adverse reactions may be more likely and more severe in older patients.

Driving and Hazardous Work: Do not drive or engage in hazardous work until you determine how the medicine affects you.

Alcohol: Avoid alcohol.

Pregnancy: Methyldopa is one of the few antihypertensive medications that can be used by pregnant women. It effectively reduces high blood pressure and has been found in several studies to be safe for both the mother and the unborn child.

Breast Feeding: Methyldopa may pass into breast milk; caution is advised. Consult your doctor for advice.

Infants and Children: No special problems are expected.

Special Concerns: Check your weight frequently and tell your doctor if you gain 5 pounds or more.

OVERDOSE
Symptoms: Weakness, fast heartbeat, dizziness, light-headedness, constipation or diarrhea, nausea, vomiting, loss of consciousness.

What to Do: Call your doctor, emergency medical services (EMS), or the nearest poison control center immediately.

▼ INTERACTIONS

DRUG INTERACTIONS
Certain drugs may interact with methyldopa. Consult your doctor for specific advice if you are taking an MAO inhibitor.

FOOD INTERACTIONS
No known food interactions.

DISEASE INTERACTIONS
Caution is advised when taking methyldopa. Consult your doctor if you have any of the following: angina, Parkinson's disease, mental depression, or pheochromocytoma. Use of methyldopa may cause complications in patients with kidney disease or liver disease, since these organs work together to remove the medication from the body.

 SIDE EFFECTS

SERIOUS
Fever shortly after starting to take this medicine, swelling of feet or lower legs, mental depression or anxiety, nightmares, dark or amber urine, stomach cramps, chills, troubled breathing, fast heartbeat, general feeling of discomfort, joint pain, skin rash or itching, yellowish tinge to eyes or skin, continued fatigue, pale stools, nausea and vomiting. Call your doctor immediately.

COMMON
Drowsiness, dry mouth, headache.

LESS COMMON
Diarrhea; dizziness or lightheadedness when getting up; decreased sexual performance; slow heartbeat; stuffy nose; swelling of breasts; unusual milk production; tingling, pain, or weakness in hands or feet.

METHYLPHENIDATE HYDROCHLORIDE

Available in: Tablets, extended-release tablets
Available OTC? No   **As Generic?** Yes
Drug Class: Central nervous system stimulant

▼ USAGE INFORMATION

WHY IT'S PRESCRIBED
To treat attention-deficit hyperactivity disorder (ADHD). It is also used to treat narcolepsy.

HOW IT WORKS
Methylphenidate is thought to stimulate the release of norepinephrine, a natural hormone that promotes the transmission of nerve impulses in the brain. It works by decreasing restlessness and increasing attention in adults and children who cannot concentrate for very long, are easily distracted, or are unusually impulsive.

▼ DOSAGE GUIDELINES

RANGE AND FREQUENCY
For ADHD— Tablets: Adults and teenagers: 5 to 20 mg, 2 to 3 times a day, taken with or after meals. Children ages 6 to 12: To start, 5 mg, 2 times a day. If needed, your doctor may increase the dose by 5 to 10 mg a week. Extended-release tablets: Adults, teenagers and children ages 6 to 12: 20 mg, 1 to 3 times a day, every 8 hours. For narcolepsy— Tablets: Adults and teenagers: 5 to 20 mg, 3 or 4 times a day, taken with or after meals. Extended-release tablets: Adults and teenagers: 20 mg, 2 to 3 times a day.

ONSET OF EFFECT
Tablets: Usually within 30 minutes. Extended-release tablets: Usually between 30 and 60 minutes.

DURATION OF ACTION
Tablets: 4 to 6 hours. Extended-release tablets: 6 hours or longer.

DIETARY ADVICE
For attention-deficit hyperactivity disorder, this medicine should be taken with or after meals. For narcolepsy, it should be taken 30 to 45 minutes before meals.

STORAGE
Store in a tightly sealed container away from heat, moisture, and direct light.

MISSED DOSE
Take it as soon as you remember. If it is near the time for the next dose, skip the missed dose and resume your regular dosage schedule. Do not double the next dose.

STOPPING THE DRUG
The decision to stop taking the drug should be made by your doctor.

PROLONGED USE
See your doctor regularly for tests and examinations.

▼ PRECAUTIONS

Over 60: No special problems are expected.

Driving and Hazardous Work: Do not drive or engage in hazardous work until you determine how the medicine affects you.

Alcohol: Avoid alcohol.

Pregnancy: Adequate human studies have not been completed. Before taking methylphenidate, tell your doctor if you are pregnant or plan to become pregnant.

Breast Feeding: It is not known whether methylphenidate passes into breast milk; caution is advised. Consult your doctor for advice.

Infants and Children: This drug is not recommended for use by children under the age of 6. Older children may be especially likely to experience side effects such as loss of appetite, stomach pain, and weight loss.

Special Concerns: To prevent insomnia, do not take methylphenidate too close to bedtime. Your prescription cannot be refilled, so you must get a new one from your doctor to obtain more medication.

OVERDOSE
Symptoms: Agitation; confusion; delirium; seizures; dry mouth; false sense of well-being; rapid, pounding, or irregular heartbeat; fever; sweating; severe headache; increased blood pressure; muscle twitching, trembling or tremors; vomiting.

What to Do: Call your doctor, emergency medical services (EMS), or the nearest poison control center immediately.

▼ INTERACTIONS

DRUG INTERACTIONS
Call your doctor for specific advice if you are taking caffeine, amantadine, appetite suppressants, tricyclic antidepressants, chlophedianol, pemoline, asthma medicine, amphetamines, medicine for colds or sinus problems or allergies, nabilone, pimozide, or MAO inhibitors.

FOOD INTERACTIONS
Do not drink large amounts of caffeinated beverages like coffee, tea, soft drinks, cocoa, or chocolate milk.

DISEASE INTERACTIONS
Consult your doctor if you have Tourette's syndrome or other tics, glaucoma, epilepsy or another seizure disorder, high blood pressure, psychosis, severe anxiety, depression, or a history of alcohol or drug abuse.

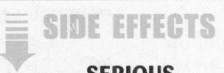
SIDE EFFECTS

SERIOUS
Fast heartbeat, unusual bleeding or bruising, chest pain, fever, joint pain, increased heartbeat, skin rash or hives, uncontrolled body movements, blurred vision or other vision changes, seizures, sore throat and fever, unusual fatigue, weight loss, mood or mental changes. Call your doctor immediately.

COMMON
Loss of appetite, insomnia, nervousness.

LESS COMMON
Dizziness, stomach pain, drowsiness, nausea, headache.

METHYLPRESOLONE

Available in: Tablets, injection, enema
Available OTC? No   **As Generic?** Yes
Drug Class: Corticosteroid

▼ USAGE INFORMATION

WHY IT'S PRESCRIBED
To treat numerous conditions that involve inflammation (a response by body tissues, producing redness, warmth, swelling, and pain). Such conditions include arthritis, allergic reactions, asthma, some skin diseases, multiple sclerosis flare-ups, and other autoimmune diseases. Also prescribed to treat deficiency of natural steroid hormones.

HOW IT WORKS
This hormone mimics the effects of the body's natural corticosteroids. It depresses the synthesis, release, and activity of inflammation-producing body chemicals. It also suppresses the activity of the immune system.

▼ DOSAGE GUIDELINES

RANGE AND FREQUENCY
Tablets: 4 to 160 mg a day, depending on condition, in 1 or more doses. Injection: 10 to 160 mg a day injected into a muscle or vein, or 4 to 120 mg as needed, injected into a muscle, joint, or lesion. Enema: 40 mg, 3 to 7 times a week. Consult your pediatrician for children's dose.

ONSET OF EFFECT
Varies widely depending on form used.

DURATION OF ACTION
30 to 36 hours with tablets; 1 to 4 weeks after muscle injection; 1 to 5 weeks after other injections.

DIETARY ADVICE
Take it with food or milk to minimize stomach upset. Your doctor may recommend a low-salt, high-potassium, high-protein diet.

STORAGE
Store in a tightly sealed container away from heat, moisture, and direct light. Do not freeze the liquid form.

MISSED DOSE
If you take several doses a day and it is close to the next dose, double the next dose. If you take 1 dose a day and you do not remember until the next day, skip the missed dose and do not double the next dose.

STOPPING THE DRUG
With long-term therapy, do not stop taking the drug abruptly; the dosage should be decreased gradually.

PROLONGED USE
Long-term use may lead to cataracts, diabetes, hypertension, or osteoporosis; see your physician for regular visits.

▼ PRECAUTIONS

Over 60: Adverse reactions may be more likely and more severe in older patients.

Driving and Hazardous Work: Avoid such activities until you determine how the medicine affects you.

Alcohol: May cause stomach problems; avoid it unless your physician approves occasional moderate drinking.

Pregnancy: Overuse during pregnancy can impair growth and development of the child.

Breast Feeding: Do not use this drug while nursing.

Infants and Children: Methylprednisolone may retard the development of bone and other tissues.

Special Concerns: This drug can lower your resistance to infection. Avoid immunizations with live vaccines. Patients undergoing long-term therapy should wear a medical-alert bracelet. Call your doctor if you develop a fever.

OVERDOSE
Symptoms: Fever, muscle or joint pain, nausea, dizziness, fainting, difficulty breathing. Prolonged overuse: Moon-face, obesity, unusual hair growth, acne, loss of sexual function, muscle wasting.

What to Do: Seek medical assistance immediately.

▼ INTERACTIONS

DRUG INTERACTIONS
Consult your doctor for specific advice if you are taking aminoglutethimide, antacids, barbiturates, carbamazepine, griseofulvin, mitotane, phenylbutazone, phenytoin, primidone, rifampin, injectable amphotericin B, oral antidiabetes agents, insulin, digitalis drugs, diuretics, or medications containing potassium or sodium.

FOOD INTERACTIONS
Avoid excess sodium.

DISEASE INTERACTIONS
Consult your doctor if you have a history of bone disease, chickenpox, measles, gastrointestinal disorders, diabetes, recent serious infection, glaucoma, heart disease, hypertension, liver or kidney disorders, high blood cholesterol, thyroid problems, myasthenia gravis, or lupus.

≡ SIDE EFFECTS ≡

SERIOUS
Vision problems, frequent urination, increased thirst, rectal bleeding, blistering skin, confusion, hallucinations, paranoia, euphoria, depression, mood swings, redness and swelling at injection site. Call your doctor immediately.

COMMON
Increased appetite, indigestion, nervousness, insomnia, greater susceptibility to infections, increased blood pressure, slowed wound healing, weight gain, easy bruising, fluid retention.

LESS COMMON
Change in skin color, dizziness, headache, increased sweating, unusual growth of body or facial hair, increased blood sugar, peptic ulcers, adrenal insufficiency, muscle weakness, cataracts, glaucoma, osteoporosis.

METHYSERGIDE MALEATE

BRAND NAME

Sansert

Available in: Tablets
Available OTC? No **As Generic?** No
Drug Class: Antimigraine/antiheadache drug

▼ USAGE INFORMATION

WHY IT'S PRESCRIBED
Used to prevent vascular headaches (those that occur in response to changes in normal blood flow within the blood vessels in the brain), such as migraines and cluster headaches. Because of the possible risk of serious, irreversible side effects, methysergide is prescribed only as a last resort for patients with frequent or disabling headaches who are unresponsive to other treatments. This medication is not useful against tension headaches or a vascular headache that has already started.

HOW IT WORKS
The exact mechanism of action is unknown, although it appears that methysergide eases vascular headaches by causing constriction of the blood vessels in the brain. It is also believed to block the effects of serotonin, a chemical messenger in the nervous system associated with vascular headaches.

▼ DOSAGE GUIDELINES

RANGE AND FREQUENCY
One 2 mg tablet, 2 or 3 times a day, with meals or milk. Do not crush methysergide tablets before taking them.

ONSET OF EFFECT
Within 1 to 2 days.

DURATION OF ACTION
From 1 to 2 days.

DIETARY ADVICE
Take methysergide with meals or milk to prevent stomach upset. A low-salt diet is advised.

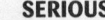

SIDE EFFECTS

SERIOUS
Chest pain or tightness; shortness of breath; extreme dizziness; difficult or painful urination; large increase or decrease in urine output; pain in the arms, legs, groin, lower back, or side; swelling of hands, ankles, feet, or lower legs; fever or chills; pale or cold hands or feet; hallucinations. Call your doctor immediately. Contact your doctor as soon as possible if you experience abdominal pain; itching; numbness or tingling of fingers, toes, or face; or weakness in the legs.

COMMON
Diarrhea; mild dizziness or lightheadedness, particularly upon arising from a lying or sitting position; drowsiness; nausea; vomiting.

LESS COMMON
Vision changes, loss of coordination, rapid or slow heartbeat, cough or hoarseness, loss of appetite or weight, raised red spots on your skin, redness or flushing of the face, skin rash.

STORAGE
Store in a tightly sealed container, away from direct light, moisture, and extremes in temperature.

MISSED DOSE
Take it as soon as you remember. However, if it is almost time for the next dose, skip the missed dose and resume your regular dosage schedule. Do not double the next dose.

STOPPING THE DRUG
Stop taking methysergide only when your doctor advises. Methysergide is usually discontinued gradually over 2 to 3 weeks to prevent rebound headaches, which may occur if the drug is discontinued abruptly.

PROLONGED USE
To reduce the risk of serious side effects, after every 4-month course of methysergide therapy, discontinue the drug for 4 weeks before starting the next course.

▼ PRECAUTIONS

Over 60: Adverse reactions may be more likely and more severe in older patients.

Driving and Hazardous Work: Do not drive or engage in hazardous work until you determine how the drug affects you.

Alcohol: Avoid alcohol, which can trigger or exacerbate vascular headaches.

Pregnancy: Avoid use during pregnancy. Consult your doctor if you become or plan to become pregnant.

Breast Feeding: Do not use methysergide while breast feeding.

Infants and Children: Methysergide is not recommended for this age group because of the potential adverse reactions associated with its long-term use.

Special Concerns: Avoid smoking, since it may increase the risk of side effects associated with decreased blood circulation.

OVERDOSE
Symptoms: Cold and pale hands or feet, severe dizziness, excitability.

What to Do: Seek emergency medical assistance right away.

▼ INTERACTIONS

DRUG INTERACTIONS
Consult your physician if you are using or plan to use any other drugs, particularly other types of ergot alkaloids, epinephrine, metaraminol, methoxamine, norepinephrine, phenylephrine, local anesthesia, or tobacco products.

FOOD INTERACTIONS
No known food interactions.

DISEASE INTERACTIONS
Tell your doctor if you have or have had any other medical problems, including arthritis; heart or blood vessel disease; high blood pressure; kidney, liver, or lung disease; stomach ulcer; severe infection; or severe itching.

METOCLOPRAMIDE HYDROCHLORIDE

Available in: Tablets, syrup, injection
Available OTC? No **As Generic?** Yes
Drug Class: Gastrointestinal stimulant

▼ USAGE INFORMATION

WHY IT'S PRESCRIBED
To prevent nausea and vomiting caused by anticancer medicines or to treat impaired emptying of food from the stomach (gastroparesis) as a complication of diabetes. Also used as a short-term treatment for heartburn (gastroesophageal reflux, a backflow of stomach acid into the esophagus).

HOW IT WORKS
Metoclopramide increases the contractions or movements of the stomach and small intestine. It decreases nausea by blocking the effect of the chemical dopamine in the vomiting center of the brain.

▼ DOSAGE GUIDELINES

RANGE AND FREQUENCY
Tablets or syrup– To treat diabetic gastroparesis: Adults and teenagers: 10 mg, 30 minutes before symptoms are likely to begin or before each meal and at bedtime, up to 4 times a day. For heartburn: Adults and teenagers: 10 to 15 mg, 30 minutes before symptoms are likely to begin or before each meal and bedtime. To increase movements of stomach and intestine: Children ages 5 to 14: 2.5 to 5 mg, 3 times a day, 30 minutes before meals. Injection– To increase movements of stomach and intestine: Adults and teenagers: 10 mg into a vein. Children: 0.45 mg per lb of body weight into a vein. Dose may be repeated after 60 minutes. To prevent vomiting and nausea caused by cancer medicines: Adults and teenagers: 1 to 2 mg per 2.2 lbs (1 kg) into a vein 30 minutes before taking cancer medicine. Children: 1 mg per 2.2 lbs (1 kg) into a vein.

ONSET OF EFFECT
Within 3 minutes of intravenous injection; 10 to 15 minutes of intramuscular injection; 30 to 60 minutes after tablets or syrup.

DURATION OF ACTION
1 to 2 hours.

DIETARY ADVICE
Take the drug 30 minutes before meals unless your doctor directs otherwise.

STORAGE
Store in a tightly sealed container away from heat, moisture, and direct light.

MISSED DOSE
Take it as soon as you remember. If it is near the time for the next dose, skip the missed dose and resume your regular dosage schedule. Do not double the next dose.

STOPPING THE DRUG
The decision to stop taking the drug should be made by your doctor.

PROLONGED USE
You should see your doctor regularly for tests and examinations if you take this drug for a prolonged period.

▼ PRECAUTIONS

Over 60: Adverse reactions may be more likely and more severe in older patients.

Driving and Hazardous Work: Do not drive or engage in hazardous work until you determine how the medicine affects you.

Alcohol: Avoid alcohol.

Pregnancy: Adequate human studies have not been completed. Before taking metoclopramide, tell your doctor if you are pregnant or plan to become pregnant.

Breast Feeding: Metoclopramide passes into breast milk; caution is advised. Consult your doctor for advice.

Infants and Children: The dosage and use should be determined by your doctor. Adverse effects are more likely to occur in infants and children.

Special Concerns: Avoid activities requiring alertness for 2 hours after each dose.

OVERDOSE
Symptoms: Drowsiness, confusion, muscle contractions, irritability, agitation.

What to Do: Call your doctor, emergency medical services (EMS), or the nearest poison control center immediately.

▼ INTERACTIONS

DRUG INTERACTIONS
Consult your doctor for specific advice if you are taking central nervous system depressants, such as antihistamines, cold medicines, sleep aids, or tranquilizers.

FOOD INTERACTIONS
No known food interactions.

DISEASE INTERACTIONS
Consult your doctor if you have a history of abdominal or stomach bleeding, asthma, high blood pressure, intestinal blockage, Parkinson's disease, epilepsy, or kidney or liver disease.

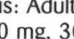

SIDE EFFECTS

SERIOUS
Muscle spasms, aching or crawling sensation in lower legs, stiffness or uncontrolled movements of arms or legs, panicky feeling, unusual nervousness, restlessness, irritability, difficulty speaking or swallowing, dizziness or fainting, fast or irregular heartbeat, general fatigue, shaking of hands and fingers, uncontrolled chewing movements, lip smacking or puckering, loss of balance, severe headache, unusual tongue movements, difficulty walking or shuffling walk. Call your doctor immediately.

COMMON
Diarrhea, restlessness, drowsiness.

LESS COMMON
Breast tenderness and swelling, increased flow of breast milk, menstrual changes, depression, constipation, nausea, skin rash, insomnia, dryness of mouth.

METOLAZONE

Available in: Tablets, extended-release tablets
Available OTC? No **As Generic?** No
Drug Class: Thiazide-like diuretic

▼ USAGE INFORMATION

WHY IT'S PRESCRIBED
To treat conditions that cause edema (swelling of body tissues resulting from excess salt and water retention). Many patients are prescribed metolazone in conjunction with other diuretics for particularly resistant fluid retention.

HOW IT WORKS
Diuretics increase the excretion of salt and water in the urine. Metolazone acts on a part of the kidney that is not affected by loop diuretics such as furosemide or bumetanide. Metolazone and a loop diuretic, when prescribed in combination, thus have a synergistic effect.

▼ DOSAGE GUIDELINES

RANGE AND FREQUENCY
Adults: 2.5 to 10 mg, 1 or 2 times per day.

ONSET OF EFFECT
Approximately 1 hour.

DURATION OF ACTION
From 12 to 24 hours.

DIETARY ADVICE
Take it with food to avoid stomach upset.

STORAGE
Store in a tightly sealed container away from heat and direct light. Keep away from moisture and extremes in temperature.

MISSED DOSE
Take it as soon as you remember. If it is near the time for the next dose, skip the missed dose and resume your regular dosage schedule. Do not double the next dose.

STOPPING THE DRUG
The decision to stop taking the drug should be made in consultation with your physician.

PROLONGED USE
See your doctor regularly for examinations and tests if you must take this medicine for an extended period.

▼ PRECAUTIONS

Over 60: Adverse reactions may be more likely and more severe in older patients.

Driving and Hazardous Work: No special precautions are necessary.

Alcohol: No special precautions are necessary.

Pregnancy: Metolazone has caused birth defects in animals. Human studies have not been done. Do not take it during pregnancy unless recommended by your doctor; other diuretics are generally preferred.

Breast Feeding: Metolazone passes into breast milk; avoid or discontinue use during the first month of nursing.

Infants and Children: No unusual side effects are expected in children. The dose must be determined by a pediatrician.

Special Concerns: Metolazone is taken once a day. To prevent it from interfering with sleep, take it in the morning. If you are taking it for high blood pressure, follow the diet and weight control measures recommended by your doctor. Avoid exposure to sunlight, use a sunblock, or wear protective clothing. This medicine may cause your body to lose potassium. Follow your doc-tor's instructions about eating potassium-rich foods or taking a potassium supplement.

OVERDOSE
Symptoms: Fainting, lethargy, dizziness, drowsiness, gastrointestinal irritation.

What to Do: Call your doctor, emergency medical services (EMS), or the nearest poison control center immediately.

▼ INTERACTIONS

DRUG INTERACTIONS
Consult your doctor for specific advice if you are taking anticoagulants, cholestyramine, colestipol, drugs for diabetes, nonsteroidal anti-inflammatory drugs, digitalis drugs, or lithium.

FOOD INTERACTIONS
No known food interactions.

DISEASE INTERACTIONS
Caution is advised when taking metolazone. Consult your doctor if you have any of the following: diabetes, gout, lupus erythematosus, pancreatitis, heart disease, blood vessel disease, liver disease, or kidney disease.

≡ SIDE EFFECTS ≡

SERIOUS
Skin rash, hives, intense itching, swelling of the mouth and throat, breathing difficulty, heart rhythm irregularities, lightheadedness, unusual bleeding or bruising. The powerful combination of metolazone and other diuretics may cause severe dehydration, possibly leading to kidney failure. Call your doctor immediately.

COMMON
Potassium depletion may lead to heart palpitations and weakness. Fluid depletion may lead to dizziness, especially upon arising from a sitting or lying position, as well as thirst, dry mouth, and constipation.

LESS COMMON
Decreased sexual ability, increased sensitivity to sunlight, loss of appetite, gout, increased blood sugar (a problem for diabetic patients), pancreatitis (rare).

METOPROLOL

Available in: Tablets, extended-release tablets (Injection is for hospital use only.)
Available OTC? No   **As Generic?** Yes
Drug Class: Beta-blocker

▼ USAGE INFORMATION

WHY IT'S PRESCRIBED
To treat mild to moderate high blood pressure or angina; also used to prevent or control heartbeat irregularities (cardiac arrhythmias). Injection is used in hospitals for emergency treatment of heart attack, followed by maintenance with oral forms.

HOW IT WORKS
Metoprolol slows the rate and force of contraction of the heart by blocking certain nerve impulses, thus reducing blood pressure. By modifying nerve impulses to the heart, the drug also helps to stabilize heart rhythm.

▼ DOSAGE GUIDELINES

RANGE AND FREQUENCY
For high blood pressure or angina– Adults: 100 to 400 mg a day in divided doses. Extended-release tablets: Up to 400 mg once a day. For treatment after a heart attack–

Initial dose is 50 mg every 6 hours, followed by a maintenance dose of 100 mg or more (up to 400 mg a day), 2 times a day for as long as the physician recommends.

ONSET OF EFFECT
Within 15 minutes.

DURATION OF ACTION
6 to 12 hours; up to 24 hours with the extended-release tablet.

DIETARY ADVICE
Take it with food. Follow your doctor's dietary restrictions, such as a low-salt or low-cholesterol diet, to improve control over high blood pressure and heart disease.

STORAGE
Store in a tightly sealed container away from heat and direct light.

MISSED DOSE
Take it as soon as you remember. However, if it is within 4 hours of your next dose (8 hours if using

extended-release tablet), skip the missed dose and resume your regular dosage schedule. Do not double the next dose.

STOPPING THE DRUG
This drug should not be stopped suddenly, as this may lead to angina and possibly a heart attack in patients with advanced heart disease. Slow reduction of the dose under doctor's close supervision for 2 to 3 weeks is advised.

PROLONGED USE
Lifelong therapy may be necessary. See your doctor regularly for examinations.

▼ PRECAUTIONS

Over 60: Adverse reactions may be more likely and more severe in older patients.

Driving and Hazardous Work: Use caution until you determine how the medicine affects you.

Alcohol: Drink in careful moderation if at all. Alcohol may interact with the drug and cause a dangerous drop in blood pressure.

Pregnancy: Discuss with your doctor the relative risks and benefits of using this drug while pregnant.

Breast Feeding: Adverse effects in infants have not been documented. Consult your doctor for advice.

Infants and Children: No special problems expected.

OVERDOSE
Symptoms: Unusually slow or rapid heartbeat, severe dizzi-

ness or fainting, poor circulation in the hands (bluish skin), breathing difficulty, seizures.

What to Do: Call your doctor, emergency medical services (EMS), or the nearest poison control center immediately.

▼ INTERACTIONS

DRUG INTERACTIONS
Consult your doctor for specific advice if you are taking amphetamines, oral antidiabetic agents, asthma medication (such as aminophylline or theophylline), calcium channel blockers, clonidine, guanabenz, halothane, immunotherapy for allergies (allergy shots), insulin, MAO inhibitors, reserpine, other beta-blockers, or any over-the-counter medicine.

FOOD INTERACTIONS
None reported.

DISEASE INTERACTIONS
Metoprolol should be used with caution in people with diabetes, especially insulin-dependent diabetes, since the drug may mask symptoms of hypoglycemia. Consult your doctor if you have allergies or asthma; heart or blood vessel disease (including congestive heart failure and peripheral vascular disease); hyperthyroidism; irregular (slow) heartbeat; myasthenia gravis; psoriasis; respiratory problems, such as bronchitis or emphysema; kidney or liver disease; or a history of mental depression.

≣ SIDE EFFECTS ≣

SERIOUS
Shortness of breath, wheezing; irregular or slow heartbeat (50 beats per minute or less); chest pain or tightness; swelling of the ankles, feet, and lower legs; mental depression. If you experience such symptoms, stop taking metoprolol and call your doctor immediately.

COMMON
Dizziness or lightheadedness, especially when rising suddenly to a standing position; decreased sexual ability; unusual fatigue, weakness, or drowsiness; insomnia.

LESS COMMON
Anxiety, irritability, nervousness; constipation; diarrhea; dry, sore eyes; itching; nausea or vomiting; nightmares or intensely vivid dreams; numbness, tingling, or other unusual sensations in the fingers, toes, or scalp.

METRONIDAZOLE

BRAND NAMES

Flagyl, Metric 21, Metro I.V., MetroGel, MetroGel Vaginal, Metrolotion, Noritate, Protostat

Available in: Cream, injection, topical and vaginal gel, tablets, extended-release tablets
Available OTC? No   **As Generic?** Yes
Drug Class: Antibacterial/antiprotozoal

▼ USAGE INFORMATION

WHY IT'S PRESCRIBED
To treat numerous bacterial infections, including certain sexually transmitted diseases, gynecological infections, amebiasis (amoeba infection in the intestine or liver), brain abscess or meningitis, pneumonia or other lung infections, blood poisoning, bone and joint infections, infections of the internal organs (including liver abscess and peritonitis), and skin infections.

HOW IT WORKS
Metronidazole kills bacteria and protozoa, probably by disrupting the organism's synthesis of DNA.

▼ DOSAGE GUIDELINES

RANGE AND FREQUENCY
The dose varies greatly depending on many factors, including the disorder being treated, the patient's age, weight, and general state of health, and the form of drug prescribed. Your doctor will determine the appropriate dosage regimen for you.

ONSET OF EFFECT
Unknown.

DURATION OF ACTION
Unknown.

DIETARY ADVICE
Oral forms of metronidazole can be taken with food to minimize stomach upset.

STORAGE
Store in a tightly sealed container away from heat, moisture, and direct light. Do not refrigerate the liquid or topical forms.

MISSED DOSE
Take it as soon as you remember. If it is near the time for the next dose, skip the missed dose and resume your regular dosage schedule. Do not double the next dose.

STOPPING THE DRUG
Take it as prescribed for the full treatment period, even if you feel better before the scheduled end of therapy.

PROLONGED USE
If your symptoms do not improve or if they become worse after a few days, consult your doctor.

▼ PRECAUTIONS

Over 60: No special advice.

Driving and Hazardous Work: Avoid such activities until you determine how the medicine affects you.

Alcohol: A serious reaction, including possible flushing, rapid heartbeat, nausea, and vomiting, may occur if alcohol is consumed while taking this drug. Alcohol-containing medications (for example, cough syrups) should also be carefully avoided, as they can cause the same reaction.

Pregnancy: Metronidazole has not caused birth defects in animals. Use of the oral forms during the first trimester is not recommended. Before you take metronidazole, tell your doctor if you are pregnant or plan to become pregnant.

Breast Feeding: Metronidazole passes into breast milk; avoid or discontinue use while nursing.

Infants and Children: The oral and injection forms are not expected to cause side effects different from or more severe than those in older persons. There is no information on the use of the topical forms by children.

Special Concerns: If you use the vaginal gel, wear cotton panties, change daily, and use a sanitary napkin to prevent leakage. Avoid using this medicine in or near the eyes. If it does get into your eyes, consult your doctor.

OVERDOSE
Symptoms: No cases of overdose have been reported.

What to Do: Emergency instructions not applicable.

▼ INTERACTIONS

DRUG INTERACTIONS
Consult your doctor for specific advice if you are taking cimetidine, lithium, anticoagulants, phenytoin, or phenobarbital. If you have taken disulfiram in the last 2 weeks, then you should not take metronidazole. Also tell your doctor if you are taking any other prescription or over-the-counter medication.

FOOD INTERACTIONS
No known food interactions.

DISEASE INTERACTIONS
Consult your doctor if you have a history of blood disease, epilepsy (or other central nervous system disorder), heart disease, or liver disease.

≣ SIDE EFFECTS ≣

SERIOUS
Oral and injection forms: Pain, tingling, numbness, or weakness in hands or feet; seizures. Call your doctor immediately.

COMMON
Oral and injection forms: Diarrhea, dizziness, lightheadedness, headache, loss of appetite, nausea, vomiting, stomach pains or cramps. Vaginal gel: Vaginal itching; painful intercourse; thick, white vaginal discharge; irritation of sexual partner's penis; burning urination; more frequent urination; redness, stinging, or itching of genital area.

LESS COMMON
Oral and injection forms: Change in taste, dry mouth, sharp metallic taste in mouth. Cream and gel: Dry skin, skin irritation, watery eyes with burning or stinging. Vaginal gel: Dizziness, lightheadedness, diarrhea, furry tongue, loss of appetite, metallic taste in the mouth, nausea, vomiting.

MEXILETINE HYDROCHLORIDE

Available in: Capsules
Available OTC? No   **As Generic?** Yes
Drug Class: Antiarrhythmic

▼ USAGE INFORMATION

WHY IT'S PRESCRIBED
To treat irregular heartbeats (cardiac arrhythmias).

HOW IT WORKS
Mexiletine slows nerve impulses in the heart and makes heart tissue less sensitive to nerve impulses, thus stabilizing heartbeat.

▼ DOSAGE GUIDELINES

RANGE AND FREQUENCY
To start, a 200 to 400 mg dose followed by 200 mg every 8 hours. The dose can be increased to 400 mg every 8 hours.

ONSET OF EFFECT
30 minutes to 2 hours.

DURATION OF ACTION
10 to 12 hours (longer in patients with liver or heart impairment).

DIETARY ADVICE
Mexiletine can be taken with food or an antacid.

STORAGE
Store in a tightly sealed container away from heat and direct light.

MISSED DOSE
Take it as soon as you remember. If it is near the time for the next dose, skip the missed dose and resume your regular dosage schedule. Do not double the next dose.

STOPPING THE DRUG
Take it as prescribed for the full treatment period, even if you begin to feel better before the scheduled end of therapy. The decision to stop taking the drug should be made by your doctor.

PROLONGED USE
Lifelong therapy may be necessary. See your doctor regularly for examinations and diagnostic tests if long-term use is required.

▼ PRECAUTIONS

Over 60: There is no specific information comparing use of this medicine in older patients to other age groups.

Driving and Hazardous Work: Do not drive or engage in hazardous work until you determine how the medicine affects you.

Alcohol: No special precautions are necessary.

Pregnancy: In animal studies mexiletine has caused a reduction in successful pregnancies but no birth defects. Before you take mexiletine, tell your physician if you are pregnant or plan to become pregnant.

Breast Feeding: Mexiletine passes into breast milk; you should avoid or discontinue usage while nursing.

Infants and Children: Safety and efficacy of mexiletine in children have not been established. Use and dose must be established by your doctor.

Special Concerns: Your doctor may want you to carry a card or wear a bracelet saying that you are taking mexiletine. Before you have any kind of surgery, tell the doctor or dentist in charge that you are taking this medicine.

OVERDOSE
Symptoms: Severe breathing difficulty, dizziness, drowsiness, burning sensation, nausea, change in mental state, seizures, abnormally slow heartbeat, unconsciousness.

What to Do: Call your doctor, emergency medical services (EMS), or the nearest poison control center immediately.

▼ INTERACTIONS

DRUG INTERACTIONS
Consult your doctor for specific advice if you are taking urinary alkalizers, such as antacids; other antiarrhythmics; hepatic enzyme inducers; metoclopramide; theophylline; rifampin; phenytoin; or phenobarbital.

FOOD INTERACTIONS
No known food interactions.

DISEASE INTERACTIONS
Caution is advised when taking mexiletine. Consult your doctor if you have any of the following: low blood pressure, congestive heart failure, a recent heart attack, or a history of seizures. Mexiletine can cause complications in patients with liver disease, since this organ works to remove the medication from the body.

 SIDE EFFECTS

SERIOUS
Chest pain, rapid or irregular heartbeat, shortness of breath, seizures, unusual bleeding or bruising, fever or chills. Call your doctor immediately.

COMMON
Dizziness or lightheadedness; nausea, vomiting, or abdominal pain; heartburn; nervousness; unsteadiness or difficulty in walking; trembling, or shaking of hands.

LESS COMMON
Confusion, blurred vision, constipation or diarrhea, headache, numbness or tingling of hands or toes, ringing in ears, skin rash, slurred speech, difficulty sleeping, unusual fatigue or weakness.

MICONAZOLE

Available in: Vaginal cream and suppositories, injection
Available OTC? Yes   **As Generic?** Yes
Drug Class: Antifungal

▼ USAGE INFORMATION

WHY IT'S PRESCRIBED
To treat severe fungal infections, including vaginal yeast infections.

HOW IT WORKS
Miconazole prevents fungal organisms from producing vital substances required for growth and function. This medication is effective only for infections caused by fungal organisms. It will not work for bacterial or viral infections.

▼ DOSAGE GUIDELINES

RANGE AND FREQUENCY
Adults and teenagers— Vaginal cream: At bedtime, insert into the vagina 1 applicatorful for 7 to 14 nights. Vaginal suppositories: At bedtime, insert one 100-mg suppository into the vagina for 7 nights, or one 200-mg or one 400-mg suppository for 3 nights. Injection: 200 to 1,200 mg into a vein 3 times a day for weeks or months. Children ages 1 to 12— Injection: 20 to 40 mg per 2.2 lbs (1 kg) of body weight per day, given in 2 or 3 doses, for weeks or months.

ONSET OF EFFECT
For cream and suppository: Unknown. For injection: Immediate.

DURATION OF ACTION
Unknown.

DIETARY ADVICE
No special restrictions.

STORAGE
Store in a tightly sealed container away from heat, moisture, and direct light. Refrigerate suppositories. Do not allow medication to freeze.

MISSED DOSE
Take it as soon as you remember. This will help keep a constant level of medication in your system. If it is near the time for the next dose, skip the missed dose and resume your regular dosage schedule. Do not double the next dose.

STOPPING THE DRUG
Take as directed for the full treatment period, even if you begin to feel better before the scheduled end of therapy. Stopping prematurely increases the risk of reinfection. Some fungal infections take many months to clear up, and some may require continuous treatment.

PROLONGED USE
Therapy with this medication may require months. Prolonged use may increase the risk of adverse effects.

▼ PRECAUTIONS

Over 60: Adverse reactions may be more likely and more severe in older patients.

Driving and Hazardous Work: Do not drive or engage in hazardous work until you determine how the medicine affects you.

Alcohol: Avoid alcohol.

Pregnancy: Adequate studies of miconazole use during pregnancy have not been done. Consult your doctor for advice if you are pregnant or are planning to become pregnant.

Breast Feeding: Miconazole passes into breast milk; caution is advised. Consult your doctor for advice.

Infants and Children: Not recommended for use by children under age 1.

Special Concerns: Sanitary napkins should be used to prevent staining of clothing. The affected area should be kept cool and dry. Do not sit for a long time in a wet bathing suit. Avoid feminine hygiene sprays. Wash daily with unscented soap and dry thoroughly with a clean towel. Tampons should not be used during therapy. The patient's sexual partner should wear a condom during intercourse. Do not stop using this medicine during your menstrual period. After urination or a bowel movement, cleanse by wiping the area from front to back to prevent reinfection.

OVERDOSE
Symptoms: An overdose with miconazole is unlikely.

What to Do: Emergency instructions not applicable.

▼ INTERACTIONS

DRUG INTERACTIONS
Tell your doctor if you are using any other vaginal prescription or over-the-counter medicine when using the vaginal forms. While taking miconazole injection, do not take astemizole, cisapride, or terfenadine. Serious side effects involving the heart may result. Do not take medications containing alcohol, such as cough syrups, elixirs, and tonics. Consult your doctor for specific advice if you are taking cyclosporine, phenytoin, or warfarin.

FOOD INTERACTIONS
No known food interactions.

DISEASE INTERACTIONS
Consult your doctor if you have a history of alcohol abuse. Use of miconazole can cause complications in patients with liver or kidney disease, since these organs work together to remove the medication from the body.

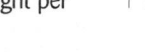

SIDE EFFECTS

SERIOUS
Skin rash or itching; fever or chills; pain at site of injection; vaginal burning, itching, discharge, or irritation not present prior to treatment. Call your doctor immediately.

COMMON
No common side effects are associated with miconazole.

LESS COMMON
Diarrhea, nausea, vomiting, constipation, dizziness, headache, redness or flushing of skin, stomach cramps or pain, burning or irritation of sexual partner's penis.

MIDODRINE HYDROCHLORIDE

Available in: Tablets
Available OTC? No   **As Generic?** No
Drug Class: Alpha-adrenergic agonist

▼ USAGE INFORMATION

WHY IT'S PRESCRIBED
To treat severe cases of orthostatic hypotension (extremely low blood pressure, causing symptoms of dizziness and faintness, especially when rising from a seated or lying position). Used when standard care, such as support stockings, fluid expansion, and lifestyle changes, is ineffective.

HOW IT WORKS
Midodrine causes constriction of the smooth muscles surrounding the blood vessels. This effect narrows the width of the blood vessels, causing blood pressure to rise, thus helping to correct low blood pressure on standing.

▼ DOSAGE GUIDELINES

RANGE AND FREQUENCY
To start, 10 mg, 3 times a day during waking hours, at intervals of 4 hours. Suggested dosage schedule is to take the medication shortly after rising, then at midday, and then late afternoon (before 6 pm). Blood pressure should be monitored while sitting and lying down at the outset of treatment for possible adjustment of doses.

ONSET OF EFFECT
Within 1 hour.

DURATION OF ACTION
From 2 to 3 hours.

DIETARY ADVICE
No special restrictions.

STORAGE
Store in a tightly sealed container away from heat, moisture, and direct light.

MISSED DOSE
Take it as soon as you remember. If it is near the time for the next dose, skip the missed dose and resume your regular dosage schedule. Do not double the next dose.

STOPPING THE DRUG
The decision to stop taking the drug should be made in consultation with your doctor.

PROLONGED USE
See your doctor regularly for measurements of blood pressure while sitting and lying down if you must take this drug for a prolonged period. Periodic tests for liver and kidney function will be done.

▼ PRECAUTIONS

Over 60: No special advice.

Driving and Hazardous Work: Do not drive or engage in hazardous work until you determine how the medicine affects you.

Alcohol: Avoid alcohol when using this medication; it may interfere with proper control of blood pressure.

Pregnancy: Adequate studies have not been done. Discuss with your doctor the relative benefits and possible risks to the unborn child when using this drug during pregnancy.

Breast Feeding: Midodrine may pass into breast milk; caution is advised. Consult your doctor for advice.

Infants and Children: The safety and effectiveness of midodrine in children have not been established.

Special Concerns: The last dose of midodrine should be taken at least 3 hours before bedtime. Use of this drug is not recommended for patients who have persistent and excessively high systolic blood pressure.

OVERDOSE
Symptoms: Goose bumps, sensation of coldness, decreased urine output, rapid heartbeat, ringing in the ears.

What to Do: It is not known whether an overdose of midodrine is life-threatening. However, if someone takes a much larger dose than prescribed, call your doctor, emergency medical services (EMS), or the nearest poison control center immediately.

▼ INTERACTIONS

DRUG INTERACTIONS
Consult your doctor for specific advice if you are taking cardiac glycosides, phenylephrine, pseudoephedrine, beta-blockers, phenylpropanolamine, dihydroergotamine, fludrocortisone acetate, prazosin, terazosin, doxazosin, metformin, cimetidine, ranitidine, procainamide, triamterene, flecainide, quinidine, or any other over-the counter or prescription drug.

FOOD INTERACTIONS
No known food interactions.

DISEASE INTERACTIONS
Caution is advised when taking midodrine. Consult your doctor if you have any of the following: urinary retention problems, severe heart disease, diabetes mellitus, vision problems, glaucoma, pheochromocytoma, or thyrotoxicosis. Use of midodrine may cause complications in patients with liver or kidney disease, since these organs work together to remove the medication from the body.

  SIDE EFFECTS

SERIOUS
Very high blood pressure, slow heartbeat, increased dizziness, fainting. Call your doctor immediately.

COMMON
Itching, numbness, or tingling, in the extremities; goose bumps; chills; urinary difficulties.

LESS COMMON
Headache, sinus pressure, redness of face, confusion, dry mouth, nervousness, anxiety, skin rash, vision problems, dizziness, dry skin, backache, gastrointestinal distress, gas, leg cramps.

MIGLITOL

Available in: Tablets
Available OTC? No **As Generic?** No
Drug Class: Antidiabetic agent

▼ USAGE INFORMATION

WHY IT'S PRESCRIBED
Used as an adjunct (supplemental) therapy to dietary measures and exercise to help control blood sugar levels in patients with type 2 diabetes mellitus. May be used in combination with a sulfonylurea when diet plus either miglitol or a sulfonylurea alone do not adequately control blood sugar levels.

HOW IT WORKS
Miglitol inhibits the activity of enzymes required to break carbohydrates down into simple sugars within the intestine. This effect delays the digestion of carbohydrates and thus reduces the rise in blood sugar that typically occurs after meals.

▼ DOSAGE GUIDELINES

RANGE AND FREQUENCY
Dosage must be determined for each patient individually, based on blood glucose levels in response to the drug. The recommended starting dosage is 25 mg taken 3 times a day with the first bite of each main meal. Four to eight weeks later, dosage may be increased by your doctor to 50 mg 3 times a day. If, after 3 months, blood sugar levels are not adequately controlled, the dosage may be increased to not more than 100 mg 3 times a day, the maxiumum recommended dose.

ONSET OF EFFECT
Unknown.

DURATION OF ACTION
Unknown.

DIETARY ADVICE
This medicine should be taken with the first bite of breakfast, lunch, and dinner. Follow your doctor's advice regarding diet, weight loss, and exercise.

STORAGE
Store in a tightly sealed container away from heat, moisture, and direct light.

MISSED DOSE
If you have finished a meal without taking the medication, skip the missed dose and resume your regular dosing schedule with the next meal. Do not double the next dose.

≡ SIDE EFFECTS ≡

SERIOUS
No serious side effects are associated with miglitol use.

COMMON
Abdominal pain, diarrhea, and flatulence.

LESS COMMON
Rash. Use in combination with sulfonylureas may cause symptoms of low blood sugar (hypoglycemia), which include sweating, tremor, anxiety, hunger, confusion, seizures, rapid heartbeat, vision changes, dizziness, headache, loss of consciousness.

STOPPING THE DRUG
Do not stop taking the drug without your doctor's consent.

PROLONGED USE
Since type 2 diabetes is a chronic condition, use of miglitol will be ongoing. Blood glucose levels should be checked regularly during treatment so that the dosage may be adjusted if necessary.

▼ PRECAUTIONS

Over 60: No special advice.

Driving and Hazardous Work: Miglitol should not impair your ability to perform such tasks safely.

Alcohol: Drink only in moderation when taking miglitol.

Pregnancy: Consult your doctor for advice. Insulin is usually the treatment of choice for pregnant diabetic patients.

Breast Feeding: Miglitol passes into breast milk, although it has not been shown to cause harm to nursing infants. Consult your doctor for specific advice.

Infants and Children: Safety and effectiveness have not been established for patients under 18 years of age. Consult your doctor for advice.

Special Concerns: Follow your doctor's advice about diet, exercise, and weight control. These aspects of treatment are just as essential to the proper control of diabetes as taking medications. Be sure to carry at all times some form of medical identification that indicates you have diabetes and that lists all of the drugs you are taking.

OVERDOSE
Symptoms: Increased gas, diarrhea, and stomach pain.

What to Do: These symptoms usually subside on their own within a short period of time. If not, consult your doctor for advice. Symptoms of hypoglycemia should not occur when taking miglitol alone, but may occur if a patient is also taking a sulfonylurea or insulin for diabetes.

▼ INTERACTIONS

DRUG INTERACTIONS
Consult your doctor for specific advice if you are taking any of the following drugs that may interact with miglitol: digestive enzyme preparations containing amylase or pancreatin, intestinal absorbents (such as charcoal), insulin, or sulfonylureas (oral antidiabetic agents).

FOOD INTERACTIONS
Avoid foods that contain large amounts of sugar (for example, cake, cookies, candy, acidic fruits). Closely follow the diet your doctor has prescribed.

DISEASE INTERACTIONS
This drug should not be taken by patients with a history of diabetic ketoacidosis, intestinal disorders (including malabsorption or obstruction), inflammatory bowel disease (for example, Crohn's disease or ulcerative colitis), or kidney dysfunction.

MILK OF MAGNESIA (MAGNESIA; MAGNESIUM HYDROXIDE)

Available in: Oral suspension, chewable tablets
Available OTC? Yes **As Generic?** Yes
Drug Class: Antacid/hyperosmotic laxative

▼ USAGE INFORMATION

WHY IT'S PRESCRIBED
To relieve symptoms of upset stomach; sometimes used also for short-term treatment of constipation.

HOW IT WORKS
As an antacid, milk of magnesia neutralizes stomach acid. As a laxative, it attracts and retains water in the intestine, increasing intestinal movement (peristalsis) and inducing the urge to defecate.

▼ DOSAGE GUIDELINES

RANGE AND FREQUENCY
As an antacid— Adults and teenagers: 5 to 15 ml of liquid form or 650 mg to 1.3 g of tablets 3 or 4 times a day. To relieve constipation— Adults and teenagers: 2.4 to 4.8 g (30 to 60 ml) daily in 1 or more doses. Children ages 6 to 12: 1.2 to 2.4 g (15 to 30 ml) daily in 1 or more doses.

ONSET OF EFFECT
30 minutes to 3 hours.

DURATION OF ACTION
Variable.

DIETARY ADVICE
Take it 1 to 3 hours after meals or at bedtime with a full glass of water.

STORAGE
Store milk of magnesia in a tightly sealed container away from heat, moisture, and direct light.

MISSED DOSE
Take it as soon as you remember. If it is near the time for the next dose, skip the missed dose and resume your regular dosage schedule. Do not double the next dose.

STOPPING THE DRUG
You may stop taking the drug whenever you choose.

PROLONGED USE
Do not take milk of magnesia for more than 2 weeks unless your doctor prescribes it.

▼ PRECAUTIONS

Over 60: No special advice.

Driving and Hazardous Work: This medicine should not impair your ability to perform such tasks safely.

Alcohol: Avoid alcohol.

Pregnancy: Extensive human studies have not been done. There have been reports of side effects in infants whose mothers took high doses of antacids for a long time during pregnancy. Before you take milk of magnesia, consult your doctor if you are pregnant or plan to become pregnant.

Breast Feeding: Milk of magnesia may pass into breast milk but has not been reported to cause problems in nursing babies. Consult your doctor for advice.

Infants and Children: Antacids and other magnesium-containing medications should not be given to children under age 6 unless prescribed by a doctor.

Special Concerns: Take milk of magnesia on a schedule that does not interfere with activities or sleep, as it produces watery stools in 3 to 6 hours. Remember that frequent or protracted use can lead to laxative dependence. Do not take milk of magnesia within 2 hours of taking other medications. Before swallowing, chew tablets well to allow the medicine to work more quickly and effectively.

OVERDOSE
Symptoms: Severe or protracted diarrhea, painful or difficult urination, muscle weakness, continuing loss of appetite, irregular heartbeat, difficulty breathing.

What to Do: An overdose of milk of magnesia is unlikely to be life threatening. However, if someone takes a much larger dose than prescribed, call your doctor, emergency medical services (EMS), or the nearest poison control center immediately.

▼ INTERACTIONS

DRUG INTERACTIONS
Consult your physician for specific advice if you are taking other antacids or laxatives, cellulose sodium phosphate, fluoroquinolones, isoniazid, ketoconazole, sodium polystyrene sulfonate resin, methenamine, mecamylamine, salicylates, or tetracyclines.

FOOD INTERACTIONS
None are known.

DISEASE INTERACTIONS
Do not use this medication if you have any symptoms of appendicitis or inflamed bowel such as lower abdominal or stomach pain, nausea or vomiting, cramping, soreness, or bloating. Consult your physician if you have any of the following: broken bones, colitis, hemorrhoids, intestinal blockage or bleeding, a recent colostomy or ileostomy, swelling of feet or lower legs, heart disease, toxemia of pregnancy, liver disease, or kidney disease.

≣ SIDE EFFECTS ≣

SERIOUS
Dizziness or lightheadedness, continuing feeling of discomfort, irregular heartbeat, loss of appetite, mood or mental changes, muscle weakness, unusual fatigue, unusual weight loss, rectal bleeding. Call your doctor immediately.

COMMON
Nausea, diarrhea.

LESS COMMON
Increased thirst, speckling or whitish color of stools, abdominal cramps.

MINOCYCLINE

Available in: Capsules, oral suspension, tablets, powder, injection
Available OTC? No   **As Generic?** Yes
Drug Class: Tetracycline antibiotic

▼ USAGE INFORMATION

WHY IT'S PRESCRIBED
To treat acne or infections caused by bacteria or protozoa (single-celled parasitic organisms).

HOW IT WORKS
Minocycline kills bacteria and protozoa by inhibiting their manufacture of certain proteins necessary for their survival.

▼ DOSAGE GUIDELINES

RANGE AND FREQUENCY
Oral forms— Adults and teenagers: 200 mg to start, then 100 mg, 2 times a day, or 100 to 200 mg to start, then 50 mg, 4 times a day. Children age 8 and over: 1.8 mg per lb of body weight to start, then 0.9 mg per lb 2 times a day. Injection— Adults and teenagers: 200 mg to start, then 100 mg, 2 times a day. Children age 8 and over: 1.8 mg per lb to start, then 0.9 mg per lb, 2 times a day.

ONSET OF EFFECT
Immediately after injection; unknown for oral forms.

DURATION OF ACTION
Unknown.

DIETARY ADVICE
Drink extra water when taking capsules or tablets.

STORAGE
Store in a tightly sealed container away from heat, moisture, and direct light.

MISSED DOSE
Take it as soon as you remember. If it is near the time for the next dose, skip the missed dose and resume your regular dosage schedule. Do not double the next dose.

STOPPING THE DRUG
Take as prescribed for the full treatment period, even if you begin to feel better before the scheduled end of therapy.

PROLONGED USE
If your symptoms do not improve within a few days (for infection) or a few weeks (for acne), see your doctor.

Prolonged use may make you more susceptible to infections caused by microorganisms resistant to antibiotics.

▼ PRECAUTIONS

Over 60: It is not known whether adverse reactions are more likely or more severe in older patients than in younger persons.

Driving and Hazardous Work: Do not drive or engage in hazardous work until you determine how the medicine affects you, since it may cause dizziness.

Alcohol: It is advisable to abstain from alcohol when fighting an infection.

Pregnancy: Use of minocycline during the second half of pregnancy should be avoided because it may discolor the unborn child's teeth, slow growth of teeth and bones, and cause liver problems in the mother.

Breast Feeding: Minocycline passes into breast milk and may be harmful to the nursing infant. The patient must choose between using the drug or breast feeding.

Infants and Children: This drug should not be used by children younger than 8 years old since it can cause permanent tooth staining.

Special Concerns: Oral contraceptives may not work when you take minocycline. Consult your doctor for specific advice. Before having surgery under a general anesthetic, tell the doctor or dentist in charge that you are taking minocycline. If minocycline increases the sensitivity of your skin to the sun, take protective measures and avoid exposure to sunlight. Do not take calcium supplements, magnesium-containing laxatives, sodium bicarbonate, or iron preparations within 2 to 3 hours of taking minocycline. Women predisposed to yeast infections may need treatment with an antifungal while taking minocycline.

OVERDOSE
Symptoms: Severe nausea and vomiting, diarrhea, difficulty swallowing.

What to Do: An overdose is unlikely to be life-threatening. However, if someone takes a much larger dose than prescribed, call your doctor, emergency medical services (EMS), or the nearest poison control center immediately.

▼ INTERACTIONS

DRUG INTERACTIONS
Other drugs may interact with minocycline. Consult your doctor for specific advice if you are taking antacids, calcium supplements, cholestyramine, choline and magnesium salicylates, medicines containing iron, laxatives containing magnesium, or oral contraceptives.

FOOD INTERACTIONS
No known food interactions.

DISEASE INTERACTIONS
Consult your doctor if you have a history of kidney disease or liver disease.

SIDE EFFECTS

SERIOUS
Increased sensitivity of skin to sunlight; abdominal pain; headache; loss of appetite; severe nausea and vomiting; yellow skin; skin discoloration; changes in vision; dizziness or loss of balance; redness, soreness, or swelling at site of injection. Call your doctor immediately.

COMMON
Cramps or burning feeling in stomach, nausea, vomiting, dizziness, lightheadedness, unsteadiness, yeast infection or oral thrush (fungal infection of the mouth or throat).

LESS COMMON
Itching in the genital area, sore tongue or mouth.

MINOXIDIL ORAL

Available in: Tablets
Available OTC? No   **As Generic?** Yes
Drug Class: Antihypertensive

▼ USAGE INFORMATION

WHY IT'S PRESCRIBED
To treat moderate to severe high blood pressure. Minoxidil is usually used after other medications have failed to achieve satisfactory results.

HOW IT WORKS
Oral minoxidil acts upon the smooth muscle tissue surrounding the arteries, causing this tissue to relax, which in turn widens the diameter of the blood vessels and thus lowers blood pressure.

▼ DOSAGE GUIDELINES

RANGE AND FREQUENCY
Adults and teenagers: 2.5 to 100 mg daily in a single dose or divided doses. Children up to 12 years of age: 200 micrograms (mcg) to 1 mg per 2.2 lbs (1 kg) of body weight daily in a single dose or divided doses.

ONSET OF EFFECT
30 minutes.

DURATION OF ACTION
2 to 5 days.

DIETARY ADVICE
Take this drug with food to minimize stomach upset. Follow a healthy diet (low-salt, low-fat, low-cholesterol) as advised by your doctor to help control blood pressure and prevent heart disease.

STORAGE
Store in a tightly sealed container away from heat and direct light.

MISSED DOSE
Take it as soon as you remember. If it is near the time for the next dose, skip the missed dose and resume your regular dosage schedule. Do not double the next dose.

STOPPING THE DRUG
The decision to stop taking the drug should be made by your doctor. Minoxidil controls your high blood pressure but does not cure it. You may have to take this medicine for the rest of your life.

PROLONGED USE
See your doctor regularly for tests and examinations if you must take this drug for a prolonged period.

▼ PRECAUTIONS

Over 60: Adverse reactions may be more likely and more severe in older patients. Minoxidil may reduce tolerance to cold temperatures in older patients.

Driving and Hazardous Work: The use of minoxidil should not impair your ability to perform such tasks safely.

Alcohol: No special precautions are necessary.

Pregnancy: Minoxidil has not been shown to cause birth defects in animals. Human studies have not been done, but there have been reports of unusual hair growth in newborn babies. High doses in animal studies have caused a reduced rate of pregnancy. Before you take minoxidil, tell your doctor if you are pregnant or are planning to become pregnant.

Breast Feeding: Minoxidil passes into breast milk; caution is advised. Consult your doctor for specific advice.

Infants and Children: Minoxidil is not expected to cause unusual problems in infants and children.

Special Concerns: Minoxidil commonly causes swelling due to fluid retention, so most patients need to take a diuretic with this medication. The drug also raises heart rate and therefore is often prescribed with a drug to stabilize heart rate. While taking minoxidil, weigh yourself every day. Contact your doctor immediately if you suddenly gain 5 pounds or more (2 pounds or more in children); you experience shortness of breath, especially when lying down; or your heart rate increases by 20 or more beats per minute while resting.

OVERDOSE
Symptoms: Very low blood pressure, fast heartbeat, buildup of fluid in the body.

What to Do: An overdose of minoxidil is unlikely to be life-threatening. However, if someone takes a much larger dose than prescribed, call your doctor, emergency medical services (EMS), or the nearest poison control center.

▼ INTERACTIONS

DRUG INTERACTIONS
The following drugs may interact with minoxidil. Consult your doctor for specific advice if you are taking guanethidine, nitrates, or any over-the-counter medicine for appetite control, asthma, colds, cough, hay fever, or sinus problems.

FOOD INTERACTIONS
No known food interactions.

DISEASE INTERACTIONS
Caution is advised when taking minoxidil. Consult your doctor for advice if you have any of the following: angina, heart disease, blood vessel disease, kidney disease, a recent heart attack or stroke, or pheochromocytoma.

≣ SIDE EFFECTS ≣

SERIOUS
Rapid heartbeat (occasionally irregular), rapid weight gain of more than 5 pounds (2 pounds in children), chest pain, shortness of breath. Call your doctor immediately.

COMMON
Swelling of lower legs or feet; increased hair growth, usually on arms, face, and back; flushing or redness of skin.

LESS COMMON
Numbness or tingling of face, hands, or feet; skin rash and itching; breast tenderness in men and women; headache.

MINOXIDIL TOPICAL

Available in: Topical solution
Available OTC? Yes **As Generic?** Yes
Drug Class: Hair growth stimulant

▼ USAGE INFORMATION

WHY IT'S PRESCRIBED
Minoxidil topical solution is prescribed to stimulate hair growth in men and women with a specific type of baldness known as "androgenetic alopecia" (popularly known as "male pattern baldness" or "female pattern baldness").

HOW IT WORKS
It is not known how minoxidil works. Although it increases the flow of blood, nutrients, and other important substances to hair follicles, other or additional poorly understood actions are believed responsible for hair growth.

▼ DOSAGE GUIDELINES

RANGE AND FREQUENCY
Adults: Apply 1 ml regardless of the size of the balding area under treatment.

ONSET OF EFFECT
At least 4 months with twice daily therapy.

DURATION OF ACTION
New hair resulting from minoxidil treatments will likely be lost 3 to 4 months following discontinuation of the medication.

DIETARY ADVICE
No special restrictions.

STORAGE
Store in a tightly sealed container away from heat and direct light. Keep away from moisture and extremes in temperature.

MISSED DOSE
Apply it as soon as you remember. If it is near the time for the next dose, skip the missed dose and resume your regular dosage schedule. Do not double the next dose.

STOPPING THE DRUG
Use it until you are able to assess changes, if any, in hair growth and cosmetic appearance. This may take at least 4 months. If you decide to abandon efforts to achieve hair regrowth, you may stop the medication at any time.

PROLONGED USE
Ongoing therapy with this medication is required for continued results. Prolonged use may increase the risk of undesirable side effects.

▼ PRECAUTIONS

Over 60: Adverse reactions may be more likely and more severe in older patients.

Driving and Hazardous Work: Do not drive or engage in hazardous work until you determine how the medicine affects you.

Alcohol: No special warnings.

Pregnancy: Avoid or discontinue topical minoxidil treatment if you are pregnant or trying to become pregnant. Consult your physician.

Breast Feeding: Minoxidil passes into breast milk; do not use it while nursing.

Infants and Children: Not recommended for children.

Special Concerns: Anyone with a history of allergy to minoxidil or other components of the product should not use this medication. Minoxidil has potentially serious side effects if absorbed in large amounts into the body. Persons with a history of heart disease should consult their doctor before using this product. Do not apply to irritated, blistered, bleeding, or broken skin. Do not use more than the recommended dose, and do not apply it more frequently than twice a day. Do not use hairdryers to accelerate drying of the medication.

OVERDOSE
Symptoms: Symptoms are the same as those listed under Serious Side Effects.

What to Do: If the above symptoms occur or someone ingests the medication, call your doctor, emergency medical services (EMS), or the nearest poison control center immediately.

▼ INTERACTIONS

DRUG INTERACTIONS
Consult your doctor for specific advice if you are taking oral minoxidil, steroids, petrolatum, or acne preparations such as tretinoin. Any person using heart or blood pressure medications should discuss minoxidil use with their doctor before starting treatment.

FOOD INTERACTIONS
No known food interactions.

DISEASE INTERACTIONS
Consult your doctor if you have any disorders affecting your skin or scalp, including rashes, sunburn, or other types of skin eruption or inflammation; heart disease; or high blood pressure.

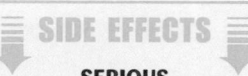

SIDE EFFECTS

SERIOUS
Rapid pulse; weakness, dizziness, or lightheaded feeling; chest pain. Notify your doctor immediately. If chest pain is present, call emergency medical services (EMS).

COMMON
Burning, tingling, or mild redness of scalp at application site; mild dryness or flaking of skin; itching.

LESS COMMON
Significant irritation or allergy with redness, itching, flaking, or rash. Tingling of hands or feet, water retention (swelling of face, hands, fingers, or legs), flushing, headache. Stop the drug and notify your doctor immediately.

MIRTAZAPINE

Available in: Tablets
Available OTC? No   **As Generic?** No
Drug Class: Antidepressant

▼ USAGE INFORMATION

WHY IT'S PRESCRIBED
To treat symptoms of major depression.

HOW IT WORKS
While the exact mechanism of action of mirtazapine is not known, it affects levels of brain chemicals (norepinephrine and serotonin) that are thought to be linked to mood, emotions, and mental state.

▼ DOSAGE GUIDELINES

RANGE AND FREQUENCY
To start, 15 mg once a day, at bedtime. The dose may be increased gradually by your doctor to no more than 45 mg a day.

ONSET OF EFFECT
Unknown.

DURATION OF ACTION
Unknown.

DIETARY ADVICE
No special restrictions.

STORAGE
Store in a tightly sealed container away from heat, moisture, and direct light.

MISSED DOSE
Take it as soon as you remember. However, if it is near the time for the next day's dose, skip the missed dose and resume your regular dosage schedule. Do not double the next day's dose.

STOPPING THE DRUG
Take as prescribed for the full treatment period, even if you begin to feel better before the scheduled end of therapy. The decision to stop taking the drug should be made in consultation with your doctor.

PROLONGED USE
You should see your doctor regularly for tests and examinations if you take this medicine for a prolonged period. Prolonged use of mirtazapine can decrease the flow of saliva, which can increase the risk of cavities, periodontal disease, and other conditions.

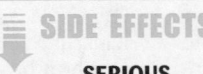

SIDE EFFECTS

SERIOUS
Mood or mental changes, confusion, breathing difficulties, increased or decreased ability to move limbs, flulike symptoms, swelling of the lower extremities, skin rash, anxiety, agitation, extreme drowsiness, disorientation, loss of memory, rapid heartbeat. Call your doctor immediately.

COMMON
Dizziness, dry mouth, drowsiness, constipation, increased appetite, weight gain.

LESS COMMON
Muscle pains, unusual dreams, fatigue, back pain, vomiting, increased thirst, nausea, dizziness or fainting when getting up suddenly, sensitivity to touch, tremor, stomach pain, increased urination.

▼ PRECAUTIONS

Over 60: No special problems have been reported.

Driving and Hazardous Work: Exercise caution until you determine how the medicine affects you. Drowsiness or lightheadedness can occur.

Alcohol: Avoid alcohol.

Pregnancy: In animal studies, mirtazapine did not cause birth defects but was shown to cause other problems. Human studies have not been done. Before you take mirtazapine, tell your doctor if you are pregnant or plan to become pregnant.

Breast Feeding: Mirtazapine may pass into breast milk; caution is advised. Consult your doctor for advice.

Infants and Children: The safety and effectiveness of mirtazapine use by infants and children have not been established.

Special Concerns: If dry mouth occurs, use sugarless candy or gum for relief.

OVERDOSE
Symptoms: Severe drowsiness, disorientation, loss of memory, rapid heartbeat.

What to Do: Call your doctor, emergency medical services (EMS), or the nearest poison control center immediately.

▼ INTERACTIONS

DRUG INTERACTIONS
Mirtazapine and MAO inhibitors should not be used within 14 days of each other. Very serious side effects such as myoclonus (uncontrolled muscle jerking), hyperthermia (excessive rise in body temperature), nausea, vomiting, seizures, and extreme stiffness may result. Other drugs may interact with mirtazapine; consult your doctor for specific advice if you are taking central nervous system depressants, high blood pressure medication, diazepam, or kidney medication.

FOOD INTERACTIONS
No known food interactions.

DISEASE INTERACTIONS
Caution is advised when taking mirtazapine. Consult your doctor if you have heart or blood vessel disease; or a history of seizures, drug abuse, or mental illness. Use of mirtazapine may cause complications in patients with liver or kidney disease, since these organs work together to remove the medication from the body.

MISOPROSTOL

Available in: Tablets
Available OTC? No   **As Generic?** No
Drug Class: Prostaglandin

▼ USAGE INFORMATION

WHY IT'S PRESCRIBED
To prevent stomach ulcers in patients taking anti-inflammatory drugs, including aspirin.

HOW IT WORKS
Ongoing therapy with anti-inflammatory drugs can irritate and damage the stomach lining, increasing the risk of ulcers. Misoprostol helps prevent ulcers and enhances the stomach's natural healing ability by increasing the production of protective mucus, as well as inhibiting the secretion of stomach acid.

▼ DOSAGE GUIDELINES

RANGE AND FREQUENCY
200 to 400 micrograms (mcg), 4 times a day, or 400 mcg, 2 times a day. The dose may be reduced to 100 mcg to prevent side effects. Treatment usually lasts 4 weeks.

ONSET OF EFFECT
30 minutes.

DURATION OF ACTION
3 hours.

DIETARY ADVICE
Misoprostol can be taken with meals to reduce the incidence of diarrhea. The last dose should be taken at bedtime.

STORAGE
Store in a tightly sealed container away from heat and direct light.

MISSED DOSE
Take it as soon as you remember. If it is near the time for the next dose, skip the missed dose and resume your regular dosage schedule. Do not double the next dose.

STOPPING THE DRUG
Take the drug as prescribed for the full treatment period, even if you begin to feel better before the scheduled end of therapy.

PROLONGED USE
You should see your doctor regularly for tests and examinations if you take this drug for a prolonged period. You should not take misoprostol for more than 4 weeks unless directed by your doctor.

▼ PRECAUTIONS

Over 60: No special problems are expected in older patients.

Driving and Hazardous Work: Avoid such activities until you determine how the medicine affects you.

Alcohol: Avoid alcohol.

Pregnancy: Misoprostol should not be used during pregnancy, because it may promote contractions and bleeding of the uterus and can cause miscarriage. Before you start taking misoprostol, you must have had a negative pregnancy test within the previous 2 weeks. You must start taking the drug only on the second or third day of your next menstrual period. An effective method of birth control should be used while you are taking misoprostol. If you suspect you are pregnant, stop taking the drug immediately and consult your doctor.

Breast Feeding: Misoprostol may pass into breast milk; avoid use while nursing because it may cause diarrhea in nursing babies.

Infants and Children: Use and dosage by anyone under the age of 18 must be determined by your doctor.

OVERDOSE
Symptoms: Tremors, sleepiness, trouble breathing, abdominal pain, severe diarrhea, fever, palpitations, extremely low blood pressure, slow heartbeat.

What to Do: An overdose of misoprostol is unlikely to be life-threatening. However, if someone takes a much larger dose than prescribed, call your doctor, emergency medical services (EMS), or the nearest poison control center.

▼ INTERACTIONS

DRUG INTERACTIONS
Before you take misoprostol, inform your doctor if you are taking any other prescription or over-the-counter medicine. Antacids may be taken with misoprostol to help relieve stomach pain, unless your doctor directs otherwise. Do not take antacids that contain magnesium, since they can cause or worsen the diarrhea that sometimes accompanies misoprostol use.

FOOD INTERACTIONS
No known food interactions.

DISEASE INTERACTIONS
Caution is advised when taking misoprostol. Consult your doctor if you have a history of blood vessel disease or epilepsy.

≡ SIDE EFFECTS ≡

SERIOUS
There are no serious side effects associated with the use of misoprostol.

COMMON
Diarrhea, mild abdominal or stomach pain.

LESS COMMON
Vaginal bleeding, constipation, cramps in lower abdomen, gas, headache, nausea and vomiting.

MITOTANE

Available in: Tablets
Available OTC? No   **As Generic?** No
Drug Class: Antineoplastic (anticancer) agent/antiadrenal

▼ USAGE INFORMATION

WHY IT'S PRESCRIBED
To treat cancer of the adrenal cortex, the outer part of the adrenal glands, which rest on top of either kidney. The adrenal cortex produces the body's natural corticosteroid hormones.

HOW IT WORKS
Mitotane appears to suppress activity (steroid production) in the adrenal cortex. For reasons that are unknown, the drug's reduction of steroid production somehow has a destructive effect on cancer cells in the adrenal cortices, and so slows the progression of cancer in that portion of the adrenal gland.

▼ DOSAGE GUIDELINES

RANGE AND FREQUENCY
2 to 6 g daily in 3 or 4 doses. The dosage can be increased to 16 g per day; the usual range is 8 to 10 g per day.

ONSET OF EFFECT
2 to 3 days.

DURATION OF ACTION
Unknown.

DIETARY ADVICE
Can be taken with or without food, according to personal preference. To minimize side effects, the last dose is best taken after the evening meal but before bedtime.

STORAGE
Store in a tightly sealed container away from heat and direct light.

MISSED DOSE
Take it as soon as you remember. If it is near the time for the next dose, skip the missed dose and resume your regular dosage schedule. Do not double the next dose.

STOPPING THE DRUG
The decision to stop taking the drug should be made by your doctor.

PROLONGED USE
See your doctor regularly for tests and examinations if you must take this drug for a prolonged period. Neurological assessments are recommended at regular intervals for persons who take mitotane for more than 2 years.

▼ PRECAUTIONS

Over 60: There is no specific information about the use of mitotane in older patients.

Driving and Hazardous Work: Do not drive or engage in hazardous work until you determine how the medicine affects you.

Alcohol: Avoid alcohol.

Pregnancy: Mitotane has not been shown to cause problems during pregnancy. Consult your doctor for specific advice if you are pregnant or plan to become pregnant.

Breast Feeding: It is unknown if mitotane passes into breast milk; caution is advised. Consult your doctor for specific advice.

Infants and Children: There is no specific information about the use of mitotane in infants and children, but it is not expected to cause different side effects or problems than it does in older patients.

Special Concerns: Initial treatment with mitotane often starts in the hospital until the dose is stabilized. Your doctor may want you to carry a card saying that you are taking mitotane. Check with your doctor if you get an infection, illness, or injury of any sort, because mitotane may weaken your body's defenses against infection and inflammation.

OVERDOSE
Symptoms: No specific ones have been reported.

What to Do: An overdose of mitotane is unlikely to be life-threatening. However, if someone takes a much larger dose than prescribed, call your doctor, emergency medical services (EMS), or the nearest poison control center immediately.

▼ INTERACTIONS

DRUG INTERACTIONS
Consult your physician for specific advice if you are taking adrenocorticoids, glucocorticoids, mineralocorticoids, corticotropin, or central nervous system depressants.

FOOD INTERACTIONS
No known food interactions.

DISEASE INTERACTIONS
Caution is advised when taking mitotane. Consult your doctor if you have any infection. Use of mitotane may cause complications in patients with liver disease, since this organ works to remove the medication from the body.

≣ SIDE EFFECTS ≣

SERIOUS
Darkening of skin, diarrhea, dizziness, drowsiness, loss of appetite, depression, severe nausea and vomiting, skin rash, unusual fatigue, blood in urine, blurred or double vision, shortness of breath, wheezing. Call your doctor immediately.

COMMON
Nausea and vomiting.

LESS COMMON
Aching muscles, dizziness or lightheadedness when rising from a sitting or lying position, fever, flushed or reddened skin, muscle twitching.

MITOXANTRONE HYDROCHLORIDE

Available in: Injection
Available OTC? No   **As Generic?** No
Drug Class: Antineoplastic (anticancer) agent

▼ USAGE INFORMATION

WHY IT'S PRESCRIBED
Mitoxantrone is combined with other chemotherapy agents in the initial first line of treatment against certain kinds of leukemias.

HOW IT WORKS
It is unknown precisely how mitoxantrone works, but it appears to interfere with the DNA of cancer cells, preventing them from reproducing. The drug may also affect the growth and development of other kinds of cells in the body, resulting in unpleasant side effects, particularly the suppression of bone marrow, which causes anemia and other blood problems.

▼ DOSAGE GUIDELINES

RANGE AND FREQUENCY
Mitoxantrone is administered intravenously in a hospital setting. Dosage will be determined by your doctor.

ONSET OF EFFECT
Unknown.

DURATION OF ACTION
Unknown.

DIETARY ADVICE
Maintain adequate food and fluid intake. Calorie, protein, and vitamin needs increase in patients with cancer. Good nutrition is essential to cope with the demands of chemotherapy.

STORAGE
Not applicable; the dose is administered only at a health care facility.

MISSED DOSE
Not applicable, since medication is given by a doctor or other health professional.

STOPPING THE DRUG
The decision to stop taking the drug should be made by your doctor.

PROLONGED USE
You should see your doctor regularly for tests and examinations if you take this drug for a prolonged period.

▼ PRECAUTIONS

Over 60: There is no specific information comparing use of mitoxantrone in older patients with use in younger persons. No special problems are expected.

Driving and Hazardous Work: The use of mitoxantrone should not impair your ability to perform such tasks safely.

Alcohol: Alcohol should be avoided while taking this medication.

Pregnancy: Mitoxantrone may cause birth defects if it is taken by either the father or the mother at the time of conception. It is best to use some kind of birth control while taking mitoxantrone. Tell your doctor immediately if you think you have become pregnant while taking mitoxantrone.

Breast Feeding: Mitoxantrone passes into breast milk; discontinue nursing before beginning treatment.

Infants and Children: There is no specific information that compares use of mitoxantrone in infants and children with use in older persons.

Special Concerns: Do not receive any immunizations without your doctor's approval while you are taking mitoxantrone. Avoid persons with infections. Be careful when using a toothbrush, dental floss, or toothpick. Take care not to cut yourself when using sharp objects such as a razor. Avoid contact sports. Before having dental work, consult your doctor. Your doctor may want you to drink extra fluids while you are taking this drug.

OVERDOSE
Symptoms: Severe infection as a result of substantial white blood cell suppression (immune system failure).

What to Do: Contact your oncologist, who will closely monitor your blood counts and symptoms and determine the course of your treatment.

▼ INTERACTIONS

DRUG INTERACTIONS
Consult your doctor for specific advice if you are taking amphotericin B, antithyroid agents, azathioprine, chloramphenicol, colchicine, flucytosine, ganciclovir, interferon, plicamycin, zidovudine, probenecid, sulfinpyrazone, or any other cancer medication.

FOOD INTERACTIONS
No known food interactions.

DISEASE INTERACTIONS
Caution is advised when taking mitoxantrone. Consult your doctor if you have a history of any of the following: chickenpox, shingles, gout, kidney stones, heart disease, or any infection. Use of mitoxantrone may cause complications in patients with liver disease, since this organ works to remove the medication from the body.

≡ SIDE EFFECTS ≡

SERIOUS
Fever; chills; black, tarry stools; cough or shortness of breath; blood in urine or stools; rapid or irregular heartbeat; red spots on skin; swelling of feet and lower legs; unusual bleeding or bruising; sores in mouth and on lips; stomach pain; decreased urination; seizures; blue skin or pain and redness at injection site; skin rash. Call your doctor immediately.

COMMON
Diarrhea, headache, nausea and vomiting, temporary hair loss, bluish-green-colored urine.

LESS COMMON
No less-common side effects are associated with the use of mitoxantrone.

MOEXIPRIL HYDROCHLORIDE

Available in: Tablets
Available OTC? No   **As Generic?** No
Drug Class: Angiotensin-converting enzyme (ACE) inhibitor

▼ USAGE INFORMATION

WHY IT'S PRESCRIBED
To control high blood pressure; to treat congestive heart failure (CHF); to treat patients with left ventricular dysfunction (damage to the pumping chamber of the heart); and to minimize further kidney damage in diabetics with mild kidney disease.

HOW IT WORKS
Angiotensin-converting enzyme (ACE) inhibitors block an enzyme that produces angiotensin, a naturally occurring substance that causes blood vessels to constrict and stimulates production of the adrenal hormone, aldosterone, which promotes sodium retention in the body. As a result, ACE inhibitors relax blood vessels (causing them to widen) and reduces sodium retention, which lowers blood pressure and so decreases the workload of the heart.

▼ DOSAGE GUIDELINES

RANGE AND FREQUENCY
To start, 7.5 mg once a day. Dosage may be increased by your doctor up to 30 mg a day, given in 1 or 2 doses.

ONSET OF EFFECT
Within 1 hour.

DURATION OF ACTION
24 hours.

DIETARY ADVICE
Take it on an empty stomach, about 1 hour before mealtime. Follow your doctor's dietary advice (such as low-salt or low-cholesterol restrictions) to improve control over high blood pressure and heart disease. Avoid high-potassium foods like bananas and citrus fruits and juices, unless you are also taking medications, such as diuretics, that lower potassium levels.

STORAGE
Store in a tightly sealed container away from heat and direct light.

MISSED DOSE
Take it as soon as you remember. If it is near the time for the next dose, skip the missed dose and resume your regular dosage schedule. Do not double the next dose.

STOPPING THE DRUG
Do not stop taking this drug abruptly, as this may cause potentially serious health problems. Dosage should be reduced gradually, according to your doctor's instructions.

PROLONGED USE
Lifelong therapy may be necessary; see your doctor for regular examinations and tests.

▼ PRECAUTIONS

Over 60: Smaller doses may be recommended.

Driving and Hazardous Work: Avoid such activities until you determine how the medicine affects you.

Alcohol: Consume alcohol only in moderation since it may increase the effect of the drug and cause an excessive drop in blood pressure. Consult your doctor for advice.

Pregnancy: Use of moexipril during the last 6 months of pregnancy may cause severe defects, even death, in the fetus. Consult your doctor.

Breast Feeding: Moexipril may pass into breast milk; caution is advised. Consult your doctor for advice.

Infants and Children: Safety and effectiveness have not been established. Benefits must be weighed against potential risks; consult your pediatrician for advice.

OVERDOSE
Symptoms: None reported.

What to Do: While overdose is unlikely, call your doctor, emergency medical services (EMS), or the nearest poison control center immediately if you suspect that someone has taken a much larger dose than prescribed.

▼ INTERACTIONS

DRUG INTERACTIONS
Consult your doctor if you are taking diuretics (especially potassium-sparing diuretics), potassium supplements or drugs containing potassium (check ingredient labels), lithium, anticoagulants (such as warfarin), indomethacin or other anti-inflammatory drugs, or any over-the-counter medications (especially cold remedies and diet pills).

FOOD INTERACTIONS
Avoid low-salt milk and salt substitutes. Many of these products contain potassium. Excessive intake of tea, coffee, cola, or other drinks that could create a diuretic effect should be avoided.

DISEASE INTERACTIONS
Consult your doctor if you have systemic lupus erythematosus (SLE) or if you have had a prior allergic reaction to ACE inhibitors. Moexipril should be used with caution by patients with severe kidney disease or renal artery stenosis (narrowing of one or both of the arteries that supply blood to the kidneys).

≡ SIDE EFFECTS ≡

SERIOUS
Fever and chills; sore throat and hoarseness; sudden difficulty breathing or swallowing; swelling of the face, mouth, or extremities; impaired kidney function (ankle swelling, decreased urination); confusion; yellow discoloration of the eyes or skin (indicating liver disorder); intense itching; chest pain or palpitations; abdominal pain. Serious side effects are very rare; contact your doctor immediately.

COMMON
Dry, persistent cough.

LESS COMMON
Dizziness or fainting; skin rash; numbness or tingling in the hands, feet, or lips; unusual fatigue or muscle weakness; nausea; drowsiness; loss of taste; headache.

MOEXIPRIL HYDROCHLORIDE/HYDROCHLOROTHIAZIDE

Available in: Tablets
Available OTC? No   **As Generic?** No
Drug Class: Angiotensin-converting enzyme (ACE) inhibitor/diuretic

BRAND NAME

Uniretic

▼ USAGE INFORMATION

WHY IT'S PRESCRIBED
To treat high blood pressure.

HOW IT WORKS
This drug combines an angiotensin-converting enzyme (ACE) inhibitor (moexipril hydrochloride) and a thiazide diuretic (hydrochlorothiazide). ACE inhibitors block an enzyme that produces angiotensin, a naturally occurring substance that causes blood vessels to constrict and stimulates production of the adrenal hormone, aldosterone, which promotes sodium retention in the body. As a result, ACE inhibitors relax blood vessels (causing them to widen) and reduces sodium retention, which lowers blood pressure and so decreases the workload of the heart. Hydrochlorothiazide (HCTZ) increases sodium and water in the urine output. By reducing the overall fluid volume in the body, diuretics reduce blood volume and so reduce blood pressure.

▼ DOSAGE GUIDELINES

RANGE AND FREQUENCY
This combination medication comes in two strengths: moexipril/hydrochlorothiazide 7.5/12.5 and 15/25. The dose ranges from 7.5 to 30 mg of moexipril and 12.5 to 50 mg of hydrochlorothiazide per day. Tablets are taken either once a day or in 2 divided doses, 1 hour before meals.

ONSET OF EFFECT
Within 1 hour.

DURATION OF ACTION
Unknown.

DIETARY ADVICE
Take it on an empty stomach, about 1 hour before meals.

STORAGE
Store in a tightly sealed container away from heat, moisture, and direct light.

MISSED DOSE
Take it as soon as you remember. If it is near the time for the next dose, skip the missed dose and resume your regular dosage schedule. Do not double the next dose.

STOPPING THE DRUG
Dosage should be reduced gradually, according to your doctor's instructions.

PROLONGED USE
Lifelong therapy may be necessary; see your regularly doctor for evaluation.

▼ PRECAUTIONS

Over 60: Adverse reactions may be more likely and more severe in older patients.

Driving and Hazardous Work: No special warnings.

Alcohol: Alcohol may increase the effect of the drug and cause an excessive drop in blood pressure; drink only in moderation.

Pregnancy: Use of this drug during the last 6 months of pregnancy may cause severe defects, even death, in the fetus. Consult your doctor.

Breast Feeding: Moexipril may pass into breast milk; consult your doctor for specific advice.

Infants and Children: Not recommended for use by children under 18.

Special Concerns: A rare complication is angioedema, characterized by swelling of the lips, tongue, and throat. It may be so severe as to cause obstruction of the airways, which could be fatal.

OVERDOSE
Symptoms: No cases of overdose have been reported; symptoms might include dizziness, faintness, or confusion.

What to Do: Seek medical assistance if you suspect that someone has taken a much larger dose than prescribed.

▼ INTERACTIONS

DRUG INTERACTIONS
Consult your doctor for specific advice if you are taking cholestyramine, colestipol, corticosteroids, digitalis drugs, antidiabetic drugs, lithium, potassium-containing medications or supplements, or any over-the-counter drug (especially cold remedies and appetite suppressants).

FOOD INTERACTIONS
Avoid low-salt milk and salt substitutes. Many of these products contain potassium.

DISEASE INTERACTIONS
Consult your doctor if you have systemic lupus erythematosus or if you have had a prior allergic reaction to ACE inhibitors. This medication should be used with caution by patients with severe kidney disease or renal artery stenosis (narrowing of one or both of the arteries that supply blood to the kidneys). This medication can increase blood triglycerides and worsen control of blood sugar in people with diabetes.

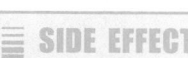 SIDE EFFECTS

SERIOUS
Fever and chills; sore throat and hoarseness; sudden difficulty breathing or swallowing; swelling of the face, mouth, or extremities; impaired kidney function (ankle swelling, decreased urination); confusion; yellow discoloration of the eyes or skin (indicating liver disorder); intense itching; chest pain or heartbeat irregularities; abdominal pain. Serious side effects are very rare; contact your doctor immediately.

COMMON
Dry, persistent cough; muscle cramps or pain; heart palpitations; dizziness (especially when rising from a sitting or lying position); dry mouth; unusual thirst; constipation.

LESS COMMON
Fainting; skin rash; numbness or tingling in the hands, feet, or lips; unusual fatigue or muscle weakness; nausea; drowsiness; loss of taste; headache; increased sensitivity to sunlight; loss of appetite; gout.

MOLINDONE

BRAND NAME

Moban

Available in: Tablets, liquid concentrate
Available OTC? No   **As Generic?** No
Drug Class: Neuroleptic; antipsychotic

▼ USAGE INFORMATION

WHY IT'S PRESCRIBED
To treat psychotic conditions (severe mental disorders characterized by distorted thoughts and perceptions), such as schizophrenia.

HOW IT WORKS
Molindone alters the activity of certain chemicals in the central nervous system, reducing aggressiveness and hyperactivity. It also appears to produce tranquilizing and antipsychotic effects.

▼ DOSAGE GUIDELINES

RANGE AND FREQUENCY
Initial dose is 50 to 75 mg a day; can be increased to 100 mg a day after 3 or 4 days. Maintenance dose may vary from 5 to 15 mg, 3 or 4 times a day, to 10 to 25 mg, 3 or 4 times a day, or 225 mg daily in several divided doses, depending on the severity of the condition being treated. Older and debilitated patients should be started on lower doses.

ONSET OF EFFECT
Sedation may occur within minutes, but onset of antipsychotic effect may take hours to occur or may not occur until days or weeks after the beginning of therapy.

DURATION OF ACTION
24 to 36 hours.

DIETARY ADVICE
No special restrictions.

STORAGE
Store in a tightly sealed container away from heat and direct light.

MISSED DOSE
Take it as soon as you remember. If it is near the time for the next dose, skip the missed dose and resume your regular dosage schedule. Do not double the next dose.

STOPPING THE DRUG
The decision to stop taking the drug should be made in consultation with your doctor.

PROLONGED USE
Prolonged use may lead to tardive dyskinesia (involuntary movements of the jaw, lips, tongue, and, in rare cases, the arms, legs, hands, or body). Consult your doctor about the need for follow-up evaluations and tests if you must take this drug for an extended period.

▼ PRECAUTIONS

Over 60: Adverse reactions are more likely and more severe in older patients.

Driving and Hazardous Work: Exercise caution until you determine how the medication affects you.

Alcohol: Avoid alcohol.

Pregnancy: Molindone has not been shown to cause birth defects in animals. Human studies have not been done. Before you take molindone, tell your doctor if you are pregnant or plan to become pregnant.

Breast Feeding: It is not known whether molindone passes into breast milk; caution is advised. Discuss potential risks and benefits with your doctor.

Infants and Children: Not recommended for use by children under age 12.

Special Concerns: Molindone is a newer drug very similar to phenothiazines (such as chlorpromazine and perphenazine), but does not appear to cause unexpected weight gain and is not as likely to cause tardive dyskinesia (an irreversible neurological disorder). The liquid concentrate form of molindone contains sulfite and so may cause severe allergic reactions in those who are highly sensitive to sulfites. Persons with asthma are incidentally at increased risk of sulfite sensitivity.

OVERDOSE
Symptoms: Extreme drowsiness, heartbeat irregularities, dry mouth, paradoxical restlessness or agitation, seizures, loss of consciousness.

What to Do: Call your doctor, emergency medical services (EMS), or the nearest poison control center immediately.

▼ INTERACTIONS

DRUG INTERACTIONS
Consult your doctor for advice if you are taking any drugs that depress the central nervous system, including antihistamines, antidepressants or other psychiatric medications, barbiturates, sedatives, cough medicines, decongestants, and painkillers. Be sure your doctor knows about any over-the-counter drugs you may take.

FOOD INTERACTIONS
None reported.

DISEASE INTERACTIONS
Consult your doctor for specific advice if you have any other medical condition.

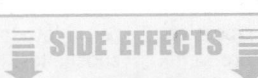
SIDE EFFECTS

SERIOUS
Restlessness; rigidity and trembling of limbs; involuntary movements of the tongue, face, mouth, or jaw; involuntary movements of the arms or legs; muscle rigidity; irregular pulse; unusually rapid heartbeat; palpitations; or other heartbeat irregularities. Call your doctor immediately.

COMMON
Drowsiness, blurred vision, palpitations, dry mouth or excessive salivation, skin rash, shaking of the hands, stiffness, stooped posture.

LESS COMMON
Increase in sexual desire, menstrual irregularities, discharge of milk from the breast, enlargement of breasts in men and women, prolonged contraction of muscles, liver abnormalities, mental depression, hyperactivity, unusual feeling of well-being (euphoria).

MOMETASONE FUROATE NASAL

Available in: Nasal spray
Available OTC? No   **As Generic?** No
Drug Class: Nasal corticosteroid

▼ USAGE INFORMATION

WHY IT'S PRESCRIBED
To prevent and treat the symptoms of allergic rhinitis (seasonal and perennial allergies, such as hay fever).

HOW IT WORKS
Respiratory corticosteroids, such as mometasone, primarily reduce or prevent inflammation of the lining of the airways, reduce the allergic response to inhaled allergens, and inhibit the secretion of mucus within the airways.

▼ DOSAGE GUIDELINES

RANGE AND FREQUENCY
Adults and teenagers: 2 sprays (50 micrograms [mcg] in each spray) in each nostril once a day, for a maximum daily dose of 200 mcg. To prevent the symptoms of allergic rhinitis from developing, it is recommended that patients with known seasonal allergies begin taking mometasone 2 to 4 weeks before the anticipated start of the pollen season.

ONSET OF EFFECT
From 11 hours to 2 days.

DURATION OF ACTION
Mometasone is effective as long as you continue to take the medication.

DIETARY ADVICE
Mometasone can be used without regard to diet.

STORAGE
Store in a tightly sealed container away from heat, moisture, and direct light.

MISSED DOSE
If you miss a dose on one day, resume your regular dosage schedule the next day. Do not double the next dose.

STOPPING THE DRUG
No special instructions.

PROLONGED USE
Consult your doctor about any need for periodic physical examinations and lab tests.

▼ PRECAUTIONS

Over 60: No special problems are expected.

Driving and Hazardous Work: Mometasone should not impair your ability to perform such tasks safely.

Alcohol: No special precautions are necessary.

Pregnancy: Nasal steroids have not been reported to cause birth defects if taken during pregnancy. Before using this drug, tell your doctor if you are pregnant or plan to become pregnant.

Breast Feeding: Mometasone may pass into breast milk; caution is advised. Consult your doctor for advice.

Infants and Children: Not recommended for use by children under age 12.

Special Concerns: Prior to your initial use of the inhaler, you must prime it by depressing the pump 10 times or until a fine mist appears. You may store the inhaler for up to 1 week without repriming. If it is unused for more than 1 week, reprime it by depressing the pump 2 times or until a fine mist appears. Avoid spraying the medication into the eyes.

OVERDOSE
Symptoms: No cases of overdose have been reported.

What to Do: An overdose with mometasone is unlikely. If someone takes a much larger dose than prescribed, call your doctor.

▼ INTERACTIONS

DRUG INTERACTIONS
Consult your doctor for advice if you are taking systemic corticosteroids, other inhaled corticosteroids, or any drugs that suppress the immune system.

FOOD INTERACTIONS
No known food interactions.

DISEASE INTERACTIONS
Consult your doctor if you have any other medical problem, particularly glaucoma, a herpes infection of the eye, a history of tuberculosis, liver disease, an underactive thyroid, or osteoporosis.

☰ SIDE EFFECTS ☰

SERIOUS
No serious side effects are associated with mometasone.

COMMON
Headache, increased susceptibility to viral infection, sore throat, nosebleeds or bloody nasal secretions.

LESS COMMON
Cough, increased susceptibility to upper respiratory infection, menstrual irregularities, bone pain, sinus pain.

MOMETASONE FUROATE TOPICAL

Available in: Cream, lotion, ointment
Available OTC? No   **As Generic?** No
Drug Class: Antipsoriasis drug; topical corticosteroid

▼ USAGE INFORMATION

WHY IT'S PRESCRIBED
For topical therapy of skin conditions associated with itching, redness, scaling and peeling, pain, and other signs of inflammation. Topical steroids come in many strengths; your physician will prescribe mometasone, a medium strength steroid, when it is the most appropriate steroid preparation for your particular skin condition.

HOW IT WORKS
Steroids interfere with the formation of natural substances within your body that are directly responsible for the process of inflammation, which produces swelling, redness, itching, and pain.

▼ DOSAGE GUIDELINES

RANGE AND FREQUENCY
Adults: Apply to the affected areas once daily. Children: Consult your pediatrician.

ONSET OF EFFECT
Soon after application. However, recognizable changes in your condition may take several days or more to develop.

DURATION OF ACTION
Unknown.

DIETARY ADVICE
Maintain your usual food and fluid intake. Increase fluids if you have a fever or diarrhea, in hot weather, or during exercise.

STORAGE
Store in a tightly sealed container away from heat and direct light. Keep away from moisture and extremes in temperature.

MISSED DOSE
Apply it as soon as you remember. If it is near the time for the next dose, skip the missed dose and resume your regular dosage schedule.

STOPPING THE DRUG
Apply it as prescribed for the full treatment period, even if you begin to feel better before the scheduled end of therapy.

PROLONGED USE
Therapy with this medication may require weeks or months. Prolonged use may increase the risk of undesirable side effects (especially thinning of the skin).

▼ PRECAUTIONS

Over 60: Adverse reactions may be more likely and more severe in older patients.

Driving and Hazardous Work: The use of topical mometasone should not impair your ability to perform such tasks safely.

Alcohol: No special precautions are necessary.

Pregnancy: Mometasone should not be used for prolonged periods by pregnant women or by women trying to become pregnant.

Breast Feeding: Mometasone may pass into breast milk; caution is advised. Consult your doctor for advice.

Infants and Children: Not recommended for prolonged use by children. Consult your pediatrician.

Special Concerns: Avoid use of this medication around the eyes. Note that mometasone is not a treatment for acne, burns, infections, or disorders of pigmentation. Do not bandage or wrap the medicated area of skin with any special dressings or coverings unless specifically told to do so by your doctor. Applying special coverings leads to increased absorption of the medication from the skin and may increase the chance of an undesirable interaction or side effect.

OVERDOSE
Symptoms: No specific ones have been reported.

What to Do: An overdose is unlikely to be life-threatening. However, if someone applies a much larger dose than prescribed, call your doctor, emergency medical services (EMS), or the nearest poison control center.

▼ INTERACTIONS

DRUG INTERACTIONS
None are known. Consult your doctor or pharmacist if you are concerned about a particular prescription or non-prescription drug.

FOOD INTERACTIONS
No known food interactions.

DISEASE INTERACTIONS
Consult your doctor if you have any of the following: diabetes, skin infection or skin sores and ulcers, infection at another site in your body, tuberculosis, unusual bleeding or bruising, glaucoma, or cataracts.

≡ SIDE EFFECTS ≡

SERIOUS
No serious side effects are associated with the use of mometasone.

COMMON
Thinning of the skin may occur with prolonged use of mometasone.

LESS COMMON
Burning or discomfort when medication is applied; blisters and pus near hair follicles; unusual bleeding or easy bruising; darkening or prominence of small skin veins; numbness or tingling of affected area, or of hands and fingers; increased susceptibility to infection; cataracts.

MONTELUKAST

Available in: Tablets, chewable tablets
Available OTC? No   **As Generic?** No
Drug Class: Leukotriene receptor antagonist

▼ USAGE INFORMATION

WHY IT'S PRESCRIBED
To prevent and treat the symptoms of chronic asthma by preventing bronchospasm (contraction of the smooth muscle tissue surrounding the airways, which results in narrowing and obstruction of the air passages). Montelukast may be used in conjunction with other asthma treatments.

HOW IT WORKS
Montelukast blocks cell receptors for leukotrienes, naturally formed substances that cause inflammation and constriction of the airways. Unlike bronchodilators, which relieve the acute symptoms of an asthma attack, montelukast is prescribed to be taken regularly when no symptoms are present to reduce the chronic inflammation of the airways that causes asthma, thus preventing asthma attacks.

▼ DOSAGE GUIDELINES

RANGE AND FREQUENCY
Adults and children age 15 and over: One 10 mg tablet, taken in the evening. Children ages 6 to 14: One 5-mg chewable tablet per day, taken in the evening. Children ages 2 to 5: One 4-mg chewable tablet, taken in the evening.

ONSET OF EFFECT
Unknown.

DURATION OF ACTION
Unknown.

DIETARY ADVICE
Montelukast can be taken without regard to diet.

STORAGE
Store in a tightly sealed container away from heat, moisture, and direct light.

MISSED DOSE
If you miss a dose one day, do not double the dose the next day. Resume your regular dosage schedule.

STOPPING THE DRUG
The decision to stop taking the drug should be made in consultation with your doctor.

PROLONGED USE
No special problems are expected.

SIDE EFFECTS

SERIOUS
Skin rash (indicating potentially life-threatening allergic reaction); gastroenteritis (causing loss of appetite, nausea, vomiting, stomach upset, fever, and diarrhea). Call your doctor immediately.

COMMON
Headache.

LESS COMMON
Weakness, fatigue, fever, abdominal pain, indigestion, mouth ulcers, dizziness, nasal congestion, cough, flulike symptoms.

▼ PRECAUTIONS

Over 60: Adverse reactions may be more likely and more severe in older patients.

Driving and Hazardous Work: No special precautions are necessary.

Alcohol: No special precautions are necessary.

Pregnancy: Adequate human studies have not been done. Before taking montelukast, tell your doctor if you are pregnant or plan to become pregnant.

Breast Feeding: Montelukast may pass into breast milk; caution is advised. Consult your doctor for advice.

Infants and Children: Not recommended for use by children under age 2.

Special Concerns: Montelukast has no effect on an asthma attack that has already started. You should have a fast-acting inhaled bronchodilator on hand to treat an acute asthma attack in progress. Consult your doctor if you need to use inhaled bronchodilators more often than usual, or if you are taking more than the maximum number of inhalations in a 24-hour period. Continue to take montelukast even when you are not experiencing any symptoms, as well as during periods of worsening asthma. In rare cases, if doses of systemic corticosteroids are reduced, montelukast may cause Churg-Strauss syndrome, a tissue disorder that sometimes strikes adult asthma patients and, if untreated, can destroy organs. Early symptoms include fever, muscle aches, and weight loss. Montelukast should not be used as the sole treatment for exercise-induced bronchospasm.

OVERDOSE
Symptoms: No cases of overdose have been reported.

What to Do: An overdose with montelukast is unlikely. If someone takes a much larger dose than prescribed, call your doctor, emergency medical services (EMS), or the nearest poison control center immediately.

▼ INTERACTIONS

DRUG INTERACTIONS
Consult your doctor for specific advice if you are already taking phenobarbital or rifampin. Before you take montelukast, tell your doctor if you are allergic to any other prescription or over-the-counter medicine.

FOOD INTERACTIONS
No known food interactions.

DISEASE INTERACTIONS
If you have phenylketonuria, you should not use the chewable tablet form of montelukast, since it contains phenylalanine. Use of montelukast may cause complications in patients with severe liver disease, since this organ works to remove the medication from the body.

MORPHINE

Available in: Capsules, tablets, oral solution, suppositories, injection
Available OTC? No   **As Generic?** Yes
Drug Class: Opioid (narcotic) analgesic

▼ USAGE INFORMATION

WHY IT'S PRESCRIBED
To relieve severe pain.

HOW IT WORKS
Opioids such as morphine relieve pain by acting on specific areas of the brain and spinal cord that process pain signals from nerves throughout the body.

▼ DOSAGE GUIDELINES

RANGE AND FREQUENCY
Adults— Capsules, tablets, oral solution: To start, 10 to 30 mg every 4 to 6 hours. Dose will be adjusted for individual needs. Extended-release capsules or tablets: Starting dose depends on individual needs and will be adjusted. Suppositories: 10 to 30 mg every 4 to 6 hours. Injection: 5 to 20 mg into a muscle or under the skin every 6 hours. Children— Dosages for all oral forms and suppositories must be determined by your doctor; for injection, 0.1 to 0.2 mg per 2.2 lbs (1 kg) of body weight, to a maximum of 15 mg, under the skin every 4 hours.

ONSET OF EFFECT
Oral forms: Within 60 minutes. Suppositories: 20 to 60 minutes. Injection: 10 to 30 minutes.

DURATION OF ACTION
Immediate-release oral forms: 4 to 5 hours. Extended-release forms: 8 to 12 hours. Suppositories and injection: 4 to 5 hours.

DIETARY ADVICE
Oral forms of morphine can be taken with food to lessen stomach upset. Long-acting tablets must be swallowed whole, without chewing.

STORAGE
Store in a tightly sealed container away from heat, moisture, and direct light. Do not allow liquid forms to freeze.

MISSED DOSE
If you are taking morphine on a fixed schedule, take it as soon as you remember. If it is near the time for the next dose, skip the missed dose and resume your regular dosage schedule. Do not double the next dose.

STOPPING THE DRUG
The decision to stop taking the drug should be made in consultation with your doctor.

PROLONGED USE
See your doctor regularly for tests and examinations if you must take this medication for a prolonged period. Prolonged use may lead to physical dependence.

▼ PRECAUTIONS

Over 60: Adverse reactions may be more likely and more severe in older patients.

Driving and Hazardous Work: Do not drive or engage in hazardous work until you determine how the medicine affects you.

Alcohol: Avoid alcohol.

Pregnancy: Avoid use during pregnancy if possible.

Breast Feeding: Morphine passes into breast milk; caution is advised. Consult your doctor for specific advice.

Infants and Children: Adverse reactions may be more likely and more severe.

Special Concerns: If you feel the medication is not working adequately after a few weeks, do not increase the dose. Consult your doctor. Before having any surgery, tell the doctor or dentist in charge you are taking morphine. Before removing the foil wrapper of the suppository, check if it is firm enough to insert. If too soft, put it in the refrigerator for 30 minutes or hold it momentarily under cold water.

OVERDOSE
Symptoms: Confusion; small, pinpoint pupils; severe drowsiness, weakness, or dizziness; slurred speech; cold, clammy skin; slow breathing; seizures; loss of consciousness.

What to Do: Call your doctor, emergency medical services (EMS), or the nearest poison control center immediately.

▼ INTERACTIONS

DRUG INTERACTIONS
Consult your doctor for specific advice if you are taking carbamazepine or other drugs for seizures, barbiturates, sedatives, cough medicines, decongestants, antidepressants, other prescription pain medicine, MAO inhibitors, naltrexone, rifampin, or zidovudine.

FOOD INTERACTIONS
None reported.

DISEASE INTERACTIONS
Consult your physician if you have a history of alcohol or drug abuse; emotional illness; brain disorders or head injury; seizures; lung disease; prostate or other problems with urination; gallstones; colitis; heart, kidney, liver, or thyroid disease.

SIDE EFFECTS

SERIOUS
Serious side effects are indistinguishable from those of overdose: Confusion; severe drowsiness, weakness, or dizziness; slurred speech; small, pinpoint pupils; cold, clammy skin; slow breathing; seizures; loss of consciousness.

COMMON
Dizziness or lightheadedness, nausea or vomiting, constipation, drowsiness, itching.

LESS COMMON
Mood swings, false sense of well-being (euphoria), urinary retention, jerking body movements (myoclonus), hallucinations, sweating.

MOXIFLOXACIN HYDROCHLORIDE

Available in: Tablets
Available OTC? No   **As Generic?** No
Drug Class: Fluoroquinolone antibiotic

▼ USAGE INFORMATION

WHY IT'S PRESCRIBED
To treat mild to severe bacterial infections, including acute sinusitis, community-acquired pneumonia, and acute bacterial complications due to chronic bronchitis.

HOW IT WORKS
Moxifloxacin inhibits the activity of a bacterial enzyme (gyrase) that is necessary for proper DNA formation and replication. This prevents bacteria from reproducing.

▼ DOSAGE GUIDELINES

RANGE AND FREQUENCY
For acute sinusitis or community-acquired pneumonia: 400 mg once a day for 10 days. For acute bacterial complications due to chronic bronchitis: 400 mg once a day for 5 days.

ONSET OF EFFECT
Varies depending on the infection being treated.

DURATION OF ACTION
Unknown.

DIETARY ADVICE
Can be taken without regard to meals. Drink plenty of fluids.

STORAGE
Store in a tightly sealed container away from heat, moisture, and direct light.

MISSED DOSE
Take it as soon as you remember. If it is near the time for the next dose, skip the missed dose and resume your regular dosage schedule. Do not double the next dose.

STOPPING THE DRUG
It is very important to take this drug as prescribed for the full treatment period, even if you begin to feel better before the scheduled end of therapy.

PROLONGED USE
If your symptoms do not improve or instead become worse after a few days, consult your doctor promptly. Moxifloxacin is typically taken for no more than 5 to 10 days.

▼ PRECAUTIONS

Over 60: No special advice.

Driving and Hazardous Work: Avoid such activities until you determine how the medicine affects you.

Alcohol: It is advisable to abstain from alcohol when fighting an infection.

Pregnancy: Moxifloxacin should be used during pregnancy only if potential benefits clearly justify the risks.

Breast Feeding: Moxifloxacin may pass into breast milk and cause serious side effects in the nursing infant; use of the drug is discouraged when nursing.

Infants and Children: Moxifloxacin is not recommended for use by persons under the age of 18.

Special Concerns: Do not take this medicine if you are allergic to any quinolone antibiotic, such as ciprofloxacin or lomefloxacin.

OVERDOSE
Symptoms: An overdose is unlikely to occur. Possible symptoms after an excessive dose may include decreased activity, drowsiness, vomiting, diarrhea, tremors, and seizures.

What to Do: Call your doctor, emergency medical services (EMS), or the nearest poison control center immediately.

▼ INTERACTIONS

DRUG INTERACTIONS
Because moxifloxacin can affect the function of the heart, it should not be used if you are taking antiarrhythmic drugs, such as amiodarone, quinidine, procainamide, or sotalol. It should be used with caution in patients taking cisapride, erythromycin, antipsychotics, tricylic antidepressants, nonsteroidal anti-inflammatory drugs (NSAIDs; including ibuprofen, aspirin, and naproxen), or digoxin. Moxifloxacin should be taken at least 4 hours before or 8 hours after using ferrous sulfate (iron supplement); dietary supplements containing zinc; didanosine; sucralfate; or antacids containing aluminum salts, magnesium salts, or calcium. Also tell your doctor if you are taking any other drug.

FOOD INTERACTIONS
No known food interactions.

DISEASE INTERACTIONS
Moxifloxacin should not be taken by people with prolongation of the QT interval on an electrocardiogram, known heart rhythm disturbances, uncorrected hypokalemia (low blood potassium levels), or those taking antiarrhythmic drugs, such as amiodarone, quinidine, procainamide, or sotalol. This drug should be used with caution in people with significant bradycardia (slow heart rate), recent myocardial ischemia, known or suspected nervous system disorders, or those who are predisposed to seizures. Use of moxifloxacin is not recommended in people with moderate or severe liver disease.

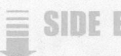
SIDE EFFECTS

SERIOUS
Serious reactions are rare and include mental confusion, nightmares, dizziness, hallucinations, anxiety, drowsiness or fainting spells, palpitations, shortness of breath, unusual swelling in the face or extremities, and loss of consciousness. Also skin burning, redness, blisters, rash, or itching on exposure to sunlight; increased risk of tendinitis or tendon rupture. Call your doctor immediately.

COMMON
Nausea, diarrhea, dizziness, headache, abdominal pain, vomiting.

LESS COMMON
Many less common side effects have been associated with moxifloxacin and may include: change in sense of taste, heartburn, weakness, insomnia, cough, dry skin, tinnitus, joint pain, dry mouth, vaginitis.

MUPIROCIN

Available in: Ointment, cream
Available OTC? No   **As Generic?** Yes
Drug Class: Antibiotic

▼ USAGE INFORMATION

WHY IT'S PRESCRIBED
Mupirocin is prescribed for topical therapy of certain bacteria-related skin infections. Mupirocin may be used alone or is occasionally used in combination with a second antibiotic (which is usually taken in an oral form).

HOW IT WORKS
Mupirocin works by preventing bacterial cells from manufacturing vital cell proteins and forming protective cell walls. This ultimately destroys the infecting bacterial organisms.

▼ DOSAGE GUIDELINES

RANGE AND FREQUENCY
Apply to affected skin 3 times a day. The site may be covered with a gauze dressing if desired.

ONSET OF EFFECT
Mupirocin begins antibacterial activity as soon as the ointment or cream is applied. Several days may be required, however, before its full effects become noticeable.

DURATION OF ACTION
Unknown.

DIETARY ADVICE
No special restrictions.

STORAGE
Store in a tightly sealed container away from heat and direct light. Keep away from moisture and extremes in temperature.

MISSED DOSE
Apply it as soon as you remember. If it is near the time for the next application, skip the missed one and resume your regular dosage schedule. Do not increase the quantity of medication with the next application.

STOPPING THE DRUG
Apply as prescribed for the full treatment period, even if you begin to feel the affected area is better before the scheduled end of therapy.

PROLONGED USE
Therapy with this medication should not require more than 14 days in most cases. Prolonged use of mupirocin may increase the risk of undesirable side effects.

▼ PRECAUTIONS

Over 60: No special precautions for older patients.

Driving and Hazardous Work: The use of mupirocin should not impair your ability to perform such tasks safely.

Alcohol: No special precautions are necessary.

Pregnancy: Mupirocin has not been evaluated in pregnant women. It is likely that mupirocin is safe for use during pregnancy in certain situations. This should be determined by your doctor.

Breast Feeding: Although not thought to be significantly absorbed into the bloodstream, if excessive amounts of mupirocin were absorbed, the drug could pass into breast milk; consult your doctor for advice.

Infants and Children: Consult your pediatrician.

Special Concerns: Mupirocin should not be used by anyone with a history of allergic reaction to mupirocin or any of the ingredients in the ointment or cream (check the label carefully). As with any other antibiotic, mupirocin is useful only against types of bacteria that are susceptible to its effects. Therefore, it is important to tell your doctor if your condition has not improved—or if it has worsened—within 3 to 5 days of starting mupirocin. The particular bacteria causing your illness may be resistant to mupirocin, and a different antibiotic may be required. Avoid using this drug near or around the eyes.

OVERDOSE

Symptoms: No cases of overdose have been reported.

What to Do: Overapplication of mupirocin is unlikely to be harmful. However, if someone swallows the medication, call your doctor, emergency medical services (EMS), or the nearest poison control center.

▼ INTERACTIONS

DRUG INTERACTIONS
No specific interactions have been reported. Consult your doctor or pharmacist if you are concerned about taking another prescription or nonprescription medication while you are using mupirocin.

FOOD INTERACTIONS
No known food interactions.

DISEASE INTERACTIONS
No disease interactions have been reported.

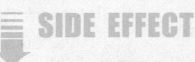

SIDE EFFECTS

SERIOUS
There are no serious side effects associated with the use of mupirocin.

COMMON
Mild stinging or burning sensation with initial application.

LESS COMMON
Persistent irritation or skin allergy with pain or discomfort (stinging or burning) at application site; itching, redness, rash, or dryness of the skin; nausea.

MUROMONAB-CD3

BRAND NAME

Orthoclone OKT3

Available in: Injection
Available OTC? No   **As Generic?** No
Drug Class: Immunosuppressant

▼ USAGE INFORMATION

WHY IT'S PRESCRIBED
To slow down or reduce the natural tendency of the immune system to reject organ transplants.

HOW IT WORKS
It suppresses the immune system's reaction against foreign tissue by inhibiting activity of white blood cells, a major component of the immune system's arsenal.

▼ DOSAGE GUIDELINES

RANGE AND FREQUENCY
Adults: 5 mg injected into a vein once a day. Muromonab-CD3 should be administered only by or under the direct supervision of your doctor. Children: The dose is determined by your doctor according to body weight.

ONSET OF EFFECT
Within minutes.

DURATION OF ACTION
One week after withdrawal of muromonab-CD3.

DIETARY ADVICE
This drug can be given without regard to meals.

STORAGE
Not applicable. Muromonab-CD3 is administered by a health care professional.

MISSED DOSE
Contact your doctor and reschedule your appointment as soon as possible.

STOPPING THE DRUG
The decision to stop taking the drug should be made by your doctor.

PROLONGED USE
See your doctor regularly for tests and examinations if you take this drug for a prolonged period. It may cause effects such as skin cancers or lymphomas that may not occur until years after the medicine is administered.

▼ PRECAUTIONS

Over 60: No special problems are expected in older patients.

Driving and Hazardous Work: Do not drive or engage in hazardous work until you determine how the medicine affects you.

Alcohol: Avoid alcohol.

Pregnancy: Studies of this medication's use during pregnancy have not been done in animals or humans. The drug may cross the placenta, but it is not known whether it harms the fetus. Before you take this drug, tell your doctor if you are pregnant or plan to become pregnant.

Breast Feeding: It is not known whether muromonab-CD3 passes into breast milk; consult your doctor for specific advice.

Infants and Children: Children are more likely to be dehydrated by the vomiting and diarrhea caused by muromonab-CD3.

Special Concerns: Treatment with muromonab-CD3 may increase the risk of other infections. Avoid persons who have received vaccinations recently or those with colds or other infections. If you think you are getting an infection, inform your doctor at once. Dental work should be done only with great caution during therapy. Practice dental hygiene and be cautious when using toothbrushes, toothpicks, and dental floss. Tell your doctor if you have had any allergic reaction to rodents, such as rats or mice; muromonab-CD3 is extracted from a mouse cell culture.

OVERDOSE
Symptoms: None reported.

What to Do: Call your doctor, emergency medical services (EMS), or the nearest poison control center immediately if you suspect an overdose.

▼ INTERACTIONS

DRUG INTERACTIONS
Consult your doctor for specific advice if you are taking azathioprine, chlorambucil, corticosteroids, cyclophosphamide, cyclosporine, cytarabine, mercaptopurine, or a live-virus vaccine.

FOOD INTERACTIONS
No known food interactions.

DISEASE INTERACTIONS
Caution is advised when taking muromonab-CD3. Consult your doctor if you have any of the following: angina, circulation problems, seizures, a history of recent heart attack, any other heart problem, kidney problems, lung problems, nervous system problems, a history of blood clots, chickenpox, shingles, or any infection.

 SIDE EFFECTS

SERIOUS
Chest pain, wheezing or shortness of breath, rapid or irregular heartbeat, swelling of the face or throat. Call your doctor immediately.

COMMON
Dizziness or faintness, diarrhea, fever and chills, general feeling of illness, headache, nausea, vomiting, muscle or joint pain.

LESS COMMON
Confusion, sensitivity of eyes to light, hallucinations, itching or tingling, stiff neck, skin rash, tremor, weakness, unusual fatigue, seizures.

MYCOPHENOLATE MOFETIL

Available in: Capsules, tablets, oral suspension
Available OTC? No   **As Generic?** No
Drug Class: Immunosuppressant

▼ USAGE INFORMATION

WHY IT'S PRESCRIBED
To slow down or reduce the natural tendency of the immune system to reject organ transplants.

HOW IT WORKS
Mycophenolate suppresses the immune system's reaction against foreign tissue by inhibiting the activity of white blood cells, a major component of the immune system's arsenal.

▼ DOSAGE GUIDELINES

RANGE AND FREQUENCY
Adults: 1 g twice a day in combination with corticosteroids and cyclosporine. Children: Dosage and frequency will be determined by your pediatrician.

ONSET OF EFFECT
Unknown.

DURATION OF ACTION
Unknown.

DIETARY ADVICE
The medication should be taken 30 minutes before or 2 hours after meals. It can be taken with a full glass of water to lessen stomach upset.

STORAGE
Store at room temperature in a tightly sealed container away from heat, moisture, and direct light. Oral suspension may be refrigerated.

MISSED DOSE
Take it as soon as you remember. However, if it is near the time for the next dose, skip the missed dose and resume your regular dosage schedule. Do not double the next dose.

STOPPING THE DRUG
The decision to stop taking the drug should be made by your doctor.

PROLONGED USE
You should see your doctor regularly for physical examinations and tests if you must take this drug for an extended period of time.

▼ PRECAUTIONS

Over 60: Information on the effects of mycophenolate in older patients as compared with younger persons is not yet available.

Driving and Hazardous Work: Do not drive or engage in hazardous work until you determine how the medicine affects you.

Alcohol: Avoid alcohol.

Pregnancy: Mycophenolate has caused birth defects in animals. Human studies have not been done, but caution is advised. A pregnancy test should be taken at least 1 week before mycophenolate treatment is started, and reliable methods of contraception should be used before, during, and 6 months after discontinuation of therapy.

Breast Feeding: It is not known whether mycophenolate passes into breast milk, but caution is advised; consult your doctor for advice.

Infants and Children: The safety and efficacy of the use of mycophenolate in infants and children have not been established.

Special Concerns: Patients should avoid contact with persons who may have infections or have recently received a vaccination. They should practice frequent oral hygiene, using a soft toothbrush. The capsules should not be opened, and the powder inside and oral suspension should not be allowed to come in contact with the skin or mucous membranes. If contact occurs, the affected area should be washed thoroughly with soap and water. If the eyes are affected, they should be rinsed with plain water. Discard any unused portion of the oral suspension 60 days after reconstitution.

OVERDOSE
Symptoms: Nausea, diarrhea, vomiting, fatigue.

What to Do: Call your doctor, emergency medical services (EMS), or the nearest poison control center immediately.

▼ INTERACTIONS

DRUG INTERACTIONS
Consult your doctor for specific advice if you are taking azathioprine, chlorambucil, corticosteroids, cyclophosphamide, cyclosporine, mercaptopurine, muromonab-CD3, a live-virus vaccine, or probenecid.

FOOD INTERACTIONS
No known food interactions.

DISEASE INTERACTIONS
Caution is advised when taking mycophenolate. Consult your doctor if you have an active digestive system disease or kidney disease.

SIDE EFFECTS

SERIOUS
Anemia; chest pain; fever or chills; cough or hoarseness; pinpoint red spots on skin; pain in lower back or side; high blood pressure; painful or difficult urination; black, tarry stools; blood in urine or stools; swelling of feet or lower legs; bloody vomit; white patches on mouth, tongue, or throat; unusual bleeding or bruising; tremor. Call your doctor immediately.

COMMON
Abdominal or stomach pain, headache, nausea, vomiting, constipation or diarrhea, heartburn, weakness.

LESS COMMON
Dizziness, skin rash, insomnia, acne.

NABUMETONE

Available in: Tablets
Available OTC? No   **As Generic?** No
Drug Class: Nonsteroidal anti-inflammatory drug (NSAID)

▼ USAGE INFORMATION

WHY IT'S PRESCRIBED
To treat mild to moderate pain and inflammation caused by tendinitis, arthritis, bursitis, gout, soft tissue injuries, migraine and other vascular headaches, menstrual cramps, and other conditions. When patients fail to respond to one NSAID, another may be tried. The greatest effectiveness often requires trial and error of several different NSAIDs.

HOW IT WORKS
NSAIDs work by interfering with prostaglandins, naturally occurring substances in the body that cause inflammation and make nerves more sensitive to pain impulses. NSAIDs also have other modes of action that are less well understood.

▼ DOSAGE GUIDELINES

RANGE AND FREQUENCY
Adults: 1,000 mg once a day. It may be increased to a maximum of 2,000 mg a day. For children's dose, consult your pediatrician.

ONSET OF EFFECT
From 30 minutes to several hours or longer.

DURATION OF ACTION
Variable.

DIETARY ADVICE
Take with food; maintain your usual food and fluid intake.

STORAGE
Store in a tightly sealed container away from heat, moisture, and direct light.

MISSED DOSE
Take it as soon as you remember. However, if it is near the time for the next dose, skip the missed dose and resume your regular dosage schedule. Do not double the next dose.

STOPPING THE DRUG
The decision to stop taking the drug should be made in consultation with your doctor.

PROLONGED USE
Prolonged use can cause gastrointestinal problems, including ulceration and bleeding, kidney dysfunction, and liver inflammation. Consult your doctor about the need for regular exams and lab tests.

▼ PRECAUTIONS

Over 60: Because of the potentially greater consequences of gastrointestinal side effects, the dose of NSAIDs for older patients, especially those over age 70, is often cut in half.

Driving and Hazardous Work: Avoid such activities until you determine how the medicine affects you.

Alcohol: Avoid alcohol when using this medication because it increases the risk of stomach irritation.

Pregnancy: Avoid or discontinue this drug if you are pregnant or plan to become pregnant.

Breast Feeding: Nabumetone passes into breast milk; avoid use while breast feeding.

Infants and Children: May be used in exceptional circumstances; consult your doctor.

Special Concerns: Because NSAIDs can interfere with blood coagulation, this drug should be stopped at least 3 days prior to any surgery.

OVERDOSE
Symptoms: Severe nausea, vomiting, headache, confusion, seizures.

What to Do: Call your doctor, emergency medical services (EMS), or the nearest poison control center immediately.

▼ INTERACTIONS

DRUG INTERACTIONS
Do not take this drug with aspirin or any other NSAIDs without your doctor's approval. In addition, consult your doctor if you are taking antihypertensives, steroids, anticoagulants, antibiotics, itraconazole or ketoconazole, plicamycin, penicillamine, valproic acid, phenytoin, cyclosporine, digitalis drugs, lithium, methotrexate, probenecid, triamterene, or zidovudine.

FOOD INTERACTIONS
No known food interactions.

DISEASE INTERACTIONS
Consult your doctor if you have any of the following: bleeding problems, inflammation or ulcers of the stomach and intestines, diabetes mellitus, systemic lupus erythematosus (SLE, lupus), anemia, asthma, epilepsy, Parkinson's disease, kidney stones, or a history of heart disease or alcohol abuse. Use of nabumetone may cause complications in patients with liver or kidney disease, since these organs work together to remove the medication from the body.

≣ SIDE EFFECTS ≣

SERIOUS
Shortness of breath or wheezing, with or without swelling of legs or other signs of heart failure; chest pain; peptic ulcer disease with vomiting of blood; black, tarry stools; decreasing kidney function. Call your doctor immediately.

COMMON
Nausea, vomiting, heartburn, diarrhea, constipation, headache, dizziness, sleepiness.

LESS COMMON
Ulcers or sores in mouth, depression, rashes or blistering of skin, ringing sound in the ears, unusual tingling or numbness of the hands or feet, seizures, blurred vision. Also elevated potassium levels, decreased blood counts; such problems can be detected by your doctor.

NADOLOL

Available in: Tablets
Available OTC? No   **As Generic?** Yes
Drug Class: Beta-blocker

▼ USAGE INFORMATION

WHY IT'S PRESCRIBED
To treat mild to moderate high blood pressure and angina. It is also used to prevent or control heartbeat irregularities (cardiac arrhythmias).

HOW IT WORKS
Nadolol slows the rate and force of contraction of the heart by blocking certain nerve impulses, thus reducing blood pressure. By modifying nerve impulses to the heart, the drug also helps to stabilize heart rhythm.

▼ DOSAGE GUIDELINES

RANGE AND FREQUENCY
For high blood pressure: 40 to 320 mg, once a day. For angina: 40 to 240 mg, once a day.

ONSET OF EFFECT
Unknown.

DURATION OF ACTION
Unknown.

DIETARY ADVICE
Follow your doctor's dietary restrictions, such as a low-salt or low-cholesterol diet, to improve control over high blood pressure and heart disease. Take with a full glass of water.

STORAGE
Store in a tightly sealed container away from heat, moisture, and direct light.

MISSED DOSE
Take it as soon as you remember. However, if it is within 8 hours of your next dose, skip the missed dose and resume your regular dosage schedule. Do not double the next dose.

STOPPING THE DRUG
This medication should not be stopped suddenly, as this may lead to angina and possibly a heart attack in patients with advanced heart disease. Slow reduction of the dose under a doctor's close supervision for 2 to 3 weeks is advised.

PROLONGED USE
Lifelong therapy may be needed. See your doctor for regular examinations and tests if you must take this medication for a prolonged period.

▼ PRECAUTIONS

Over 60: Adverse reactions may be more likely and more severe in older patients.

Driving and Hazardous Work: This drug may impair alertness, especially in the early stages of treatment. Do not drive or engage in hazardous work until you determine how the medication affects you.

Alcohol: Drink in careful moderation if at all. Alcohol may interact with the drug and cause a dangerous drop in blood pressure.

Pregnancy: Discuss with your doctor the relative risks and benefits of using this drug while pregnant.

Breast Feeding: Trace amounts of nadolol can be found in breast milk, but adverse effects in infants have not been documented. Consult your doctor for advice.

Infants and Children: No special problems expected.

OVERDOSE
Symptoms: Unusually slow or rapid heartbeat, severe dizziness or fainting, poor circulation in the hands (bluish skin), breathing difficulty, seizures.

What to Do: Call your doctor, emergency medical services (EMS), or the nearest poison control center immediately.

▼ INTERACTIONS

DRUG INTERACTIONS
Consult your doctor for specific advice if you are taking amphetamines, oral antidiabetic agents, asthma medication (such as aminophylline or theophylline), calcium channel blockers, clonidine, guanabenz, halothane, immunotherapy for allergies (allergy shots), insulin, MAO inhibitors, reserpine, other beta-blockers, or any over-the-counter medicine.

FOOD INTERACTIONS
None reported.

DISEASE INTERACTIONS
Nadolol should be used with caution in people with diabetes, especially insulin-dependent diabetes, since the drug may mask symptoms of hypoglycemia. Consult your doctor for special advice if you have allergies or asthma; heart or blood vessel disease (including congestive heart failure and peripheral vascular disease); hyperthyroidism; irregular (slow) heartbeat; myasthenia gravis; psoriasis; respiratory problems, such as bronchitis or emphysema; kidney or liver disease; or a history of depression.

SIDE EFFECTS

SERIOUS
Shortness of breath, wheezing; irregular or slow heartbeat (50 beats per minute or less); pain or feelings of tightness or pressure in the chest; swelling of the ankles, feet, and lower legs; mental depression. If you experience any such symptoms, stop taking nadolol and contact your doctor right away.

COMMON
Dizziness or lightheadedness, especially when rising suddenly to a standing position; rapid heartbeat or palpitations; decreased sexual ability; unusual fatigue, weakness, or drowsiness; insomnia.

LESS COMMON
Anxiety, irritability, nervousness; constipation; diarrhea; dry, sore eyes; itching; nausea or vomiting; nightmares or intensely vivid dreams; numbness, tingling, or other unusual sensations in the fingers, toes, or scalp.

NAFARELIN ACETATE

Available in: Nasal spray
Available OTC? Yes   **As Generic?** No
Drug Class: Gonadotropin-releasing hormone

▼ USAGE INFORMATION

WHY IT'S PRESCRIBED
To relieve the pain and discomfort of endometriosis.

HOW IT WORKS
Nafarelin decreases the production of estrogen by the ovaries. Reduced blood estrogen levels lead to shrinking of endometrial tissue (uterine lining), which eases flare-ups of endometriosis.

▼ DOSAGE GUIDELINES

RANGE AND FREQUENCY
One spray of 200 micrograms into 1 nostril in the morning and 1 spray into the other nostril in the evening, beginning on day 2, 3, or 4 of the menstrual period.

ONSET OF EFFECT
After 4 weeks.

DURATION OF ACTION
3 to 6 months.

DIETARY ADVICE
No special restrictions.

STORAGE
Store container upright away from heat and direct light.

MISSED DOSE
Take it as soon as you remember. However, if it is near the time for the next dose, skip the missed dose and resume your regular dosage schedule. Do not double the next dose.

STOPPING THE DRUG
The decision to stop taking the drug should be made by your doctor.

PROLONGED USE
Your doctor should check your progress regularly during prolonged use.

▼ PRECAUTIONS

Over 60: This medicine is generally not used by older patients.

Driving and Hazardous Work: The use of nafarelin should not impair your ability to perform such tasks safely.

Alcohol: Avoid alcohol.

Pregnancy: Nafarelin is not recommended during pregnancy. When taking the drug, women should use nonhormonal contraception (that is, methods other than birth control pills). If you think you are pregnant, stop taking the medicine and call your doctor immediately.

Breast Feeding: Nafarelin may pass into breast milk; caution is advised. Consult your doctor for advice.

Infants and Children: This drug is not recommended for use by children under the age of puberty.

Special Concerns: Tell your doctor if you smoke cigarettes or consume a lot of alcohol or caffeine. When using a new bottle of nafarelin spray, point the bottle away from you and pump about 7 times to prime it. Each time you use the spray, wipe the tip with a clean tissue or cloth. Every 3 or 4 days, rinse the tip with warm water and wipe the tip for about 15 seconds, then dry. To take a dose of nafarelin, first blow your nose gently. Hold your head forward a little, put the spray tip in the nostril, and aim for the back. Close the other nostril by pressing with 1 finger. After the spray, tilt your head back for a few seconds. Do not blow your nose.

OVERDOSE
Symptoms: No specific ones have been reported.

What to Do: An overdose of nafarelin is unlikely to be life-threatening. However, if someone takes a much larger dose than prescribed, call your doctor, emergency medical services (EMS), or the nearest poison control center immediately.

▼ INTERACTIONS

DRUG INTERACTIONS
Consult your doctor for specific advice if you are taking any nasal spray decongestant, adrenocorticoids, or anticonvulsant medication.

FOOD INTERACTIONS
No known food interactions.

DISEASE INTERACTIONS
Caution is advised when taking nafarelin. Consult your doctor if you have any menstrual disorder.

  SIDE EFFECTS

SERIOUS
Vaginal bleeding between menstrual periods; longer or heavier menstrual periods; shortness of breath, chest pain, joint pain, and hives caused by an allergic reaction; bloating or tenderness of the lower abdomen; unexpected or excess flow of milk. Call your doctor immediately.

COMMON
Acne, decreased sex drive, dryness of vagina, hot flashes, pain during intercourse, decreased breast size, palpitations, oily skin, cessation of menstrual periods.

LESS COMMON
Breast pain, headache, runny nose, mental depression, mood swings, rash, weight changes.

NALBUPHINE HYDROCHLORIDE

Available in: Injection
Available OTC? No   **As Generic?** Yes
Drug Class: Opioid (narcotic) analgesic

▼ USAGE INFORMATION

WHY IT'S PRESCRIBED
To relieve moderate to severe pain.

HOW IT WORKS
Opioids such as nalbuphine relieve pain by acting on specific areas of the spinal cord and brain that process pain signals from nerves throughout the body.

▼ DOSAGE GUIDELINES

RANGE AND FREQUENCY
For pain: 10 mg every 3 to 6 hours, into a vein or muscle or under the skin. Children: Dosages must be determined by your doctor.

ONSET OF EFFECT
Into a vein: 2 to 3 minutes. Into a muscle or under the skin: Within 15 minutes

DURATION OF ACTION
3 to 6 hours.

DIETARY ADVICE
This drug can be taken without regard to diet.

STORAGE
Store in a tightly sealed container away from heat, moisture, and direct light. Do not allow it to freeze.

MISSED DOSE
If you are taking nalbuphine on a fixed schedule, take it as soon as you remember. If it is near the time for the next dose, skip the missed dose and resume your regular dosage schedule. Do not double the next dose.

STOPPING THE DRUG
The decision to stop taking the drug should be made by your doctor.

PROLONGED USE
See your doctor regularly for tests and examinations if you take this medication for a prolonged period. Prolonged use can cause mental or physical dependence.

▼ PRECAUTIONS

Over 60: Adverse reactions may be more likely and more severe in older patients.

Driving and Hazardous Work: Do not drive or engage in hazardous work until you determine how the medicine affects you.

Alcohol: Avoid alcohol.

Pregnancy: Nalbuphine has not been shown to cause birth defects in animals. Human studies have not been done. Before you use this medication, tell your doctor if you are pregnant or plan to become pregnant. Overuse during pregnancy can cause drug dependence in the fetus.

Breast Feeding: Nalbuphine may pass into breast milk; caution is advised. Consult your doctor for advice.

Infants and Children: Adverse reactions may be more likely and more severe in children. Consult your doctor for advice.

Special Concerns: If you feel the medication is not working properly after a few weeks, do not increase the dose. Consult your doctor. Before having any surgery, tell the doctor or dentist in charge that you are taking this drug.

OVERDOSE
Symptoms: Confusion; severe drowsiness, weakness or dizziness; slurred speech; small, pinpoint pupils; cold, clammy skin; slow breathing; seizures; loss of consciousness.

What to Do: Call your doctor, emergency medical services (EMS), or the nearest poison control center immediately.

▼ INTERACTIONS

DRUG INTERACTIONS
Consult your physician for specific advice if you are taking carbamazepine or other medicine for seizures, barbiturates, sedatives, cough medicines, decongestants, antidepressants, other prescription pain medications, MAO inhibitors, naltrexone, rifampin, or zidovudine (AZT).

FOOD INTERACTIONS
No known food interactions.

DISEASE INTERACTIONS
Consult your doctor if you have any of the following: history of alcohol or drug abuse; emotional illness; brain disorders or head injury; seizures; lung disease; prostate problems or other problems with urination; gallstones; colitis; heart, kidney, liver, or thyroid disease.

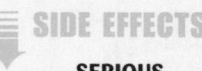
SIDE EFFECTS

SERIOUS
Serious side effects of nalbuphine are indistinguishable from those of overdose: Confusion; severe drowsiness, weakness, or dizziness; slurred speech; small, pinpoint pupils; cold, clammy skin; slow breathing; seizures; loss of consciousness.

COMMON
Dizziness or lightheadedness, nausea or vomiting, constipation, drowsiness, itching.

LESS COMMON
Mood swings or false sense of well-being (euphoria), hallucinations.

NALIDIXIC ACID

Available in: Suspension, tablets
Available OTC? No **As Generic?** No
Drug Class: Anti-infective

▼ USAGE INFORMATION

WHY IT'S PRESCRIBED
To treat urinary tract infections (UTIs).

HOW IT WORKS
By interfering with the genetic material of bacteria, nalidixic acid prevents them from reproducing. Eventually the bacteria die out, eliminating the infection.

▼ DOSAGE GUIDELINES

RANGE AND FREQUENCY
Adults and teenagers: 1,000 mg every 6 hours for 1 to 2 weeks, then 500 mg every 6 hours for long-term use. Children 3 months to 12 years: 55 mg per 2.2 lbs (1 kg) of body weight per day in equal doses every 6 hours for 1 to 2 weeks, then 33 mg per 2.2 lbs per day for long-term use.

ONSET OF EFFECT
3 to 4 hours.

DURATION OF ACTION
Unknown.

DIETARY ADVICE
Take it with a full glass of water on an empty stomach, at least 1 hour before or 2 hours after eating. However, if nalidixic acid causes stomach upset, it may be taken with food or milk.

STORAGE
Store in a tightly sealed container away from heat and direct light.

MISSED DOSE
Take it as soon as you remember. However, if it is near the time for the next dose, skip the missed dose and resume your regular dosage schedule. Do not double the next dose.

STOPPING THE DRUG
Take it as prescribed for the full treatment period, even if you feel better before the scheduled end of therapy.

PROLONGED USE
See your doctor for regular tests and evaluation if you must take this drug for more than 2 weeks.

SIDE EFFECTS

SERIOUS
Blurred, double, or decreased vision; change in color vision; seeing halos around lights; seizures; dark urine; hallucinations; bulging of the fontanel (soft spot) on top of an infant's head; severe headache; mood changes; pale skin; pale stools; skin rash and itching; severe stomach pain; unusual bleeding or bruising; unusual fatigue; yellow eyes or skin. Call your doctor immediately.

COMMON
Dizziness, diarrhea, drowsiness, headache, nausea or vomiting, stomach pain.

LESS COMMON
Increased sensitivity of skin to sunlight.

▼ PRECAUTIONS

Over 60: No special problems are expected.

Driving and Hazardous Work: Do not drive or engage in hazardous work until you determine how the medicine affects you.

Alcohol: Drink only in strict moderation, if at all.

Pregnancy: Nalidixic acid should not be used during pregnancy because in animal tests it has been shown to cause birth defects.

Breast Feeding: Nalidixic acid passes into breast milk and causes problems in babies with glucose-6-phosphate dehydrogenase (G6PD) deficiency. Problems with other nursing children have not been reported. Consult your doctor for specific individual advice on nursing while you take this medicine.

Infants and Children: This drug is not recommended for use by infants under the age of 3 months.

Special Concerns: Avoid exposure to sunlight until you determine how this medicine affects you. Photosensitivity may last up to 3 months after the last dose. Nalidixic acid may cause false results on tests of blood sugar.

OVERDOSE
Symptoms: Lethargy, psychosis, nausea, vomiting, seizures, severe headache (caused by increased pressure within the skull).

What to Do: Call your doctor, emergency medical services (EMS), or the nearest poison control center immediately.

▼ INTERACTIONS

DRUG INTERACTIONS
Certain drugs may interact adversely with nalidixic acid. Consult your doctor for specific advice, especially if you are taking anticoagulants.

FOOD INTERACTIONS
No known food interactions.

DISEASE INTERACTIONS
Caution is advised when taking nalidixic acid. Consult your doctor if you have any of the following: hardening of the arteries in the brain, G6PD deficiency, or a seizure disorder such as epilepsy. Use of nalidixic acid may cause complications in patients with liver or kidney disease, since these organs work together to remove the medication from the body.

NALTREXONE

BRAND NAME

ReVia

Available in: Tablets
Available OTC? No   **As Generic?** Yes
Drug Class: Opioid antagonist

▼ USAGE INFORMATION

WHY IT'S PRESCRIBED
To aid in the treatment of narcotic and alcohol dependence, in conjunction with psychological and social counseling. Naltrexone is not effective in treating dependency on cocaine or other nonopioid drugs.

HOW IT WORKS
Naltrexone blocks the euphoric effects of opioid narcotics (such as morphine and heroin) by competitive binding to opioid receptors in the brain. While the precise mechanism of action for alcohol dependence is unknown, naltrexone has been shown to reduce alcohol craving and consumption.

▼ DOSAGE GUIDELINES

RANGE AND FREQUENCY
For alcoholism: 50 mg (1 tablet) once a day. For narcotic dependence: Treatment should not be initiated unless the patient has been opioid-free for at least 7 to 10 days. To start, 25 mg (½ tablet) for the first day. If symptoms of narcotic withdrawal do not appear, dose will be increased to 50 mg once a day. Your doctor may increase or alter the dosage and frequency if necessary.

ONSET OF EFFECT
Within 60 minutes.

DURATION OF ACTION
24 to 72 hours.

DIETARY ADVICE
No special recommendations.

STORAGE
Store in a tightly sealed container away from heat, moisture, and direct light.

MISSED DOSE
If you take naltrexone once a day, take the missed dose as soon as possible. However, if you do not remember until the next day, skip the missed dose and resume your regular dosage schedule. Do not double the next dose. If your dosage schedule is different, consult your doctor for advice.

STOPPING THE DRUG
The decision to stop taking the drug should be made in consultation with your doctor.

PROLONGED USE
See your doctor regularly for tests of liver function and examinations.

▼ PRECAUTIONS

Over 60: No special advice.

Driving and Hazardous Work: Avoid such activities until you determine how the medicine affects you.

Alcohol: Avoid alcohol.

Pregnancy: Naltrexone should be given during pregnancy only if potential benefits outweigh the risks to the unborn child.

Breast Feeding: Naltrexone may pass into breast milk; caution is advised.

Infants and Children: Safety and effectiveness have not been established for children under the age of 18.

Special Concerns: Naltrexone will not prevent you from becoming intoxicated upon consumption of alcohol. Carry an identification card indicating you are taking naltrexone. It is of fundamental importance that patients using naltrexone abstain completely from opioid narcotics. If you have not been opioid-free for 7 to 10 days prior to taking naltrexone, it may induce symptoms of acute withdrawal. Also, the effects of naltrexone may be overcome by taking large doses of narcotics, but this poses a serious risk of a fatal narcotic overdose.

OVERDOSE
Symptoms: No cases of overdose have been reported. However, overdose symptoms may resemble Serious Side Effects.

What to Do: If you suspect an overdose or if someone takes a much larger dose than prescribed, call your doctor, emergency medical services (EMS), or the nearest poison control center immediately.

▼ INTERACTIONS

DRUG INTERACTIONS
Naltrexone should not be used at the same time as narcotic pain relievers, such as meperidine, morphine, and methadone. Studies with other types of medications have not be done. Consult your doctor for advice if you are taking any other prescription or over-the-counter drugs.

FOOD INTERACTIONS
No known food interactions.

DISEASE INTERACTIONS
Do not take naltrexone if you have acute hepatitis or liver failure.

≡ SIDE EFFECTS ≡

SERIOUS
Naltrexone may cause liver damage when taken in excess or by people with liver disease due to other causes. Call your doctor immediately if you develop abdominal pain lasting more than a few days, white bowel movements, dark urine, or a yellow discoloration of the eyes or skin.

COMMON
For alcoholism: Nausea, headache, dizziness, nervousness, fatigue. For narcotic addiction: Difficulty sleeping, nervousness, anxiety, abdominal pain or cramps, nausea, vomiting, decreased energy, muscle and joint pain, headache.

LESS COMMON
For alcoholism: Insomnia, vomiting, anxiety, drowsiness. For narcotic addiction: Loss of appetite, constipation, diarrhea, increased thirst, increased energy, depression, irritability, dizziness, skin rash, erectile dysfunction, chills.

NAPROXEN

Available in: Tablets, oral suspension, gelcaps
Available OTC? Yes   **As Generic?** Yes
Drug Class: Nonsteroidal anti-inflammatory drug (NSAID)

▼ USAGE INFORMATION

WHY IT'S PRESCRIBED
To relieve minor pain or inflammation associated with headaches, the common cold, toothache, muscle aches, backache, arthritis, tendinitis, bursitis, or menstrual cramps; also, to reduce fever. When patients fail to respond to one NSAID, others may be tried.

HOW IT WORKS
NSAIDs work by interfering with the formation of prostaglandins, naturally occurring substances in the body that cause inflammation and make nerves more sensitive to pain impulses. NSAIDs also have other modes of action that are less well understood.

▼ DOSAGE GUIDELINES

RANGE AND FREQUENCY
Adults: 440 to 1,500 mg daily. Maximum dose is 1,500 mg a day, taken in 2 to 3 evenly divided doses.

ONSET OF EFFECT
Rapid; relieves pain within 1 hour. However, it may take up to 2 weeks to suppress inflammation.

DURATION OF ACTION
Up to 12 hours.

DIETARY ADVICE
Take with food; maintain your usual food and fluid intake.

STORAGE
Store tablets in a tightly sealed container away from heat, moisture, and direct light. Store oral suspension in refrigerator, but do not freeze.

MISSED DOSE
Take it as soon as you remember. However, if it is near the time for the next dose, skip the missed dose and resume your regular dosage schedule. Do not double the next dose.

STOPPING THE DRUG
If you are taking this drug by prescription, do not stop taking it without first consulting your doctor.

PROLONGED USE
Prolonged use can cause gastrointestinal problems, including ulceration and bleeding, kidney dysfunction, and liver inflammation. Consult your doctor about the need for medical examinations and laboratory studies.

▼ PRECAUTIONS

Over 60: Because of the potentially greater consequences of gastrointestinal side effects, the dose of NSAIDs for older patients, especially those over age 70, is often cut in half.

Driving and Hazardous Work: Avoid such activities until you determine how the medication affects you.

Alcohol: Avoid alcohol when taking this drug; the combination of naproxen and alcohol can be highly toxic to the liver.

Pregnancy: Avoid this drug if you are pregnant or plan to become pregnant.

Breast Feeding: Naproxen passes into breast milk; avoid use while nursing.

Infants and Children: Naproxen may be used in exceptional circumstances; consult your pediatrician for specific advice.

Special Concerns: Because NSAIDs can interfere with blood coagulation, this drug should be stopped at least 3 days prior to any surgery.

OVERDOSE
Symptoms: Severe nausea, vomiting, headache, confusion, seizures.

What to Do: Call your doctor, emergency medical services (EMS), or the nearest poison control center immediately.

▼ INTERACTIONS

DRUG INTERACTIONS
Do not take this drug with aspirin or any other NSAIDs without your doctor's approval. In addition, consult your doctor if you are taking antihypertensives, steroids, anticoagulants, antibiotics, itraconazole or ketoconazole, plicamycin, penicillamine, valproic acid, phenytoin, cyclosporine, digitalis drugs, lithium, methotrexate, probenecid, triamterene, or zidovudine.

FOOD INTERACTIONS
No known food interactions.

DISEASE INTERACTIONS
Consult your doctor if you have any of the following: bleeding problems, inflammation or ulcers of the stomach and intestines, diabetes mellitus, systemic lupus erythematosus (SLE, lupus), anemia, asthma, epilepsy, Parkinson's disease, kidney stones, or a history of heart disease or alcohol abuse. Use of naproxen may cause complications in patients with liver or kidney disease, since these organs work together to remove the medication from the body.

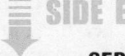

SIDE EFFECTS

SERIOUS
Shortness of breath or wheezing, with or without swelling of legs or other signs of heart failure; chest pain; peptic ulcer disease with vomiting of blood; black, tarry stools; decreasing kidney function. Call your doctor immediately.

COMMON
Nausea, vomiting, heartburn, diarrhea, constipation, headache, dizziness, sleepiness.

LESS COMMON
Ulcers or sores in mouth, depression, rashes or blistering of skin, ringing sound in the ears, unusual tingling or numbness of the hands or feet, seizures, blurred vision. Also elevated potassium levels, decreased blood counts; such problems can be detected by your doctor.

NARATRIPTAN HYDROCHLORIDE

Available in: Tablets
Available OTC? No   **As Generic?** No
Drug Class: Antimigraine/antiheadache drug

▼ USAGE INFORMATION

WHY IT'S PRESCRIBED
To treat severe, acute migraine headaches. Naratriptan is not intended as a migraine preventive or for use against any other kinds of pain or headache, including basilar and hemiplegic migraines. Your doctor will determine whether this medication is appropriate in your particular case.

HOW IT WORKS
The exact mechanism of action is unknown.

▼ DOSAGE GUIDELINES

RANGE AND FREQUENCY
A single tablet of 1 or 2.5 mg taken with water is generally effective. If the migraine returns or there is only partial relief, the dose may be repeated once after 4 hours, but no more than 5 mg should be taken in a 24-hour period. Since individuals may vary in response to naratriptan, your experience with the drug will determine the most appropriate initial dosage.

ONSET OF EFFECT
Within 1 to 3 hours.

DURATION OF ACTION
Up to 24 hours.

DIETARY ADVICE
The medication can be taken with or without food.

STORAGE
Store in a tightly sealed container away from heat, moisture, and direct light.

MISSED DOSE
Not applicable, since the drug is taken only when necessary.

STOPPING THE DRUG
Consult your doctor before discontinuing naratriptan.

PROLONGED USE
No special problems are expected. However, if you are at risk for coronary artery disease (see Special Concerns), you should undergo periodic medical tests and evaluation.

▼ PRECAUTIONS

Over 60: Naratriptan is not recommended for use in older patients.

Driving and Hazardous Work: Some people feel drowsy or dizzy during or following a migraine attack or after taking naratriptan. Avoid driving or other tasks requiring concentration if you have such symptoms.

Alcohol: No special warnings, although alcohol may trigger or exacerbate migraine headaches.

Pregnancy: Adequate human studies have not been done. Discuss with your doctor the relative risks and benefits of using the drug while pregnant.

Breast Feeding: Naratriptan may pass into breast milk; caution is advised. Consult your doctor for advice.

Infants and Children: The safety and effectiveness of naratriptan have not been established for patients under age 18. Consult your pediatrician for advice.

Special Concerns: Serious, but rare, heart-related problems may occur after naratriptan use. Anyone at risk for unrecognized coronary artery disease, such as postmenopausal women, men over age 40, or those with risk factors for coronary artery disease (hypertension, high blood cholesterol levels, obesity, diabetes, strong family history of heart disease, or cigarette smoking) should have the first dose of naratriptan administered in a doctor's office. Naratriptan should not be used by anyone with any symptoms of heart disease (chest pain or tightness, shortness of breath).

OVERDOSE
Symptoms: Increase in blood pressure resulting in lightheadedness, tension in the neck, fatigue, and loss of coordination.

What to Do: An overdose with naratriptan is unlikely. If someone takes a much larger dose than prescribed, call your doctor, emergency medical services (EMS), or the nearest poison control center immediately.

▼ INTERACTIONS

DRUG INTERACTIONS
Do not take naratriptan within 24 hours of taking dihydroergotamine mesylate or methysergide mesylate. Oral contraceptives may interact with naratriptan. Consult your doctor for specific advice.

FOOD INTERACTIONS
No known food interactions.

DISEASE INTERACTIONS
You should not take naratriptan if you have a history of angina, heart disease, stroke, uncontrolled hypertension, heartbeat irregularities, peripheral vascular disease, or severely impaired kidney or liver function.

▼ SIDE EFFECTS

SERIOUS
Chest pain or tightness; sudden or severe abdominal pain; shortness of breath; wheezing; heartbeat irregularities or palpitations; skin rash; hives; swelling of the eyelids, face, or lips. Call your doctor immediately.

COMMON
Tingling, hot flashes, flushing, weakness, drowsiness or dizziness, fatigue, general feeling of illness.

LESS COMMON
There are no less-common side effects associated with the use of naratriptan.

NATAMYCIN

Available in: Ophthalmic suspension
Available OTC? No   **As Generic?** No
Drug Class: Antifungal

▼ USAGE INFORMATION

WHY IT'S PRESCRIBED
To treat several types of fungal infections of the eye, including fungal blepharitis (inflammation of the eyelid), conjunctivitis (inflammation of the mucous membranes that line the inner surface of the eyelids and whites of the eyes), and keratitis (inflammation of the cornea).

HOW IT WORKS
Natamycin binds to and alters the fungal cell membrane so that vital structures inside the cell pass though the membrane and out of the cell. Without these structures, the fungal cells cannot survive.

▼ DOSAGE GUIDELINES

RANGE AND FREQUENCY
Fungal blepharitis or conjunctivitis: 1 drop every 4 to 6 hours. Fungal keratitis: 1 drop every 1 to 2 hours for the first 3 or 4 days, and 1 drop 6 to 8 times a day thereafter.

ONSET OF EFFECT
Unknown.

DURATION OF ACTION
Unknown.

DIETARY ADVICE
No special restrictions.

STORAGE
Store in a tightly sealed container away from heat, moisture, and direct light. You may store it at room temperature or in the refrigerator, but do not allow it to freeze.

MISSED DOSE
Apply natamycin as soon as you remember and then resume your regular dosage schedule. Do not double the next dose.

STOPPING THE DRUG
Use it as prescribed for the full treatment period, even if you begin to feel better before the scheduled end of therapy.

PROLONGED USE
Therapy is generally continued for up to 14 to 21 days, depending on the type and severity of infection, or until the infection has been checked. However, no signs of improvement within 7 to 10 days may indicate that a microorganism not susceptible to natamycin is causing the infection; check with your doctor if symptoms do not improve within this amount of time. Your doctor should check your progress regularly, which may be as often as 3 times a week for certain eye infections.

▼ PRECAUTIONS

Over 60: No special problems are expected.

Driving and Hazardous Work: Avoid such activities until you determine how the medicine affects your vision.

Alcohol: No special warnings.

Pregnancy: Adequate human studies have not been completed. Before taking natamycin, tell your doctor if you are pregnant or plan to become pregnant.

Breast Feeding: Natamycin may pass into breast milk; caution is advised. Consult your doctor for advice.

Infants and Children: Proper use of natamycin should be determined by your doctor.

Special Concerns: To use the eye drops, first wash your hands. Tilt your head back. Gently apply pressure to the inside corner of the eyelid and with the index finger of the same hand, pull downward on the lower eyelid to make a space. Drop the medicine into this space and close your eye. Apply gentle pressure for 1 or 2 minutes while keeping the eye closed without blinking. Then wash your hands again. Make sure the tip of the dropper does not touch your eye, finger, or any other surface. Shake the container well before each dose.

OVERDOSE
Symptoms: No specific ones have been reported.

What to Do: An overdose of natamycin is unlikely to be life-threatening. However, if someone applies a much larger dose than prescribed or accidentally ingests the medicine, call your doctor, emergency medical services (EMS), or the nearest poison control center immediately.

▼ INTERACTIONS

DRUG INTERACTIONS
None known.

FOOD INTERACTIONS
None known.

DISEASE INTERACTIONS
None known.

≡ SIDE EFFECTS ≡

SERIOUS
Eye redness, swelling or irritation not present before applying natamycin. Call your doctor as soon as possible.

COMMON
No common side effects are associated with natamycin.

LESS COMMON
No less-common side effects are associated with natamycin.

NEDOCROMIL SODIUM INHALANT

Available in: Inhalation aerosol
Available OTC? No   **As Generic?** No
Drug Class: Respiratory inhalant

▼ USAGE INFORMATION

WHY IT'S PRESCRIBED
To prevent the symptoms of asthma and to prevent bronchospasm (contraction of the smooth muscle tissue surrounding the airways, which results in narrowing and obstruction of air passages). It cannot relieve an asthma attack once it has started.

HOW IT WORKS
Nedocromil prevents inflammatory cells in the lungs from releasing substances that cause asthma symptoms or bronchospasm. Unlike bronchodilators that are taken to relieve the acute symptoms of an asthma attack, nedocromil is generally prescribed to be taken on a regular basis when no symptoms are present, to reduce the chronic inflammation of the airways that underlies asthma. Nedocromil may also be used preventively just prior to exposure to certain conditions or substances (cold air, exercise, chemicals, air pollution, or allergens such as pollen or dust mites) that may trigger an acute asthma attack.

▼ DOSAGE GUIDELINES

RANGE AND FREQUENCY
For prevention of asthma symptoms, adults and teenagers: 2 puffs (3.5 to 4 mg) twice a day at regularly spaced times. To prevent bronchospasm, adults and teenagers: 2 puffs up to 30 minutes before exercise or exposure to anything that can trigger bronchospasm. Children: Consult pediatrician for proper dose.

ONSET OF EFFECT
Several days to 4 weeks.

DURATION OF ACTION
6 to 12 hours.

DIETARY ADVICE
No special recommendations.

STORAGE
Store in a tightly sealed container away from heat and direct light. Do not allow the medication to freeze. Do not puncture, break, or incinerate the aerosol canister, even if it is empty.

MISSED DOSE
Take it as soon as you remember. If it is near the time for the next dose, skip the missed dose and resume your regular dosage schedule. Do not double the next dose.

STOPPING THE DRUG
The decision to stop taking the drug should be made by your doctor.

PROLONGED USE
You should see your doctor regularly for tests and examinations if you take this drug for a prolonged period.

▼ PRECAUTIONS

Over 60: No special problems are expected.

Driving and Hazardous Work: The use of nedocromil should not impair your ability to perform such tasks safely.

Alcohol: No special warnings.

Pregnancy: Nedocromil has not caused birth defects in animals. Human studies have not been done. Before you take nedocromil, tell your doctor if you are pregnant or plan to become pregnant.

Breast Feeding: Nedocromil may pass into breast milk; caution is advised. Mothers who wish to breast feed while taking nedocromil should consult their doctor for specific advice.

Infants and Children: No special problems expected. Use and dose must be determined by your doctor.

Special Concerns: Shake the inhaler well and test before using. Remember to clean the inhaler at least twice a week.

OVERDOSE
Symptoms: No specific ones have been reported.

What to Do: An overdose of nedocromil is unlikely to be life-threatening. However, if someone takes a much larger dose than prescribed, call your doctor, emergency medical services (EMS), or the nearest poison control center.

▼ INTERACTIONS

DRUG INTERACTIONS
Before you take nedocromil, tell your doctor if you are taking any prescription or over-the-counter medicine.

FOOD INTERACTIONS
No known food interactions.

DISEASE INTERACTIONS
No disease interactions have been reported.

≋ SIDE EFFECTS ≋

SERIOUS
Increased wheezing, tightness or pain in the chest, or breathing difficulty. Call your doctor right away.

COMMON
There are no common side effects associated with the use of nedocromil.

LESS COMMON
Cough; headache; nausea or vomiting; runny or stuffy nose; throat irritation, soreness, or difficulty swallowing; unpleasant taste.

NEDOCROMIL SODIUM OPHTHALMIC

Available in: Ophthalmic solution
Available OTC? No   **As Generic?** No
Drug Class: Antihistamine

▼ USAGE INFORMATION

WHY IT'S PRESCRIBED
For temporary relief of itching of the eye due to allergic conjunctivitis (inflammation of the mucous membranes that line the inner surface of the eyelids and whites of the eyes).

HOW IT WORKS
Nedocromil inhibits the release and blocks the effects of histamine, a substance that causes swelling, itching, sneezing, watery eyes, hives, and other symptoms of allergic reaction.

▼ DOSAGE GUIDELINES

RANGE AND FREQUENCY
1 or 2 drops in each affected eye twice a day.

ONSET OF EFFECT
Unknown.

DURATION OF ACTION
Unknown.

DIETARY ADVICE
No special restrictions.

STORAGE
Store in a tightly sealed container away from heat, moisture, and direct light. Do not allow it to freeze.

MISSED DOSE
Apply the next dose as needed; do not double the next dose.

STOPPING THE DRUG
This medication is to be used throughout the period of exposure (the duration of the pollen season or until the cause of the conjunctivitis is no longer present), even when symptoms are absent.

PROLONGED USE
See your doctor regularly for tests and examinations if you must take this drug for a prolonged period.

▼ PRECAUTIONS

Over 60: No special problems are expected.

Driving and Hazardous Work: Do not drive or engage in hazardous work until you determine how the medicine affects your vision.

Alcohol: No special warnings.

Pregnancy: In animal studies, large doses of nedocromil did not cause birth defects. Human studies have not been done. Nedocromil should be used by pregnant women only if the potential benefit to the mother justifies the potential risk to the embryo or fetus. Consult your doctor for specific advice.

Breast Feeding: Nedocromil may pass into breast milk; caution is advised. Consult your doctor for advice.

Infants and Children: The safety and effectiveness of nedocromil in infants and children under the age of 3 have not been established.

Special Concerns: To use the eye drops, first wash your hands. Tilt your head back. Gently apply pressure to the inside corner of the eyelid and with the index finger of the same hand, pull downward on the lower eyelid to make a space. Drop the medicine into this space and close your eye. Apply pressure for 1 or 2 minutes while keeping the eye closed without blinking. Then wash your hands again. Make sure the tip of the dropper does not touch your eye, finger, or any other surface. If you use contact lenses, do not wear them while administering nedocromil.

OVERDOSE
Symptoms: No specific ones have been reported.

What to Do: An overdose of nedocromil is unlikely to be life-threatening. However, if someone applies a much larger dose than prescribed or accidentally ingests the medicine, call your doctor, emergency medical services (EMS), or the nearest poison control center immediately.

▼ INTERACTIONS

DRUG INTERACTIONS
Do not use with any other eye medication. Consult your doctor for specific advice.

FOOD INTERACTIONS
No known food interactions.

DISEASE INTERACTIONS
Caution is advised when taking nedocromil. Consult your doctor if you have any medical condition, especially one affecting the eyes.

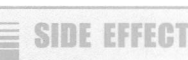

SIDE EFFECTS

SERIOUS
No serious side effects are associated with nedocromil.

COMMON
Headache, temporary burning and stinging of the eye, unpleasant taste, nasal congestion.

LESS COMMON
Asthma, conjunctivitis, eye redness, increased eye sensitivity to light, runny nose.

NEFAZODONE HYDROCHLORIDE

Available in: Tablets
Available OTC? No   **As Generic?** No
Drug Class: Antidepressant

▼ USAGE INFORMATION

WHY IT'S PRESCRIBED
To treat symptoms of major depression.

HOW IT WORKS
Nefazodone affects the levels of serotonin and norepinephrine, brain chemicals that are thought to be linked to mood, emotions, and mental state.

▼ DOSAGE GUIDELINES

RANGE AND FREQUENCY
Adults: To start, 100 mg once a day. The dose may be gradually increased by your doctor to a maximum of 600 mg a day. Older adults: To start, 50 mg 1 or 2 times a day. The dose may be gradually increased by your doctor.

ONSET OF EFFECT
The full effect may take several weeks.

DURATION OF ACTION
Unknown.

DIETARY ADVICE
Nefazodone can be taken without regard to diet.

STORAGE
Store in a tightly sealed container away from heat, moisture, and direct light.

MISSED DOSE
Take it as soon as you remember. However, if it is near the time for the next dose, skip the missed dose and resume your regular dosage schedule. Do not double the next dose.

STOPPING THE DRUG
Take it as prescribed for the full treatment period, even if you begin to feel better before the scheduled end of therapy. The decision to stop taking the drug should be made in consultation with your doctor.

PROLONGED USE
The usual course of therapy lasts 6 months to 1 year; some patients benefit from additional therapy.

≡ SIDE EFFECTS ≡

SERIOUS
Blurred, partial loss of, or changes in vision; unsteadiness or clumsiness; skin rash; lightheadedness; ringing in the ears; prolonged or painful erection (lasting more than 4 hours). Call your doctor immediately.

COMMON
Drowsiness or dizziness, agitation, dry mouth, confusion, constipation or diarrhea, unusual dreams, heartburn, fever or chills, insomnia, loss of memory, headache, flushing, nausea or vomiting, increased appetite.

LESS COMMON
Joint pain, increased thirst, breast pain, cough, swelling of lower extremities, sore throat, trembling. Also unusual tingling, burning, or prickling sensations.

▼ PRECAUTIONS

Over 60: Adverse reactions may be more likely and more severe in older patients. A lower dose may be warranted.

Driving and Hazardous Work: Proceed with caution until you determine how the medicine affects you. Drowsiness may occur.

Alcohol: Avoid alcohol.

Pregnancy: Nefazodone has not been shown to cause birth defects in animals. Adequate human studies have not been done. Before you take this medication, tell your doctor if you are pregnant or plan to become pregnant.

Breast Feeding: Nefazodone may pass into breast milk; caution is advised.

Infants and Children: Safety and effectiveness of the drug in children under age 18 have not been established.

Special Concerns: Use sugarless gum or candy for relief of dry mouth.

OVERDOSE
Symptoms: Lightheadedness, dizziness, confusion, fainting, nausea, vomiting, drowsiness.

What to Do: Call your doctor, emergency medical services (EMS), or the nearest poison control center immediately.

▼ INTERACTIONS

DRUG INTERACTIONS
Do not take nefazodone if you are taking terfenadine or astemizole. Nefazodone and

MAO inhibitors should not be used within 14 days of each other. Very serious side effects such as myoclonus (uncontrolled muscle jerking), hyperthermia (excessive rise in body temperature), and extreme stiffness may result. For many patients, especially the elderly, the use of nefazodone in combination with triazolam is not recommended. Other drugs may also interact with nefazodone; consult your doctor if you are taking alprazolam, high blood pressure medication (antihypertensives), central nervous system depressants (including cold medications, allergy drugs, narcotic pain relievers, and muscle relaxants), or tricyclic antidepressants.

FOOD INTERACTIONS
No known food interactions.

DISEASE INTERACTIONS
Consult your doctor if you have a history of drug or alcohol abuse, any heart condition, a history of seizures, any condition affecting blood vessels of the brain, symptoms of dehydration (confusion, irritability, flushed, dry skin, decreased urine output, extreme thirst), or a history of mental disorders.

NELFINAVIR

Available in: Oral powder, tablets
Available OTC? No   **As Generic?** No
Drug Class: Antiviral/protease inhibitor

▼ USAGE INFORMATION

WHY IT'S PRESCRIBED
To treat HIV (human immunodeficiency virus) infection. While not a cure for HIV, this drug may suppress the replication of the virus and delay the progression of the disease.

HOW IT WORKS
Nelfinavir blocks the activity of a viral protease, an enzyme that is needed by HIV to reproduce. Blocking the protease produces HIV copies that cannot infect new cells.

▼ DOSAGE GUIDELINES

RANGE AND FREQUENCY
Adults: 750 mg, 3 times a day. Children: 20 to 30 mg per 2.2 lbs (1 kg) of body weight, 3 times a day. Instead of tablets, children can be given the oral powder mixed with water, milk, formula, soy milk, or a dietary supplement. Citrus or other acidic foods or juices are not recommended since they may produce a bit-ter taste when mixed with the medication. Other antiretroviral drugs are prescribed in combination with nelfinavir.

ONSET OF EFFECT
Initial response: Several days. Maximum therapeutic effect: 12 to 16 weeks.

DURATION OF ACTION
Unknown.

DIETARY ADVICE
Nelfinavir should be taken with a light meal or snack.

STORAGE
Store in a tightly sealed container away from heat and direct light. Once oral powder is mixed with liquid, it should not be stored for more than 6 hours; taking the full dose immediately is recommended.

MISSED DOSE
Take it as soon as you remember. If it is near the time for the next dose, skip the missed dose and resume your regular dosage schedule. Do not double the next dose.

STOPPING THE DRUG
The decision to stop taking the drug should be made in consultation with your doctor.

PROLONGED USE
See your doctor regularly for tests and examinations.

▼ PRECAUTIONS

Over 60: It is not known whether nelfinavir causes different or more severe side effects in older patients.

Driving and Hazardous Work: Avoid such activities until you determine how the medicine affects you.

Alcohol: Avoid alcohol if liver function is impaired.

Pregnancy: Nelfinavir has been shown to cause birth defects in animal studies; however, it is increasingly being used along with other drugs to treat pregnant HIV-infected women.

Breast Feeding: It is unknown whether nelfinavir passes into breast milk; however, to avoid transmitting the virus to an uninfected child, women infected with HIV should not breast feed.

Infants and Children: The safety and effectiveness of nelfinavir have not been established for children under 2 years of age.

Special Concerns: Use of nelfinavir does not eliminate the risk of passing the AIDS virus to other persons. You should take appropriate preventive measures.

OVERDOSE

Symptoms: No cases of overdose have been reported.

What to Do: An overdose is unlikely to occur. Nonetheless, if you have any reason to suspect an overdose, call your doctor, emergency medical services (EMS), or the nearest poison control center.

▼ INTERACTIONS

DRUG INTERACTIONS
Nelfinavir should not be used concurrently with certain other drugs, because the combination could cause life-threatening heart abnormalities or prolonged loss of consciousness. These drugs include astemizole, cisapride, midazolam, oral contraceptives, rifampin, amiodarone, quinidine, ergot derivatives (found in certain migraine medications), and triazolam. Other drugs may interact with nelfinavir, requiring some change in your drug regimen. Consult your doctor for specific advice if you are taking any other prescription or over-the-counter medication, especially anticonvulsants (carbamazepine, phenobarbital, phenytoin), indinavir, ritonavir, or rifabutin.

FOOD INTERACTIONS
Food improves the absorption of nelfinavir.

DISEASE INTERACTIONS
Consult your doctor for advice if you have any other medical condition, especially hemophilia. Use of nelfinavir can cause complications in patients with liver disease, as this organ works to remove the drug from the body.

≡ SIDE EFFECTS ≡

SERIOUS
High blood sugar (diabetes) has occurred in patients taking drugs of this class, although a cause-and-effect relationship has not been established. Contact your doctor if you develop increased thirst or excessive urination.

COMMON
Diarrhea, abdominal pain, low-grade fever, nausea, gas, skin rash.

LESS COMMON
Back pain, headache, loss of appetite, gastrointestinal bleeding, mouth ulcers, vomiting, arthritis, cramps, muscle pain, anxiety, depression, dizziness, insomnia, migraine headache, seizures, drowsiness, breathing difficulty, skin problems, eye disorders, loss of sexual function.

NEOMYCIN/POLYMYXIN B/BACITRACIN OPHTHALMIC

Available in: Ophthalmic ointment
Available OTC? No   **As Generic?** Yes
Drug Class: Antibiotic combination

▼ USAGE INFORMATION

WHY IT'S PRESCRIBED
To treat or prevent bacterial infections of the eye.

HOW IT WORKS
Ophthalmic neomycin/polymyxin B/bacitracin antibiotic combination kills bacteria by interfering with the genetic material of bacterial cells, thus preventing them from multiplying.

▼ DOSAGE GUIDELINES

RANGE AND FREQUENCY
Apply a thin strip of ointment every 3 to 4 hours for 7 to 10 days.

ONSET OF EFFECT
Unknown.

DURATION OF ACTION
Unknown.

DIETARY ADVICE
This medication can be used without regard to diet.

STORAGE
Store this medication in a tightly sealed container away from heat, moisture, and direct light.

MISSED DOSE
Apply it as soon as you remember. If it is near the time for the next dose, skip the missed dose and resume your regular dosage schedule. Do not double the next dose.

STOPPING THE DRUG
Use this drug as prescribed for the full treatment period, even if you begin to feel better before the scheduled end of therapy.

PROLONGED USE
You should see your doctor regularly for tests and examinations if you use this drug for a prolonged period.

▼ PRECAUTIONS

Over 60: No special problems are expected.

Driving and Hazardous Work: Do not drive or engage in hazardous work until you determine how the medicine affects your vision.

Alcohol: No special precautions are necessary.

Pregnancy: This combination antibiotic has not been shown to cause birth defects or other problems during pregnancy. Before taking this medication, tell your doctor if you are pregnant or plan to become pregnant.

Breast Feeding: This combination antibiotic has not been shown to cause problems in nursing babies.

Infants and Children: There is no information comparing the use of this combination antibiotic in infants and children with use in adults.

Special Concerns: To use the ointment, first wash your hands. Tilt your head back. Gently apply pressure to the inside corner of the eyelid and with the index finger of the same hand, pull downward on the lower eyelid to make a space. Put a short strip of ointment (about ⅓ inch long) into this space and close your eye. Apply pressure for 1 or 2 minutes while keeping the eye closed without blinking. Then wash your hands again. Make sure the tip of the applicator does not touch your eye, finger, or any other surface. If your symptoms do not improve in a few days or if they become worse, check with your doctor. Before you use this medication, tell your doctor if you have had an allergic reaction to neomycin, polymyxin B, bacitracin, or any related antibiotic.

OVERDOSE
Symptoms: No specific ones have been reported.

What to Do: An overdose of this combination antibiotic is unlikely to be life-threatening. If someone accidentally ingests the medicine, call your doctor, emergency medical services (EMS), or the nearest poison control center.

▼ INTERACTIONS

DRUG INTERACTIONS
Other drugs may interact with this combination antibiotic. Consult your doctor for specific advice if you are taking any other prescription or over-the-counter medication.

FOOD INTERACTIONS
No known food interactions.

DISEASE INTERACTIONS
Caution is advised when taking this combination antibiotic. Consult your doctor if you have any other medical condition.

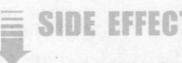

SIDE EFFECTS

SERIOUS
Itching, rash, redness, swelling, or other eye irritation that was not present before therapy. Stop using the medication and call your doctor immediately.

COMMON
Blurred vision for up to 30 minutes after application.

LESS COMMON
There are no less-common side effects associated with ophthalmic neomycin/polymyxin B/ bacitracin.

NEOMYCIN/POLYMYXIN B/BACITRACIN TOPICAL

Available in: Ointment
Available OTC? Yes **As Generic?** Yes
Drug Class: Antibiotic combination

▼ USAGE INFORMATION

WHY IT'S PRESCRIBED
To help prevent bacterial skin infections following minor cuts, abrasions, or burns.

HOW IT WORKS
This is a combination drug containing three distinct antibiotics that each attack and kill bacteria in a different way. Their combined, overlapping effect is capable of warding off infection by a variety of bacterial organisms.

▼ DOSAGE GUIDELINES

RANGE AND FREQUENCY
The usual treatment is to apply the ointment 2 to 5 times a day to areas of the skin that have suffered a minor injury. If you are using the prescription-strength form of the medication, follow your doctor's orders carefully; for over-the-counter forms, follow the directions on the label.

ONSET OF EFFECT
Unknown.

DURATION OF ACTION
Unknown.

DIETARY ADVICE
This medication can be used without regard to diet.

STORAGE
Store in a tightly sealed container away from heat and direct light. Keep away from moisture and extremes in temperature.

MISSED DOSE
Apply it as soon as you remember. However, if it is near the time for the next dose, skip the missed dose and resume your regular dosage schedule. Do not apply a double dose.

STOPPING THE DRUG
Use as prescribed for the full treatment period, even if the affected area begins to look and feel better before the scheduled end of therapy. If you stop treatment prematurely, the heartier strains of bacteria are likely to survive, reproduce, and cause a worse infection later (known as a "rebound infection").

PROLONGED USE
Consult your physician if you must use this medicine for a prolonged period.

▼ PRECAUTIONS

Over 60: No special precautions for older patients.

Driving and Hazardous Work: No special precautions are necessary.

Alcohol: No special precautions are necessary.

Pregnancy: Clinical studies of the use of this medication during pregnancy have not been done. Consult your doctor if you become or are planning to become pregnant.

Breast Feeding: It is not known whether this combination antibiotic passes into breast milk; caution is advised. Consult your doctor for specific advice.

Infants and Children: There is no information about use of this combination antibiotic in infants and children. However, no special problems are expected.

Special Concerns: Do not use this medication if you have a history of allergic reaction to any of the active or inactive ingredients in the ointment. If you use this medicine without a prescription, do not use it to treat puncture wounds, deep wounds, serious burns, or raw areas unless you have first consulted your doctor. Do not use this medicine in the eyes. Before you apply the medication, wash the affected area with soap and water and dry thoroughly. You may cover the treated area with a gauze bandage if you desire.

OVERDOSE
Symptoms: No specific ones have been reported.

What to Do: While no cases of overdose have been reported, if someone accidentally ingests this medicine, call your doctor, emergency medical services (EMS), or the nearest poison control center.

▼ INTERACTIONS

DRUG INTERACTIONS
Do not use other topical medications with this preparation unless otherwise instructed by your doctor.

FOOD INTERACTIONS
No known food interactions.

DISEASE INTERACTIONS
No disease interactions have been reported with the use of this combination antibiotic.

≡ SIDE EFFECTS ≡

SERIOUS
Rare, severe allergic reaction that may cause breathing difficulty or, at the extreme, total closure of the airways with potentially fatal anaphylactic shock. Contact emergency medical services (EMS) immediately. In very rare cases hearing loss may occur; if so, call your doctor immediately.

COMMON
No common side effects are associated with this medicine.

LESS COMMON
Irritation or skin allergy with burning, stinging, itching, redness, or rash. Contact your doctor as soon as possible if such side effects persist.

NEOMYCIN/POLYMYXIN B/HYDROCORTISONE OPHTHALMIC AND OTIC

Available in: Ophthalmic suspension, otic solution and suspension
Available OTC? No   **As Generic?** Yes
Drug Class: Antibiotic/corticosteroid combination

▼ USAGE INFORMATION

WHY IT'S PRESCRIBED
To treat or prevent bacterial infections of the eye or ear and to provide relief from eye or ear irritation and discomfort.

HOW IT WORKS
Ophthalmic and otic neomycin/polymyxin B/hydrocortisone kills bacteria by interfering with the genetic material of bacterial cells, preventing them from multiplying.

▼ DOSAGE GUIDELINES

RANGE AND FREQUENCY
Ophthalmic suspension—1 drop every 3 to 4 hours. Otic solution and suspension, for ear canal infection—Adults: 4 drops in the ear 3 to 4 times a day. Children: 3 drops in the ear 3 to 4 times a day.

ONSET OF EFFECT
Unknown.

DURATION OF ACTION
Unknown.

DIETARY ADVICE
No special restrictions.

SIDE EFFECTS

SERIOUS
Itching, rash, redness, swelling, or other eye or ear irritation that was not present before therapy. Call your doctor immediately.

COMMON
No common side effects have been reported with neomycin/polymyxin B/hydrocortisone.

LESS COMMON
Burning or stinging from the eye drops. There are no less-common side effects associated with the ear preparation.

STORAGE
Store in a tightly sealed container away from heat, moisture, and direct light. Do not allow it to freeze.

MISSED DOSE
Apply it as soon as you remember. However, if it is near the time for the next dose, skip the missed dose and resume your regular dosage schedule. Do not double the next dose.

STOPPING THE DRUG
Use this drug as prescribed for the full treatment period, even if you begin to feel better before the scheduled end of therapy.

PROLONGED USE
Do not use the ear medication for more than 10 days unless your doctor directs otherwise. If you use the eye medication for a prolonged period, you should see your doctor regularly for tests and examinations.

▼ PRECAUTIONS

Over 60: No special problems are expected.

Driving and Hazardous Work: Do not drive or engage in hazardous work until you determine how the medicine affects your vision.

Alcohol: No special precautions are necessary.

Pregnancy: This medication is not likely to cause problems unless absorbed into the bloodstream; consult your doctor for advice.

Breast Feeding: This combination medication has not been shown to cause problems in nursing babies.

Infants and Children: No special precautions.

Special Concerns: To use the eye drops, first wash your hands. Tilt your head back. Gently apply pressure to the inside corner of the eyelid and with the index finger of the same hand, pull downward on the lower eyelid to make a space. Drop the medicine into this space and close your eye. Apply pressure for 1 or 2 minutes while keeping the eye closed without blinking. To use the ear drops, lie down or tilt your head so the infected ear faces up. Gently pull the earlobe up and back for adults (down and back for children) to straighten the ear canal. Drop the medicine into the ear. Keep the ear facing upward for 5 minutes (2 minutes for children) after inserting the drops to allow the medicine to reach the infection. If necessary, insert a cotton ball to prevent the medicine from leaking out. Make sure the applicator for eye or ear drops does not touch your eye, ear, finger, or any other surface. If your symptoms do not improve in a few days or if they become worse, contact your doctor.

OVERDOSE

Symptoms: No specific ones have been reported.

What to Do: An overdose of this combination medication is unlikely to be life-threatening. If a large volume enters the eye, flush with water. If a large volume enters the ear or someone accidentally ingests the medicine, call your doctor, emergency medical services (EMS), or the nearest poison control center.

▼ INTERACTIONS

DRUG INTERACTIONS
Consult your doctor for specific advice if you are taking any other prescription or over-the-counter medication.

FOOD INTERACTIONS
No known food interactions.

DISEASE INTERACTIONS
Caution is advised when taking this combination antibiotic. Consult your doctor if you have any other eye or ear infection or medical problem.

NEOSTIGMINE

Available in: Tablets, injection
Available OTC? No   **As Generic?** Yes
Drug Class: Antimyasthenic; muscle stimulant

▼ USAGE INFORMATION

WHY IT'S PRESCRIBED
To provide temporary relief of the muscle weakness and fatigability associated with myasthenia gravis. It is also used sometimes to improve bladder or bowel function, particularly after surgery.

HOW IT WORKS
Neostigmine inhibits the activity of the enzyme cholinesterase, which breaks up acetylcholine, a neurotransmitter involved in muscle activity. Consequently, neostigmine increases the amount of available acetylcholine, which in turn improves muscle strength and endurance in patients with milder forms of myasthenia gravis. The drug's effect also improves the tone of the muscles controlling bladder or bowel activity.

▼ DOSAGE GUIDELINES

RANGE AND FREQUENCY
For myasthenia gravis— Adults and teenagers: Initial dose of tablets (neostigmine bromide) is 15 mg every 3 or 4 hours; maintenance dose is 150 mg every 24 hours in 1 or more doses. Injection (neostigmine methylsulfate): 500 micrograms (mcg) every few hours. Children: With tablets, 2 mg per 2.2 lbs (1 kg) of body weight per day in 6 to 8 doses; or by injection, 10 to 40 mcg per 2.2 lbs every 2 or 3 hours. For bowel and bladder conditions— Adults and teenagers: By injection, 250 to 500 mcg, as needed. Children's use and dosage must be determined by your pediatrician.

ONSET OF EFFECT
From 4 to 30 minutes for injection; 45 to 75 minutes for tablets.

DURATION OF ACTION
2 to 4 hours.

DIETARY ADVICE
Tablets should be taken with food or milk to reduce gastrointestinal upset.

STORAGE
Store in a tightly sealed container away from heat and direct light.

MISSED DOSE
Take it as soon as you remember. If it is near the time for the next dose, skip the missed dose and resume your regular dosage schedule. Do not double the next dose.

STOPPING THE DRUG
The decision to stop taking the drug should be made by your doctor.

PROLONGED USE
You should see your doctor regularly for tests and examinations if you take this drug for a prolonged period.

▼ PRECAUTIONS

Over 60: No special problems are expected.

Driving and Hazardous Work: Use of neostigmine should not impair your ability to perform such tasks safely.

Alcohol: No special warnings.

Pregnancy: Temporary muscle weakness has occurred in some babies whose mothers took neostigmine during pregnancy. Before you take neostigmine, tell your doctor if you are pregnant or plan to become pregnant.

Breast Feeding: Neostigmine is not believed to pass into breast milk. Consult your doctor for advice.

Infants and Children: No special problems are expected to occur with younger patients.

Special Concerns: Myasthenia gravis patients may be asked to keep a diary of when muscle weakness or other symptoms occur, to allow adjustment of dose size and timing.

OVERDOSE
Symptoms: Abdominal cramps, anxiety, blurred vision, clumsiness or unsteadiness, diarrhea, sweating, excessive salivation, panic attack, progressive muscle weakness leading to paralysis, muscle cramps or twitching, unusual irritability or nervousness, unusual tiredness or weakness, urgent need to urinate.

What to Do: Call your doctor, emergency medical services (EMS), or the nearest poison control center immediately.

▼ INTERACTIONS

DRUG INTERACTIONS
Consult your physician for specific advice if you are taking demecarium, echothiophate, isoflurophate, malathion, guanadrel, guanethidine, procainamide, or trimethaphan.

FOOD INTERACTIONS
No known food interactions.

DISEASE INTERACTIONS
Caution is advised when taking neostigmine. Consult your doctor if you have a history of intestinal blockage, urinary tract blockage, or a current urinary tract infection.

 SIDE EFFECTS

SERIOUS
Skin rash; itching; hives; breathing difficulty; asthmatic wheezing; swelling of the tongue, lips, and throat. Call your doctor right away.

COMMON
Diarrhea, increased sweating, increased watering of mouth, nausea or vomiting, stomach pain or cramps.

LESS COMMON
Increased bronchial secretions, unusual watering of eyes, unusually constricted pupils, gas, increased urination, flushing, weakness.

NEVIRAPINE

Available in: Tablets
Available OTC? No   **As Generic?** No
Drug Class: Antiviral

BRAND NAME

Viramune

▼ USAGE INFORMATION

WHY IT'S PRESCRIBED
To treat HIV infection in combination with other drugs. While not a cure for HIV, such drugs may suppress the replication of the virus and delay the progression of the disease.

HOW IT WORKS
Nevirapine interferes with the activity of enzymes needed for the replication of DNA in viral cells, thus preventing the human immunodeficiency virus (HIV) from reproducing.

▼ DOSAGE GUIDELINES

RANGE AND FREQUENCY
To start, 200 mg once a day, for 14 days; then 200 mg, 2 times a day. Nevirapine should be given in combination with other drugs for HIV, to delay the development of resistant strains of the virus.

ONSET OF EFFECT
Unknown. With most antiretroviral drugs, an early response can be seen within the first few days of therapy, but the maximum effect may take 12 to 16 weeks.

DURATION OF ACTION
Unknown. Effects of the drug may be prolonged if nevirapine is used in combination with other effective drugs and the virus is maximally suppressed.

DIETARY ADVICE
May be taken with or without food. Drink plenty of fluids.

STORAGE
Store in a tightly sealed container away from heat and direct light.

MISSED DOSE
Take it as soon as you remember. If it is near the time for the next dose, skip the missed dose and resume your regular dosage schedule. Do not double the next dose.

STOPPING THE DRUG
The decision to stop taking the drug should be made in consultation with your doctor.

PROLONGED USE
See your doctor regularly for tests and examinations if you must use this medicine for a prolonged period.

▼ PRECAUTIONS

Over 60: It is not known whether nevirapine causes different or more severe side effects in older patients than it does in younger persons.

Driving and Hazardous Work: Do not drive or engage in hazardous work until you determine how the medicine affects you.

Alcohol: Avoid alcohol if liver function is impaired.

Pregnancy: Nevirapine has been shown to cause birth defects in animals. Adequate human studies have not been done. Nevertheless, nevirapine is increasingly being used in combination with other antiretroviral drugs to treat HIV-infected women who are pregnant.

Breast Feeding: Women infected with HIV should not breast feed, to avoid transmitting the virus to an uninfected child.

Infants and Children: Safety and effectiveness of nevirapine in infants and children have not been established. Use and dose must be determined by your pediatrician.

Special Concerns: Patients who stop nevirapine therapy for more than 7 days should resume with 200 mg once a day for 7 days, then 200 mg once a day for 14 days, then 200 mg, twice a day. Patients taking nevirapine should not use oral contraceptives, but should use another method of birth control, such as condoms.

OVERDOSE
Symptoms: No cases of overdose have been reported.

What to Do: An overdose of nevirapine is unlikely to occur. Nonetheless, if you have any reason to suspect an overdose, call your doctor, emergency medical services (EMS), or the nearest poison control center.

▼ INTERACTIONS

DRUG INTERACTIONS
Consult your doctor for specific advice if you are taking cimetidine, estrogen-containing oral contraceptives, macrolide antibiotics, rifabutin, rifampin, methadone, or any other prescription or over-the-counter drug.

FOOD INTERACTIONS
No known food interactions.

DISEASE INTERACTIONS
Consult your physician if you have any other medical condition. Use of nevirapine may cause complications in patients with liver or kidney disease, since these organs work together to remove the medication from the body.

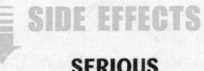

SIDE EFFECTS

SERIOUS
Severe skin rash, sometimes with peeling of skin and mucous membranes; yellowish tinge to eyes or skin (indicating liver damage); muscle or joint pain; inflammation of the tissue surrounding the eye. If such symptoms arise, call your doctor immediately.

COMMON
Mild to moderate skin rash (often with itching), abdominal pain or discomfort, diarrhea, nausea, headache.

LESS COMMON
Fever; mouth sores or ulcers; general ill feeling (malaise); inflammation of the tissue surrounding the eye; numbness, tingling, or prickling in the extremities.

NICARDIPINE HYDROCHLORIDE ORAL

Available in: Capsules, sustained-release capsules
Available OTC? No   **As Generic?** Yes
Drug Class: Calcium channel blocker

▼ USAGE INFORMATION

WHY IT'S PRESCRIBED
To prevent attacks of angina (chest pain associated with heart disease) and to control high blood pressure.

HOW IT WORKS
Nicardipine interferes with the movement of calcium into heart muscle cells and the smooth muscle cells in the walls of the arteries. This action relaxes blood vessels (causing them to widen), which lowers blood pressure, increases the blood supply to the heart, and decreases the heart's overall workload.

▼ DOSAGE GUIDELINES

RANGE AND FREQUENCY
For angina— Capsules: 20 mg, 3 times a day to start. For high blood pressure— Capsules: 20 to 40 mg, 3 times a day. Sustained-release capsules: 30 mg, 2 times a day. The dose may need to be increased.

ONSET OF EFFECT
Within 20 minutes.

DURATION OF ACTION
Capsules: 6 to 8 hours. Sustained-release capsules: Up to 12 hours.

DIETARY ADVICE
Nicardipine can be taken with or without food.

STORAGE
Store in a tightly sealed container away from heat and direct light.

MISSED DOSE
Take it as soon as you remember. If it is near the time for the next dose, skip the missed dose and resume your regular dosage schedule. Do not double the next dose.

STOPPING THE DRUG
Do not stop taking this drug suddenly, as this may cause potentially serious health problems. If therapy is to be discontinued, dosage should be reduced gradually, according to doctor's instructions.

PROLONGED USE
You should see your doctor regularly for examinations and tests if you take this medicine for a prolonged period. Remember that this medica-tion controls your high blood pressure but does not cure it. You may have to take nicardipine for the rest of your life.

▼ PRECAUTIONS

Over 60: Adverse reactions may be more likely and more severe in older patients.

Driving and Hazardous Work: Do not drive or engage in hazardous work until you determine how the medicine affects you.

Alcohol: Avoid alcohol.

Pregnancy: In animal studies, large doses of nicardipine have caused birth defects. Human studies have not been done. Before you take nicardipine, tell your doctor if you are pregnant or plan to become pregnant.

Breast Feeding: Nicardipine may pass into breast milk; caution is advised. Consult your doctor for advice.

Infants and Children: Safety and effectiveness have not been determined for young patients.

Special Concerns: In addition to taking nicardipine, be sure to follow all special instructions on weight control and diet. Your doctor will tell you which specific factors are most important for you. Check with your doctor before changing your diet.

OVERDOSE
Symptoms: Dizziness, slurred speech, nausea, vomiting, weakness, drowsiness, confu-sion, heart palpitations, nervousness or excitability.

What to Do: Call your doctor, emergency medical services (EMS), or the nearest poison control center immediately.

▼ INTERACTIONS

DRUG INTERACTIONS
Consult your physician for specific advice if you are taking acetazolamide, amphotericin B, corticosteroids, dichlorphenamide, diuretics, methazolamide, beta-blockers, carbamazepine, cyclosporine, procainamide, quinidine, digitalis drugs, disopyramide or the following eye medicines: betaxolol, levobunolol, metipranolol, or timolol.

FOOD INTERACTIONS
Avoid foods high in sodium.

DISEASE INTERACTIONS
Consult your doctor if you have abnormal heart rhythm or other disorders of the heart and blood vessels, mental depression, or Parkinson's disease. Use of nicardipine may cause complications in patients with liver or kidney disease, since these organs work together to remove the medication from the body.

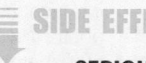

SIDE EFFECTS

SERIOUS
Breathing difficulty, coughing, or wheezing; irregular or pounding heartbeat; chest pain; fainting. Call your doctor immediately.

COMMON
Headache; dizziness; skin flushing and feeling of warmth; swelling in the feet, ankles, or calves; palpitations.

LESS COMMON
Constipation or diarrhea, nausea, unusual fatigue and weakness, skin rash, increased urination.

NICOTINE

Available in: Chewing gum, skin patch, nasal spray, inhaler
Available OTC? Yes **As Generic?** Yes
Drug Class: Smoking deterrent

▼ USAGE INFORMATION

WHY IT'S PRESCRIBED
To reduce nicotine withdrawal symptoms as part of a comprehensive smoking cessation program.

HOW IT WORKS
It replaces the nicotine that would otherwise be taken in by tobacco use.

▼ DOSAGE GUIDELINES

RANGE AND FREQUENCY
Used when you have the desire to smoke. Chewing gum: 20 to 24 mg a day; not to exceed 24 pieces of gum a day. Number of sticks is gradually reduced. Skin patch: To start, 1 patch supplying 22 to 24 mg a day. Dose is gradually reduced over 2 to 5 months. Nasal spray: 1 squirt (0.5 mg each, for a total dose of 1 mg) in each nostril as needed, no more than 80 times (40 mg) a day, for 3 to 6 months. Inhaler: Initially (up to 12 weeks), 6 to 16 cartridges a day. The number of cartridges per day is then gradually reduced over the next 6 to 12 weeks.

ONSET OF EFFECT
30 minutes to 2 hours.

DURATION OF ACTION
3 to 6 hours.

DIETARY ADVICE
Gum should be chewed slowly over 30 minutes. Other forms can be used without regard to diet.

STORAGE
Store in a tightly sealed container away from heat and direct light.

MISSED DOSE
If you are on a specific regimen, take a missed dose as soon as you remember. If it is near the time for the next dose, skip the missed dose and resume your regular dosage schedule. Otherwise, nicotine is taken as needed.

STOPPING THE DRUG
The decision to stop taking the drug should be made in consultation with your doctor. Dose for the patch should be tapered as directed.

PROLONGED USE
Treatment should generally not exceed 2 to 6 months. If relapse of smoking occurs, treatment may be repeated.

▼ PRECAUTIONS

Over 60: Adverse reactions are not expected to be more severe in older patients than in younger persons.

Driving and Hazardous Work: The use of nicotine should not impair your ability to perform such tasks safely.

Alcohol: No special warnings.

Pregnancy: Nicotine should not be used during pregnancy. Before you use nicotine, tell your doctor if you are pregnant or plan to become pregnant.

Breast Feeding: Nicotine passes into breast milk; do not use it while nursing.

Infants and Children: Should not be used. Even small amounts of nicotine can cause serious problems in infants and children.

Special Concerns: When disposing of patches, inhaler, or gum, be sure to use a method that keeps them out of the reach of children and animals. You should not smoke while being treated with nicotine. Do not apply a patch in the same place for at least a week. Do not inhale while spraying the nasal spray.

OVERDOSE
Symptoms: Nausea, vomiting, increased salivation, severe abdominal or stomach pain, diarrhea, severe headache, cold sweats, severe dizziness, hearing and vision disturbances, confusion, weakness, breathing difficulty, heartbeat irregularities, seizures, loss of consciousness.

What to Do: Call your doctor, emergency medical services (EMS), or the nearest poison control center immediately.

▼ INTERACTIONS

DRUG INTERACTIONS
Other drugs may interact with nicotine. Consult your doctor for specific advice if you are taking aminophylline, insulin, oxtriphylline, propoxyphene, or theophylline.

FOOD INTERACTIONS
No known food interactions.

DISEASE INTERACTIONS
Caution is advised when taking nicotine. Consult your doctor if you have a history of diabetes, dental problems (with gum), sinus problems or nasal allergies (with nasal spray), heart or blood vessel disease, inflamed mouth or throat (with gum), skin allergies (with patch), an overactive thyroid, pheochromocytoma, or stomach ulcer.

  SIDE EFFECTS

SERIOUS
With gum: Injury to mouth, dental work, or teeth. Call your dentist. With patch: Hives, itching, skin rash, or swelling. Call your doctor immediately.

COMMON
Mild headache; rapid heartbeat; increased appetite; increased salivation (with gum); sore mouth or throat; pain in jaw or neck; tooth problems (with gum and inhaler); belching (with gum); redness, burning, or itching at site of application (with patch); stinging in the nose (nasal spray).

LESS COMMON
Constipation, diarrhea, lightheadedness, dry mouth, hiccups (with gum), coughing (with inhaler), hoarseness (with gum and nasal spray), nervousness, irritability, loss of appetite, menstrual pain, joint or muscle pain, stomach upset, sweating, insomnia, unusual dreams, runny nose (with inhaler).

NIFEDIPINE

Available in: Extended-release tablets, capsules
Available OTC? No   **As Generic?** Yes
Drug Class: Calcium channel blocker

BRAND NAMES

Adalat, Adalat CC,
Procardia, Procardia XL

▼ USAGE INFORMATION

WHY IT'S PRESCRIBED
To treat high blood pressure and to prevent attacks of angina pectoris (chest pain associated with coronary artery disease).

HOW IT WORKS
Nifedipine interferes with the movement of calcium into heart muscle cells and the smooth muscle cells in the walls of the arteries. This action relaxes blood vessels (causing them to widen), which lowers blood pressure, increases the blood supply to the heart, and decreases the heart's overall workload.

▼ DOSAGE GUIDELINES

RANGE AND FREQUENCY
Extended-release tablets: 30 or 60 mg once a day. The doses may be increased as determined by your doctor.

ONSET OF EFFECT
Within 20 minutes.

DURATION OF ACTION
Extended-release tablets: 12 to 24 hours.

DIETARY ADVICE
Nifedipine can be taken with or without food.

STORAGE
Store in a tightly sealed container away from heat and direct light.

MISSED DOSE
Take it as soon as you remember. If it is near the time for the next dose, skip the missed dose and resume your regular dosage schedule. Do not double the next dose.

STOPPING THE DRUG
Do not stop taking this drug suddenly, as this may cause potentially serious health problems. If therapy is to be discontinued, the dosage should be reduced gradually, according to your doctor's instructions.

PROLONGED USE
You should see your doctor regularly for examinations and tests if you take this medicine for a prolonged period. Remember that this medication controls high blood pressure but does not cure it. You may have to take nifedipine for the rest of your life.

▼ PRECAUTIONS

Over 60:
Adverse reactions may be more likely and more severe in older patients.

Driving and Hazardous Work:
Do not drive or engage in hazardous work until you determine how the medicine affects you.

Alcohol:
Avoid alcohol.

Pregnancy:
In animal studies, large doses of nifedipine have been shown to cause birth defects. Human studies have not been done. Before you take nifedipine, tell your doctor if you are pregnant or plan to become pregnant.

Breast Feeding:
Nifedipine passes into breast milk but has not been reported to cause problems; caution is advised. Consult your doctor for specific advice.

Infants and Children:
While there is no specific information on the use of this medication in younger patients, the use of the capsules is not recommended.

Special Concerns:
In addition to taking nifedipine, be sure to follow all special instructions on weight control and diet. Your doctor will tell you which specific factors are most important for you. Check with your doctor before changing your diet.

OVERDOSE

Symptoms: Dizziness, slurred speech, nausea, weakness, drowsiness, confusion, abnormal heartbeat.

What to Do: Call your doctor, emergency medical services (EMS), or the nearest poison control center immediately.

▼ INTERACTIONS

DRUG INTERACTIONS
Consult your physician for specific advice if you are taking acetazolamide, amphotericin B, corticosteroids, dichlorphenamide, diuretics, methazolamide, beta-blockers, carbamazepine, cyclosporine, procainamide, quinidine, digitalis drugs, disopyramide or the following eye medicines: betaxolol, levobunolol, metipranolol, or timolol.

FOOD INTERACTIONS
Avoid foods high in sodium.

DISEASE INTERACTIONS
Caution is advised when taking nifedipine. Consult your doctor if you have any of the following: abnormal heart rhythm, other disorders of the heart and blood vessels, mental depression, or Parkinson's disease. Use of nifedipine may cause complications in patients with liver or kidney disease, since these organs work together to remove the medication from the body.

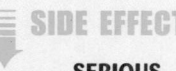

SIDE EFFECTS

SERIOUS
Breathing difficulty, coughing, or wheezing; irregular or pounding heartbeat; chest pain; fainting. Call your doctor immediately.

COMMON
Headache; dizziness; skin flushing and feeling of warmth; swelling in the feet, ankles, or calves; palpitations.

LESS COMMON
Constipation or diarrhea, nausea, unusual fatigue and weakness, skin rash, increased urination, vision problems.

NILUTAMIDE

Available in: Tablets
Available OTC? No   **As Generic?** No
Drug Class: Antiandrogen

▼ USAGE INFORMATION

WHY IT'S PRESCRIBED
Used in conjunction with surgical castration to treat cancer of the prostate.

HOW IT WORKS
The growth of some types of prostate tumors is stimulated by the hormone testosterone. Nilutamide blocks the activity of testosterone, thus slowing or halting the growth of such tumors. Testosterone is primarily manufactured in the testicles; surgical castration thus further reduces testosterone levels in the body.

▼ DOSAGE GUIDELINES

RANGE AND FREQUENCY
Adult males: To start, 300 mg once a day for 30 days; then 150 mg once a day.

ONSET OF EFFECT
Within hours.

DURATION OF ACTION
Unknown.

DIETARY ADVICE
No special restrictions.

STORAGE
Store in a tightly sealed container away from heat, moisture, and direct light.

MISSED DOSE
This drug is prescribed to be taken once a day. If you miss a day, skip the missed dose and resume your regular dosage schedule. Do not double the next dose.

STOPPING THE DRUG
Take it as prescribed for the full treatment period, even if you begin to feel better before the scheduled end of therapy. The decision to stop taking this drug should be made by your doctor.

PROLONGED USE
Nilutamide is not intended to be used on a long-term, ongoing basis. See your doctor regularly for evaluation of your condition for the duration of therapy with this drug.

▼ PRECAUTIONS

Over 60: The dosage may be reduced, because the medication takes longer to be eliminated from the body in older patients, but nilutamide is not otherwise expected to cause different side effects or problems in older persons than it does in younger people.

Driving and Hazardous Work: Do not drive or engage in hazardous work until you determine how the medicine affects you.

Alcohol: Avoid alcohol while using this medication.

Pregnancy: Not applicable; prostate cancer occurs only in men.

Breast Feeding: Not applicable; prostate cancer occurs only in men.

Infants and Children: Not applicable.

Special Concerns: Nilutamide treatment must start on the day of or the day after surgical castration is performed.

OVERDOSE
Symptoms: No specific ones have been reported.

What to Do: An overdose with nilutamide is unlikely to occur. If someone takes a much larger dose than prescribed, call your doctor, emergency medical services (EMS), or the nearest poison control center.

▼ INTERACTIONS

DRUG INTERACTIONS
The following drugs may interact with nilutamide. Consult your doctor for specific advice if you are taking vitamin K antagonists, phenytoin, or theophylline. Also tell your doctor if you are taking any other prescription or over-the-counter medication.

FOOD INTERACTIONS
No known food interactions.

DISEASE INTERACTIONS
Caution is advised when taking nilutamide. Consult your doctor for advice if you have severe respiratory problems or any other chronic or significant medical condition. Use of nilutamide may cause complications in patients with liver disease, since this organ works to remove the medication from the body.

SIDE EFFECTS

SERIOUS
Chest pain, difficulty breathing, fever, bone pain, cough, pneumonia. Call your physician immediately.

COMMON
Abdominal pain, headache, loss of appetite, decreased sex drive, nausea, constipation, difficulty of eyes adjusting to darkness, flushing or sensations of warmth.

LESS COMMON
Indigestion, flulike symptoms, vomiting, dry skin, rash, sweating, loss of body hair, difficulty of eyes adjusting to light, color blindness.

NIMODIPINE

Available in: Capsules
Available OTC? No   **As Generic?** No
Drug Class: Calcium channel blocker

▼ USAGE INFORMATION

WHY IT'S PRESCRIBED
To minimize neurological damage in the aftermath of a type of stroke known as subarachnoid hemorrhage (a ruptured blood vessel that spills blood into the space between the protective layers of membranes surrounding the brain).

HOW IT WORKS
Nimodipine prevents the constriction of smooth muscle tissue that surrounds the blood vessels, especially the arteries in the brain. This helps to keep cerebral arteries open, thus maintaining blood supply to brain tissue, preventing nerve cell death, and preserving function in the areas of the brain affected by the stroke.

▼ DOSAGE GUIDELINES

RANGE AND FREQUENCY
Adults: 60 mg every 4 hours, for 21 consecutive days.

ONSET OF EFFECT
Peak effects within 1 hour.

DURATION OF ACTION
Up to 4 hours.

DIETARY ADVICE
Nimodipine can be taken with or without food.

STORAGE
Store in a tightly sealed container away from heat and direct light.

MISSED DOSE
It is imperative to try not to miss a dose of nimodipine. However, if you do miss a dose, take it as soon as you remember. If it is near the time for the next dose, skip the missed dose and resume your regular dosage schedule. Do not double the next dose. If you miss more than one dose, contact your doctor.

STOPPING THE DRUG
Do not stop taking this drug suddenly, as this may cause potentially serious health problems. Therapy with nimodipine typically ends after 21 days, or as determined by your doctor.

PROLONGED USE
Prolonged use is not common; regular medical examinations and tests are necessary if you are required to take this medication for an extended period.

▼ PRECAUTIONS

Over 60: Adverse reactions may be more likely and more severe in older patients.

Driving and Hazardous Work: Do not drive or engage in hazardous work until you determine how the medicine affects you.

Alcohol: Avoid alcohol.

Pregnancy: Large doses of nimodipine have been shown to cause birth defects in animals. Human studies have not been done. Before you take nimodipine, tell your doctor if you are pregnant or plan to become pregnant.

Breast Feeding: Nimodipine may pass into breast milk but has not been reported to cause problems; caution is advised. Consult your doctor for advice.

Infants and Children: While there is no specific information on use of this medication in younger patients, no special problems are expected.

Special Concerns: To be effective, it is crucial to take nimodipine at the regularly scheduled times without fail.

OVERDOSE
Symptoms: Overdose of nimodipine has not been reported. Symptoms would likely be dizziness, confusion, or fainting.

What to Do: If someone takes a much larger dose than prescribed, call your doctor, emergency medical services (EMS), or the nearest poison control center right away.

▼ INTERACTIONS

DRUG INTERACTIONS
Some drugs may interact adversely with nimodipine. Consult your doctor for specific advice if you are taking antihypertensive drugs (beta-blockers or other calcium channel blockers), cimetidine, or fentanyl.

FOOD INTERACTIONS
No known food interactions.

DISEASE INTERACTIONS
Caution is advised when taking nimodipine. Consult your doctor if you have any of the following: abnormal heart rhythm or other disorders of the heart and blood vessels, mental depression, or Parkinson's disease. Use of nimodipine may cause complications in patients with liver or kidney disease, since these organs work together to remove the medication from the body.

≡ SIDE EFFECTS ≡

SERIOUS
Slow or irregular heartbeat, extreme dizziness, fainting, swelling of the extremities, breathing difficulty. Such side effects are rare but serious; call your doctor or emergency medical services (EMS) immediately.

COMMON
Flushing and feeling of warmth, headache.

LESS COMMON
Constipation or diarrhea, dizziness or lightheadedness, nausea, unusual fatigue.

NITROFURANTOIN

BRAND NAMES
Furadantin, Furalan, Furatoin, Macrobid, Macrodantin, Nitrofuracot

Available in: Capsules, oral suspension, tablets, extended-release capsules
Available OTC? No   **As Generic?** Yes
Drug Class: Anti-infective

▼ USAGE INFORMATION

WHY IT'S PRESCRIBED
To treat urinary tract infections (UTIs).

HOW IT WORKS
Nitrofurantoin interferes with bacterial metabolism and cell wall formation. Eventually the bacteria die out, bringing an end to the infection.

▼ DOSAGE GUIDELINES

RANGE AND FREQUENCY
Adults and teenagers— Capsules, oral suspension, tablets: 50 to 100 mg every 6 hours. Extended-release capsules: 100 mg every 12 hours. Children up to 12 years— Dosage must be determined by your doctor.

ONSET OF EFFECT
Within 1 hour.

DURATION OF ACTION
Capsules, oral suspension, tablets: 6 hours. Extended-release capsules: 24 hours.

DIETARY ADVICE
Nitrofurantoin should be taken with food or milk.

STORAGE
Store in a tightly sealed container away from heat and direct light. Keep the oral suspension from freezing.

MISSED DOSE
Take it as soon as you remember. If it is near the time for the next dose, skip the missed dose and resume your regular dosage schedule. Do not double the next dose.

STOPPING THE DRUG
Take as prescribed for the full treatment period, even if you begin to feel better before the scheduled end of therapy.

PROLONGED USE
See your doctor regularly if you must take this drug for a prolonged period.

▼ PRECAUTIONS

Over 60: Adverse reactions may be more likely and more severe in older patients.

Driving and Hazardous Work: Do not drive or engage in hazardous work until you determine how the medicine affects you.

Alcohol: Avoid alcohol.

Pregnancy: Nitrofurantoin should not be taken within several weeks of the delivery date or during labor.

Breast Feeding: Nitrofurantoin passes into breast milk; avoid use while breast feeding.

Infants and Children: Nitrofurantoin is not recommended for use by infants under 1 month old.

Special Concerns: Nitrofurantoin may cause false results in some urine sugar tests for diabetes. If your symptoms do not improve or instead become worse within a few days, check with your doctor. When taking the oral suspension, be sure to shake the container forcefully before each dose. Use a specially marked measuring spoon or other device to dispense each dose. A household teaspoon might not hold the correct amount. Tell your doctor if you have ever had an allergic reaction to nitrofurantoin or any related medicine, such as furazolidone, or if you are allergic to any other substance. When taking the extended-release capsule, swallow it whole without chewing.

OVERDOSE
Symptoms: Severe nausea, vomiting, diarrhea, loss of appetite.

What to Do: An overdose of nitrofurantoin is unlikely to be life-threatening. However, if someone takes a much larger dose than prescribed, call your doctor, emergency medical services (EMS), or the nearest poison control center.

▼ INTERACTIONS

DRUG INTERACTIONS
Consult your doctor for specific advice if you are taking acetohydroxamine, oral diabetes medicine, dapsone, furazolidone, methyldopa, procainamide, quinidine, sulfonamides, vitamin K, carbamazepine, chloroquine, cisplatin, cytarabine, vaccine for diphtheria, tetanus, and pertussis (DTP), disulfiram, ethotoin, hydrochloroquine, lindane, lithium, mephenytoin, mexiletine, pemoline, phenytoin, pyridoxine, vincristine, probenecid, sulfinpyrazone, quinine, or any other anti-infective agent.

FOOD INTERACTIONS
No known food interactions.

DISEASE INTERACTIONS
Consult your doctor if you have any of the following: glucose-6-phosphate dehydrogenase (G6PD) deficiency, kidney disease, lung disease, or nerve damage.

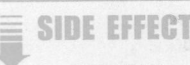
SIDE EFFECTS

SERIOUS
Chest pain, chills, cough, fever, troubled breathing, dizziness, drowsiness, tingling or burning of face or mouth, sore throat, unusual weakness, unusual fatigue. Call your doctor immediately.

COMMON
Abdominal pain or stomach upset, diarrhea, nausea, vomiting, loss of appetite.

LESS COMMON
Dark yellow or brownish urine.

NITROGLYCERIN

Available in: Capsules, tablets, ointment, skin patch, aerosol
Available OTC? No   **As Generic?** Yes
Drug Class: Nitrate

▼ USAGE INFORMATION

WHY IT'S PRESCRIBED
To prevent or relieve attacks of angina (chest pain associated with heart disease).

HOW IT WORKS
Nitroglycerin relaxes the smooth muscle that surrounds the blood vessels and increases the supply of blood and oxygen to the heart. It also reduces the heart's workload and demand for oxygen.

▼ DOSAGE GUIDELINES

RANGE AND FREQUENCY
Ointment: 15 to 30 mg applied to skin every 6 to 8 hours. Skin patch: 1 patch applied every day, left on for 12 to 14 hours. Aerosol: 1 or 2 doses on or under the tongue at 5-minute intervals to relieve angina attack. Extended-release capsules: 2.5, 6.5, or 9 mg every 12 hours; can be taken every 8 hours. Extended-release tablets: 1.3, 2.6, or 6.5 mg every 12 hours; can be taken every 8 hours. Sublingual (under tongue) or buccal (inside the cheek) tablets: 0.15 to 0.6 mg repeated at 5-minute intervals to treat angina attack. If 3 tablets do not relieve pain, consult your doctor.

ONSET OF EFFECT
Sublingual: 2 to 4 minutes. Buccal: 3 minutes. Oral: 20 to 45 minutes. Ointment and skin patch: 30 minutes.

DURATION OF ACTION
Sublingual: 30 to 60 minutes. Buccal: 5 hours. Oral: 8 to 12 hours. Ointment: 4 to 8 hours. Skin patch: Up to 24 hours.

DIETARY ADVICE
Oral forms used as a preventive should be taken 30 minutes before or 1 to 2 hours after meals.

STORAGE
Store in a tightly sealed container away from heat, moisture, and direct light.

MISSED DOSE
Take it as soon as you remember. If it is near the time for the next dose, skip the missed dose and resume your regular dosage schedule, as prescribed. Do not double the next dose.

STOPPING THE DRUG
The decision to stop taking nitroglycerin should be made by your doctor.

PROLONGED USE
You should see your doctor regularly for examinations and tests if you take this medicine for a prolonged period.

▼ PRECAUTIONS

Over 60: Adverse reactions may be more likely and more severe in older patients.

Driving and Hazardous Work: Do not drive or engage in hazardous work until you determine how the medicine affects you.

Alcohol: Avoid alcohol.

Pregnancy: Not recommended during pregnancy. Before taking nitroglycerin, be sure to tell your doctor if you are pregnant or plan to become pregnant.

Breast Feeding: Nitroglycerin may pass into breast milk; caution is advised. Consult your doctor for advice.

Infants and Children: No studies in infants and children have been done.

Special Concerns: Skin patch should be applied to different sites to prevent skin irritation.

OVERDOSE
Symptoms: Fast heartbeat, red and perspiring skin, headache, dizziness, palpitations, vision disturbances, nausea, vomiting, confusion, difficulty breathing.

What to Do: Call your doctor, emergency medical services (EMS), or the nearest poison control center immediately.

▼ INTERACTIONS

DRUG INTERACTIONS
Do not take nitroglycerin within 24 hours of taking sildenafil citrate. Sildenafil can enhance the action of nitrates (such as nitroglycerin), causing potentially dangerous decreases in blood pressure. Consult your doctor for specific advice if you are taking other heart medicines or drugs for hypertension.

FOOD INTERACTIONS
No known food interactions.

DISEASE INTERACTIONS
Consult your physician if you have any of the following: anemia, glaucoma, a recent head injury or stroke, a recent heart attack, or an overactive thyroid. Use of nitroglycerin may cause complications in patients with severe liver or kidney disease, since these organs work together to remove the medication from the body.

SIDE EFFECTS

SERIOUS
Blurred vision, severe or prolonged headache, skin rash, dry mouth. Call your doctor immediately.

COMMON
Flushing of face and neck, headache, nausea or vomiting, dizziness or lightheadedness when getting up, rapid heartbeat, restlessness.

LESS COMMON
Sore, reddened skin.

NIZATIDINE

Available in: Capsules, tablets
Available OTC? Yes   **As Generic?** No
Drug Class: Histamine (H2) blocker

▼ USAGE INFORMATION

WHY IT'S PRESCRIBED
To treat and prevent the return of ulcers of the stomach and duodenum, as well as conditions that cause increased stomach acid production (such as Zollinger-Ellison syndrome), gastroesophageal reflux (backwash of stomach acid into the esophagus, resulting in heartburn), and minor episodes of heartburn.

HOW IT WORKS
Nizatidine blocks the action of histamine (a compound produced in the body's cells), which in turn decreases the stomach's secretion of hydrochloric acid. Once stomach acid production has been decreased, the body is better able to heal itself.

▼ DOSAGE GUIDELINES

RANGE AND FREQUENCY
Adults and teenagers— To treat stomach ulcers: 300 mg once a day at bedtime, or 150 mg twice a day. To prevent the recurrence of duodenal ulcers: 150 mg once a day at bedtime. To treat gastroesophageal reflux: 150 mg, 2 times a day. To prevent minor cases of heartburn, acid indigestion, and sour stomach: 75 mg taken 30 to 60 minutes before a meal, once a day.

ONSET OF EFFECT
Within 30 minutes.

DURATION OF ACTION
Up to 12 hours.

DIETARY ADVICE
If you are taking two doses of nizatidine a day, the first dose can be taken after breakfast. Avoid foods that cause stomach irritation.

STORAGE
Store in a tightly sealed container away from heat and direct light.

MISSED DOSE
Take it as soon as you remember. If it is near the time for the next dose, skip the missed dose and resume your regular dosage schedule. Do not double the next dose.

STOPPING THE DRUG
Take the prescription-strength form for the full treatment period, even if you begin to feel better before the scheduled end of therapy.

PROLONGED USE
Do not take the maximum daily dosage continually for more than 2 weeks unless directed by your doctor.

▼ PRECAUTIONS

Over 60: Adverse reactions may be more likely and more severe in older patients.

Driving and Hazardous Work: Do not drive or engage in hazardous work until you determine how the medicine affects you.

Alcohol: Avoid alcohol.

Pregnancy: Risks vary, depending on patient and dosage. Consult your doctor.

Breast Feeding: Nizatidine passes into breast milk and may pose harm to the child; avoid or discontinue use while nursing.

Infants and Children: Nizatidine is not recommended for young patients, although it has not been shown to cause side effects or problems different from those in adults when used for short periods of time.

Special Concerns: Avoid cigarette smoking because it may increase stomach acid secretion and thus worsen the disease. Do not take nizatidine if you have ever had an allergic reaction to a histamine H2 blocker. If stomach pain becomes worse while using the drug, be sure to tell your doctor right away.

OVERDOSE

Symptoms: No cases of overdose have been reported.

What to Do: Although an overdose is unlikely, if someone takes a much larger dose than prescribed, call your doctor, emergency medical services (EMS), or the nearest poison control center right away.

▼ INTERACTIONS

DRUG INTERACTIONS
No significant drug interactions have been identified. However, nizatidine may increase blood levels of aspirin. Consult your doctor for specific advice if you are taking aspirin.

FOOD INTERACTIONS
Tomato-based mixed vegetable juices, carbonated drinks, citrus fruits and juices, caffeine-containing beverages, and other acidic foods or liquids may irritate the stomach or interfere with the therapeutic action of nizatidine.

DISEASE INTERACTIONS
Patients with kidney disease should not use nizatidine or should use it in smaller, limited doses under careful supervision by a physician.

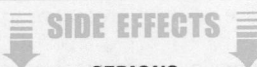

SIDE EFFECTS

SERIOUS
Irregular heart rhythm (palpitations); slowed heartbeat; severe blood problems, resulting in unusual bleeding, bruising, fever, chills, and increased susceptibility to infection. Call your doctor immediately.

COMMON
Headache, fatigue, drowsiness, dizziness, nausea, vomiting, abdominal pain, diarrhea, constipation.

LESS COMMON
Blurred vision, decreased sexual desire or function, swelling of breasts in males and females, temporary hair loss, hallucinations, depression, insomnia, skin rash, hives, or redness.

NORETHINDRONE

Available in: Tablets
Available OTC? No   **As Generic?** No
Drug Class: Progestin (hormone)

▼ USAGE INFORMATION

WHY IT'S PRESCRIBED
To prevent pregnancy; also used to treat menstrual disorders, such as amenorrhea (unexpected cessation of menstrual periods) and abnormal uterine bleeding, and to treat endometriosis.

HOW IT WORKS
Norethindrone prevents ovulation, probably by inhibiting secretion of pituitary hormones that in turn regulate menstrual and reproductive cycles. Norethindrone also alters activity of uterine cells, resulting in, among other changes, thickening of the cervical mucus. These changes make it less likely for a partner's sperm to reach and fertilize an egg.

▼ DOSAGE GUIDELINES

RANGE AND FREQUENCY
For contraception: 0.35 mg every day at the same time beginning on the first day of the menstrual period (28 days from the first day of the last menstrual period). For amenorrhea or abnormal uterine bleeding: 2.5 to 10 mg on days 5 through 25 of the menstrual cycle. For endometriosis: To start, 5 mg a day for 14 days. Your doctor may gradually increase your dose up to 15 mg a day for 6 to 9 months. Contact your physician as soon as your menstrual period begins.

ONSET OF EFFECT
Unknown.

DURATION OF ACTION
Unknown.

DIETARY ADVICE
No special restrictions.

STORAGE
Store in a tightly sealed container away from heat and direct light.

MISSED DOSE
When you are 3 hours or more late or miss 1 day's dose, take the missed dose immediately, resume your regular dosage schedule and use another method of contraception for 2 days. If you miss 2 doses, take 1 tablet immediately and use another method of birth control for 7 days. Do not double the next dose. For amenorrhea, abnormal uterine bleeding, and endometriosis: Take it as soon as you remember. If it is near the time for the next dose, skip the missed dose and resume your regular dosage schedule. Do not double the next dose.

STOPPING THE DRUG
If the medication was given to treat amenorrhea, abnormal uterine bleeding, or endometriosis, the decision to stop taking it should be made by your doctor.

PROLONGED USE
See your doctor regularly, usually every 6 to 12 months, for examinations and tests.

▼ PRECAUTIONS

Over 60: No special problems are expected.

Driving and Hazardous Work: The use of this drug should not impair your ability to perform such tasks safely.

Alcohol: No special precautions are necessary.

Pregnancy: This drug should not be taken during pregnancy. Problems including genital defects and smaller-than-normal body size have been reported in babies born to women who took progestins during pregnancy.

Breast Feeding: Norethindrone passes into breast milk but has not been shown to cause problems in the nursing child. Norethindrone may increase or decrease the quality or amount of breast milk. Low-dose progestins are recommended for contraception during breast feeding. Consult your doctor for specific advice.

Infants and Children: Progestins can been used for contraception by teenagers with no unusual adverse effects.

Special Concerns: Check with your doctor if vaginal bleeding continues for an unusually long time or if your menstrual period has not started within 45 days of the previous one.

OVERDOSE
Symptoms: None are known; no cases of overdose have been reported.

What to Do: An overdose with norethindrone is unlikely to occur. Emergency instructions are not applicable.

▼ INTERACTIONS

DRUG INTERACTIONS
Other drugs may interact with norethindrone. Consult your doctor for specific advice if you are taking aminoglutethimide, carbamazepine, phenobarbital, phenytoin, rifabutin, or rifampin.

FOOD INTERACTIONS
No known food interactions.

DISEASE INTERACTIONS
Consult your doctor if you have a history of any of the following: breast cancer (known or suspected), liver disease, thrombophlebitis, or thromboembolic disease.

SIDE EFFECTS

SERIOUS
Changes in menstrual bleeding pattern, mental depression, skin rash, unexpected or increased flow of breast milk. Call your doctor immediately.

COMMON
Abdominal pain or cramps; swollen face, ankles, or feet; mood changes; mild headache; nervousness; unusual fatigue; weight gain.

LESS COMMON
Acne, breast pain or tenderness, brown spots on skin, hot flashes, loss or gain of hair on body or scalp, loss of sexual desire, nausea, insomnia.

NORFLOXACIN

Available in: Eye drops, tablets
Available OTC? No   **As Generic?** No
Drug Class: Fluoroquinolone antibiotic

▼ USAGE INFORMATION

WHY IT'S PRESCRIBED
To treat urinary tract infections, sexually transmitted diseases, or eye infections caused by bacteria.

HOW IT WORKS
Norfloxacin inhibits the activity of a bacterial enzyme (gyrase) that is necessary for proper DNA formation and replication. This prevents bacteria cells from reproducing.

▼ DOSAGE GUIDELINES

RANGE AND FREQUENCY
For urinary tract infections: Adults: 400 mg, 2 times a day, for 3 to 21 days. For sexually transmitted diseases: 800 mg in a single one-time dose. For eye infections: 1 drop in each affected eye, 4 times a day, for 7 days.

ONSET OF EFFECT
Varies depending on the infection being treated.

DURATION OF ACTION
Unknown.

DIETARY ADVICE
Tablets should be taken on an empty stomach, 1 hour before or 2 hours after meals, with a full glass of water. Drink plenty of fluids, especially citrus juices or cranberry juice, but avoid milk and dairy derivatives.

STORAGE
Store in a tightly sealed container away from heat, moisture, and direct light.

MISSED DOSE
Take it as soon as you remember. If it is near the time for the next dose, skip the missed dose and resume your regular dosage schedule. Do not double the next dose.

STOPPING THE DRUG
It is very important to take this drug afor the full treatment period, even if you begin to feel better before the scheduled end of therapy.

PROLONGED USE
If your symptoms do not improve or instead become worse after a few days, consult your doctor promptly.

▼ PRECAUTIONS

Over 60: No special problems are expected.

Driving and Hazardous Work: Do not drive or engage in hazardous work until you determine how the medicine affects you.

Alcohol: It is advisable to abstain from alcohol when fighting an infection.

Pregnancy: In some animal tests, norfloxacin has caused birth defects. Adequate studies in humans have not been done. It should be used during pregnancy only if potential benefits clearly justify the risks. Before you take norfloxacin, tell your doctor if you are pregnant or plan to become pregnant.

Breast Feeding: Norfloxacin passes into breast milk and may cause serious side effects in the nursing infant; use of the drug is discouraged when nursing.

Infants and Children: Oral forms of fluoroquino-lones such as norfloxacin should not be used by persons under the age of 18. Norfloxacin eye drops should not be used by children under 1 year old.

Special Concerns: If norfloxacin makes your skin or eyes more sensitive to sunlight, wear sunglasses and protective clothing, use a sunscreen with an SPF (sun protection factor) of 15 or higher, and avoid excessive exposure to the sun.

OVERDOSE
Symptoms: Nausea, headache, dizziness, vomiting, drowsiness, seizures.

What to Do: Call your doctor, emergency medical services (EMS), or the nearest poison control center immediately.

▼ INTERACTIONS

DRUG INTERACTIONS
Consult your doctor for specific advice if you are taking aminophylline, antacids, cancer drugs, cyclosporine, didanosine, iron supplements, sucralfate, theophylline, or zinc salts.

FOOD INTERACTIONS
The effects of caffeine may be magnified by this drug. Milk and dairy products can reduce blood levels of norfloxacin by as much as half.

DISEASE INTERACTIONS
Caution is advised when taking norfloxacin. Consult your doctor if you have a disorder of the central nervous system or any other medical condition. Use of norfloxacin may cause complications in patients with kidney disease, since this organ works to remove the medication from the body.

≡ SIDE EFFECTS ≡

SERIOUS
Serious reactions to norfloxacin are rare and include seizures, mental confusion, hallucinations, agitation, nightmares, depression, shortness of breath, unusual swelling in the face or extremities, and loss of consciousness. Also skin burning, redness, blisters, rash, or itching on exposure to sunlight. Call your doctor immediately.

COMMON
Increased sensitivity to sunlight (and increased risk of sunburn) for days following therapy.

LESS COMMON
Diarrhea, nausea and vomiting, stomach pain and upset, gas, headache, dizziness, restlessness, insomnia, changes in taste perception, drowsiness, itching, dry mouth, unusual body aches or pains.

NORTRIPTYLINE HYDROCHLORIDE

Available in: Capsules, oral solution
Available OTC? No **As Generic?** Yes
Drug Class: Tricyclic antidepressant

▼ USAGE INFORMATION

WHY IT'S PRESCRIBED
To relieve symptoms of major depression, anxiety disorders, panic disorder, or chronic pain.

HOW IT WORKS
Nortriptyline affects levels of norepinephrine, a brain chemical that is thought to be linked to mood, emotions, and mental state.

▼ DOSAGE GUIDELINES

RANGE AND FREQUENCY
Adults: 25 mg, 3 to 4 times a day; may be increased to a maximum dose of 150 mg a day. Teenagers: 25 to 50 mg a day. Children ages 6 to 12: 10 to 20 mg a day. Older adults: 25 to 100 mg a day; may be increased gradually by your doctor. Dosage is usually determined by blood level monitoring.

ONSET OF EFFECT
1 to 6 weeks.

DURATION OF ACTION
Unknown.

DIETARY ADVICE
To lessen stomach upset, take with food, unless your doctor instructs otherwise. Increase intake of fiber and fluids.

STORAGE
Store in a tightly sealed container away from heat, moisture, and direct light. Do not allow solution to freeze.

MISSED DOSE
If you take a one-time daily bedtime dose, do not take the missed dose in the morning because it may cause drowsiness. Call your doctor for specific advice. If you take more than 1 dose a day, take it as soon as you remember. If it is near the time for the next dose, skip the missed dose and resume your regular dosage schedule. Do not double the next dose.

STOPPING THE DRUG
Take as prescribed for the full treatment period, even if you begin to feel better before the scheduled end of therapy. The decision to stop taking the drug should be made in consultation with your doctor.

PROLONGED USE
The usual course of therapy lasts 6 months to 1 year; some patients benefit from additional therapy.

▼ PRECAUTIONS

Over 60: Adverse reactions may be more likely and more severe in older patients. A lower dose may be warranted.

Driving and Hazardous Work: Use caution when driving or engaging in hazardous work until you determine how the medication affects you. Drowsiness or lightheadedness can occur.

Alcohol: Avoid alcohol.

Pregnancy: Adequate human studies have not been done. Consult your doctor for specific advice.

Breast Feeding: Nortriptyline passes into breast milk; do not use it while nursing.

Infants and Children: Not prescribed for children under the age of 6 years.

Special Concerns: This is a potentially dangerous drug, especially if taken in excess. Tricyclic antidepressants should not be within easy reach of suicidal patients. If dry mouth occurs, use candy or sugarless gum for relief.

OVERDOSE
Symptoms: Difficulty breathing, severe fatigue, seizures, confusion, hallucinations, dilated pupils, irregular heartbeat, fever, impaired concentration.

What to Do: Call your doctor, emergency medical services (EMS), or the nearest poison control center immediately.

▼ INTERACTIONS

DRUG INTERACTIONS
Consult your doctor for specific advice if you are taking antithyroid agents, cimetidine, clonidine, guanadrel, guanethidine, metrizamide, appetite suppressants, isoproterenol, ephedrine, epinephrine, amphetamines, phenylephrine, antipsychotic drugs, pimozide, methyldopa, metyrosine, metoclopramide, pemoline, promethazine, trimeprazine, rauwolfia alkaloids, MAO inhibitors, or any drugs that depress the central nervous system.

FOOD INTERACTIONS
No known food interactions.

DISEASE INTERACTIONS
Consult your doctor if you have any of the following: a history of alcohol abuse, difficulty urinating, asthma, bipolar disorder, high blood pressure, stomach or intestinal problems, glaucoma, overactive thyroid, enlarged prostate, schizophrenia, seizures, a blood disorder, or kidney, heart, or liver disease.

SIDE EFFECTS

SERIOUS
Confusion, heartbeat irregularities, hallucinations, seizures, extreme fatigue or drowsiness, blurred or altered vision, breathing difficulty, constipation, staring and absence of facial expression, impaired concentration, difficult urination, fever, extreme and persistent restlessness, loss of coordination and balance, difficulty swallowing or speaking, dilated pupils, eye pain, fainting. Also trembling, shaking, weakness, and stiffness in the extremities; shuffling gait. Call your doctor immediately.

COMMON
Drowsiness or dizziness, headache, dry mouth or unpleasant taste, fatigue, heightened sensitivity to light, weight gain, nausea, increased appetite.

LESS COMMON
Heartburn, sleeping difficulty, diarrhea, increased or profuse sweating, vomiting.

NYSTATIN

Available in: Lozenges, oral suspension, cream, ointment, powder, vaginal tablets
Available OTC? No   **As Generic?** Yes
Drug Class: Antifungal

▼ USAGE INFORMATION

WHY IT'S PRESCRIBED
To treat fungal infections of the skin, mouth, and vagina.

HOW IT WORKS
Nystatin prevents fungal organisms from producing vital substances required for growth and function. This medication is effective only for infections caused by fungal organisms. It will not work for bacterial or viral infections.

▼ DOSAGE GUIDELINES

RANGE AND FREQUENCY
Lozenges— Adults and children age 5 and older: 1 or 2 lozenges 4 to 5 times a day for up to 14 days. Lozenges should be allowed to dissolve in the mouth, which may take 15 to 30 minutes. Do not swallow. Suspension— Adults and children age 5 and older: 4 to 6 ml (1 teaspoon), 4 times a day. Children up to 5 years: 2 ml, 4 times a day. Premature and low-birth-weight infants: 1 ml, 4 times a day. Follow doctor's instructions for correct use. Cream, ointment, or powder— Adults and children: Apply to the affected area 2 to 3 times a day. Vaginal tablets— Adults and teenagers: Insert one 100,000-unit tablet into the vagina 1 or 2 times a day for 14 days.

ONSET OF EFFECT
Not applicable.

DURATION OF ACTION
Unknown.

DIETARY ADVICE
No special restrictions.

STORAGE
Store in a tightly sealed container away from heat, moisture, and direct light. Lozenges should be kept in the refrigerator, but keep them from freezing.

MISSED DOSE
Take it as soon as you remember. However, if it is near the time for the next dose, skip the missed dose and resume your regular dosage schedule. Do not double the next dose.

STOPPING THE DRUG
Take it as prescribed for the full treatment period, even if you begin to feel better before the scheduled end of therapy. The decision to stop taking the drug should be made by your doctor.

PROLONGED USE
Nystatin is generally prescribed for short-term therapy (1 to 3 weeks). Consult your doctor if your condition does not improve, or instead becomes worse, within 1 to 2 weeks of beginning therapy.

▼ PRECAUTIONS

Over 60: There have been no specific studies of the use of nystatin in older patients.

Driving and Hazardous Work: The use of nystatin should not impair your ability to perform such tasks safely.

Alcohol: No special precautions are necessary.

Pregnancy: Adequate studies of use during pregnancy have not been done. Consult your doctor for specific advice if you are pregnant or plan to become pregnant.

Breast Feeding: Nystatin may pass into breast milk; caution is advised. Consult your doctor for specific advice.

Infants and Children: The oral suspension should be used for children up to 5 years of age, rather than the lozenges. There have been no specific studies evaluating the use of the other forms of nystatin in children.

Special Concerns: Patients with dentures may have to soak them each night in nystatin to kill the fungus on the dentures. In some cases new dentures may be necessary.

OVERDOSE
Symptoms: Nausea, vomiting, diarrhea.

What to Do: Call your doctor, emergency medical services (EMS), or the nearest poison control center immediately.

▼ INTERACTIONS

DRUG INTERACTIONS
Other drugs may interact with nystatin. Consult your doctor for specific advice if you are taking any other prescription or over-the-counter drug.

FOOD INTERACTIONS
None known.

DISEASE INTERACTIONS
Consult your doctor for specific advice if you have any other medical condition.

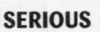 **SIDE EFFECTS**

SERIOUS
No serious side effects are associated with the use of nystatin.

COMMON
No common side effects are associated with the use of nystatin.

LESS COMMON
Nausea, vomiting, diarrhea, stomach pain, skin or vaginal irritation not present prior to therapy.

OCTREOTIDE ACETATE

Available in: Injection
Available OTC? No   **As Generic?** No
Drug Class: Hormone

▼ USAGE INFORMATION

WHY IT'S PRESCRIBED
To treat severe, chronic diarrhea that occurs with certain intestinal tumors (carcinoid tumors and vasoactive intestinal peptide tumors). Also used to treat acromegaly, a disease caused by the overproduction of human growth hormone during adulthood, and characterized by thick, bulky overgrowth of the bones in the hands, feet, forehead, and face.

HOW IT WORKS
Octreotide mimics the activity of the hormone somatostatin, which suppresses the release of certain chemicals that trigger diarrhea. The drug does not attack or cure intestinal cancer, but helps ease symptoms, allowing the patient to lead a more normal life. By suppressing the release of human growth hormone, octreotide slows the progression of acromegaly.

▼ DOSAGE GUIDELINES

RANGE AND FREQUENCY
For carcinoid tumor diarrhea: 100 to 600 micrograms (mcg) a day, administered subcutaneously (under the skin) in 2 to 4 doses. For vasoactive intestinal peptide tumors: 200 to 300 mcg a day in 2 to 4 doses. For acromegaly: From 50 to 300 mcg, 3 times a day. The dose is based on body weight.

ONSET OF EFFECT
Within 30 minutes.

DURATION OF ACTION
Up to 12 hours.

DIETARY ADVICE
No restrictions apply.

STORAGE
Store in a tightly sealed container away from heat and direct light. Keep away from moisture and extremes in temperature.

MISSED DOSE
Take it as soon as you remember. If it is near the time for the next dose, skip the missed dose and resume your regular dosage schedule. Do not double the next dose.

STOPPING THE DRUG
The decision to stop taking the drug should be made by your doctor.

PROLONGED USE
You should see your doctor regularly for tests and examinations if you take this drug for a prolonged period.

▼ PRECAUTIONS

Over 60: No special problems are expected.

Driving and Hazardous Work: Do not drive or engage in hazardous work until you determine how the medicine affects you.

Alcohol: Avoid alcohol.

Pregnancy: In animal studies, octreotide has not been shown to cause birth defects, even when given at high doses. Human studies have not been done. Consult your doctor for specific advice if you are pregnant or plan to become pregnant.

Breast Feeding: It is not known whether octreotide passes into breast milk; caution is advised. Consult your doctor for specific advice.

Infants and Children: Octreotide has not been shown to cause different side effects in infants and children than it does in other patients.

Special Concerns: Octreotide can cause either high or low blood sugar levels. Blood sugar should be monitored carefully. Follow your doctor's instructions about selecting and rotating injection sites to help prevent skin problems.

OVERDOSE
Symptoms: Very high or very low blood sugar levels.

What to Do: An overdose of octreotide is unlikely to be life-threatening. However, if someone takes a much larger dose than prescribed, call your doctor, emergency medical services (EMS), or the nearest poison control center.

▼ INTERACTIONS

DRUG INTERACTIONS
Consult your doctor for specific advice if you are taking antidiabetic agents, such as glucagon or insulin, or growth hormone.

FOOD INTERACTIONS
No known food interactions.

DISEASE INTERACTIONS
Consult your physician if you have diabetes mellitus, gallbladder disease, or gallstones. Use of octreotide may cause complications in patients with kidney disease, since this organ works to remove the medication from the body.

≡ SIDE EFFECTS ≡

SERIOUS
High blood sugar levels causing drowsiness, dry mouth, flushed and dry skin, fruity breath odor, increased urination, loss of appetite, severe stomach pain, nausea, or vomiting, rapid and deep breathing, unusual thirst, unusual fatigue, rapid weight loss. Low blood sugar levels causing anxiety, chills, cool and pale skin, difficulty concentrating, headache, nausea, nervousness, shakiness, sweating, unusual fatigue, weakness. Call your doctor immediately.

COMMON
Stomach or abdominal pain or discomfort; diarrhea, nausea and vomiting; pain, stinging, tingling, or burning at injection site; redness and swelling at the site of injection.

LESS COMMON
Dizziness or lightheadedness, unusual fatigue, headache, red or flushed face, swelling of feet and lower legs.

OFLOXACIN OPHTHALMIC

Available in: Ophthalmic solution
Available OTC? No   **As Generic?** No
Drug Class: Antibiotic

▼ USAGE INFORMATION

WHY IT'S PRESCRIBED
To treat bacterial conjunctivitis (infection of the mucous membranes that line the inner surface of the eyelids and whites of the eyes) or bacterial keratitis (infection of the cornea).

HOW IT WORKS
Ofloxacin kills bacteria by interfering with genetic material of bacterial cells, thus preventing them from multiplying.

▼ DOSAGE GUIDELINES

RANGE AND FREQUENCY
The exact dosing of ophthalmic ofloxacin varies depending on the nature of the infection and its response to treatment. Follow your doctor's instructions precisely. The following dosing example is for conjunctivitis. Adults and children 1 year of age and older: 1 drop in each eye every 2 to 4 hours, while awake, for 2 days, then 1 drop in each eye 4 times a day for up to 5 days.

ONSET OF EFFECT
Unknown.

DURATION OF ACTION
Unknown.

DIETARY ADVICE
No special restrictions.

STORAGE
Store in a tightly sealed container away from heat, moisture, and direct light. Do not refrigerate or allow it to freeze.

MISSED DOSE
Apply it as soon as you remember. If it is near the time for the next dose, skip the missed dose and resume your regular dosage schedule. Do not double the next dose.

STOPPING THE DRUG
Use it as prescribed for the full treatment period, even if you feel better before the scheduled end of therapy.

PROLONGED USE
You should see your doctor regularly for tests and examinations if you take this drug for a prolonged period.

▼ PRECAUTIONS

Over 60: No special problems are expected.

Driving and Hazardous Work: Do not drive or engage in hazardous work until you determine how the medicine affects your vision.

Alcohol: No special precautions are necessary.

Pregnancy: Large doses of ophthalmic ofloxacin have caused birth defects and other problems in animals. Human studies have not been done. Before you take ophthalmic ofloxacin, tell your doctor if you are pregnant or plan to become pregnant.

Breast Feeding: Ophthalmic ofloxacin may pass into breast milk; caution is advised. Consult your doctor for advice.

Infants and Children: Not recommended for use on children under age 1.

Special Concerns: To use the eye drops, first wash your hands. Tilt your head back. Gently apply pressure to the inside corner of the eyelid and with the index finger of the same hand, pull downward on the lower eyelid to make a space. Drop the medicine into this space and close your eye. Apply gentle pressure for 1 or 2 minutes while keeping the eye closed without blinking. Then wash your hands again. Make sure the tip of the dropper does not touch your eye, finger, or any other surface. If your symptoms do not improve in a few days or if they become worse, check with your doctor.

OVERDOSE
Symptoms: No specific ones have been reported.

What to Do: An overdose of ophthalmic ofloxacin is unlikely to be life-threatening. If a large volume enters the eye, flush with water. If someone accidentally ingests the medicine, call your doctor, emergency medical services (EMS), or the nearest poison control center immediately.

▼ INTERACTIONS

DRUG INTERACTIONS
Other drugs may interact with ophthalmic ofloxacin. Consult your doctor for specific advice if you are taking any other prescription or over-the-counter medication.

FOOD INTERACTIONS
No known food interactions.

DISEASE INTERACTIONS
Caution is advised when taking ophthalmic ofloxacin. Consult your physician if you have any other medical condition.

≡ SIDE EFFECTS ≡

SERIOUS
Itching, swelling, hives, difficulty breathing. If these signs of allergy develop, stop using the drug and call your doctor immediately.

COMMON
Burning eyes.

LESS COMMON
Increased sensitivity of eyes to light; stinging, itching, tearing, redness, or drying of the eye.

OFLOXACIN ORAL

Available in: Tablets
Available OTC? No   **As Generic?** No
Drug Class: Fluoroquinolone antibiotic

▼ USAGE INFORMATION

WHY IT'S PRESCRIBED
To treat mild to severe bacterial infections, including those of the urinary tract, lower respiratory tract (such as pneumonia), and the skin. It is also used to treat certain sexually transmitted diseases (chlamydia and gonorrhea) and prostatitis (infection and inflammation of the prostate).

HOW IT WORKS
Ofloxacin inhibits the activity of a bacterial enzyme (gyrase) that is necessary for proper DNA formation and replication. This fights infection by preventing bacteria cells from reproducing.

▼ DOSAGE GUIDELINES

RANGE AND FREQUENCY
For most infections: 200 to 400 mg, 2 times a day, for 3 to 10 days. For gonorrhea: 400 mg in a single one-time dose.

ONSET OF EFFECT
Varies depending on the infection being treated.

DURATION OF ACTION
Unknown.

DIETARY ADVICE
Take it on an empty stomach, 1 hour before or 2 hours after meals, with a full glass of water. Drink plenty of fluids.

STORAGE
Store in a tightly sealed container away from heat and direct light.

MISSED DOSE
Take it as soon as you remember. If it is near the time for the next dose, skip the missed dose and resume your regular dosage schedule. Do not double the next dose.

STOPPING THE DRUG
Take it as prescribed for the full treatment period, even if you begin to feel better before the scheduled end of therapy.

PROLONGED USE
See your doctor regularly for tests and examinations if you must take this medicine for a prolonged period. If your symptoms do not improve or instead get worse in a few days, consult your doctor.

▼ PRECAUTIONS

Over 60: No special problems are expected.

Driving and Hazardous Work: Do not drive or engage in hazardous work until you determine how the medicine affects you.

Alcohol: It is advisable to abstain from alcohol when fighting an infection.

Pregnancy: In some animal tests, ofloxacin has caused birth defects. Adequate studies in humans have not been done. It should be used during pregnancy only if potential benefits clearly justify the risks. Before you take ofloxacin, tell your doctor if you are pregnant or plan to become pregnant.

Breast Feeding: Ofloxacin passes into breast milk and may cause serious side effects in the nursing infant; use of the drug is discouraged when nursing.

Infants and Children: Ofloxacin is generally not recommended for use by persons under the age of 18, as it has been shown to interfere with bone development. But ofloxacin may be used by teenagers and younger persons if no alternative treatment is available.

Special Concerns: If ofloxacin causes unusual sensitivity to sunlight, wear protective clothing, use a sunblock and try to avoid exposure to sunlight, especially between 10 am and 3 pm. Do not take any antacid 2 hours before or 2 hours after taking ofloxacin.

OVERDOSE
Symptoms: Nausea, headache, dizziness, vomiting, drowsiness, seizures.

What to Do: Call your doctor, emergency medical services (EMS), or the nearest poison control center immediately.

▼ INTERACTIONS

DRUG INTERACTIONS
Consult your doctor for specific advice if you are taking aminophylline, antacids, didanosine, iron supplements, sucralfate, or zinc salts. Also tell your doctor if you are taking any other prescription or over-the-counter drug.

FOOD INTERACTIONS
No known food interactions.

DISEASE INTERACTIONS
Consult your doctor if you have any disease of the brain or spinal cord. Use of ofloxacin may cause complications in patients with liver or kidney disease, since these organs work together to remove the medication from the body.

SIDE EFFECTS

SERIOUS
Serious reactions to ofloxacin are rare and include seizures, mental confusion, hallucinations, agitation, nightmares, depression, shortness of breath, unusual swelling in the face or extremities, and loss of consciousness. Also skin burning, redness, blisters, rash, or itching on exposure to sunlight. Call your doctor immediately.

COMMON
Increased sensitivity to sunlight (and increased risk of sunburn) for days following therapy.

LESS COMMON
Diarrhea, nausea and vomiting, stomach pain and upset, gas, headache, dizziness, restlessness, insomnia, changes in taste perception, drowsiness, itching, dry mouth, unusual body aches or pains.

OFLOXACIN OTIC

Available in: Otic solution
Available OTC? No   **As Generic?** No
Drug Class: Antibiotic

▼ USAGE INFORMATION

WHY IT'S PRESCRIBED
To treat bacterial infections of the ear canal and the middle ear.

HOW IT WORKS
Ofloxacin inhibits the activity of a bacterial enzyme (gyrase) that is necessary for proper DNA replication and repair. Inhibition of this enzyme fights infection by preventing bacteria cells from reproducing.

▼ DOSAGE GUIDELINES

RANGE AND FREQUENCY
Ear drops should be administered 2 times a day, 12 hours apart, in the affected ear for 10 days (14 days for adults with chronic middle ear infection). Adults and teenagers should receive 10 drops in the affected ear per dose. Children ages 1 to 12 should receive 5 drops in the affected ear per dose.

ONSET OF EFFECT
Unknown.

DURATION OF ACTION
Unknown.

DIETARY ADVICE
The drug can be applied without regard to diet.

STORAGE
Store in a tightly sealed container away from heat, moisture, and direct light.

MISSED DOSE
Instill it as soon as you remember. If it is near the time for the next dose, skip the missed dose and resume your regular dosage schedule. Do not double the next dose unless your physician has instructed you to do otherwise.

STOPPING THE DRUG
Take it as prescribed for the full treatment period, even if your symptoms improve before the scheduled end of therapy.

PROLONGED USE
Ofloxacin is prescribed only for short-term use.

▼ PRECAUTIONS

Over 60:
No special problems are expected.

Driving and Hazardous Work:
No special precautions are necessary.

Alcohol:
No special precautions are necessary.

Pregnancy:
Adequate human studies have not been done. Before taking ofloxacin, discuss with your doctor the relative risks and benefits of using this drug while pregnant.

Breast Feeding:
It is not known whether ofloxacin passes into breast milk after administration to the ear; caution is advised. Consult your doctor for advice.

Infants and Children:
Not recommended for use by children under 1 year of age.

Special Concerns:
Gently clean any discharge from the outer ear prior to instilling the drops. Do not insert any object or swab into the ear canal. To use the ear drops, lie down or tilt your head so the infected ear faces up. For middle ear infections, the person instilling the drops should gently press the tragus (the small projection of cartilage in front of the ear canal) 4 times in a pumping motion to aid in the passage of the drops through the eardrum and into the middle ear. For ear canal infections, gently pull the earlobe up and back for adults (down and back for children) to straighten the ear canal. Drop the medicine into the ear. Keep the ear facing upward for 5 minutes after inserting the drops to allow the medicine to flow down into the ear canal and reach the infection. You may insert a cotton ball to prevent the medicine from leaking out. Make sure the applicator for the ear drops does not touch your ear, finger, or any other surface. When bathing, avoid getting the affected ear(s) wet. Avoid swimming unless your doctor has given you permission to do so.

OVERDOSE
Symptoms: An overdose with ofloxacin otic is unlikely to occur.

What to Do: If someone instills a much larger dose than prescribed or accidentally swallows ofloxacin otic, call your doctor.

▼ INTERACTIONS

DRUG INTERACTIONS
Do not take ofloxacin otic if you are allergic to ofloxacin or other fluoroquinolone antibiotics.

FOOD INTERACTIONS
None reported.

DISEASE INTERACTIONS
None reported.

≡ SIDE EFFECTS ≡

SERIOUS
No serious side effects are associated with the use of ofloxacin.

COMMON
Bitter taste in the mouth.

LESS COMMON
Earache, itching, skin rash, dizziness or lightheadedness, discomfort upon application.

OLANZAPINE

Available in: Tablets
Available OTC? No   **As Generic?** No
Drug Class: Neuroleptic; antipsychotic

▼ USAGE INFORMATION

WHY IT'S PRESCRIBED
To treat psychotic conditions (severe mental disorders characterized by distorted thoughts and perceptions, such as schizophrenia.

HOW IT WORKS
While the exact mechanism of action of olanzapine is unknown, it appears to alter the activity of certain chemicals in the central nervous system to produce a tranquilizing and antipsychotic effect.

▼ DOSAGE GUIDELINES

RANGE AND FREQUENCY
Initial dose is 5 to 10 mg, once daily. Dose may be increased by your doctor to a maximum of 20 mg a day.

ONSET OF EFFECT
Sedation may occur within minutes, but onset of antipsychotic effect may take hours to occur or may not occur until days or weeks after the beginning of therapy.

DURATION OF ACTION
12 to 24 hours, but effects may persist for several days.

DIETARY ADVICE
No special restrictions.

STORAGE
Store in a tightly sealed container away from heat, moisture, and direct light.

MISSED DOSE
Take it as soon as you remember. However, if it is near the time for the next dose, skip the missed dose and resume your regular dosage schedule. Do not double the next dose.

STOPPING THE DRUG
The decision to stop taking the drug should be made in consultation with your physician.

PROLONGED USE
Consult your doctor about the need for follow-up evaluations and tests if you must take this drug for an extended period. Because olanzapine is a recently released drug, its risk of inducing potentially irreversible tardive dyskinesia (involuntary movements of the jaw, lips, tongue, and body) is unknown.

▼ PRECAUTIONS

Over 60: No special problems are expected.

Driving and Hazardous Work: Do not drive or engage in hazardous work until you determine how the medicine affects you.

Alcohol: Avoid alcohol.

Pregnancy: Large doses of olanzapine reduced fetal survival in animal tests. Before you take olanzapine, tell your doctor if you are pregnant or plan to become pregnant.

Breast Feeding: Olanzapine may pass into breast milk; avoid use while breast feeding.

Infants and Children: The safety and effectiveness of olanzapine in children under 18 have not been established.

Special Concerns: Avoid prolonged exposure to high temperatures or hot climates. Drink plenty of fluids and stay cool in the summertime. Avoid overexposure to sunlight until you determine if the drug heightens your skin's sensitivity to ultraviolet light.

OVERDOSE
Symptoms: Extreme drowsiness, slurred speech.

What to Do: Call your doctor, emergency medical services (EMS), or the nearest poison control center immediately.

▼ INTERACTIONS

DRUG INTERACTIONS
The following drugs may interact with olanzapine. Consult your doctor for specific advice if you are taking carbamazepine, omeprazole, rifampin, high blood pressure medication, or any drugs that depress the central nervous system, including antihistamines, antidepressants or other psychiatric medications, barbiturates, sedatives, cough medicines, decongestants, and painkillers. Be sure your doctor knows about any over-the-counter medication you may take.

FOOD INTERACTIONS
No known food interactions.

DISEASE INTERACTIONS
Consult your doctor if you have Parkinson's disease or any movement disorder, glaucoma, epilepsy, liver disease, or kidney disease.

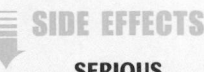

SIDE EFFECTS

SERIOUS
Stiffness; shuffling gait; difficulty swallowing or speaking; persistent, uncontrolled chewing, lip-smacking, or tongue movements; fever. Call your doctor immediately.

COMMON
Drowsiness, headache, dizziness, constipation, dry mouth, blurred vision, runny nose.

LESS COMMON
Stomach pain, unclear speech or stuttering, muscle tightness, faintness, increased appetite, increased cough, watering of mouth, insomnia, joint pain, nausea, sore throat, rapid heartbeat, increased thirst, urinary incontinence, vomiting, weight loss.

OLOPATADINE

BRAND NAME

Patanol

Available in: Ophthalmic solution
Available OTC? No   **As Generic?** No
Drug Class: Antihistamine

▼ USAGE INFORMATION

WHY IT'S PRESCRIBED
For temporary relief of itching of the eye due to allergic conjunctivitis (inflammation of the mucous membranes that line the inner surface of the eyelids and whites of the eyes).

HOW IT WORKS
Olopatadine inhibits the release and blocks the effects of histamine, a substance that causes swelling, itching, sneezing, watery eyes, hives, and other symptoms of allergic reaction.

▼ DOSAGE GUIDELINES

RANGE AND FREQUENCY
1 drop in each affected eye every 6 to 8 hours as needed.

ONSET OF EFFECT
Immediate.

DURATION OF ACTION
6 to 8 hours.

DIETARY ADVICE
No special restrictions.

STORAGE
Store in a tightly sealed container away from heat, moisture, and direct light. Do not allow it to freeze.

MISSED DOSE
Apply the next dose as needed; do not double the next dose.

STOPPING THE DRUG
This medication is to be used as needed for relief of itching associated with allergic inflammation. If you are not experiencing symptoms, do not apply the medication.

PROLONGED USE
See your doctor regularly for tests and examinations if you must take this drug for a prolonged period.

▼ PRECAUTIONS

Over 60: No special problems are expected.

Driving and Hazardous Work: Do not drive or engage in hazardous work until you determine how the medicine affects your vision.

Alcohol: Avoid alcohol.

Pregnancy: In animal studies, large doses of olopatadine did not cause birth defects. Human studies have not been done. Olopatadine should be used by pregnant women only if the potential benefit to the mother justifies the potential risk to the embryo or fetus. Consult your doctor for specific advice.

Breast Feeding: Olopatadine may pass into breast milk; caution is advised. Consult your doctor for advice.

Infants and Children: The safety and effectiveness of olopatadine in infants and children under the age of 3 have not been established.

Special Concerns: To use the eye drops, first wash your hands. Tilt your head back. Gently apply pressure to the inside corner of the eyelid and with the index finger of the same hand, pull downward on the lower eyelid to make a space. Drop the medicine into this space and close your eye. Apply pressure for 1 or 2 minutes while keeping the eye closed without blinking. Then wash your hands again. Make sure the tip of the dropper does not touch your eye, finger, or any other surface. If you use contact lenses, you should not wear them while administering olopatadine.

OVERDOSE
Symptoms: No specific ones have been reported.

What to Do: An overdose of olopatadine is unlikely to be life-threatening. However, if someone applies a much larger dose than prescribed or accidentally ingests the medicine, call your doctor, emergency medical services (EMS), or the nearest poison control center immediately.

▼ INTERACTIONS

DRUG INTERACTIONS
Other drugs may interact with olopatadine. Consult your doctor for specific advice if you are taking any other medication.

FOOD INTERACTIONS
No known food interactions.

DISEASE INTERACTIONS
Caution is advised when taking olopatadine. Consult your doctor if you have any medical condition, especially one affecting the eyes.

SIDE EFFECTS

SERIOUS
No serious side effects are associated with olopatadine.

COMMON
Headache, temporary burning and stinging of the eye.

LESS COMMON
Dry eyes, sensation of something in the eye, vomiting, swollen eyelids, itching of eyes.

OLSALAZINE SODIUM

Available in: Capsules
Available OTC? No   **As Generic?** No
Drug Class: Gastrointestinal anti-inflammatory

▼ USAGE INFORMATION

WHY IT'S PRESCRIBED
The first line of drug therapy for ulcerative colitis is usually sulfasalazine, but some patients cannot take it because of intolerable side effects. Olsalazine is a chemically similar drug that can be given instead to such patients. It is generally prescribed as maintenance therapy for those who have ulcerative colitis in a state of remission (absence of recent symptom flareups).

HOW IT WORKS
The exact mechanism of action is uncertain, although it appears that olsalazine inhibits production of substances such as arachidonic acid that produce inflammation in the digestive tract.

▼ DOSAGE GUIDELINES

RANGE AND FREQUENCY
500 mg, 2 times a day.

ONSET OF EFFECT
Unknown.

DURATION OF ACTION
Unknown.

DIETARY ADVICE
Olsalazine should be taken with meals to minimize stomach upset. If stomach or intestinal problems persist, consult your doctor.

STORAGE
Store in a tightly sealed container away from heat and direct light.

MISSED DOSE
Take it as soon as you remember, but only with meals. If it is near the time for the next dose, skip the missed dose and resume your regular dosage schedule. Do not double the next dose.

STOPPING THE DRUG
Take it as prescribed for the full treatment period, even if you begin to feel better before the end of therapy.

PROLONGED USE
You should see your doctor regularly for tests and examinations if you must take this drug for a prolonged period.

▼ PRECAUTIONS

Over 60: Olsalazine is not expected to cause different problems in older persons than in younger patients.

Driving and Hazardous Work: Do not drive or engage in hazardous work until you determine how the medicine affects you.

Alcohol: Avoid alcohol when taking this drug.

Pregnancy: Large doses of olsalazine have been shown to cause birth defects in animals. Human studies have not been done. The drug should be used during pregnancy only if its benefits clearly outweigh the potential risks. Before you take olsalazine, be sure to tell your doctor if you are pregnant or plan to become pregnant.

Breast Feeding: Olsalazine may pass into breast milk; caution is advised. In animal studies, olsalazine has been shown to cause slowed growth and other problems during nursing. Consult your doctor for specific advice about stopping breast feeding or switching to another drug.

Infants and Children: There is no information comparing use of olsalazine in infants and children with other age groups. Use and dosage must be determined by your pediatrician.

OVERDOSE

Symptoms: No cases of overdose with olsalazine have been reported.

What to Do: While an overdose is unlikely, call your doctor, emergency medical services (EMS), or the nearest poison control center immediately if you suspect someone has taken a dose much larger than prescribed.

▼ INTERACTIONS

DRUG INTERACTIONS
Consult your doctor for advice if you are taking any other prescription or over-the-counter medication. Olsalazine should not be used by patients who have had prior allergic reactions to aspirin or other salicylate drugs.

FOOD INTERACTIONS
No known food interactions.

DISEASE INTERACTIONS
Caution is advised when taking olsalazine. Consult your doctor if you have high blood pressure or kidney disease.

SIDE EFFECTS

SERIOUS
Severe pain in the back or stomach, bloody diarrhea, rapid heartbeat, fever, nausea or vomiting, rash, abdominal swelling or stiffness, yellowish tinge to the eyes or skin (jaundice). Call your doctor immediately if such symptoms occur.

COMMON
Abdominal pain or upset, an increase in the number of loose stools, diarrhea, loss of appetite.

LESS COMMON
Joint and muscle pain; acne; depression or anxiety; dizziness; drowsiness; headache; insomnia; skin sensitivity to sunlight; bruising; bleeding in the intestinal tract, causing bloody stools.

OMEPRAZOLE

Available in: Capsules
Available OTC? No　**As Generic?** No
Drug Class: Antacid/proton pump inhibitor

▼ USAGE INFORMATION

WHY IT'S PRESCRIBED
To treat duodenal (intestinal) ulcers, as well as conditions that cause increased stomach acid production (such as Zollinger-Ellison syndrome), erosive esophagitis (severe, chronic inflammation of the esophagus), and gastroesophageal reflux (backwash of stomach acid into the esophagus, resulting in heartburn).

HOW IT WORKS
Omeprazole blocks the action of a specific enzyme in the cells that line the stomach, thereby decreasing the production of stomach acid. Reduction of stomach acid promotes healing of ulcers.

▼ DOSAGE GUIDELINES

RANGE AND FREQUENCY
For duodenal ulcer, esophagitis, or gastroesophageal reflux: 20 mg per day. For Zollinger-Ellison syndrome or similar conditions: 60 mg per day.

ONSET OF EFFECT
Within 1 to 3 hours.

DURATION OF ACTION
At least 72 hours.

DIETARY ADVICE
Take omeprazole immediately before a meal. Capsules should be swallowed whole.

STORAGE
Store in a tightly sealed container away from heat and direct light.

MISSED DOSE
Take it as soon as you remember. If it is near the time for the next dose, skip the missed dose and resume your regular dosage schedule. Do not double the next dose.

STOPPING THE DRUG
Take it as prescribed for the full treatment period, even if you begin to feel better before the scheduled end of therapy. The decision to stop taking the drug should be made in consultation with your doctor.

PROLONGED USE
Omeprazole should not be used indefinitely as maintenance therapy for duodenal ulcer or esophagitis; it is generally taken for a limited period of 4 to 8 weeks. Do not take it for a longer period unless instructed to do so by your doctor. See your doctor regularly for tests and examinations if you must take this drug for an extended period of time.

▼ PRECAUTIONS

Over 60: No specific problems for older people have been reported.

Driving and Hazardous Work: Do not drive or engage in hazardous activities until you determine how the drug affects you.

Alcohol: Avoid alcohol while taking this medication, as it may aggravate your condition.

Pregnancy: In animal tests, omeprazole has not caused problems. Human tests have not been done. Before you take omeprazole, tell your doctor if you are pregnant or plan to become pregnant.

Breast Feeding: Omeprazole may pass into breast milk; caution is advised. Consult your doctor for advice.

Infants and Children: Use and dose for anyone under 18 should be determined by your doctor or pediatrician.

Special Concerns: Tell any doctor or dentist whom you see for treatment that you are taking omeprazole. Do not chew the capsules. If you have trouble swallowing them, you may open them and sprinkle the contents on applesauce or similar food. If your doctor directs, you may take an antacid along with omeprazole.

OVERDOSE
Symptoms: Blurred vision, confusion, profuse sweating, drowsiness, dry mouth, flushing of the face, head-ache, nausea, palpitations or unusually rapid heartbeat.

What to Do: Call your doctor, emergency medical services (EMS), or the nearest poison control center immediately.

▼ INTERACTIONS

DRUG INTERACTIONS
The following drugs may interact with omeprazole. Consult your doctor for specific advice if you are taking: ampicillin, sucralfate, iron salts or supplements, cyclosporine, diazepam, disulfiram, ketoconazole, phenytoin, or theophylline.

FOOD INTERACTIONS
No significant food interactions have been reported.

DISEASE INTERACTIONS
Caution is advised when taking omeprazole. Consult your doctor if you have liver disease, since it may increase the risk of side effects.

⬇ SIDE EFFECTS ⬇

SERIOUS
No serious side effects are associated with this medication.

COMMON
Diarrhea, constipation, vomiting, headache, dizziness, stomach pain. Consult your physician if such side effects persist or interfere with daily activities.

LESS COMMON
Bloody or cloudy urine, persistent or recurring sores or ulcers in the mouth, painful or very frequent urination, sore throat, fever, unusual bruising or bleeding, unusual weakness or tiredness, muscle pain, chest pain, nausea. Consult your doctor if such symptoms occur.

ONDANSETRON HYDROCHLORIDE

Available in: Tablets, oral solution, injection
Available OTC? No   **As Generic?** No
Drug Class: Antiemetic

▼ USAGE INFORMATION

WHY IT'S PRESCRIBED
To prevent nausea and vomiting that may occur after surgery or after treatment with anticancer medicine or radiation.

HOW IT WORKS
Ondansetron interferes with the chemical receptor sites and nerve pathways involved in the mechanisms that stimulate feelings of nausea and that induce vomiting.

▼ DOSAGE GUIDELINES

RANGE AND FREQUENCY
Tablets and oral solution— To prevent nausea and vomiting after anticancer medicine: Adults and teenagers: 8 mg or 2 teaspoons, 30 minutes before anticancer medicine is given, followed by 8 mg or 2 teaspoons, 8 hours after the first dose, then 8 mg or 2 teaspoons every 12 hours for 1 to 2 days. Children ages 4 to 12: 4 mg or 1 teaspoon, 30 minutes before anticancer medicine is given, followed by 4 mg or 1 teaspoon, 4 and 8 hours later, then 4 mg or 1 teaspoon every 8 hours for 1 to 2 days. To prevent nausea and vomiting after surgery: 16 mg or 4 teaspoons, 1 hour before anesthesia. To prevent nausea and vomiting after radiation treatment: 8 mg or 2 teaspoons, 1 to 2 hours before undergoing treatment; 8 mg or 2 teaspoons every 8 hours each day that radiation treatment is administered. Injection— To prevent nausea and vomiting after anticancer medicine: Adults: 32 mg (or 68 micrograms [mcg] per lb of body weight) into a vein over 15 minutes starting 30 minutes before an anticancer drug is given. Inject again 4 hours and then 8 hours after the initial dose. Children ages 4 to 18: 68 mcg per lb of body weight into a vein over 15 minutes starting 30 minutes before the anticancer medicine is given. To prevent nausea and vomiting after surgery: 4 mg into a vein or muscle from 30 seconds to 5 minutes before anesthesia.

ONSET OF EFFECT
Unknown.

DURATION OF ACTION
Unknown.

DIETARY ADVICE
Take the tablets with food.

STORAGE
Store in a tightly sealed container away from heat, moisture, and direct light.

MISSED DOSE
Take it as soon as you remember. If it is near the time for the next dose, skip the missed dose and resume your regular dosage schedule. Do not double the next dose.

STOPPING THE DRUG
The decision to stop taking the drug should be made by your doctor.

PROLONGED USE
You should see your doctor regularly for tests and examinations if you take this medicine for a prolonged period.

▼ PRECAUTIONS

Over 60: This drug has not been shown to cause different side effects or problems in older patients.

Driving and Hazardous Work: Do not drive or engage in hazardous work until you determine how the medicine affects you.

Alcohol: Avoid alcohol.

Pregnancy: Adequate human studies have not been completed. Before taking ondansetron, tell your doctor if you are pregnant or plan to become pregnant.

Breast Feeding: Ondansetron may pass into breast milk; caution is advised. Consult your doctor for advice.

Infants and Children: The dosage for children up to the age of 4 must be determined by your doctor.

OVERDOSE
Symptoms: No specific ones have been reported.

What to Do: An overdose of ondansetron is unlikely to be life-threatening. However, if someone takes a much larger dose than prescribed, call your doctor, emergency medical services (EMS), or the nearest poison control center.

▼ INTERACTIONS

DRUG INTERACTIONS
Consult your doctor for specific advice if you are taking drugs that alter liver function, such as phenobarbital or cimetidine. They may interact with ondansetron.

FOOD INTERACTIONS
No known food interactions.

DISEASE INTERACTIONS
Caution is advised when taking ondansetron. Consult your doctor if you have had recent abdominal surgery or have liver disease.

≋ SIDE EFFECTS ≋

SERIOUS
Chest pain, shortness of breath, skin rash, itching or hives, troubled breathing, tightness in chest, wheezing. Call your doctor immediately.

COMMON
Constipation or diarrhea, fever, headache.

LESS COMMON
Abdominal pain, stomach cramps, dizziness or lightheadedness, dry mouth, unusual fatigue or weakness.

ORLISTAT

BRAND NAME

Xenical

Available in: Capsules
Available OTC? No   **As Generic?** No
Drug Class: Lipase inhibitor

▼ USAGE INFORMATION

WHY IT'S PRESCRIBED
To achieve weight loss and weight maintenance in the maintenance of obesity when used in conjunction with a reduced-calorie diet and appropriate physical activity. Orlistat is indicated for patients with an initial body mass index (BMI) of 30 or greater and in those with a BMI greater than 27 (see Special Concerns for information on BMI calculation) who also have other risk factors, such as high blood pressure, high blood cholesterol, and diabetes.

HOW IT WORKS
Orlistat inhibits the activity of lipases, intestinal enzymes required for the digestion of dietary fats. Orlistat prevents the breakdown of a portion of ingested fat. The undigested fat cannot be absorbed and is excreted in the feces. Full doses of orlistat reduce the absorption of fat by about 30%.

▼ DOSAGE GUIDELINES

RANGE AND FREQUENCY
120 mg (one capsule) 3 times a day at mealtime.

ONSET OF EFFECT
Within 24 to 48 hours.

DURATION OF ACTION
48 to 72 hours.

DIETARY ADVICE
Take with liquid during or up to one hour after each main meal containing fat. Follow a balanced, reduced-calorie diet. The daily intake of fat (approximately ⅓ of the calories), carbohydrate, and protein should be spread out over the three meals. If a meal is missed or contains no fat, the dose of orlistat can be skipped. Since orlistat can also reduce the absorption of fat-soluble vitamins, a multivitamin supplement (containing vitamins A, D, and E and beta-carotene) should also be taken once a day at least two hours before or after ingesting orlistat.

STORAGE
Store in a tightly sealed container away from heat, moisture, and direct light.

MISSED DOSE
If you miss a dose, take it if you remember within 1 hour of eating. However, if more than 1 hour has passed, skip the missed dose and return to your regular schedule. Do not double the next dose.

STOPPING THE DRUG
The decision to stop taking the drug should be made in consultation with your doctor.

PROLONGED USE
The safety and effectiveness of orlistat have not been determined beyond 2 years of use.

▼ PRECAUTIONS

Over 60: No studies have been done specifically on older patients.

Driving and Hazardous Work: The use of orlistat should not impair your ability to perform such tasks safely.

Alcohol: No special precautions are necessary.

Pregnancy: Adequate human studies have not been done. Before taking orlistat, tell your doctor if you are pregnant or plan to become pregnant.

Breast Feeding: It is unknown whether orlistat passes into breast milk. However, do not take the drug while nursing. Consult your doctor for advice.

Infants and Children: Safety and effectiveness have not been established for children under age 18.

Special Concerns: A medical cause for obesity (such as hypothyroidism) should be ruled out before taking orlistat. Consult your doctor or a nutritionist for information on a nutritionally balanced, reduced-calorie diet and an exercise program. The BMI can be calculated by dividing your weight in pounds by your height in inches squared, and then multiplying by 705.

OVERDOSE
Symptoms: No cases of overdose have been reported.

What to Do: An overdose with orlistat is unlikely. If someone takes a much larger dose than prescribed, call your doctor.

▼ INTERACTIONS

DRUG INTERACTIONS
The following drugs may interact with orlistat. Consult your doctor for specific advice if you are taking: cyclosporine, statin (cholesterol-lowering) drugs, warfarin, another weight-loss medication (such as sibutramine or phentermine), or any other prescription or over-the-counter medications.

FOOD INTERACTIONS
Orlistat reduces the absorption of fat-soluble vitamins A, D, E, and K and beta-carotene. Gastrointestinal side effects may increase following the consumption of high-fat foods or with a diet high in fat (more than 30% of the day's total calories from fat).

DISEASE INTERACTIONS
This drug should not be used if you have chronic malabsorption or gallbladder problems. Consult your doctor if you have an eating disorder (anorexia or bulimia).

 SIDE EFFECTS

SERIOUS
No serious side effects have yet been reported.

COMMON
Oily spotting, gas with discharge, fecal urgency, oily stool, anal leakage, increased defecation, fecal incontinence.

LESS COMMON
Abdominal pain or discomfort.

ORPHENADRINE CITRATE

Available in: Extended-release tablets, injection
Available OTC? No **As Generic?** Yes
Drug Class: Muscle relaxant

▼ USAGE INFORMATION

WHY IT'S PRESCRIBED
To relieve the stiffness, pain, and discomfort caused by sprains and strains, muscle spasms, or other muscle problems; sometimes used to ease the trembling associated with Parkinson's disease. Orphenadrine may be prescribed in conjunction with other treatment methods, such as physical therapy.

HOW IT WORKS
Orphenadrine depresses activity in the central nervous system (brain and spinal cord), which in turn interferes with the transmission of nerve impulses from the spinal cord to the muscles.

▼ DOSAGE GUIDELINES

RANGE AND FREQUENCY
Adults and teenagers— Extended-release tablets: 100 mg, 2 times a day, in the morning and evening. Injection: 60 mg injected into a muscle or vein every 12 hours as needed. Children— Use and dosage must be determined by your doctor.

ONSET OF EFFECT
With tablets, 1 hour; with injection, 5 minutes.

DURATION OF ACTION
More than 6 hours.

DIETARY ADVICE
It can be taken with or between meals. To avoid dry mouth, maintain adequate fluid intake and suck on ice chips if desired.

STORAGE
Store in a tightly sealed container away from heat and direct light.

MISSED DOSE
Take it as soon as you remember. If it is near the time for the next dose, skip the missed dose and resume your regular dosage schedule. Do not double the next dose.

STOPPING THE DRUG
The decision to stop taking the drug should be made by your doctor.

PROLONGED USE
See your doctor regularly for tests and examinations if you must take this drug for a prolonged period.

▼ PRECAUTIONS

Over 60: There is no specific information comparing use of orphenadrine in older patients with use in younger persons.

Driving and Hazardous Work: Avoid such activities until you determine how the medicine affects you.

Alcohol: Avoid alcohol while taking this drug because it may compound the sedative effect and may cause liver damage.

Pregnancy: Orphenadrine has not been reported to cause problems in pregnancy. Before you take orphenadrine, tell your doctor if you are pregnant or plan to become pregnant.

Breast Feeding: Orphenadrine may pass into breast milk but has not been reported to cause problems in nursing babies. Consult your doctor for advice.

Infants and Children: There is no specific information comparing use of orphenadrine in infants and children with use in older persons.

Special Concerns: If dry mouth occurs, use sugarless candy or gum, bits of ice, or a saliva substitute. If dry mouth persists for more than 2 weeks, consult your dentist. Do not take orphenadrine if you are allergic to any other skeletal muscle relaxant. Orphenadrine will intensify the effect of alcohol, sedatives, and other central nervous system depressants.

OVERDOSE
Symptoms: Heart rhythm disturbances, changes in mental state, drowsiness, seizures, pale or clammy skin, diminished urine output, loss of consciousness.

What to Do: Call your doctor, emergency medical services (EMS), or the nearest poison control center immediately.

▼ INTERACTIONS

DRUG INTERACTIONS
Consult your doctor for specific advice if you are taking tricyclic antidepressants or drugs that depress the central nervous system.

FOOD INTERACTIONS
No known food interactions.

DISEASE INTERACTIONS
Consult your doctor if you have a history of any of the following: disease of the digestive tract, enlarged prostate, rapid or irregular heartbeat, glaucoma, myasthenia gravis, urinary tract blockage, heart disease, or kidney or liver disease.

≡ SIDE EFFECTS ≡

SERIOUS
Fainting; palpitations or rapid heartbeat; fever; hives and severe swelling of face, lips, or tongue along with shortness of breath, chest tightness, or wheezing (indicating a potentially life-threatening allergic reaction); low blood counts. Seek medical help immediately.

COMMON
Dry mouth, drowsiness, dizziness.

LESS COMMON
Inability to pass urine; sores on lips, ulcers in mouth; abdominal cramps or pain; clumsiness; unsteady gait; confusion; constipation; diarrhea; nervousness or irritability; flushing or redness of face; headache; heartburn; hiccups; muscle weakness; nausea and vomiting; trembling; insomnia or fitful sleep; burning, red eyes; stuffy nose.

OSELTAMIVIR PHOSPHATE

Available in: Capsules
Available OTC? No   **As Generic?** No
Drug Class: Antiviral

▼ USAGE INFORMATION

WHY IT'S PRESCRIBED
To treat influenza type A or B. Oseltamivir can reduce the severity of symptoms and shorten the duration of flu episodes.

HOW IT WORKS
Oseltamivir is believed to interfere with the synthesis of the viral enzyme neuraminidase, which is needed in order for the virus to infect cells in the respiratory tract and elsewhere in the body. The drug affects only certain susceptible strains of the influenza type A or B viruses.

▼ DOSAGE GUIDELINES

RANGE AND FREQUENCY
75 mg twice a day for 5 days. Treatment should be initiated as soon as possible, and no longer than 2 days after the onset of signs or symptoms of the flu.

ONSET OF EFFECT
Unknown.

DURATION OF ACTION
Unknown.

DIETARY ADVICE
No special restrictions.

STORAGE
Store in a tightly sealed container away from heat, moisture, and direct light.

MISSED DOSE
Take it as soon as you remember. If it is near (within 2 hours) the time for the next dose, skip the missed dose and resume your regular dosage schedule. Do not double the next dose.

STOPPING THE DRUG
It is important to take oseltamivir for the full treatment period as prescribed. Do not stop taking the drug before the scheduled end of therapy even if you begin to feel better, as this may lead to a relapse.

PROLONGED USE
If your symptoms do not improve or if they become worse in a few days, consult your doctor for further evaluation.

▼ PRECAUTIONS

Over 60: No special problems are expected in older patients.

Driving and Hazardous Work: Do not drive or engage in hazardous work until you determine how the medication affects you.

Alcohol: No special precautions are necessary.

Pregnancy: Adequate studies have not been completed. Discuss with your doctor the relative risks and benefits of using this drug while pregnant.

Breast Feeding: Oseltamivir may pass into breast milk, although it is unknown if this poses any risks to the nursing infant. Consult your doctor for specific advice.

Infants and Children: The safety and effectiveness of this drug have not been established for children under the age of 18.

Special Concerns: This medication is not a substitute for a flu shot. Continue to receive your annual flu shot.

OVERDOSE
Symptoms: No cases of overdose have been reported. However, nausea and vomiting would be likely symptoms in the event of an overdose.

What to Do: If you have any reason to suspect an overdose, call your doctor, emergency medical services (EMS), or the nearest poison control center as soon as possible.

▼ INTERACTIONS

DRUG INTERACTIONS
No known drug interactions.

FOOD INTERACTIONS
No known food interactions.

DISEASE INTERACTIONS
The dose of oseltamivir should be lowered in patients with significant kidney disease. Safety has not been determined in people with liver disease.

≡ SIDE EFFECTS ≡

SERIOUS
No serious side effects are associated with oseltamivir.

COMMON
Nausea and vomiting.

LESS COMMON
Bronchitis, insomnia, dizziness.

OXACILLIN

Available in: Capsules, oral suspension, injection
Available OTC? No   **As Generic?** Yes
Drug Class: Penicillin antibiotic

▼ USAGE INFORMATION

WHY IT'S PRESCRIBED
To treat a variety of bacterial infections, especially those caused by staphylococcus bacteria. Oxacillin is effective only against infections caused by bacteria; it is ineffective against those caused by viruses, fungi, or other microorganisms.

HOW IT WORKS
Oxacillin blocks the formation of bacterial cell walls, rendering bacteria unable to multiply and spread.

▼ DOSAGE GUIDELINES

RANGE AND FREQUENCY
Oral forms– Adults and children weighing more than 88 lbs: 500 to 1,000 mg every 4 to 6 hours. Children up to 88 lbs: 5.7 to 11.4 mg per lb of body weight every 6 hours. Injection– Adults and children weighing more than 88 lbs: 250 to 1,000 mg every 4 to 6 hours. Children under 88 lbs: 5.7 to 11.4 mg per lb of body weight every 4 to 6 hours. Infants: 2.8 mg per lb of body weight every 6 hours.

ONSET OF EFFECT
Immediate after intravenous injection; unknown for other forms.

DURATION OF ACTION
Unknown.

DIETARY ADVICE
Oral doses should be given at least 1 hour before or 2 hours after meals.

STORAGE
Store in a tightly sealed container away from heat and direct light. Liquid forms can be refrigerated but not frozen.

MISSED DOSE
Take it as soon as you remember. If it is near the time for the next dose, skip the missed dose and resume your regular dosage schedule. Do not double the next dose.

STOPPING THE DRUG
Take it as prescribed for the full treatment period, even if you begin to feel better before the scheduled end of therapy. Stopping the drug prematurely may slow your recovery or lead to a rebound infection, also known as superinfection, in which the heartier strains of bacteria survive and multiply, leading to a more serious and drug-resistant infection.

PROLONGED USE
Prolonged use of any antibiotic increases the risk of superinfection; caution is advised.

▼ PRECAUTIONS

Over 60: Oxacillin is not expected to cause different or more severe side effects in older patients than it does in younger persons.

Driving and Hazardous Work: The use of oxacillin should not impair your ability to perform such tasks safely.

Alcohol: No special warnings.

Pregnancy: Oxacillin and other penicillins have not caused birth defects in animals. Human studies have not been done. Before you take oxacillin, tell your doctor if you are pregnant or plan to become pregnant.

Breast Feeding: Oxacillin passes into breast milk; avoid use while nursing.

Infants and Children: No special problems expected.

Special Concerns: Before you have any medical test, tell the doctor in charge that you are taking oxacillin. It can cause false results on some urine sugar tests for diabetics. Oral contraceptives may not be effective while you are taking oxacillin. Use other methods of contraception to avoid an unplanned pregnancy.

OVERDOSE
Symptoms: Unusual muscle excitability, agitation, confusion, hallucinations, seizures, loss of consciousness, coma.

What to Do: Call your doctor, emergency medical services (EMS), or the nearest poison control center immediately.

▼ INTERACTIONS

DRUG INTERACTIONS
Consult your physician for specific advice if you are taking aminoglycosides, ACE inhibitors, diuretics, potassium supplements or potassium-containing medications, anticoagulants or other anti-clotting drugs, nonsteroidal anti-inflammatory drugs, sulfinpyrazone, cholestyramine, colestipol, oral contraceptives, methotrexate, probenecid, or rifampin.

FOOD INTERACTIONS
No known food interactions.

DISEASE INTERACTIONS
Consult your doctor if you have a history of allergies, congestive heart failure, gastrointestinal disorders (especially colitis associated with the use of antibiotics), or impaired kidney function.

  SIDE EFFECTS

SERIOUS
Irregular or fast breathing; fever; joint pain, lightheadedness; fainting; severely decreased urination; severe or bloody diarrhea; puffiness of face; redness of skin; shortness of breath; severe rash, hives, and itching; depression; unusual bleeding or bruising; yellow discoloration of the eyes or skin. Call your doctor immediately.

COMMON
Rash, mild diarrhea, nausea, vomiting, headache, sore tongue, sore mouth, vaginal discharge and itching, white patches in mouth.

LESS COMMON
Diminished urine output, chills, weakness, fatigue.

OXAPROZIN

Available in: Caplets
Available OTC? No   **As Generic?** No
Drug Class: Nonsteroidal anti-inflammatory drug (NSAID)

▼ USAGE INFORMATION

WHY IT'S PRESCRIBED
To treat mild to moderate pain and inflammation caused by tendinitis, arthritis, bursitis, gout, soft tissue injuries, migraine and other vascular headaches, menstrual cramps, and other conditions. When patients fail to respond to one NSAID, another may be tried. The greatest effectiveness often requires trial and error of several different NSAIDs.

HOW IT WORKS
NSAIDs work by interfering with the formation of prostaglandins, natural substances in the body that cause inflammation and make nerves more sensitive to pain impulses. NSAIDs also have other modes of action that are less well understood.

▼ DOSAGE GUIDELINES

RANGE AND FREQUENCY
Adults: 1,200 mg once a day. Maximum daily dose is 1,800 mg divided into smaller amounts taken 2 or 3 times a day. Children: Consult your pediatrician.

ONSET OF EFFECT
From 30 minutes to several hours or longer.

DURATION OF ACTION
Varies.

DIETARY ADVICE
Take with food; maintain your usual food and fluid intake.

STORAGE
Store in a tightly sealed container away from heat, moisture, and direct light.

MISSED DOSE
Take it as soon as you remember. If it is near the time for the next dose, skip the missed dose and resume your regular dosage schedule. Do not double the next dose.

STOPPING THE DRUG
The decision to stop taking the drug should be made in consultation with your doctor.

PROLONGED USE
Prolonged use can cause gastrointestinal problems, including ulceration and bleeding, kidney dysfunction, and liver inflammation. Consult your doctor about the need for medical examinations and laboratory tests.

▼ PRECAUTIONS

Over 60: Because of the potentially greater consequences of gastrointestinal side effects, the dose of NSAIDs for older patients, especially those over age 70, is often cut in half.

Driving and Hazardous Work: Avoid such activities until you determine how the medicine affects you.

Alcohol: Avoid alcohol when using this medication because it increases the risk of stomach irritation.

Pregnancy: Avoid or discontinue this drug if you are pregnant or plan to become pregnant.

Breast Feeding: Oxaprozin passes into breast milk; avoid use while nursing.

Infants and Children: May be used in exceptional circumstances; consult your doctor.

Special Concerns: Because NSAIDs can interfere with blood coagulation, this drug should be stopped at least 3 days prior to any surgery.

OVERDOSE
Symptoms: Severe nausea, vomiting, headache, confusion, seizures.

What to Do: Call your doctor, emergency medical services (EMS), or the nearest poison control center immediately.

▼ INTERACTIONS

DRUG INTERACTIONS
Do not take this drug with aspirin or any other NSAIDs without your doctor's approval. In addition, consult your doctor if you are taking antihypertensives, steroids, anticoagulants, antibiotics, itraconazole or ketoconazole, plicamycin, penicillamine, valproic acid, phenytoin, cyclosporine, digitalis drugs, lithium, methotrexate, probenecid, triamterene, or zidovudine.

FOOD INTERACTIONS
No known food interactions.

DISEASE INTERACTIONS
Consult your doctor if you have any of the following: bleeding problems, inflammation or ulcers of the stomach and intestines, diabetes mellitus, systemic lupus erythematosus (SLE, lupus), anemia, asthma, epilepsy, Parkinson's disease, kidney stones, or a history of heart disease or alcohol abuse. Use of oxaprozin may cause complications in patients with liver or kidney disease, since these organs work together to remove the medication from the body.

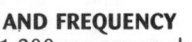 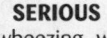

≣ SIDE EFFECTS ≣

SERIOUS
Shortness of breath or wheezing, with or without swelling of legs or other signs of heart failure; chest pain; peptic ulcer disease with vomiting of blood; black, tarry stools; decreasing kidney function. Call your doctor immediately.

COMMON
Nausea, vomiting, heartburn, diarrhea, constipation, headache, dizziness, sleepiness.

LESS COMMON
Ulcers or sores in mouth, depression, rashes or blistering of skin, ringing sound in the ears, unusual tingling or numbness of the hands or feet, seizures, blurred vision. Also elevated potassium levels, decreased blood counts; such problems can be detected by your doctor.

OXAZEPAM

Available in: Capsules, tablets
Available OTC? No   **As Generic?** Yes
Drug Class: Benzodiazepine tranquilizer; antianxiety agent

▼ USAGE INFORMATION

WHY IT'S PRESCRIBED
To treat anxiety and panic disorder. Also used to prevent alcohol withdrawal symptoms.

HOW IT WORKS
In general, oxazepam produces mild sedation by depressing activity in the central nervous system (brain and spinal cord). In particular, oxazepam appears to enhance the effect of gamma-aminobutyric acid (GABA), a natural chemical that inhibits the firing of neurons and dampens the transmission of nerve signals, thus decreasing nervous excitation.

▼ DOSAGE GUIDELINES

RANGE AND FREQUENCY
For anxiety— Adults: 10 to 30 mg, 3 or 4 times a day. Older adults: Initial dose of 10 mg, 3 times a day. The dose may be increased to a maximum of 15 mg, 4 times a day. For alcohol withdrawal symptoms— Dosage will be adjusted by your doctor on an individual basis.

ONSET OF EFFECT
30 minutes to 2 hours.

DURATION OF ACTION
8 to 12 hours.

DIETARY ADVICE
Oxazepam can be taken with food to prevent gastrointestinal upset.

STORAGE
Store in a tightly sealed container away from heat, moisture, and direct light.

MISSED DOSE
Take it as soon as you remember. If it is near the time for the next dose, skip the missed dose and resume your regular dosage schedule. Do not double the next dose.

STOPPING THE DRUG
Discontinuing the drug abruptly may produce withdrawal symptoms. The dosage should be reduced gradually according to your doctor's instructions.

PROLONGED USE
Short-term therapy (8 weeks or less) is typical; do not take it for a longer period unless so advised by your doctor.

▼ PRECAUTIONS

Over 60: A lower dose may be warranted.

Driving and Hazardous Work: Oxazepam can impair mental alertness and physical coordination. Adjust your activities accordingly.

Alcohol: Avoid alcohol.

Pregnancy: Use during pregnancy should be avoided if possible. Be sure to tell your doctor if you are pregnant or plan to become pregnant.

Breast Feeding: Oxazepam passes into breast milk; do not take it while nursing.

Infants and Children: Oxazepam should be used by children only under close medical supervision.

Special Concerns: Oxazepam use can lead to psychological or physical dependence. Never take more than the prescribed daily dose.

OVERDOSE
Symptoms: Extreme drowsiness, confusion, slurred speech, slow reflexes, poor coordination, staggering gait, tremor, slowed breathing, loss of consciousness.

What to Do: Call your doctor, emergency medical services (EMS), or the nearest poison control center immediately.

▼ INTERACTIONS

DRUG INTERACTIONS
Other drugs may interact with oxazepam. Consult your doctor for specific advice if you are taking any drugs that depress the central nervous system; these include antihistamines, antidepressants or other psychiatric medications, barbiturates, sedatives, cough medicines, decongestants, and painkillers. Be sure your doctor knows about any over-the-counter medication you may take.

FOOD INTERACTIONS
None known.

DISEASE INTERACTIONS
Consult your doctor if you have a history of alcohol or drug abuse, stroke or other brain disease, any chronic lung disease, hyperactivity, depression or other mental illness, myasthenia gravis, sleep apnea, epilepsy, porphyria, kidney disease, or liver disease.

≣ SIDE EFFECTS ≣

SERIOUS
Difficulty concentrating, outbursts of anger, other behavior problems, depression, hallucinations, low blood pressure (causing faintness or confusion), memory impairment, muscle weakness, skin rash or itching, sore throat, fever and chills, sores or ulcers in throat or mouth, unusual bruising or bleeding, extreme fatigue, yellowish tinge to eyes or skin. Call your doctor immediately.

COMMON
Drowsiness, loss of coordination, unsteady gait, dizziness, lightheadedness, slurred speech.

LESS COMMON
Change in sexual desire or ability, constipation, false sense of well-being, nausea and vomiting, urinary problems, unusual fatigue.

OXCARBAZEPINE

Available in: Tablets
Available OTC? No   **As Generic?** No
Drug Class: Anticonvulsant

▼ USAGE INFORMATION

WHY IT'S PRESCRIBED
To control partial seizures (those which begin with an abnormal burst of electrical activity in a small portion of the brain, often resulting in twitching or numbness in a localized part of the body), either alone or in conjunction with other anticonvulsant drugs, in people with epilepsy.

HOW IT WORKS
The mechanism of action is not well understood. It is believed that oxcarbazepine inhibits activity in certain parts of the brain and suppresses the abnormal firing of neurons that causes seizures.

▼ DOSAGE GUIDELINES

RANGE AND FREQUENCY
Adults— The drug should be taken in 2 equal doses per day. Monotherapy (use of oxcarbazepine alone): To start, 600 mg a day; dose should be increased by 300 mg a day every third day to a dose of 1,200 mg a day. Adjunctive therapy (use with other anticonvulsants): To start, 600 mg a day. If necessary, dose may be increased at weekly intervals by an additional 600 mg a day, up to 1,200 mg a day. Converting to monotherapy: This should be done in close consultation with your doctor. To start, 600 mg a day while simultaneously reducing dose of the other anticonvulsant. If necessary, oxcarbazepine's dose may be increased by a maximum of 600 mg a day at weekly intervals, up to 2,400 mg a day. Children ages 4 to 16— The drug should be taken in 2 equal doses per day. To start, 8 to 10 mg per 2.2 lbs (1 kg), but no more than 600 mg a day. The maintenance dose is dependent upon body weight. Your doctor will determine the appropriate dosage.

ONSET OF EFFECT
At least 2 to 3 days.

DURATION OF ACTION
Unknown.

DIETARY ADVICE
Can be taken without regard to meals.

≡ SIDE EFFECTS ≡

SERIOUS
No serious side effects are associated with the use of oxcarbazepine.

COMMON
Dizziness, drowsiness, fatigue, nausea, vomiting, indigestion, abdominal pain, double vision or other visual disturbances, coordination difficulties, abnormal gait, tremor.

LESS COMMON
Muscle weakness, insomnia, nervousness, speech and language difficulties, impaired hand-eye coordination, impaired concentration, acne.

STORAGE
Store in a tightly sealed container away from heat, moisture, and direct light.

MISSED DOSE
Take it as soon as you remember. If it is near the time for the next dose, skip the missed dose and resume your regular dosage schedule. Do not double the next dose.

STOPPING THE DRUG
Never stop this drug abruptly; this may cause seizures. The dose is typically tapered over a period of weeks.

PROLONGED USE
See your physician for periodic checkups.

▼ PRECAUTIONS

Over 60: Adverse reactions may be more likely and more severe in older patients.

Driving and Hazardous Work: This drug may cause drowsiness or dizziness, particularly in the first few weeks it is used. Exercise caution.

Alcohol: Avoid alcohol; it may contribute to excessive drowsiness.

Pregnancy: Oxcarbazepine has caused birth defects in animal studies. Human studies with this drug have not been done, but other anticonvulsants are known to increase the risk of birth defects. However, seizures during pregnancy can also increase the risks to the fetus. Discuss with your doctor the potential risks and benefits of using this drug during pregnancy.

Breast Feeding: Oxcarbazepine passes into breast milk. Discuss with your doctor the relative risks and benefits of using it while breast feeding.

Infants and Children: Not recommended for use by children under age 4.

Special Concerns: See your doctor for regular check-ups to detect the onset of any serious side effects. Periodic measurements of serum sodium may be required because the drug can lower sodium levels in the blood. Your doctor may advise you to carry an ID card or bracelet that says you are taking this drug. Oxcarbazepine may reduce the effectiveness of oral contraceptives; other means of contraception should be considered.

OVERDOSE
Symptoms: Few overdoses have been reported.

What to Do: If an excessive dose is taken, call your doctor, emergency medical services (EMS), or poison control center immediately.

▼ INTERACTIONS

DRUG INTERACTIONS
During combination therapy, it may be necessary to lower the dose of phenytoin.

FOOD INTERACTIONS
No known food interactions.

DISEASE INTERACTIONS
A lower dose of oxcarbazepine may be needed in patients with decreased kidney function or severe liver disease.

OXYBUTYNIN CHLORIDE

Available in: Syrup, tablets, extended-release tablets
Available OTC? No   **As Generic?** Yes
Drug Class: Antispasmodic

▼ USAGE INFORMATION

WHY IT'S PRESCRIBED
To decrease muscle spasms of the bladder and the frequent urination caused by the spasms.

HOW IT WORKS
Oxybutynin relaxes the muscle cells of the urinary tract and increases urinary bladder capacity.

▼ DOSAGE GUIDELINES

RANGE AND FREQUENCY
Syrup or tablets— Adults: 5 mg, 2 or 3 times a day. Children ages 5 to 12: 5 mg, 2 times a day. Dose may be gradually increased by your doctor to a maximum dose of 20 mg a day. Extended-release tablets— Adults: 5 mg once a day. Dose may be gradually increased by your doctor to a maximum dose of 30 mg a day.

ONSET OF EFFECT
30 to 60 minutes.

DURATION OF ACTION
6 to 10 hours. Extended-release: up to 24 hours.

DIETARY ADVICE
Take it with water on an empty stomach. It can, however, be taken with food to prevent stomach upset.

STORAGE
Store in a tightly sealed container away from heat and direct light. Keep the syrup form refrigerated, but do not allow it to freeze.

MISSED DOSE
Take it as soon as you remember. If it is near the time for the next dose, skip the missed dose and resume your regular dosage schedule. Do not double the next dose.

STOPPING THE DRUG
The decision to stop taking the drug should be made by your doctor.

PROLONGED USE
See your doctor periodically if you must take this drug for a prolonged period.

▼ PRECAUTIONS

Over 60:
Adverse reactions may be more likely and more severe in older patients.

Driving and Hazardous Work:
Avoid such activities until you determine how the medicine affects you.

Alcohol:
Avoid alcohol.

Pregnancy:
Oxybutynin has not been shown to cause birth defects in animals. Adequate human studies have not been done. Consult your doctor for advice.

Breast Feeding:
Oxybutynin has not been reported to affect nursing infants. However, nursing may be difficult since the medication can reduce the flow of breast milk.

Infants and Children:
The proper dose for children under the age of 5 has not been determined. The safety and effectiveness of the extended-release form have not been established in children under the age of 18.

Special Concerns:
Wear sunglasses and avoid exposure to bright light if the drug increases your sensitivity to sunlight. Use extra care not to become overheated during warm weather or exercise, since oxybutynin may interfere with the ability to sweat, increasing the risk of heat stroke. Use sugarless gum, candy, or ice chips to relieve dryness in the mouth, nose, and throat. If dryness persists for more than 2 weeks, check with your doctor or dentist.

OVERDOSE

Symptoms: Flushing, fever, confusion, clumsiness, severe drowsiness, rapid heartbeat, hallucinations, breathing difficulty, unusual nervousness, restlessness or irritability.

What to Do: An overdose of oxybutynin is unlikely to be life-threatening. However, if someone takes a much larger dose than prescribed, call your doctor, emergency medical services (EMS), or the nearest poison control center.

▼ INTERACTIONS

DRUG INTERACTIONS
Consult your doctor for specific advice if you are taking amantadine, anticholinergics, antidepressants, antidyskinetics (such as medication for Parkinson's disease or other movement disorders), antihistamines, antipsychotic medications, buclizine, carbamazepine, cyclizine, cyclobenzaprine, disopyramide, flavoxate, ipratropium, meclizine, methylphenidate, orphenadrine, procainamide, promethazine, quinidine, or trimeprazine.

FOOD INTERACTIONS
No known food interactions.

DISEASE INTERACTIONS
Consult your doctor if you have any of the following: severe bleeding, colitis, enlarged prostate, glaucoma, heart disease, severe and constant dryness of the mouth, hiatal hernia, high blood pressure, any intestinal or stomach problem, myasthenia gravis, toxemia of pregnancy, any problem with urination, or an overactive thyroid. Use of oxybutynin may cause complications in patients with liver or kidney disease, since these organs work together to remove the medication from the body.

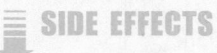

≡ SIDE EFFECTS ≡

SERIOUS
Eye pain, skin rash or hives. Call your doctor immediately.

COMMON
Constipation; decreased sweating; drowsiness; dry mouth, nose, and throat.

LESS COMMON
Blurred vision, decreased sexual ability, difficulty urinating, difficulty swallowing, headache, increased sensitivity of eyes to light, nausea or vomiting, insomnia, unusual fatigue, reduced flow of breast milk.

OXYCODONE HYDROCHLORIDE

Available in: Oral solution, tablets, controlled-release tablets
Available OTC? No   **As Generic?** No
Drug Class: Opioid (narcotic) analgesic

▼ USAGE INFORMATION

WHY IT'S PRESCRIBED
To relieve moderate to severe pain.

HOW IT WORKS
Opioids analgesics such as oxycodone relieve pain by acting upon specific areas of the central nervous system (the brain and spinal cord) that process pain signals from nerves throughout the body.

▼ DOSAGE GUIDELINES

RANGE AND FREQUENCY
5 mg every 3 to 6 hours, or 10 mg, 3 to 4 times a day as needed. Children: Dosages must be determined by your pediatrician. Controlled-release tablets: Your physician will determine the proper dosage.

ONSET OF EFFECT
10 to 15 minutes.

DURATION OF ACTION
3 to 6 hours.

DIETARY ADVICE
This medication can be taken with food or milk to lessen stomach upset.

STORAGE
Store in a tightly sealed container away from heat, moisture, and direct light. Do not freeze the liquid form.

MISSED DOSE
If you are taking oxycodone on a fixed schedule, take it as soon as you remember. If it is near the time for the next dose, skip the missed dose and resume your regular dosage schedule. Do not double the next dose.

STOPPING THE DRUG
The decision to stop taking the drug should be made by your doctor.

PROLONGED USE
You should see your doctor regularly for tests and examinations if you must take this medication for an extended period. Prolonged use can cause physical dependence.

▼ PRECAUTIONS

Over 60: Adverse reactions may be more likely and more severe in older patients.

Driving and Hazardous Work: Avoid such activities until you determine how the medicine affects you.

Alcohol: Avoid alcohol.

Pregnancy: Human studies have not been done. Before using this drug, tell your doctor if you are pregnant or plan to become pregnant. Overuse during pregnancy can cause drug dependence in the fetus.

Breast Feeding: Oxycodone may pass into breast milk; caution is advised. Consult your doctor for specific advice.

Infants and Children: Adverse reactions to oxycodone may be more likely and more severe in children. Consult your doctor for specific advice.

Special Concerns: If you feel the medication is not working properly after a few weeks, do not increase the dose. Consult your doctor. Before having any surgery, tell the doctor or dentist in charge that you are taking this drug. The controlled-release tablets are prescribed for use only in opioid-tolerant patients requiring daily doses of 160 mg or more.

OVERDOSE
Symptoms: Confusion; severe drowsiness, weakness, or dizziness; slurred speech; constricted pupils; cold, clammy skin; slow breathing; seizures; loss of consciousness.

What to Do: Call your doctor, emergency medical services (EMS), or the nearest poison control center immediately.

▼ INTERACTIONS

DRUG INTERACTIONS
Consult your doctor for specific advice if you are taking carbamazepine or other medicine for seizures, barbiturates, sedatives, cough medicines, decongestants, antidepressants, other prescription pain medications, MAO inhibitors, naltrexone, rifampin, or zidovudine.

FOOD INTERACTIONS
No known food interactions.

DISEASE INTERACTIONS
Consult your doctor if you have any of the following: a history of alcohol or drug abuse; emotional illness; brain disorders or head injury; seizures; lung disease; prostate problems or other problems with urination; gallstones; colitis; heart, kidney, liver, or thyroid disease.

SIDE EFFECTS

SERIOUS
Serious side effects of oxycodone are indistinguishable from those of overdose: Confusion; severe drowsiness, weakness, or dizziness; slurred speech; small, pinpoint pupils; cold, clammy skin; slow breathing; seizures; loss of consciousness.

COMMON
Dizziness or lightheadedness, nausea or vomiting, drowsiness, constipation, itching.

LESS COMMON
Swelling in the feet, sweating, false sense of well-being (euphoria), urinary retention.

OXYCODONE/ACETAMINOPHEN

Available in: Capsules, oral solution, tablets
Available OTC? No   **As Generic?** Yes
Drug Class: Opioid (narcotic) analgesic

▼ USAGE INFORMATION

WHY IT'S PRESCRIBED
To relieve moderate to severe pain when nonprescription pain relievers prove inadequate. A narcotic analgesic such as oxycodone, in combination with acetaminophen, may provide better pain relief than either medicine used alone. Used together, relief may be achieved at lower doses of the two drugs.

HOW IT WORKS
Opioids such as oxycodone relieve pain by acting on specific areas of the central nervous system (brain and spinal cord) that process pain signals from nerves throughout the body. Acetaminophen appears to interfere with the action of prostaglandins, naturally occurring substances in the body that cause inflammation and make nerves more sensitive to pain impulses.

▼ DOSAGE GUIDELINES

RANGE AND FREQUENCY
Adults: 1 capsule or tablet every 4 to 6 hours, or 1 teaspoon of the oral solution every 4 to 6 hours.

ONSET OF EFFECT
Unknown.

DURATION OF ACTION
Unknown.

DIETARY ADVICE
This medication can be taken with food or milk to lessen stomach irritation.

STORAGE
Store in a tightly sealed container away from heat, moisture, and direct light.

MISSED DOSE
If you are taking the drug on a fixed schedule, take it as soon as you remember. However, if it is near the time for the next dose, skip the missed dose and resume your regular dosage schedule. Do not double the next dose.

STOPPING THE DRUG
The decision to stop taking the drug should be made by your doctor.

PROLONGED USE
See your doctor regularly for examinations and laboratory tests if long-term therapy is required. Prolonged use of narcotic drugs can cause physical dependence; prolonged use of acetaminophen at high doses can cause liver damage.

▼ PRECAUTIONS

Over 60: Adverse reactions may be more likely and more severe in older patients.

Driving and Hazardous Work: Do not drive or engage in hazardous work until you determine how the medicine affects you.

Alcohol: Avoid alcohol.

Pregnancy: Human studies have not been done. Before you use this drug, tell your doctor if you are pregnant or plan to become pregnant. Overuse of the medication during pregnancy can cause drug dependence in the fetus.

Breast Feeding: It is not known whether this medication passes into breast milk; caution is advised. Consult your doctor for advice.

Infants and Children: Adverse reactions may be more likely and more severe in children.

Special Concerns: If you feel the medication is not working properly after a few weeks, do not increase the dose. Consult your doctor.

OVERDOSE
Symptoms: Severe dizziness or drowsiness; cold, clammy skin; difficult or slow breathing or shortness of breath; severe confusion; seizures; stomach cramps or pain; diarrhea; low blood pressure; increased sweating; constricted pupils of eyes; nausea or vomiting; irregular heartbeat; severe weakness.

What to Do: Call your doctor, emergency medical services (EMS), or the nearest poison control center immediately.

▼ INTERACTIONS

DRUG INTERACTIONS
Consult your doctor for specific advice if you are taking any prescription or over-the-counter drugs, especially drugs with acetaminophen; central nervous system depressants such as antihistamines or medicine for hay fever, allergies, or colds; barbiturates; seizure medicine; muscle relaxants; anesthetics; tranquilizers, sedatives, or sleep aids.

FOOD INTERACTIONS
No known food interactions.

DISEASE INTERACTIONS
Consult your physician if you have a head injury or brain disease, an underactive thyroid, an enlarged prostate, seizures, kidney or liver disease, gallbladder problems, a blood disorder, or a history of alcohol or drug abuse.

SIDE EFFECTS

SERIOUS
Bloody, dark, or cloudy urine; severe pain in lower back or side; pale or black, tarry stools; yellowish tinge to the eyes or skin; hallucinations; frequent urge to urinate; painful or difficult urination; sudden decrease in amount of urine; unusual bleeding or bruising; irregular heartbeat; skin rash, hives, or itching; unusual excitement; swelling of face; confusion; trembling or uncontrolled muscle movements; redness or flushing of face. Call your doctor immediately.

COMMON
Dizziness, lightheadedness, nausea or vomiting, drowsiness, constipation.

LESS COMMON
Allergic reaction, false sense of well-being (euphoria), depression, loss of appetite, blurring or change in vision, headache, sweating.

OXYCODONE/ASPIRIN

Available in: Tablets
Available OTC? No   **As Generic?** Yes
Drug Class: Opioid (narcotic) analgesic

▼ USAGE INFORMATION

WHY IT'S PRESCRIBED
To relieve moderate to severe pain when nonprescription pain relievers prove inadequate. A narcotic analgesic, such as oxycodone, in combination with aspirin, may provide better pain relief than either medication used alone. Used together, pain relief may be achieved at lower doses of the two medications.

HOW IT WORKS
Opioids, such as oxycodone, relieve pain by acting on specific areas of the central nervous system (brain and spinal cord) that process pain signals from nerves throughout the body. Nonsteroidal anti-inflammatory drugs (NSAIDs), such as aspirin, inhibit the release of chemicals in the body called "prostaglandins," which play a role in inflammation.

▼ DOSAGE GUIDELINES

RANGE AND FREQUENCY
Adults: 1 or 2 half-strength tablets or 1 full-strength tablet every 4 to 6 hours as needed. Teenagers: ½ half-strength tablet every 6 hours as needed. Children age 6 to 12: ¼ half-strength tablet every 6 hours as needed.

ONSET OF EFFECT
Unknown.

DURATION OF ACTION
Unknown.

DIETARY ADVICE
This drug can be taken with food or a full glass of water to lessen stomach irritation.

STORAGE
Store in a tightly sealed container away from heat, moisture, and direct light.

MISSED DOSE
If you are taking the drug on a fixed schedule, take it as soon as you remember. However, if it is near the time for the next dose, skip the missed dose and resume your regular dosage schedule. Do not double the next dose.

STOPPING THE DRUG
The decision to stop taking the drug should be made in consultation with your doctor.

PROLONGED USE
See your doctor regularly for examinations and laboratory tests if long-term therapy is required.

≡ SIDE EFFECTS ≡

SERIOUS
Serious side effects are indistinguishable from those of overdose. See Overdose.

COMMON
Lightheadedness, dizziness, drowsiness, nausea, vomiting.

LESS COMMON
Euphoric feeling, depression, constipation, itching.

▼ PRECAUTIONS

Over 60: Adverse reactions may be more likely and more severe in older patients.

Driving and Hazardous Work: Avoid such activities until you determine how the medicine affects you.

Alcohol: Avoid alcohol.

Pregnancy: Before you use this drug, tell your doctor if you are pregnant or plan to become pregnant. Overuse of the medication during pregnancy can cause drug dependence in the fetus.

Breast Feeding: It is not known whether this medication passes into breast milk; caution is advised. Consult your doctor for advice.

Infants and Children: Adverse reactions may be more likely and more severe in children. This drug should not be given to children who have or recently recovered from a viral infection such as chickenpox or the flu. Aspirin has been linked to a rare, but potentially fatal illness called Reye's syndrome. Consult your doctor for information.

Special Concerns: If you feel the medication is not working properly after a few weeks, do not increase the dose. Consult your doctor. Prolonged use of narcotics can cause psychological and physical dependence.

OVERDOSE
Symptoms: Loss of hearing; blood in urine; cold, clammy skin; confusion; seizures; diarrhea; severe dizziness or lightheadedness; severe drowsiness; extreme excitement, nervousness, or restlessness; fever; hallucinations; severe or ongoing headache; increased sweating or thirst; severe or continuing nausea or vomiting; pinpoint pupils of eyes; tinnitus (ringing or buzzing in the ears); shortness of breath or breathing difficulty; slowed heartbeat; abdominal pain; vision problems; severe weakness.

What to Do: Call your doctor, emergency medical services (EMS), or the nearest poison control center immediately.

▼ INTERACTIONS

DRUG INTERACTIONS
Consult your doctor for specific advice if you are taking any prescription or over-the-counter drugs, especially those containing aspirin or other NSAIDs (such as ibuprofen, ketoprofen, or naproxen); acetaminophen; central nervous system depressants, such as antihistamines or medicine for hay fever, allergies, or colds; barbiturates; seizure medicine; muscle relaxants; anesthetics; tranquilizers, sedatives, or sleep aids.

FOOD INTERACTIONS
No known food interactions.

DISEASE INTERACTIONS
Consult your physician if you have a head injury or brain disease, an underactive thyroid, an enlarged prostate, seizures, kidney or liver disease, gallbladder problems, asthma, diarrhea caused by antibiotics or poisoning, a blood disorder, or a history of alcohol or drug abuse.

OXYMETAZOLINE NASAL

Available in: Nasal drops, nasal spray
Available OTC? Yes   **As Generic?** Yes
Drug Class: Decongestant

▼ USAGE INFORMATION

WHY IT'S PRESCRIBED
To relieve nasal congestion caused by allergies, colds, or sinus conditions.

HOW IT WORKS
Oxymetazoline constricts blood vessels to reduce the blood flow to swollen nasal passages and other tissues, which reduces nasal secretions and improves nasal airflow.

▼ DOSAGE GUIDELINES

RANGE AND FREQUENCY
Adults and children 6 years of age and older: 2 or 3 drops or sprays of 0.05% solution in each nostril 2 times a day, in the morning and evening. Children ages 2 to 6: 2 or 3 drops of 0.025% solution in each nostril 2 times a day, in the morning and evening.

ONSET OF EFFECT
Rapid.

DURATION OF ACTION
Unknown.

DIETARY ADVICE
Drink plenty of fluids.

STORAGE
Store in a tightly sealed container away from heat and direct light.

MISSED DOSE
Take it as soon as you remember. If it is near the time for the next dose, skip the missed dose and resume your regular dosage schedule. Do not double the next dose.

STOPPING THE DRUG
Do not use this medicine for more than 3 days without consulting your doctor.

PROLONGED USE
Using this medicine for more than 3 days may lead to rebound congestion (more severe congestion as a result of the body's adaptation to the drug).

▼ PRECAUTIONS

Over 60: Although no studies have specifically examined the use of this drug in older patients, no special problems are expected.

Driving and Hazardous Work: Do not drive or engage in hazardous work until you determine how the medicine affects you.

Alcohol: Avoid alcohol.

Pregnancy: Oxymetazoline has not been shown to cause birth defects or other problems when taken during pregnancy.

Breast Feeding: It is not known whether oxymetazoline passes into breast milk; caution is advised. Consult your doctor for advice.

Infants and Children: This drug is not recommended for children under the age of 2.

Special Concerns: Each container of medicine should be used by only one person to avoid spread of infection. Blow your nose gently before using this medicine. To use the nose drops, tilt your head back or lie down on a bed and hang your head over the side. Keep your head tilted back for a few minutes after instilling the drops. To use the nasal spray, keep your head upright and sniff briskly while spraying. For best results, spray again in 3 to 5 minutes.

OVERDOSE
Symptoms: Rapid, irregular, or pounding heartbeat; headache or dizziness; increased sweating; nervousness; trembling; paleness; insomnia. Such symptoms are more likely to be seen in young children.

What to Do: If someone takes a much larger dose than recommended, call your doctor, emergency medical services (EMS), or the nearest poison control center immediately.

▼ INTERACTIONS

DRUG INTERACTIONS
Before you take oxymetazoline, tell your doctor if you are taking maprotiline or tricyclic antidepressants.

FOOD INTERACTIONS
No known food interactions.

DISEASE INTERACTIONS
Consult your doctor if you have a history of any of the following: high blood pressure, diabetes mellitus, heart disease, blood vessel disease, or an overactive thyroid gland.

≣ SIDE EFFECTS ≣

SERIOUS
No serious side effects have been reported.

COMMON
Burning, dryness, or stinging inside the nose. An increase in nasal discharge or congestion may occur after 3 to 5 days of continuous use.

LESS COMMON
Headache, rapid or irregular heartbeat, unusual excitability, restlessness.

OXYMETAZOLINE OPHTHALMIC

BRAND NAMES

OcuClear, Visine L.R.

Available in: Ophthalmic solution
Available OTC? Yes   **As Generic?** No
Drug Class: Ophthalmic decongestant

▼ USAGE INFORMATION

WHY IT'S PRESCRIBED
To reduce redness of the eye caused by minor irritation.

HOW IT WORKS
Ophthalmic oxymetazoline reduces redness by constricting the superficial blood vessels in the whites (sclera) of the eye.

▼ DOSAGE GUIDELINES

RANGE AND FREQUENCY
Adults and children age 6 and older: 1 drop in the affected eye every 6 hours, as needed.

ONSET OF EFFECT
Rapid, within 5 minutes.

DURATION OF ACTION
About 6 hours.

DIETARY ADVICE
No special restrictions.

STORAGE
Store in a tightly sealed container away from heat, moisture, and direct light. Do not allow the medicine to freeze.

MISSED DOSE
Apply it as soon as you remember. However, if it is near the time for the next dose, skip the missed dose and resume your regular dosage schedule. Do not double the next dose.

STOPPING THE DRUG
Do not use this medicine for more than 3 days without consulting your doctor.

PROLONGED USE
Consult your doctor if you intend to use this medicine for more than 3 days.

▼ PRECAUTIONS

Over 60: Although no studies have specifically examined the use of this drug in older patients, no special problems are expected.

Driving and Hazardous Work: Do not drive or engage in hazardous work until you determine how the medicine affects you.

Alcohol: No special warnings.

Pregnancy: No problems are expected, but studies of effects in pregnancy have not been done in humans. Consult your physician.

Breast Feeding: No problems are expected, but studies of effects in breast feeding have not been done in humans. Consult your doctor.

Infants and Children: Dosage for children under the age of 6 should be determined by a pediatrician.

Special Concerns: To use the eye drops, first wash your hands. Tilt your head back. Gently apply pressure to the inside corner of the eyelid and with the index finger of the same hand, pull downward on the lower eyelid to make a space. Drop the medicine into this space and close your eye. Apply pressure for 1 or 2 minutes while keeping the eye closed without blinking. Then wash your hands again. Make sure the tip of the dropper does not touch your eye, finger, or any other surface.

OVERDOSE
Symptoms: Dizziness; headache; rapid, irregular, or pounding heartbeat; trembling; insomnia.

What to Do: Call your doctor, emergency medical services (EMS), or the nearest poison control center immediately.

▼ INTERACTIONS

DRUG INTERACTIONS
Before you take oxymetazoline, tell your doctor if you are taking maprotiline or tricyclic antidepressants.

FOOD INTERACTIONS
No known food interactions.

DISEASE INTERACTIONS
Caution is advised when taking oxymetazoline. Consult your doctor if you have a history of any of the following: high blood pressure; eye disease, infection, or injury; narrow-angle glaucoma; heart disease; blood vessel disease; or an overactive thyroid gland.

≣ SIDE EFFECTS ≣

SERIOUS
No serious side effects have been reported.

COMMON
No common side effects have been reported.

LESS COMMON
Headache, rapid or irregular heartbeat, excitability, restlessness, increase in redness of the eye.

PACLITAXEL INJECTION

Available in: Injection
Available OTC? No   **As Generic?** No
Drug Class: Antineoplastic (anticancer) agent

▼ USAGE INFORMATION

WHY IT'S PRESCRIBED
To treat cancers of the ovary, breast, lung, head, and neck, and to treat melanoma (a type of skin cancer that can spread to other organs). Paclitaxel is also used as secondary treatment for AIDS-related Kaposi's sarcoma.

HOW IT WORKS
Paclitaxel interferes with essential phases of cell division in cancer cells, preventing them from multiplying. The drug may also affect the health and development of other kinds of cells in the body, resulting in unpleasant side effects.

▼ DOSAGE GUIDELINES

RANGE AND FREQUENCY
135 to 175 mg per square meter of body surface, either as a 24-hour infusion or as a 3-hour infusion administered every 3 to 4 hours. AIDS-related Kaposi's sarcoma: 135 mg per square meter of body surface as a 3-hour infusion administered every 3 weeks or 100 mg per square meter of body surface as a 3-hour infusion every 2 weeks. Your oncologist will determine the proper dosage schedule.

ONSET OF EFFECT
Unknown.

DURATION OF ACTION
Unknown.

DIETARY ADVICE
Maintain adequate food and fluid intake. Calorie, protein, and vitamin needs increase in patients with cancer.

STORAGE
Not applicable; the dose is administered only at a health care facility.

MISSED DOSE
Not applicable, since it is given by a doctor or other health care professional.

STOPPING THE DRUG
The decision to stop taking the drug should be made by your doctor.

PROLONGED USE
You should see your doctor regularly for tests and examinations if you must take this drug for a prolonged period.

▼ PRECAUTIONS

Over 60: No special problems are expected.

Driving and Hazardous Work: Do not drive or engage in hazardous work until you determine how the medicine affects you.

Alcohol: Avoid alcohol.

Pregnancy: Paclitaxel has caused fetal death and miscarriage in animals. Tell your doctor at once if you become pregnant while taking paclitaxel.

Breast Feeding: Paclitaxel may pass into breast milk; avoid or discontinue usage while nursing.

Infants and Children: There is no specific information comparing the use of paclitaxel in infants and children with its use in older persons.

Special Concerns: While taking paclitaxel, do not receive any immunizations without consulting your doctor. Avoid persons with infections. Be careful when using a toothbrush, dental floss, or toothpick. Check with your doctor before having any dental work. Do not touch your eyes or the inside of your nose unless you have just washed your hands. Be careful not to cut yourself when using sharp objects such as a razor. Avoid contact sports and other activities during which bruising could occur.

OVERDOSE
Symptoms: Excessive dosages over an extended period of time may cause weakness, fatigue, and low resistance to infections (due to anemia), numbness or tingling in the extremities (due to peripheral nerve damage), and increased inflammation of the mucous membranes.

What to Do: Notify your doctor right away if you develop such symptoms.

▼ INTERACTIONS

DRUG INTERACTIONS
Consult your doctor for specific advice if you are taking amphotericin B, antithyroid agents, azathioprine, chloramphenicol, colchicine, flucytosine, ganciclovir, ketoconazole, interferon, plicamycin, or zidovudine.

FOOD INTERACTIONS
No known food interactions.

DISEASE INTERACTIONS
Caution is advised when taking paclitaxel. Consult your doctor if you have a history of any of the following: chicken pox, shingles, heart rhythm problems, or any recent infection.

 SIDE EFFECTS

SERIOUS
Black, tarry, or bloody stools; blood-tinged (pink or maroon) urine; cough or hoarseness; fever and chills; lower back or flank pain; painful, difficult urination; tiny bright red spots on skin; bleeding from gums, nose, other unusual places; easy bruising; shortness of breath. These side effects may mean that normal blood cells and special blood-clotting cells have been affected, or that normal immune cells have been affected and an infection is developing somewhere in your body. See your doctor as soon as possible if any of these side effects occur.

COMMON
Diarrhea, nausea, and vomiting; numbness, burning, or tingling in hands or feet; pain in the joints and muscles, especially in the limbs; total but temporary loss of body hair (hair begins to regrow after therapy is discontinued).

LESS COMMON
Dizziness or lightheadedness, slowed heartbeat.

PANCRELIPASE

Available in: Capsules, delayed-release capsules, powder, tablets
Available OTC? No   **As Generic?** Yes
Drug Class: Pancreatic enzyme

▼ USAGE INFORMATION

WHY IT'S PRESCRIBED
The pancreas secretes various substances—including digestive enzymes, insulin, and glucagon—that are essential to good health. Pancrelipase is prescribed to replace the enzymes needed for digestion in patients for whom the pancreas is not functioning properly.

HOW IT WORKS
Pancrelipase contains the enzymes that would otherwise be manufactured by the pancreas to digest proteins, starches, and fats.

▼ DOSAGE GUIDELINES

RANGE AND FREQUENCY
Capsules— Adults and teenagers: 1 to 3 capsules before or with meals and snacks. Children: Contents of 1 to 3 capsules sprinkled on food with each meal. Delayed-release capsules— Adults and teenagers: 1 to 2 capsules before or with meals and

snacks. Children: 1 to 2 capsules with meals. Powder— Adults and teenagers: ¼ teaspoon (0.7 gram) with meals and snacks. Children: ¼ teaspoon with meals. Tablets— Adults and teenagers: 1 to 3 tablets before or with meals and snacks. Children: 1 to 2 tablets with meals. Doses may be altered as determined by your doctor.

ONSET OF EFFECT
Variable.

DURATION OF ACTION
Variable.

DIETARY ADVICE
Take before or with meals and snacks as directed.

STORAGE
Store in a tightly sealed container away from heat, moisture, and direct light.

MISSED DOSE
Take it as soon as you remember. However, if it is near the time for the next dose, skip the missed dose and resume your regular

dosage schedule. Do not double the next dose.

STOPPING THE DRUG
The decision to stop taking the drug should be made by your doctor.

PROLONGED USE
You should see your doctor regularly for tests and examinations while taking this medicine. Lifetime therapy with pancrelipase may be required.

▼ PRECAUTIONS

Over 60: No special problems are expected.

Driving and Hazardous Work: No special precautions are necessary.

Alcohol: No special precautions are necessary.

Pregnancy: Animal and human studies have not been done. Before you take pancrelipase, tell your doctor if you are pregnant or plan to become pregnant.

Breast Feeding: It is not known whether pancrelipase passes into breast milk. Problems have not been reported. Consult your doctor for specific advice.

Infants and Children: The dosage for children under 6 months of age has not been established.

Special Concerns: Be careful not to inhale the powder form or powder from capsules; it may cause stuffy nose, shortness of breath, troubled breathing, wheezing, or tightness in the chest. Do not

change brands or forms of pancrelipase without consulting your physician; different products may work in different ways. If your physician prescribes a personal diet for you, be careful to observe it.

OVERDOSE
Symptoms: Nausea, vomiting, abdominal cramps, diarrhea.

What to Do: Call your doctor, emergency medical services (EMS), or the nearest poison control center immediately.

▼ INTERACTIONS

DRUG INTERACTIONS
Consult your doctor for specific advice if you are taking any prescription or over-the-counter medication.

FOOD INTERACTIONS
No known food interactions.

DISEASE INTERACTIONS
Consult your doctor if you have any other medical problem, especially pancreatitis, which is sudden and severe inflammation of the pancreas.

≡ SIDE EFFECTS ≡

SERIOUS
Serious side effects are not likely with normal doses. With high doses, side effects may include diarrhea, intestinal blockage, nausea, and stomach cramps or pain. Very high doses may cause blood in urine, joint pain, or swelling of feet or lower legs. If the powder form is accidentally inhaled, breathing problems, tightness in the chest, and wheezing may occur. Call your doctor immediately.

COMMON
No common side effects have been reported with the recommended dosage.

LESS COMMON
Skin rash or hives.

PANTOPRAZOLE SODIUM

Available in: Delayed-release tablets
Available OTC? No **As Generic?** No
Drug Class: Antacid/proton pump inhibitor

▼ USAGE INFORMATION

WHY IT'S PRESCRIBED
For the short-term treatment of erosive esophagitis (severe, chronic inflammation or ulceration of the esophagus) associated with gastroesophageal reflux disease (GERD; backwash of stomach acid into the esophagus).

HOW IT WORKS
Pantoprazole blocks the action of a specific enzyme in the cells that line the stomach, thereby decreasing the production of stomach acid.

▼ DOSAGE GUIDELINES

RANGE AND FREQUENCY
Adults: 40 mg once a day for up to 8 weeks.

ONSET OF EFFECT
Within 1 to 3 hours.

DURATION OF ACTION
Unknown.

DIETARY ADVICE
Pantoprazole may be taken without regard to meals. Tablets should be swallowed whole.

STORAGE
Store in a tightly sealed container away from heat, moisture, and direct light.

MISSED DOSE
Take it as soon as you remember. However, if it is near the time for the next dose, skip the missed dose and resume your regular dosage schedule. Do not double the next dose.

STOPPING THE DRUG
Take it as prescribed for the full treatment period, even if your symptoms improve before the scheduled end of therapy. The decision to stop taking the drug should be made in consultation with your doctor.

PROLONGED USE
Pantoprazole should not be used indefinitely as maintenance therapy for esophagitis; it is generally taken for a limited period of up to 8 weeks. For those who have not healed within this period, an additional 8 weeks of therapy may be considered by your doctor.

▼ PRECAUTIONS

Over 60: No special problems are expected.

Driving and Hazardous Work: No special precautions are necessary.

Alcohol: Avoid alcohol while taking this medication, as it may aggravate your condition.

Pregnancy: In animal tests, pantoprazole has not caused problems. Human tests have not been done. Before you take pantoprazole, tell your doctor if you are pregnant or plan to become pregnant.

Breast Feeding: Pantoprazole may pass into breast milk; caution is advised. Consult your doctor for advice. Discuss with your doctor the relative risks and benefits of using this drug while nursing.

Infants and Children: Safety and effectiveness have not been established for patients under age 18.

Special Concerns: Do not chew, crush, or split the tablets. If your doctor directs, you may take an antacid along with pantoprazole.

OVERDOSE
Symptoms: Few cases of overdose have been reported.

What to Do: An overdose is unlikely to be life-threatening. However, if someone takes a much larger dose than prescribed, call your doctor, emergency medical services (EMS), or the nearest poison control center immediately.

▼ INTERACTIONS

DRUG INTERACTIONS
Drug interactions are unlikely. Consult your doctor for specific advice if you are taking ampicillin, iron salts or supplements, or ketoconazole.

FOOD INTERACTIONS
No significant food interactions have been reported.

DISEASE INTERACTIONS
Consult your doctor if you have severe liver disease, which may increase the risk of side effects.

 SIDE EFFECTS

SERIOUS
No serious side effects are associated with the use of pantoprazole.

COMMON
Diarrhea.

LESS COMMON
Rash, raised blood sugar levels. Many additional side effects can occur; consult your doctor if you are concerned about any adverse or unusual reactions you experience while taking this drug.

PAPAVERINE HYDROCHLORIDE

Available in: Tablets, extended-release capsules, injection
Available OTC? No   **As Generic?** Yes
Drug Class: Vasodilator

▼ USAGE INFORMATION

WHY IT'S PRESCRIBED
To treat problems caused by poor blood circulation. The injectable form of papaverine has recently been approved to treat erectile dysfunction (impotence) in men.

HOW IT WORKS
Papaverine causes dilation of blood vessels, improving blood flow to the tissues supplied by the affected vessels. When injected into the penis, papaverine causes the penile arteries to dilate, thus promoting erection.

▼ DOSAGE GUIDELINES

RANGE AND FREQUENCY
To treat poor blood circulation (average adult dose)– Tablets: 100 to 300 mg, 3 to 5 times a day. Extended-release capsules: 150 mg every 12 hours. May be increased by your doctor to 150 mg every 8 hours, or 300 mg every 12 hours. Injection: 30 to 120 mg into a vein or muscle every 3 hours. (Dose for children will be determined by pediatrician.) For erectile dys-

function– Injection: 30 mg, self-administered at the base of penis as needed, just prior to sexual activity. Patients with erectile dysfunction due to nerve damage (as opposed to circulatory problems) may require lower doses. It should not be administered more than once per day, more than 2 days in a row, or more than 3 times a week. Dose may be increased to 60 mg a day based on patient response.

ONSET OF EFFECT
For circulation: Rapid. For erectile dysfunction: Variable; usually 10 to 15 minutes.

DURATION OF ACTION
Call your doctor immediately if erection persists for more than 4 hours.

DIETARY ADVICE
Oral forms can be taken with meals, milk, or antacids to minimize stomach upset.

STORAGE
Store in a tightly sealed container away from heat, moisture, and direct light. Do not refrigerate or freeze injectable forms of pure papaverine. Various mixtures of papaver-

ine with other agents may require refrigeration.

MISSED DOSE
Oral forms: Take the medicine as soon as you remember. If it is near the time for the next dose, skip the missed dose and resume your regular dosage schedule. Do not double the next dose. Injection: Use as needed.

STOPPING THE DRUG
The decision to stop taking the drug should be made in consultation with your doctor.

PROLONGED USE
See your doctor regularly for tests and examinations to evaluate your condition and make any necessary adjustments in therapy.

▼ PRECAUTIONS

Over 60: Oral forms may reduce older patients' tolerance to cold temperatures.

Driving and Hazardous Work: No special precautions are necessary.

Alcohol: Avoid alcohol.

Pregnancy: Adequate studies on the use of oral papaverine during pregnancy have not been done; consult your doctor for specific advice.

Breast Feeding: Oral papaverine may pass into breast milk; caution is advised. Consult a doctor.

Infants and Children: Lower doses of oral papaverine are needed for young patients; consult your pediatrician.

Special Concerns: Oral forms: Papaverine may cause dizziness; get up slowly from a seated or prone position. If you have glaucoma, you should have regular eye examinations. If you have difficulty swallowing the whole capsule, you can mix its contents with jelly or jam and swallow the mixture without chewing. Avoid smoking. Injection: Your doctor should instruct you on how to administer the papaverine before you attempt to do it yourself.

OVERDOSE
Symptoms: Oral forms: Blurred or double vision, drowsiness, fatigue. Injection: Painful erection or erection that persists for more than 4 hours. This may cause permanent damage to the tissues of the penis and may result in the inability to achieve subsequent erections.

What to Do: Seek medical assistance immediately.

▼ INTERACTIONS

DRUG INTERACTIONS
Consult your doctor for specific advice if you are taking any other prescription or over-the-counter drug.

FOOD INTERACTIONS
No known food interactions.

DISEASE INTERACTIONS
Consult your doctor if you have had heart disease, glaucoma, or a recent heart attack or stroke.

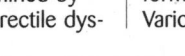

SIDE EFFECTS

SERIOUS
Oral forms: Blurred or double vision, drowsiness, fatigue. Injection: Lumps in penis, painful or prolonged erection (lasting more than 4 hours). Call your doctor immediately.

COMMON
Oral forms: None. Injection for erectile dysfunction: Mild pain or burning along the penis.

LESS COMMON
Oral forms: Dizziness, rapid heartbeat, flushing of face, difficult breathing. Injection: Bruising, bleeding, or tingling at injection site; impaired ejaculation; dizziness.

PAROXETINE HYDROCHLORIDE

Available in: Tablets, oral suspension
Available OTC? No   **As Generic?** No
Drug Class: Selective serotonin reuptake inhibitor (SSRI) antidepressant

▼ USAGE INFORMATION

WHY IT'S PRESCRIBED
To treat symptoms of major depression, obsessive-compulsive disorder, panic disorder, and social anxiety disorder.

HOW IT WORKS
Paroxetine affects levels of serotonin, a brain chemical that is thought to be linked to mood, emotions, and mental state.

▼ DOSAGE GUIDELINES

RANGE AND FREQUENCY
Adults: To start, 20 mg once a day, usually taken in the morning; dose may be gradually increased by your doctor to 50 mg a day. Older adults: To start, 10 mg once a day; may be gradually increased by your doctor to 40 mg a day.

ONSET OF EFFECT
From 1 to 4 weeks.

DURATION OF ACTION
Unknown.

DIETARY ADVICE
This drug can be taken without regard to diet.

STORAGE
Store in a tightly sealed container away from heat, moisture, and direct light.

MISSED DOSE
Take it as soon as you remember. If it is near the time for the next dose, skip the missed dose and resume your regular dosage schedule. Do not double the next dose.

STOPPING THE DRUG
Take as prescribed for the full treatment period even if you begin to feel better before the scheduled end of therapy. The decision to stop taking the drug should be made in consultation with your doctor. Dosage should be gradually tapered over 1 to 2 weeks.

PROLONGED USE
Usual course of therapy for depression lasts 6 months to 1 year; some patients may benefit from additional therapy.

▼ PRECAUTIONS

Over 60: Adverse reactions may be more likely and more severe in older patients. A lower dose may be warranted.

Driving and Hazardous Work: Use caution when driving or engaging in hazardous work until you determine how the medicine affects you.

Alcohol: Avoid alcohol.

Pregnancy: Adequate studies of paroxetine use during pregnancy have not been done. Before you take paroxetine, tell your doctor if you are pregnant or plan to become pregnant.

Breast Feeding: Paroxetine passes into breast milk; caution is advised. Consult your doctor for advice.

Infants and Children: The safety and effectiveness of paroxetine use in children have not been established.

Special Concerns: Take paroxetine at least 6 hours before bedtime to prevent insomnia, unless it causes drowsiness.

OVERDOSE
Symptoms: Agitation or irritability, severe drowsiness, dilated pupils, severe dry mouth, rapid heartbeat, trembling, severe nausea and vomiting.

What to Do: Call your doctor, emergency medical services (EMS), or the nearest poison control center immediately.

▼ INTERACTIONS

DRUG INTERACTIONS
Paroxetine and MAO inhibitors should not be used within 14 days of each other. Very serious side effects such as myoclonus (uncontrolled muscle spasms), hyperthermia (excessive rise in body temperature), and extreme stiffness may result. Tryptophan, warfarin, sumatriptan, naratriptan, rizatriptan, and zolmitriptan may also interact with paroxetine; consult your doctor for advice.

FOOD INTERACTIONS
No known food interactions.

DISEASE INTERACTIONS
Caution is advised when taking paroxetine. Consult your doctor if you have a history of alcohol or drug abuse or a seizure disorder. Use of paroxetine may cause complications in patients with liver or kidney disease, since these organs work together to remove the drug from the body.

≡ SIDE EFFECTS ≡

SERIOUS
Muscle pain or fatigue, lightheadedness or fainting, rash, agitation or irritability, severe drowsiness, dilated pupils, severe dry mouth, rapid heartbeat, trembling, severe nausea or vomiting. Call your doctor immediately.

COMMON
Insomnia, dizziness, sexual dysfunction, unusual fatigue, loss of initiative, nausea or vomiting, constipation, difficulty urinating, headache, trembling.

LESS COMMON
Decreased sexual desire, blurred vision, increased or decreased appetite, weight gain or loss, heartbeat irregularities, change in sense of taste. Also tingling, prickling, or burning feeling.

PEMOLINE

Available in: Tablets, chewable tablets
Available OTC? No **As Generic?** No
Drug Class: Central nervous system stimulant

▼ USAGE INFORMATION

WHY IT'S PRESCRIBED
To treat attention-deficit hyper-activity disorder (ADHD) in children and adults. Because of the risk of serious side effects, pemoline is generally not considered appropriate as first-line therapy.

HOW IT WORKS
Pemoline is thought to stimu-late the release of norepi-nephrine, a natural hormone that promotes the transmis-sion of nerve impulses in the central nervous system. It works by decreasing restless-ness and increasing attention in adults and children who cannot concentrate for very long, are easily distracted, or are impulsive.

▼ DOSAGE GUIDELINES

RANGE AND FREQUENCY
Adults and children age 6 and older: To start, 37.5 mg every morning. Dose may be increased by your doctor in increments of 18.75 mg weekly, up to a maximum of 112.5 mg a day.

ONSET OF EFFECT
Significant benefit may not be evident until the third or fourth week of therapy.

DURATION OF ACTION
8 to 12 hours.

DIETARY ADVICE
No special restrictions.

STORAGE
Store in a tightly sealed con-tainer away from heat, mois-ture, and direct light.

MISSED DOSE
Pemoline is generally pre-scribed for once-daily use. If you are unable to take it on a particular day, resume your regular scheduled dose the following morning.

STOPPING THE DRUG
The decision to stop taking the drug should be made in consultation with your doctor.

PROLONGED USE
You should see your doctor regularly for tests and exami-nations if you take this medi-cine for a prolonged period. Liver function tests should be performed every 2 weeks

after starting pemoline for as long as you remain on the medication. The drug should be discontinued if no clinical benefit is observed 3 weeks after dosage has been increased to 112.5 mg daily.

▼ PRECAUTIONS

Over 60: No special prob-lems are expected.

Driving and Hazardous Work: Avoid such activities until you determine how the medicine affects you.

Alcohol: Avoid alcohol.

Pregnancy: In animal studies, pemoline has been shown to cause stillbirths and decreased survival; however, it has not been shown to cause birth defects in humans. Before you take pemoline, tell your doctor if you are pregnant or plan to become pregnant, so that you may weigh the potential risks and benefits.

Breast Feeding: Pemoline may pass into breast milk; caution is advised. Consult your doctor for advice.

Infants and Children: There have been reports of slowed growth in children who have taken pemoline for long peri-ods. Consult your pediation.

Special Concerns: After you stop taking pemoline, you may exhibit unusual behavior and experience severe mental depression or unusual fatigue. Consult your doctor if you develop these symptoms. Pemoline can cause physical or mental dependence if taken for a long time. Signs of

dependence include a strong desire to continue taking the medicine, a need to increase the dose to attain the same effect, and withdrawal symp-toms when you stop taking the drug. Check with your doctor if you have such symptoms.

OVERDOSE
Symptoms: Agitation, muscle trembling or twitching, confu-sion, high blood pressure, seizures, false sense of well-being, rapid heartbeat, halluci-nations, enlarged pupils, restlessness, vomiting, high fever with sweating, uncon-trolled movements of the eyes or parts of the body, severe headache.

What to Do: Call your doctor, emergency medical services (EMS), or the nearest poison control center immediately.

▼ INTERACTIONS

DRUG INTERACTIONS
Consult your doctor for spe-cific advice if you are taking any other prescription or over-the-counter medication.

FOOD INTERACTIONS
Avoid coffee, tea, cola, and other drinks that are high in caffeine.

DISEASE INTERACTIONS
Pemoline should not be used by patients with liver disease. Use of pemoline may cause complications in patients with kidney disease. Consult your doctor if you have Tourette's syndrome or other tic disorders.

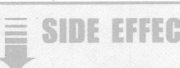

SIDE EFFECTS

SERIOUS
The most serious potential side effect is liver toxicity, which can cause jaundice (characterized by yellowish discoloration of the skin and eyes), nausea, vomiting, abdominal pain, fatigue, loss of appetite, and dark urine. Call your doctor immediately.

COMMON
Insomnia, loss of appetite, weight loss.

LESS COMMON
Dizziness, stomachache, drowsiness, mental depression, increased irritability, nausea, skin rash.

PENBUTOLOL SULFATE

Available in: Tablets
Available OTC? No **As Generic?** No
Drug Class: Beta-blocker

▼ USAGE INFORMATION

WHY IT'S PRESCRIBED
To treat mild to moderate high blood pressure.

HOW IT WORKS
Penbutolol sulfate slows the rate and force of contraction of the heart by blocking certain nerve impulses, thus reducing blood pressure.

▼ DOSAGE GUIDELINES

RANGE AND FREQUENCY
20 mg once a day.

ONSET OF EFFECT
Within 1 hour.

DURATION OF ACTION
Up to 24 hours.

DIETARY ADVICE
Follow your doctor's dietary restrictions, such as a low-salt or low-cholesterol diet, to improve control over hypertension and heart disease.

STORAGE
Store in a tightly sealed container away from heat and direct light.

MISSED DOSE
Take the medicine as soon as you remember. If it is within 8 hours of your next dose, skip the missed dose and resume your regular schedule. Do not double the next dose.

STOPPING THE DRUG
This drug should not be stopped suddenly, as this may lead to angina and possibly a heart attack in patients with advanced heart disease. Slow reduction of the dose under your doctor's close supervision for 2 to 3 weeks is advised.

PROLONGED USE
Regular visits to your doctor are needed to evaluate the drug's ongoing, long-term effectiveness.

▼ PRECAUTIONS

Over 60: Adverse reactions may be more likely and more severe in older patients.

Driving and Hazardous Work: Do not drive or engage in hazardous work until you determine how the medicine affects you.

Alcohol: Drink in careful moderation if at all. Alcohol may interact with the drug and cause a dangerous drop in blood pressure.

Pregnancy: Discuss with your doctor the relative risks and benefits of using this drug while pregnant.

Breast Feeding: Trace amounts of penbutolol sulfate can be found in breast milk, but adverse effects in infants have not been documented. Consult your doctor for specific advice.

Infants and Children: No special problems.

OVERDOSE
Symptoms: Unusually slow or rapid heartbeat, severe dizziness or fainting, poor circulation in the hands (bluish skin), breathing difficulty, seizures.

What to Do: Call your doctor, emergency medical services (EMS), or the nearest poison control center immediately.

▼ INTERACTIONS

DRUG INTERACTIONS
Consult your doctor for specific advice if you are taking amphetamines, oral antidiabetic agents, asthma medication (such as aminophylline or theophylline), calcium channel blockers, clonidine, guanabenz, halothane, immunotherapy for allergies (allergy shots), insulin, MAO inhibitors, reserpine, other beta-blockers, or any over-the-counter medicine.

FOOD INTERACTIONS
None reported.

DISEASE INTERACTIONS
Penbutolol sulfate should be used with caution in people with diabetes, especially insulin-dependent diabetes, since the drug may mask symptoms of hypoglycemia. Consult your doctor if you have allergies or asthma, heart or blood vessel disease (including congestive heart failure and peripheral vascular disease), hyperthyroidism, irregular (slow) heartbeat, myasthenia gravis, psoriasis, respiratory problems, such as bronchitis or emphysema, kidney or liver disease, or a history of mental depression.

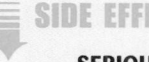

SIDE EFFECTS

SERIOUS
Shortness of breath, wheezing; irregular or slow heartbeat (50 beats per minute or less); pain or feelings of tightness or pressure in the chest; swelling of the ankles, feet, and lower legs; mental depression. If you experience such symptoms, stop taking penbutolol sulfate and call your doctor immediately.

COMMON
Dizziness or lightheadedness, especially when rising suddenly to a standing position; decreased sexual ability; unusual fatigue, weakness, or drowsiness; insomnia.

LESS COMMON
Anxiety, irritability, nervousness; constipation; diarrhea; dry, sore eyes; itching; nausea; vomiting; nightmares or intensely vivid dreams; numbness, tingling, or other unusual sensations in the fingers, toes, or scalp.

PENCICLOVIR

Available in: Topical cream
Available OTC? No   **As Generic?** No
Drug Class: Antiviral

▼ USAGE INFORMATION

WHY IT'S PRESCRIBED
To treat herpes labialis infection (cold sores) of the lips and face in adults with healthy immune systems. (Other treatments are recommended for those with impaired immune function.)

HOW IT WORKS
Penciclovir interferes with the activity of enzymes needed for the replication of viral DNA in cells, thus preventing the virus from multiplying.

▼ DOSAGE GUIDELINES

RANGE AND FREQUENCY
Apply it every 2 hours during waking hours, for 4 days. Start treatment as early as possible, when the first lesions appear on the face.

ONSET OF EFFECT
Unknown.

DURATION OF ACTION
Unknown.

DIETARY ADVICE
There are no special dietary recommendations, but before eating, be sure to wash your hands thorough-ly after applying penciclovir.

STORAGE
Store in a tightly sealed container away from heat and direct light.

MISSED DOSE
Apply it as soon as you remember. If it is near the time for the next dose, skip the missed dose and resume your regular dosage schedule. Do not double the next dose.

STOPPING THE DRUG
The decision to stop using this medication should be made in consultation with your doctor.

PROLONGED USE
See your doctor regularly for tests and examinations if you must use this medicine for a prolonged period.

▼ PRECAUTIONS

Over 60: In human tests penciclovir did not cause more side effects in older patients than it did in younger users.

Driving and Hazardous Work: The use of penciclovir should not impair your ability to perform such tasks safely.

Alcohol: No special precautions are necessary.

Pregnancy: Penciclovir has not been shown to cause birth defects in animals. Human studies have not been done. Before you take penciclovir, tell your doctor if you are pregnant or planning to become pregnant. Use this medication during pregnancy only if its benefits clearly outweigh potential risks.

Breast Feeding: In animal studies, penciclovir given orally was shown to pass into breast milk, and in fact to be present in higher concentrations than those found in the blood. While there is no information on whether penciclovir passes into human breast milk after topical application, you should consult your doctor to help you decide whether to discontinue breast feeding (if the drug is determined to be necessary to the mother) or to discontinue the drug.

Infants and Children: The safety and effectiveness of penciclovir in infants and children have not been established. This medication should be used only under close medical supervision.

Special Concerns: Be careful not to apply penciclovir to the mucous membranes of the mouth and nose. Apply it with care near the eyes, since it can cause pain and irritation if it enters them. You should not use penciclovir if you are allergic to it or to any of its chemical components.

OVERDOSE
Symptoms: None reported.

What to Do: An overdose of penciclovir is very unlikely to occur. However, if someone accidentally ingests a large quantity of the medicine, call your doctor, emergency medical services (EMS), or the nearest poison control center.

▼ INTERACTIONS

DRUG INTERACTIONS
Other drugs may interact with penciclovir. Consult your doctor for specific advice if you are taking any other prescription or over-the-counter drug.

FOOD INTERACTIONS
No known food interactions.

DISEASE INTERACTIONS
Consult your doctor for advice if you have any other medical condition.

≡ SIDE EFFECTS ≡

SERIOUS
No serious side effects have been reported.

COMMON
Headache, allergic reaction at site of application.

LESS COMMON
Numbness or deadening of feeling in skin at application sites, skin rash, odd taste or changes in taste perception.

PENICILLAMINE

Available in: Capsules, tablets
Available OTC? No   **As Generic?** No
Drug Class: Chelating agent; antirheumatic; antiurolithic

▼ USAGE INFORMATION

WHY IT'S PRESCRIBED
To treat Wilson's disease (excessive accumulation of copper in the body tissues) and rheumatoid arthritis, and to prevent or treat kidney stones in patients with excessive amounts of the amino acid cystine in the urine or who have a history of recurrent cystine kidney stones. It can also be used to treat heavy metal (mercury, lead) poisoning.

HOW IT WORKS
Penicillamine is a chelating (chemical binding) agent that removes excess copper (the underlying problem in Wilson's disease), mercury, and lead from the body. It is not clear how penicillamine improves rheumatoid arthritis, but it may suppress the body's release of certain chemicals that cause inflammation. Penicillamine also binds with cystine and eliminates it from the body; high concentrations of cystine can cause kidney stone formation.

▼ DOSAGE GUIDELINES

RANGE AND FREQUENCY
For Wilson's disease— Adults and teenagers: To start, 250 mg, 4 times a day; may be increased to 500 mg, 4 times a day. Children: To start, 250 mg once a day; may be increased. For rheumatoid arthritis— Adults: To start, 125 to 250 mg once a day; may be increased to 500 mg, 3 times a day. To prevent cystine kidney stones— Adults: To start, 500 mg, 4 times a day; may be increased to 1,000 mg, 4 times a day. Children: To start, 3.5 mg per lb of body weight, 4 times a day; may be increased. To treat heavy metal poisoning— 500 mg to 1.5 g a day in adults for 1 to 2 months.

ONSET OF EFFECT
For Wilson's disease: Within 1 to 3 months. For rheumatoid arthritis: Within 2 to 3 months. For kidney stones: Unknown.

DURATION OF ACTION
Unknown.

DIETARY ADVICE
For Wilson's disease or rheumatoid arthritis: Take on an empty stomach. For rheumatoid arthritis, take at least 1 hour before or after any other food, milk, or medicine. For prevention or treatment of kidney stones: Drink at least 2 full glasses of water at bedtime and another 2 glasses of water during the night.

STORAGE
Store in a tightly sealed container away from heat, moisture, and direct light.

MISSED DOSE
Take it as soon as you remember. If it is near the time for the next dose, skip the missed dose and resume your regular dosage schedule. Do not double the next dose.

STOPPING THE DRUG
Take it as prescribed for the full treatment period.

PROLONGED USE
See your doctor regularly for tests and examinations.

▼ PRECAUTIONS

Over 60: Adverse reactions may be more likely and more severe in older patients.

Driving and Hazardous Work: No special warnings.

Alcohol: No special warnings.

Pregnancy: Penicillamine may cause birth defects if taken during pregnancy.

Breast Feeding: Penicillamine may pass into breast milk; do not use it while nursing.

Infants and Children: No special warnings.

Special Concerns: Do not take any iron-containing medication or supplement within 2 hours of taking penicillamine. Patients should take 25 mg a day of vitamin B6 during therapy, since the drug increases the need for this vitamin. Patients may also take a multivitamin, but those with Wilson's disease must ensure it is copper-free.

OVERDOSE
Symptoms: None known.

What to Do: If someone takes a much larger dose than prescribed, seek medical assistance immediately.

▼ INTERACTIONS

DRUG INTERACTIONS
Do not take gold compounds or phenylbutazone if you are taking penicillamine. Also, tell your doctor if you are taking any other prescription or over-the-counter medication.

FOOD INTERACTIONS
Patients with Wilson's disease should not eat foods high in copper, such as chocolate, nuts, shellfish, mushrooms, liver, molasses, and broccoli.

DISEASE INTERACTIONS
Consult your doctor if you have a history of blood problems or kidney disease. Persons sensitive to penicillin may have allergic reactions to penicillamine.

≡ SIDE EFFECTS ≡

SERIOUS
Joint pain, wheezing or tightness in chest, hives, skin rash or itching, cloudy or bloody urine, shortness of breath, unusual fatigue, sore throat and fever, painful or swollen glands, weight gain, unusual bleeding. Also white spots, sores, or ulcers in mouth; swollen face, feet, or lower legs. Call your doctor immediately.

COMMON
Diarrhea, nausea or vomiting, loss of taste, mild stomach pain, loss of appetite.

LESS COMMON
No less-common side effects are associated with this drug.

PENICILLIN G

Available in: Capsules, oral solution, injection
Available OTC? No   **As Generic?** No
Drug Class: Penicillin antibiotic

▼ USAGE INFORMATION

WHY IT'S PRESCRIBED
To treat a variety of bacterial infections, including those of the ear, nose, and throat, skin and soft tissues, genitourinary tract, and the respiratory tract. It is also prescribed preventively before surgery or dental work in patients at risk for endocarditis (infection of the interior lining of the heart, which may damage the heart's valves). It may also be given to treat meningitis and syphilis.

HOW IT WORKS
Penicillin G blocks the formation of bacterial cell walls, rendering bacteria unable to multiply and spread.

▼ DOSAGE GUIDELINES

RANGE AND FREQUENCY
Oral forms— Adults and teenagers: 200,000 to 500,000 units every 4 to 6 hours. Children: 189 to 13,636 units per lb of body weight every 4 to 8 hours. Injection (benzathine form)— Adults and teenagers: 1,200,000 to 2,400,000 units in 1 dose. Children: 300,000 to 1,200,000 units in 1 dose. Injection (procaine form)— Adults and teenagers: 600,000 to 1,200,000 units once a day. Children: 22,727 units per lb of body weight once a day. Other injection forms— Adults and teenagers: 1,000,000 to 5,000,000 units injected every 4 to 6 hours. Children: 3,788 to 11,363 units per lb of body weight every 4 to 6 hours. Infants: 13,636 units per lb of body weight every 12 hours.

ONSET OF EFFECT
Immediate after intravenous injection; unknown for other forms of the drug.

DURATION OF ACTION
Unknown.

DIETARY ADVICE
Oral doses should be given at least 1 hour before or 2 hours after meals.

STORAGE
Store in a tightly sealed container away from heat and direct light. Liquid forms can be refrigerated but not frozen.

MISSED DOSE
Take it as soon as you remember. If it is near the time for the next dose, skip the missed dose and resume your regular dosage schedule. Do not double the next dose.

STOPPING THE DRUG
Take this drug as prescribed for the full treatment period, even if you feel better before the scheduled end of therapy.

PROLONGED USE
See your doctor regularly for tests and examinations if you must take this medicine for a prolonged period.

▼ PRECAUTIONS

Over 60: No special advice.

Driving and Hazardous Work: The use of penicillin G should not impair your ability to perform such tasks safely.

Alcohol: No special precautions are necessary.

Pregnancy: Adequate studies of use of this drug during pregnancy have not been done; however, no problems have been reported.

Breast Feeding: Penicillin G may pass into breast milk and cause problems in the nursing infant; avoid use while nursing.

Infants and Children: No special problems are expected.

Special Concerns: Penicillin G can cause false results on some urine sugar tests for patients with diabetes. Those who are prone to asthma, hay fever, hives, or allergies may be more likely to have an allergic reaction to a penicillin antibiotic. If severe diarrhea occurs as a side effect of this drug, do not take antidiarrheal medications; call your doctor.

OVERDOSE
Symptoms: Severe nausea, vomiting, diarrhea, seizures.

What to Do: Call your doctor, emergency medical services (EMS), or the nearest poison control center immediately.

▼ INTERACTIONS

DRUG INTERACTIONS
Consult your physician for specific advice if you are taking aminoglycosides, ACE inhibitors, diuretics, potassium supplements or potassium-containing medications, anticoagulants or other anti-clotting drugs, nonsteroidal anti-inflammatory drugs, sulfinpyrazone, cholestyramine, colestipol, oral contraceptives, methotrexate, probenecid, or rifampin.

FOOD INTERACTIONS
No known food interactions.

DISEASE INTERACTIONS
Consult your doctor if you have a history of allergies, asthma, bleeding disorders (such as hemophilia), congestive heart failure, cystic fibrosis, gastrointestinal disorders (especially colitis associated with the use of antibiotics), infectious mononucleosis, or impaired kidney function.

≡ SIDE EFFECTS ≡

SERIOUS
Irregular, rapid, or labored breathing; lightheadedness or sudden fainting; joint pain; fever; severe abdominal pain and cramping with watery or bloody stools; severe allergic reaction (marked by sudden swelling of the lips, tongue, face, or throat; breathing difficulty; skin rash, itching, or hives); unusual bleeding or bruising; yellowish tinge to eyes or skin. Call your doctor immediately.

COMMON
Mild rash, mild diarrhea, nausea, vomiting, headache, vaginal discharge and itching, pain or white patches in the mouth or on the tongue.

LESS COMMON
Diminished urine output, chills, weakness, fatigue.

PENICILLIN V

BRAND NAMES

Abocillin VK,
Apo-Pen VK, Beepen-VK,
Betapen-VK, Ledercillin
VK, Napopen-V,
Pen Vee, Robocillin VK,
V-Cillin K, Veetids

Available in: Tablets, delayed-release tablets, liquid
Available OTC? No   **As Generic?** Yes
Drug Class: Penicillin antibiotic

▼ USAGE INFORMATION

WHY IT'S PRESCRIBED
To treat a variety of bacterial infections, including those of the ear, nose, and throat, skin and soft tissues, genitourinary tract, and the respiratory tract. It is also prescribed before surgery or dental work in patients at risk for endocarditis (infection of the lining of the heart, which may damage the heart's valves).

HOW IT WORKS
Penicillin V destroys susceptible bacteria by interfering with their ability to produce cell walls as they multiply.

▼ DOSAGE GUIDELINES

RANGE AND FREQUENCY
Adults: 500 to 2,000 mg a day for infections; 2,000 mg to prevent bacterial endocarditis; or as ordered by physician. Children: 15 to 50 mg per 2.2 lbs (1 kg) of body weight per day in divided doses to treat infections. To prevent infection after dental surgery, 2 g (1 g for children), 30 to 60 minutes before procedure, then 1 g (500 mg for children) 6 hours afterward.

ONSET OF EFFECT
Unknown.

DURATION OF ACTION
Up to 6 hours.

DIETARY ADVICE
Take it on an empty stomach, 1 to 2 hours before or 3 to 4 hours after a meal.

STORAGE
Store in a tightly sealed container away from heat and direct light.

MISSED DOSE
Take it as soon as you remember. If it is near the time for the next dose, skip the missed dose and resume your regular dosage schedule. Do not double the next dose.

STOPPING THE DRUG
It is very important to take this drug as prescribed for the full treatment period. Stopping the drug prematurely may lead to serious complications.

PROLONGED USE
Prolonged use of any antibiotic increases the risk of superinfection (a more severe and drug-resistant infection); caution is advised.

▼ PRECAUTIONS

Over 60: No special problems are expected.

Driving and Hazardous Work: The use of penicillin should not impair your ability to perform such tasks safely.

Alcohol: No special precautions are necessary.

Pregnancy: Adequate studies of penicillin antibiotic use during pregnancy have not been done; however, no problems have been reported.

Breast Feeding: Penicillin V may pass into breast milk and cause problems in the nursing infant; avoid use while nursing.

Infants and Children: No special problems expected.

Special Concerns: Penicillin V can cause false results on some urine sugar tests for patients with diabetes. If severe diarrhea occurs as a side effect of this drug, do not take antidiarrheal medications; call your doctor. Oral contraceptives may not be effective while you are taking penicillin; consider other methods of birth control. Those who are prone to asthma, hay fever, hives, or allergies may be more likely to have an allergic reaction to a penicillin antibiotic.

OVERDOSE
Symptoms: Severe nausea, vomiting, diarrhea, seizures.

What to Do: An overdose is unlikely to be life-threatening. However, if someone takes a much larger dose than prescribed, call your doctor or emergency medical services (EMS) right away.

▼ INTERACTIONS

DRUG INTERACTIONS
Consult your physician for specific advice if you are taking aminoglycosides, ACE inhibitors, diuretics, potassium supplements or potassium-containing medications, anticoagulants or other anti-clotting drugs, nonsteroidal anti-inflammatory drugs, sulfinpyrazone, cholestyramine, colestipol, oral contraceptives, methotrexate, probenecid, or rifampin.

FOOD INTERACTIONS
Acidic foods or juices can reduce the antibiotic effect.

DISEASE INTERACTIONS
Consult your doctor if you have a history of allergies, asthma, congestive heart failure, gastrointestinal disorders (especially colitis associated with the use of antibiotics), or impaired kidney function.

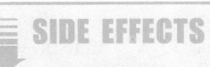

≡ SIDE EFFECTS ≡

SERIOUS
Irregular, rapid, or labored breathing; lightheadedness or sudden fainting; joint pain; fever; severe abdominal pain and cramping with watery or bloody stools; severe allergic reaction (marked by sudden swelling of the lips, tongue, face, or throat; breathing difficulty; skin rash, itching, or hives); unusual bleeding or bruising; yellowish tinge to eyes or skin. Call your doctor immediately.

COMMON
Mild rash, mild diarrhea, nausea, vomiting, headache, vaginal discharge and itching, pain or white patches in the mouth or on the tongue.

LESS COMMON
Diminished urine output, chills, weakness, fatigue.

PENTAMIDINE ISETHIONATE

BRAND NAMES

NebuPent, Pentam 300

Available in: Inhalation, injection
Available OTC? No   **As Generic?** Yes
Drug Class: Anti-infective; antiprotozoal

▼ USAGE INFORMATION

WHY IT'S PRESCRIBED
To prevent and treat Pneumo-cystis carinii pneumonia (PCP). This serious type of pneumonia is prevalent among AIDS patients. The inhalation form is used to attempt to prevent PCP. The injection form is used to treat PCP. It may also be used for other types of infection as determined by your doctor.

HOW IT WORKS
The exact way in which pen-tamidine works is unknown.

▼ DOSAGE GUIDELINES

RANGE AND FREQUENCY
To prevent PCP– Inhalation (using the Respirgard II nebu-lizer by Marquest), adults and children age 5 and older: 300 mg once every 4 weeks. To treat PCP– Injection: 3 to 4 mg per 2.2 lbs (1 kg) of body weight into a vein over a period of 1 to 2 hours once a day for 21 days.

ONSET OF EFFECT
Unknown.

DURATION OF ACTION
Unknown.

DIETARY ADVICE
No special restrictions.

STORAGE
Not applicable; the dose is administered only at a health care facility.

MISSED DOSE
Be sure to receive treatment as soon as possible. Contact your doctor.

STOPPING THE DRUG
Take it as prescribed for the full treatment period. The decision to stop taking the drug should be made in con-sultation with your physician.

PROLONGED USE
See your doctor regularly for tests and examinations if you must take this medicine for a prolonged period.

▼ PRECAUTIONS

Over 60: No studies have been done specifically on older patients.

Driving and Hazardous Work: Do not drive or engage in hazardous work until you determine how the medicine affects you.

Alcohol: Avoid alcohol.

Pregnancy: Adequate human studies have not been done. Before taking this drug, tell your doctor if you are cur-rently pregnant or plan to become pregnant.

Breast Feeding: Pentamidine may pass into breast milk; avoid use while breast feeding.

Infants and Children: Ade-quate studies on the use of pentamidine in children younger than 4 months have not been done. Consult your doctor for more information.

Special Concerns: Do not mix the inhalation solution with any other drugs or use any other drug in the nebu-lizer. Injectable pentamidine can cause a sudden drop in blood pressure. Lie down while taking it. The drug may also increase the chance of infection because it can lower the number of white blood cells in your blood. Consult your doctor at once if you detect signs of an infection (fever, sore throat). Use an electric shaver rather than a razor, as pentamidine may increase the risk of uncon-trolled bleeding. Consult your dentist about ways to safely clean your teeth.

OVERDOSE
Symptoms: See Serious Side Effects.

What to Do: An overdose is unlikely. However, if you sus-pect an overdose, call your doctor, emergency medical services (EMS), or the nearest control center immediately.

▼ INTERACTIONS

DRUG INTERACTIONS
Other drugs may interact with pentamidine. Consult your doctor if you are taking bone marrow depressants, didano-sine, macrolide antibiotics, foscarnet, or any drugs that may damage the kidney. Also consult your doctor if you are undergoing radiation therapy.

FOOD INTERACTIONS
No known food interactions.

DISEASE INTERACTIONS
Consult your doctor if you have heart, kidney, or liver disease, tuberculosis, a bleed-ing disorder, low blood pres-sure, diabetes mellitus, or low blood sugar. PCP prevention by inhalation may be less effective in those with chronic obstructive pulmonary dis-ease (emphysema).

SIDE EFFECTS

SERIOUS
Inhalation: Chest pain or congestion, difficulty breathing or swallowing, wheezing, skin rash, burning pain, dryness or feeling of lump in throat, cough. Injection: Decreased uri-nation, unusual bruising or bleeding due to reduced num-ber of platelets (clotting agents) in the blood, sore throat and fever; symptoms of high blood sugar or diabetes melli-tus (flushed, dry skin, drowsiness, fruity breath, increased urination and thirst, loss of appetite); symptoms of low blood sugar (nausea, headache, anxiety, cold sweats or chills, shakiness, cool, pale skin, increased appetite); signs of low blood pressure (dizziness, confusion, fatigue, blurred vision, fainting or lightheadedness); dry, red, or itchy skin; vomiting or nausea; fast or irregular pulse; abdominal pain; pain or redness at injection site. Serious side effects occur commonly; call your doctor immediately.

COMMON
Injection: Loss of appetite, diarrhea, unpleasant metallic taste, nausea and vomiting.

LESS COMMON
There are no less-common side effects.

PENTAZOCINE

Available in: Injection
Available OTC? No   **As Generic?** No
Drug Class: Opioid agonist-antagonist analgesic

▼ USAGE INFORMATION

WHY IT'S PRESCRIBED
To relieve moderate to severe pain.

HOW IT WORKS
Opioids such as pentazocine relieve pain by acting on areas of the brain that process pain signals from nerves throughout the body.

▼ DOSAGE GUIDELINES

RANGE AND FREQUENCY
Adults: 25 to 50 mg every 3 or 4 hours. Maximum dose is 360 mg a day. Children: The dose must be determined by your pediatrician.

ONSET OF EFFECT
Into a vein: Within 2 to 3 minutes. Into a muscle: Within 15 to 20 minutes.

DURATION OF ACTION
From 2 to 3 hours.

DIETARY ADVICE
Drink 2 to 3 quarts of fluid a day, if possible, to help prevent constipation.

STORAGE
Not applicable; the dose is administered only in a health care facility.

MISSED DOSE
Not applicable; the dose is administered by a health care professional.

STOPPING THE DRUG
The decision to stop taking the drug should be made by your doctor.

PROLONGED USE
You should see your doctor regularly for tests and examinations if you take this medication for a prolonged period. Prolonged use can cause physical dependence.

▼ PRECAUTIONS

Over 60: Adverse reactions may be more likely and more severe in older patients.

Driving and Hazardous Work: Do not drive or engage in hazardous work until you determine how the medicine affects you.

Alcohol: Avoid alcohol while using this medication.

Pregnancy: In animal studies, pentazocine has not been shown to cause birth defects; adequate human studies have not been done. Before using this drug, tell your doctor if you are pregnant or plan to become pregnant. Overuse during pregnancy can cause drug dependence in the fetus.

Breast Feeding: Pentazocine may pass into breast milk; caution is advised. Consult your doctor for specific advice.

Infants and Children: Adverse reactions may be more likely and more severe in children. Consult your doctor for specific advice. Not recommended for use by children under the age of 12.

Special Concerns: If you feel the medication is not working properly after a few weeks, consult your doctor about other treatment options. Before undergoing any surgical procedure (including dental surgery), be sure to tell the doctor or dentist in charge that you are taking pentazocine.

OVERDOSE
Symptoms: Confusion; severe drowsiness, weakness, or dizziness; slurred speech; small, pinpoint (constricted) pupils; cold, clammy skin; slow breathing; seizures; loss of consciousness.

What to Do: Call your doctor, emergency medical services (EMS), or the nearest poison control center immediately.

▼ INTERACTIONS

DRUG INTERACTIONS
Consult your physician for specific advice if you are taking carbamazepine or other medicine for seizures, barbiturates, sedatives, cough medicines, decongestants, antidepressants, other prescription pain medications, MAO inhibitors, naltrexone, rifampin, or zidovudine (AZT).

FOOD INTERACTIONS
No known food interactions.

DISEASE INTERACTIONS
Consult your doctor if you have any of the following: a history of alcohol or drug abuse, emotional illness, brain disorders or head injury, seizures, lung disease, prostate disorders or other problems with urination, gallstones, colitis, or heart, kidney, liver, or thyroid disease.

SIDE EFFECTS

SERIOUS
Serious side effects of pentazocine are indistinguishable from those of overdose: Confusion; severe drowsiness, weakness, or dizziness; slurred speech; small, pinpoint pupils; cold, clammy skin; slow breathing; seizures; loss of consciousness.

COMMON
Dizziness or lightheadedness, nausea or vomiting, constipation, itching.

LESS COMMON
Mood swings or false sense of well-being and euphoria, hallucinations, nightmares.

PENTOBARBITAL SODIUM

Available in: Capsules, elixir, injection, suppositories
Available OTC? No   **As Generic?** Yes
Drug Class: Barbiturate

▼ USAGE INFORMATION

WHY IT'S PRESCRIBED
Primarily for sedation before surgery and to control certain types of seizures. With the availability of newer sleep-inducing drugs, pentobarbital is now rarely used for short-term treatment of insomnia.

HOW IT WORKS
Barbiturates such as pentobarbital act as powerful sedatives by reducing activity in the central nervous system.

▼ DOSAGE GUIDELINES

RANGE AND FREQUENCY
Sedation before surgery—Adult oral dosage: 100 mg. Children's oral dosage: 0.9 mg to 2.7 mg per lb of body weight, usually not more than 100 mg. To control seizures—Usually given intravenously by a doctor. Pentobarbital injection (into a vein or muscle) is only done under the direction of a physician. For insomnia—Adult oral dosage: 100 mg taken at bedtime.

ONSET OF EFFECT
Within 30 minutes.

DURATION OF ACTION
1 to 4 hours for oral or rectal forms, 15 minutes for injection.

DIETARY ADVICE
Oral forms can be taken with fluid or food.

STORAGE
Store in a tightly sealed container away from heat, moisture, and direct light.

MISSED DOSE
Take it as soon as you remember. If it is near the time for the next dose, skip the missed dose and resume your regular dosage schedule. Do not double the next dose.

STOPPING THE DRUG
The decision to stop taking the drug should be made by your doctor. There is a risk of withdrawal side effects when the drug is stopped suddenly.

PROLONGED USE
Barbiturates may be habit-forming, and prolonged use may increase the risk of dependency. Pentobarbital, as well as other barbiturates, when used for insomnia, is only prescribed on a short-term basis. It is not usually effective when used for longer than 2 weeks.

▼ PRECAUTIONS

Over 60:
Adverse reactions may be more likely and more severe in older patients and may require that smaller doses be used.

Driving and Hazardous Work:
Because of sedative effects, do not drive or engage in hazardous work until you determine how the medicine affects you.

Alcohol:
Avoid alcohol; its sedative effects are additive to those of the drug.

Pregnancy:
Pentobarbital can cause birth defects and problems during pregnancy. Before taking pentobarbital, be sure to tell your doctor if you are pregnant or plan to become pregnant.

Breast Feeding:
Pentobarbital passes into breast milk in small amounts and can cause side effects in breast-feeding infants. Consult your doctor for advice.

Infants and Children:
As with older patients, infants and children are more sensitive to the effects of pentobarbital. A lower dose may be warranted.

Special Concerns:
Pentobarbital may cause physical or mental dependence. Check with your doctor at once if you feel overly sedated or if you suffer withdrawal side effects when you stop taking the medication.

OVERDOSE
Symptoms: Severe sedation or excessive drowsiness, confusion, irritability, shortness of breath or troubled breathing, slurred speech, staggering walk, severe weakness.

What to Do: Call your doctor, emergency medical services (EMS), or the nearest poison control center immediately.

▼ INTERACTIONS

DRUG INTERACTIONS
Consult your doctor for specific advice if you are taking other seizure medicines, central nervous system depressants, warfarin (blood thinner), or oral contraceptives. Pentobarbital may make oral contraceptives less effective.

FOOD INTERACTIONS
No known food interactions.

DISEASE INTERACTIONS
Caution is advised when taking pentobarbital. Consult your doctor if you have any of the following: kidney disease, liver disease, porphyria, hyperactivity, mental depression, or a history of alcohol or drug abuse.

SIDE EFFECTS

SERIOUS
Excitability, confusion, or excessive sedation to the point you cannot be awakened. Also yellowish tinge to the eyes or skin; swollen eyelids, face, or lips; wheezing; or rash (these may be signs of drug allergy); sores on lips or mouth. Call your doctor immediately.

COMMON
Clumsiness, unsteadiness, persistent drowsiness, dizziness or lightheadedness.

LESS COMMON
Anxiety or nervousness, nightmares, insomnia, constipation, feeling faint, irritability, headache, nausea or vomiting.

PENTOSAN POLYSULFATE SODIUM

Available in: Capsules
Available OTC? No **As Generic?** No
Drug Class: Synthetic sulfated polysaccharide

▼ USAGE INFORMATION

WHY IT'S PRESCRIBED
To relieve bladder pain or discomfort caused by interstitial cystitis, an inflammatory bladder condition predominantly affecting women, marked by frequent and painful urination.

HOW IT WORKS
The exact mechanism of action is unknown, but pentosan is believed to adhere to the mucosal lining of the bladder, acting as a coating to prevent irritating substances in the urine from reaching the bladder wall.

▼ DOSAGE GUIDELINES

RANGE AND FREQUENCY
100 mg, 3 times a day.

ONSET OF EFFECT
Unknown.

DURATION OF ACTION
Unknown.

DIETARY ADVICE
Pentosan should be taken with a full glass of water on an empty stomach, at least 1 hour before or 2 hours after meals, and at least 1 hour before or after any other food, milk or milk-based product, or medication.

STORAGE
Store in a tightly sealed container away from heat, moisture, and direct light.

MISSED DOSE
Take it as soon as you remember. If it is near the time for the next dose, skip the missed dose and resume your regular dosage schedule. Do not double the next dose.

STOPPING THE DRUG
Take it as prescribed for the full treatment period, even if you begin to feel better before the scheduled end of therapy. The decision to stop taking the drug should be made by your doctor.

PROLONGED USE
Therapy generally lasts for 3 months. You should be reassessed by your doctor at that time. If your condition has not improved and there are few side effects, your doctor may continue therapy for an additional 3 months.

▼ PRECAUTIONS

Over 60: Adverse reactions may be more likely and more severe in older patients.

Driving and Hazardous Work: Do not drive or engage in hazardous work until you determine how the medicine affects you.

Alcohol: Avoid alcohol when taking this medication, since it may provoke further bladder irritation.

Pregnancy: Adequate studies of the use of this drug during pregnancy have not been done. Before taking pentosan, be sure to tell your doctor if you are pregnant or plan to become pregnant.

Breast Feeding: Pentosan may pass into breast milk; caution is advised. Consult your doctor for advice.

Infants and Children: The safety and effectiveness of pentosan use by patients under age 16 have not been established.

Special Concerns: This drug may increase your susceptibility to sunburn. Use measures to protect your skin from ultraviolet light until you determine how the medicine affects you.

OVERDOSE
Symptoms: An overdose of pentosan is unlikely; no cases of overdose have been reported.

What to Do: Emergency instructions not applicable.

▼ INTERACTIONS

DRUG INTERACTIONS
The following drugs may interact with pentosan. Consult your doctor for specific advice if you are taking alteplase, aspirin, warfarin or any other anticoagulant, heparin, or streptokinase.

FOOD INTERACTIONS
No known food interactions.

DISEASE INTERACTIONS
Caution is advised when taking pentosan. Consult your doctor if you have any of the following conditions: hemophilia, low platelet count or any bleeding problems, blockage or obstruction of the intestine, stomach or intestinal ulcers, polyps, liver disease, or blood vessel disease.

SIDE EFFECTS

SERIOUS
Fever, unusual tiredness or fatigue, chills, itching, skin rash or hives, difficulty breathing, sore throat, unusual bleeding or bruising. Call your doctor immediately.

COMMON
No common side effects are associated with the use of pentosan.

LESS COMMON
Abdominal pain, hair loss, diarrhea, nausea, stomach distress, dizziness, rash, headache.

PENTOXIFYLLINE

Available in: Extended-release tablets
Available OTC? No   **As Generic?** Yes
Drug Class: Hemorheologic agent

▼ USAGE INFORMATION

WHY IT'S PRESCRIBED
To improve blood flow and reduce leg pain in patients with poor circulation.

HOW IT WORKS
It decreases the viscosity (or thickness) of blood, permitting easier red blood cell movement throughout the circulatory system.

▼ DOSAGE GUIDELINES

RANGE AND FREQUENCY
400 mg, 2 or 3 times a day.

ONSET OF EFFECT
Unknown. The full effect may take 2 to 4 weeks or longer.

DURATION OF ACTION
Unknown.

DIETARY ADVICE
Pentoxifylline should be taken with meals to minimize the risk of gastrointestinal (stomach) upset. Taking an antacid may also help.

STORAGE
Store in a tightly sealed container away from heat and direct light.

MISSED DOSE
Take a missed dose as soon as you remember. If it is near the time for the next dose, skip the missed dose and resume your regular dosage schedule, as prescribed. Do not double the next dose.

STOPPING THE DRUG
The decision to stop taking the drug should be made by your doctor. Take as prescribed for the full treatment period, even if you are feeling better before the scheduled end of therapy.

PROLONGED USE
You should see your doctor regularly for tests and physical examinations if you must take this drug for a prolonged period of time.

▼ PRECAUTIONS

Over 60: Adverse reactions may be more likely and more severe in older patients.

Driving and Hazardous Work: Do not drive or engage in hazardous work until you determine how the medicine affects you.

Alcohol: Avoid alcohol.

SIDE EFFECTS

SERIOUS
Chest pain, heartbeat irregularities. Call your doctor or emergency medical services (EMS) immediately.

COMMON
No common side effects have been reported.

LESS COMMON
Dizziness, headache, stomach pain or upset, nausea or vomiting.

Pregnancy: Pentoxifylline has not been shown to cause birth defects, but in animal studies it has caused other harmful effects. Human studies have not been done. Before you take pentoxifylline, be sure to tell your doctor if you are pregnant or plan to become pregnant.

Breast Feeding: Pentoxifylline passes into breast milk; caution is advised. Consult your doctor for specific advice.

Infants and Children: There is no specific information comparing use of pentoxifylline in infants and children with other age groups. Use and dosage must be determined by your doctor.

Special Concerns: In addition to taking pentoxifylline, you should practice such measures as weight control and exercise. Bathe your feet daily in lukewarm water, applying lanolin afterward, and wear clean cotton socks. Do not smoke cigarettes, since smoking can make your condition worse by narrowing blood vessels; indeed, tobacco of all types must be avoided. Tablets should be swallowed whole, without breaking, crushing, or chewing.

OVERDOSE
Symptoms: Flushing, very low blood pressure, nervousness, agitation, tremors, seizures, fever, agitation, loss of consciousness, very slow heartbeat. Symptoms usually appear 4 to 5 hours following an overdose.

What to Do: Discontinue the medication and call your doctor, emergency medical services (EMS), or the nearest poison control center right away.

▼ INTERACTIONS

DRUG INTERACTIONS
Consult your doctor for specific advice if you are taking anticoagulants, theophylline, drugs for hypertension, or any other prescription or over-the-counter drugs.

FOOD INTERACTIONS
No known food interactions.

DISEASE INTERACTIONS
Caution is advised when taking pentoxifylline. Consult your doctor if you have any condition in which there is a risk of bleeding, such as a recent stroke. Use of pentoxifylline may cause complications in patients with liver or kidney disease, since these organs work together to remove the medication from the body.

PERGOLIDE MESYLATE

Available in: Tablets
Available OTC? No   **As Generic?** No
Drug Class: Antiparkinsonism drug

▼ USAGE INFORMATION

WHY IT'S PRESCRIBED
Pergolide is used in conjunction with levodopa/carbidopa to treat Parkinson's disease or Parkinson-like syndromes, which can occur following injury to or infection of the nervous system, damage to the blood vessels in the brain, or exposure to certain toxins.

HOW IT WORKS
Pergolide directly stimulates receptor cells that act with the brain chemical dopamine to initiate and enhance smooth control of voluntary muscle movement.

▼ DOSAGE GUIDELINES

RANGE AND FREQUENCY
Adults: Initial dose is 0.05 mg, once a day. This is gradually increased over the course of 12 days to 0.25 mg per day. The dose can then be increased every 3 days until the ideal therapeutic response is achieved. The usual adult maintenance dose is 3 mg a day, usually given in 3 divided doses. The maximum dose is 5 mg a day. Children: This medication is generally not prescribed for children.

ONSET OF EFFECT
Unknown.

DURATION OF ACTION
Unknown.

DIETARY ADVICE
No special restrictions.

STORAGE
Store in a tightly sealed container away from heat, moisture, and direct light.

MISSED DOSE
Take it as soon as you remember. If it is near the time for the next dose, skip the missed dose and resume your regular dosage schedule. Do not double the next dose.

STOPPING THE DRUG
Consult your doctor before stopping the drug. The dosage should be tapered gradually over the course of 7 to 14 days.

PROLONGED USE
It is not known whether long-term use of pergolide presents any special problems; study of the drug's long-term effects is very limited.

▼ PRECAUTIONS

Over 60: No special problems are expected, but use this drug with caution.

Driving and Hazardous Work: Pergolide may cause drowsiness or confusion. Do not drive or engage in hazardous work until you determine how the medicine affects you.

Alcohol: Avoid alcohol.

Pregnancy: Adequate human studies have not been done. This drug should not be used in pregnant women.

Breast Feeding: Pergolide may inhibit the secretion of breast milk and so should not be used by nursing mothers.

Infants and Children: The safety and effectiveness of this medication for infants and children have not been established; consult your pediatrician.

Special Concerns: This drug should be used with special caution by those with any gastrointestinal disorders or any urinary difficulty, for example, problems when urinating, pain with urination, or urinary tract infection.

OVERDOSE
Symptoms: There have been very few reports of pergolide mesylate overdose. Signs and symptoms include low blood pressure and agitation.

What to Do: Call your doctor, emergency medical services (EMS), or the nearest poison control center immediately.

▼ INTERACTIONS

DRUG INTERACTIONS
Pergolide may interact with phenothiazine antipsychotic drugs such as chlorpromazine hydrochloride, thio-ridazine hydrochloride, or prochlorperazine. Consult your doctor for advice.

FOOD INTERACTIONS
No known food interactions.

DISEASE INTERACTIONS
Consult your doctor if you have any of the following: a gastrointestinal disorder, a urinary tract disorder, or heart disease (especially a condition associated with heart rhythm abnormalities).

≣ SIDE EFFECTS ≣

SERIOUS
Confusion, hallucinations, unusual or abnormal muscle movements, low blood pressure (causing dizziness, lightheadedness, fainting, or confusion) pain or burning while urinating (symptoms of a urinary tract infection).

COMMON
Dizziness or lightheadedness when standing or sitting up suddenly is particularly common when the drug is first started but usually subsides with continued use.

LESS COMMON
High blood pressure, diarrhea, dry mouth, facial swelling.

PERINDOPRIL ERBUMINE

Available in: Tablets
Available OTC? No   **As Generic?** No
Drug Class: Angiotensin-converting enzyme (ACE) inhibitor

▼ USAGE INFORMATION

WHY IT'S PRESCRIBED
To control high blood pressure (hypertension).

HOW IT WORKS
Angiotensin-converting enzyme (ACE) inhibitors block an enzyme that produces angiotensin, a naturally occurring substance that causes blood vessels to constrict and stimulates production of the adrenal hormone, aldosterone, which promotes sodium retention in the body. As a result, ACE inhibitors relax blood vessels (causing them to widen) and reduces sodium retention, which lowers blood pressure and so decreases the workload of the heart.

▼ DOSAGE GUIDELINES

RANGE AND FREQUENCY
To start, 4 mg once a day. Doses may be increased to a maximum of 16 mg a day in 1 or 2 doses. The usual main-tenance dose is 4 to 8 mg a day. Patients over the age of 65 should start with a dose of 2 mg and not take more than 8 mg a day without consulting their doctor.

ONSET OF EFFECT
Within 1 to 2 hours.

DURATION OF ACTION
Up to 24 hours.

DIETARY ADVICE
Perindopril can be taken without regard to meals. Follow your doctor's dietary advice (such as low-salt or low-cholesterol restrictions) to improve control over high blood pressure and heart disease. Avoid high-potassium foods like bananas and citrus fruits and juices, unless you are also taking medications, such as diuretics, that lower potassium levels.

STORAGE
Store in a tightly sealed container away from heat, moisture, and direct light.

MISSED DOSE
Take it as soon as you remember. If it is near the time for the next dose, skip the missed dose and resume your regular dosage schedule. Do not double the next dose.

STOPPING THE DRUG
Do not stop taking this drug abruptly, as this may cause potentially serious health problems. Dosage should be reduced gradually, according to your doctor's instructions.

PROLONGED USE
See your doctor regularly for examinations and tests if you must take this medicine for a prolonged period. Remember that perindopril helps control high blood pressure but does not cure it. Lifelong therapy may be necessary.

▼ PRECAUTIONS

Over 60: Some elderly patients may be more sensitive to the effects of this drug; smaller doses may be warranted.

Driving and Hazardous Work: Avoid such activities until you determine how the medicine affects you.

Alcohol: Consume alcohol only in moderation since it may increase the effect of the drug and cause an excessive drop in blood pressure. Consult your doctor for advice.

Pregnancy: Use of perindopril during the last 6 months of pregnancy may cause severe defects, even death, in the fetus. The drug should be discontinued if you are pregnant or plan to become pregnant.

Breast Feeding: Perindopril may pass into breast milk; caution is advised. Consult your doctor for advice.

Infants and Children: Safety and effectiveness have not been established for patients under age 18.

Special Concerns: Perindopril has to be stopped if blood liver enzymes become markedly elevated.

OVERDOSE
Symptoms: Dizziness or fainting due to extremely low blood pressure.

What to Do: Few cases of overdose have been reported. However, call your doctor, emergency medical services (EMS), or the nearest poison control center immediately if you suspect that someone has taken a much larger dose than prescribed.

▼ INTERACTIONS

DRUG INTERACTIONS
Consult your doctor if you are taking diuretics (especially potassium-sparing diuretics), potassium supplements or drugs containing potassium (check ingredient labels), lithium, or gentamicin.

FOOD INTERACTIONS
Avoid low-salt milk and salt substitutes. Many of these products contain potassium.

DISEASE INTERACTIONS
Consult your doctor if you have had a prior allergic reaction to an ACE inhibitor, congestive heart failure, other types of heart disease, liver disease, or kidney failure.

 SIDE EFFECTS

SERIOUS
Fever and chills; sore throat and hoarseness; sudden difficulty breathing or swallowing; swelling of the face, mouth, or extremities; impaired kidney function (ankle swelling, decreased urination); confusion; yellow discoloration of the eyes or skin (indicating liver dysfunction); intense itching, chest pain or palpitations; abdominal pain. Serious side effects are very rare; contact your doctor immediately.

COMMON
Dry, persistent cough.

LESS COMMON
Dizziness or fainting; skin rash; numbness or tingling in the hands, feet, or lips; unusual fatigue or muscle weakness; nausea; drowsiness; loss of taste; headache.

PERMETHRIN

Available in: Lotion
Available OTC? Yes **As Generic?** Yes
Drug Class: Topical antiparasitic

▼ USAGE INFORMATION

WHY IT'S PRESCRIBED
To treat head lice infestations.

HOW IT WORKS
Permethrin is absorbed into the bodies of lice, where it blocks nerve activity, ultimately causing paralysis and death of the lice. (The drug has no such toxic effect on humans.)

▼ DOSAGE GUIDELINES

RANGE AND FREQUENCY
For treatment of head lice (pediculus humanus capitis): After the hair has been washed with shampoo, rinsed with water, and dried with a towel, apply a sufficient amount (approximately 25 mL) of liquid. Allow it to remain on the hair for 10 minutes, then rinse off with water. Rinse thoroughly and dry with a clean towel. Use a fine-tooth comb to remove any remaining nits or nit shells. If lice are found after 7 days, repeat the treatment.

ONSET OF EFFECT
Within 10 minutes.

DURATION OF ACTION
Up to 10 days.

DIETARY ADVICE
Permethrin can be used without regard to diet.

STORAGE
Store in a tightly sealed container away from heat and direct light.

MISSED DOSE
If a second dose is needed and you do not administer it after 7 days, do so as soon as you remember.

STOPPING THE DRUG
You need not take the second dose if no lice are found after 7 days.

PROLONGED USE
If lice recur, consult your physcian.

▼ PRECAUTIONS

Over 60: No special problems are expected.

Driving and Hazardous Work: The use of permethrin should not impair your ability to perform such tasks safely.

Alcohol: No special warnings.

Pregnancy: In animal studies, permethrin has not caused problems or birth defects. Human studies have not been done. Before you use permethrin, tell your doctor if you are pregnant or plan to become pregnant.

Breast Feeding: Permethrin may pass into breast milk; caution is advised. Consult your doctor for advice.

Infants and Children: Use and dosage in children up to 2 years of age must be determined by your doctor.

Special Concerns: All members of your household should be examined for lice and given treatment if necessary. Any sexual partner should be examined and treated if necessary. Clothing, household linen, hairbrushes, combs, and bedding should be thoroughly cleaned by machine washing with hot water and machine drying for at least 20 minutes, using the hot cycle. Seal nonwashable items in a plastic bag for at least 2 weeks or spray them with a product designed to eliminate lice and their nits. You should not use this drug if you are hypersensitive to chrysanthemums. Treatment with permethrin may temporarily worsen the itching and other symptoms of head lice infestation.

OVERDOSE
Symptoms: No cases of overdose have been reported.

What to Do: Although overdose is unlikely, if someone accidentally ingests the drug, call your doctor, emergency medical services (EMS), or the nearest poison control center immediately.

▼ INTERACTIONS

DRUG INTERACTIONS
Before you use this medicine, tell your doctor if you are using any other prescription or over-the-counter medication that is to be applied to the scalp.

FOOD INTERACTIONS
No known food interactions.

DISEASE INTERACTIONS
Consult your doctor if you have severe inflammation of the skin.

≡ SIDE EFFECTS ≡

SERIOUS
No serious side effects have been reported.

COMMON
Burning, itching, numbness, rash, redness, stinging, swelling, or tingling of scalp. In most cases, such symptoms are mild and temporary; notify your doctor if they are more troublesome or if they persist.

LESS COMMON
No less-common side effects have been reported.

PERPHENAZINE

Available in: Oral solution, tablets, injection
Available OTC? No   **As Generic?** Yes
Drug Class: Neuroleptic; antipsychotic

▼ USAGE INFORMATION

WHY IT'S PRESCRIBED
To treat psychotic conditions (severe mental disorders characterized by distorted thoughts and perceptions, such as schizophrenia.

HOW IT WORKS
Perphenazine blocks receptors of dopamine (a chemical that aids in the transmission of nerve impulses) in the central nervous system. Presumably, this produces a tranquilizing or antipsychotic effect.

▼ DOSAGE GUIDELINES

RANGE AND FREQUENCY
Usual adult dose: Initially, 4 to 8 mg a day. Your doctor may gradually increase the dose as needed and tolerated, not to exceed 64 mg a day.

ONSET OF EFFECT
Sedation may occur within minutes, but onset of antipsy-chotic effect may take hours to occur or may not occur until days or weeks after the beginning of therapy.

DURATION OF ACTION
12 to 24 hours, but effects may persist for several days.

DIETARY ADVICE
Can be taken with food or a full glass of milk or water.

STORAGE
Store in a tightly sealed container away from heat, moisture, and direct light.

MISSED DOSE
Take it as soon as you remember. However, if it is near the time for the next dose, skip the missed dose and resume your regular dosage schedule. Do not double the next dose.

STOPPING THE DRUG
The decision to stop taking the drug should be made in consultation with your doctor.

PROLONGED USE
Consult your doctor about the need for follow-up evaluations and tests if you must take this drug for an extended period.

▼ PRECAUTIONS

Over 60: Adverse reactions are more likely and more severe in older patients.

Driving and Hazardous Work: Avoid such activities until you determine how the medicine affects you.

Alcohol: Avoid alcohol.

Pregnancy: Avoid using per-phenazine if you are pregnant or plan to become pregnant.

Breast Feeding: Either avoid taking the drug if possible or refrain from breast feeding.

Infants and Children: Adverse reactions may be more likely and more severe in children.

Special Concerns: Avoid prolonged exposure to high temperatures or hot climates. Drink plenty of fluids and stay cool in the summertime. Avoid overexposure to sunlight until you determine if the drug heightens your skin's sensitivity to ultraviolet light.

OVERDOSE
Symptoms: Extreme drowsiness, heartbeat irregularities, dry mouth, paradoxical restlessness or agitation, seizures, loss of consciousness.

What to Do: Call your doctor, emergency medical services (EMS), or the nearest poison control center immediately.

▼ INTERACTIONS

DRUG INTERACTIONS
Consult your doctor for specific advice if you are taking amantadine, high blood pressure medication, bromocriptine, deferoxamine, diuretics, levobunolol, heart medication, metipranolol, nabilone, other psychiatric drugs, pentamidine, pimozide, promethazine, trimeprazine, a thyroid agent, central nervous system depressants, epinephrine, lithium, levodopa, methyldopa, metoclopramide, metyrosine, pemoline, a rauwolfia alkaloid, or metrizamide.

FOOD INTERACTIONS
No known food interactions.

DISEASE INTERACTIONS
Consult your doctor if you have Parkinson's disease or any movement disorder, glaucoma, epilepsy, liver disease, or kidney disease.

SIDE EFFECTS

SERIOUS
Rapid heartbeat, profuse sweating, seizures, difficulty breathing, neck stiffness, swelling of the tongue, difficulty swallowing. Also a rare condition can develop called neuroleptic malignant syndrome, characterized by stiffness or spasms of the muscles, high fever, and confusion or disorientation. Call your doctor immediately.

COMMON
Nausea, reduced sweating, dry mouth, blurred vision, drowsiness, shaking of hands, stiffness, stooped posture.

LESS COMMON
Difficult urination, menstrual irregularities, breast pain or swelling, unexpected weight gain, uncontrolled movements of the tongue, fever, chills, sore throat, unusual bruising or bleeding, heart palpitations, skin rash, itching, increased sensitivity of the skin to sunlight.

PHENAZOPYRIDINE HYDROCHLORIDE

Available in: Tablets
Available OTC? Yes   **As Generic?** Yes
Drug Class: Urinary analgesic

▼ USAGE INFORMATION

WHY IT'S PRESCRIBED
For short-term relief of symptoms caused by irritation of the urinary tract. Such symptoms include burning, pain, and discomfort during urination, as well as an increased urge to urinate with only small amounts of urine passed on each occasion. Irritation of the urinary tract commonly occurs as a result of bladder infection; phenazopyridine can ease symptoms but will not cure such an infection.

HOW IT WORKS
Phenazopyridine passes through—and has a local anesthetic effect upon the lining of—the urinary tract, thus relieving the discomfort associated with infection or inflammation.

▼ DOSAGE GUIDELINES

RANGE AND FREQUENCY
Adults: 200 mg, 3 times a day. Children: 1.8 mg per lb of body weight, 3 times a day.

ONSET OF EFFECT
Unknown.

DURATION OF ACTION
Unknown.

DIETARY ADVICE
This medication is best taken with or after meals to minimize stomach upset.

STORAGE
Store in a tightly sealed container away from heat, moisture, and direct light.

MISSED DOSE
Take it as soon as you remember. If it is near the time for the next dose, skip the missed dose and resume your regular dosage schedule. Do not double the next dose.

STOPPING THE DRUG
The decision to stop taking the drug should be made by your doctor. If it is being taken with an antibiotic, it should be taken for only 2 days (6 doses).

PROLONGED USE
Phenazopyridine is intended only for short-term use.

▼ PRECAUTIONS

Over 60: No special problems are expected.

Driving and Hazardous Work: Do not drive or engage in hazardous work until you determine how the medicine affects you.

Alcohol: No special precautions are necessary.

Pregnancy: Adequate human studies have not been done. Before taking phenazopyridine, tell your doctor if you are pregnant or plan to become pregnant.

Breast Feeding: Phenazopyridine may pass into breast milk; caution is advised. Consult your doctor for advice.

Infants and Children: No special problems are expected.

Special Concerns: Phenazopyridine causes the urine to turn reddish orange. This is harmless, but it may stain clothing. The drug may also cause permanent staining or discoloration of soft contact lenses; it is best to wear glasses while taking the drug. For diabetic patients, phenazopyridine may cause false test results with sugar and urine ketone tests. Do not chew the tablets; chewing may cause permanent discoloration of teeth. Do not use any leftover medicine for future urinary tract infections without consulting your doctor.

OVERDOSE
Symptoms: Fatigue, paleness, shortness of breath, heart palpitations, bloody or cloudy urine, decreased urine output, swelling of the ankles and calves, lower back or flank pain, nausea or vomiting.

What to Do: While an overdose is unlikely, call your doctor, emergency medical services (EMS), or the nearest poison control center immediately if symptoms of overdose occur.

▼ INTERACTIONS

DRUG INTERACTIONS
Some drugs may interact with phenazopyridine. Consult your doctor for specific advice if you are taking any prescription or over-the-counter medication.

FOOD INTERACTIONS
No known food interactions.

DISEASE INTERACTIONS
Caution is advised when taking phenazopyridine. Consult your doctor if you have any of the following: glucose-6-phosphate dehydrogenase deficiency (G6PD), hepatitis, uremia, pyelonephritis (kidney infection) during pregnancy, or other kidney disease.

≣ SIDE EFFECTS ≣

SERIOUS
Serious side effects are rare. Call your doctor immediately if you experience any of the following: difficulty breathing; swelling of the face, fingers, feet, or lower legs; blue or purple-blue skin color; unusual fatigue; fever; confusion; sudden decrease in urine output; shortness of breath; tightness in the chest; skin rash; yellow discoloration of the eyes or skin; unusual weight gain.

COMMON
Reddish-orange urine.

LESS COMMON
Indigestion, dizziness, stomach cramps or pain, headache.

PHENELZINE SULFATE

Available in: Tablets
Available OTC? No **As Generic?** No
Drug Class: Monoamine oxidase (MAO) inhibitor antidepressant

▼ USAGE INFORMATION

WHY IT'S PRESCRIBED
To treat symptoms of major mental depression.

HOW IT WORKS
Phenelzine inhibits the activity of monoamine oxidase, an enzyme that renders certain brain chemicals (epinephrine, norepinephrine, and dopamine) inactive. Consequently, this drug increases the availability of these chemicals in the nervous system; this is thought to have an antidepressant effect.

▼ DOSAGE GUIDELINES

RANGE AND FREQUENCY
Adults: To start, 15 mg, 3 times a day; may be increased to 90 mg a day. Older adults: To start, 15 mg once a day; may be increased to 60 mg a day.

ONSET OF EFFECT
7 to 10 days; it may take up to 8 weeks for full effect.

DURATION OF ACTION
Up to 10 days after treatment is stopped.

DIETARY ADVICE
See Food Interactions.

STORAGE
Store in a tightly sealed container away from heat and direct light.

MISSED DOSE
Take it as soon as you remember. If it is near the time for the next dose, skip the missed dose and resume your regular dosage schedule. Do not double the next dose.

STOPPING THE DRUG
The decision to stop taking the drug should be made in consultation with your doctor.

PROLONGED USE
The usual course of therapy lasts 6 months to 1 year; some patients benefit from additional therapy. See your doctor regularly for tests and examinations if long-term therapy is required.

▼ PRECAUTIONS

Over 60: Adverse reactions may be more likely and more severe in older patients.

Driving and Hazardous Work: Exercise caution until you determine how the medicine affects you.

Alcohol: Avoid alcohol.

Pregnancy: Using this drug during pregnancy may increase the risk of birth defects.

Breast Feeding: Phenelzine may pass into breast milk; caution is advised. Consult your doctor for advice.

Infants and Children: Phenelzine is not recommended for children 16 years of age and under.

Special Concerns: Before having any surgical procedure, emergency treatment, or dental work, tell the doctor or dentist in charge that you are taking phenelzine. Your doctor may advise you to carry a card or wear a bracelet saying that you use phenelzine.

▼ OVERDOSE
Symptoms: Profound anxiety, confusion, seizures, cold, clammy skin, severe drowsiness, irregular pulse, hallucinations, severe headache, fainting, stiff muscles, sweating, breathing difficulty.

What to Do: Call your doctor, emergency medical services (EMS), or the nearest poison control center immediately.

▼ INTERACTIONS

DRUG INTERACTIONS
Consult your doctor for specific advice if you are taking or have recently taken amphetamines, blood pressure medications, diet pills, cyclobenzaprine, fluoxetine, levodopa, maprotiline, asthma medication, cold or allergy medication, meperidine, methylphenidate, another MAO inhibitor, paroxetine, sertraline, a tricyclic antidepressant, an oral diabetes drug, insulin, bupropion, buspirone, carbamazepine, any central nervous system depressant, dextromethorphan, trazodone, or tryptophan.

FOOD INTERACTIONS
Do not eat foods with a high tyramine content, such as cheeses; yeast or meat extracts; pickled or smoked meat, poultry, or fish; processed meats like bologna, salami, and pepperoni; and sauerkraut. Do not drink red wine or alcohol-free or reduced-alcohol beer. Do not drink beverages or eat food with a high caffeine content, such as coffee and chocolate.

DISEASE INTERACTIONS
Caution is advised when taking phenelzine. Consult your doctor if you have any of the following: a history of alcohol abuse, angina, frequent headaches, asthma, bronchitis, diabetes, epilepsy, heart disease or a recent heart attack, blood vessel disease, liver disease, Parkinson's disease, a recent stroke, kidney disease, an overactive thyroid, or pheochromocytoma.

SIDE EFFECTS

SERIOUS
Severe headache, high blood pressure, severe chest pain, dilated pupils, irregular heartbeat, sensitivity of eyes to light (photophobia), fever and sweating, nausea and vomiting, stiff neck, extreme dizziness. Call your doctor immediately.

COMMON
Blurring of vision; decreased urination; sexual dysfunction; dizziness or lightheadedness; mild headache; appetite changes, including cravings for sweets; weight gain; increase in sweating; muscle twitching during sleep; restlessness; shakiness; fatigue; insomnia.

LESS COMMON
Chills, constipation, decrease in appetite, dry mouth, swelling in the lower extremities.

PHENOBARBITAL

Available in: Capsules, elixir, tablets, injection
Available OTC? No   **As Generic?** Yes
Drug Class: Barbiturate

▼ USAGE INFORMATION

WHY IT'S PRESCRIBED
Primarily used for sedation before surgery and to control certain types of seizures. With the availability of newer sleep-inducing drugs, it is now rarely used for the short-term treatment of insomnia.

HOW IT WORKS
Barbiturates such as pheno-barbital act as powerful sedatives by reducing activity in the central nervous system (the brain and spinal cord).

▼ DOSAGE GUIDELINES

RANGE AND FREQUENCY
For sedation— Adult oral dose: 30 to 120 mg, 2 or 3 times a day (not to exceed 400 mg a day). Children's oral dose: 2 mg per 2.2 lbs (1 kg) of body weight, 3 times a day. For seizures— Adult oral dose: 60 to 250 mg a day. Children's oral dose: 1 to 6 mg per 2.2 lbs of body weight per day. For insomnia— Adult oral dose: 100 to 320 mg at bedtime.

Dosages for injectable forms of the drug will be determined by your doctor.

ONSET OF EFFECT
About 1 hour.

DURATION OF ACTION
10 to 12 hours.

DIETARY ADVICE
Tablets may be crushed and taken with fluid or food.

STORAGE
Store in a tightly sealed container away from heat, moisture, and direct light.

MISSED DOSE
If you are taking phenobarbital regularly, take the missed dose as soon as you remember. If it is near the time for the next dose, skip the missed dose and resume your regular dosage schedule. Do not double the next dose.

STOPPING THE DRUG
The decision to stop taking the drug should be made by your doctor. There is a risk of withdrawal side effects when the drug is stopped suddenly.

PROLONGED USE
Barbiturates may be habit-forming, and prolonged use may increase the risk of dependency. Phenobarbital, as well as other barbiturates, is used only for short-term treatment of insomnia. It is not usually effective when used for longer than 14 days.

▼ PRECAUTIONS

Over 60: Adverse reactions may be more likely and more severe in older patients and may require that smaller doses be used.

Driving and Hazardous Work: Because of sedative effects, do not drive or engage in hazardous work until you determine how the medicine affects you.

Alcohol: Avoid alcohol; its sedative effects are additive to those of the drug.

Pregnancy: Phenobarbital can cause birth defects and problems during pregnancy. Before you take phenobarbital, be sure to tell your doctor if you are pregnant or plan to become pregnant.

Breast Feeding: Phenobarbital passes into breast milk in small amounts and can cause side effects in breast-feeding infants. Consult your doctor for advice.

Infants and Children: As with older patients, infants and children are sensitive to the effects of phenobarbital.

Special Concerns: Phenobarbital may cause physical or mental dependence. Check with your doctor if you feel overly sedated or if you suffer withdrawal side effects when you stop taking the drug.

OVERDOSE
Symptoms: Severe sedation or excessive drowsiness, |confusion, severe weakness, slurred speech, staggering walk, shortness of breath or troubled breathing.

What to Do: Call your doctor, emergency medical services (EMS), or the nearest poison control center immediately.

▼ INTERACTIONS

DRUG INTERACTIONS
Consult your doctor for specific advice if you are taking other seizure medications, central nervous system depressants, warfarin (blood thinner), or oral contraceptives. Phenobarbital may make oral contraceptives less effective.

FOOD INTERACTIONS
No known food interactions.

DISEASE INTERACTIONS
Caution is advised when taking phenobarbital. Consult your doctor if you have any of the following: kidney disease, liver disease, porphyria, anemia, hyperactivity, mental depression, or a history of alcohol or drug abuse.

SIDE EFFECTS

SERIOUS
Excitability, confusion, or excessive sedation to the point you cannot be awakened. Also yellow discoloration of eyes or skin; swollen eyelids, face, or lips; wheezing; or rash (may be signs of drug allergy); sores on the lips or mouth. Call your doctor immediately.

COMMON
Clumsiness, unsteadiness, persistent drowsiness, dizziness or lightheadedness.

LESS COMMON
Anxiety or nervousness, nightmares, insomnia, constipation, feeling faint, irritability, headache, nausea or vomiting.

PHENOXYBENZAMINE HYDROCHLORIDE

Available in: Capsules
Available OTC? No   **As Generic?** No
Drug Class: Centrally acting antihypertensive

▼ USAGE INFORMATION

WHY IT'S PRESCRIBED
To treat high blood pressure caused by pheochromocytoma, a rare type of tumor that develops inside the adrenal glands, small hormone-producing glands located atop the kidneys.

HOW IT WORKS
Phenoxybenzamine acts upon certain areas of the central nervous system (the brain and spinal cord) that regulate the activity of the heart and the smooth muscle tissue surrounding the arteries. The drug causes the blood vessels to relax and widen, which lowers blood pressure.

▼ DOSAGE GUIDELINES

RANGE AND FREQUENCY
Adults: To start, 10 mg, 2 times a day. It may be increased to 20 to 40 mg, 2 or 3 times a day. Children: To start, 0.2 mg per 2.2 lbs (1 kg) of body weight once a day. It may be increased to 0.4 to 1.2 mg per 2.2 lbs in 3 or 4 daily doses.

ONSET OF EFFECT
Several hours.

DURATION OF ACTION
3 to 4 days.

DIETARY ADVICE
Take it with milk to avoid gastrointestinal irritation. Follow a healthy diet (low-salt, low-fat, low-cholesterol) as advised by your doctor to help control blood pressure and prevent heart disease.

STORAGE
Store in a tightly sealed container away from heat and direct light.

MISSED DOSE
Take it as soon as you remember. If it is near the time for the next dose, skip the missed dose and resume your regular dosage schedule. Do not double the next dose.

STOPPING THE DRUG
The decision to stop taking the drug should be made by your doctor.

PROLONGED USE
You should see your doctor regularly for tests and examinations if you take this drug for a prolonged period.

▼ PRECAUTIONS

Over 60: Adverse reactions, especially dizziness and lightheadedness, may be more likely and more severe in older patients. Phenoxybenzamine may reduce tolerance to cold temperatures in older patients.

Driving and Hazardous Work: Do not drive or engage in hazardous work until you determine how the medicine affects you.

Alcohol: Alcohol should be avoided while taking this medication.

Pregnancy: Animal and human studies of phenoxybenzamine have not been done. Before you take phenoxybenzamine, tell your doctor if you are pregnant or plan to become pregnant.

Breast Feeding: It is not known if phenoxybenzamine passes into breast milk. It has not been reported to cause problems in breast-fed babies. Consult your doctor about its use while nursing.

Infants and Children: No special problems expected.

Special Concerns: Before you have any kind of dental or surgical procedure, be sure to tell the doctor or dentist in charge that you take phenoxybenzamine. If dryness of the mouth continues for more than 2 weeks, consult your doctor or dentist. Be cautious in hot weather, as well as during exercise, or if you must stand for long periods of time, since these situations may increase the chances that you will become dizzy or lightheaded.

OVERDOSE
Symptoms: Dizziness, faintness, rapid heartbeat, vomiting, lethargy, loss of consciousness.

What to Do: Call your doctor, emergency medical services (EMS), or the nearest poison control center immediately.

▼ INTERACTIONS

DRUG INTERACTIONS
Consult your doctor for specific advice if you are taking diazoxide, dopamine, guanadrel, guanethidine, epinephrine, metaraminol, methoxamine, phenylephrine, or any over-the-counter medicines for appetite control, asthma, colds, hay fever, cough, or sinus problems.

FOOD INTERACTIONS
No known food interactions.

DISEASE INTERACTIONS
Caution is advised when taking phenoxybenzamine. Consult your doctor if you have cerebrovascular insufficiency, coronary artery disease, congestive heart failure, kidney disease, or a lung infection, or if you have had a recent heart attack or stroke.

  SIDE EFFECTS

SERIOUS
In laboratory animals, high and repeated doses of phenoxybenzamine have caused tumors. Whether such effects occur in humans is unknown.

COMMON
Dizziness or lightheadedness, especially when getting up from a sitting or lying position; rapid heartbeat; constricted pupils; stuffy nose.

LESS COMMON
Drowsiness, confusion, dry mouth, headache, lack of energy, male sexual problems, unusual fatigue.

PHENTERMINE

Available in: Tablets, capsules
Available OTC? No **As Generic?** Yes
Drug Class: Appetite suppressant

▼ USAGE INFORMATION

WHY IT'S PRESCRIBED
To suppress appetite in obese patients. It should be used in conjunction with a strict diet and should not be prescribed as the sole method for achieving weight loss.

HOW IT WORKS
Researchers believe that the appetite-control center for the body may be found in a part of the brain called the hypothalamus. Phentermine probably affects the transmission of nerve impulses in this area.

▼ DOSAGE GUIDELINES

RANGE AND FREQUENCY
15 to 37.5 mg once a day.

ONSET OF EFFECT
Within 1 hour.

DURATION OF ACTION
12 to 14 hours.

DIETARY ADVICE
Phentermine can be taken before breakfast or 1 to 2 hours after breakfast.

STORAGE
Store in a tightly sealed container away from heat and direct light.

MISSED DOSE
Take it as soon as you remember. If it is near the time for the next dose, skip the missed dose and resume your regular dosage schedule. Do not double the next dose.

STOPPING THE DRUG
Take as prescribed for the full treatment period, even if you begin to observe favorable results before the scheduled end of therapy.

PROLONGED USE
Prolonged use of phentermine may result in drug tolerance or occasionally drug dependence.

▼ PRECAUTIONS

Over 60: Adverse reactions may be more likely and more severe in older patients, especially when taken in combination with drugs that act on the central nervous system.

Driving and Hazardous Work: Do not drive or engage in hazardous work until you determine how the medicine affects you.

Alcohol: Avoid alcohol.

Pregnancy: Phentermine has not been shown to cause birth defects in humans. Before you take this drug, be sure to tell your doctor if you are pregnant or planning to become pregnant.

Breast Feeding: Phentermine may pass into breast milk; caution is advised. Consult your doctor for advice.

Infants and Children: Not recommended for use by children under age 16.

Special Concerns: After you stop taking this drug, your body may need time to adjust. Phentermine may affect blood sugar levels; consult your doctor if you have any concern. Notify your doctor if you experience mental depression, nausea or vomiting, unusual fatigue, or trembling after you stop taking phentermine. Before you have medical or dental treatment, be sure to tell your doctor or dentist that you are taking phentermine.

OVERDOSE
Symptoms: Stomach cramps, severe diarrhea, fever, hallucinations, unusual high or low blood pressure, irregular heartbeat, severe nausea or vomiting, feeling of panic, restlessness, tremor.

What to Do: An overdose of phentermine is unlikely to be life-threatening. However, if someone takes a much larger dose than recommended, call your doctor, emergency medical services (EMS), or the nearest poison control center immediately.

▼ INTERACTIONS

DRUG INTERACTIONS
The following drugs may interact with phentermine. Consult your doctor for specific advice if you are taking amantadine, amphetamines, chlophenadiol, medicine for asthma, colds, sinus problems, or allergies, methyl-phenidate, nabilone, pemoline, selective serotonin reuptake inhibitors (SSRIs), or MAO inhibitors.

FOOD INTERACTIONS
Avoid caffeine-containing foods or beverages.

DISEASE INTERACTIONS
Caution is advised when taking phentermine. Consult your doctor if you have any of the following: a history of drug or alcohol abuse, diabetes, epilepsy, glaucoma, heart disease, blood vessel disease, high blood pressure, an overactive thyroid, or kidney disease.

SIDE EFFECTS

SERIOUS
Confusion or mental depression, skin rash or hives, high blood pressure, sore throat and fever, unusual bleeding or bruising. Call your doctor immediately.

COMMON
Irritability, nervousness, restlessness, insomnia.

LESS COMMON
Blurred vision, change in sexual desire, constipation or diarrhea, difficult or painful urination, dizziness, lightheadedness, drowsiness, dry mouth, rapid heartbeat, increased urination, headache, increased sweating, nausea or vomiting, stomach cramps, unpleasant taste in the mouth.

PHENYLEPHRINE HYDROCHLORIDE OPHTHALMIC

Available in: Ophthalmic solution
Available OTC? Yes   **As Generic?** Yes
Drug Class: Adrenergic agent

▼ USAGE INFORMATION

WHY IT'S PRESCRIBED
The 2.5% and 10% solutions are used to dilate the pupil of the eye (prior to eye exams or ophthalmologic procedures) and to treat certain eye conditions. The 0.12% solution is used to reduce redness of the eye caused by minor irritation.

HOW IT WORKS
Ophthalmic phenylephrine affects the muscles that control the pupils, causing them to dilate, which helps the doctor view the interior structures of the eye. The drug reduces redness by constricting the superficial blood vessels in the whites of the eye.

▼ DOSAGE GUIDELINES

RANGE AND FREQUENCY
For redness— Adults and children: 1 drop of 0.12% solution every 3 or 4 hours as needed. For certain eye conditions— Adults and teenagers: 1 drop of 2.5% or 10% solution from 1 to 3 times a day. Children: 1 drop of 2.5% solution from 1 to 3 times a day.

ONSET OF EFFECT
Rapid.

DURATION OF ACTION
From 2 to 7 hours depending on the strength of the solution.

DIETARY ADVICE
This medication can be used without regard to diet.

STORAGE
Store in a tightly sealed container away from heat, moisture, and direct light. Do not allow the medicine to freeze.

MISSED DOSE
Apply it as soon as you remember. However, if it is near the time for the next dose, skip the missed dose and resume your regular dosage schedule. Do not double the next dose.

STOPPING THE DRUG
The decision to stop using the drug should be made by your doctor.

PROLONGED USE
You should see your doctor regularly for tests and examinations if you must use this drug for an extended period of time.

▼ PRECAUTIONS

Over 60: No special advice.

Driving and Hazardous Work: Do not drive or engage in hazardous work until you determine how the medicine affects your vision.

Alcohol: No special precautions are necessary.

Pregnancy: No problems are expected, but studies of effects in pregnancy have not been done in humans. Consult your physician.

Breast Feeding: No problems are expected, but studies of effects in breast feeding have not been done in humans. Consult your doctor.

Infants and Children: Adverse reactions may be more likely and more severe in infants and children. The 10% solution should not be used on infants. The other strengths should not be used on low-birth-weight infants.

Special Concerns: To use the eye drops, first wash your hands. Tilt your head back. Gently apply pressure to the inside corner of the eyelid and with the index finger of the same hand, pull downward on the lower eyelid to make a space. Drop the medicine into this space and close your eye. Apply pressure for 1 or 2 minutes while keeping the eye closed without blinking. Then wash your hands again. Make sure the tip of the dropper does not touch your eye, finger, or any other surface. Phenylephrine will make your eyes more sensitive to sunlight. If this occurs, wear sunglasses or avoid bright light as comfort dictates. If this effect continues for more than 12 hours after you have stopped using the medicine, consult your doctor. Ophthalmic phenylephrine is available over the counter only in the 0.12% solution. The 2.5% and 10% solutions are by doctor's prescription only.

OVERDOSE
Symptoms: Dizziness; paleness; rapid, irregular, or pounding heartbeat; trembling; profuse sweating; vomiting; coma; shock.

What to Do: Call your doctor, emergency medical services (EMS), or the nearest poison control center immediately.

▼ INTERACTIONS

DRUG INTERACTIONS
Be sure to tell your doctor if you are using any other prescription or over-the-counter medication.

FOOD INTERACTIONS
No known food interactions.

DISEASE INTERACTIONS
Consult your doctor if you have a history of heart disease, blood vessel disease, diabetes mellitus, high blood pressure, or idiopathic orthostatic hypotension (low blood pressure). This drug should not be used by those with a history of closed-angle glaucoma.

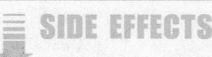

SIDE EFFECTS

SERIOUS
Dizziness; paleness; rapid, irregular, or pounding heartbeat; trembling; increased sweating. Call your doctor immediately.

COMMON
Unusually large pupils; burning, stinging, or watering of eyes; sensitivity of eyes to light; headache or brow ache.

LESS COMMON
Eye irritation not present prior to therapy.

PHENYLEPHRINE HYDROCHLORIDE SYSTEMIC

Available in: Nasal jelly, nasal drops, nasal spray
Available OTC? Yes   **As Generic?** Yes
Drug Class: Decongestant

▼ USAGE INFORMATION

WHY IT'S PRESCRIBED
To relieve nasal congestion caused by allergies, colds, or sinus conditions; to relieve congestion associated with ear infections.

HOW IT WORKS
Phenylephrine constricts blood vessels to reduce blood flow to swollen nasal passages, which reduces nasal secretions and improves airflow.

▼ DOSAGE GUIDELINES

RANGE AND FREQUENCY
Adults and children 12 and over: 2 to 3 drops of 0.25% to 0.5% solution, or 1 to 2 sprays, or a small amount of jelly in each nostril every 4 hours. Children 6 to 12 years: 2 to 3 drops or 1 to 2 sprays of a 0.25% solution in each nostril every 4 hours. Children under 6 years: 2 to 3 drops of 0.125% solution every 4 hours.

ONSET OF EFFECT
Rapid.

DURATION OF ACTION
From 30 minutes to 4 hours.

DIETARY ADVICE
Drink plenty of fluids.

STORAGE
Store in a tightly sealed container away from heat and direct light.

MISSED DOSE
Take it as soon as you remember. If it is near the time for the next dose, skip the missed dose and resume your regular dosage schedule. Do not double the next dose.

STOPPING THE DRUG
Do not use this medicine for more than 3 days without consulting your doctor.

PROLONGED USE
Using this medicine for more than 3 days may lead to rebound congestion (more severe congestion caused by the body's adaptation to the drug).

▼ PRECAUTIONS

Over 60: Although no studies have specifically examined the use of this drug in older patients, no special problems are expected.

Driving and Hazardous Work: Do not drive or engage in hazardous work until you determine how the medicine affects you.

Alcohol: Avoid alcohol.

Pregnancy: Phenylephrine hydrochloride has not been shown to cause birth defects or other problems if taken during pregnancy.

Breast Feeding: It is not known whether phenylephrine passes into breast milk; caution is advised. Consult your doctor for advice.

Infants and Children: Adverse reactions may be more likely and more severe in infants and children.

Special Concerns: Each container of medicine should be used by only one person to avoid spread of infection. Blow your nose gently before using this medicine. To use the nose drops, tilt your head back or lie down on a bed and hang your head over the side. Keep your head tilted back for a few minutes after instilling the drops. To use the nasal spray, keep your head upright and sniff briskly while spraying. For best results, spray again in 3 to 5 minutes. To use the nasal jelly, first wash your hands, then place an amount of jelly about the size of a pea into each nostril and sniff it well back into the nose.

OVERDOSE
Symptoms: Rapid, irregular, or pounding heartbeat; headache or dizziness; increased sweating; nervousness; trembling; paleness; insomnia. Such symptoms are more likely to be seen in young children.

What to Do: If someone takes a much larger dose than recommended, call your doctor, emergency medical services (EMS), or the nearest poison control center immediately.

▼ INTERACTIONS

DRUG INTERACTIONS
Before you take phenylephrine, tell your doctor if you are taking any other prescription or over-the-counter drug.

FOOD INTERACTIONS
No known food interactions.

DISEASE INTERACTIONS
Consult your doctor if you have a history of any of the following: high blood pressure, diabetes mellitus, heart disease, blood vessel (vascular) disease, or an overactive thyroid gland.

≣ SIDE EFFECTS ≣

SERIOUS
No serious side effects have been reported.

COMMON
Burning, dryness, or stinging inside the nose. An increase in nasal discharge or congestion may occur after 3 to 5 days of continuous use.

LESS COMMON
Headache, rapid or irregular heartbeat, excitability, restlessness.

PHENYLPROPANOLAMINE HYDROCHLORIDE

Available in: Capsules, tablets, extended-release capsules and tablets
Available OTC? Yes **As Generic?** Yes
Drug Class: Decongestant; appetite suppressant

▼ USAGE INFORMATION

WHY IT'S PRESCRIBED
To treat nasal congestion. Also works as an appetite suppressant. Note: Due to safety concerns, The Food and Drug Administration (FDA) is taking steps to remove phenylpropanolamine (PPA) from all drug products and has requested that all drug companies discontinue marketing products containing PPA.

HOW IT WORKS
PPA constricts blood vessels to reduce blood flow to swollen nasal passages and other tissues, which reduces nasal secretions; it also suppresses the appetite control center of the brain.

▼ DOSAGE GUIDELINES

RANGE AND FREQUENCY
For nasal congestion. Capsules and tablets— Adults and children 12 to 18 years of age: 25 mg every 4 hours as needed; no more than 150 mg per day. Children 6 to 12 years of age: 12.5 mg every 4 hours as needed; no more than 75 mg per day. Children 2 to 6 years of age: 6.25 mg every 4 hours as needed; no more than 37.5 mg per day. Extended-release capsules— Adults: 75 mg every 12 hours. Children: Use and dosage must be determined by a doctor. For appetite control. Capsules and tablets— Adults: 25 mg 3 times a day. Children 12 to 18 years of age: Use and dosage must be determined by a doctor. Children up to 12 years of age: Use is not recommended. Extended-release capsules and tablets— Adults: 75 mg once a day, taken in the morning. Children 12 to 18 years of age: Use and dosage must be determined by a doctor.

ONSET OF EFFECT
15 to 30 minutes.

DURATION OF ACTION
Capsules and tablets: 3 hours. Extended-release capsules and tablets: 12 to 16 hours.

DIETARY ADVICE
For appetite suppression, take it 30 minutes before meals; extended-release form, take it after breakfast. Be sure to drink plenty of fluids.

STORAGE
Store in a tightly sealed container away from heat and direct light.

MISSED DOSE
Take it as soon as you remember. If it is near the time for the next dose (12 hours for extended-release form), skip the missed dose and resume your regular dosage schedule. Do not double the next dose.

STOPPING THE DRUG
The decision to stop taking the drug should be made by your doctor.

PROLONGED USE
If cold symptoms do not improve within 7 days or if you have a high fever, check with your doctor. For appetite suppression: Do not take this drug for more than a few weeks without the approval of your doctor.

▼ PRECAUTIONS

Over 60: No special advice.

Driving and Hazardous Work: No special warnings.

Alcohol: No special warnings.

Pregnancy: There is no evidence of harm to the fetus, although women who have used this drug during pregnancy appear to be at greater risk for postpartum psychiatric disorders.

Breast Feeding: No problems have been reported.

Infants and Children: Phenylpropanolamine should not be used for weight control in children under 12. Its use for weight control in children 12 to 18 should be closely supervised by your doctor or pediatrician.

OVERDOSE
Symptoms: Abdominal pain, rapid or irregular heartbeat, severe headache, increased sweating, nausea, vomiting, severe nervousness and restlessness, confusion, seizures, rapid or irregular pulse, hallucinations, hostile behavior, trembling.

What to Do: Call your doctor, emergency medical services (EMS), or the nearest poison control center immediately.

▼ INTERACTIONS

DRUG INTERACTIONS
Consult your doctor for if you are taking amantadine, amphetamines, chlophedianol, asthma medicine, methylphenidate, nabilone, other appetite suppressants, cold medicines, pemoline, beta-blockers, digitalis drugs, MAO inhibitors, or rauwolfia alkaloids.

FOOD INTERACTIONS
Avoid large amounts of caffeinated beverages.

DISEASE INTERACTIONS
Consult your physician if you have diabetes mellitus, glaucoma, high blood pressure, heart disease, blood vessel disease, an overactive thyroid, or a history of mental illness.

SIDE EFFECTS

SERIOUS
Severe increase in blood pressure, with symptoms including severe headache, dizziness, double vision, ringing in the ears, and distended neck veins; tightness in chest; difficult or painful urination. Call your doctor immediately.

COMMON
No common side effects have been reported.

LESS COMMON
Dizziness, dry nose or mouth, mild headache, mild nausea, nervousness, restlessness, insomnia, euphoria.

PHENYLPROPANOLAMINE HYDROCHLORIDE/GUAIFENESIN

Available in: Tablets, extended-release tablets
Available OTC? Yes   **As Generic?** Yes
Drug Class: Nasal decongestant/expectorant

▼ USAGE INFORMATION

WHY IT'S PRESCRIBED
To relieve nasal congestion associated with minor upper respiratory conditions including the common cold, bronchitis, and sinus and throat infections. Note: Due to safety concerns, The Food and Drug Administration (FDA) is taking steps to remove phenylpropanolamine (PPA) from all drug products and has requested that all drug companies discontinue marketing products containing PPA.

HOW IT WORKS
Phenylpropanolamine narrows and constricts blood vessels to reduce the blood flow to swollen nasal passages and other tissues, which reduces nasal secretions and helps open up the airways. Guaifenesin purportedly breaks up, liquefies, and loosens mucus secretions in the respiratory tract, making it easier to cough up phlegm and thus breathe easier.

▼ DOSAGE GUIDELINES

RANGE AND FREQUENCY
Adults– Tablets: 25 mg phenylpropanolamine and 100 to 440 mg guaifenesin every 4 hours. Extended-release tablets: 75 mg phenylpropanolamine and 100 to 600 mg guaifenesin every 12 hours. Children– 6.25 to 12.5 mg phenylpropanolamine and 50 to 200 mg guaifenesin every 4 hours.

ONSET OF EFFECT
Unknown.

DURATION OF ACTION
Up to 24 hours.

DIETARY ADVICE
Drink plenty of fluids.

STORAGE
Store in a tightly sealed container away from heat and direct light.

MISSED DOSE
Take it as soon as you remember. If it is near the time for the next dose, skip the missed dose and resume your regular dosage schedule. Do not double the next dose.

STOPPING THE DRUG
The decision to stop taking the drug should be made when you begin to note improvement.

PROLONGED USE
Tell your doctor if your symptoms persist for more than a week, recur, or are accompanied by fever, rash, or a persistent headache.

▼ PRECAUTIONS

Over 60: Adverse reactions may be more likely and more severe in older patients.

Driving and Hazardous Work: Do not drive or engage in hazardous work until you determine how the medicine affects you.

Alcohol: Avoid alcohol.

Pregnancy: Before taking this medicine, be sure to tell your doctor if you are pregnant or plan to become pregnant.

Breast Feeding: This medicine may pass into breast milk; caution is advised. Consult your doctor for specific advice.

Infants and Children: Blood pressure changes and mental changes are likely to occur in children. Consult your doctor for advice.

Special Concerns: Be sure to take adequate amounts of fluids to help make mucus thin. This medicine should not be taken for a persistent or chronic cough associated with cigarette smoking, asthma, or emphysema. Do not crush or chew the extended-release form of the medication.

OVERDOSE
Symptoms: Restlessness, tremor, confusion, seizures, hallucinations, heart arrhythmias, unusually high or low blood pressure, nausea, vomiting, drowsiness, lethargy.

What to Do: Call your doctor, emergency medical services (EMS), or the nearest poison control center immediately.

▼ INTERACTIONS

DRUG INTERACTIONS
Consult your doctor for specific advice if you are taking MAO inhibitors or other sympathomimetic medications.

FOOD INTERACTIONS
No known food interactions.

DISEASE INTERACTIONS
Caution is advised when taking this medicine. Consult your physician if you have any of the following: anemia, gout, hemophilia, ulcers or other stomach problems, brain disease, colitis, seizures, diarrhea, gallbladder disease, gallstones, cystic fibrosis, diabetes, any chronic lung disease, an enlarged prostate, difficulty urinating, glaucoma, heart or blood vessel disease, or thyroid disease. Use of phenylpropanolamine with guaifenesin may cause complications in patients with liver or kidney disease, since those organs work together to remove the medication from the body.

≡ SIDE EFFECTS ≡

SERIOUS
Heart arrhythmias, palpitations, unusually slow or rapid heartbeat. Call your doctor immediately.

COMMON
Nervousness, insomnia, restlessness, headache, nausea, malaise, stomach irritation.

LESS COMMON
There are no less-common side effects associated with the use of this medication.

PHENYTOIN

Available in: Prompt and extended capsules, chewable tablets, oral suspension
Available OTC? No **As Generic?** Yes
Drug Class: Anticonvulsant

▼ USAGE INFORMATION

WHY IT'S PRESCRIBED
To prevent or control seizures in the treatment of certain types of epilepsy and other conditions.

HOW IT WORKS
Phenytoin is thought to depress the activity of certain parts of the brain and suppress the irregular and uncontrolled firing of neurons that causes seizures.

▼ DOSAGE GUIDELINES

RANGE AND FREQUENCY
Adults: 200 to 500 mg a day, as a single dose or in 2 divided doses. Children: 5 to 300 mg a day, as a single dose or in 2 divided doses. Some patients require higher doses. A low dose is used to start, then gradually increased by your doctor.

ONSET OF EFFECT
Several hours.

DURATION OF ACTION
Maximum effect lasts for 24 hours or longer; effectiveness then gradually decreases.

DIETARY ADVICE
Take with food to minimize stomach upset. Tablets may be crushed, chewed, or swallowed whole.

STORAGE
Store in a tightly sealed container away from heat, moisture, and direct light.

MISSED DOSE
Take it as soon as you remember. Be especially attentive about not missing a dose if you are taking this drug only once daily.

STOPPING THE DRUG
This medication should never be stopped abruptly because this may cause seizures. The dose is typically tapered over a period of weeks under the supervision of your doctor.

PROLONGED USE
This drug is often taken for prolonged periods. See your doctor for periodic checkups.

▼ PRECAUTIONS

Over 60: Older patients may require lower doses to minimize side effects.

Driving and Hazardous Work: Do not drive or engage in hazardous work until you determine how the medicine affects you.

Alcohol: May contribute to excessive drowsiness.

Pregnancy: Anticonvulsants are associated with an increased risk of birth defects. However, seizures during pregnancy can also increase the risks to the unborn child. Discuss with your doctor the potential risks and benefits of using this drug during pregnancy. Folate supplementation is recommended beginning 1 to 2 months before conception and throughout pregnancy.

Breast Feeding: Phenytoin passes into breast milk, although at low levels. Consult your doctor for advice.

Infants and Children: No special problems expected.

Special Concerns: The generic version of this drug is not recommended. Do not change the brand of phenytoin you are taking without consulting your doctor. The suspension form of phenytoin should be shaken well before you take it. Your doctor may advise you to wear a medical bracelet or carry an identification card saying that you are taking this medication.

OVERDOSE
Symptoms: Blurred or double vision, difficulty walking, severe clumsiness or unsteadiness, severe confusion, dizziness or drowsiness.

What to Do: Call your doctor, emergency medical services (EMS), or the nearest poison control center immediately.

▼ INTERACTIONS

DRUG INTERACTIONS
Many other drugs may interact with phenytoin, including other anticonvulsants (carbamazepine, phenobarbital, primidone, valproic acid), allopurinol, amiodarone, anticancer drugs, chloramphenicol, chlorpheniramine, cimetidine, diazoxide, dicumarol, disulfiram, isoniazid, loxapine, phenylbutazone, rifampin, sulfonamides, trazodone, trimethoprim.

FOOD INTERACTIONS
No known food interactions.

DISEASE INTERACTIONS
Caution is advised in those with liver or kidney disease, since these organs work together to remove the medication from the body.

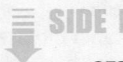
SIDE EFFECTS

SERIOUS
Fever, sore throat, swollen glands, pointlike rash on the skin or mucous membranes, blistering or peeling, mouth sores or bleeding gums, easy bruising, pallor, weakness, confusion, or seizures may be a sign of a potentially fatal blood disorder or other complication. Call your doctor immediately.

COMMON
Sedation, lethargy, nervousness, dizziness, thickened gums, excessive growth of body and facial hair. High doses may cause abnormal movements of the eyes, mouth, tongue, or limbs. Prolonged use may cause mild nerve impairment in the arms or legs.

LESS COMMON
Constipation, acne, mild skin rash, incoordination. There are numerous additional possible side effects; consult your doctor if you are concerned about any adverse or unusual reactions.

PILOCARPINE OPHTHALMIC

Available in: Ophthalmic solution and gel, ocular system
Available OTC? No   **As Generic?** Yes
Drug Class: Antiglaucoma agent

▼ USAGE INFORMATION

WHY IT'S PRESCRIBED
To treat glaucoma and to constrict the pupil.

HOW IT WORKS
Glaucoma, a sight-threatening disorder, occurs when aqueous humor (the fluid inside the eye) cannot drain properly, causing an increase in pressure within the eyeball (intraocular pressure). This can damage the optic nerve and lead to a gradually progressive loss of vision. Pilocarpine contracts the muscles that constrict the pupil; this action appears to help open the structures that allow drainage of the aqueous humor, thereby decreasing eye pressure.

▼ DOSAGE GUIDELINES

RANGE AND FREQUENCY
Ophthalmic solution– Adults and children: Chronic glaucoma: 1 drop into the eye 1 to 4 times a day. Acute closed-angle glaucoma: 1 drop into the eye every 5 to 10 minutes for 3 to 6 doses, then 1 drop every 1 to 3 hours. Ophthalmic gel–

Adults and teenagers: Once a day at bedtime. Children: Use and dosage must be determined by your doctor. Ocular system: Adults and children: 1 insert every 7 days. Infants: Use and dosage must be determined by your doctor.

ONSET OF EFFECT
10 to 60 minutes.

DURATION OF ACTION
Ophthalmic solution: 4 to 14 hours. Ophthalmic gel: Up to 24 hours; Ocular system: Up to 7 days.

DIETARY ADVICE
No special restrictions.

STORAGE
Store in a tightly sealed container away from heat, moisture, and direct light. Store the ophthalmic solution and the 3.5 g size of the ophthalmic gel at room temperature. The 5 g size of the ophthalmic gel and the ocular system should be refrigerated until used, but do not allow either to freeze.

MISSED DOSE
Apply it as soon as you remember. If it is near the time for the next dose, skip the missed dose and resume your regular dosage schedule. Do not double the next dose.

STOPPING THE DRUG
The decision to stop using the drug should be made by your doctor.

PROLONGED USE
See your doctor regularly for tests and examinations if you take this medication for a prolonged period.

▼ PRECAUTIONS

Over 60: No special problems are expected.

Driving and Hazardous Work: Do not drive or engage in hazardous work until you determine how the medicine affects your vision.

Alcohol: No special precautions are necessary.

Pregnancy: No specific studies in humans have been done. Consult your doctor for specific advice.

Breast Feeding: No specific studies in humans have been done. Consult your doctor for specific advice.

Infants and Children: No special precautions.

Special Concerns: To use the eye drops or the gel, first wash your hands. Tilt your head back. Gently apply pressure to the inside corner of the eyelid and with your index finger, pull downward on the lower eyelid to make a space. Drop the medicine or put a short strip of gel (about ½ inch long) into this space and close your eye. Apply pressure for 1 or 2 minutes while keeping the eye closed without blinking. Wash hands again. Make sure the tip of the dropper or the applicator does not touch your eye, finger, or any other surface. To use the eye insert, follow the package directions carefully. The unit should be inserted at bedtime unless your doctor instructs otherwise.

OVERDOSE
Symptoms: Sweating, nausea, vomiting, diarrhea, trouble breathing.

What to Do: An overdose of ophthalmic pilocarpine is unlikely to be life-threatening. If a large volume enters the eye, flush with water. If someone accidentally ingests the medicine, call your doctor, emergency medical services (EMS), or the nearest poison control center immediately.

▼ INTERACTIONS

DRUG INTERACTIONS
Consult your doctor for specific advice if you are taking any other prescription or over-the-counter medication.

FOOD INTERACTIONS
No known food interactions.

DISEASE INTERACTIONS
Consult your doctor if you have asthma or any other eye disease or problem. This medicine should not be used if iritis (inflammation in the eye) is present or develops.

SIDE EFFECTS

SERIOUS
Increased sweating; muscle tremors; nausea, vomiting, or diarrhea; troubled breathing or wheezing; watering of mouth; eye pain. Call your doctor immediately.

COMMON
Decreased night vision, blurred vision, change in near or far vision, eyebrow pain (usually disappears within a week).

LESS COMMON
Headache, eye irritation.

PILOCARPINE SYSTEMIC

Available in: Tablets
Available OTC? No   **As Generic?** No
Drug Class: Cholinergic parasympathomimetic agent

▼ USAGE INFORMATION

WHY IT'S PRESCRIBED
To treat dryness of the mouth and throat that occurs after radiation therapy for cancer of the head and neck.

HOW IT WORKS
Pilocarpine stimulates the activity of salivary glands.

▼ DOSAGE GUIDELINES

RANGE AND FREQUENCY
Adults: 5 mg, 3 times a day. If needed, dose may be increased to 10 mg, 3 times a day.

ONSET OF EFFECT
Unknown.

DURATION OF ACTION
Unknown.

DIETARY ADVICE
Take it with food to reduce stomach upset. Otherwise, no special restrictions.

STORAGE
Store in a tightly sealed container away from heat, moisture, and direct light.

MISSED DOSE
Take it as soon as you remember. If it is near the time for the next dose, skip the missed dose and resume your regular dosage schedule. Do not double the next dose.

STOPPING THE DRUG
Take it as prescribed for the full treatment period, even if you begin to feel better before the scheduled end of therapy. The decision to stop taking the drug should be made by your doctor.

PROLONGED USE
See your physician and your dentist regularly for tests and examinations if you must take this drug for a prolonged period. A dry mouth condition increases the likelihood of dental cavities or other mouth problems.

▼ PRECAUTIONS

Over 60: No special problems have been reported.

Driving and Hazardous Work: Do not drive or engage in hazardous work until you determine how the medicine affects you.

Alcohol: Moderate alcohol intake is acceptable.

Pregnancy: Adequate human studies have not been done. Before taking pilocarpine, tell your physician if you are pregnant or plan to become pregnant.

Breast Feeding: Pilocarpine may pass into breast milk; avoid or discontinue use while nursing, unless approved by your doctor.

Infants and Children: The safety and effectiveness of pilocarpine use in infants and children have not been established.

Special Concerns: See your dentist regularly while taking pilocarpine. If the drug causes increased sweating, consume more fluids to prevent dehydration. Consult your doctor if you have any concerns about the proper amount of fluid intake.

OVERDOSE
Symptoms: Chest pain, heartbeat irregularities, severe or ongoing diarrhea, confusion, nausea or vomiting, severe headache, stomach pain or cramps, difficulty breathing, vision problems, severe trembling or shaking, severe fatigue.

What to Do: Call your doctor, emergency medical services (EMS), or the nearest poison control center immediately.

▼ INTERACTIONS

DRUG INTERACTIONS
Other drugs may interact with pilocarpine. Consult your doctor for specific advice if you are taking anticholinergics, antiglaucoma agents, bethanechol, cholinergics, or beta-blockers.

FOOD INTERACTIONS
No known food interactions.

DISEASE INTERACTIONS
Pilocarpine should not be used if you have uncontrolled asthma, narrow-angle closure glaucoma, acute iritis, or major heart, blood vessel, or lung disease. Consult your doctor if you have any of the following: controlled asthma, chronic bronchitis or any other breathing problem, gallbladder problems, heart or blood vessel disease, psychological disorders, detached retina, or another retinal disease.

≡ SIDE EFFECTS ≡

SERIOUS
Serious side effects of pilocarpine are indistinguishable from those of overdose and include chest pain, heartbeat irregularities, severe or ongoing diarrhea, confusion, nausea or vomiting, headache, stomach pain or cramps, difficulty breathing, severe or persistent vision problems, severe trembling or shaking, and fatigue. Call your doctor immediately.

COMMON
Increased sweating.

LESS COMMON
Bloating or fluid retention, chills, nausea or vomiting, diarrhea, runny nose, dizziness, rapid heartbeat, headache, indigestion, frequent urination, redness of face or feeling of warmth, trembling or shaking, difficulty swallowing, excessive tearing, change in voice.

PINDOLOL

Available in: Tablets
Available OTC? No   **As Generic?** Yes
Drug Class: Beta-blocker

BRAND NAME

Visken

▼ USAGE INFORMATION

WHY IT'S PRESCRIBED
To treat mild to moderate high blood pressure.

HOW IT WORKS
Pindolol slows the rate and force of contraction of the heart by blocking certain nerve impulses, thus reducing blood pressure.

▼ DOSAGE GUIDELINES

RANGE AND FREQUENCY
Adults: 5 mg, 2 times a day. Dosage may be increased to a maximum of 30 mg, 2 times a day.

ONSET OF EFFECT
Within 1 hour.

DURATION OF ACTION
Up to 12 hours.

DIETARY ADVICE
Pindolol can be taken without regard to diet.

STORAGE
Store in a tightly sealed container away from heat and direct light.

MISSED DOSE
Take it as soon as you remember. If it is near the time for the next dose, skip the missed dose and resume your regular dosage schedule. Do not double the next dose.

STOPPING THE DRUG
The decision to stop taking the drug should be made by your doctor. Slow reduction of the dose under doctor's close supervision for 2 to 3 weeks is advised.

PROLONGED USE
Lifelong therapy with pindolol may be necessary; prolonged use may be associated with a greater incidence of side effects. Regular monitoring and evaluation by your doctor is advised.

▼ PRECAUTIONS

Over 60: Adverse reactions may be more likely and more severe in older patients. Resistance to cold temperatures may be decreased in older patients.

Driving and Hazardous Work: Use caution when driving or engaging in hazardous work until you determine how the medicine affects you.

Alcohol: Drink in careful moderation if at all. Alcohol may interact with the drug and cause a dangerous drop in blood pressure.

Pregnancy: Pindolol was shown to cause fetal harm in some animal studies. Before you take it, tell your doctor if you are pregnant or plan to become pregnant.

Breast Feeding: Pindolol passes into breast milk; consult your doctor about its use during nursing.

Infants and Children: The dosage must be determined by your pediatrician.

Special Concerns: Take extra care during exercise or hot weather, as taking this drug may contribute to dizziness. Check your pulse regularly while taking pindolol. If it is slower than your usual rate or less than 50 beats a minute, check with your doctor.

OVERDOSE
Symptoms: Unusually slow or rapid heartbeat, severe dizziness or fainting, poor circulation in the hands (bluish skin), breathing difficulty; seizures.

What to Do: An overdose of pindolol is unlikely to be life-threatening. However, if someone takes a much larger dose than prescribed, call your doctor, emergency medical services (EMS), or the nearest poison control center immediately.

▼ INTERACTIONS

DRUG INTERACTIONS
Consult your doctor for specific advice if you are taking allergy shots, aminophylline, caffeine, oxtriphylline, theophylline, oral antidiabetics, insulin, calcium channel blockers, clonidine, guanabenz, or MAO inhibitors.

FOOD INTERACTIONS
No known food interactions.

DISEASE INTERACTIONS
Pindolol should be used with caution in people with diabetes, especially insulin-dependent diabetes, since the drug may mask symptoms of hypoglycemia. Use of pindolol may cause complications in patients with liver or kidney disease, since these organs work together to remove the medication from the body. Also consult your doctor if you have any of the following: any allergy (including hay fever), bronchitis, emphysema, heart disease, blood vessel disease, mental depression, myasthenia gravis, psoriasis, or hyperthyroidism.

SIDE EFFECTS

SERIOUS
Shortness of breath, wheezing; irregular or slow heartbeat (50 beats per minute or less); pain or feelings of tightness or pressure in the chest; swelling of the ankles, feet, and lower legs; mental depression. If you experience any such symptoms, stop taking pindolol and contact your doctor right away.

COMMON
Dizziness or lightheadedness, especially when rising suddenly to a standing position; decreased sexual ability; unusual fatigue, weakness, or drowsiness; insomnia.

LESS COMMON
Anxiety, irritability, nervousness; constipation; diarrhea; dry, sore eyes; itching; nausea or vomiting; nightmares or intensely vivid dreams; numbness, tingling, or other unusual sensations in the fingers, toes, or scalp.

PIOGLITAZONE HYDROCHLORIDE

Available in: Tablets
Available OTC? No   **As Generic?** No
Drug Class: Thiazolidinedione/antidiabetic agent

▼ USAGE INFORMATION

WHY IT'S PRESCRIBED
As a single therapeutic agent or as an adjunct (supplemental) therapy to a sulfonylurea, metformin, or insulin to control blood glucose levels in patients with non-insulin-dependent (type 2) diabetes.

HOW IT WORKS
Pioglitazone increases the body's sensitivity and response to insulin.

▼ DOSAGE GUIDELINES

RANGE AND FREQUENCY
To start, 15 to 30 mg once a day. For people taking only pioglitazone and who do not respond adequately, the dose may be increased by a doctor to no more than 45 mg once a day. If monotherapy does not control blood glucose, combination therapy should be considered. If hypoglycemia occurs when taking pioglitazone in combination with a sulfonylurea or insulin, it may be necessary to decrease the dose of the sulfonylurea or insulin.

ONSET OF EFFECT
Within 1 week.

DURATION OF ACTION
Unknown.

DIETARY ADVICE
Pioglitazone may be taken with or without food.

STORAGE
Store in a tightly sealed container away from heat, moisture, and direct light.

MISSED DOSE
If it is the same day, take the missed dose as soon as you remember. If you miss an entire day's dose, resume your regular dosage schedule the following day and do not double the next dose.

STOPPING THE DRUG
The decision to stop taking pioglitazone should be made in consultation with your physician.

PROLONGED USE
See your doctor regularly for liver function tests if you must take pioglitazone for an extended period of time.

▼ PRECAUTIONS

Over 60:
No special problems are expected.

Driving and Hazardous Work:
Pioglitazone should not impair your ability to perform such tasks safely.

Alcohol:
Drink only in moderation, if at all.

Pregnancy:
Adequate studies of pioglitazone use during pregnancy have not been done. In general, insulin is the treatment of choice for controlling blood glucose levels during pregnancy. Pioglitazone should not be used during pregnancy unless your doctor believes the potential benefit justifies the potential risk to the fetus. Pioglitazone may stimulate ovulation in premenopausal women who have stopped ovulating. Contraception may be advised.

Breast Feeding:
Pioglitazone may pass into breast milk; do not use it while nursing.

Infants and Children:
Safety and effectiveness of pioglitazone have not been established in children.

Special Concerns:
Another thiazolidinedione drug, troglitazone, has been associated with rare, serious, and sometimes fatal, liver-related side effects. Although no similar side effects have been reported for pioglitazone, liver function tests are recommended just prior to treatment, every two months for the first year, and periodically thereafter. If you develop unexplained symptoms of liver dysfunction, such as nausea, vomiting, abdominal pain, fatigue, loss of appetite, or dark urine, call your doctor immediately. It is important to follow your doctor's advice on diet, exercise, and other measures to help control diabetes.

OVERDOSE

Symptoms: No specific ones have been reported.

What to Do: While no cases of overdose have been reported, if someone takes a much larger dose than prescribed, call your doctor, emergency medical services (EMS), or the nearest poison control center immediately.

▼ INTERACTIONS

DRUG INTERACTIONS
No known drug interactions.

FOOD INTERACTIONS
No known food interactions.

DISEASE INTERACTIONS
Pioglitazone should not be taken by those with type 1 diabetes or for the treatment of diabetic ketoacidosis. Caution is advised if you have edema or heart failure. Consult your doctor prior to using pioglitazone if you have any type of liver abnormality.

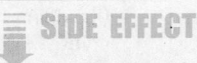
SIDE EFFECTS

SERIOUS
No serious side effects have been associated with the use of pioglitazone.

COMMON
Upper respiratory tract infection, sore throat.

LESS COMMON
Headache, sinusitis, muscle pain, tooth disorder, edema (swelling).

PIPERAZINE

Available in: Tablets
Available OTC? No   **As Generic?** Yes
Drug Class: Anthelmintic

▼ USAGE INFORMATION

WHY IT'S PRESCRIBED
To treat various worm infections, including ascariasis (common roundworm) and enterobiasis (pinworm), as an alternative to more standard lines of therapy. It is also used to treat partial intestinal obstruction by the common roundworm, a condition primarily occurring in children.

HOW IT WORKS
Piperazine paralyzes the worm; it is then expelled from the body in the stool.

▼ DOSAGE GUIDELINES

RANGE AND FREQUENCY
For common roundworms—Adults: 3.5 g a day for 2 days. Treatment may be repeated after a week. Children: 75 mg per 2.2 lbs (1 kg) of body weight a day for 2 days. Treatment may be repeated after 2 weeks. For pinworms— Adults and children: 65 mg per 2.2 lbs for 7 days. Treatment may be repeated after a week.

ONSET OF EFFECT
Unknown.

DURATION OF ACTION
Unknown.

DIETARY ADVICE
No special restrictions.

STORAGE
Store in a tightly sealed container away from heat, moisture, and direct light.

MISSED DOSE
Take it as soon as possible. If it is near the time for the next dose, skip the missed dose and resume your regular dosage schedule. Do not double the next dose.

STOPPING THE DRUG
Take as prescribed for the full treatment period, even if you begin to feel better before the scheduled end of therapy.

PROLONGED USE
See your doctor regularly for tests and examinations.

▼ PRECAUTIONS

Over 60: Adverse reactions may be more likely and more severein older patients.

Driving and Hazardous Work: No special precautions are necessary.

SIDE EFFECTS

SERIOUS
Joint pain, skin rash, fever, itching. Call your physician as soon as possible.

COMMON
No common side effects are associated with the use of piperazine.

LESS COMMON
Headache, diarrhea, stomach cramps or pain, dizziness, muscle fatigue, trembling, drowsiness, nausea or vomiting.

Alcohol: No special precautions are necessary.

Pregnancy: Adequate studies of piperazine use during pregnancy have not been done. Consult your doctor for specific advice if you are pregnant or plan to become pregnant.

Breast Feeding: Piperazine may pass into breast milk; caution is advised. Consult your doctor for specific advice.

Infants and Children: Adverse reactions may be more likely and more severe in children.

Special Concerns: For pinworm infection, clothing, bedding, and towels should be washed daily. All members of the family may have to be treated to eradicate the infestation. A second treatment for all household members may be necessary after 2 or 3 weeks. All bedding and nightclothes should be washed after treatment. To prevent reinfection, you should wash the anal region daily, change your underwear and bedding every day, and wash your hands and fingernails before each meal and after bowel movements. If your symptoms do not improve after a full course of treatment, consult your doctor.

OVERDOSE
Symptoms: Muscle fatigue, seizures, difficulty breathing.

What to Do: An overdose of piperazine is unlikely to be life-threatening. However, if someone takes a much larger dose than prescribed, call your doctor, emergency medical services (EMS), or the nearest poison control center.

▼ INTERACTIONS

DRUG INTERACTIONS
Other drugs may interact with piperazine. Consult your doctor for specific advice if you are taking phenothiazines or pyrantel. Also tell your doctor if you are taking any other prescription or over-the-counter medication.

FOOD INTERACTIONS
No known food interactions.

DISEASE INTERACTIONS
Caution is advised when taking piperazine. This drug should not be used if you have a seizure disorder, especially a history of epilepsy. Use of piperazine may cause complications in patients with kidney disease, since this organ works to remove the medication from the body.

PIRBUTEROL ACETATE

Available in: Inhalation aerosol
Available OTC? No **As Generic?** No
Drug Class: Bronchodilator/sympathomimetic

▼ USAGE INFORMATION

WHY IT'S PRESCRIBED
To dilate air passages in the lungs that have become narrowed as a result of disease or inflammation. It is used in the treatment of asthma and chronic obstructive pulmonary disease (COPD).

HOW IT WORKS
Pirbuterol widens constricted airways in the lungs by relaxing the smooth muscle tissue that surrounds the bronchial passages.

▼ DOSAGE GUIDELINES

RANGE AND FREQUENCY
May be used when needed to relieve breathing difficulty. Adults and children 12 years and older, by inhalation aerosol: 1 to 2 inhalations every 4 to 6 hours. Do not exceed more than 12 inhala-tions per day. Infants and children less than 12 years of age: Consult your pediatrician.

ONSET OF EFFECT
Within 5 minutes.

DURATION OF ACTION
5 hours.

DIETARY ADVICE
Maintain your usual food and fluid intake.

STORAGE
Store in a tightly sealed container away from heat and direct light. Do not refrigerate inhalation solutions.

MISSED DOSE
Skip the missed dose and resume your regular dosage schedule. Do not double the next dose.

STOPPING THE DRUG
It may not be necessary to finish the recommended course of therapy. Consult your doctor for advice.

PROLONGED USE
Therapy may require months or years. Excessive use may result in temporary loss of effectiveness.

▼ PRECAUTIONS

Over 60: Adverse reactions may be more likely and more severe in older patients.

Driving and Hazardous Work: Do not drive or engage in hazardous work until you determine how the medicine affects you.

Alcohol: No special precautions are necessary.

Pregnancy: Adequate studies have not been done; the benefits must be weighed against potential risks. Consult your doctor for advice.

Breast Feeding: It is not known if pirbuterol passes into breast milk. Mothers who wish to breast-feed while taking this drug should discuss the matter with their doctor.

Infants and Children: Use of the inhalation aerosol requires special coordination skills and is not recommended in young children. Dosage in children younger than 12 has not been established.

Special Concerns: Pay heed to any asthma attack or other breathing problem that does not improve after your usual nebulizer treatment or usual number of puffs. Seek help immediately if you feel your lungs are persistently constricted, if you are using more than the recommended number of treatments or puffs per day, or if you feel a recent attack is somehow different from others. Do not use with other mouthpieces or canisters.

OVERDOSE
Symptoms: Chest pain or heaviness; irregular, racing, fluttering, or pounding heartbeat; dizziness; lightheadedness; fainting; severe weakness; severe headache.

What to Do: Call your doctor, emergency medical services (EMS), or the nearest poison control center immediately.

▼ INTERACTIONS

DRUG INTERACTIONS
Consult your doctor for specific advice if you are taking a beta-blocker, ergotamine or ergotamine-like medications, antidepressants, digitalis drugs, or an MAO inhibitor.

FOOD INTERACTIONS
No known food interactions.

DISEASE INTERACTIONS
Consult your doctor if you have a history of substance abuse (especially cocaine), seizures, brain damage, heart disease, heartbeat irregularities, high blood pressure, anxiety disorders, or a thyroid condition.

SIDE EFFECTS

SERIOUS
Pirbuterol may become ineffective if used too often, resulting in more-severe breathing difficulty that does not improve. Signs include persistent wheezing, coughing, or shortness of breath; confusion; bluish color to lips or fingernails; inability to speak. Other side effects include chest pain or heaviness; irregular, racing, fluttering, or pounding heartbeat; lightheadedness; fainting; severe weakness; severe headache.

COMMON
Sleeping difficulty, dry mouth, sore throat, nervousness, excitability, restlessness.

LESS COMMON
Trembling; sweating; headache; nausea or vomiting; flushing or redness to cheeks or other skin; mood changes; unusual bruising; numbness, tingling, or other change in sensation of hands and feet; loss of appetite; changes in sense of smell and taste.

PIROXICAM

Available in: Capsules
Available OTC? No **As Generic?** Yes
Drug Class: Nonsteroidal anti-inflammatory drug (NSAID)

▼ USAGE INFORMATION

WHY IT'S PRESCRIBED
To treat mild to moderate pain and inflammation caused by tendinitis, arthritis, bursitis, gout, soft tissue injuries, migraine and other vascular headaches, menstrual cramps, and other conditions. When patients fail to respond to one NSAID, another may be tried. The greatest effectiveness often requires trial and error of several different NSAIDs.

HOW IT WORKS
NSAIDs work by interfering with the formation of prostaglandins, natural substances in the body that cause inflammation and make nerves more sensitive to pain impulses. NSAIDs also have other modes of action that are less well understood.

▼ DOSAGE GUIDELINES

RANGE AND FREQUENCY
Adults: 20 mg once a day. The dose may be increased to 20 mg, 2 times a day. For children's dose, consult your pediatrician.

ONSET OF EFFECT
Several hours for analgesic relief; up to 2 weeks for anti-inflammatory effects.

DURATION OF ACTION
Varies.

DIETARY ADVICE
Take with food; maintain your usual food and fluid intake.

STORAGE
Store in a tightly sealed container away from heat, moisture, and direct light.

MISSED DOSE
Take it as soon as you remember. If it is near the time for the next dose, skip the missed dose and resume your regular dosage schedule. Do not double the next dose.

STOPPING THE DRUG
The decision to stop taking the drug should be made in consultation with your doctor.

PROLONGED USE
Prolonged use can cause gastrointestinal problems, including ulceration and bleeding, kidney dysfunction, and liver inflammation. Consult your doctor about the need for medical examinations and lab tests.

▼ PRECAUTIONS

Over 60: Because of the potentially greater consequences of gastrointestinal side effects, the dose of NSAIDs for older patients, especially those over age 70, is often cut in half.

Driving and Hazardous Work: Avoid such activities until you determine how the medicine affects you.

Alcohol: Avoid alcohol when using this medication because it increases the risk of stomach irritation.

Pregnancy: Avoid or discontinue this drug if you are pregnant or plan to become pregnant.

Breast Feeding: Piroxicam passes into breast milk; avoid use while nursing.

Infants and Children: May be used in exceptional circumstances; consult your doctor.

Special Concerns: Because NSAIDs can interfere with blood coagulation, this drug should be stopped at least 3 days prior to any surgery.

OVERDOSE
Symptoms: Severe nausea, vomiting, headache, confusion, seizures.

What to Do: Call your doctor, emergency medical services (EMS), or the nearest poison control center immediately.

▼ INTERACTIONS

DRUG INTERACTIONS
Do not take this drug with aspirin or any other NSAIDs without your doctor's approval. In addition, consult your doctor if you are taking antihypertensives, steroids, anticoagulants, antibiotics, itraconazole or ketoconazole, plicamycin, penicillamine, valproic acid, phenytoin, cyclosporine, digitalis drugs, lithium, methotrexate, probenecid, triamterene, or zidovudine.

FOOD INTERACTIONS
No known food interactions.

DISEASE INTERACTIONS
Caution is advised when taking piroxicam. Consult your doctor if you have any of the following: bleeding problems, inflammation or ulcers of the stomach and intestines, diabetes mellitus, systemic lupus erythematosus (SLE, lupus), anemia, asthma, epilepsy, Parkinson's disease, kidney stones, or a history of heart disease or alcohol abuse. Use of piroxicam may cause complications in patients with liver or kidney disease, since these organs work together to remove the medication from the body.

≣ SIDE EFFECTS ≣

SERIOUS
Shortness of breath or wheezing, with or without swelling of legs or other signs of heart failure; chest pain; peptic ulcer disease with vomiting of blood; black, tarry stools; decreasing kidney function. Call your doctor immediately.

COMMON
Nausea, vomiting, heartburn, diarrhea, constipation, headache, dizziness, sleepiness.

LESS COMMON
Ulcers or sores in mouth, depression, rashes or blistering of skin, ringing sound in the ears, unusual tingling or numbness of the hands or feet, seizures, blurred vision. Also elevated potassium levels, decreased blood counts; such problems can be detected by your doctor.

PNEUMOCOCCAL VACCINE

Available in: Injection
Available OTC? No   **As Generic?** No
Drug Class: Vaccine

▼ USAGE INFORMATION

WHY IT'S PRESCRIBED
To prevent pneumococcal bacteria infections, such as pneumonia, meningitis, and bacteremia (a severe bacterial blood infection).

HOW IT WORKS
Pneumococcal vaccine stimulates the body's immune system to produce its own protective antibodies against the bacteria.

▼ DOSAGE GUIDELINES

RANGE AND FREQUENCY
Adults and children age 2 and older: A single injection under the skin or into a muscle of the upper arm or midthigh.

ONSET OF EFFECT
2 to 3 weeks.

DURATION OF ACTION
5 to 10 years.

DIETARY ADVICE
No special restrictions.

STORAGE
Not applicable; the dose is administered only at a health care facility.

MISSED DOSE
Not applicable.

STOPPING THE DRUG
Not applicable.

PROLONGED USE
Not applicable.

▼ PRECAUTIONS

Over 60: Pneumococcal vaccine is particularly recommended for persons over the age of 50. It is not expected to cause different or more severe side effects in older persons than it does in younger people.

Driving and Hazardous Work: Do not drive or engage in hazardous work until you determine how the medicine affects you.

Alcohol: No special precautions are necessary.

Pregnancy: Studies on the effects of pneumococcal vaccine in pregnant women have not been done. However, if needed, it should be given only after the first trimester of pregnancy. It should be given only to women who have a condition that makes them more vulnerable to infection or more likely to develop serious problems from a pneumococcal infection. Before you receive pneumococcal vaccine, tell your doctor if you are pregnant or plan to become pregnant.

Breast Feeding: Pneumococcal vaccine may pass into breast milk; caution is advised. Consult your doctor for specific advice.

Infants and Children: This vaccine is not recommended for use by children under the age of 2.

Special Concerns: If you have more than one doctor, be sure they all know that you have received this vaccine. In general, only one shot of the vaccine is needed for protection. Revaccination is recommended for persons who received the pneumococcal vaccine that was distributed between 1977 and 1983 if they are at high risk for infection. A second vaccination, 3 to 5 years after the first, may be necessary for children under age 10 with nephrotic syndrome, asplenia, or sickle-cell anemia.

OVERDOSE
Symptoms: An overdose with this vaccine is unlikely.

What to Do: No cases of overdose have been reported.

▼ INTERACTIONS

DRUG INTERACTIONS
Other drugs may interact with pneumococcal vaccine. Consult your doctor for advice if you are taking any prescription or over-the-counter medication. Tell your doctor if you have had any pneumococcal vaccine in the past.

FOOD INTERACTIONS
No known food interactions.

DISEASE INTERACTIONS
Consult your doctor if you have any severe illness that is causing fever. The vaccine should be given with caution to patients receiving anticoagulant therapy. Patients who have received extensive chemotherapy or radiation treatment for Hodgkin's disease should not receive the pneumococcal vaccine.

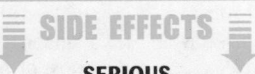

SIDE EFFECTS

SERIOUS
Serious allergic reaction involving difficulty swallowing or breathing; reddened skin, especially around the ears; itching, particularly of the hands or feet; hives; unusual and severe fatigue; swollen face, eyes, or nasal passages; and fever over 102°F. Call your doctor immediately.

COMMON
Pain, redness, swelling, or the formation of a hard lump at the site of the injection.

LESS COMMON
Fever, aches and pains in the joints or muscles, skin rash, unusual fatigue, general feeling of illness or discomfort, swollen glands.

PODOFILOX

BRAND NAME

Condylox

Available in: Topical gel, solution
Available OTC? No   **As Generic?** No
Drug Class: Antimitotic

▼ USAGE INFORMATION

WHY IT'S PRESCRIBED
To treat external condylomata acuminata (genital and peri-anal warts) in adults. Genital and perianal warts are caused by the human papillomavirus (HPV).

HOW IT WORKS
The exact mechanism of action is unknown.

▼ DOSAGE GUIDELINES

RANGE AND FREQUENCY
Apply a thin layer with the supplied cotton-tipped applicator (topical solution) or with the applicator tip or finger (topical gel) to the affected area(s) 2 times a day, in the morning and evening, for 3 consecutive days. Then discontinue treatment for 4 consecutive days. This cycle of treatment may be repeated until there are no more visible warts or for a maximum of 4 cycles. Your doctor should demonstrate the proper technique prior to the initial application.

ONSET OF EFFECT
Unknown.

DURATION OF ACTION
Unknown.

DIETARY ADVICE
Podofilox can be used without regard to diet.

STORAGE
Store in a tightly sealed container away from moisture, direct light, and extremes in temperature.

MISSED DOSE
Apply it as soon as you remember. If it is near the time for the next dose, skip the missed dose and resume your regular dosage schedule. Do not apply more than directed. It will not make the medicine work better and may increase side effects.

STOPPING THE DRUG
Apply podofilox in one-week cycles until there is no visible wart tissue or for a maximum of 4 cycles. Consult your doctor for specific advice if further treatment is needed.

PROLONGED USE
Safety and effectiveness beyond 4 weeks have not been determined. If response to therapy is incomplete after 4 one-week cycles, discontinue treatment and contact your physician.

▼ PRECAUTIONS

Over 60: No special problems are expected.

Driving and Hazardous Work: The use of podofilox should not impair your ability to perform such tasks safely.

Alcohol: No special precautions are necessary.

Pregnancy: Adequate human studies have not been done. Before taking podofilox, discuss with your doctor the relative risks and benefits of using this drug while pregnant.

Breast Feeding: Podofilox may pass into breast milk; caution is advised. Consult your doctor for advice.

Infants and Children: The safety and effectiveness of podofilox use in children under the age of 12 have not been established. Genital and perianal warts are contracted by people who are sexually active.

Special Concerns: Let the treated areas dry before allowing contact with unaffected skin. Wash your hands before and after each application. Podofilox is for external use only; do not apply to the urethra, rectum, or vagina. Do not apply the topical solution to the perianal (around the anus) area. Avoid getting podofilox into your eyes. If eye contact occurs, flush the eye at once with large quantities of water, and contact your doctor. Do not have sexual intercourse during the 3 days you are applying podofilox. Condoms may help protect new sexual partners from contracting HPV as well as other sexually transmitted diseases, such as herpes and HIV. However, they are not 100% effective. If the warts reappear, contact your doctor.

OVERDOSE
Symptoms: An overdose with podofilox is unlikely.

What to Do: If someone applies a much larger dose than prescribed or accidentally ingests podofilox, call your doctor.

▼ INTERACTIONS

DRUG INTERACTIONS
None reported.

FOOD INTERACTIONS
None reported.

DISEASE INTERACTIONS
None reported.

≡ SIDE EFFECTS ≡

SERIOUS
No serious side effects are associated with the use of podofilox.

COMMON
Burning, inflammation, pain, itching, sores, stinging, redness at the application sites.

LESS COMMON
Local tingling, blisters, dryness, crusting, swelling, scarring, bleeding, or chafing at the application sites. Vomiting, headache, insomnia, painful intercourse.

POLIOVIRUS VACCINE

Available in: Injection, oral solution
Available OTC? No   **As Generic?** Yes
Drug Class: Vaccine

▼ USAGE INFORMATION

WHY IT'S PRESCRIBED
To prevent poliomyelitis
(polio).

HOW IT WORKS
Poliovirus vaccine stimulates
the body's immune system to
produce its own protective
antibodies against the virus
that causes polio.

▼ DOSAGE GUIDELINES

RANGE AND FREQUENCY
Injection (inactivated vaccine)– All doses are given
under the skin, in either the
upper arm (adults) or midthigh (infants and children).
First dose is given at initial
visit. For children, this is usually at 6 to 8 weeks of age.
Second dose is given 8 weeks
later. Third dose is given 8
weeks to 12 months after the
second dose. Fourth dose,
when needed, is given 6 to
12 months after the third
dose. First booster dose, for
children, is usually administered upon entering school,
usually between ages 4 and 6.
Oral solution (live vaccine)–
Follow the same dosage
schedule as used for the
injection form.

ONSET OF EFFECT
Within 7 to 10 days.

DURATION OF ACTION
Up to 12 years.

DIETARY ADVICE
No special restrictions.

STORAGE
Not applicable; the dose is
administered only at a health
care facility.

MISSED DOSE
If your child misses a scheduled vaccination, contact your
pediatrician.

STOPPING THE DRUG
The full schedule of vaccinations should be followed
unless a medical problem
intervenes.

PROLONGED USE
No special problems are
expected.

≡ SIDE EFFECTS ≡

SERIOUS
Serious allergic reaction involving difficulty swallowing or
breathing; reddened skin, especially around the ears; itching, particularly of the hands or feet; hives; unusual and
severe fatigue; and swollen face, eyes, or nasal passages.
Call your doctor immediately.

COMMON
No common side effects are associated with the use
of poliovirus vaccine.

LESS COMMON
Injection: Fever; soreness, rash, tenderness, or pain at
injection site. There are no less-common side effects associated with the oral suspension.

▼ PRECAUTIONS

Over 60: Poliovirus vaccine is
not expected to cause different or more severe side
effects in older patients than
it does in younger persons.
Inactivated poliovirus vaccine
is preferred in adults.

**Driving and Hazardous
Work:** No special advice.

Alcohol: No warnings.

Pregnancy: Studies on the
effects of poliovirus vaccine
in pregnant women have not
been done. However, if
needed, it should be given
only to pregnant women at
great risk of acquiring polio.
Consult your doctor for
specific advice.

Breast Feeding: Poliovirus
vaccine has not been
reported to cause problems
during breast feeding. Consult
your doctor for advice. If your
child has taken the oral solution, refrain from breast feeding for 2 to 3 hours before
and after immunization.

Infants and Children: This
vaccine is not recommended
for use by infants under the
age of 6 weeks.

Special Concerns: Immunization with inactivated polio
vaccine is recommended for
any adult at risk of the disease, such as those traveling
to countries where polio is
not under control, those who
have not had the complete
series of immunizations, those
who work in medical facilities
or day-care centers, and
those working in laboratories
where poliovirus samples may
be handled.

OVERDOSE
Symptoms: An overdose of
poliovirus vaccine is unlikely.

What to Do: No cases of
overdose have been reported.

▼ INTERACTIONS

DRUG INTERACTIONS
Consult your doctor for
advice if you are undergoing
chemotherapy for cancer or
taking corticosteroids.

FOOD INTERACTIONS
No known food interactions.

DISEASE INTERACTIONS
Except under special circumstances, you should not
receive the poliovirus vaccine
if you have ongoing diarrhea,
any moderate or severe illness causing fever or vomiting, any immune deficiency
condition, such as HIV, a
family history of immune
deficiency, or a household
member with an immunodeficiency. Consult your doctor.

POLYETHYLENE GLYCOL SOLUTION (PEG)

Available in: Oral solution, powder for oral solution
Available OTC? No **As Generic?** No
Drug Class: Stimulant laxative

▼ USAGE INFORMATION

WHY IT'S PRESCRIBED
To clean the colon and rectum prior to diagnostic tests or surgical procedures involving the colon.

HOW IT WORKS
Polyethylene glycol (PEG) solution induces mild diarrhea to flush solid material from the colon.

▼ DOSAGE GUIDELINES

RANGE AND FREQUENCY
Adults and teenagers: Drink 1 full glass (8 oz) of PEG rapidly every 10 minutes until at least 4 liters have been consumed. Children: 11.3 to 18.2 mL per pound of body weight per hour.

ONSET OF EFFECT
Within 1 hour.

DURATION OF ACTION
Variable.

DIETARY ADVICE
Consume no food for 4 hours before taking PEG. Afterward, drink only clear fluids like water, ginger ale, decaffeinated cola, decaffeinated tea, or broth.

STORAGE
Store in a tightly sealed container away from heat, moisture, and direct light. Refrigerate the solution but do not allow it to freeze.

MISSED DOSE
Take it as soon as you remember. If it is near the time for the next dose, skip the missed dose and resume your regular dosage schedule. Do not double the next dose.

STOPPING THE DRUG
Continue drinking the solution until your stools are watery, clear and free of solid material. The decision to stop taking the drug should be made by your doctor.

PROLONGED USE
PEG is not intended for prolonged use.

▼ PRECAUTIONS

Over 60: No special problems are expected in older patients.

Driving and Hazardous Work: Do not drive or engage in hazardous work until you determine how the medicine affects you.

Alcohol: Avoid alcohol.

Pregnancy: Adequate human studies have not been done. Before taking PEG, tell your doctor if you are pregnant or plan to become pregnant.

Breast Feeding: PEG may pass into breast milk; caution is advised. Consult your doctor for specific advice.

Infants and Children: There is no specific information comparing use of PEG in children with use in other age groups. However, no special problems are expected.

Special Concerns: It will take up to 3 hours to consume the full recommended dose of PEG. The first bowel movement may start in 1 hour. Patients using the powder form of PEG should first mix the powder with water and add enough lukewarm water to reach the fill mark on the bottle. Shake well until all the ingredients are dissolved. Do not add any flavorings or other ingredients to the solution. Do not drink the solution chilled. Cases of hypothermia have been reported following ingestion of chilled solutions. Use the mixed solution within 48 hours.

OVERDOSE
Symptoms: Diarrhea, abdominal pain, bloating.

What to Do: An overdose of PEG is unlikely to occur. However, if you are concerned about the possibility of an overdose, call a doctor, emergency medical services (EMS), or the nearest poison control center.

▼ INTERACTIONS

DRUG INTERACTIONS
Any other oral medication taken within 1 hour of PEG may be flushed from the body. Consult your doctor for advice if you are taking any other medication.

FOOD INTERACTIONS
Do not consume any food for at least 4 hours before taking PEG.

DISEASE INTERACTIONS
Caution is advised when taking PEG. Consult your doctor if you have a history of any of the following: blockage or obstruction of the intestine, paralytic ileus, perforated bowel, toxic colitis, or toxic megacolon.

SIDE EFFECTS

SERIOUS
Skin rash. Call your doctor immediately should this occur.

COMMON
Bloating, nausea.

LESS COMMON
Stomach upset or abdominal cramps, vomiting, irritation of the anal region.

POTASSIUM CHLORIDE

Available in: Liquid, soluble granules, powder, tablets, sustained-release capsules
Available OTC? No   **As Generic?** Yes
Drug Class: Electrolyte

▼ USAGE INFORMATION

WHY IT'S PRESCRIBED
To restore or maintain proper potassium levels in the body. Potassium is an electrolyte, a mineral that helps maintain proper fluid balance. It is also vital in the transmission of nerve impulses.

HOW IT WORKS
Potassium chloride is absorbed in the body fluids and taken into the cells where it is part of a number of metabolic actions, especially those that involve the release of energy. It also aids in the conduction of nerve impulses responsible for muscle movement and heart contraction.

▼ DOSAGE GUIDELINES

RANGE AND FREQUENCY
20 milliequivalents (mEq) to 100 mEq daily in divided doses. A single dose should not exceed 20 mEq.

ONSET OF EFFECT
Unknown.

DURATION OF ACTION
Unknown.

DIETARY ADVICE
Must be taken after meals or with food and a glass of water or other liquid. Follow all special dietary guidelines as outlined by your doctor.

STORAGE
Store in a tightly sealed container away from heat and direct light. Keep liquid forms of potassium refrigerated, but do not allow to freeze.

MISSED DOSE
If you remember within 2 hours, take the missed dose with food or liquids and resume your regular dosage schedule. If you remember after 2 hours, skip the missed dose and return to your regular dosage schedule. Do not double the next dose.

STOPPING THE DRUG
Do not stop taking potassium without first consulting your doctor. Be especially careful not to stop taking potassium abruptly if you are also taking digitalis drugs (digoxin).

PROLONGED USE
Requires periodic testing of blood potassium levels by your doctor.

≡ SIDE EFFECTS ≡

SERIOUS
Numbness or tingling in the hands, feet, or lips; slowed or irregular heartbeat; breathing difficulty; unusual fatigue or weakness; confusion. Stop taking the drug and consult your doctor at once.

COMMON
Diarrhea, abdominal discomfort, gas, nausea and vomiting.

LESS COMMON
Black or bloody stools, pain when swallowing. Consult your doctor if such symptoms persist.

▼ PRECAUTIONS

Over 60: Elderly people may be at greater risk of retaining too much potassium owing to age-related changes in the ability of the kidneys to excrete it. Older patients should have their potassium levels checked regularly.

Driving and Hazardous Work: No special problems are expected.

Alcohol: No special problems are expected.

Pregnancy: Potassium supplements are considered safe during pregnancy if used exactly as prescribed.

Breast Feeding: Potassium may pass into breast milk. Consult your doctor for specific advice.

Infants and Children: Although the safety and effectiveness of potassium use by children have not been established, no specific problems have been documented.

Special Concerns: Remember that the foods in your diet must also be considered when calculating your total intake of potassium. Be certain to read all labels carefully, especially on all products labeled "low-sodium," such as canned foods and some breads, many of which contain potassium. Do not crush sustained-release forms. Swallow tablets without chewing, sucking, or crushing. Be sure the powder form is completely dissolved before ingesting.

OVERDOSE

Symptoms: Irregular heartbeat; muscle weakness, which may progress to paralysis of the diaphragm and interfere with breathing.

What to Do: Call your doctor, emergency medical services (EMS), or the nearest poison control center immediately.

▼ INTERACTIONS

DRUG INTERACTIONS
The following drugs may interact adversely with potassium chloride. Consult your doctor for advice if you are taking digitalis drugs, potassium-sparing diuretics, thiazide diuretics, NSAIDs, beta-blockers, heparin, triamterene, anticholinergics, or ACE inhibitors.

FOOD INTERACTIONS
To prevent ingestion of too much potassium, discuss your diet with your doctor. Foods high in potassium include avocados, bananas, broccoli, dried fruits, grapefruit, beans, meats, nuts, spinach, low-salt milk, squash, melon, brussels sprouts, zucchini, frozen orange juice, and tomatoes.

DISEASE INTERACTIONS
Consult your doctor if you have any of the following: intestinal obstruction, dehydration, severe diarrhea, compression of the esophagus, delayed gastric emptying, peptic ulcer, heart block, or a predisposition to retaining potassium.

PRAMIPEXOLE DIHYDROCHLORIDE

Available in: Tablets
Available OTC? No   **As Generic?** No
Drug Class: Dopamine agonist

▼ USAGE INFORMATION

WHY IT'S PRESCRIBED
To treat the symptoms of Parkinson's disease.

HOW IT WORKS
The exact mechanism of action is unknown, but pramipexole is believed to help increase the release of certain neurological chemicals that improve control over movement.

▼ DOSAGE GUIDELINES

RANGE AND FREQUENCY
Initial dose (for first week of therapy): 0.125 mg, 3 times a day. The dose is gradually increased (usually once a week for 7 weeks) up to 1.5 mg, taken 3 times a day, for a total dose of 4.5 mg a day.

ONSET OF EFFECT
Unknown.

DURATION OF ACTION
Unknown.

DIETARY ADVICE
Pramipexole may be taken with meals, if desired, to minimize the incidence of nausea or stomach upset.

STORAGE
Store in a tightly sealed container away from heat and direct light. Keep away from moisture and extremes in temperature.

MISSED DOSE
Take it as soon as you remember. If it is near the time for the next dose, skip the missed dose and resume your regular dosage schedule. Do not double the next dose.

STOPPING THE DRUG
The decision to stop taking the drug should be made in consultation with your doctor. Do not stop taking pramipexole suddenly; it is recommended that the dose be reduced gradually over a period of at least 1 week, according to your doctor's instructions.

PROLONGED USE
Lifetime therapy with pramipexole may be necessary; prolonged use may be associated with a greater incidence of side effects. Regular monitoring and evaluation by your doctor is advised.

▼ PRECAUTIONS

Over 60: Adverse reactions (especially hallucinations) may be more likely and more severe in older patients. Lower doses may be advised.

Driving and Hazardous Work: Pramipexole may cause sudden and extreme drowsiness. Do not drive or engage in hazardous work until you determine how the medicine affects you.

Alcohol: Avoid alcohol.

Pregnancy: Pramipexole should not be used by pregnant women.

Breast Feeding: Pramipexole should not be taken while nursing. The patient must choose between using the drug or breast feeding.

Infants and Children: Pramipexole should not be taken by children.

Special Concerns: This drug may cause dizziness and faintness, especially when getting up out of a chair or sitting up after lying down (a condition known as postural orthostatic hypertension, characterized by temporary episodes of excessively low blood pressure). Be cautious and move slowly when arising.

OVERDOSE
Symptoms: No cases of overdose have been reported.

What to Do: An overdose of pramipexole is unlikely to occur. However, if someone takes a much larger dose than prescribed, call your doctor, emergency medical services (EMS), or the nearest poison control center right away.

▼ INTERACTIONS

DRUG INTERACTIONS
Consult your doctor for specific advice if you are taking antiulcer drugs (specifically, histamine H2 blockers such as cimetidine and ranitidine), calcium channel blockers (such as diltiazem and verapamil), potassium-sparing diuretics (such as triamterene), or other dopamine agonists (such as phenothiazines, butyrophenones, thioxanthenes, and metoclopramide).

FOOD INTERACTIONS
No known food interactions.

DISEASE INTERACTIONS
Use of pramipexole may cause complications in patients with a history of kidney disease, since this medication is eliminated from the body through the kidneys.

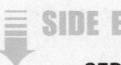
SIDE EFFECTS

SERIOUS
Excessively low blood pressure (orthostatic hypotension), causing extreme dizziness, confusion, nausea, fainting, or blackouts, especially when rising from a seated or lying position; hallucinations; impaired control over voluntary movements (dyskinesia).

COMMON
Mild to moderate dizziness or faintness (caused by a less severe drop in blood pressure) upon standing or sitting up, drowsiness, dry mouth.

LESS COMMON
Increased sweating, vision abnormalities, joint pain, increased urine output, weakness, pneumonia, increased incidence of accidental injury, tooth disease, leg cramps.

PRAVASTATIN

Available in: Tablets
Available OTC? No   **As Generic?** No
Drug Class: Antilipidemic (cholesterol-lowering agent)

▼ USAGE INFORMATION

WHY IT'S PRESCRIBED
To treat high cholesterol. Usually prescribed after first lines of treatment—including diet, weight loss, and exercise—fail to reduce total and low-density lipoprotein (LDL) cholesterol to acceptable levels.

HOW IT WORKS
Pravastatin blocks the action of an enzyme required for the manufacture of cholesterol, thereby interfering with its formation. By lowering the amount of cholesterol in the liver cells, pravastatin increases the formation of receptors for LDL, and thereby reduces blood levels of total and LDL cholesterol. In addition to lowering LDL cholesterol, pravastatin also modestly reduces triglyceride levels and raises HDL (the so-called good) cholesterol.

▼ DOSAGE GUIDELINES

RANGE AND FREQUENCY
Initial dose is 10 to 20 mg once a day. The dose may be increased to a maximum of 40 mg per day. Pravastatin is most effective when taken in the evening.

ONSET OF EFFECT
2 to 4 weeks.

DURATION OF ACTION
The effect persists for the duration of therapy.

DIETARY ADVICE
Cholesterol-lowering drugs are only one part of a total program that should include regular exercise and a healthy diet. The American Heart Association publishes a "Healthy Heart" diet, which is recommended.

STORAGE
Store in a tightly sealed container away from heat and direct light.

MISSED DOSE
Take it as soon as you remember. Take the next scheduled dose at the proper time and resume your regular dosage schedule, as prescribed. Do not double the next dose.

STOPPING THE DRUG
The decision to stop taking the drug should be made in consultation with your doctor. Once the medication is discontinued, blood cholesterol is likely to return to original elevated levels.

PROLONGED USE
Side effects are more likely with prolonged use. As you continue with pravastatin, your doctor will periodically order blood tests to evaluate liver function.

▼ PRECAUTIONS

Over 60: No special problems are expected.

Driving and Hazardous Work: The use of pravastatin should not impair your ability to perform such tasks safely.

Alcohol: No special precautions are necessary.

Pregnancy: Pravastatin should not be used during pregnancy or by women who plan to become pregnant in the near future.

Breast Feeding: This drug is not recommended for women who are nursing.

Infants and Children: Long-term effects of pravastatin in children have not been determined. Rarely used in young patients; consult your doctor.

Special Concerns: Important elements of treatment for high cholesterol include proper diet, weight loss, regular moderate exercise, and the avoidance of certain medications that may increase cholesterol levels. Because pravastatin has potential side effects, it is important that you maintain a recommended healthy diet and cooperate with other treatments your physician may suggest.

OVERDOSE
Symptoms: Overdose is unlikely to occur.

What to Do: Emergency instructions not applicable.

▼ INTERACTIONS

DRUG INTERACTIONS
Consult your doctor if you are taking cyclosporine, gemfibrozil, niacin, antibiotics, especially erythromycin, or medications for fungus infections. All of these drugs may increase the risk of myositis (muscle inflammation) when taken with pravastatin and may lead to kidney failure.

FOOD INTERACTIONS
No known food interactions.

DISEASE INTERACTIONS
Consult your doctor if you have any of the following problems: liver, kidney, or muscle disease, or a medical history involving organ transplant or recent surgery.

  SIDE EFFECTS

SERIOUS
Fever, unusual or unexplained muscle aches and tenderness. Call your doctor right away.

COMMON
Side effects occur in only 1% to 2% of patients. These include constipation or diarrhea, dizziness, gas, headache, heartburn, nausea, skin rash, stomach pain, rise in liver enzymes (detectable by your doctor).

LESS COMMON
Insomnia.

PRAZIQUANTEL

Available in: Tablets
Available OTC? No   **As Generic?** No
Drug Class: Anthelmintic

▼ USAGE INFORMATION

WHY IT'S PRESCRIBED
To treat trematode (fluke) infections, such as clonorchiasis, caused by Clonorchis sinensis (Chinese or Oriental liver fluke); opisthorchiasis, caused by Opisthorchis viverrini and O. felineus (liver flukes); and schistosomiasis, caused by Schistosoma mekongi, S. japonicum, S. mansoni, and S. hematobium (blood flukes). Praziquantel may be prescribed to treat other types of parasite-related disease as determined by your physician.

HOW IT WORKS
Praziquantel works by causing severe spasms and paralysis of the worm's muscles. The body's immune system can then better attack and expel the worm.

▼ DOSAGE GUIDELINES

RANGE AND FREQUENCY
For clonorchiasis, opisthorchiasis, and lung or intestinal fluke infection— Adults and children age 4 and older: 25 mg per 2.2 lbs (1 kg) of body weight, 3 times a day for 1 day. For schistosomiasis— Adults and children age 4 and older: 20 mg per 2.2 lbs, 2 to 3 times for 1 day. (Different doses may be prescribed in conjunction with corticosteroids to treat certain other parasite-related diseases.)

ONSET OF EFFECT
Unknown.

DURATION OF ACTION
Unknown.

DIETARY ADVICE
Praziquantel is best taken during meals with liquid. Do not chew the tablets.

STORAGE
Store in a tightly sealed container away from heat, moisture, and direct light.

MISSED DOSE
Take it as soon as you remember. However, if it is near the time for the next dose, skip the missed dose and resume your regular dosage schedule. Do not double the next dose.

STOPPING THE DRUG
Take it as prescribed for the full treatment period.

PROLONGED USE
See your doctor regularly for tests and examinations if you must take this medicine for a prolonged period. If your condition has not improved by the end of the course of therapy, consult your doctor.

▼ PRECAUTIONS

Over 60: Adverse reactions may be more likely and more severe in older patients.

Driving and Hazardous Work: Avoid such activities until you determine how the medicine affects you. If it does cause problems, do not drive or engage in hazardous activities the day you take praziquantel and for 24 hours after treatment.

Alcohol: No special warnings.

Pregnancy: Adequate human studies have not been done. Before taking praziquantel, be sure to tell your doctor if you are pregnant or plan to become pregnant.

Breast Feeding: Praziquantel passes into breast milk. Stop nursing the day you start therapy. Do not restart breast feeding until 72 hours after therapy is completed. All breast milk during this time should be extracted with a breast pump or squeezed out and thrown away.

Infants and Children: Use and dosage for children under age 4 must be determined by your pediatrician.

Special Concerns: Praziquantel has a bitter taste that can cause gagging or vomiting, especially if the pills are chewed. Swallow the pills whole with a small amount of liquid during meals.

OVERDOSE
Symptoms: An overdose with praziquantel is unlikely.

What to Do: An overdose with praziquantel is unlikely to be life-threatening. However, if you take a much larger dose than prescribed, take a fast-acting laxative and call your doctor.

▼ INTERACTIONS

DRUG INTERACTIONS
Consult your doctor for advice if you are taking any other prescription or over-the-counter medication, especially corticosteroids (used concurrently with praziquantel in the treatment of some parasite-related diseases), cimetidine, ketoconazole, or miconazole.

FOOD INTERACTIONS
No known food interactions.

DISEASE INTERACTIONS
Praziquantel should not be used when Taenia solium worm cysts are present in the eye. The death of the worm cysts by praziquantel may cause irreparable damage to the eyes. Caution is advised when taking praziquantel. If you have liver disease, you may be at greater risk for side effects. Consult your doctor for specific advice.

SIDE EFFECTS

SERIOUS
No serious side effects are associated with the use of praziquantel.

COMMON
Stomach pain or cramps, dizziness, drowsiness, bloody diarrhea, fever, nausea or vomiting, headache, increased sweating, loss of appetite, general discomfort. These symptoms are likely to occur as allergic reactions to dead worms and usually resolve on their own.

LESS COMMON
Hives, skin rash, itching.

PRAZOSIN

Available in: Capsules
Available OTC? No   **As Generic?** Yes
Drug Class: Peripherally acting antihypertensive

▼ USAGE INFORMATION

WHY IT'S PRESCRIBED
To treat high blood pressure (hypertension).

HOW IT WORKS
Prazosin causes the blood vessels to relax and widen, which in turn lowers blood pressure.

▼ DOSAGE GUIDELINES

RANGE AND FREQUENCY
Adults: To start, 0.5 to 1 mg, 2 or 3 times a day. The dose may be increased slowly to 6 to 15 mg a day divided into 2 or 3 doses. Children: 50 to 400 micrograms (mcg) per 2.2 lbs (1 kg) of body weight divided into 2 or 3 doses.

ONSET OF EFFECT
30 to 90 minutes. The full effect may not be realized for 3 to 4 weeks.

DURATION OF ACTION
7 to 10 hours.

DIETARY ADVICE
Follow a healthy diet (low-salt, low-fat, low-cholesterol) as advised by your doctor to help control blood pressure and prevent heart disease.

STORAGE
Store in a tightly sealed container away from heat and direct light.

MISSED DOSE
Take it as soon as you remember. If it is near the time for the next dose, skip the missed dose and resume your regular dosage schedule. Do not double the next dose.

STOPPING THE DRUG
The decision to stop taking the drug should be made by your doctor. Prazosin controls high blood pressure but does not cure it.

PROLONGED USE
Lifelong therapy may be necessary. See your doctor for regular tests and examinations if you must take this drug for a prolonged period.

▼ PRECAUTIONS

Over 60:
Adverse reactions, particularly dizziness, lightheadedness, and fainting, may be more likely and more severe in older patients. This medication may reduce tolerance to cold temperatures in older patients.

Driving and Hazardous Work:
Do not drive or engage in hazardous work until you determine how the medicine affects you.

Alcohol:
Avoid alcohol.

Pregnancy:
In animal studies and limited human studies, prazosin has not caused birth defects. High doses in animal studies have caused reduced birth weight. Before you take prazosin, tell your doctor if you are pregnant or plan to become pregnant.

Breast Feeding:
Prazosin passes into breast milk; caution is advised. Consult your doctor for advice.

Infants and Children:
There is no information comparing use of prazosin by infants and children with use by older patients. Consult your doctor for specific advice.

Special Concerns:
Be careful when you start using this medication or when the dose is increased, since you may be more likely to experience dizziness or lightheadedness at these times. For the same reason, as you continue to take prazosin use extra care in hot weather, as well as during exercise or if you must stand for a long time.

OVERDOSE
Symptoms: Drowsiness, slowed reflexes, extremely low blood pressure.

What to Do: An overdose of prazosin is unlikely to be life-threatening. However, if someone takes a much larger dose than prescribed, call your doctor, emergency medical services (EMS), or the nearest poison control center immediately.

▼ INTERACTIONS

DRUG INTERACTIONS
Consult your doctor for advice if you are taking non-steroidal anti-inflammatory drugs (NSAIDs), estrogens, sympathomimetics, propranolol or other beta-blockers, or any over-the-counter drug for appetite control, asthma, colds, cough, hay fever, or sinus problems.

FOOD INTERACTIONS
No known food interactions.

DISEASE INTERACTIONS
Caution is advised when taking prazosin. Consult your doctor if you have angina, severe heart disease, or kidney disease.

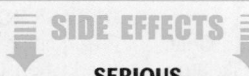

≡ SIDE EFFECTS ≡

SERIOUS
Dizziness or lightheadedness, especially when getting up from a sitting or lying position; fainting; loss of bladder control; pounding heartbeat; swelling of feet and lower legs; chest pain; continuing inappropriate and painful erections; shortness of breath. Call your doctor immediately.

COMMON
Drowsiness, headache, lack of energy.

LESS COMMON
Dry mouth, unusual fatigue, nervousness, nausea, frequent urge to urinate.

PREDNISOLONE OPHTHALMIC

Available in: Ophthalmic solution, suspension
Available OTC? No   **As Generic?** Yes
Drug Class: Corticosteroid

▼ USAGE INFORMATION

WHY IT'S PRESCRIBED
To control inflammation and prevent potentially permanent damage that may result from eye problems such as conjunctivitis, herpes of the eye, and cornea injuries. It is also used to help relieve redness, irritation, and discomfort in the eye, and may be used after eye surgery to control any inflammatory response.

HOW IT WORKS
Ophthalmic prednisolone inhibits the release of natural substances that stimulate an inflammatory reaction and pain in eye tissues.

▼ DOSAGE GUIDELINES

RANGE AND FREQUENCY
Solution or suspension: 1 or 2 drops in each eye up to 16 times a day.

ONSET OF EFFECT
Unknown.

DURATION OF ACTION
Unknown.

DIETARY ADVICE
No special restrictions.

STORAGE
Store in a tightly sealed container away from heat, moisture, and direct light. Do not allow it to freeze.

MISSED DOSE
Apply it as soon as you remember. If it is near the time for the next dose, skip the missed dose and resume your regular dosage schedule. Do not double the next dose.

STOPPING THE DRUG
It is very important to use this drug as prescribed for the full treatment period, even if symptoms improve before the scheduled end of therapy.

PROLONGED USE
You should see your doctor regularly for tests and examinations if you use this drug for a prolonged period.

▼ PRECAUTIONS

Over 60: No special problems are expected.

Driving and Hazardous Work: Do not drive or engage in hazardous work until you determine how the medicine affects your vision.

Alcohol: No special warnings.

Pregnancy: Adequate human studies have not been done, though no birth defects have been reported. Before taking ophthalmic prednisolone, be sure to tell your doctor if you are pregnant or plan to become pregnant.

Breast Feeding: Ophthalmic prednisolone has not been reported to cause problems in nursing babies. Consult your doctor for advice.

Infants and Children: Children under 2 years of age may be especially sensitive to the effects of ophthalmic prednisolone.

Special Concerns: To use the eye drops, first wash your hands. Tilt your head back. Gently apply pressure to the inside corner of the eyelid and with the index finger of the same hand, pull downward on the lower eyelid to make a space. Drop the medicine into this space and close your eye. Apply pressure for 1 or 2 minutes while keeping the eye closed without blinking. Then wash your hands again. Make sure the tip of the dropper does not touch your eye, finger, or any other surface. If your symptoms do not improve in 5 to 7 days or if they become worse, check

with your doctor. Wearing contact lenses while using this medication may increase the risk of infection. Your doctor may tell you not to wear contact lenses during and for a day or two after treatment.

OVERDOSE

Symptoms: When used topically, an overdose is very unlikely. Inadvertent oral ingestion, however, may cause fever, muscle pain, loss of appetite, dizziness, fainting, and trouble breathing.

What to Do: An overdose of this drug is unlikely to be life-threatening. However, if someone applies a much larger dose than prescribed or accidentally ingests the medicine, call your doctor, emergency medical services (EMS), or the nearest poison control center.

▼ INTERACTIONS

DRUG INTERACTIONS
Consult your doctor for specific advice if you are taking any other prescription or over-the-counter medication.

FOOD INTERACTIONS
No known food interactions.

DISEASE INTERACTIONS
Caution is advised when taking ophthalmic prednisolone. Consult your doctor if you have any of the following: cataracts, diabetes, glaucoma, herpes infection of the eye, tuberculosis of the eye, or any other eye infection.

▼ SIDE EFFECTS

SERIOUS
Decreased vision or blurring of vision (from cataract); eye pain, nausea, vomiting (from increased eye pressure); pain, redness, sensitivity to bright light, discharge (from eye infection). Call your doctor immediately if you experience any of these signs or symptoms. The drug may trigger a recurrence of herpes infection of the eye; mention any previous herpes infection to your doctor.

COMMON
Increased eye pressure (especially with the topical prednisolone acetate form); this is usually reversed once the drug is stopped.

LESS COMMON
Burning, stinging, redness, or watering of eyes.

PREDNISOLONE SYSTEMIC

Available in: Solution, syrup, tablets, injection
Available OTC? No **As Generic?** Yes
Drug Class: Corticosteroid

▼ USAGE INFORMATION

WHY IT'S PRESCRIBED
To treat numerous conditions that involve inflammation (a response by body tissues, producing redness, warmth, swelling, and pain). Such conditions include arthritis, allergic reactions, asthma, some skin diseases, multiple sclerosis flare-ups, and other autoimmune diseases. Also prescribed to treat deficiency of natural steroid hormones.

HOW IT WORKS
This hormone mimics the effects of the body's natural corticosteroids. It depresses the synthesis, release, and activity of inflammation-producing body chemicals. It also suppresses the activity of the immune system.

▼ DOSAGE GUIDELINES

RANGE AND FREQUENCY
Oral dosage: 5 to 200 mg a day, depending on condition, in 1 or several doses. Injection: 2 to 100 mg a day injected into a muscle, joint, vein, or lesion depending on condition. Consult pediatrician for children's dose.

ONSET OF EFFECT
Within 1 hour of taking oral forms or after injection into a muscle or vein; 1 to 2 days after injection into a lesion.

DURATION OF ACTION
30 to 36 hours for tablets; 3 to 4 days for injection.

DIETARY ADVICE
It can be taken with food or milk to minimize stomach upset. Your doctor may recommend a special diet.

STORAGE
Store in a tightly sealed container away from heat, moisture, and direct light. Do not allow liquid forms to freeze.

MISSED DOSE
If you take several doses a day and it is close to the next dose, double the next dose. If you take 1 dose a day and you do not remember until the next day, skip the missed dose and do not double the next dose.

STOPPING THE DRUG
With long-term therapy, do not stop taking the drug abruptly; the dosage should be decreased gradually.

PROLONGED USE
Long-term use may lead to cataracts, diabetes, hypertension, or osteoporosis; see your doctor for regular visits.

▼ PRECAUTIONS

Over 60: Adverse reactions may be more likely and more severe in older patients.

Driving and Hazardous Work: Avoid such activities until you determine how the medicine affects you.

Alcohol: May cause stomach problems; avoid it unless your physician approves occasional moderate drinking.

Pregnancy: Overuse during pregnancy can impair growth and development of the child.

Breast Feeding: Do not use this drug while nursing.

Infants and Children: Prednisolone may retard the development of bone and other tissues.

Special Concerns: This drug can lower resistance to infection. Avoid immunizations with live vaccines. Patients undergoing long-term therapy should wear a medical-alert bracelet. Call your doctor if you develop a fever.

OVERDOSE
Symptoms: Fever, muscle or joint pain, nausea, dizziness, fainting, difficulty breathing. Prolonged overuse: Moonface, obesity, unusual hair growth, acne, loss of sexual function, muscle wasting.

What to Do: Call your doctor, emergency medical services (EMS), or the nearest poison control center immediately.

▼ INTERACTIONS

DRUG INTERACTIONS
Consult your doctor for advice if you are taking aminoglutethimide, antacids, barbiturates, carbamazepine, griseofulvin, mitotane, phenylbutazone, phenytoin, primidone, rifampin, injectable amphotericin B, oral antidiabetes agents, insulin, digitalis drugs, diuretics or drugs containing potassium or sodium.

FOOD INTERACTIONS
Avoid excess sodium.

DISEASE INTERACTIONS
Consult your doctor if you have a history of bone disease, chickenpox, measles, gastrointestinal disorders, diabetes, recent serious infection, glaucoma, heart disease, hypertension, liver or kidney disorders, high blood cholesterol, thyroid problems, myasthenia gravis, or lupus.

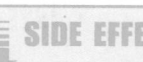
SIDE EFFECTS

SERIOUS
Vision problems, frequent urination, increased thirst, rectal bleeding, blistering skin, confusion, hallucinations, paranoia, euphoria, depression, mood swings, redness and swelling at injection site. Call your doctor immediately.

COMMON
Increased appetite, indigestion, nervousness, insomnia, greater susceptibility to infections, increased blood pressure, slowed wound healing, weight gain, easy bruising, fluid retention.

LESS COMMON
Change in skin color, dizziness, headache, increased sweating, unusual growth of body or facial hair, increased blood sugar, peptic ulcers, adrenal insufficiency, muscle weakness, cataracts, glaucoma, osteoporosis.

PREDNISONE

Available in: Oral suspension, syrup, tablets
Available OTC? No   **As Generic?** Yes
Drug Class: Corticosteroid

▼ USAGE INFORMATION

WHY IT'S PRESCRIBED
To treat numerous conditions that involve inflammation (a response by body tissues, producing redness, warmth, swelling, and pain). Such conditions include arthritis, allergic reactions, asthma, some skin diseases, multiple sclerosis flare-ups, and other autoimmune diseases. Also prescribed to treat deficiency of natural steroid hormones.

HOW IT WORKS
Prednisone mimics the body's natural corticosteroid hormones. It depresses the synthesis, release, and activity of inflammation-producing body chemicals. It also suppresses the activity of the immune system.

▼ DOSAGE GUIDELINES

RANGE AND FREQUENCY
Adults and teenagers— For severe inflammation or to suppress the immune system: 5 to 100 mg a day in divided doses. For multiple sclerosis: 200 mg daily for 1 week, then 80 mg every other day for 1 month. Children— Consult your pediatrician.

ONSET OF EFFECT
Variable.

DURATION OF ACTION
Variable.

DIETARY ADVICE
It can be taken with food or milk to minimize stomach upset. Your doctor may recommend a low-salt, high-potassium, high-protein diet.

STORAGE
Store in a tightly sealed container away from heat, moisture, and direct light. Do not allow liquid forms to freeze.

MISSED DOSE
Take it as soon as you remember. If you take several doses a day and it is close to the next dose, double the next dose. If you take 1 dose a day and you do not remember until the next day, skip the missed dose and do not double the next dose.

STOPPING THE DRUG
With long-term therapy, do not stop taking the drug abruptly; the dosage should be decreased gradually.

PROLONGED USE
Long-term use may lead to cataracts, diabetes, hypertension, or osteoporosis; see your doctor for regular examinations.

▼ PRECAUTIONS

Over 60: Adverse reactions may be more likely and more severe.

Driving and Hazardous Work: Avoid such activities until you determine how the medicine affects you.

Alcohol: May cause stomach problems; avoid it unless your physician approves occasional moderate drinking.

Pregnancy: Overuse during pregnancy can retard the child's growth and cause other developmental problems. Consult your doctor.

Breast Feeding: Do not use this drug while nursing.

Infants and Children: Prednisone may retard the growth and development of bone and other tissues.

Special Concerns: This drug can lower resistance to infection. Avoid immunizations with live vaccines. Patients undergoing long-term therapy should wear a medical-alert bracelet. Call your doctor if you develop a fever.

OVERDOSE
Symptoms: Fever, muscle or joint pain, nausea, dizziness, fainting, difficulty breathing. Prolonged overuse: Moonface, obesity, unusual hair growth, acne, loss of sexual function, muscle wasting.

What to Do: Call your doctor, emergency medical services (EMS), or the nearest poison control center immediately.

▼ INTERACTIONS

DRUG INTERACTIONS
Consult your doctor for specific advice if you are taking aminoglutethimide, antacids, barbiturates, carbamazepine, griseofulvin, mitotane, phenylbutazone, phenytoin, primidone, rifampin, injectable amphotericin B, oral antidiabetes agents, insulin, digitalis drugs, diuretics, or medications containing potassium or sodium.

FOOD INTERACTIONS
Avoid excess sodium.

DISEASE INTERACTIONS
Consult your doctor if you have a history of bone disease, chickenpox, measles, gastrointestinal disorders, diabetes, recent serious infection, glaucoma, heart disease, hypertension, liver or kidney disorders, high blood cholesterol, thyroid problems, myasthenia gravis, or lupus.

SIDE EFFECTS

SERIOUS
Vision problems, frequent urination, increased thirst, rectal bleeding, blistering skin, confusion, hallucinations, paranoia, euphoria, depression, mood swings, redness and swelling at injection site. Call your doctor immediately.

COMMON
Increased appetite, indigestion, nervousness, insomnia, greater susceptibility to infections, increased blood pressure, slowed wound healing, weight gain, easy bruising, fluid retention.

LESS COMMON
Change in skin color, dizziness, headache, increased sweating, unusual growth of body or facial hair, increased blood sugar, peptic ulcers, adrenal insufficiency, muscle weakness, cataracts, glaucoma, osteoporosis.

PRIMAQUINE

Available in: Tablets
Available OTC? No **As Generic?** Yes
Drug Class: Anti-infective/antimalarial

▼ USAGE INFORMATION

WHY IT'S PRESCRIBED
To prevent relapses of malaria caused by the protozoans Plasmodium vivax and Plasmodium ovale. It is used after chloroquine treatment has been completed, or following preventive therapy with chloroquine in people who have had heavy exposure to these forms of malaria.

HOW IT WORKS
Primaquine interferes with the energy-producing biological processes of the protozoa.

▼ DOSAGE GUIDELINES

RANGE AND FREQUENCY
Adults and teenagers: One 26.3 mg tablet (15 mg base) once a day for 14 days; in patients with mild G6PD deficiency, 3 tablets (45 mg base) weekly for 8 weeks; in patients with severe G6PD deficiency, 2 tablets (30 mg base) weekly for 30 weeks. Some strains of P. vivax (particularly those from Southeast Asia), may require a higher dose of 39.4 to 52.6 mg once a day for 14 days. Consult your doctor. Children age 12 and under: 0.68 mg (0.39 mg base) per 2.2 lbs (1 kg) of body weight once a day for 14 days.

ONSET OF EFFECT
Unknown.

DURATION OF ACTION
Unknown.

DIETARY ADVICE
Primaquine can be taken with food or juice to minimize stomach upset. Notify your doctor if you experience persistent stomach upset with pain, nausea, or vomiting.

STORAGE
Store in a tightly sealed container away from heat, moisture, and direct light.

MISSED DOSE
Take it as soon as you remember. However, if it is near the time for the next dose, skip the missed dose and resume your regular dosage schedule. Do not double the next dose.

STOPPING THE DRUG
Take it as prescribed for the full treatment period, even if you begin to feel better before the scheduled end of therapy.

PROLONGED USE
See your doctor regularly for blood tests and examinations if you must take this medicine for a prolonged period.

▼ PRECAUTIONS

Over 60: Adverse reactions may be more likely and more severe in older patients.

Driving and Hazardous Work: Do not drive or engage in hazardous work until you determine how the medicine affects you.

Alcohol: No special precautions are necessary.

Pregnancy: Primaquine should not be used during pregnancy. Before you take primaquine, tell your doctor if you are pregnant or plan to become pregnant.

Breast Feeding: Primaquine may pass into breast milk; caution is advised. Consult your doctor for advice.

Infants and Children: Adverse reactions may be more likely and more severe in children.

Special Concerns: You should not take primaquine if you are taking or have taken quinacrine within the previous 3 months. If you are of Mediterranean, African, or East Asian ancestry, you may be at higher risk for side effects due to a deficiency of the enzyme glucose-6-phosphate dehydrogenase (G6PD); consult your doctor.

OVERDOSE
Symptoms: Weakness, pale, sickly appearance, shortness of breath, severe abdominal cramps, vomiting, heartbeat irregularities.

What to Do: Call your doctor, emergency medical services (EMS), or the nearest poison control center immediately.

▼ INTERACTIONS

DRUG INTERACTIONS
Consult your physician for specific advice if you are taking quinacrine or any drugs that may cause anemia (such as sulfonamides and nitrofurans) or bone marrow suppression (including methotrexate, phenylbutazone, and chloramphenicol). Also, tell your physician if you are taking any other prescription or over-the-counter drug.

FOOD INTERACTIONS
No known food interactions.

DISEASE INTERACTIONS
You should not take primaquine if you are acutely ill with a disease that may reduce white blood cell counts, such as rheumatoid arthritis or lupus erythematosus. Consult your doctor if you have a family history of favism or hemolytic anemia, G6PD deficiency, or a deficiency of nicotinamide adenine dinucleotide (NADH).

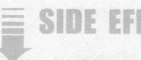

SIDE EFFECTS

SERIOUS
Discontinue taking primaquine and consult your doctor immediately if your urine is markedly darker than usual. Other serious side effects include unusual fatigue; pain in the back, legs, or stomach; loss of appetite; pale skin; fever; blue fingernails, lips, or skin; difficulty breathing; dizziness or lightheadedness. Call your doctor immediately.

COMMON
Stomach cramps or pain, nausea and vomiting.

LESS COMMON
Low white blood cell counts causing sore throat, fever, or other signs of infection (rare).

PRIMIDONE

Available in: Tablets, suspension
Available OTC? No   **As Generic?** Yes
Drug Class: Anticonvulsant

▼ USAGE INFORMATION

WHY IT'S PRESCRIBED
To control certain types of seizures due to epilepsy.

HOW IT WORKS
Primidone is thought to depress the activity of certain parts of the brain and suppress the abnormal firing of neurons that causes seizures.

▼ DOSAGE GUIDELINES

RANGE AND FREQUENCY
Adults: 500 to 1,000 mg (or more) a day, in 3 or 4 divided doses. Children: 10 to 20 mg a day, in 3 or 4 divided doses. A low dose is used to start, and gradually increased.

ONSET OF EFFECT
Several hours.

DURATION OF ACTION
Maximum effectiveness:12 hours or longer; effectiveness then gradually decreases.

DIETARY ADVICE
Take with food to help avoid stomach upset.

STORAGE
Store in a tightly sealed container away from heat, moisture, and direct light. Do not freeze the liquid form.

MISSED DOSE
Take it as soon as you remember. If it is close to the next dose, skip the missed dose and resume regular dosage schedule. Do not double the next dose, unless so advised by your doctor.

STOPPING THE DRUG
Never stop this drug abruptly; seizures may ensue. Your doctor will taper the dose gradually over a period of weeks to months.

PROLONGED USE
This drug is typically taken for prolonged periods. See your doctor regularly for tests and examinations.

≣ SIDE EFFECTS ≣

SERIOUS
Fever, sore throat, swollen glands, red or purple pointlike rash on the skin or mucous membranes, blistering or peeling skin lesions, mouth sores, easy bruising, paleness, weakness, confusion, lethargy, or seizures may be a sign of a potentially fatal blood reaction or other complication. Call your doctor immediately.

COMMON
Drowsiness, dizziness, loss of coordination, double vision, hyperactivity (in children).

LESS COMMON
Loss of appetite, mental or mood changes, nausea or vomiting, impotence, mild rash, lethargy followed by insomnia. There are numerous additional side effects associated with this drug; consult your doctor if you are concerned about any adverse or unusual reactions.

▼ PRECAUTIONS

Over 60: Older patients may require lower doses to minimize side effects.

Driving and Hazardous Work: This drug may cause drowsiness or dizziness. Do not drive or engage in hazardous work until you determine how it affects you.

Alcohol: May contribute to excessive drowsiness.

Pregnancy: Birth defects and bleeding problems in the mother have been reported in association with primidone use during pregnancy. Scientific studies are incomplete. However, seizures during pregnancy also increase the risks to the fetus. Discuss with your doctor the potential risks and benefits of using this drug during pregnancy. Folate supplementation is recommended beginning 1 to 2 months before conception and throughout the course of pregnancy.

Breast Feeding: Primidone passes into breast milk, although at low levels. Consult your doctor for advice.

Infants and Children: Adverse reactions may be more likely and more severe in children.

Special Concerns: The generic version of this drug is not recommended. Do not change the brand of primidone you are taking without consulting your doctor. The suspension form of primidone should be shaken well before you take it. Your doctor may want you to carry an ID card or bracelet saying that you are taking this drug.

OVERDOSE
Symptoms: Drowsiness, breathing problems, loss of consciousness.

What to Do: Call your doctor, emergency medical services (EMS), or the nearest poison control center immediately.

▼ INTERACTIONS

DRUG INTERACTIONS
Primidone may interact with other drugs, including other anticonvulsants (phenytoin, carbamazepine, clonazepam, valproic acid), benzodiazepines, caffeine, calcium channel blockers, corticosteroids, corticotropin, cyclophosphamide, cyclosporine, dacarbazine, digitoxin, disopyramide, doxycycline, general anesthetics, griseofulvin, H1 blockers, haloperidol, isoniazid, ketamine, levothyroxine, loxapine, maprotiline, metoprolol, mexiletine, phenytoin, propranolol, quinidine, theophylline, tricyclic antidepressants, vitamin D, and warfarin. May decrease the effectiveness of oral contraceptives, causing contraceptive failure.

FOOD INTERACTIONS
No known food interactions.

DISEASE INTERACTIONS
Caution is advised if you have asthma, chronic lung disease, hyperactivity (in children), kidney or liver disease, or porphyria.

PROBENECID

Available in: Tablets
Available OTC? No **As Generic?** Yes
Drug Class: Antigout drug; adjunct to antibiotic therapy

▼ USAGE INFORMATION

WHY IT'S PRESCRIBED
To treat chronic gout and gouty arthritis—specifically, to lower the uric acid level in hopes of preventing future gout attacks. Probenecid is also prescribed to enhance the action of certain antibiotics when treating infections.

HOW IT WORKS
Gout occurs when excessive amounts of uric acid build up in the blood. This leads to the formation of uric-acid-based crystals that are deposited in the joints, causing inflammation and leading to the sharp, excruciating pain of a gout attack. Probenecid promotes excretion of excess uric acid from the body and so eases or prevents gout attacks. Probenecid also slows the body's removal of antibiotics, thus increasing their levels in the blood and prolonging their duration of action.

▼ DOSAGE GUIDELINES

RANGE AND FREQUENCY
For gout— 250 mg, 2 times a day for first week, then 500 mg, 2 times a day, to maximum of 2,000 mg per day. For antibiotic therapy with penicillin— 500 mg, 4 times a day. Children ages 2 to 14: 25 mg per 2.2 lbs (1 kg) of body weight to start, then 25 mg per 2.2 lbs in 4 daily doses. To treat gonorrhea— 1 g of probenecid with or before 3.5 mg of ampicillin or 4.8 million units of injected penicillin.

ONSET OF EFFECT
To ease gout: Several months of therapy may be required before probenecid begins to prevent gout attacks. To suppress the excretion of antibiotics: 2 hours.

DURATION OF ACTION
For gout: Unknown. For enhancement of antibiotic therapy: 2 hours.

DIETARY ADVICE
It can be taken with food or antacids to reduce stomach upset. Drink 8 to 10 full glasses of water a day.

STORAGE
Store in a tightly sealed container away from heat and direct light.

MISSED DOSE
Take it as soon as you remember. If it is near the time for the next dose, skip the missed dose and resume your regular dosage schedule. Do not double the next dose.

STOPPING THE DRUG
The decision to stop taking the drug should be made by your doctor.

PROLONGED USE
See your doctor regularly for tests and examinations if you take this drug for a prolonged period. Gout attacks may continue for a while after you start taking probenecid.

▼ PRECAUTIONS

Over 60: No special problems are expected.

Driving and Hazardous Work: Avoid such activities until you determine how the medicine affects you.

Alcohol: Avoid alcohol.

Pregnancy: Probenecid has not been shown to cause problems during pregnancy.

Breast Feeding: Probenecid may pass into breast milk; caution is advised. Consult your doctor for advice.

Infants and Children: Not recommended for use by children under age 2.

Special Concerns: Before you have any medical tests, be sure to tell the doctor you are taking probenecid.

OVERDOSE
Symptoms: Nausea, vomiting, diarrhea, seizures.

What to Do: Call your doctor, emergency medical services (EMS), or the nearest poison control center immediately.

▼ INTERACTIONS

DRUG INTERACTIONS
Consult your doctor for specific advice if you are taking anticancer (chemotherapy) medications, aspirin or other salicylates, heparin, indomethacin, ketoprofen, methotrexate, medicine for any type of infection, nitrofurantoin, or zidovudine.

FOOD INTERACTIONS
None are likely, but a low-purine diet is recommended to reduce the risk of gout attacks. Foods high in purines include anchovies, sardines, legumes, poultry, sweetbreads, liver, kidneys, and other organ meats.

DISEASE INTERACTIONS
Caution is advised when taking probenecid. Consult your doctor if you have a blood disease, cancer, kidney disease or kidney stones, or a stomach ulcer.

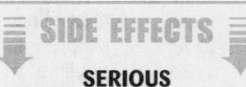

SIDE EFFECTS

SERIOUS
Rapid or irregular heartbeat; puffiness or swelling around eyes; trouble breathing; tightness in chest; changes in skin color; rash, hives, or itching; bloody or cloudy urine; difficult urination; lower back or side pain; sores, ulcers, or white spots on lips or in mouth; sore throat and fever; sudden decrease in urine; swollen face, fingers, feet, or lower legs; swollen or painful glands; unusual bleeding or bruising; unusual fatigue; yellow discoloration of the eyes or skin; unusual weight gain. Call your doctor immediately.

COMMON
Headache, redness, pain or swelling in joints, loss of appetite, nausea or vomiting.

LESS COMMON
Dizziness, reddened face, frequent urge to urinate, red or sore gums.

PROCAINAMIDE HYDROCHLORIDE

Available in: Capsules, tablets, extended-release tablets, injection
Available OTC? No **As Generic?** Yes
Drug Class: Antiarrhythmic

▼ USAGE INFORMATION

WHY IT'S PRESCRIBED
To treat irregular heartbeats (cardiac arrhythmias).

HOW IT WORKS
Procainamide hydrochloride slows nerve impulses in the heart and reduces the sensitivity of heart tissue to certain nerve impulses, thus stabilizing the heartbeat.

▼ DOSAGE GUIDELINES

RANGE AND FREQUENCY
Tablets and capsules– Adults: 500 to 1,000 mg every 4 to 6 hours. Children: 12.5 mg per 2.2 lbs (1 kg) of body weight 4 times a day. Extended-release tablets– 1,000 to 2,000 mg every 12 hours.

ONSET OF EFFECT
Oral: 60 to 90 minutes. Injection: immediate.

DURATION OF ACTION
From 3 to 8 hours (longer in patients with kidney disease or heart failure).

DIETARY ADVICE
Procainamide should be taken with a glass of water on an empty stomach 1 hour before or 2 hours after meals.

STORAGE
Store in a tightly sealed container away from heat and direct light.

MISSED DOSE
Take a missed dose as soon as you remember. If it is near the time for the next dose, skip the missed dose and resume your regular dosage schedule. Do not double the next dose.

STOPPING THE DRUG
Take as prescribed for the full treatment period, even if you begin to feel better before the scheduled end of therapy. The decision to stop taking the drug should be made by your doctor.

PROLONGED USE
Lifelong therapy may be necessary. See your doctor regularly for examinations and diagnostic tests if you must take this medicine for a prolonged period.

▼ PRECAUTIONS

Over 60: Adverse reactions may be more likely and more severe in older patients.

Driving and Hazardous Work: Do not drive or engage in hazardous work until you determine how the medicine affects you.

Alcohol: Avoid alcohol.

Pregnancy: Procainamide has not been shown to cause problems during pregnancy. In any case, if you are taking this drug, be sure to tell your doctor if you are pregnant or plan to become pregnant.

Breast Feeding: Procainamide passes into breast milk. Consult your doctor for specific advice.

Infants and Children: Procainamide has not been shown to cause problems in limited use in children.

Special Concerns: Your doctor may want you to carry a medical identification card or bracelet saying you use procainamide. Before having any kind of surgical procedure or medical test, tell the doctor or dentist in charge that you are taking procainamide.

OVERDOSE
Symptoms: Confusion, severe dizziness, fainting, rapid or irregular heartbeat, decrease in urination, nausea or vomiting.

What to Do: Call your doctor, emergency medical services (EMS), or the nearest poison control center immediately.

▼ INTERACTIONS

DRUG INTERACTIONS
Consult your doctor for specific advice if you are taking other antiarrhythmics, drugs for high blood pressure, antimyasthenics, pimozide, or antihistamines.

FOOD INTERACTIONS
No known food interactions.

DISEASE INTERACTIONS
Consult your doctor if you have any of the following: heart block, asthma, myasthenia gravis, or systemic lupus erythematosus. Use of procainamide may cause complications in patients with liver or kidney disease, since these organs work together to remove the medication from the body.

⬇ SIDE EFFECTS ⬇

SERIOUS
Fainting; rapid or irregular heartbeat (palpitations); fever and chills; joint pain or swelling; painful breathing; skin rash or itching; confusion; sore mouth, gums, or throat; hallucinations; depression; unusual bleeding or bruising; unusual fatigue. Call your doctor immediately.

COMMON
Diarrhea, abdominal pain, nausea, vomiting, loss of appetite.

LESS COMMON
Dizziness, lightheadedness, weakness, dry mouth.

PROCARBAZINE HYDROCHLORIDE

Matulane

Available in: Capsules
Available OTC? No   **As Generic?** No
Drug Class: Antineoplastic (anticancer) agent

▼ USAGE INFORMATION

WHY IT'S PRESCRIBED
To treat Hodgkin's disease (a cancer affecting the spleen and lymph nodes). Procarbazine is usually only one drug of several given in combination with other chemotherapy agents to fight cancer.

HOW IT WORKS
Procarbazine kills cancer cells by interfering with the activity of their genetic material, which prevents the cells from reproducing. The drug may also affect the growth and development of other kinds of cells in the body, resulting in unpleasant side effects. Procarbazine is also a weak inhibitor of the enzyme known as mono-amine oxidase (MAO); MAO inhibitors are routinely prescribed to treat depression, although this has no impact on procarbazine's function as a cancer-fighting drug.

▼ DOSAGE GUIDELINES

RANGE AND FREQUENCY
Adults: 2 to 4 mg per 2.2 lbs (1 kg) of body weight per day for first week. Then 4 to 6 mg per 2.2 lbs per day until the blood cell count falls substantially. Then 1 to 2 mg per 2.2 lbs per day. Children: 50 mg per square meter of body surface per day for first week, then 100 mg per square meter of body surface per day until toxicity occurs, then 50 mg per square meter of body surface per day.

ONSET OF EFFECT
Unknown.

DURATION OF ACTION
Unknown.

DIETARY ADVICE
Maintain adequate food and fluid intake. Calorie, protein, and vitamin needs increase in patients with cancer. Good nutrition is essential to cope with the demands of chemotherapy. Foods high in the substance tyramine must be eliminated from the diet during therapy with procarbazine; see Special Concerns and Food Interactions for further information.

STORAGE
Store in a tightly sealed container away from heat and direct light. Unopened vials should be refrigerated but not allowed to freeze.

MISSED DOSE
If you miss a dose, take it as soon as you remember. If it is near the time for the next dose, skip the missed dose and resume your regular dosage schedule. Do not double the next dose.

STOPPING THE DRUG
The decision to stop taking the drug should be made by your doctor.

PROLONGED USE
You should see your doctor regularly for tests and examinations if you take this drug for a prolonged period.

▼ PRECAUTIONS

Over 60: Adverse reactions may be more likely and more severe in older patients.

Driving and Hazardous Work: Do not drive or engage in hazardous work until you determine how the medicine affects you.

Alcohol: Avoid alcohol.

Pregnancy: Procarbazine can cause birth defects if either the father or mother takes it. Consult your doctor for specific advice if you are pregnant or plan to become pregnant. Use of a reliable method of birth control is recommended throughout the duration of therapy with procarbazine.

Breast Feeding: Procarbazine passes into breast milk; avoid or discontinue use of this drug while breast feeding.

Infants and Children: Procarbazine is not expected to cause different problems in infants and children than it does in older persons.

Special Concerns: Like all drugs categorized as MAO inhibitors, procarbazine prevents the liver and other body tissues from neutralizing a substance called tyramine, which, in the bloodstream, causes a sudden increase in blood pressure. Therefore, foods high in tyramines must be avoided while undergoing therapy with procarbazine. Such foods include aged cheeses, processed meats, many varieties of dried or preserved foods, as well as

▤ SIDE EFFECTS ▤

SERIOUS
Severe chest pain; dilated pupils; rapid or slowed heartbeat; severe headache; sensitivity of eyes to light; increased sweating; stiff neck; black, tarry stools; blood in urine or stools; bloody vomit; cough or hoarseness; fever and chills; pain in lower back or flanks; painful or difficult urination; tiny bright red spots on skin; unusual bleeding or bruising; confusion; seizures; hallucinations; absent menstrual periods; shortness of breath; thickened bronchial (lung) secretions; diarrhea; sores in mouth and on the lips; tingling or numbness of fingers or toes; incoordination or unsteady gait; yellowish tinge to eyes or skin. Such side effects may mean that normal blood cells and special blood-clotting cells have been affected, or that the immune system has been affected and an infection is developing. See your doctor immediately.

COMMON
Drowsiness, muscle or joint pain, muscle twitching, nausea or vomiting, nervousness, restlessness, nightmares, insomnia, unusual fatigue.

LESS COMMON
Constipation, darkened skin, difficulty swallowing, lightheadedness when arising, dry mouth, loss of appetite, depression, flushing of the face.

PROCARBAZINE HYDROCHLORIDE (continued)

certain kinds of liquor and wine (especially red wine). See Food Interactions for a more complete list of foods and beverages high in tyramines. While taking procarbazine, do not receive any immunizations without consulting your doctor. Avoid people with infections and those who have recently had oral polio vaccine. Be careful when using a toothbrush, dental floss, or toothpick. Check with your doctor before having any dental work done. If you are going to have surgery, tell the doctor or dentist in charge that you are taking procarbazine. Do not touch your eyes or the inside of your nose unless you have just washed your hands. Be careful not to cut yourself when using sharp objects such as a razor.

Avoid contact sports and other activities during which bruising could occur.

OVERDOSE
Symptoms: Nausea, vomiting, diarrhea, tremors, seizures, loss of consciousness, very low blood pressure, coma.

What to Do: Call your doctor, emergency medical services (EMS), or the nearest poison control center immediately.

▼ INTERACTIONS

DRUG INTERACTIONS
Consult your doctor for specific advice if you are taking amantadine, anticholinergics, diabetes medicine, antidyskinetics, antihistamines, antipsychotics, buclizine, central nervous system depressants, cyclizine, disopyramide, flavoxate, ipratropium, meclizine, orphenadrine, oxybutynin, procainamide, promethazine, quinidine, trimeprazine, amphetamines, diet pills, dextromethorphan, levodopa, asthma or cold medicine, methyldopa, methylphenidate, narcotic pain medicine, amphotericin B, antithyroid agents, azathioprine, chloramphenicol, colchicine, flucytosine, interferon, plicamycin, zidovudine, buspirone, carbamazepine, cyclobenzaprine, maprotiline, other MAO inhibitors, antidepressants, fluoxetine, guanadrel, guanethidine, or rauwolfia alkaloids.

FOOD INTERACTIONS
Avoid tyramine-rich foods, which include aged cheeses, avocados, banana skins, bean curd, bologna and other processed lunch meats, chicken livers, chocolate, figs, canned or dried fish, pickled herring, meat extracts, pepperoni, raisins, raspberries, unpasteurized beer, Chianti, sherry, vermouth, and red wines in general. Also avoid caffeine-rich beverages or foods.

DISEASE INTERACTIONS
Caution is advised when taking procarbazine. Consult your doctor if you have a history of any of the following: alcoholism, angina, recent heart attack or stroke, chicken pox, shingles, epilepsy, frequent headaches, infection, kidney disease, liver disease, mental illness, overactive thyroid, Parkinson's disease, or pheochromocytoma.

PROCHLORPERAZINE

Available in: Extended-release capsules, syrup, tablets, suppositories, injection
Available OTC? No   **As Generic?** Yes
Drug Class: Neuroleptic; antiemetic

▼ USAGE INFORMATION

WHY IT'S PRESCRIBED
To treat severe nausea and vomiting.

HOW IT WORKS
Prochlorperazine suppresses activity in the trigger zones of the brain and gastrointestinal tract that govern the vomiting reflex.

▼ DOSAGE GUIDELINES

RANGE AND FREQUENCY
Usual adult dose: Initially, 5 to 10 mg, 3 or 4 times a day. Injection: 10 to 20 mg injected into a muscle every 4 to 6 hours. Your doctor may increase the dose as needed and tolerated.

ONSET OF EFFECT
30 to 40 minutes for oral forms; 60 minutes for suppository; 10 to 20 minutes after injection.

DURATION OF ACTION
3 to 4 hours; 12 hours for extended-release capsules.

DIETARY ADVICE
Can be taken with food or a full glass of milk or water.

STORAGE
Store in a tightly sealed container away from heat and direct light.

MISSED DOSE
Take it as soon as you remember. If it is near the time for the next dose, skip the missed dose and resume your regular dosage schedule. Do not double the next dose.

STOPPING THE DRUG
The decision to stop taking the drug should be made by your doctor.

PROLONGED USE
See your doctor regularly for tests and examinations if you must take this medicine for a prolonged period.

▼ PRECAUTIONS

Over 60: Adverse reactions are more common in elderly patients. A lower dose may be warranted.

Driving and Hazardous Work: Do not drive or engage in hazardous work until you determine how the medicine affects you.

Alcohol: Avoid alcohol.

Pregnancy: Avoid using this drug if you are pregnant or plan to become pregnant.

Breast Feeding: Either avoid taking the drug if possible or refrain from breast feeding.

Infants and Children: Adverse reactions may be more likely and more severe in children.

Special Concerns: Avoid prolonged exposure to high temperatures or hot climates while taking prochlorperazine. Drink plenty of fluids and try to stay cool in the summertime. Avoid overexposure to sunlight until you determine if the drug heightens your skin's sensitivity to ultraviolet radiation and increases your risk of sunburn.

OVERDOSE
Symptoms: Extreme drowsiness, heartbeat irregularities, dry mouth, paradoxical restlessness or agitation, seizures, loss of consciousness.

What to Do: Call your doctor, emergency medical services (EMS), or the nearest poison control center immediately.

▼ INTERACTIONS

DRUG INTERACTIONS
Consult your doctor for specific advice if you are taking anticholinergics; anticonvulsants; antidepressants; antihistamines; antihypertensives; bupropion; central nervous system depressants, such as barbiturates; clozapine; dronabinol; ethinamate; fluoxetine; guanethidine; guanfacine; lithium; methyldopa; carbamazepine; rifampin; or trihexyphenidyl.

FOOD INTERACTIONS
None known.

DISEASE INTERACTIONS
Consult your doctor if you have a history of alcohol abuse, any blood disorder, breast cancer, benign prostatic hyperplasia (BPH), epilepsy or seizures, glaucoma, heart, lung, or blood vessel disease, liver disease, Parkinson's disease, peptic ulcer, or urinary difficulty.

≡ SIDE EFFECTS ≡

SERIOUS
Rapid heartbeat, profuse sweating, seizures, difficulty breathing, neck stiffness, swelling of the tongue, difficulty swallowing. Also a rare condition can develop called neuroleptic malignant syndrome, characterized by stiffness or spasms of the muscles, high fever, and confusion or disorientation. Call your doctor immediately.

COMMON
Nausea, reduced sweating, dry mouth, blurred vision, drowsiness, shaking of hands, stiffness, stooped posture.

LESS COMMON
Difficult urination, menstrual irregularities, breast pain or swelling, unexpected weight gain, uncontrolled movements of the tongue, fever, chills, sore throat, unusual bruising or bleeding, heart palpitations, skin rash, itching, increased sensitivity of the skin to sunlight.

PROCYCLIDINE

Available in: Tablets
Available OTC? No   **As Generic?** No
Drug Class: Antiparkinsonism drug

BRAND NAME
Kemadrin

▼ USAGE INFORMATION

WHY IT'S PRESCRIBED
To treat Parkinson's disease and Parkinson-like syndromes, which can occur as a result of injury to or infection of the central nervous system, damage to blood vessels in the brain, or exposure to certain toxins.

HOW IT WORKS
Procyclidine promotes the release of dopamine in the brain. Dopamine is a chemical that is necessary for both the initiation and smooth control of voluntary muscle movement.

▼ DOSAGE GUIDELINES

RANGE AND FREQUENCY
Adults: To start, 2.5 mg, 3 times a day. The dosage is increased gradually to 5 mg, 3 times a day. Children: Consult a pediatrician.

ONSET OF EFFECT
Within 1 hour.

DURATION OF ACTION
From 6 to 12 hours.

DIETARY ADVICE
Procyclidine should be taken after meals to prevent nausea.

STORAGE
Store in a tightly sealed container away from heat, moisture, and direct light.

MISSED DOSE
Take it as soon as you remember, unless the time for your next scheduled dose is within the next 2 hours. If so, skip the missed dose and resume your regular dosage schedule. Do not double the next dose.

STOPPING THE DRUG
The decision to stop taking the drug should be made in consultation with your doctor. The dosage should be decreased gradually.

PROLONGED USE
No special difficulties are expected with long-term use of procyclidine.

▼ PRECAUTIONS

Over 60: Adverse reactions may be more likely and more severe in older patients. Procyclidine should be used cautiously in patients in this age group. If higher doses are needed, it is best to increase the dose very gradually.

Driving and Hazardous Work: Procyclidine can cause drowsiness or confusion. Exercise caution until you determine how it affects you.

Alcohol: Avoid alcohol; combined with the medication, alcohol is likely to cause or worsen confusion.

Pregnancy: This medication should not be used in pregnant women.

Breast Feeding: It is not known to what degree procyclidine passes into breast milk. Nursing mothers should avoid use of this medication.

Infants and Children: There is little known about the safety and effectiveness of procyclidine in infants and children. Consult your pediatrician to discuss the use of this drug in children.

Special Concerns: Procyclidine can cause or worsen glaucoma (the buildup of excessive pressure within the eye). See your ophthalmologist regularly for periodic monitoring of eye pressure.

OVERDOSE
Symptoms: Clumsiness, seizures, severe mouth dryness, drowsiness, hallucinations, loss of consciousness.

What to Do: Call your doctor, emergency medical services (EMS), or the nearest poison control center immediately.

▼ INTERACTIONS

DRUG INTERACTIONS
Procyclidine may interact with many drugs, in particular drugs that depress the central nervous system (such as alcohol, barbiturates, and other sleep-inducing drugs) and MAO inhibitor antidepressants (such as phenelzine sulfate and tranylcypromine sulfate). Consult your doctor if you are taking these drugs.

FOOD INTERACTIONS
No known food interactions.

DISEASE INTERACTIONS
Caution is advised when taking procyclidine. Consult your doctor if you have any of the following: irregular heartbeat or heart rhythm abnormalities, glaucoma, intestinal obstruction, urinary retention or trouble urinating, or enlarged prostate (benign prostatic hyperplasia).

SIDE EFFECTS

SERIOUS
Confusion, severe drowsiness, rapid heartbeat, hallucinations, glaucoma.

COMMON
Blurred vision; constipation; dry mouth, nose, and throat.

LESS COMMON
Dizziness and lightheadedness, loss of memory, nausea.

PROGESTERONE INTRAUTERINE SYSTEM

Available in: Intrauterine device
Available OTC? No   **As Generic?** Yes
Drug Class: Progestin (hormone)

▼ USAGE INFORMATION

WHY IT'S PRESCRIBED
As a contraceptive (birth control method).

HOW IT WORKS
Progesterone inhibits the secretion of pituitary hormones that in turn regulate menstrual and reproductive cycles; it also alters the activity of uterine cells.

▼ DOSAGE GUIDELINES

RANGE AND FREQUENCY
1 intrauterine device (IUD) is inserted into the vagina by a health professional and replaced within 12 months.

ONSET OF EFFECT
Within days.

DURATION OF ACTION
1 year.

DIETARY ADVICE
The IUD can be used without regard to diet.

STORAGE
Not applicable.

MISSED DOSE
Not applicable; the IUD remains implanted in the body for the entire duration of use.

STOPPING THE DRUG
Consult your gynecologist if you decide you no longer wish to use the IUD.

PROLONGED USE
You should check for the IUD thread every month, especially after each menstrual period. Wash your hands thoroughly before checking. Use your middle fingers to find the thread inside the cervix. Do not pull on the thread. If you cannot find the thread, call your gynecologist.

▼ PRECAUTIONS

Over 60: Not applicable to patients over 60.

Driving and Hazardous Work: The use of a progesterone IUD should not impair your ability to perform such tasks safely.

Alcohol: No special precautions are necessary.

Pregnancy: This IUD should not be used during pregnancy or by a woman who has had an ectopic pregnancy.

Breast Feeding: The progesterone IUD has not been shown to cause problems in nursing babies. Its use is recommended for women who require contraception while breast-feeding.

Infants and Children: Sexually active teenagers are urged to use a contraceptive method (for example, condoms) that protects them against sexually transmitted diseases; this IUD does not. Teenagers who have not given birth generally have more side effects than teenagers or adults who have. The IUD may move out of place, harming the uterus or cervix. Abdominal pain and increased menstrual bleeding are more common in teenagers than in older women.

Special Concerns: It is possible for pregnancy to occur while using the progesterone-containing IUD. Notify your doctor immediately if you feel the changes that can occur with pregnancy, such as enlarged or tender breasts, lack of menstrual period, unusual uterine bleeding, or pain and cramping in the lower abdomen. Until your doctor can see you, use another birth control method, such as condoms. If you think that the IUD has moved out of place, call your doctor immediately. If you think you are pregnant, do a home pregnancy test. Do not try to put the IUD in place inside the uterus yourself, nor try to remove it yourself.

OVERDOSE
Symptoms: Not applicable.

What to Do: Emergency instructions not applicable.

▼ INTERACTIONS

DRUG INTERACTIONS
The following drugs may interact with progesterone. Consult your doctor for specific advice if you are taking aminoglutethimide, carbamazepine, phenytoin, rifabutin, or rifampin.

FOOD INTERACTIONS
No known food interactions.

DISEASE INTERACTIONS
Caution is advised when using the progesterone IUD. Consult your doctor if you have any of the following conditions: uterine abnormalities or bleeding problems, acquired immunodeficiency syndrome (AIDS), a blood disorder, a heart defect, insulin-dependent diabetes, a recent sexually transmitted disease, abnormally slow heartbeat, or any recent surgery involving the uterus or fallopian tubes.

⇊ SIDE EFFECTS ⇊

SERIOUS
Severe abdominal pain or cramping; faintness, dizziness, or sharp pain at time of IUD insertion; heavy or unexpected uterine bleeding between periods; fever; odorous discharge; unusual fatigue; any unusual uterine bleeding. Call your doctor immediately.

COMMON
No common side effects are associated with use of the progesterone IUD.

LESS COMMON
There are no less-common side effects associated with use of the progesterone IUD.

PROGESTERONE SYSTEMIC AND TOPICAL

BRAND NAMES

Crinone, Gesterol 50, Prometrium

Available in: Injection, vaginal gel, capsules, suppositories
Available OTC? No   **As Generic?** Yes
Drug Class: Progestin (hormone)

▼ USAGE INFORMATION

WHY IT'S PRESCRIBED
To treat amenorrhea (cessation of menstrual periods) and abnormal uterine bleeding in the absence of structural pathology, such as uterine fibroids or uterine cancer. The vaginal gel is used as part of Assisted Reproductive Technology for infertile women with progesterone deficiency, and to promote menstruation in women with premature cessation of menses.

HOW IT WORKS
Progesterone inhibits the secretion of pituitary hormones that regulate a woman's menstrual and reproductive cycles.

▼ DOSAGE GUIDELINES

RANGE AND FREQUENCY
Injection— For amenorrhea and abnormal uterine bleeding: 5 to 10 mg injected into a muscle daily for 6 to 10 days, or 150 mg injected into a muscle as a single dose. (Progesterone vaginal suppositories may be provided by a pharmacist in lieu of injections.) Vaginal gel— For amenorrhea: 45 mg (Crinone 4%) every other day, up to 6 doses. For progesterone supplementation: 90 mg (Crinone 8%), once a day. For progesterone replacement: 90 mg, 2 times a day. Capsules— For secondary amenorrhea: 400 mg once a day in the evening for 10 days.

ONSET OF EFFECT
Injection— For amenorrhea: 48 to 70 hours after the last injection. For uterine bleeding: Within 6 days. Treatment will be stopped if bleeding continues or recurs during the therapy. Vaginal gel and capsules— Unknown.

DURATION OF ACTION
Unknown.

DIETARY ADVICE
No special restrictions.

STORAGE
Store in a tightly sealed container away from heat and direct light. Do not allow the gel form to freeze.

MISSED DOSE
Injection: Take it as soon as you remember. However, if it is near the time for the next dose, skip the missed dose and resume your regular dosage schedule. Do not double the next dose. Vaginal gel: If you miss a dose on one day, do not apply an excessive amount the next day. Resume your regular dosage schedule. Capsules: Skip the missed dose and resume your regular dosage schedule. Do not double the next dose.

STOPPING THE DRUG
The decision to stop taking the drug should be made in conjunction with your doctor.

PROLONGED USE
Consult your doctor about the need for periodic examinations and laboratory tests.

▼ PRECAUTIONS

Over 60: No special advice.

Driving and Hazardous Work: No special warnings.

Alcohol: No special warnings.

Pregnancy: This hormone should not be used during pregnancy. If you suspect a pregnancy, stop taking progesterone immediately and call your doctor. The vaginal gel may be used safely as part of Assisted Reproductive Technology in progesterone-deficient women.

Breast Feeding: Progesterone passes into breast milk and may change the quality or quantity of milk. Discuss risks and benefits with your doctor.

Infants and Children: Safety and effectiveness have not been determined.

Special Concerns: You should have a Pap test at least every 6 months.

OVERDOSE
Symptoms: None.

What to Do: An overdose is unlikely to be life-threatening. However, if someone takes a much larger dose than prescribed or accidentally ingests the gel, seek emergency medical attention right away

▼ INTERACTIONS

DRUG INTERACTIONS
Consult your doctor for specific advice if you are taking aminoglutethimide, carbamazepine, phenytoin, rifabutin, or rifampin.

FOOD INTERACTIONS
Do not take the capsules if you are allergic to peanuts. The capsules contain peanut oil. No other food interactions have been reported.

DISEASE INTERACTIONS
Consult your doctor if you have any of the following: asthma, epilepsy, cardiovascular problems, migraine headaches, breast disease, bleeding problems, diabetes, high blood cholesterol, or central nervous system disorders such as depression. Use of progesterone may cause complications in patients with liver or kidney disease, since these organs work together to remove drugs from the body.

≣ SIDE EFFECTS ≣

SERIOUS
Changes in or cessation of menstrual bleeding; unexpected or increased flow of breast milk; mental depression; skin rash; loss of or change in speech, coordination, or vision; severe and sudden shortness of breath; severe headache. Call your doctor immediately.

COMMON
Stomach pain or cramping; swelling of face, ankles, or feet; mild headache; mood changes; unusual fatigue; weight gain; pain or irritation at site of injection.

LESS COMMON
Acne, breast pain or tenderness, hot flashes, insomnia, loss of sexual desire, loss or gain of scalp hair or body hair, brown spots on skin.

PROMETHAZINE HYDROCHLORIDE

Available in: Tablets, syrup, injection, suppositories
Available OTC? No   **As Generic?** Yes
Drug Class: Antihistamine

▼ USAGE INFORMATION

WHY IT'S PRESCRIBED
To relieve the symptoms of hay fever and other allergies, to prevent motion sickness, and to treat nausea and vomiting. Promethazine may also be used in some patients for its sedative effect.

HOW IT WORKS
Promethazine interferes with, but does not block, the release and action of histamine, a naturally occurring substance in the body that causes swelling, itching, sneezing, watery eyes, hives, and other symptoms of allergic reaction. Promethazine also has an anticholinergic effect, meaning it blocks the transmission of certain nerve impulses, which in turn relaxes the smooth muscle tissue controlling activity in the bladder, stomach, intestine, lungs, and other organ systems. This effect thereby helps to ease the symptoms of motion sickness, nausea, gastrointestinal upset, and anxiety.

▼ DOSAGE GUIDELINES

RANGE AND FREQUENCY
Tablets or syrup– For allergies: Adults and teenagers: 10 to 12.5 mg, 4 times a day before meals and at bedtime, or 25 mg at bedtime. Children 2 and older: 5 to 12.5 mg, 3 times a day, or 25 mg at bedtime. For nausea and vomiting: Adults and teenagers: 25 mg for first dose, then 10 to 25 mg every 4 to 6 hours as needed. Children 2 and older: 10 to 25 mg every 4 to 6 hours. To prevent motion sickness: Adults and teenagers: 25 mg taken 30 to 60 minutes before traveling. Children 2 and older: 10 to 25 mg, 30 to 60 minutes before traveling. For dizziness: Adults and teenagers: 25 mg, 2 times a day. Children 2 and older: 10 to 25, mg 2 times a day. As a sedative: Adults and teenagers: 25 to 50 mg. Children 2 and older: 10 to 25 mg. Injection– For allergies: Adults and teenagers: 25 mg into a vein or muscle. Children 2 and older: 6.25 to 12.5 mg, 3 times a day into a muscle, or 25 mg at bedtime. For nausea and vomiting: Adults and teenagers: 12.5 to 25 mg every 4 hours into a vein or muscle. Children 2 and older: 12.5 to 25 mg every 4 to 6 hours into a muscle. As a sedative: Adults and teenagers: 25 to 50 mg injected into a vein or muscle. Children 2 and older: 12.5 to 25 mg into a muscle. Suppositories– For allergies: Adults and teenagers: 25 mg at first; 25 mg, 2 hours later if needed. Children 2 and older: 6.25 to 12.5 mg, 3 times a day, or 25 mg at bedtime. For nausea and vomiting: Adults and teenagers: 25 mg at first, then 12.5 to 25 mg every 4 to 6 hours if needed. Children 2 and older: 12.5 to 25 mg every 4 to 6 hours. For dizziness: Adults and teenagers: 25 mg, 2 times a day. Children 2 and older: 12.5 to 25 mg, 2 times a day. As a sedative: Adults and teenagers: 25 to 50 mg. Children 2 and older: 12.25 to 25 mg.

ONSET OF EFFECT
15 to 60 minutes orally or by suppository; 20 minutes after injection.

DURATION OF ACTION
Up to 12 hours.

DIETARY ADVICE
Take it with food or milk to lessen stomach irritation.

STORAGE
Store in a tightly sealed container away from heat and direct light at room temperature. Do not store the tablets in a place with excessive moisture, such as the bathroom medicine cabinet. Do not allow the syrup or injection to freeze.

MISSED DOSE
Take it as soon as you remember. If it is near the time for the next dose, skip the missed dose and resume your regular dosage schedule. Do not double the next dose.

STOPPING THE DRUG
You should take it as prescribed for the full treatment period, but you may stop taking the drug if you are feeling better before the scheduled end of therapy.

PROLONGED USE
See your doctor regularly if you take this medicine for a prolonged period. Prolonged use of this antihistamine may decrease salivary flow, which may lead to thrush (white, furry patches in the mouth caused by fungal infection), periodontal disease (disease and decay of the teeth, gums, jaw, and other supportive structures in the mouth), dental caries (cavities), and gingivitis (gum disease). Practice good oral hygiene to prevent these disorders.

▼ PRECAUTIONS

Over 60: Adverse reactions may be more likely and more severe in older patients.

≋ SIDE EFFECTS ≋

SERIOUS
Sore throat and fever, unusual fatigue, unusual bleeding or bruising. Call your doctor immediately.

COMMON
Drowsiness, thickening of mucus.

LESS COMMON
Blurred vision; confusion; difficult or painful urination; dizziness; dry mouth, nose, or throat; increased sensitivity of skin to sunlight; faintness; increased sweating; stinging or burning of rectum (suppository form); loss of appetite; ringing or buzzing in ears; skin rash; fast heartbeat; unusual excitement or irritability.

Driving and Hazardous Work: Do not drive or engage in hazardous work until you determine how the medicine affects you.

Alcohol: Avoid alcohol.

Pregnancy: Promethazine has not been shown to cause birth defects in animals. Thorough human studies have not been done. However, if the mother takes the drug within 2 weeks of delivery, the baby may have jaundice or problems with blood clotting. Before you take it, tell your doctor if you are pregnant or plan to become pregnant.

Breast Feeding: Promethazine passes into breast milk; avoid or discontinue use while nursing. The flow of breast milk may be decreased as a result of the medication.

Infants and Children: Adverse reactions, such as seizures, may be more common and more severe in infants and children. It is not recommended for children with a history of breathing difficulty while sleeping or with a family history of sudden infant death syndrome (SIDS). Children and adolescets with signs of Reye's syndrome should not take promethazine, especially by injection. Promethazine's side effects may be mistaken for symptoms of Reye's syndrome.

Special Concerns: If you have an allergy test, stop taking promethazine 4 days before the test and tell the doctor that you were taking promethazine.

OVERDOSE

Symptoms: Clumsiness; insomnia; seizures; severe dryness of mouth, nose, or throat; redness of face; hallucinations; muscle spasms; trouble breathing; jerky movements of head and face; dizziness; trembling and shaking of hands.

What to Do: Call your doctor, emergency medical services (EMS), or the nearest poison control center immediately.

▼ INTERACTIONS

DRUG INTERACTIONS

Consult your doctor for specific advice if you are taking amoxapine, antipsychotics, medications containing alcohol, barbiturates, methyldopa, metoclopramide, metyrosine, epinephrine, metrizamide, pemoline, pimozide, rauwolfia alkaloids, anticholinergics, central nervous system depressants, maprotiline, other antihistamines, tricyclic antidepressants, levodopa, or MAO inhibitors.

FOOD INTERACTIONS

No known food interactions.

DISEASE INTERACTIONS

Consult your doctor if you have any of the following: blood disease, heart or blood vessel disease, enlarged prostate, urinary tract blockage, epilepsy, glaucoma, Reye's syndrome, jaundice, or liver disease.

PROPAFENONE

Available in: Tablets
Available OTC? No   **As Generic?** No
Drug Class: Antiarrhythmic

▼ USAGE INFORMATION

WHY IT'S PRESCRIBED
To correct heartbeat irregularities (cardiac arrhythmias).

HOW IT WORKS
Propafenone slows the conduction of nerve impulses in the heart and reduces the sensitivity of heart tissue to specific nerve impulses, which helps to stabilize heartbeat. It also has weak beta-blocking properties.

▼ DOSAGE GUIDELINES

RANGE AND FREQUENCY
Adults: 150 mg every 8 hours. It may be increased after 3 or 4 days to 225 mg every 8 hours, or 300 mg every 12 hours, up to a maximum of 300 mg every 8 hours. The maintenance dose will be determined by careful follow-up, including ECG and blood pressure monitoring. Lower doses may be required for the elderly and those with liver or heart disease.

ONSET OF EFFECT
1 hour.

DURATION OF ACTION
8 to 12 hours.

DIETARY ADVICE
Propafenone can be taken with food to minimize stomach upset.

STORAGE
Store in a tightly sealed container away from heat, moisture, and direct light.

MISSED DOSE
Take it as soon as you remember, unless the time for your next scheduled dose is within the next 4 hours. If so, skip the missed dose and resume your regular dosage schedule. Do not double the next dose.

STOPPING THE DRUG
The decision to stop taking the drug should be made in conjnction with your doctor.

PROLONGED USE
Lifelong therapy may be necessary. See your doctor regularly for examinations and diagnostic tests if you must take this medicine for a prolonged period.

▼ PRECAUTIONS

Over 60: The dose may need to be reduced.

Driving and Hazardous Work: Avoid such activities until you determine how the medication affects you.

Alcohol: Avoid alcohol.

Pregnancy: Adequate studies on the use of this drug during pregnancy have not been done. Before taking propafenone, tell your doctor if you are pregnant or plan to become pregnant.

Breast Feeding: Propafenone passes into breast milk; caution is advised. Consult your doctor for advice.

Infants and Children: The safety and efficacy of propafenone in infants and children have not been established. Limited use in young patients indicates that the incidence of side effects in younger persons is the same as for older patients. Consult your pediatrician for advice.

Special Concerns: Wearing a medical bracelet or carrying an identification card saying that you take this medication is recommended. Before having any kind of surgery, tell the doctor or dentist in charge that you use this drug.

OVERDOSE
Symptoms: Dizziness or faintness, drowsiness, slowed heartbeat, seizures, heart palpitations.

What to Do: Call your doctor, emergency medical services (EMS), or the nearest poison control center immediately.

▼ INTERACTIONS

DRUG INTERACTIONS
Consult your doctor for specific advice if you are taking warfarin, local anesthetics, other antiarrhythmic agents, digitalis drugs, beta-blockers, ritonavir, rifampin, cimetidine, or quinidine.

FOOD INTERACTIONS
No known food interactions.

DISEASE INTERACTIONS
Consult your doctor if you have had a recent heart attack or if you have any of the following: asthma, bronchitis, emphysema, slow heartbeat, or congestive heart failure. Use of propafenone may cause complications in patients with liver or kidney disease, since these organs work together to remove the medication from the body.

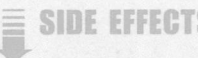
SIDE EFFECTS

SERIOUS
Fast or irregular heartbeat, chest pain, shortness of breath, swelling of feet or lower legs. Call your doctor immediately.

COMMON
Dizziness, change in taste, bitter or metallic taste.

LESS COMMON
Blurred vision, headache, constipation or diarrhea, skin rash, dry mouth, nausea or vomiting, unusual fatigue.

PROPANTHELINE BROMIDE

Available in: Tablets
Available OTC? No **As Generic?** Yes
Drug Class: Anticholinergic; antispasmodic

▼ USAGE INFORMATION

WHY IT'S PRESCRIBED
To help treat peptic (stomach and intestinal) ulcers, usually in conjunction with other forms of therapy.

HOW IT WORKS
Propantheline inhibits nerve receptor sites that stimulate both the secretion of stomach acid and the smooth muscle activity in the digestive tract. This, in turn, promotes healing of ulcers.

▼ DOSAGE GUIDELINES

RANGE AND FREQUENCY
Adults and teenagers: 7.5 to 15 mg, 3 times a day 30 minutes before meals, and 30 mg at bedtime. The dose may be changed. Older adults: 7.5 mg, 3 times a day before meals. Children: 170 micrograms per lb of body weight 4 times a day. The dose may be changed.

ONSET OF EFFECT
Unknown.

DURATION OF ACTION
6 hours.

DIETARY ADVICE
Take it 30 minutes before meals unless your doctor advises otherwise.

STORAGE
Store in a tightly sealed container away from heat and direct light.

MISSED DOSE
Take it as soon as you remember. If it is near the time for the next dose, skip the missed dose and resume your regular dosage schedule. Do not double the next dose.

STOPPING THE DRUG
The decision to stop taking the drug should be made by your doctor. Your doctor may reduce the dosage gradually; stopping abruptly can cause withdrawal side effects.

PROLONGED USE
See your doctor regularly for tests and examinations if you use it for a prolonged period.

▼ PRECAUTIONS

Over 60: Adverse reactions may be more likely and more severe in older patients.

Driving and Hazardous Work: Do not drive or engage in hazardous work until you determine how the medicine affects you.

Alcohol: Avoid alcohol.

Pregnancy: Studies of propantheline in animals or humans have not been done. Before you take propantheline, tell your doctor if you are pregnant or plan to become pregnant.

Breast Feeding: Propantheline may pass into breast milk; caution is advised. Consult your doctor for advice.

Infants and Children: Use and dosage for infants and children should be determined by your doctor.

Special Concerns: Propantheline increases the risk of heat prostration; take special care not to become overheated by exercise or during hot weather.

OVERDOSE
Symptoms: Dry mouth; thirst; difficulty swallowing; muscular weakness or paralysis; restlessness; vomiting; fever; dizziness; headache; anxiety; rapid pulse and respiration; shallow breathing; abnormal heartbeat; increased need to urinate; blurred vision; flushed, hot, and dry skin; skin rash; decreased level of consciousness or loss of consciousness.

What to Do: Call your doctor, emergency medical services (EMS), or the nearest poison control center immediately.

▼ INTERACTIONS

DRUG INTERACTIONS
Consult your doctor for specific advice if you are taking antacids, diarrhea medicine containing kaolin or attapulgite, ketoconazole, other anticholinergics, tricyclic antidepressants, or potassium chloride.

FOOD INTERACTIONS
No known food interactions.

DISEASE INTERACTIONS
Caution is advised when taking propantheline. Consult your doctor if you have any of the following: bleeding problems, glaucoma, colitis, severe dryness of mouth, enlarged prostate, glaucoma, heart disease, hiatal hernia, high blood pressure, any intestinal problem, chronic lung disease, myasthenia gravis, toxemia of pregnancy, urinary difficulty, Down syndrome, overactive thyroid, or, in children, spastic paralysis. Use of propantheline may cause complications in patients with liver or kidney disease, since these organs work together to remove the drug from the body.

▽ SIDE EFFECTS ▽

SERIOUS
Confusion, persistent lightheadedness, dizziness, fainting, eye pain, skin rash or hives. Call your doctor immediately.

COMMON
Constipation; decreased sweating; dryness of the mouth, nose, throat, or skin.

LESS COMMON
Blurred vision, bloated feeling, difficult urination, drowsiness, headache, sensitivity of eyes to light, memory loss, nausea or vomiting, unusual fatigue.

PROPOXYPHENE

Available in: Capsules, oral suspension, tablets
Available OTC? No   **As Generic?** Yes
Drug Class: Opioid (narcotic) analgesic

▼ USAGE INFORMATION

WHY IT'S PRESCRIBED
To relieve mild to moderate pain.

HOW IT WORKS
Opioids such as propoxyphene relieve pain by acting on specific areas of the central nervous system (spinal cord and brain) that process pain signals from nerves throughout the body.

▼ DOSAGE GUIDELINES

RANGE AND FREQUENCY
There are two forms of propoxyphene: propoxyphene hydrochloride and propoxyphene napsylate, which is less powerful. Adults— Propoxyphene hydrochloride: 65 mg every 4 hours; no more than 390 mg a day. Propoxyphene napsylate: 100 mg every 4 hours; no more than 600 mg a day. Children— Dose will be determined by a pediatrician.

ONSET OF EFFECT
15 to 60 minutes.

DURATION OF ACTION
4 to 6 hours.

DIETARY ADVICE
It can be taken with food to lessen stomach upset.

STORAGE
Store in a tightly sealed container away from heat, moisture, and direct light. Do not freeze the liquid form.

MISSED DOSE
If you are taking propoxyphene on a fixed schedule, take it as soon as you remember. If it is near the time for the next dose, skip the missed dose and resume your regular dosage schedule. Do not double the next dose.

STOPPING THE DRUG
The decision to stop taking the drug should be made in consultation with your doctor.

PROLONGED USE
You should see your doctor regularly for tests and examinations if you take this medication for an extended period. Prolonged use can cause nerve damage or physical dependence.

▼ PRECAUTIONS

Over 60: Adverse reactions may be more likely and more severe in older patients.

Driving and Hazardous Work: Do not drive or engage in hazardous work until you determine how the medicine affects you.

Alcohol: Avoid alcohol.

Pregnancy: Propoxyphene has not caused birth defects in animals. Human studies have not been done. Before you use this medication, tell your doctor if you are pregnant or plan to become pregnant. Overuse during pregnancy can cause drug dependence in the fetus.

Breast Feeding: Propoxyphene passes into breast milk; caution is advised. Consult your doctor for specific advice.

Infants and Children: Adverse reactions may be more likely and more severe in children. Consult your doctor for advice.

Special Concerns: If you feel the medication is not working properly after a few weeks, do not increase the dose. Consult your doctor. Before having any surgery, tell the doctor or dentist in charge that you are taking this drug.

OVERDOSE

Symptoms: Confusion; sleepiness; slurred speech; unconsciousness; small, pinpoint pupils; cold, clammy skin; slow breathing; seizures; severe drowsiness, weakness, or dizziness.

What to Do: Call your doctor, emergency medical services (EMS), or the nearest poison control center immediately.

▼ INTERACTIONS

DRUG INTERACTIONS
Consult your doctor for specific advice if you are taking carbamazepine or other medicine for seizures, barbiturates, sedatives, cough medicines, decongestants, antidepressants, other prescription pain medications, MAO inhibitors, naltrexone, rifampin, or zidovudine.

FOOD INTERACTIONS
No known food interactions.

DISEASE INTERACTIONS
Consult your doctor if you have any of the following: a history of alcohol or drug abuse; emotional illness; brain disorders or a head injury; seizures; lung disease; prostate problems or other problems with urination; gallstones; colitis; heart, kidney, liver, or thyroid disease.

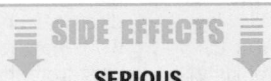

SIDE EFFECTS

SERIOUS
Some serious side effects of propoxyphene are indistinguishable from those of overdose: Confusion; sleepiness; slurred speech; unconsciousness; small, pinpoint pupils; cold, clammy skin; slow breathing; seizures; severe drowsiness, weakness, or dizziness. Other serious side effects include dark urine, yellow discoloration of eyes or skin, and pale stools.

COMMON
Dizziness or lightheadedness, nausea or vomiting, constipation, itching.

LESS COMMON
Mood swings or false sense of well-being (euphoria), hallucinations.

PROPOXYPHENE/ACETAMINOPHEN

Available in: Tablets
Available OTC? No   **As Generic?** Yes
Drug Class: Opioid (narcotic) analgesic

▼ USAGE INFORMATION

WHY IT'S PRESCRIBED
To relieve mild to moderate pain.

HOW IT WORKS
Opioids such as propoxyphene relieve pain by acting on specific areas of the spinal cord and brain that process pain signals from nerves throughout the body. Acetaminophen appears to interfere with the action of prostaglandins, naturally occurring substances in the body that cause inflammation and make nerves more sensitive to pain impulses.

▼ DOSAGE GUIDELINES

RANGE AND FREQUENCY
Adults: 1 or 2 tablets, depending on strength, every 4 to 6 hours. Children: Dose must be determined individually by your pediatrician.

ONSET OF EFFECT
Within 2 hours.

DURATION OF ACTION
Unknown.

DIETARY ADVICE
It can be taken with food to lessen stomach irritation.

STORAGE
Store in a tightly sealed container away from heat, moisture, and direct light.

MISSED DOSE
If you are taking the drug on a fixed schedule, take it as soon as you remember. If it is near the time for the next dose, skip the missed dose and resume your regular dosage schedule. Do not double the next dose.

STOPPING THE DRUG
The decision to stop taking the drug should be made by your doctor.

PROLONGED USE
You should see your doctor regularly for tests and examinations if you take this medication for a prolonged period. Prolonged use can cause nerve damage as well as physical dependence.

▼ PRECAUTIONS

Over 60: Adverse reactions may be more likely and more severe in older patients.

Driving and Hazardous Work: Avoid such activities until you determine how the medication affects you.

Alcohol: Avoid alcohol.

Pregnancy: Propoxyphene has not caused birth defects in animals. Human studies have not been done. Before you use this medication, tell your doctor if you are pregnant or plan to become pregnant. Overuse of the medication during pregnancy can cause physical dependence in the newborn.

Breast Feeding: Propoxyphene and acetaminophen pass into breast milk and may cause sedation in the nursing infant; caution is advised. Consult your doctor for specific advice.

Infants and Children: Adverse reactions may be more likely and more severe in children. Consult your pediatrician for advice.

Special Concerns: If you feel the medication is not working properly after a few weeks, do not increase the dose. Consult your doctor.

OVERDOSE
Symptoms: Severe dizziness or drowsiness; cold, clammy skin; difficult or slow breathing or shortness of breath; severe confusion; seizures; stomach cramps or pain; diarrhea; low blood pressure; increased sweating; constricted pupils; nausea or vomiting; irregular heartbeat; severe weakness.

What to Do: Call your doctor, emergency medical services (EMS), or the nearest poison control center immediately.

▼ INTERACTIONS

DRUG INTERACTIONS
Consult your doctor for specific advice if you are taking any prescription or over-the-counter drugs, especially other drugs containing acetaminophen, or central nervous system depressants which include: antihistamines or decongestants for hay fever, allergies, or colds; barbiturates; seizure medication; muscle relaxants; anesthetics; tranquilizers, sedatives, or sleep-inducing medications.

FOOD INTERACTIONS
No known food interactions.

DISEASE INTERACTIONS
Consult your doctor if you have a head injury or brain disease, an underactive thyroid, an enlarged prostate, seizures, kidney or liver disease, gall bladder problems, a blood disorder, or a history of alcohol or drug abuse.

▒ SIDE EFFECTS ▒

SERIOUS
Bloody, dark, or cloudy urine; severe pain in the lower back or side; pale or black, tarry stools; yellow discoloration of eyes or skin (jaundice); hallucinations; frequent urge to urinate; painful or difficult urination; sudden decrease in urine output; increased sweating; unusual bleeding or bruising; irregular heartbeat; skin rash, hives, or itching; excitability; ringing or buzzing in the ears; pinpoint red spots on skin; sore throat and fever; confusion; trembling or uncontrolled muscle movements; redness, flushing, or swelling of the face. Call your doctor immediately.

COMMON
Dizziness, lightheadedness, constipation, nausea, vomiting, drowsiness, unusual fatigue.

LESS COMMON
Stomach pain, false sense of well-being (euphoria), depression, loss of appetite, blurred vision, nightmares or unusual dreams, dry mouth, headache, nervousness, insomnia.

PROPRANOLOL HYDROCHLORIDE

Available in: Extended-release capsules, oral solution, tablets, injection
Available OTC? No   **As Generic?** Yes
Drug Class: Beta-blocker

▼ USAGE INFORMATION

WHY IT'S PRESCRIBED
To treat angina, mild to moderate high blood pressure, irregular heartbeat (cardiac arrhythmias), hypertrophic cardiomyopathy (weakness of the heart muscle), heart attack, pheochromocytoma, tremors, and migraine headaches.

HOW IT WORKS
Propranolol blocks nerve impulses to various parts of the body, which accounts for its many effects. For example, it slows the heart's rate and force of the contraction (which helps lower blood pressure), decreases the heart's oxygen requirement (which helps prevent angina), and helps stabilize heart rhythm.

▼ DOSAGE GUIDELINES

RANGE AND FREQUENCY
Adults— For angina: 80 to 320 mg a day in 2, 3, or 4 doses. For high blood pressure: 40 mg, 2 times a day; may be increased up to 640 mg a day. For irregular heartbeat: 10 to 30 mg, 3 or 4 times a day. For cardiomyopathy: 20 to 40 mg, 3 or 4 times a day. For pheochromocytoma: 30 to 160 mg a day in divided doses. For preventing migraine headache: 20 mg, 4 times a day; may be increased to 240 mg a day. For trembling: 40 mg, 2 times a day; may be increased to 320 mg a day. Children— For high blood pressure: 0.5 mg to 4 mg per 2.2 lbs (1 kg) of body weight a day. For irregular heartbeat: 0.5 to 4 mg per 2.2 lbs of body weight a day in divided doses.

ONSET OF EFFECT
Within 30 minutes.

DURATION OF ACTION
Up to 12 hours.

DIETARY ADVICE
Mix the concentrated oral solution with water, juice, or a carbonated drink.

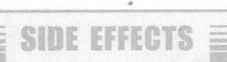

SIDE EFFECTS

SERIOUS
Shortness of breath, wheezing; irregular or slow heartbeat (50 beats per minute or less); pain or feelings of tightness or pressure in the chest; swelling of the ankles, feet, and lower legs; depression. Call your doctor immediately.

COMMON
Dizziness or lightheadedness, especially when rising suddenly to a standing position; decreased sexual ability; unusual fatigue, weakness, or drowsiness; insomnia.

LESS COMMON
Anxiety, irritability; constipation; diarrhea; dry eyes; itching; nausea or vomiting; nightmares or intensely vivid dreams; numbness, tingling, or prickling in the fingers, toes, or scalp.

STORAGE
Store in a tightly sealed container away from heat and direct light.

MISSED DOSE
Take it as soon as you remember. If it is near the time for the next dose, skip the missed dose and resume your regular dosage schedule. Do not double the next dose.

STOPPING THE DRUG
Do not stop taking this drug suddenly; the dosage must be slowly tapered under your physician's close supervision.

PROLONGED USE
Lifelong therapy with propranolol may be necessary; prolonged use may be associated with a greater incidence of side effects. Regular monitoring and evaluation by your doctor is advised.

▼ PRECAUTIONS

Over 60: Adverse reactions may be more likely and more severe in older patients.

Driving and Hazardous Work: Avoid such activities until you determine how the drug affects you.

Alcohol: Avoid alcohol.

Pregnancy: Consult your doctor to weigh the risks and benefits of using propranolol during pregnancy.

Breast Feeding: Propranolol passes into breast milk; caution is advised.

Infants and Children: Dosage will be determined by your pediatrician.

Special Concerns: Take extra care during exercise or hot weather to avoid dizziness and fainting. Check your pulse often; if it is slower than usual or less than 50 beats a minute, call your doctor.

OVERDOSE
Symptoms: Unusually slow or rapid heartbeat, severe dizziness or fainting, poor circulation in the hands (bluish skin), breathing difficulty; seizures.

What to Do: Call your doctor, emergency medical services (EMS), or the nearest poison control center immediately.

▼ INTERACTIONS

DRUG INTERACTIONS
Consult your doctor for specific advice if you are taking allergy shots, aminophylline, caffeine, oxtriphylline, theophylline, oral antidiabetics, insulin, calcium channel blockers, clonidine, guanabenz, or MAO inhibitors.

FOOD INTERACTIONS
No known food interactions.

DISEASE INTERACTIONS
Must be used with caution in people with diabetes, especially insulin-dependent diabetes, since the drug may mask symptoms of hypoglycemia. Consult your doctor if you have allergies, bronchitis, emphysema, heart or blood vessel disease (including congestive heart failure and peripheral vascular disease), mental depression, myasthenia gravis, psoriasis, hyperthyroidism, kidney disease, or liver disease.

PROPRANOLOL/HYDROCHLOROTHIAZIDE

BRAND NAMES

Inderide, Inderide LA

Available in: Extended-release capsules, tablets
Available OTC? No   **As Generic?** Yes
Drug Class: Beta-blocker/thiazide diuretic; antihypertensive

▼ USAGE INFORMATION

WHY IT'S PRESCRIBED
To control hypertension (high blood pressure).

HOW IT WORKS
Propranolol, a beta-blocker, blocks nerve impulses to various parts of the body, which accounts for its many effects. For example, it reduces the heart rate and force of the heart's contractions (which helps to lower blood pressure), decreases the heart's oxygen requirement (which helps prevent angina) and helps stabilize heart rhythm. Hydrochlorothiazide, a diuretic, increases the excretion of salt and water in the urine. By reducing the overall amount of fluid in the body, diuretics reduce pressure within the blood vessels.

▼ DOSAGE GUIDELINES

RANGE AND FREQUENCY
Adults— Extended-release capsules: 1 capsule a day. Tablets: 1 or 2 tablets, 2 times a day.

ONSET OF EFFECT
Unknown.

DURATION OF ACTION
Unknown.

DIETARY ADVICE
No special restrictions.

STORAGE
Store in a tightly sealed container away from heat, moisture, and direct light.

MISSED DOSE
Take it as soon as you remember. If it is near the time for the next dose, skip the missed dose and resume your regular dosage schedule. Do not double the next dose.

STOPPING THE DRUG
The decision to stop taking the drug should be made in consultation with your physician. Do not stop taking this drug abruptly; your dose must be gradually tapered before stopping completely.

PROLONGED USE
Propranolol/hydrochlorothiazide is used to control high blood pressure, but it cannot cure it. Lifelong therapy may be necessary. See your doctor regularly for tests and examinations if you must take this drug for a prolonged period of time.

▼ PRECAUTIONS

Over 60: Adverse reactions, especially dizziness, lightheadedness, and reduced tolerance to cold, may be more likely and more severe in older patients.

Driving and Hazardous Work: Do not drive or engage in hazardous work until you determine how the medicine affects you.

Alcohol: Avoid alcohol.

Pregnancy: Beta-blockers and thiazide diuretics may cause problems during pregnancy. Before taking this medication, tell your doctor if you are pregnant or plan to become pregnant.

Breast Feeding: This drug passes into breast milk; caution is advised. Consult your doctor for specific advice.

Infants and Children: Adequate studies of the use of this drug by children have not been done. No special problems are expected. Consult your pediatrician for advice.

Special Concerns: In addition to taking this medicine, follow your doctor's instructions on weight control and diet for reduction of blood pressure. Protect yourself from sunlight until you determine how this medicine affects you.

OVERDOSE

Symptoms: Slow heartbeat, severe dizziness or fainting, difficulty breathing, bluish colored fingernails or palms of hands, seizures.

What to Do: Call your doctor, emergency medical services (EMS), or the nearest poison control center immediately.

▼ INTERACTIONS

DRUG INTERACTIONS
Consult your doctor for specific advice if you are receiving allergy shots or skin tests, or are taking oral diabetes medications, insulin, calcium channel blockers, digitalis drugs, clonidine, lithium, MAO inhibitors, xanthines, or guanabenz.

FOOD INTERACTIONS
Avoid foods high in sodium.

DISEASE INTERACTIONS
Consult your doctor if you have any of the following: any allergic condition, bronchial asthma, emphysema, slow heartbeat, heart or blood vessel disease, diabetes mellitus, congestive heart failure, kidney disease, liver disease, depression, or an overactive thyroid (hyperthyroidism).

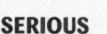

SIDE EFFECTS

SERIOUS
Slow heartbeat; difficulty breathing; mental depression; cold hands and feet; swelling of ankles, feet, or lower legs. Call your doctor immediately.

COMMON
Dizziness or lightheadedness, decreased sexual ability, drowsiness, insomnia.

LESS COMMON
Anxiety, loss of appetite, upset stomach, nervousness or excitability, constipation or diarrhea, increased sensitivity of the skin to sunlight, numbness and tingling in the fingers and toes, stuffy nose.

PROPYLTHIOURACIL

Available in: Tablets
Available OTC? No   **As Generic?** Yes
Drug Class: Antithyroid agent

▼ USAGE INFORMATION

WHY IT'S PRESCRIBED
To treat conditions in which the thyroid gland produces too much thyroid hormone (hyperthyroidism).

HOW IT WORKS
Propylthiouracil interferes with the body's ability to use iodine in the manufacture of thyroid hormone.

▼ DOSAGE GUIDELINES

RANGE AND FREQUENCY
Adults: To start, 300 to 900 mg a day, with doses every 8 hours. Maximum dose: 1,200 mg a day. Usual maintenance dose is 50 to 600 mg a day. Children ages 6 to 10: To start, 50 to 150 mg a day in 3 doses. The dose can be adjusted later. Children ages 10 and older: 50 to 300 mg per day, in 3 doses. To treat a thyroid crisis: 400 mg or more (up to 900 mg a day) for the first day, reduced gradually over subsequent days.

ONSET OF EFFECT
5 days or more.

DURATION OF ACTION
Unknown.

DIETARY ADVICE
Take it with meals to minimize stomach upset.

STORAGE
Store in a tightly sealed container away from heat and direct light.

MISSED DOSE
Take it as soon as you remember. If it is near the time for the next dose, skip the missed dose and resume your regular dosage schedule. Do not double the next dose.

STOPPING THE DRUG
The decision to stop taking the drug should be made by your doctor.

PROLONGED USE
No special problems are expected. It may be necessary to take this medication for several years.

⬇ SIDE EFFECTS ⬇

SERIOUS
Cough, continuing or severe fever or chills; hoarseness; mouth sores; pain, swelling, or redness in joints; throat infection; yellowish tinge (jaundice) in skin or eyes; general feeling of discomfort, weakness, or illness. Call your doctor immediately.

COMMON
Mild and temporary fever, rash or itching.

LESS COMMON
Backache; black and tarry stools; blood in urine or stools; shortness of breath; increased or decreased urination; swelling of feet or lower legs; swollen lymph or salivary glands; numbness or tingling of face, fingers, or toes; dizziness; nausea; stomach pain; vomiting.

▼ PRECAUTIONS

Over 60: Adverse reactions may be more common and more severe in older patients.

Driving and Hazardous Work: The use of propylthiouracil should not impair your ability to perform such tasks safely.

Alcohol: Consult your doctor about consuming alcohol while taking this drug.

Pregnancy: Too large a dose during pregnancy may cause problems in the fetus. The prescribed dose, with careful monitoring, is not likely to cause problems.

Breast Feeding: Although propylthiouracil passes into breast milk, your doctor may allow you to continue breast feeding if the dose is kept low and the infant is checked regularly.

Infants and Children: This medicine has not been shown to cause different side effects or problems in children than it does in adults.

Special Concerns: Before undergoing any kind of medical or dental procedure, be sure to tell the doctor or dentist in charge that you are taking propylthiouracil. During and after treatment, do not receive any immunizations without your doctor's approval, and avoid persons who have recently taken oral polio vaccine.

OVERDOSE
Symptoms: Nausea, vomiting, coldness, constipation, changes in menstrual period, dry and puffy skin, headache, listlessness, muscle aches, sleepiness, swollen neck, unusual weight gain.

What to Do: An overdose of propylthiouracil is unlikely to be life-threatening. However, if someone takes a much larger dose than prescribed, call your doctor, emergency medical services (EMS), or local poison control center.

▼ INTERACTIONS

DRUG INTERACTIONS
Consult your doctor for advice if you are taking amiodarone, iodinated glycerol, potassium iodide, anticoagulants, or digitalis drugs.

FOOD INTERACTIONS
Consult your doctor about the need for a special low-iodine diet.

DISEASE INTERACTIONS
Use of propylthiouracil may cause complications in patients who have liver disease, since this organ works to remove medications from the body.

PROTRIPTYLINE HYDROCHLORIDE

Available in: Tablets
Available OTC? No **As Generic?** Yes
Drug Class: Tricyclic antidepressant

▼ USAGE INFORMATION

WHY IT'S PRESCRIBED
To relieve symptoms of major depression.

HOW IT WORKS
Protriptyline affects levels of norepinephrine, a brain chemical that is thought to be linked to mood, emotions, and mental state.

▼ DOSAGE GUIDELINES

RANGE AND FREQUENCY
Adults: To start, 5 to 10 mg, 3 to 4 times a day; may be increased to 60 mg a day. Teenagers: To start, 5 mg, 3 times a day; may be increased gradually by your doctor. Older adults: To start, 5 mg, 3 times a day; may be increased gradually by your doctor.

ONSET OF EFFECT
1 to 6 weeks.

DURATION OF ACTION
Unknown.

DIETARY ADVICE
To reduce the likelihood of stomach upset, take with food, unless your doctor instructs otherwise. Increase intake of fiber and fluids.

STORAGE
Store in a tightly sealed container away from heat, moisture, and direct light.

MISSED DOSE
If you take a one-time daily bedtime dose, do not take the missed dose in the morning because it may cause drowsiness. Call your doctor. If you take more than 1 dose a day, take it as soon as you remember. However, if it is near the time for the next dose, skip the missed dose and resume your regular dosage schedule. Do not double the next dose.

STOPPING THE DRUG
Take as prescribed for the full treatment period, even if you begin to feel better before the scheduled end of therapy. The decision to stop taking the drug should be made in consultation with your doctor.

PROLONGED USE
The usual course of therapy lasts 6 months to 1 year; some patients benefit from additional therapy.

▼ PRECAUTIONS

Over 60: Adverse reactions may be more likely and more severe in older patients. A lower dose may be warranted.

Driving and Hazardous Work: Use caution when driving or engaging in hazardous work until you know how the medication affects you. Drowsiness or lightheadedness can occur.

Alcohol: Avoid alcohol.

Pregnancy: Adequate human studies have not been done. Consult your doctor for specific advice.

Breast Feeding: Protriptyline passes into breast milk; do not use it while nursing.

Infants and Children: This drug is not prescribed for children under age 6.

Special Concerns: This is a potentially dangerous drug, especially if taken in excess. Tricyclic antidepressants should not be within easy reach of suicidal patients. If dry mouth occurs, use candy or sugarless gum for relief.

OVERDOSE
Symptoms: Difficulty breathing, severe fatigue, seizures, confusion, hallucinations, dilated pupils, irregular heartbeat, fever, impaired ability to concentrate.

What to Do: Call your doctor, emergency medical services (EMS), or the nearest poison control center immediately.

▼ INTERACTIONS

DRUG INTERACTIONS
Consult your doctor for specific advice if you are taking antithyroid agents, cimetidine, cisapride, clonidine, guanadrel, guanethidine, metrizamide, appetite suppressants, isoproterenol, ephedrine, epinephrine, amphetamines, phenylephrine, antipsychotic drugs, pimozide, methyldopa, metyrosine, metoclopramide, pemoline, promethazine, trimeprazine, rauwolfia alkaloids, MAO inhibitors, or any drugs that depress the central nervous system.

FOOD INTERACTIONS
No known food interactions.

DISEASE INTERACTIONS
Consult your doctor if you have any of the following: a history of alcohol abuse, difficulty urinating, asthma, bipolar disorder, high blood pressure, stomach or intestinal problems, glaucoma, overactive thyroid, enlarged prostate, schizophrenia, seizures, a blood disorder, or kidney, heart, or liver disease.

≡ SIDE EFFECTS ≡

SERIOUS
Confusion, heartbeat irregularities, hallucinations, seizures, extreme fatigue or drowsiness, blurred or altered vision, breathing difficulty, constipation, staring and absence of facial expression, impaired concentration, difficult urination, fever, extreme and persistent restlessness, loss of coordination and balance, difficulty swallowing or speaking, dilated pupils, eye pain, fainting. Also trembling, shaking, weakness, and stiffness in the extremities; shuffling gait. Call your doctor immediately.

COMMON
Drowsiness or dizziness, headache, dry mouth or unpleasant taste, fatigue, heightened sensitivity to light, weight gain, increased appetite, nausea, excitability.

LESS COMMON
Heartburn or indigestion, sleeping difficulty, diarrhea, increased sweating, vomiting.

PSEUDOEPHEDRINE

Available in: Extended-release capsules, oral solution, syrup, tablets
Available OTC? Yes   **As Generic?** Yes
Drug Class: Decongestant/cough drug

▼ USAGE INFORMATION

WHY IT'S PRESCRIBED
To relieve nasal or sinus congestion caused by colds, sinus infection, hay fever, or other respiratory allergies.

HOW IT WORKS
Pseudoephedrine narrows and constricts blood vessels to reduce the blood flow to swollen nasal passages and other tissues, which reduces nasal secretions, shrinks swollen nasal mucous membranes, and improves airflow in nasal passages.

▼ DOSAGE GUIDELINES

RANGE AND FREQUENCY
Short-acting forms— Adults and teenagers: 60 mg every 4 to 6 hours; not more than 240 mg in 24 hours. Children 6 to 12 years of age: 30 mg every 4 to 6 hours; not more than 120 mg in 24 hours. Children 2 to 6 years of age: 15 mg every 4 hours; not more than 60 mg in 24 hours. Extended-release form— Adults and teenagers: 120 mg every 12 hours or 240 mg every 24 hours.

ONSET OF EFFECT
15 to 30 minutes.

DURATION OF ACTION
3 to 4 hours for short-acting forms, 8 to 12 hours for extended-release form.

DIETARY ADVICE
Drink plenty of fluids.

STORAGE
Store in a tightly sealed container away from heat and direct light. Do not allow the liquid form to freeze.

MISSED DOSE
Take it as soon as you remember. If it is near the time for the next dose, skip the missed dose and resume your regular dosage schedule. Do not double the next dose.

STOPPING THE DRUG
Do not take this drug longer than recommended on the label unless directed to do so by your doctor.

PROLONGED USE
Consult your doctor about taking pseudoephedrine for more than 5 to 7 days.

▼ PRECAUTIONS

Over 60: Side effects may be more likely and more severe in elderly patients.

Driving and Hazardous Work: Avoid such activities until you determine how the medicine affects you.

Alcohol: No special precautions are necessary.

Pregnancy: Safety has not been established; it should be used only if clearly necessary. Consult your doctor for specific advice.

Breast Feeding: Pseudoephedrine passes into breast milk; avoid or discontinue use while nursing.

Infants and Children: Use of extended-release forms of pseudoephedrine is not recommended for children under the age of 12.

Special Concerns: If your symptoms do not improve within 7 days, check with your doctor. To help prevent insomnia, take the last dose at least 2 hours before your bedtime.

OVERDOSE
Symptoms: Drowsiness, sedation, profuse sweating, pale or clammy skin, low blood pressure, diminished urine output, dizziness, changes in mental state, hallucinations, seizures, loss of consciousness.

What to Do: In some cases an overdose can be fatal, especially among elderly patients. At the first sign of overdose, call your doctor, emergency medical services (EMS), or the nearest poison control center immediately.

▼ INTERACTIONS

DRUG INTERACTIONS
Consult your doctor for specific advice if you are taking beta-blockers or MAO inhibitors.

FOOD INTERACTIONS
No known food interactions.

DISEASE INTERACTIONS
Caution is advised when taking pseudoephedrine. Consult your doctor if you have any of the following: diabetes, enlarged prostate, heart disease, blood vessel disease, high blood pressure, or an overactive thyroid gland.

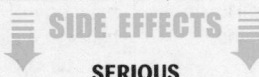
SIDE EFFECTS

SERIOUS
Seizures, irregular or slowed heartbeat, shortness of breath, breathing difficulty, hallucinations. Stop taking the medication and call your doctor right away.

COMMON
Nervousness, restlessness, insomnia.

LESS COMMON
Difficult or painful urination, dizziness or lightheadedness, rapid or pounding heartbeat, increased sweating, nausea or vomiting, trembling, trouble breathing, paleness, weakness.

PSEUDOEPHEDRINE/GUAIFENESIN

Available in: Capsules, oral solution, syrup, tablets, extended-release forms
Available OTC? Yes   **As Generic?** No
Drug Class: Decongestant/cough drug

▼ USAGE INFORMATION

WHY IT'S PRESCRIBED
To relieve nasal or sinus congestion caused by colds, influenza (flu), hay fever, and other respiratory allergies. Also intended to break up congestion in the lungs to promote better breathing.

HOW IT WORKS
Pseudoephedrine narrows and constricts blood vessels to reduce the blood flow to swollen nasal passages and other tissues, which reduces nasal secretions, shrinks swollen nasal mucous membranes, and improves airflow. Guaifenesin purportedly breaks up, liquefies, and loosens mucus secretions in the respiratory tract, making it easier to cough up phlegm and thus breathe easier. (There is some debate however as to whether guaifenesin is actually effective in this regard.)

▼ DOSAGE GUIDELINES

RANGE AND FREQUENCY
Take the drug as directed to relieve symptoms.

ONSET OF EFFECT
Within 1 hour.

DURATION OF ACTION
Unknown.

DIETARY ADVICE
No special restrictions.

STORAGE
Store in a tightly sealed container away from heat and direct light.

MISSED DOSE
Take it as soon as you remember. If it is near the time for the next dose, skip the missed dose and resume your regular dosage schedule. Do not double the next dose.

STOPPING THE DRUG
The decision to stop taking the drug should be made by your doctor or when you note improvement.

PROLONGED USE
Check with your doctor if symptoms do not improve within 5 days.

▼ PRECAUTIONS

Over 60: Adverse reactions may be more likely and more severe in older patients.

Driving and Hazardous Work: Do not drive or engage in hazardous work until you determine how the medicine affects you.

Alcohol: Avoid alcohol.

Pregnancy: Before taking pseudoephedrine and guaifenesin, tell your doctor if you are pregnant or plan to become pregnant.

Breast Feeding: Pseudoephedrine passes into breast milk; avoid or discontinue use while nursing.

Infants and Children: Check the package label or with your doctor before giving it to infants or children.

Special Concerns: If you have trouble sleeping, take the last dose of pseudoephedrine and guaifenesin a few hours before bedtime. Before having any surgery, tell your doctor or dentist that you are taking this drug. Be sure your doctor knows if you have high blood pressure.

OVERDOSE
Symptoms: Rapid, pounding, or irregular heartbeat, continuing and severe headache, severe nausea or vomiting, severe nervousness or restlessness, severe shortness of breath or troubled breathing.

What to Do: Call your doctor, emergency medical services (EMS), or the nearest poison control center immediately.

▼ INTERACTIONS

DRUG INTERACTIONS
Consult your doctor if you are taking any prescription or nonprescription medication. Do not take any drug for diet or appetite control unless you have checked with your doctor first.

FOOD INTERACTIONS
No known food interactions.

DISEASE INTERACTIONS
Caution is advised when taking pseudoephedrine and guaifenesin. Consult your doctor if you have any of the following: anemia, gout, hemophilia, stomach problems, brain disease, colitis, seizures, diarrhea, gallbladder disease or gallstones, cystic fibrosis, diabetes mellitus, any chronic lung disease, enlarged prostate, difficult urination, glaucoma, heart or blood vessel disease, thyroid disease, or high blood pressure. Use of pseudoephedrine and guaifenesin may cause complications in persons with liver or kidney disease, since these organs work together to remove the medication from the body.

SIDE EFFECTS

SERIOUS
Skin rash, hives, itching, rapid or irregular heartbeat, persistent headache, nervousness or restlessness, shortness of breath or breathing difficulty, seizures, unusual fear and anxiety. Call your doctor or emergency medical services (EMS) right away.

COMMON
Constipation; decreased sweating; difficult urination; dizziness or lightheadedness; drowsiness; dry mouth, nose, or throat; increased sensitivity of skin to sun; nausea or vomiting; nightmares; stomach pain; thickened mucus; insomnia; unusual excitement or restlessness; unusual tiredness or weakness. Contact your doctor if these symptoms persist or interfere with your daily activities.

LESS COMMON
There are no less-common side effects associated with the use of this drug.

PSYLLIUM

Available in: Caramels, granules, powder
Available OTC? Yes   **As Generic?** Yes
Drug Class: Bulk-forming laxative

▼ USAGE INFORMATION

WHY IT'S PRESCRIBED
To relieve constipation. It also may be prescribed for treatment of diarrhea.

HOW IT WORKS
Psyllium is a natural soluble fiber derived from the husks of a seed grain. It absorbs liquid in the intestines and swells to form a soft, bulky stool. The increased bulk of the stool stimulates bowel activity and triggers the urge to defecate. Psyllium has also been shown in studies to improve the ratio of HDL ("good") cholesterol to LDL ("bad") cholesterol in the blood. For this reason, it is sometimes prescribed as part of a program to reduce high cholesterol levels before resorting to drug therapy.

▼ DOSAGE GUIDELINES

RANGE AND FREQUENCY
Adults: 1 to 2 rounded teaspoons or 1 packet dissolved in water, 1, 2, or 3 times a day, followed by a second glass of liquid. Children over 6: 1 level teaspoon in half a glass of water.

ONSET OF EFFECT
Usually, 12 to 24 hours. In some cases, up to 3 days.

DURATION OF ACTION
Variable.

DIETARY ADVICE
Take psyllium with a full glass of cold liquid, such as fruit juice or water, and follow with another full glass.

STORAGE
Store in a tightly sealed container away from heat, moisture, and direct light.

MISSED DOSE
Take it as soon as you remember. If it is near the time for the next dose, skip the missed dose and resume your regular dosage schedule. Do not double the next dose.

STOPPING THE DRUG
Take it as prescribed for the full treatment period. However, you may stop taking it if you are feeling better before the scheduled end of therapy.

PROLONGED USE
Do not take psyllium for more than 1 week unless your doctor has ordered a special schedule for you.

▼ PRECAUTIONS

Over 60: No special advice.

Driving and Hazardous Work: No special warnings.

Alcohol: Avoid alcohol; it can irritate the gastrointestinal tract and interfere with proper digestion.

Pregnancy: Discuss with your doctor the relative risks and benefits of using psyllium while pregnant.

Breast Feeding: Psyllium may pass into breast milk; caution is advised. Consult your doctor for advice.

Infants and Children: Not recommended for use by children under age 6.

Special Concerns: You should have an adequate amount of fiber-containing food in your diet, such as cereals, fresh fruit, and vegetables. Before taking psyllium, tell your doctor if you have had any unusual or allergic reaction to laxatives. Make sure that your doctor knows if you are on any special diet. Do not take any other medicine within 2 hours of taking psyllium. Drink from 6 to 8 eight-ounce glasses of water every day.

OVERDOSE
Symptoms: Intestinal blockage if psyllium is taken in excessive doses.

What to Do: An overdose of psyllium is unlikely. However, if someone takes a much larger dose than prescribed, seek medical help promptly.

▼ INTERACTIONS

DRUG INTERACTIONS
Consult your doctor for advice if you are taking oral tetracyclines.

FOOD INTERACTIONS
Psyllium may interfere with the absorption of certain minerals, especially in high doses or with regular use.

DISEASE INTERACTIONS
Consult your doctor if you have any of the following: heart disease, a colostomy or ileostomy, diabetes mellitus, high blood pressure, kidney disease, rectal bleeding of unknown cause, difficulty swallowing, or any signs of appendicitis.

≡ SIDE EFFECTS ≡

SERIOUS
Difficulty breathing, intestinal blockage (resulting in severe, painful constipation), skin rash or itching, difficulty swallowing. Call your doctor immediately.

COMMON
No common side effects have been reported.

LESS COMMON
Nausea, vomiting, partial intestinal obstruction, abdominal pain or cramping.

PYRANTEL PAMOATE

Available in: Oral suspension
Available OTC? Yes   **As Generic?** Yes
Drug Class: Anthelmintic

▼ USAGE INFORMATION

WHY IT'S PRESCRIBED
To treat various worm infections, including ascariasis (common roundworm) and enterobiasis or oxyuriasis (pinworm). It may be used to treat more than one worm infection at a time. It may also be used for other types of infection as determined by your doctor.

HOW IT WORKS
Pyrantel paralyzes the worm. While it is paralyzed, the worm is expelled from the body in the stool.

▼ DOSAGE GUIDELINES

RANGE AND FREQUENCY
Adults and children age 2 and older— For roundworms: 1 dose of 11 mg per 2.2 lbs (1 kg) of body weight. Maximum dose is 1,000 mg. If necessary, the dose may be repeated in 2 to 3 weeks. For pinworms: 1 dose of 11 mg per 2.2 lbs of body weight. Maximum dose is 1,000 mg. Repeat the dose in 2 to 3 weeks.

ONSET OF EFFECT
Variable.

DURATION OF ACTION
Variable.

DIETARY ADVICE
Pyrantel can be taken with fruit juice, milk, or food.

STORAGE
Store in a tightly sealed container away from heat, moisture, and direct light. Do not allow it to freeze.

MISSED DOSE
Take a missed dose as soon as you remember.

STOPPING THE DRUG
The decision to stop taking the drug should be made in consultation with your doctor.

PROLONGED USE
Pyrantel is generally prescribed for one-time use (two-time use for pinworms).

▼ PRECAUTIONS

Over 60: Adverse reactions may be more likely and more severe in older patients.

Driving and Hazardous Work: Do not drive or engage in hazardous work until you determine how the medicine affects you.

Alcohol: No special precautions are necessary.

Pregnancy: Pyrantel is not recommended for use in pregnant women. Consult your doctor for specific advice if you are pregnant or plan to become pregnant.

Breast Feeding: Pyrantel may pass into breast milk; caution is advised. Consult your doctor for advice.

Infants and Children: Use and dosage for children under the age of 2 should be determined by your doctor. Not recommended for use by children under the age of 1.

Special Concerns: For pinworm infection, clothing, bedding, and towels should be washed daily. All members of the family may have to be treated to eradicate the infestation. A second treatment for all household members may be necessary after 2 or 3 weeks. All bedding and nightclothes should be washed after treatment. To prevent reinfection, you should wash the anal region daily, change your underwear and bedding every day, and wash your hands and fingernails before each meal and after bowel movements. Consult your doctor if your condition has not improved upon completion of therapy.

OVERDOSE

Symptoms: An overdose with pyrantel is unlikely to occur.

What to Do: If someone takes a much larger dose than prescribed, call your doctor, emergency medical services (EMS), or the nearest poison control center right away.

▼ INTERACTIONS

DRUG INTERACTIONS
Do not take piperazine when taking pyrantel. The effectiveness of both drugs may be reduced. Consult your doctor for specific advice. Also tell your doctor if you are taking any other prescription or over-the-counter medication.

FOOD INTERACTIONS
No known food interactions.

DISEASE INTERACTIONS
Caution is advised when taking pyrantel. Consult your doctor for specific advice if you have any other medical condition.

▼ SIDE EFFECTS

SERIOUS
Skin rash. Stop using the drug and call your doctor as soon as possible.

COMMON
No common side effects are associated with the use of pyrantel.

LESS COMMON
Pain or cramps in abdomen or stomach, headache, dizziness, diarrhea, drowsiness, insomnia, nausea or vomiting, loss of appetite.

PYRAZINAMIDE

Available in: Tablets
Available OTC? No **As Generic?** Yes
Drug Class: Anti-infective/antitubercular agent

▼ USAGE INFORMATION

WHY IT'S PRESCRIBED
To treat active tuberculosis; it must be used in conjunction with other antitubercular agents, such as isoniazid, streptomycin, and rifampin.

HOW IT WORKS
Pyrazinamide kills the tuberculosis bacteria.

▼ DOSAGE GUIDELINES

RANGE AND FREQUENCY
Adults: 1.5 to 2.5 g (6.8 to 13.6 mg per lb of body weight) per day. Children: 6.8 to 13.6 mg per lb once a day; not more than 2,000 mg daily. It may also be given to adults or children 2 to 3 times a week in a dose of 22.7 to 31.8 mg per lb. If the schedule is twice a week, adults should take no more than 4,000 mg per dose; if the schedule is 3 times a week, no more than 2,500 mg per dose. Children should receive not more than 2,000 mg per day, even if it is taken only 2 or 3 times a week.

ONSET OF EFFECT
Unknown.

DURATION OF ACTION
Unknown.

DIETARY ADVICE
Take it with food to minimize stomach irritation.

STORAGE
Store in a tightly sealed container away from heat, moisture, and direct light.

MISSED DOSE
Take it as soon as you remember. This will help keep a constant level of medication in your system. If it is near the time for the next dose, skip the missed dose and resume your regular dosage schedule. Do not double the next dose.

STOPPING THE DRUG
Take it as prescribed for the full treatment period, even if you begin to feel better before the scheduled end of therapy. Treatment may continue for months or years. The decision to stop taking the drug should be made by your doctor.

PROLONGED USE
Consult your doctor about the need for periodic medical examinations and laboratory tests. If your symptoms do not improve or instead become worse in 2 to 3 weeks, consult your doctor.

▼ PRECAUTIONS

Over 60: Adverse reactions may be more likely and more severe in older patients.

Driving and Hazardous Work: The use of pyrazinamide should not impair your ability to perform such tasks safely.

Alcohol: Avoid alcohol.

Pregnancy: Adequate human studies have not been done. Before taking pyrazinamide, tell your doctor if you are pregnant or are planning to become pregnant.

Breast Feeding: Pyrazinamide passes into breast milk; caution is advised. Consult your doctor for specific advice.

Infants and Children: Pyrazinamide has not been shown to cause different or more severe side effects in children. However, owing to the serious nature of the side effects, it should be used only under the strict supervision of your doctor. Discuss with your pediatrician the relative risks and benefits of your child's using this drug.

Special Concerns: Pyrazinamide may cause false results on urine ketone tests for diabetes. Check with your doctor before adjusting your medication dosage or diet. Patients with HIV may require a longer period of treatment.

OVERDOSE
Symptoms: Abnormal results on tests of liver function. This problem can be detected by your doctor.

What to Do: An overdose of pyrazinamide is unlikely to be life-threatening. However, if someone takes a much larger dose than prescribed, call your doctor, emergency medical services (EMS), or the nearest poison control center.

▼ INTERACTIONS

DRUG INTERACTIONS
Consult your doctor for specific advice if you are taking any other prescription or over-the-counter medication.

FOOD INTERACTIONS
No known food interactions.

DISEASE INTERACTIONS
Consult your doctor if you have a history of alcohol abuse, diabetes, or gout. The use of pyrazinamide may cause complications in patients who have liver disease, since this organ works to remove the medication from the body.

≡ SIDE EFFECTS ≡

SERIOUS
Joint pain or swelling, especially in leg and foot joints; nausea, vomiting, weakness, fatigue, yellow discoloration of the eyes or skin (may be signs of hepatitis). Call your doctor immediately.

COMMON
Joint pain, hepatitis (see above).

LESS COMMON
Skin rash, itching, stomach upset.

PYRETHRINS/PIPERONYL BUTOXIDE

Available in: Gel, solution shampoo, topical solution
Available OTC? Yes   **As Generic?** Yes
Drug Class: Topical antiparasitic

▼ USAGE INFORMATION

WHY IT'S PRESCRIBED
To treat head, body, and pubic lice infestations. Although this drug is available without a prescription, your doctor may have special instructions regarding its proper use.

HOW IT WORKS
Pyrethrins and piperonyl butoxide are a combination of active ingredients. The medication is absorbed into the bodies of lice, where it blocks nerve activity, ultimately causing paralysis and death of the lice. (The drug has no such toxic effect on humans.)

▼ DOSAGE GUIDELINES

RANGE AND FREQUENCY
Use 1 time, then repeat one more time in 7 to 10 days. Gel or solution: Apply enough medicine to thoroughly wet hair, scalp, or skin. Allow the medicine to remain on the affected areas for 10 minutes, then wash with warm water and soap or regular shampoo. Rinse thoroughly and dry with a clean towel. Shampoo: Apply enough medicine to wet the hair, scalp, or skin. Allow the medicine to remain on the affected areas for 10 minutes, then use a small amount of water to work shampoo more thoroughly into affected area. Rinse and dry with a clean towel. With either method, use a nit-removal comb to remove dead lice and eggs from hair.

ONSET OF EFFECT
Within 10 minutes.

DURATION OF ACTION
Up to 10 days.

DIETARY ADVICE
This medication can be used without regard to diet.

STORAGE
Store in a tightly sealed container away from heat and direct light, and away from children.

MISSED DOSE
If you do not administer the second dose within 10 days after the initial dose, do so as soon as you remember.

STOPPING THE DRUG
Take both recommended doses, even if you are feeling better before the scheduled end of therapy.

PROLONGED USE
If lice recur, consult your doctor.

▼ PRECAUTIONS

Over 60: No special problems are expected in older patients.

Driving and Hazardous Work: The use of pyrethrins and piperonyl butoxide should not impair your ability to perform such tasks safely.

Alcohol: No special precautions are necessary.

Pregnancy: This drug has not been shown to cause birth defects or other problems during pregnancy. Before you use pyrethrins and piperonyl butoxide, tell your doctor if you are pregnant or plan to become pregnant.

Breast Feeding: Pyrethrins and piperonyl butoxide may pass into breast milk; caution is advised. Consult your doctor for specific information.

Infants and Children: No special problems are expected in younger patients.

Special Concerns: All members of your household should be examined for lice and given treatment if necessary. Clothing, household linen, hairbrushes, combs, and bedding should be thoroughly cleaned. Furniture, rugs, and floors should be vacuumed thoroughly. Toilet seats should be scrubbed frequently. If you use this medicine for pubic lice, your sexual partner may also need to be treated. Keep this medicine away from the mouth and do not inhale it. Apply it in a well-ventilated room to help prevent inhalation. Keep the medicine away from the eyes and other mucous membranes, such as the inside of the nose or vagina.

OVERDOSE
Symptoms: If accidentally ingested, pyrethrins and piperonyl butoxide can cause nausea, vomiting, muscle paralysis, and central nervous system depression.

What to Do: Call your doctor, emergency medical services (EMS), or the nearest poison control center immediately.

▼ INTERACTIONS

DRUG INTERACTIONS
Before you use this medicine, tell your doctor if you are using any other prescription or over-the-counter drugs.

FOOD INTERACTIONS
No known food interactions.

DISEASE INTERACTIONS
Consult your doctor if you have any severe inflammation of the skin.

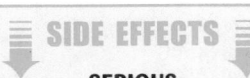
SIDE EFFECTS

SERIOUS
Skin irritation not present before use of the medicine, skin rash or infection, sudden attacks of sneezing, stuffy or runny nose, wheezing or difficulty breathing. Call your doctor immediately.

COMMON
No common side effects are associated with the use of pyrethrins and piperonyl butoxide.

LESS COMMON
No less-common side effects are associated with the use of pyrethrins and piperonyl butoxide.

QUAZEPAM

Available in: Tablets
Available OTC? No   **As Generic?** No
Drug Class: Benzodiazepine tranquilizer

▼ USAGE INFORMATION

WHY IT'S PRESCRIBED
To treat insomnia.

HOW IT WORKS
In general, quazepam produces mild sedation by depressing activity in the central nervous system. In particular, quazepam appears to enhance the effect of gamma-aminobutyric acid (GABA), a natural chemical that inhibits the firing of neurons and dampens the transmission of nerve signals, thus decreasing nervous excitation.

▼ DOSAGE GUIDELINES

RANGE AND FREQUENCY
Adults: 7.5 to 15 mg in 1 dose at bedtime. Use and dose for children under the age of 18 must be determined by your doctor.

ONSET OF EFFECT
Unknown.

DURATION OF ACTION
Unknown.

DIETARY ADVICE
Quazepam should be taken 30 to 60 minutes before bedtime with a full glass of water. It can be taken with food to prevent gastrointestinal upset.

STORAGE
Store in a tightly sealed container away from heat and direct light.

MISSED DOSE
Take it as soon as you remember, unless it is late at night. Do not take the medicine unless your schedule allows a full night's sleep.

STOPPING THE DRUG
Discontinuing the drug abruptly may produce withdrawal symptoms (sleep disruption, nervousness, irritability, diarrhea, abdominal cramps, muscle aches, memory impairment). Dosage may need to be reduced gradually.

PROLONGED USE
Do not take quazepam for more than 8 weeks without consulting your doctor.

▼ PRECAUTIONS

Over 60: Adverse reactions are more likely and may be more severe. A lower dose may be warranted.

Driving and Hazardous Work: Quazepam can impair mental alertness and physical coordination. Adjust your activities accordingly.

Alcohol: Avoid alcohol.

Pregnancy: Use during pregnancy should be avoided if possible. Consult your doctor for specific advice.

Breast Feeding: Quazepam passes into breast milk; do not take it while nursing.

Infants and Children: Safety and effectiveness have not been established for children under age 18.

Special Concerns: Quazepam use can lead to psychological or physical dependence. Never take more than the prescribed daily dose. Never stop taking the drug abruptly.

OVERDOSE
Symptoms: Extreme drowsiness, confusion, slurred speech, slow reflexes, poor coordination, staggering gait, tremor, slowed breathing, loss of consciousness.

What to Do: Call your doctor, emergency medical services (EMS), or the nearest poison control center immediately.

▼ INTERACTIONS

DRUG INTERACTIONS
Other drugs may interact with quazepam. Consult your doctor for specific advice if you are taking any drugs that depress the central nervous system; these include antihistamines, antidepressants or other psychiatric medications, barbiturates, sedatives, cough medicines, decongestants, and painkillers. Be sure your doctor knows about any over-the-counter medication you may take.

FOOD INTERACTIONS
None reported.

DISEASE INTERACTIONS
Caution is advised when taking quazepam. Consult your doctor if you have a history of alcohol or drug abuse, stroke or other brain disease, any chronic lung disease, hyperactivity, depression or other mental illness, myasthenia gravis, sleep apnea, epilepsy, porphyria, kidney disease, or liver disease.

  SIDE EFFECTS

SERIOUS
Difficulty concentrating, outbursts of anger, other behavior problems, depression, hallucinations, low blood pressure (causing faintness or confusion), memory impairment, muscle weakness, skin rash or itching, sore throat, fever and chills, sores or ulcers in throat or mouth, unusual bruising or bleeding, extreme fatigue, yellowish tinge to eyes or skin. Call your doctor immediately.

COMMON
Drowsiness, loss of coordination, unsteady gait, dizziness, lightheadedness, slurred speech.

LESS COMMON
Change in sexual desire or ability, constipation, false sense of well-being, nausea and vomiting, urinary problems, unusual fatigue.

QUETIAPINE FUMARATE

Available in: Tablets
Available OTC? No   **As Generic?** No
Drug Class: Antipsychotic

▼ USAGE INFORMATION

WHY IT'S PRESCRIBED
To treat psychotic conditions (severe mental disorders characterized by distorted thoughts, perceptions, and emotions), such as schizophrenia.

HOW IT WORKS
While the exact mechanism of action of quetiapine is unknown, it appears to interfere with receptors for certain critical natural substances (neurotransmitters) in the brain to produce a tranquilizing and antipsychotic effect.

▼ DOSAGE GUIDELINES

RANGE AND FREQUENCY
Initial dose is 25 mg twice a day. On the second and third days, the dose should be increased by 25 to 50 mg, 2 to 3 times a day, if tolerated. On the fourth day, the dosage should be 300 to 400 mg a day in 2 or 3 divided doses. If needed, further adjustments in dose should occur at least 2 days apart in increments or decrements of 25 to 50 mg, 2 times a day. Clinical trials have not evaluated daily doses greater than 800 mg.

ONSET OF EFFECT
Unknown.

DURATION OF ACTION
Unknown.

DIETARY ADVICE
Quetiapine can be taken without regard to food intake.

STORAGE
Store in a tightly sealed container away from heat, moisture, and direct light.

MISSED DOSE
Take it as soon as you remember. If it is near the time for the next dose, skip the missed dose and resume your regular dosage schedule. Do not double the next dose.

STOPPING THE DRUG
Take it as prescribed for the full treatment period. The decision to stop taking the drug should be made in consultation with your physician.

PROLONGED USE
Prolonged use may lead to a potentially irreversible condition called "tardive dyskinesia" (involuntary movements of the jaw, lips, and tongue). Your doctor must periodically evaluate the drug's effectiveness if it is used for an extended period. Examinations of the eyes for possible development of cataracts are recommended at the onset of treatment and at 6-month intervals during chronic treatment.

▼ PRECAUTIONS

Over 60: Adverse reactions are more likely and more severe. A lower dose may be warranted.

Driving and Hazardous Work: The use of quetiapine may impair your ability to perform such tasks safely. Do not drive or engage in hazardous work until you determine how the medicine affects you.

Alcohol: Avoid alcohol.

Pregnancy: Adequate human studies have not been completed. Discuss with your doctor the relative risks and benefits of using this drug while pregnant.

Breast Feeding: Quetiapine may pass into breast milk; avoid or discontinue breast feeding while taking this drug.

Infants and Children: Not recommended for use by children under age 18.

Special Concerns: Avoid prolonged exposure to high temperatures or hot climates. Drink plenty of fluids and stay cool in the summertime.

OVERDOSE
Symptoms: Few cases of overdose have been reported. In clinical studies, excessive doses appear to exacerbate quetiapine's known side effects.

What to Do: Call your doctor, emergency medical services (EMS), or the nearest poison control center immediately.

▼ INTERACTIONS

DRUG INTERACTIONS
Consult your doctor for specific advice if you are taking phenytoin, ketoconazole, itraconazole, fluconazole, erythromycin, antihypertensives, antiparkinsonism drugs, central nervous system depressants, or any other prescription or over-the-counter drug.

FOOD INTERACTIONS
No known food interactions.

DISEASE INTERACTIONS
Caution is advised when taking quetiapine if you have a history of liver disease, severe kidney dysfunction, symptomatic reactions to low blood pressure (dizziness, lightheadedness, or fainting, especially when rising from a sitting or lying position), heart disease, stroke, or seizures.

  SIDE EFFECTS

SERIOUS
Tardive dyskinesia (involuntary movements of the jaw, lips, and tongue), amnesia, psychosis, hallucinations, paranoia, delusions, manic episodes, suicidal impulses, catatonic reaction, stroke, shortness of breath, asthma, paralysis of one side of the body. Call your doctor immediately. Neuroleptic malignant syndrome, characterized by high fever, muscle rigidity, altered mental status, and heart rhythm abnormalities, is a potentially fatal condition.

COMMON
Drowsiness, headache, dizziness, constipation.

LESS COMMON
Dry mouth, lightheadedness when rising from a sitting or lying position (orthostatic hypotension), rapid heartbeat, indigestion, weakness, abdominal pain, skin rash, unexpected weight gain.

QUINACRINE HYDROCHLORIDE

Available in: Tablets
Available OTC? No   **As Generic?** No
Drug Class: Anti-infective/antimalarial/anthelmintic

▼ USAGE INFORMATION

WHY IT'S PRESCRIBED
Used as a primary agent in the treatment of gardiasis (traveler's diarrhea), a protozoal infection of the intestinal tract, usually contracted by consuming water that is contaminated with Giardia lamblia cysts.

HOW IT WORKS
The exact way in which quinacrine works is unknown. It appears to interfere with the parasite's metabolism.

▼ DOSAGE GUIDELINES

RANGE AND FREQUENCY
Adults and teenagers: 100 mg, 3 times a day for 5 to 7 days. Children under age 12: 2 mg per 2.2 lbs (1 kg) of body weight 3 times a day, not to exceed 300 mg daily, for 5 to 7 days.

ONSET OF EFFECT
Unknown.

DURATION OF ACTION
Unknown.

DIETARY ADVICE
This medication is best taken after meals with a full glass of water, fruit juice, or tea, unless your doctor instructs otherwise. Tablets may be crushed and mixed with chocolate syrup, honey, or jam for persons who cannot stand the bitter taste or have difficulty swallowing tablets.

STORAGE
Store in a tightly sealed container away from heat, moisture, and direct light.

MISSED DOSE
Take it as soon as you remember. If it is near the time for the next dose, skip the missed dose and resume your regular dosage schedule. Do not double the next dose.

STOPPING THE DRUG
Take it as prescribed for the full treatment period, even if you feel better before the scheduled end of therapy.

PROLONGED USE
See your doctor regularly for tests and examinations. The dosage may need to be adjusted.

▼ PRECAUTIONS

Over 60: Adverse reactions may be more likely and more severe. A lower dose may be warranted.

Driving and Hazardous Work: The use of quinacrine may impair your ability to perform such tasks safely. Exercise caution until you determine how this medication affects you.

Alcohol: Avoid all forms of alcohol, including medications such as cough syrup.

Pregnancy: Do not take quinacrine while pregnant; treatment should be delayed until after childbirth. If you are planning to become pregnant, consult your physician.

Breast Feeding: Quinacrine passes into breast milk and may be harmful to the nursing infant; consult your doctor for specific advice.

Infants and Children: Adverse reactions may be more likely and more severe. Quinacrine's bitter taste may cause vomiting in children. Tablets may be crushed and mixed with chocolate syrup, honey, or jam to cover the taste. Discuss with your pediatrician the relative risks and benefits of your child using this medication.

OVERDOSE
Symptoms: Fainting, seizures, heart rhythm irregularities.

What to Do: Stop taking the drug and call your doctor, emergency medical services (EMS), or the nearest poison control center.

▼ INTERACTIONS

DRUG INTERACTIONS
Other drugs may interact with quinacrine. Do not take primaquine for up to 3 months after taking quinacrine. Also tell your doctor if you are taking any other prescription or over-the-counter medication.

FOOD INTERACTIONS
No known food interactions.

DISEASE INTERACTIONS
Consult your doctor for specific advice if you have any of the following: a history of mental illness or alcoholism, porphyria, or psoriasis. Also tell your doctor if you have any other medical condition.

SIDE EFFECTS

SERIOUS
Hallucinations; mental or mood changes; irritability; nervousness; skin rash; reddening, itching or peeling of skin; nightmares. Call your doctor immediately.

COMMON
Yellow color of the skin and urine, stomach or abdominal cramps, loss of appetite, dizziness, headache, nausea or vomiting, diarrhea.

LESS COMMON
No less-common side effects are associated with the use of quinacrine.

QUINAPRIL HYDROCHLORIDE

Available in: Tablets
Available OTC? No   **As Generic?** No
Drug Class: Angiotensin-converting enzyme (ACE) inhibitor

▼ USAGE INFORMATION

WHY IT'S PRESCRIBED
To control high blood pressure (hypertension); to treat congestive heart failure (CHF); to treat patients with left ventricular dysfunction (damage to the pumping chamber of the heart); and to minimize further kidney damage in diabetics with mild kidney disease.

HOW IT WORKS
Angiotensin-converting enzyme (ACE) inhibitors block an enzyme that produces angiotensin, a naturally occurring substance that causes blood vessels to constrict and stimulates production of the adrenal hormone, aldosterone, which promotes sodium retention in the body. As a result, ACE inhibitors relax blood vessels (causing them to widen) and reduces sodium retention, which lowers blood pressure and so decreases the workload of the heart.

▼ DOSAGE GUIDELINES

RANGE AND FREQUENCY
10 mg once a day. Dose may be increased to 20 to 80 mg a day, taken in 1 or 2 doses.

ONSET OF EFFECT
Within 1 hour.

DURATION OF ACTION
24 hours.

DIETARY ADVICE
Take quinapril on an empty stomach, about 1 hour before mealtime. Follow your doctor's dietary advice (such as low-salt or low-cholesterol restrictions) to improve control over high blood pressure and heart disease. Avoid high-potassium foods like bananas and citrus fruits and juices, unless you are also taking drugs such as diuretics that lower potassium levels.

STORAGE
Store in a tightly sealed container away from heat and direct light.

MISSED DOSE
Take it as soon as you remember. If it is near the time for the next dose, skip the missed dose and resume your regular dosage schedule. Do not double the next dose.

STOPPING THE DRUG
Do not stop taking this drug abruptly, as this may cause potentially serious health problems. Dosage should be reduced gradually, according to your doctor's instructions.

PROLONGED USE
Lifelong therapy may be necessary. See your doctor for regular evaluation.

▼ PRECAUTIONS

Over 60: No special advice.

Driving and Hazardous Work: Avoid such activities until you determine how the medicine affects you.

Alcohol: Consume alcohol only in moderation since it may increase the effect of the drug and cause an excessive drop in blood pressure.

Pregnancy: Use of quinapril during the last 6 months of pregnancy may cause severe defects, even death, to the fetus. Discontinue the drug if you are pregnant or plan to become pregnant.

Breast Feeding: Quinapril may pass into breast milk; caution is advised. Consult your doctor for advice.

Infants and Children: The safety and efficacy of quinapril use by infants and children have not been estab-lished. Benefits must be weighed against potential risks; consult your pediatrician for specific advice.

OVERDOSE
Symptoms: None reported.

What to Do: While overdose is unlikely, call your doctor, emergency medical services (EMS), or the nearest poison control center immediately if you suspect that someone has taken a much larger dose than prescribed.

▼ INTERACTIONS

DRUG INTERACTIONS
Consult your doctor if you are taking diuretics (especially potassium-sparing diuretics), potassium supplements or drugs containing potassium (check ingredient labels), lithium, anticoagulants (such as warfarin), indomethacin or other anti-inflammatory drugs, or any over-the-counter medications (especially cold remedies and diet pills).

FOOD INTERACTIONS
Avoid low-salt milk and salt substitutes. Many of these products contain potassium. Avoid large servings of high-potassium foods like bananas and citrus fruits or juices.

DISEASE INTERACTIONS
Consult your doctor if you have systemic lupus erythematosus (SLE) or if you have had a prior allergic reaction to ACE inhibitors. Quinapril should be used with caution by patients with severe kidney disease or renal artery stenosis (narrowing of one or both of the arteries that supply blood to the kidneys).

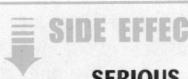
SIDE EFFECTS

SERIOUS
Fever and chills; sore throat and hoarseness; sudden difficulty breathing or swallowing; swelling of the face, mouth, or extremities; impaired kidney function (ankle swelling, decreased urination); confusion; yellow discoloration of the eyes or skin (indicating liver disorder);, intense itching; chest pain or palpitations; abdominal pain. Serious side effects are very rare; contact your doctor immediately.

COMMON
Dry, persistent cough.

LESS COMMON
Dizziness or fainting; skin rash; numbness or tingling in the hands, feet, or lips; unusual fatigue or muscle weakness; nausea; drowsiness; loss of taste; headache.

QUINAPRIL HYDROCHLORIDE/HYDROCHLOROTHIAZIDE

Available in: Tablets
Available OTC? No   **As Generic?** No
Drug Class: Angiotensin-converting enzyme (ACE) inhibitor/diuretic

▼ USAGE INFORMATION

WHY IT'S PRESCRIBED
To treat high blood pressure (hypertension). Used in patients for whom both quinapril and hydrochlorothiazide have been prescribed.

HOW IT WORKS
Angiotensin-converting enzyme (ACE) inhibitors such as quinapril relax blood vessels (causing them to widen) and reduce sodium retention, which lowers blood pressure and so decreases the workload of the heart. Hydrochlorothiazide (HCTZ), a diuretic, increases sodium and water in the urine output. By reducing the overall fluid volume in the body, diuretics reduce blood volume and so reduce blood pressure.

▼ DOSAGE GUIDELINES

RANGE AND FREQUENCY
This combination medication comes in three strengths: quinapril/hydrochlorothiazide 10/12.5, 20/12.5, and 20/25. Your doctor will determine the appropriate dose.

ONSET OF EFFECT
Within 1 hour for quinapril; within 2 hours for HCTZ.

DURATION OF ACTION
24 hours for quinapril; 6 to 12 hours for HCTZ.

DIETARY ADVICE
Follow your doctor's dietary advice (such as low-salt or low-cholesterol restrictions) to improve control over high blood pressure and prevent heart disease.

STORAGE
Store in a tightly sealed container away from heat, moisture, and direct light.

MISSED DOSE
If you do not remember until the next day, skip the missed dose and resume your regular dosage schedule. Do not double the next dose.

SIDE EFFECTS

SERIOUS
Fever and chills; sore throat; sudden difficulty breathing or swallowing; swelling of the face, mouth, or extremities; impaired kidney function (ankle swelling, decreased urination); confusion; jaundice; intense itching; chest pain or heartbeat irregularities; abdominal pain. Serious side effects are very rare; contact your doctor immediately.

COMMON
Dry, persistent cough, drowsiness.

LESS COMMON
Dizziness or fainting; skin rash; numbness or tingling in the hands, feet, or lips; change in color of the hands from white to blue to red (Raynaud's phenomenon) in cold weather; unusual fatigue or muscle weakness; nausea; loss of taste; headache; unusual dreams.

STOPPING THE DRUG
Discontinuing this drug abruptly may cause potentially serious problems. The dosage should be reduced gradually, according to your doctor's instructions.

PROLONGED USE
Lifelong therapy may be necessary; see your doctor regularly for regular evaluation.

▼ PRECAUTIONS

Over 60: Adverse reactions may be more likely and more severe in older patients.

Driving and Hazardous Work: Avoid such activities until you determine how the medicine affects you.

Alcohol: Consume alcohol only in moderation since it may increase the effect of the drug and cause an excessive drop in blood pressure. Consult your doctor for advice.

Pregnancy: Before taking this medication, tell your doctor if you are pregnant or plan to become pregnant. Use of this drug during the last 6 months of pregnancy may cause severe defects, even death, in the fetus.

Breast Feeding: Quinapril and hydrochlorothiazide may pass into breast milk; caution is advised. Consult your doctor for specific advice.

Infants and Children: Not recommended for use by children under 18.

Special Concerns: A rare complication is angioedema, characterized by swelling of the lips, tongue, and throat. It may be so severe as to cause obstruction of the airways, which could be fatal.

OVERDOSE
Symptoms: Overdose has not been reported; symptoms might include dizziness, faintness, or confusion.

What to Do: While overdose is unlikely, call your doctor, emergency medical services (EMS), or the nearest poison control center immediately if you suspect that someone has taken a much larger dose than prescribed.

▼ INTERACTIONS

DRUG INTERACTIONS
Consult your doctor for specific advice if you are taking cholestyramine, colestipol, corticosteroids, digitalis drugs, antidiabetic drugs, lithium, potassium-containing medications or supplements, or any over-the-counter drug (especially cold remedies and appetite suppressants).

FOOD INTERACTIONS
Avoid low-salt milk and salt substitutes. Many of these products contain potassium.

DISEASE INTERACTIONS
Consult your doctor if you have systemic lupus erythematosus or if you have had a prior allergic reaction to ACE inhibitors. This medication should be used with caution by patients with abnormal liver function and is not recommended for those with severe kidney disease. This drug can increase blood triglycerides and worsen control of blood sugar in people with diabetes.

QUINIDINE

Available in: Capsules, tablets, extended-release tablets
Available OTC? No   **As Generic?** Yes
Drug Class: Antiarrhythmic

▼ USAGE INFORMATION

WHY IT'S PRESCRIBED
To correct irregular heartbeats (cardiac arrhythmias).

HOW IT WORKS
Quinidine slows nerve impulses in the heart and reduces the sensitivity of heart tissue to certain nerve impulses, thus stabilizing heartbeat.

▼ DOSAGE GUIDELINES

RANGE AND FREQUENCY
Capsules and tablets— Adults: 300 to 600 mg, 4 times a day. Children: 6 to 8.5 mg per 2.2 lbs (1 kg) of body weight, 5 times a day. Extended-release tablets— Adults: 300 to 660 mg every 6 to 12 hours.

ONSET OF EFFECT
Oral forms, 1 to 2 hours.

DURATION OF ACTION
6 to 8 hours.

DIETARY ADVICE
Oral forms are usually taken with a full glass of water 1 hour before or 2 hours after meals. The medication can be taken with food or milk to lessen stomach upset.

STORAGE
Store in a tightly sealed container away from heat and direct light.

MISSED DOSE
If you miss a dose, take it as soon as you remember. If it is close to the next dose, skip the missed dose and resume your regular dosage schedule, as prescribed. Do not double the next dose.

STOPPING THE DRUG
Take as prescribed for the full treatment period, even if you begin to feel better before the scheduled end of therapy. The decision to stop taking the drug should be made by your doctor.

PROLONGED USE
Lifelong therapy may be necessary. See your doctor regularly for examinations and diagnostic tests if you must take this medicine for a prolonged period.

SIDE EFFECTS

SERIOUS
Dizziness, lightheadedness, or fainting; any change in vision; fever; severe headache; ringing or buzzing in the ears; hearing loss; skin rash or hives; shortness of breath or wheezing; rapid heartbeat; unusual bleeding or bruising; unexplained fatigue. Call your doctor immediately.

COMMON
Diarrhea, loss of appetite, bitter taste, flushing and itching skin, nausea, vomiting, stomach pain or cramps.

LESS COMMON
Mental confusion, rash.

▼ PRECAUTIONS

Over 60: Adverse reactions may be more likely and more severe in older patients.

Driving and Hazardous Work: Do not drive or engage in hazardous work until you determine how the medicine affects you.

Alcohol: No special precautions are required.

Pregnancy: In animal studies, quinine, a closely related drug, has caused birth defects. Tests of quinidine have not been done. Before you take quinidine, tell your doctor if you are pregnant or plan to become pregnant.

Breast Feeding: Quinidine passes into breast milk; caution is advised. Consult your doctor for specific advice.

Infants and Children: The long-acting oral dosage form is not recommended for use in children.

Special Concerns: You may have to wear dark glasses both indoors and outside if quinidine makes you sensitive to light.

OVERDOSE
Symptoms: Lethargy, confusion, headache, seizures, dizziness, vomiting, stomach pain, hearing and vision disturbances, fainting, severe weakness or fatigue, breathing difficulty, loss of consciousness.

What to Do: Call your doctor, emergency medical services (EMS), or the nearest poison control center immediately.

▼ INTERACTIONS

DRUG INTERACTIONS
Avoid diuretics if possible to prevent lowering of blood potassium levels. Consult your doctor for specific advice if you are taking digoxin, phenobarbital, phenytoin, anticoagulants, other heart medications, antacids, acetazolamide, or pimozide.

FOOD INTERACTIONS
No known food interactions.

DISEASE INTERACTIONS
Consult your doctor if you have any of the following: asthma, emphysema, an infection of any kind, myasthenia gravis, hyperthyroidism, or psoriasis. Use of quinidine may cause complications in patients with liver or kidney disease, since these organs work together to remove the medication from the body.

RABEPRAZOLE SODIUM

Available in: Delayed-release tablets
Available OTC? No   **As Generic?** No
Drug Class: Antacid/proton pump inhibitor

▼ USAGE INFORMATION

WHY IT'S PRESCRIBED
To treat duodenal (intestinal) ulcers, as well as conditions that cause extreme increases in stomach acid production (such as Zollinger-Ellison syndrome), erosive esophagitis (severe, chronic inflammation or ulceration of the esophagus), and heartburn due to gastroesophageal reflux (backwash of stomach acid into the esophagus).

HOW IT WORKS
Rabeprazole blocks the action of a specific enzyme in the cells that line the stomach, thereby decreasing the production of stomach acid. Reduction of stomach acid promotes healing of ulcers.

▼ DOSAGE GUIDELINES

RANGE AND FREQUENCY
For ulcer, esophagitis, or gastroesophageal reflux: 20 mg a day. For Zollinger-Ellison syndrome or similar conditions: 60 to 100 mg a day, up to 60 mg twice a day.

ONSET OF EFFECT
Within 1 hour.

DURATION OF ACTION
At least 24 hours.

DIETARY ADVICE
Take rabeprazole after the morning meal. Tablets should be swallowed whole.

STORAGE
Store in a tightly sealed container away from heat, moisture, and direct light.

MISSED DOSE
Take it as soon as you remember. However, if it is near the time for the next dose, skip the missed dose and resume your regular dosage schedule. Do not double the next dose.

STOPPING THE DRUG
Take it as prescribed for the full treatment period, even if your symptoms improve before the scheduled end of therapy. The decision to stop taking the drug should be made in consultation with your doctor.

PROLONGED USE
Rabeprazole should not be used indefinitely as maintenance therapy for esophagitis; it is generally taken for a limited period of 4 to 8 weeks. For those who have not healed within this period, an additional 8 weeks of therapy may be considered by your doctor. People with duodenal ulcer generally heal within 4 weeks of therapy. Some people with Zollinger-Ellison syndrome have been treated for up to one year. See your doctor regularly for tests and examinations if you must take this drug for an extended period of time.

▼ PRECAUTIONS

Over 60: No specific problems for older people have been reported.

Driving and Hazardous Work: Avoid such activities until you determine how the drug affects you.

Alcohol: Avoid alcohol while taking this medication, as it may aggravate your condition.

Pregnancy: In animal tests, rabeprazole has not caused problems. Human tests have not been done. Before you take rabeprazole, tell your doctor if you are pregnant or plan to become pregnant.

Breast Feeding: Rabeprazole may pass into breast milk; caution is advised. Consult your doctor for advice.

Infants and Children: Safety and effectiveness have not been established for patients under age 18.

Special Concerns: Do not chew, crush, or split the tablets. If your doctor directs, you may take an antacid along with rabeprazole.

OVERDOSE
Symptoms: Few cases of overdose have been reported.

What to Do: An overdose is unlikely to be life-threatening. However, if someone takes a much larger dose than prescribed, call your doctor, emergency medical services (EMS), or the nearest poison control center immediately.

▼ INTERACTIONS

DRUG INTERACTIONS
Consult your doctor for specific advice if you are taking ketoconazole or digoxin.

FOOD INTERACTIONS
No significant food interactions have been reported.

DISEASE INTERACTIONS
Consult your doctor if you have severe liver disease, since it may increase the risk of side effects.

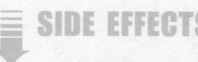

SERIOUS
No serious side effects have been reported in association with the use of rabeprazole.

COMMON
Headache.

LESS COMMON
Weakness, fever, chills, allergic reaction, diarrhea, nausea, vomiting, abdominal pain, dry mouth, change in appetite, difficulty swallowing, muscle or joint pain. Many additional side effects can occur; consult your doctor if you are concerned about any adverse or unusual reactions you experience while taking this drug.

RALOXIFENE HYDROCHLORIDE

Available in: Tablets
Available OTC? No   **As Generic?** No
Drug Class: Selective estrogen receptor modulator (SERM)

BRAND NAME
Evista

▼ USAGE INFORMATION

WHY IT'S PRESCRIBED
For the treatment and prevention of osteoporosis in postmenopausal women. Unlike estrogen, raloxifene does not stimulate overgrowth of the endometrium (the tissue lining the uterus) and thus does not increase the risk of uterine cancer.

HOW IT WORKS
Healthy bone tissue is continuously remodeled (broken down and then reformed); the minerals and other components of bone are reabsorbed by certain cells and then replaced by new bone formation. Raloxifene suppresses the activity of the cells that resorb bone; consequently, the breakdown of bone tissue occurs more slowly than the laying down of new bone. This action preserves bone density and strength.

▼ DOSAGE GUIDELINES

RANGE AND FREQUENCY
One 60-mg tablet a day.

ONSET OF EFFECT
Unknown.

DURATION OF ACTION
Unknown.

DIETARY ADVICE
Raloxifene may be taken at any time of day without regard to meal schedule. Patients are generally advised to take calcium and vitamin D supplements to aid bone formation.

STORAGE
Store in a tightly sealed container away from heat, moisture, and direct light.

MISSED DOSE
If you miss a dose on one day, do not double the dose the next day.

STOPPING THE DRUG
The decision to stop taking the drug should be made in consultation with your doctor.

PROLONGED USE
Safety and effectiveness beyond three years of use have not been determined.

▼ PRECAUTIONS

Over 60: No special advice.

Driving and Hazardous Work: No special warnings.

Alcohol: Alcohol should be restricted in high-risk women because it is a risk factor for osteoporosis.

Pregnancy: Raloxifene is normally not used in premenopausal women. Raloxifene should not be given to pregnant women.

Breast Feeding: Raloxifene should not be used by nursing mothers.

Infants and Children: Not for use by children.

Special Concerns: Patients taking raloxifene are encouraged to engage in regular weight-bearing exercise and should avoid cigarettes and limit alcohol, which inhibit healthy bone production. Unlike estrogen replacement therapy, raloxifene does not reduce hot flashes in postmenopausal women.

OVERDOSE
Symptoms: No cases of overdose have been reported.

What to Do: An overdose with raloxifene is unlikely. If someone takes a much larger dose than prescribed, call your doctor.

▼ INTERACTIONS

DRUG INTERACTIONS
Estrogen should not be taken concurrently with raloxifene. Since cholestyramine reduces absorption of raloxifene, the two drugs should not be taken at the same time of day. Consult your doctor if you are taking any of the following drugs that may interact with raloxifene: warfarin, clofibrate, indomethacin, naproxen, ibuprofen, diazepam, or diazoxide.

FOOD INTERACTIONS
No known food interactions.

DISEASE INTERACTIONS
You should not take raloxifene if you have a history of thromboembolic disease, including deep vein thrombosis, pulmonary embolism, and retinal vein thrombosis. Raloxifene must be used with caution by patients with impaired liver function; consult your doctor for specific advice.

≡ SIDE EFFECTS ≡

SERIOUS
No serious side effects have been reported.

COMMON
Increased incidence of infections, flulike symptoms, hot flashes, joint pain, sinusitis, unexpected weight gain.

LESS COMMON
Leg cramps, mild chest pain, fever, migraine, indigestion, vomiting, flatulence, stomach upset, swelling of the legs and feet, muscle pain, insomnia, sore throat, increased cough, pneumonia, laryngitis, rash, sweating, yeast infection, urinary tract infection, white vaginal discharge.

RAMIPRIL

Available in: Tablets
Available OTC? No   **As Generic?** No
Drug Class: Angiotensin-converting enzyme (ACE) inhibitor

▼ USAGE INFORMATION

WHY IT'S PRESCRIBED
To control high blood pressure (hypertension); to treat congestive heart failure; to treat patients with left ventricular dysfunction (damage to the pumping chamber of the heart); and to minimize further kidney damage in diabetics with mild kidney disease.

HOW IT WORKS
Angiotensin-converting enzyme (ACE) inhibitors block an enzyme that produces angiotensin, a naturally occurring substance that causes blood vessels to constrict and stimulates production of the adrenal hormone, aldosterone, which promotes sodium retention in the body. As a result, ACE inhibitors relax blood vessels (causing them to widen) and reduces sodium retention, which lowers blood pressure and so decreases the workload of the heart.

▼ DOSAGE GUIDELINES

RANGE AND FREQUENCY
2.5 mg to 20 mg per day, taken in 1 or 2 doses.

ONSET OF EFFECT
Within 1 to 2 hours.

DURATION OF ACTION
24 hours.

DIETARY ADVICE
Take it on an empty stomach, about 1 hour before mealtime. Follow your doctor's dietary advice (such as low-salt or low-cholesterol restrictions) to improve control over high blood pressure and heart disease. Avoid high-potassium foods like bananas and citrus fruits and juices, unless you are also taking medications, such as diuretics, that lower potassium levels.

STORAGE
Store in a tightly sealed container away from heat and direct light.

MISSED DOSE
Take it as soon as you remember. If it is near the time for the next dose, skip the missed dose and resume your regular dosage schedule. Do not double the next dose.

STOPPING THE DRUG
Do not stop taking this drug abruptly, as this may cause potentially serious health problems. Dosage should be reduced gradually, according to your doctor's instructions.

PROLONGED USE
Lifelong therapy may be necessary. See your doctor regularly for examinations and tests if you must take this medicine for a prolonged period of time.

▼ PRECAUTIONS

Over 60: No special advice.

Driving and Hazardous Work: Do not drive or engage in hazardous work until you determine how the medicine affects you.

Alcohol: Consume alcohol only in moderation since it may increase the effect of the drug and cause an excessive drop in blood pressure. Consult your doctor for advice.

Pregnancy: Use of ramipril during the last 6 months of pregnancy may cause severe defects, even death, in the fetus. The drug should be discontinued if you are pregnant or plan to become pregnant.

Breast Feeding: Ramipril may pass into breast milk; caution is advised. Consult your doctor for advice.

Infants and Children: Children may be especially sensitive to the effects of ramipril. Benefits must be weighed against potential risks; consult your pediatrician for advice.

OVERDOSE
Symptoms: Dizziness or fainting due to extremely low blood pressure.

What to Do: Seek emergency medical assistance right away.

▼ INTERACTIONS

DRUG INTERACTIONS
Consult your doctor if you are taking diuretics (especially potassium-sparing diuretics), potassium supplements or drugs containing potassium (check ingredient labels), lithium, anticoagulants (such as warfarin), indomethacin or other anti-inflammatory drugs, or any over-the-counter medications (especially cold remedies and diet pills).

FOOD INTERACTIONS
Avoid low-salt milk and salt substitutes. Many of these products contain potassium. Avoid consuming large servings of high-potassium foods like bananas and citrus fruits or juices.

DISEASE INTERACTIONS
Consult your doctor if you have systemic lupus erythematosus (SLE) or if you have had a prior allergic reaction to ACE inhibitors. Ramipril should be used with caution by patients with severe kidney disease or renal artery stenosis (narrowing of one or both of the arteries that supply blood to the kidneys).

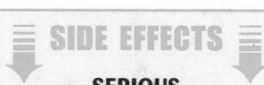

SIDE EFFECTS

SERIOUS
Fever and chills; sore throat and hoarseness; sudden difficulty breathing or swallowing; swelling of the face, mouth, or extremities; impaired kidney function (ankle swelling, decreased urination); confusion; yellow discoloration of the eyes or skin (indicating liver disorder); intense itching; chest pain or palpitations; abdominal pain. Serious side effects are very rare; contact your doctor immediately.

COMMON
Dry, persistent cough.

LESS COMMON
Dizziness or fainting; skin rash; numbness or tingling in the hands, feet, or lips; unusual fatigue or muscle weakness; nausea; drowsiness; loss of taste; headache.

RANITIDINE

Available in: Capsules, tablets, injection, syrup, granules
Available OTC? Yes   **As Generic?** Yes
Drug Class: Histamine (H2) blocker

▼ USAGE INFORMATION

WHY IT'S PRESCRIBED
To treat ulcers of the stomach and duodenum, conditions that cause increased stomach acid production (such as Zollinger-Ellison syndrome), erosive esophagitis (severe, chronic inflammation of the esophagus), and gastroesophageal reflux (backwash of stomach acid into the esophagus, resulting in heartburn).

HOW IT WORKS
Ranitidine blocks the action of histamine (a compound produced in the body's cells), which in turn decreases the stomach's secretion of hydrochloric acid. Once stomach acid production is decreased, the body is better able to heal itself.

▼ DOSAGE GUIDELINES

RANGE AND FREQUENCY
Adults— Oral dose: 150 mg, 2 times a day, in the morning and at bedtime, or 300 mg once daily before bedtime.

Injection: 50 mg every 6 to 8 hours. Patients with Zollinger-Ellison syndrome may require up to 6 g per day, taken orally. For treatment of heartburn with the over-the-counter form: 75 mg, as needed, not to exceed 150 mg a day. Children— Consult your pediatrician for appropriate individual dosage.

ONSET OF EFFECT
30 to 60 minutes.

DURATION OF ACTION
Up to 13 hours.

DIETARY ADVICE
Avoid foods that cause stomach irritation.

STORAGE
Store away from heat and direct light. Keep liquid form from freezing.

MISSED DOSE
Take it as soon as you remember. If it is near the time for the next dose, skip the missed dose and resume your regular dosage schedule. Do not double the next dose.

STOPPING THE DRUG
Take the prescription-strength medication for the full treatment period, even if you begin to feel better before the scheduled end of therapy.

PROLONGED USE
Do not take nonprescription-strength ranitidine for more than 2 weeks unless you have been otherwise instructed by your doctor.

▼ PRECAUTIONS

Over 60: Adverse reactions may be more likely and more severe in older patients.

Driving and Hazardous Work: Do not drive or engage in hazardous work until you determine how the medicine affects you.

Alcohol: Avoid alcohol. Ranitidine may increase blood alcohol levels.

Pregnancy: Risks vary, depending on the patient and dosage. Consult your doctor.

Breast Feeding: Ranitidine passes into breast milk and may pose harm to the child; avoid or discontinue use while nursing.

Infants and Children: Ranitidine is not recommended for young patients, although it has not been shown to cause any side effects or problems different from those in adults when used for short periods of time.

Special Concerns: Avoid cigarette smoking because it may increase stomach acid secretion and thus worsen

the disease. Do not take ranitidine if you have ever had an allergic reaction to a histamine (H2) blocker. If stomach pain becomes worse while using the drug, be sure to tell your doctor right away.

OVERDOSE
Symptoms: Vomiting, diarrhea, breathing problems, slurred speech, rapid heartbeat, delirium.

What to Do: Call your doctor, emergency medical services (EMS), or the nearest poison control center immediately.

▼ INTERACTIONS

DRUG INTERACTIONS
Consult your doctor for specific advice if you are taking antacids, antidepressants, aspirin, beta-blockers, caffeine, diazepam, glipizide, ketoconazole, lidocaine, phenytoin, procainamide, theophylline, or warfarin.

FOOD INTERACTIONS
Carbonated drinks, citrus fruits and juices, caffeine-containing beverages, and other acidic foods or liquids may irritate the stomach or interfere with the therapeutic action of ranitidine.

DISEASE INTERACTIONS
Patients with kidney disease should not use ranitidine or should use it in smaller, limited doses under careful supervision by a physician.

≡ SIDE EFFECTS ≡

SERIOUS
Irregular heart rhythm (palpitations), slowed heartbeat, severe blood problems resulting in unusual bleeding, bruising, fever, chills, and increased susceptibility to infection. Call your doctor immediately.

COMMON
Headache, fatigue, drowsiness, dizziness, nausea, vomiting, abdominal pain, diarrhea, constipation.

LESS COMMON
Blurred vision, decreased sexual desire or function, swelling of breasts in males or females, temporary hair loss, hallucinations, depression, insomnia, skin rash, hives, or redness.

RANITIDINE BISMUTH CITRATE

BRAND NAME

Tritec

Available in: Tablets
Available OTC? No **As Generic?** No
Drug Class: Antiulcer drug

▼ USAGE INFORMATION

WHY IT'S PRESCRIBED
To treat duodenal ulcers caused by infection with Helicobacter pylori bacteria. Therapy with ranitidine bismuth citrate is done in combination with the antibiotic clarithromycin.

HOW IT WORKS
Research has shown that the majority of peptic ulcers are caused by infection with a bacterium known as H. pylori. Clarithro-mycin kills bacteria; ranitidine bismuth citrate enhances clarithromycin's antibiotic effect to help eradicate H. pylori. Ranitidine bismuth citrate also inhibits the secretion of stomach acid, thereby facilitating the healing of ulcers.

▼ DOSAGE GUIDELINES

RANGE AND FREQUENCY
400 mg of ranitidine bismuth citrate 2 times a day for 4 weeks with 500 mg of clarithromycin, 3 times a day for the first 2 weeks. Ranitidine bismuth citrate should never be taken alone for treatment of active duodenal ulcers.

ONSET OF EFFECT
Unknown.

DURATION OF ACTION
Unknown.

DIETARY ADVICE
This drug is best taken at least 30 minutes after meals.

STORAGE
Store in a tightly sealed container away from heat and direct light.

MISSED DOSE
Take it as soon as you remember. If it is near the time for the next dose, skip the missed dose and resume your regular dosage schedule. Do not double the next dose.

STOPPING THE DRUG
Take it as prescribed for the full treatment period, even if you begin to feel better before the scheduled end of therapy.

PROLONGED USE
Not applicable. This drug is not intended for prolonged use. Healing of the ulcer should occur within 4 weeks, and a second course of therapy is not warranted if the first proves ineffective.

▼ PRECAUTIONS

Over 60: Ranitidine bismuth citrate does not cause more side effects and problems in older patients than it does in younger people.

Driving and Hazardous Work: The use of this drug should not impair your ability to perform such tasks safely.

Alcohol: Avoid alcohol.

Pregnancy: In animal studies, ranitidine bismuth citrate has not caused problems; human studies have not been done. However, ranitidine bismuth citrate taken with clarithromycin may cause problems during pregnancy. Before you take this drug combination, be sure to tell your doctor if you are pregnant or plan to become pregnant.

Breast Feeding: It is not known whether ranitidine bismuth citrate passes into breast milk; caution is advised. Consult your doctor for specific advice.

Infants and Children: The safety and effectiveness of ranitidine bismuth citrate and clarithromycin for use by infants and children have not been established.

Special Concerns: Patients whose Helicobacter pylori infections are not eradicated after treatment with ranitidine bismuth citrate and clarithromycin should be considered to be infected with bacteria that are resistant to clarithromycin. They should not be treated with clarithromycin again. The bismuth component of this drug may cause a temporary and harmless darkening of the tongue and the stools.

OVERDOSE
Symptoms: No specific ones have been reported.

What to Do: An overdose of ranitidine bismuth citrate is unlikely to be life-threatening. However, if someone takes a much larger dose than prescribed, call your doctor, emergency medical services (EMS), or the nearest poison control center immediately.

▼ INTERACTIONS

DRUG INTERACTIONS
Drug interactions with ranitidine bismuth citrate have not been established. Before you take the medication, tell your doctor if you are taking any prescription or over-the-counter drug.

FOOD INTERACTIONS
No known food interactions.

DISEASE INTERACTIONS
Caution is advised when taking ranitidine bismuth citrate. Tell your doctor if you have any other medical condition. Use of this drug may cause problems in patients with kidney disease, because this organ works to remove the medication from the body.

 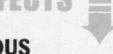 **SIDE EFFECTS**

SERIOUS
No serious side effects have been reported.

COMMON
Diarrhea, nausea and vomiting, headache, changes in taste perception, sleep disorders, chest symptoms, skin itching.

LESS COMMON
Abdominal discomfort, tremors.

REPAGLINIDE

Available in: Tablets
Available OTC? No   **As Generic?** No
Drug Class: Antidiabetic agent

▼ USAGE INFORMATION

WHY IT'S PRESCRIBED
Used as an adjunct (supplemental) therapy to dietary measures and exercise to help control blood sugar levels in patients with type 2 diabetes mellitus. Repaglinide is the first in a new class of oral antidiabetic drugs designed to control blood glucose levels following meals.

HOW IT WORKS
Repaglinide stimulates the pancreas to produce more insulin. Increased insulin levels reduce blood glucose by promoting the transport of glucose into muscle cells and other tissues, where it is used as a source of energy. The rapid onset and short duration of repaglinide's action make it effective in controlling glucose levels after a meal.

▼ DOSAGE GUIDELINES

RANGE AND FREQUENCY
Dosage must be determined for each patient individually, based on blood glucose levels

and response to the drug. The recommended dosage range is 0.5 to 4 mg taken 15 to 30 minutes before meals. Repaglinide may be taken before meals 2, 3, or 4 times a day depending on the patient's meal pattern. The maximum recommended daily dose is 16 mg.

ONSET OF EFFECT
30 to 60 minutes.

DURATION OF ACTION
1 to 2 hours.

DIETARY ADVICE
Doses should be taken 15 to 30 minutes before meals.

STORAGE
Store in a tightly sealed container away from heat, moisture, and direct light.

MISSED DOSE
If you miss a dose, take it with the next meal. Do not double the next dose.

STOPPING THE DRUG
Do not stop taking the drug without your doctor's approval.

PROLONGED USE
Prolonged use increases the risk of adverse effects. Periodic physical examinations and blood tests to monitor glucose levels are needed.

▼ PRECAUTIONS

Over 60: Older patients may be more susceptible to adverse effects, especially hypoglycemia.

Driving and Hazardous Work: Caution is advised until you have reached a stable dosing regimen that does not produce episodes of hypoglycemia.

Alcohol: Limit alcohol intake; hypoglycemia is more likely to occur after the consumption of alcohol.

Pregnancy: Repaglinide is not usually given during pregnancy. Insulin is the treatment of choice for pregnant diabetic patients.

Breast Feeding: Repaglinide may pass into breast milk; consult your doctor for advice.

Infants and Children: Safety and effectiveness have not been established.

Special Concerns: Follow your doctor's advice about diet, exercise, and weight control carefully. These aspects of treatment are just as essential to the proper control of diabetes as taking the medication. Be sure to carry at all times some form of medical identification that indicates you have diabetes and that lists all of the drugs you are taking.

OVERDOSE
Symptoms: Excessive hunger, nausea, anxiety, cold sweats, drowsiness, rapid heartbeat, weakness, changes in mental state, loss of consciousness (indications of hypoglycemia). Overdose is most likely to occur when caloric intake is deficient, following or during more exercise than usual, or after consuming more than a small amount of alcohol.

What to Do: Call your doctor, emergency medical services (EMS), or local hospital immediately.

▼ INTERACTIONS

DRUG INTERACTIONS
Consult your doctor if you are taking antifungal agents, such as ketoconazole or miconazole; also, antibiotics, rifampin, barbiturates, carbamazepine, aspirin or other NSAIDs, sulfonamides, chloramphenicol, probenecid, MAO inhibitors, beta-blockers, diuretics, corticosteroids, phenothiazines, estrogens, oral contraceptives, phenytoin, calcium channel blockers, sympathomimetics, or isoniazid.

FOOD INTERACTIONS
A special diet is essential for proper control of blood glucose levels.

DISEASE INTERACTIONS
Do not use repaglinide if you have type 1 diabetes mellitus. Use of repaglinide may cause complications in patients with impaired liver or kidney function, since these organs are both involved in removing the medication from the body.

SIDE EFFECTS

SERIOUS
Hypoglycemia (blood sugar levels that are too low), resulting in shakiness, headache, cold sweats, anxiety, and changes in mental state. Immediately ingest sugar-containing food or drink. Inform your doctor about the frequency and timing of hypoglycemic events.

COMMON
Increased incidence of upper respiratory or sinus infection, headache, back pain, joint pain, diarrhea.

LESS COMMON
Constipation, indigestion, urinary tract infection, mild allergic reaction.

RESORCINOL

Available in: Lotion, cream, stick
Available OTC? Yes   **As Generic?** Yes
Drug Class: Acne drug

▼ USAGE INFORMATION

WHY IT'S PRESCRIBED
To treat acne and seborrheic dermatitis. Resorcinol is also infrequently used to treat eczema, psoriasis, corns, calluses, warts, and other skin conditions.

HOW IT WORKS
Resorcinol fights fungal and bacterial organisms and promotes softening, dissolution, and peeling of the skin.

▼ DOSAGE GUIDELINES

RANGE AND FREQUENCY
For acne and seborrheic dermatitis: Apply once or twice daily as recommended or as tolerated. Wash your hands thoroughly after applying resorcinol.

ONSET OF EFFECT
Unknown.

DURATION OF ACTION
Unknown.

DIETARY ADVICE
No special restrictions.

STORAGE
Store in a tightly sealed container away from heat and direct light.

MISSED DOSE
Skip the missed application and resume your regular dosage schedule. Do not double the next dose.

STOPPING THE DRUG
If you are using resorcinol by prescription, the decision to stop using the drug should be made by your doctor. If you are using it without a prescription, you may stop using it whenever your acne clears; however, it is likely that discontinuing use of the drug will lead to a recurrence of acne.

PROLONGED USE
Do not use resorcinol for longer than prescribed.

▼ PRECAUTIONS

Over 60: No special advice.

Driving and Hazardous Work: No special precautions are necessary.

Alcohol: No special precautions are necessary.

Pregnancy: Resorcinol has not been shown to cause birth defects or other problems during pregnancy. However, it may be absorbed through the skin. Consult your doctor for specific advice if you are pregnant or plan to become pregnant.

Breast Feeding: Resorcinol may be absorbed into the body through the skin; caution is advised. Consult your doctor for advice.

Infants and Children: Resorcinol should not be used on large areas of the body of children.

Special Concerns: Anyone with a history of allergy to resorcinol or any other ingredients in the specific product should not use this medication. Resorcinol should not be used on wounds, because it may cause methemoglobinemia, a blood disorder. It should not be applied over large areas of the body, especially when used in high concentrations. Avoid contact of resorcinol with the eyes. This medication is generally not recommended for black persons, since it may significantly darken treated areas of skin. Resorcinol may darken light-colored hair.

OVERDOSE
Symptoms: If ingested, diarrhea, nausea, abdominal pain, vomiting, drowsiness, dizziness, severe or persistent headache, breathing difficulty, unusual tiredness or weakness, slow heartbeat, and profuse sweating may occur.

What to Do: In case of ingestion, call your doctor, emergency medical services (EMS), or the nearest poison control center.

▼ INTERACTIONS

DRUG INTERACTIONS
The following drugs or other products may irritate the skin and therefore should not be used with resorcinol unless recommended by your doctor: abrasive soaps or cleansers, alcohol-containing preparations (including astringents, aftershave lotions, other perfumed toiletries), any other acne agent, any preparation containing a peeling agent such as benzoyl peroxide, salicylic acid, alpha hydroxy acids, sulfur, or vitamin A, and soaps, medicated cosmetics, or other cosmetics that dry the skin.

FOOD INTERACTIONS
No known food interactions.

DISEASE INTERACTIONS
You should not use resorcinol if you have had a prior allergic reaction to it.

≣ SIDE EFFECTS ≣

SERIOUS
No serious side effects are associated with resorcinol during normal use (as prescribed).

COMMON
Mild redness and peeling of the skin. Such side effects tend to occur at the beginning of therapy and diminish as your body adjusts to the medication; notify your doctor if such symptoms persist or interfere with daily activities.

LESS COMMON
More-severe irritation or allergy with redness, peeling, burning, stinging, itching, or rash. Call your doctor.

RIFABUTIN

Available in: Capsules
Available OTC? No   **As Generic?** No
Drug Class: Anti-infective

▼ USAGE INFORMATION

WHY IT'S PRESCRIBED
A tuberculosis (TB)-like disease known as "Mycobacterium avium complex (MAC)" is common in people with advanced AIDS. Rifabutin is used to prevent MAC and can be used with other drugs to treat MAC infection. It is occasionally used to treat TB.

HOW IT WORKS
Rifabutin interferes with the activity of enzymes needed for the replication of RNA (ribonucleic acid) in bacterial cells, thus preventing the bacteria from reproducing.

▼ DOSAGE GUIDELINES

RANGE AND FREQUENCY
Adults and teenagers: 300 mg once a day, or 150 mg, 2 times a day.

ONSET OF EFFECT
Unknown.

DURATION OF ACTION
Unknown.

DIETARY ADVICE
Take it on an empty stomach, 1 hour before or 2 hours after meals. If nausea and vomiting develop or you are unable to swallow the pills, the contents of the capsules can be mixed with food such as applesauce.

STORAGE
Store in a tightly sealed container away from heat, moisture, and direct light.

MISSED DOSE
Take the drug as soon as you remember. This will help keep a constant level of medication in your system. If it is near the time for the next dose, skip the missed dose and resume your regular dosage schedule. Do not double the next dose.

STOPPING THE DRUG
Take it as prescribed for the full treatment period, even if you begin to feel better before the scheduled end of therapy. Treatment may continue for months or years. The decision to stop taking the drug should be made by your doctor.

PROLONGED USE
Long-term therapy is often required; consult your doctor about the need for periodic medical examinations and laboratory tests.

▼ PRECAUTIONS

Over 60: No special problems are expected.

Driving and Hazardous Work: Do not drive or engage in hazardous work until you determine how the medicine affects you.

Alcohol: Avoid alcohol.

Pregnancy: Adequate studies of rifabutin use during pregnancy have not been done. This drug should be given during pregnancy only if potential benefits clearly outweigh the risks to the unborn child. There is no evidence that the drug will reduce the risk of transmitting the virus from the mother to the fetus.

Breast Feeding: It is not known whether rifabutin passes into breast milk; caution is advised. Women who are infected with HIV should not breast feed, to avoid transmitting the virus to an uninfected child.

Infants and Children: Use and dose for infants and children must be determined by your doctor. It is not known whether rifabutin causes different or more severe side effects in infants and children than it does in older persons.

Special Concerns: Soft contact lenses may become permanently discolored. If you have been using oral contraceptives, you should use a different method of birth control while taking rifabutin.

OVERDOSE
Symptoms: An overdose with rifabutin is unlikely.

What to Do: If someone takes a much larger dose than prescribed, call your doctor, emergency medical services (EMS), or the nearest poison control center right away.

▼ INTERACTIONS

DRUG INTERACTIONS
Rifabutin should not be taken if you are also taking the protease inhibitor ritonavir, and it should be used with caution if you are taking other protease inhibitors (a class of drugs used to treat AIDS). Consult your doctor for specific advice if you are taking ketoconazole, phenytoin, prednisone, propranolol, quinidine, oral contraceptives, sulfonylureas (oral antidiabetics), warfarin, or zidovudine. Also tell your doctor if you are taking any other prescription or over-the-counter medication.

FOOD INTERACTIONS
No known food interactions.

DISEASE INTERACTIONS
Caution is advised when taking rifabutin. Consult your doctor if you have active TB. If you have to take rifabutin and have active TB, you must take other medications to cure TB. Rifabutin, if used alone, may cause drug-resistant strains of the TB bacterium to thrive, resulting in a TB infection that is very hard to treat.

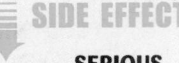
SIDE EFFECTS

SERIOUS
No serious side effects are associated with the use of rifabutin.

COMMON
Reddish-orange or brown discoloration of urine, saliva, phlegm, stools, sweat, skin, and tears; skin rash; nausea and vomiting; low white blood cell count.

LESS COMMON
Joint aches, eye irritation, blurred or decreased vision.

RIFAMPIN

Available in: Capsules, injection
Available OTC? No   **As Generic?** Yes
Drug Class: Anti-infective/antitubercular agent

▼ USAGE INFORMATION

WHY IT'S PRESCRIBED
To treat all forms of tuberculosis (TB); must be used in conjunction with other antitubercular agents. Also to prevent the spread of TB by people who are carriers of it but who do not have active disease, and to treat other bacterial infections and persons who have been exposed to certain types of meningitis-causing bacteria.

HOW IT WORKS
Rifampin interferes with the activity of enzymes needed for the replication of RNA (ribonucleic acid) in bacterial cells, preventing the bacteria from reproducing.

▼ DOSAGE GUIDELINES

RANGE AND FREQUENCY
To treat TB— Adults and teenagers: 600 mg once a day. Children ages 5 to 12: 4.5 to 9 mg per lb of body weight once a day (not more than 600 mg a day). Older adults: 4.5 mg per lb once a day. It may be decreased to twice a week. To prevent meningitis— Adults and teenagers: 600 mg twice a day for 2 days. Children 1 month to 12 years: 9 mg per lb twice a day for 2 days, or 9 to 18 mg per lb once a day for 4 days.

ONSET OF EFFECT
Unknown.

DURATION OF ACTION
Unknown.

DIETARY ADVICE
Take the capsules on an empty stomach at least 1 hour before or 2 hours after meals. If you experience nausea and vomiting from taking the medication, or you have trouble swallowing the pills, mix the contents of the capsules in with food, such as applesauce.

STORAGE
Store in a tightly sealed container away from heat, moisture, and direct light.

MISSED DOSE
Take the drug as soon as you remember. This will help keep a constant level of medication in your system. However, if it is near the time for the next dose, skip the missed dose and resume your regular dosage schedule. Do not double the next dose.

STOPPING THE DRUG
Take it as prescribed for the full treatment period, even if you feel better before the scheduled end of therapy.

PROLONGED USE
Consult your doctor about the need for periodic medical examinations and laboratory tests. If symptoms do not improve or instead become worse in 2 to 3 weeks, consult your doctor.

▼ PRECAUTIONS

Over 60: No special advice.

Driving and Hazardous Work: Do not drive or engage in hazardous work until you determine how the medicine affects you.

Alcohol: Avoid alcohol.

Pregnancy: Rifampin, in conjunction with other antitubercular agents, can be used to treat tuberculosis in pregnant women. Be suer to tell your doctor if you are pregnant or plan to become pregnant.

Breast Feeding: Rifampin passes into breast milk; caution is advised. Consult your doctor for specific advice.

Infants and Children: No special problems expected.

Special Concerns: Rifampin can lower your white blood cell count and the number of platelets in your blood, temporarily increasing the risk of infection, slowing healing, and making your gums more susceptible to bleeding. Try to delay dental work until after therapy. Soft contact lenses may become permanently discolored. Oral contraceptives containing estrogen may be ineffective during use.

OVERDOSE
Symptoms: Whole-body itching, facial swelling, changes in mental state, reddish-orange discoloration of skin, eyes, and mouth.

What to Do: Call your doctor, emergency medical services (EMS), or the nearest poison control center immediately.

▼ INTERACTIONS

DRUG INTERACTIONS
Consult your doctor for advice if you are taking theophylline, anticoagulants, oral antidiabetics, azole antifungal agents, anticancer agents, estrogens, cortico-steroids, digitalis drugs, antiarrhythmics, antitubercular agents, methadone, phenytoin, verapamil, protease inhibitors, cyclosporine, or tacrolimus (FK506).

FOOD INTERACTIONS
No known food interactions.

DISEASE INTERACTIONS
Consult your doctor if you have a history of alcohol abuse. Use of rifampin may cause complications in patients with liver disease, since this organ works to remove the medication from the body.

≡ SIDE EFFECTS ≡

SERIOUS
Difficulty breathing, chills, pain in muscles and bones, dizziness, headache, itching, fever, shivering, skin rash and redness, nausea and vomiting, diarrhea, yellow discoloration of the skin or eyes. Call your doctor immediately.

COMMON
Reddish-orange or brown discoloration of urine, saliva, phlegm, stools, sweat, skin, and tears; stomach cramps.

LESS COMMON
There are no less-common side effects associated with the use of rifampin.

RIFAPENTINE

Available in: Tablets
Available OTC? No **As Generic?** No
Drug Class: Anti-infective/antitubercular agent

▼ USAGE INFORMATION

WHY IT'S PRESCRIBED
To treat active pulmonary tuberculosis; must be used in conjunction with other antitubercular agents (such as isoniazid, pyrazinamide, ethambutol, and streptomycin) to which the bacteria is susceptible.

HOW IT WORKS
Rifapentine interferes with the activity of enzymes needed for the formation of RNA (ribonucleic acid) in the bacteria that causes tuberculosis, thus preventing them from reproducing.

▼ DOSAGE GUIDELINES

RANGE AND FREQUENCY
For first 2 months of treatment: 600 mg (four 150-mg tablets) twice a week (with no more than 3 days between doses) in combination with other antitubercular agents. For the next 4 months of treatment: 600 mg once a week in conjunction with other antitubercular agents.

ONSET OF EFFECT
Unknown.

DURATION OF ACTION
Unknown.

DIETARY ADVICE
This medication may be taken with liquid or food to minimize stomach irritation.

STORAGE
Store in a tightly sealed container away from heat, moisture, and direct light.

MISSED DOSE
It is critical to take each dose to prevent the development of bacteria resistant to the drug's action. If you do miss a dose, take it as soon as you remember. This will help keep a constant level of medication in your system. However, if it is near the time for the next dose, skip the missed dose and resume your regular dosage schedule. Do not double the next dose.

STOPPING THE DRUG
Take it as prescribed for the full treatment period. Treatment may continue for months or years.

PROLONGED USE
Tuberculosis bacteria must be tested for sensitivity to the drug (and other tuberculosis medications) before starting treatment and throughout the course of therapy. If symptoms do not improve or instead become worse in 2 to 3 weeks, consult your doctor.

▼ PRECAUTIONS

Over 60: No special advice.

Driving and Hazardous Work: No special warnings.

Alcohol: Avoid alcohol.

Pregnancy: Adequate studies have not been done. This drug should be taken during pregnancy only if potential benefits clearly outweigh the risks to the unborn child.

Breast Feeding: It is not known whether rifapentine passes into breast milk; consult your doctor for advice.

Infants and Children: Safety and effectiveness for use by children under the age of 12 have not been determined.

Special Concerns: Rifapentine can lower your white blood cell count and the number of platelets in your blood, temporarily increasing the risk of infection, slowing healing, and making your gums more susceptible to bleeding. Try to delay dental work until after therapy. Soft contact lenses may become permanently discolored. Oral hormone contraceptives may be ineffective during treatment with rifapentine.

▼ OVERDOSE

Symptoms: No cases of overdose have been reported.

What to Do: If someone takes a much larger dose than prescribed, call your doctor, emergency medical services (EMS), or the nearest poison control center right away.

▼ INTERACTIONS

DRUG INTERACTIONS
Rifapentine should be used with extreme caution, if at all, with protease inhibitors, such as indinavir. Consult your doctor for advice if you are taking hormonal contraceptives, anticonvulsants, antiarrythmics, antibiotics, theophylline, anticoagulants, oral antidiabetic drugs, azole antifungal agents, barbiturates, benzodiazepines, beta-blockers, calcium channel blockers, clofibrate, haloperidol, estrogens and progestins, corticosteroids, digitalis drugs, other antitubercular agents, levothyroxine, narcotic analgesics, quinine, zidovudine, delavirdine, lamivudine, sildenafil citrate, tricyclic antidepressants, cyclosporine, or tacrolimus (FK506).

FOOD INTERACTIONS
No known food interactions.

DISEASE INTERACTIONS
Consult your doctor if you have a history of alcohol abuse. Use of rifapentine may cause complications in patients with liver disease, since this organ works to remove the medication from the body.

≡ SIDE EFFECTS ≡

SERIOUS
Pain or swelling in joints, fever, dizziness, headache, itching, skin rash and redness, loss of appetite, nausea, vomiting, diarrhea, yellow discoloration of the skin or eyes, dark urine. Call your doctor immediately.

COMMON
Reddish-orange or brown discoloration of urine, saliva, phlegm, stools, sweat, skin, and tears; stomach cramps.

LESS COMMON
There are no less-common side effects associated with the use of rifapentine.

RILUZOLE

Available in: Tablets
Available OTC? No   **As Generic?** No
Drug Class: Neuroprotective

▼ USAGE INFORMATION

WHY IT'S PRESCRIBED
To treat amyotrophic lateral sclerosis (ALS, more commonly known as "Lou Gehrig's disease"). Riluzole is not a cure for the disease, but it is the first and currently only drug approved for the treatment of ALS. It can extend the life of the patient in the early stages of the disease and delay the time before a tracheostomy (surgical opening of the throat) is required to permit breathing.

HOW IT WORKS
ALS is a disease marked by degeneration of the motor nerve cells of the spinal cord, lower brain stem, and cortex, resulting in gradual loss of muscle control; the senses and mental faculties are not affected. The deterioration of the muscles governing crucial body functions—especially swallowing and breathing—eventually proves fatal. The exact way in which riluzole works is unclear, but it appears to protect nerve tissue against degenerative changes, which slows the course of ALS.

▼ DOSAGE GUIDELINES

RANGE AND FREQUENCY
Usual adult dose: 50 mg every 12 hours. It should be taken at the same time each day. Do not change the dosage on your own without consulting your doctor.

ONSET OF EFFECT
Unknown.

DURATION OF ACTION
Unknown.

DIETARY ADVICE
Riluzole works best when taken at the same time each day, with a full glass of water, at least 1 hour before or 2 hours after eating.

STORAGE
Store in a tightly sealed container away from heat, moisture, and direct light.

MISSED DOSE
Skip the missed dose and resume your regular dosage schedule the next day. Do not double the next dose.

STOPPING THE DRUG
No special problems are expected.

≡ SIDE EFFECTS ≡

SERIOUS
No serious side effects are known to be associated with the use of riluzole.

COMMON
Elevated liver enzymes (detectable by your doctor); occurrence of some of the symptoms of ALS, including weakness, muscle fatigue, lack of energy, nausea, vomiting.

LESS COMMON
Dizziness, numbness or tingling around the mouth, drowsiness, loss of appetite, diarrhea.

PROLONGED USE
Prolonged use of riluzole is often necessary.

▼ PRECAUTIONS

Over 60: No special problems are expected.

Driving and Hazardous Work: Avoid such activities until you determine how this medication affects you.

Alcohol: Avoid alcohol.

Pregnancy: Adequate studies of the use of riluzole during pregnancy have not been done. Consult your doctor for specific advice.

Breast Feeding: It is not known if riluzole passes into breast milk, but in light of the potentially serious risks to nursing infants, it is recommended that women using this medication refrain from breast feeding.

Infants and Children: Riluzole is generally not prescribed for children; safety and effectiveness for patients in this age group have not been established.

OVERDOSE
Symptoms: No cases of overdose have been reported.

What to Do: Emergency instructions not applicable.

▼ INTERACTIONS

DRUG INTERACTIONS
Consult your doctor for specific advice if you are taking any other prescription or over-the-counter medication.

FOOD INTERACTIONS
No known food interactions.

DISEASE INTERACTIONS
No disease interactions have been reported.

RIMANTADINE HYDROCHLORIDE

Available in: Syrup, tablets
Available OTC? No **As Generic?** No
Drug Class: Antiviral

▼ USAGE INFORMATION

WHY IT'S PRESCRIBED
To prevent or treat influenza type A.

HOW IT WORKS
Rimantadine interferes with the activity of the virus's genetic material, blocking an essential step in the the process of viral replication. The drug affects only certain susceptible strains of the influenza type A virus.

▼ DOSAGE GUIDELINES

RANGE AND FREQUENCY
Adults and children age 10 years and older: 100 mg, 2 times a day, or 200 mg once a day. Children up to age 10: 2.3 mg per lb of body weight, once a day; the dose should not exceed a total of 150 mg daily. Frail, older adults or those with impaired liver or kidney function: 100 mg once a day. The drug should be continued for about 7 days.

ONSET OF EFFECT
Unknown. For prevention of flu, take rimantadine prior to or immediately after exposure to others with influenza.

DURATION OF ACTION
Unknown.

DIETARY ADVICE
Take it on an empty stomach at least 1 hour before or 2 hours after a meal.

STORAGE
Store in a tightly sealed container away from heat and direct light. Do not allow the syrup to freeze.

MISSED DOSE
Take it as soon as you remember. If it is near the time for the next dose, skip the missed dose and resume your regular dosage schedule. Do not double the next dose.

STOPPING THE DRUG
It is important to take rimantadine for the full treatment period as prescribed, whether for treatment or prevention of influenza. If you have the flu, do not stop taking the drug before the scheduled end of therapy even if you begin to feel better, as this may lead to a relapse.

PROLONGED USE
If your symptoms do not improve or if they become worse in a few days, you should consult your doctor. You should see your doctor

regularly for tests and examinations if you take this medicine for a prolonged period.

▼ PRECAUTIONS

Over 60: Adverse reactions may be more likely and more severe; a smaller dose is commonly prescribed.

Driving and Hazardous Work: Do not drive or engage in hazardous work until you determine how the medicine affects you.

Alcohol: Avoid alcohol.

Pregnancy: Rimantadine has been shown to cause birth defects in animals. Human studies have not been done. Before you take rimantadine, tell your physician if you are pregnant or plan to become pregnant.

Breast Feeding: Rimantadine may pass into breast milk, although it is unknown if this poses any risks to the nursing infant. Consult your doctor for specific advice.

Infants and Children: In tests, rimantadine was not demonstrated to cause unusual side effects or problems in children over 1 year of age. Tests in children under 1 year of age have not been done. Consult your pediatrician for advice.

Special Concerns: Ask your doctor about receiving an influenza vaccine (flu shot) if you have not yet had one. If you are taking the syrup form of rimantadine, use a special measuring spoon to dispense the dose accurately. If the

medicine causes insomnia, take it several hours before going to bed.

OVERDOSE
Symptoms: Agitation, heart rhythm abnormalities.

What to Do: An overdose of rimantadine is unlikely to be life-threatening. However, if someone takes a much larger dose than prescribed, call your doctor, emergency medical services (EMS), or the nearest poison control center.

▼ INTERACTIONS

DRUG INTERACTIONS
Other drugs may interact with rimantadine; consult your doctor for specific advice if you are taking any other prescription or over-the-counter medication.

FOOD INTERACTIONS
No known food interactions.

DISEASE INTERACTIONS
Consult your doctor if you have a history of epilepsy or other seizures. Use of rimantadine may cause complications in patients with liver or kidney disease, since these organs work together to remove the medication from the body.

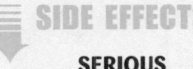

≣ SIDE EFFECTS ≣

SERIOUS
No serious side effects are associated with rimantadine.

COMMON
Nausea and vomiting, mild diarrhea.

LESS COMMON
Dizziness, trouble concentrating, nervousness, dry mouth, loss of appetite, stomach pain, unusual fatigue, insomnia.

RIMEXOLONE

Available in: Ophthalmic suspension
Available OTC? No   **As Generic?** No
Drug Class: Corticosteroid

▼ USAGE INFORMATION

WHY IT'S PRESCRIBED
To control inflammation and prevent potentially permanent damage that may result from conditions involving inflammation in the tissues of the eye. Such conditions may occur in the aftermath of eye surgery or in association with uveitis (inflammation of the uvea, the central portion of the eye).

HOW IT WORKS
Rimexolone inhibits the release of natural substances that stimulate an inflammatory reaction and pain or scarring in eye tissues.

▼ DOSAGE GUIDELINES

RANGE AND FREQUENCY
For treatment of postoperative eye inflammation: Instill 1 or 2 drops into affected eye(s) 4 times a day or as directed by your doctor. For uveitis: Instill 1 or 2 drops every hour during waking hours for the first week. The dose is then gradually tapered according to the doctor's instructions until uveitis resolves. Always shake the medicine well before using it.

ONSET OF EFFECT
Unknown.

DURATION OF ACTION
Unknown.

DIETARY ADVICE
No special restrictions.

STORAGE
Store in a tightly sealed container away from heat, moisture, and direct light. Do not allow it to freeze.

MISSED DOSE
Apply it as soon as you remember. If it is near the time for the next dose, skip the missed dose and resume your regular dosage schedule. Do not double the next dose.

STOPPING THE DRUG
Take this drug as prescribed for the full treatment period, even if symptoms begin to improve before the scheduled end of therapy.

PROLONGED USE
See your doctor regularly for tests and examinations if you must take this drug for a prolonged period.

▼ PRECAUTIONS

Over 60: No special problems are expected.

Driving and Hazardous Work: Do not drive or engage in hazardous work until you determine how the medicine affects your vision.

Alcohol: No special precautions are necessary.

Pregnancy: Adequate human studies have not been done; rimexolone should be used during pregnancy only if benefits clearly outweigh potential risks.

Breast Feeding: It is unknown if rimexolone passes into breast milk; caution is advised. Consult your doctor for specific advice.

Infants and Children: Safety and effectiveness have not been established for children.

Special Concerns: To use the eye drops, first wash your hands. Tilt your head back. Gently apply pressure to the inside corner of the eyelid and with the index finger of the same hand, pull downward on the lower eyelid to make a space. Drop the medicine into this space and close your eye. Apply pressure for 1 or 2 minutes while keeping the eye closed without blinking. Then wash your hands again. Make sure the tip of the dropper does not touch your eye, finger or any other surface. If your symptoms do not improve in 5 to 7 days or if they become worse, check with your doctor. Wearing contact lenses while using this medication may increase the risk of infection. Your doctor may tell you not to wear contact lenses during treatment and for a day or two afterward.

OVERDOSE
Symptoms: When used topically, an overdose of rimexolone is very unlikely. Inadvertent oral ingestion, however, may cause fever, muscle pain, loss of appetite, dizziness, fainting, and breathing trouble.

What to Do: In case of accidental ingestion, call your doctor, emergency medical services (EMS), or the nearest poison control center right away.

▼ INTERACTIONS

DRUG INTERACTIONS
No drug interactions have been reported. Nonetheless, it is wise to consult your doctor before taking any other prescription or over-the-counter eye medication.

FOOD INTERACTIONS
No food interactions have been reported.

DISEASE INTERACTIONS
Consult your doctor if you have a history of cataracts, diabetes mellitus, glaucoma, herpes infection of the eye, fungal infection of the eye, or any other eye infection.

≡ SIDE EFFECTS ≡

SERIOUS
Decreased or blurred vision (from cataract); eye pain, nausea, vomiting (from increased eye pressure); pain, redness, sensitivity to bright light, discharge (from eye infection). Call your doctor immediately if you experience any of these signs or symptoms. This drug may trigger a recurrence of herpes infection of the eye; mention any previous herpes infection to your doctor.

COMMON
Increased eye pressure; this is usually reversed once the drug is stopped.

LESS COMMON
Burning, stinging, redness, or watering of eyes.

RISEDRONATE SODIUM

Available in: Tablets
Available OTC? No   **As Generic?** No
Drug Class: Bisphosphonate inhibitor of bone resorption

▼ USAGE INFORMATION

WHY IT'S PRESCRIBED
To treat and prevent osteoporosis in postmenopausal women. Also used to prevent and treat steroid-induced osteoporosis in men and women who are either beginning or continuing treatment with steroids (such as prednisone) for chronic diseases. To treat Paget's disease, a disorder characterized by rapid breakdown and reformation of bone, which can lead to fragility and malformation of bones.

HOW IT WORKS
Healthy bones are continuously remodeled (broken down and then reformed); the minerals and other components of bones are reabsorbed by one set of cells (osteoclasts) and replaced by another set of cells to form new bone. Risedronate suppresses the activity of osteoclasts; consequently, the breakdown of bone tissue occurs more slowly than the laying down of new bone. As a result, bone density and strength are preserved.

▼ DOSAGE GUIDELINES

RANGE AND FREQUENCY
For treatment and prevention of osteoporosis (postmenopausal and steroid-induced): 5 mg a day. For Paget's disease: 30 mg once a day for 2 months.

ONSET OF EFFECT
Unknown.

DURATION OF ACTION
Unknown.

DIETARY ADVICE
Take it with a full glass of plain water. Taking risedronate with food or beverages (including mineral water) other than plain water is likely to reduce the absorption of the drug from the intestine. Take the tablets at least 30 minutes before the first food or drink of the day (other than plain water). The drug must be taken in an upright position. Maintain adequate vitamin D and calcium intake; however, vitamin or mineral supplements should be taken no sooner than 2 hours after taking risedronate.

STORAGE
Store in a tightly sealed container away from heat, moisture, and direct light.

MISSED DOSE
If you miss a dose on one day, do not double the dose the next day. Resume your regular dosage schedule.

STOPPING THE DRUG
Take it as prescribed for the full treatment period. The decision to stop taking the drug should be made in consultation with your physician.

PROLONGED USE
For Paget's disease: Risedronate is generally prescribed for a 2-month course of therapy. A second round of treatment may be considered after this 2-month period. Consult your doctor.

▼ PRECAUTIONS

Over 60: No special problems are expected.

Driving and Hazardous Work: Do not drive or engage in hazardous work until you determine how the medicine affects you.

Alcohol: No special precautions are necessary.

Pregnancy: Consult your doctor about whether the benefits of taking the medicine outweigh the potential risks to the unborn child.

Breast Feeding: Risedronate may pass into breast milk; caution is advised. Consult your doctor for specific advice.

Infants and Children: Safety and effectiveness have not been established for children under age 18.

Special Concerns: Remain upright for at least 30 minutes after taking this medication. If you develop symptoms of esophageal disease (such as difficulty or pain when swallowing; chest pain, specifically behind the sternum; or severe or persistent heartburn), contact your doctor before continuing risedronate.

OVERDOSE
Symptoms: No cases of overdose have been reported.

What to Do: If someone takes a much larger dose than prescribed, call your doctor, emergency medical services (EMS), or a poison control center.

▼ INTERACTIONS

DRUG INTERACTIONS
Aluminum-, calcium-, or magnesium-containing antacids, if needed, should be taken no sooner than 2 hours after taking risedronate.

FOOD INTERACTIONS
No known food interactions, although risedronate works best when taken on an empty stomach.

DISEASE INTERACTIONS
Kidney impairment or a gastrointestinal disease may increase the risk of side effects. Low blood calcium levels and vitamin D deficiency must be treated before using risedronate.

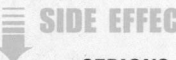 SIDE EFFECTS

SERIOUS
Serious side effects are rare and may include chest pain; swelling of the arms, legs, face, lips, tongue, or throat.

COMMON
Flulike symptoms, diarrhea, abdominal pain, nausea, constipation, joint pain, headache, dizziness, skin rash.

LESS COMMON
Weakness, growth of tumors, belching, bone pain, leg cramps, muscle weakness, bronchitis, sinus infection, ringing in the ears, dry eye.

RISPERIDONE

Available in: Tablets, oral solution
Available OTC? No   **As Generic?** No
Drug Class: Antipsychotic

BRAND NAME
Risperdal

▼ USAGE INFORMATION

WHY IT'S PRESCRIBED
To treat psychotic conditions (severe mental disorders characterized by distorted thoughts, perceptions, and emotions), such as schizophrenia.

HOW IT WORKS
While the exact mechanism of action of risperidone is unknown, it appears to alter the activity of certain chemicals in the central nervous system to produce a tranquilizing and antipsychotic effect.

▼ DOSAGE GUIDELINES

RANGE AND FREQUENCY
Adults and teenagers– 2 to 6 mg a day in 1 or 2 divided doses. Dosage may be adjusted by your doctor, if needed, at intervals of not less than one week. Older adults– To start, 0.5 mg, 2 times a day; may be increased to 3 mg a day.

ONSET OF EFFECT
Sedation may occur within minutes, but onset of antipsychotic effect may take hours to occur or may not occur until days or weeks after the beginning of therapy.

DURATION OF ACTION
At least 12 to 24 hours, although effects may persist for several days.

DIETARY ADVICE
No special restrictions.

STORAGE
Store in a tightly sealed container away from heat, moisture, and direct light.

MISSED DOSE
Take it as soon as you remember. However, if it is near the time for the next dose, skip the missed dose and resume your regular dosage schedule. Do not double the next dose.

STOPPING THE DRUG
The decision to stop taking the drug should be made in consultation with your doctor.

PROLONGED USE
Prolonged use may lead to tardive dyskinesia (involuntary movements of the jaw, lips, tongue, and, in rare cases, the arms, legs, hands, or body). Consult your doctor about the need for follow-up evaluations and tests if you must take this drug for an extended period.

▼ PRECAUTIONS

Over 60: Adverse reactions may be more likely and more severe in older patients.

Driving and Hazardous Work: Do not drive or engage in hazardous work until you determine how the medicine affects you.

Alcohol: Avoid alcohol.

Pregnancy: Adequate studies have not been done. Before you take risperidone, tell your doctor if you are pregnant or plan to become pregnant.

Breast Feeding: It is not known if risperidone passes into breast milk; caution is advised. Consult your doctor for specific advice.

Infants and Children: Risperidone is not commonly prescribed for patients under age 18 years of age.

Special Concerns: Avoid prolonged exposure to high temperatures or hot climates. Drink plenty of fluids and stay cool in the summertime. Avoid overexposure to sunlight until you determine if the drug heightens your skin's sensitivity to ultraviolet light.

OVERDOSE
Symptoms: Drowsiness, rapid heartbeat, low blood pressure, seizures.

What to Do: Call your doctor, emergency medical services (EMS), or the nearest poison control center immediately.

▼ INTERACTIONS

DRUG INTERACTIONS
Other drugs may interact ith risperidone. Consult your doctor for advice if you are taking an antidepressant, bromocriptine, carbamazepine, clozapine, high blood pressure medication, levodopa, pergolide, or any medications that depress the central nervous system, including antihistamines, cold remedies, decongestants, and tranquilizers.

FOOD INTERACTIONS
No known food interactions.

DISEASE INTERACTIONS
Consult your doctor if you have Parkinson's disease or any movement disorder, glaucoma, epilepsy, liver disease, kidney disease, heart disease.

SIDE EFFECTS

SERIOUS
Rapid heartbeat, profuse sweating, seizures, difficulty breathing, neck stiffness, swelling of the tongue, difficulty swallowing. Also a rare condition can develop called neuroleptic malignant syndrome, characterized by stiffness or spasms of the muscles, high fever, and confusion or disorientation. Call your doctor immediately.

COMMON
Nausea, reduced perspiration, dry mouth, blurred vision, drowsiness, shaking of the hands, muscle stiffness, stooped posture.

LESS COMMON
Difficult urination, menstrual irregularities, breast pain or swelling, unexpected weight gain, uncontrolled movements of the tongue, fever, chills, sore throat, unusual bruising or bleeding, heart palpitations, skin rash, itching, increased sensitivity of the skin to sunlight.

RITONAVIR

Available in: Capsules, oral solution
Available OTC? No   **As Generic?** No
Drug Class: Antiviral/protease inhibitor

▼ USAGE INFORMATION

WHY IT'S PRESCRIBED
To treat HIV (human immun-odeficiency virus), often in combination with other drugs. While not a cure for HIV, this drug may suppress replication of the virus and delay the progression of the disease.

HOW IT WORKS
Ritonavir blocks the activity of viral protease, an enzyme needed by HIV to reproduce. Blocking the protease causes HIV to make copies that cannot infect new cells.

▼ DOSAGE GUIDELINES

RANGE AND FREQUENCY
Adults and children 12 and over: 600 mg, 2 times a day. Dose should be started lower and increased gradually, starting with 300 mg, 2 times a day for 1 to 2 days, then 400 mg, 2 times a day for 1 to 3 days, then 500 mg, 2 times a day for 1 to 8 days, then 600 mg, 2 times a day thereafter.

The full dose should be reached in no later than 14 days. Lower doses (400 to 500 mg, 2 times a day) are sometimes used when ritonavir is combined with other drugs such as saquinavir. Children ages 2 to 12: 400 mg per square meter of body mass 2 times a day, not to exceed 600 mg 2 times a day. Dose should be started lower and increased gradually, starting with 250 mg per square meter and increased at 2- to 3-day intervals by 50 mg per square meter 2 times a day.

ONSET OF EFFECT
Unknown. Maximum effect may take 12 to 16 weeks.

DURATION OF ACTION
Unknown.

DIETARY ADVICE
Take it with food. The solution can be mixed with chocolate milk to improve taste; take it within 1 hour after mixing.

STORAGE
Store oral solution at room temperature in a tightly sealed container. Refrigerate capsules.

MISSED DOSE
Take it as soon as you remember. If it is near the time for the next dose, skip the missed dose and resume your regular dosage schedule. Do not double the next dose.

STOPPING THE DRUG
The decision to stop taking the drug should be made in consultation with your doctor.

PROLONGED USE
See your doctor regularly for tests and examinations.

▼ PRECAUTIONS

Over 60: No special advice.

Driving and Hazardous Work: Avoid such activities until you determine how the medicine affects you.

Alcohol: Avoid alcohol if liver function is impaired.

Pregnancy: Adequate studies of use during pregnancy have not been done; consult your doctor for specific advice. There is no evidence that the drug will reduce the risk of transmitting the virus from the mother to the fetus.

Breast Feeding: Women with HIV should not breast feed, to avoid transmitting the virus to an uninfected child.

Infants and Children: Not recommended for use by children under age 2.

Special Concerns: Do not switch between the capsules and solution without consult-ing your doctor; the body absorbs them at different rates. Taking ritonavir does not eliminate the risk of passing the AIDS virus to other persons. Take appropriate preventive measures.

OVERDOSE
Symptoms: Temporary numb-ness, tingling, or prickling.

What to Do: An overdose is unlikely to occur or be life-threatening. If, however, someone takes a much larger dose than prescribed, seek medical assistance right away.

▼ INTERACTIONS

DRUG INTERACTIONS
Do not take ritonavir with the following drugs because serious or life-threatening adverse effects, such as heartbeat irregularities, breathing difficulties, or excessive sedation could occur: amiodarone, astemi-zole, bepridil, cisapride, flecainide, propafenone, quinidine, terfenadine, mid-azolam, triazolam, pimozide, ergotamine, or dihydroergot-amine. Use of ritonavir with the cholesterol-lowering statin medications is not recom-mended. Consult your doctor for specific advice if you are taking any other prescription or over-the-counter drug.

FOOD INTERACTIONS
Increasing the amount of fat in the diet can help to reduce side effects.

DISEASE INTERACTIONS
Consult your doctor if you have liver disease or any other medical condition.

⩩ SIDE EFFECTS ⩩

SERIOUS
High blood sugar (diabetes) has occurred in patients taking drugs of this class, although a cause-and-effect relationship has not been established. Contact your doctor if you develop increased thirst or excessive urination.

COMMON
Diarrhea, abdominal pain, low-grade fever, nausea, gas, skin rash, fatigue, numbness or tingling around the mouth or in the arms and legs.

LESS COMMON
Back pain, fever, headache or migraines, loss of appetite, gastrointestinal bleeding, mouth ulcers, vomiting, joint pain, muscle pain or cramps, anxiety, depression, dizzi-ness, insomnia, seizures, drowsiness, breathing difficulty, skin problems, eye disorders, impaired sexual function.

RIVASTIGMINE TARTRATE

Available in: Capsules, oral solution
Available OTC? No **As Generic?** No
Drug Class: Reversible cholinesterase inhibitor

▼ USAGE INFORMATION

WHY IT'S PRESCRIBED
To treat mild to moderate Alzheimer's disease.

HOW IT WORKS
The exact mechanism of action is unknown. However, rivastigmine is believed to work by inhibiting acetyl-cholinesterase enzymes, which reduces the breakdown of acetylcholine, a brain chemical crucial to memory. Acetylcholine deficiency is thought to result in memory loss associated with Alzheimer's disease.

▼ DOSAGE GUIDELINES

RANGE AND FREQUENCY
To start, 1.5 mg twice a day. After two weeks of treatment, your doctor may increase the dose to 3 mg twice a day. The dose may be further increased at no less than 2-week intervals to 4.5 mg twice a day and then to the maximum dose of 6 mg twice a day, if tolerated.

ONSET OF EFFECT
Unknown.

DURATION OF ACTION
Unknown.

DIETARY ADVICE
Take with food in the morning and evening. The oral solution may be swallowed directly from the syringe or mixed with a small glass of water, cold fruit juice, or soda.

STORAGE
Store in a tightly sealed container away from heat, moisture, and direct light. Do not freeze the oral solution.

MISSED DOSE
Take it as soon as you remember, unless the time for your next scheduled dose is within the next 2 hours. If so, do not take the missed dose. Take your next scheduled dose at the proper time and resume your regular dosage schedule. Do not double the next dose.

STOPPING THE DRUG
The decision to stop taking the drug should be made in consultation with your doctor.

PROLONGED USE
No problems are expected with long-term use.

▼ PRECAUTIONS

Over 60:
No special problems are expected.

Driving and Hazardous Work:
Do not drive or engage in hazardous work until you determine how the medicine affects you.

Alcohol:
Avoid alcohol.

Pregnancy:
In some animal studies, large doses of rivastigmine were shown to cause problems. Before you take rivastigmine, tell your doctor if you are pregnant or plan to become pregnant.

Breast Feeding:
It is not known whether rivastigmine passes into breast milk; caution is advised. Consult your doctor for specific advice.

Infants and Children:
Rivastigmine is not intended for use in children.

Special Concerns:
Before you have any surgery or dental or emergency treatment, tell the doctor or dentist in charge that you are taking rivastigmine. Rivastigmine will not cure Alzheimer's disease and will not stop the disease from getting worse, but it will improve cognitive ability of some patients. Caretakers should be instructed in the correct way to administer the oral solution of rivastigmine.

OVERDOSE
Symptoms: Severe nausea, vomiting, increased salivation, sweating, slow heartbeat, low blood pressure, irregular breathing, unconsciousness, increased muscle weakness, death.

What to Do: Call your doctor, emergency medical services (EMS), or the nearest poison control center immediately.

▼ INTERACTIONS

DRUG INTERACTIONS
Nonsteroidal anti-inflammatory drugs (NSAIDs) may increase the risk of peptic ulcer or gastrointestinal bleeding when taken with rivastigmine.

FOOD INTERACTIONS
No known food interactions.

DISEASE INTERACTIONS
Caution is advised when taking rivastigmine. Consult your doctor if you have asthma, epilepsy or a history of seizures, heart problems, intestinal blockage, stomach or duodenal ulcer, liver disease, or urinary problems.

 SIDE EFFECTS

SERIOUS
Possible gastrointestinal bleeding. No other serious side effects are associated with the use of rivastigmine.

COMMON
Significant nausea, vomiting, loss of appetite, and weight loss. Other common side effects include heartburn, weakness, dizziness, diarrhea, abdominal pain.

LESS COMMON
Increased sweating, fatigue, malaise, headache, drowsiness, tremor, flatulence, insomnia, depression, anxiety.

RIZATRIPTAN BENZOATE

BRAND NAMES

Maxalt, Maxalt-MLT

Available in: Tablets, orally disintegrating wafers
Available OTC? No   **As Generic?** No
Drug Class: Antimigraine/antiheadache drug

▼ USAGE INFORMATION

WHY IT'S PRESCRIBED
To treat severe, acute migraine headaches. Rizatriptan is not intended as a migraine preventive or for use against any other kinds of pain or headache, including basilar and hemiplegic migraines. Your doctor will determine whether this drug is appropriate in your particular case.

HOW IT WORKS
The exact mechanism of rizatriptan's action is unknown.

▼ DOSAGE GUIDELINES

RANGE AND FREQUENCY
A single dose ranging from 5 to 10 mg is generally effective. If the migraine returns or there is only partial relief, the dose may be repeated once after 2 hours, but no more than 30 mg should be taken in a 24-hour period. Since individual response to rizatriptan may vary, your doctor will determine the appropriate dosage.

ONSET OF EFFECT
Within 2 hours.

DURATION OF ACTION
Up to 24 hours.

DIETARY ADVICE
The medication can be taken with or without food.

STORAGE
Store in a tightly sealed container away from heat, moisture, and direct light.

MISSED DOSE
Not applicable, since the drug is taken only when necessary.

STOPPING THE DRUG
Consult your doctor before discontinuing rizatriptan.

PROLONGED USE
No special problems are expected. Patients at risk for heart disease should undergo periodic medical tests and evaluation.

▼ PRECAUTIONS

Over 60: This drug should not be used unless the presence of coronary heart disease has been ruled out through appropriate tests.

Driving and Hazardous Work: Some people feel drowsy or dizzy during or following a migraine attack or after taking rizatriptan. Avoid driving or other tasks requiring concentration if you have such symptoms.

Alcohol: No special warnings, although alcohol may trigger or exacerbate migraines.

Pregnancy: Adequate human studies have not been done. Discuss with your doctor the relative risks and benefits of using it while pregnant.

Breast Feeding: Rizatriptan may pass into breast milk; consult your doctor.

Infants and Children: Safety and effectiveness have not been established for children under age 18.

Special Concerns: Serious, but rare, heart-related problems may occur after taking rizatriptan. Rizatriptan should not be used by anyone with any symptoms of coronary artery disease (chest pain or tightness, shortness of breath). Anyone at risk for unrecognized CAD—such as postmenopausal women, men over the age of 40, or those with known risk factors for heart disease—should have the first dose administered in a doctor's office, and then only after tests show they are probably free of coronary artery disease.

OVERDOSE
Symptoms: No overdoses have been reported.

What to Do: Although overdose is unlikely, if you take a much larger dose than prescribed, call your doctor, emergency medical services (EMS), or the nearest poison control center immediately.

▼ INTERACTIONS

DRUG INTERACTIONS
Do not take rizatriptan within 24 hours of taking naratriptan, sumatriptan, zolmitriptan, ergotamine-containing medication, dihydroergotamine mesylate, or methysergide mesylate. Rizatriptan and MAO inhibitors should not be used within 14 days of each other. Rizatriptan should be used with caution in patients taking SSRIs (selective serotonin reuptake inhibitors).

FOOD INTERACTIONS
No known food interactions.

DISEASE INTERACTIONS
You should not take rizatriptan if you have a history of angina, heart disease, stroke, uncontrolled hypertension, heartbeat irregularities, or peripheral vascular disease. Rizatriptan should be used with caution in patients with liver disease or severely impaired kidney function.

SIDE EFFECTS

SERIOUS
Serious side effects with rizatriptan are rare. However, rizatriptan may cause a heart attack; chest pain or tightness; sudden or severe abdominal pain; shortness of breath; wheezing; heartbeat irregularities; swelling of eyelids, face, or lips; skin rash; or hives. Call your doctor immediately.

COMMON
Sensations of cold or warmth, dizziness, drowsiness, fatigue, hot flashes, diarrhea, vomiting, flushing, difficulty concentrating, tremor, false sense of well-being, prickling or tingling sensations.

LESS COMMON
Chills; sensitivity to heat; weakness; stiffness; muscle pain, spasms, and cramps; bone and joint pain; indigestion; increased thirst; flatulence; nervousness; insomnia; anxiety; mental depression; confusion; sore throat; nasal irritation; nose bleeds; ringing in the ears; vision difficulties; increased sweating; itching; mild rash; frequent urination.

ROFECOXIB

Available in: Tablets, oral suspension
Available OTC? No   **As Generic?** No
Drug Class: Nonsteroidal anti-inflammatory drug (NSAID)/COX-2 inhibitor

▼ USAGE INFORMATION

WHY IT'S PRESCRIBED
For the management of chronic osteoarthritis pain. Rofecoxib is also used in the short-term relief of acute general and menstrual pain.

HOW IT WORKS
By inhibiting the activity of the enzyme cyclooxygenase-2 (COX-2), rofecoxib reduces the synthesis of prostaglandins that play a role in causing arthritis pain and inflammation. It does not inhibit the activity of COX-1, the enzyme involved in the synthesis of prostaglandins that help protect against stomach ulcers and other health problems.

▼ DOSAGE GUIDELINES

RANGE AND FREQUENCY
For osteoarthritis: To start, 12.5 mg once a day. Your doctor may increase the dose to 25 mg once a day if adequate relief is not achieved with the lower dose. For acute or menstrual pain: 50 mg once a day. To minimize potential gastrointestinal side effects, the lowest effective dose should be used for the shortest possible time. Use of rofecoxib for more than 5 days for relief of acute pain has not been studied.

ONSET OF EFFECT
For acute pain: Within 45 minutes. For osteoarthritis: Unknown.

DURATION OF ACTION
Unknown.

DIETARY ADVICE
Rofecoxib may be taken with or without food.

STORAGE
Store in a tightly sealed container away from heat, moisture, and direct light. Do not refrigerate the oral suspension.

MISSED DOSE
If you do not remember until the next day, skip the missed dose and resume your regular dosage schedule. Do not double the next dose.

STOPPING THE DRUG
The decision to stop taking the drug should be made in consultation with your doctor.

PROLONGED USE
The risk of gastrointestinal side effects may be increased with extended use.

▼ PRECAUTIONS

Over 60: No special problems are expected. Therapy should be started with the lowest recommended dose.

Driving and Hazardous Work: No special problems are expected.

Alcohol: Avoid alcohol when using this medication because it increases the risk of stomach irritation.

Pregnancy: Discuss with your doctor the relative risks and benefits of using this drug while pregnant. Do not use rofecoxib during the last trimester.

Breast Feeding: Rofecoxib may pass into breast milk; caution is advised. Consult your doctor for advice on whether to discontinue nursing or discontinue the drug.

Infants and Children: The safety and effectiveness of this drug have not been established for children under the age of 18.

OVERDOSE
Symptoms: No cases of overdose have been reported. Symptoms may include lethargy; drowsiness; nausea; vomiting; abdominal pain; black, tarry stools; breathing difficulty; and coma.

What to Do: If you suspect an overdose or if someone takes a much larger dose than prescribed, call your doctor, emergency medical services (EMS), or the nearest poison control immediately.

▼ INTERACTIONS

DRUG INTERACTIONS
Do not take this drug with aspirin or any other NSAIDs without your doctor's approval. In addition, consult your doctor if you are taking furosemide, ACE inhibitors, methotrexate, lithium, rifampin, or warfarin.

FOOD INTERACTIONS
No known food interactions.

DISEASE INTERACTIONS
Rofecoxib should not be taken by people who have experienced asthma, hives, or allergic-type reactions after taking aspirin or other NSAIDs. Consult your doctor if you have any of the following: bleeding problems, inflammation or ulcers of the stomach and intestines, asthma, high blood pressure, or heart failure. Use of rofecoxib may cause complications in patients with liver or kidney disease, since these organs both work to remove the drug from the body.

▼ SIDE EFFECTS

SERIOUS
Stomach ulcers. Black, tarry stools may signal stomach bleeding. Symptoms of liver disease (nausea, fatigue, lethargy, itching, yellowish discoloration of the eyes or skin, fluid retention). Call your doctor immediately.

COMMON
Indigestion, mild swelling, heartburn, nausea, increased blood pressure.

LESS COMMON
Flatulence, sore throat, upper respiratory tract infection, back pain, and mild abdominal pain.

ROPINIROLE HYDROCHLORIDE

Available in: Tablets
Available OTC? No   **As Generic?** No
Drug Class: Antiparkinsonism drug

▼ USAGE INFORMATION

WHY IT'S PRESCRIBED
To treat signs and symptoms of Parkinson's disease.

HOW IT WORKS
Ropinirole is believed to act by stimulating specific dopamine receptors in the brain, enhancing control over voluntary movements.

▼ DOSAGE GUIDELINES

RANGE AND FREQUENCY
Week 1: 0.25 mg, 3 times a day. Doses may be gradually increased on an individual basis to achieve maximal benefit with the least side effects. Week 2: 0.5 mg, 3 times a day. Week 3: 0.75 mg, 3 times a day. Week 4: 1 mg, 3 times a day. After week 4, if necessary, daily dosage may be increased by 1.5 mg per day on a weekly basis up to a dose of 9 mg a day, and then by 3 mg per day weekly to a total dose of 24 mg a day.

ONSET OF EFFECT
Unknown.

DURATION OF ACTION
Unknown.

DIETARY ADVICE
Ropinirole can be taken without regard to meals. However, taking it with food may help to reduce the risk of stomach upset.

STORAGE
Store in a tightly sealed container away from heat, moisture, and direct light.

MISSED DOSE
Take it as soon as you remember. If it is near the time for the next dose, skip the missed dose and resume your regular dosage schedule. Do not double the next dose.

STOPPING THE DRUG
Ropinirole should be discontinued gradually over a 7-day period. The frequency of dosage should be reduced from 3 times a day to 2 times a day for 4 days. For the remaining 3 days, the frequency should be reduced to once a day before completely discontinuing the drug.

PROLONGED USE
Side effects are more likely with prolonged use.

▼ PRECAUTIONS

Over 60: Adverse effects, such as hallucinations, are more likely and may be more severe in older patients. A reduced dose may be necessary.

Driving and Hazardous Work: Do not drive or engage in dangerous work until you determine how ropinirole affects you.

Alcohol: Alcohol should be avoided because this medicine increases its effects.

Pregnancy: Adequate human studies have not been done. Before taking ropinirole, tell your doctor if you are or plan to become pregnant. Discuss with your doctor the relative risks and benefits of using this drug while pregnant.

Breast Feeding: Ropinirole may pass into breast milk; caution is advised. Consult your doctor for advice.

Infants and Children: Ropinirole is not recommended for children under the age of 18.

Special Concerns: This drug may cause dizziness and faintness, especially when getting up out of a chair or sitting up after lying down (a condition known as postural or orthostatic hypertension, characterized by temporary episodes of excessively low blood pressure). Be cautious and move slowly when arising.

OVERDOSE
Symptoms: An overdose is unlikely to occur. Possible symptoms after an excessive dose may include mild facial paralysis or spasticity, nausea, agitation, drowsiness, sedation, orthostatic hypotension, chest pain, confusion, and vomiting.

What to Do: If someone takes a much larger dose than prescribed, call your doctor, emergency medical services (EMS), or the nearest poison control immediately.

▼ INTERACTIONS

DRUG INTERACTIONS
Consult your doctor if you are taking any of the following drugs that may interact with ropinirole: ciprofloxacin, metoclopramide, or any sedatives, tranquilizers, or analgesics.

FOOD INTERACTIONS
None reported.

DISEASE INTERACTIONS
None reported.

≡ SIDE EFFECTS ≡

SERIOUS
Chest pain, heart rhythm irregularities, confusion, hallucinations. Call your doctor immediately.

COMMON
Nausea, dizziness, faintness, sweating, or loss of consciousness, caused by a significant drop in blood pressure that occurs when rising from a seated or lying position (orthostatic hypotension). Also unusual drowsiness, fatigue, indigestion, vomiting, increased susceptibility to viral infection, headache, impaired ability to execute voluntary movements.

LESS COMMON
Flushing, dry mouth, increased sweating, weakness, swelling of the legs or feet, general feeling of illness, pain, decreased reflexes, abdominal pain, loss of appetite, flatulence, amnesia, impaired concentration, yawning, erectile dysfunction, bronchitis, sore throat, shortness of breath, vision abnormalities, increased incidence of accidental injury, tremor, constipation, diarrhea, joint pain, arthritis, anxiety, nervousness.

ROPIVACAINE HYDROCHLORIDE MONOHYDRATE

Available in: Injection
Available OTC? No **As Generic?** No
Drug Class: Local anesthetic

▼ USAGE INFORMATION

WHY IT'S PRESCRIBED
As a local (site specific) anesthetic to help manage pain during or after surgery and during childbirth (both conventional childbirth and cesarean section).

HOW IT WORKS
Ropivacaine interferes with the ability of certain nerves to conduct electrical signals, thereby blocking the transmission of nerve impulses that carry pain messages.

▼ DOSAGE GUIDELINES

RANGE AND FREQUENCY
Dosage range and frequency vary considerably based on the reason the drug is being used and the status of the individual patient.

ONSET OF EFFECT
1 to 30 minutes, depending on the concentration and dose of the drug, as well as the site of administration.

DURATION OF ACTION
Depends on the concentration and dose of the drug, as well as the site of administration. Duration ranges from 30 minutes to 8 hours.

DIETARY ADVICE
No special restrictions.

STORAGE
Not applicable; this drug is administered only in a hospital setting.

MISSED DOSE
Not applicable; your doctor will decide when to administer doses.

STOPPING THE DRUG
The decision to stop taking the drug should be made by your doctor.

PROLONGED USE
Ropivacaine is not intended for prolonged use.

▼ PRECAUTIONS

Over 60: Adverse reactions may be more likely and more severe in older patients.

Driving and Hazardous Work: Not applicable; this drug is used only in a hospital setting.

Alcohol: Not applicable; this drug is used exclusively in a hospital setting.

Pregnancy: Ropivacaine has been shown in scientific study to cross the placenta, although sufficient studies of whether this poses harm to the fetus have not been done. Use of ropivacaine during the first phase of labor may delay or prolong the second stage by interfering with the mother's reflex urge to push or by reducing the mother's ability to push. If ropivacaine is to be used for surgical purposes (that is, other than childbirth), be sure to tell your doctor if you are pregnant or plan to become pregnant.

Breast Feeding: Ropivacaine may pass into breast milk; however, no problems have been documented. Consult your doctor for advice.

Infants and Children: Safety and efficacy of ropivacaine in children under the age of 12 have not been established.

Special Concerns: Blood pressure, heart rate, neurological status, and respiratory status should be monitored carefully during therapy.

OVERDOSE
Symptoms: Bluish lips or skin, dizziness, seizures.

What to Do: Since ropivacaine is generally used in hospital situations only, emergency procedures will be carried out by hospital personnel if an accidental overdose were to occur.

▼ INTERACTIONS

DRUG INTERACTIONS
Consult your doctor for specific advice if you are taking other local anesthetics, fluvoxamine, imipramine, theophylline, or verapamil.

FOOD INTERACTIONS
No known food interactions.

DISEASE INTERACTIONS
Caution is advised when taking ropivacaine. Consult your doctor if you have heart disease. Use of ropivacaine may cause complications in patients with liver or kidney disease, since these organs work together to remove the medication from the body.

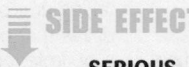
SIDE EFFECTS

SERIOUS
Dizziness, nausea, back pain, fever, headache, burning or prickling sensation, vomiting, anxiety, blurred vision, drowsiness, incoherent speech, metallic taste, numbness or tingling of mouth or lips, itching, restlessness, tremors, twitching, difficulty urinating. Call your doctor immediately.

COMMON
No common side effects have been reported.

LESS COMMON
No less-common side effects have been reported.

ROSIGLITAZONE MALEATE

Available in: Tablets
Available OTC? No   **As Generic?** No
Drug Class: Thiazolidinedione/antidiabetic agent

▼ USAGE INFORMATION

WHY IT'S PRESCRIBED
As a single therapeutic agent or as an adjunct (supplemental) therapy to metformin to control blood glucose (sugar) levels in patients with non-insulin-dependent (type 2) diabetes.

HOW IT WORKS
Rosiglitazone increases the body's sensitivity and response to its own insulin.

▼ DOSAGE GUIDELINES

RANGE AND FREQUENCY
To start, 4 mg, once a day (in the morning) or in two divided doses (in the morning and evening). Patients not responding adequately to 4 mg a day after 12 weeks may have their dose increased by their doctor to 8 mg once a day or in two divided doses.

ONSET OF EFFECT
Within 2 to 4 weeks.

DURATION OF ACTION
Unknown.

DIETARY ADVICE
Rosiglitazone may be taken with or without food.

STORAGE
Store in a tightly sealed container away from heat, moisture, and direct light.

MISSED DOSE
Take it as soon as you remember. If it is near the time for the next dose, skip the missed dose and resume your regular dosage schedule. Do not double the next dose.

STOPPING THE DRUG
The decision to stop taking the drug should be made in consultation with your doctor.

PROLONGED USE
See your doctor regularly for liver function tests if you take rosiglitazone for an extended period.

▼ PRECAUTIONS

Over 60: No special problems are expected.

Driving and Hazardous Work: The use of rosiglitazone should not impair your ability to perform such tasks safely.

Alcohol: Drink alcohol only in moderation.

Pregnancy: Adequate studies of rosiglitazone use during pregnancy have not been done. In general, insulin is the treatment of choice for controlling blood glucose levels during pregnancy. Rosiglitazone should not be used during pregnancy unless your doctor believes the potential benefit justifies the potential risk to the fetus. Rosiglitazone may stimulate ovulation in premenopausal women who have stopped ovulating. Contraception may be advised.

Breast Feeding: Rosiglitazone may pass into breast milk; do not use it while nursing.

Infants and Children: Safety and effectiveness of rosiglitazone have not been established in children.

Special Concerns: Another thiazolidinedione drug, troglitazone, has been associated with rare, serious, and sometimes fatal, liver-related side effects. Although no similar side effects have been reported for rosiglitazone, liver function tests are recommended just prior to treatment, every two months for the first year, and periodically thereafter. If you develop unexplained symptoms of liver dysfunction, such as nausea, vomiting, abdominal pain, fatigue, loss of appetite, or dark urine, call your doctor immediately. It is important to follow your doctor's advice on diet, exercise, and other measures to help control diabetes.

OVERDOSE
Symptoms: No specific ones have been reported.

What to Do: While no cases of overdose have been reported, if someone takes a much larger dose than prescribed, call your doctor, emergency medical services (EMS), or the nearest poison control center immediately.

▼ INTERACTIONS

DRUG INTERACTIONS
No known drug interactions.

FOOD INTERACTIONS
No known food interactions.

DISEASE INTERACTIONS
Rosiglitazone should not be taken by those with type 1 diabetes or for the treatment of diabetic ketoacidosis. Caution is advised if you have edema or heart failure. Consult your doctor prior to using rosiglitazone if you have any type of liver abnormality.

SIDE EFFECTS

SERIOUS
No serious side effects have been associated with rosiglitazone.

COMMON
Weight gain.

LESS COMMON
Upper respiratory tract infection, headache, edema (swelling).

SALMETEROL XINAFOATE

Available in: Inhalation aerosol, inhalation powder
Available OTC? No   **As Generic?** No
Drug Class: Bronchodilator/sympathomimetic

▼ USAGE INFORMATION

WHY IT'S PRESCRIBED
Salmeterol is used to dilate air passages in the lungs that have become narrowed as a result of disease or inflammation. It is used in the treatment of asthma and chronic obstructive pulmonary disease.

HOW IT WORKS
Salmeterol widens constricted airways in the lungs by relaxing the smooth muscles that surround the bronchial passages.

▼ DOSAGE GUIDELINES

RANGE AND FREQUENCY
This drug may be used when needed to relieve breathing difficulty. Adults and teenagers– By inhalation aerosol: Two inhalations twice daily, approximately 12 hours apart. By inhalation powder: One inhalation twice a day, approximately 12 hours apart.

ONSET OF EFFECT
Within 15 minutes.

DURATION OF ACTION
Up to 12 hours.

DIETARY ADVICE
Maintain your usual food and fluid intake. Increase fluids if you have a fever or diarrhea, in hot weather, or during exercise.

STORAGE
Store in a tightly sealed container away from heat, moisture, and direct light.

MISSED DOSE
Take it as soon as you remember. If it is near the time for the next dose, skip the missed dose and resume your regular dosage schedule. Do not double the next dose.

STOPPING THE DRUG
The decision to stop taking the drug should be made by your doctor.

PROLONGED USE
It may not be necessary to finish the recommended course of therapy. Consult your doctor.

▼ PRECAUTIONS

Over 60: Adverse reactions may be more likely and more severe in older patients.

Driving and Hazardous Work: Do not drive or engage in hazardous work until you determine how the medicine affects you.

Alcohol: No special warnings.

Pregnancy: Safety of use during pregnancy has not been established. Consult your doctor.

Breast Feeding: It is not known if salmeterol passes into breast milk. Mothers who wish to breast-feed while taking this drug should discuss the matter with their doctor.

Infants and Children: Use of salmeterol inhalation aerosol is not recommended in children younger than 12.

Special Concerns: This medication takes 15 minutes to work. Do not use salmeterol for acute or sudden attacks, or for worsening asthma. Pay heed to any asthma attack or other breathing difficulty that does not improve after your usual rescue treatment. Seek help immediately if you feel your lungs are persistently constricted, if you are using more than the recommended number of treatments or puffs per day, or if you feel a recent attack is somehow different from others. Do not wash the device for the inhalation powder. Keep it dry.

OVERDOSE
Symptoms: Chest pain or heaviness; irregular, racing, fluttering, or pounding heartbeat; dizziness; lightheadedness; severe weakness; fainting; severe headache; muscle tremors or shaking.

What to Do: Call your doctor, emergency medical services (EMS), or the nearest poison control center immediately.

▼ INTERACTIONS

DRUG INTERACTIONS
Consult your doctor for specific advice if you are taking beta-blockers.

FOOD INTERACTIONS
No known food interactions.

DISEASE INTERACTIONS
Consult your doctor if you have a history of any of the following: heart disease or heartbeat irregularities, high blood pressure, anxiety disorders, or a thyroid condition.

SIDE EFFECTS

SERIOUS
Salmeterol may become ineffective if used too often, resulting in more-severe breathing difficulty that does not improve. Signs include persistent wheezing, coughing, or shortness of breath; confusion; bluish color to lips or fingernails; inability to speak. Other side effects include chest pain or heaviness; irregular, racing, fluttering, or pounding heartbeat; lightheadedness; fainting; severe weakness; severe headache.

COMMON
Headache, sore throat, runny or stuffy nose.

LESS COMMON
Abdominal pain, diarrhea, nausea, cough, muscle aches.

SALSALATE

Available in: Capsules, tablets
Available OTC? No **As Generic?** Yes
Drug Class: Salicylate/nonsteroidal anti-inflammatory drug (NSAID)

▼ USAGE INFORMATION

WHY IT'S PRESCRIBED
To treat rheumatoid arthritis, osteoarthritis, and other rheumatic (joint) disorders.

HOW IT WORKS
Salsalate appears to work by interfering with the action of prostaglandins, naturally occurring substances in the body that cause inflammation and make nerves more sensitive to pain impulses.

▼ DOSAGE GUIDELINES

RANGE AND FREQUENCY
Adults and teenagers: To start, 500 to 1,000 mg, 2 or 3 times a day. The dose may be adjusted later.

ONSET OF EFFECT
Unknown.

DURATION OF ACTION
Unknown.

DIETARY ADVICE
Salsalate should be taken with food or milk, to minimize stomach upset, and a large glass of water.

STORAGE
Store in a tightly sealed container away from heat, moisture, and direct light.

MISSED DOSE
Take it as soon as you remember. If it is near the time for the next dose, skip the missed dose and resume your regular dosage schedule. Do not double the next dose.

STOPPING THE DRUG
Take as directed for the full treatment period, even if you begin to feel better before the scheduled end of therapy.

PROLONGED USE
See your doctor regularly for tests and examinations if you must take this medicine for a prolonged period.

▼ PRECAUTIONS

Over 60: Adverse reactions may be more likely and more severe in older patients.

Driving and Hazardous Work: Do not drive or engage in hazardous work until you determine how the medicine affects you.

Alcohol: Avoid alcohol.

Pregnancy: Adequate studies have not been done. Consult your doctor if you are pregnant or plan to become pregnant.

Breast Feeding: Salsalate passes into breast milk; caution is advised.

Infants and Children: Do not give salsalate to a child or teenager with a fever or other signs of a viral infection like the flu or chicken pox without consulting your doctor.

Special Concerns: Salsalate may cause false urine-sugar-test results for diabetics if you are taking 4 or more 500-mg doses, or 3 or more 750-mg doses, per day.

OVERDOSE
Symptoms: Confusion, dizziness, ringing or buzzing in the ears, severe drowsiness or fatigue, excitability or nervousness, rapid or heavy breathing, sweating, diarrhea, vomiting, fever, dehydration, loss of consciousness.

What to Do: Call your doctor, emergency medical services (EMS), or the nearest poison control center immediately. To prevent further absorption of salsalate, take ipecac syrup.

▼ INTERACTIONS

DRUG INTERACTIONS
Consult your doctor for advice if you are taking NSAIDs, carbonic anhydrase inhibitors, citrates, sodium bicarbonate, antacids, anticoagulants, heparin, thrombolytic agents, oral antidiabetic agents or insulin, cefamandole, cefoperazone, cefotetan, plicamycin, valproic acid, methotrexate, vancomycin, probenecid, or sulfinpyrazone.

FOOD INTERACTIONS
No known food interactions.

DISEASE INTERACTIONS
Caution is advised when taking salsalate. Consult your doctor if you have any of the following: anemia, stomach ulcer or other stomach problems, hyperthyroidism, glucose-6-phosphate dehydrogenase (G6PD) deficiency, high blood pressure, gout, heart disease, any bleeding problems, or a history of asthma or allergies. Use of this drug may cause complications in patients with liver or kidney disease, since these organs work together to remove the medication from the body.

≣ SIDE EFFECTS ≣

SERIOUS
Hearing loss; blood in the urine; severe diarrhea; difficulty swallowing; dizziness; lightheadedness; severe drowsiness; extreme nervousness or excitability; confusion; seizures; change in skin color; hallucinations; increased sweating and thirst; severe nausea or vomiting; shortness of breath; tightness in the chest; severe stomach pain; swollen eyelids, face, or lips; fever; bloody or black, tarry stools; severe headache; buzzing or ringing in the ears; vomiting of blood or dark material. Call your doctor immediately.

COMMON
Mild stomach or abdominal cramps, pains, or discomfort; indigestion; heartburn; nausea or vomiting; skin rash; hives; or itching.

LESS COMMON
None reported.

SAQUINAVIR

Available in: Capsules
Available OTC? No   **As Generic?** No
Drug Class: Antiviral/protease inhibitor

▼ USAGE INFORMATION

WHY IT'S PRESCRIBED
To treat HIV (human immuno-deficiency virus) infection in combination with other drugs. While not a cure for HIV infection, saquinavir may suppress replication of the virus and delay progression of the disease.

HOW IT WORKS
Saquinavir blocks the activity of a viral protease, an enzyme that is needed by HIV to reproduce. Blocking the protease causes HIV to make copies that cannot infect new cells.

▼ DOSAGE GUIDELINES

RANGE AND FREQUENCY
Adults and teenagers 16 and over: 600 mg, 3 times a day, in combination with other antiretroviral drugs. Higher doses (up to 1,200 mg, 3 times a day) are sometimes used. Lower doses (400 mg,

2 times a day) are used when saquinavir is combined with ritonavir, a similar drug.

ONSET OF EFFECT
Unknown. With most anti-retroviral drugs, an early response can be seen within the first few days of therapy, but the maximum effect may take 12 to 16 weeks.

DURATION OF ACTION
Unknown.

DIETARY ADVICE
It should be taken within 2 hours after a full meal.

STORAGE
Capsules should be refrigerated. If brought to room temperature, store in a tightly sealed container away from heat and direct light and use within 3 months.

MISSED DOSE
Take it as soon as you remember. However, if it is

near the time for the next dose, skip the missed dose and resume your regular dosage schedule. Do not double the next dose.

STOPPING THE DRUG
The decision to stop taking the drug should be made in consultation with your doctor.

PROLONGED USE
See your doctor regularly for tests and examinations.

▼ PRECAUTIONS

Over 60: No special studies have been done.

Driving and Hazardous Work: Do not drive or engage in hazardous work until you determine how the medicine affects you.

Alcohol: Avoid alcohol if liver function is impaired.

Pregnancy: Human studies have not been done. Nevertheless, the drug is being used increasingly in combination with other antiretroviral drugs to treat pregnant HIV-infected women.

Breast Feeding: It is unknown whether saquinavir passes into breast milk; however, women infected with HIV should not breast-feed, to avoid transmitting the virus to an uninfected child.

Infants and Children: The safety and effectiveness in children under the age of 16 have not been established.

Special Concerns: Use of saquinavir does not eliminate the risk of passing the AIDS

virus to other persons. You should take appropriate preventive measures. Do not substitute one brand of saquinavir for another without consulting your doctor. They are not equal in strength.

OVERDOSE
Symptoms: No cases of overdose have been reported.

What to Do: An overdose is unlikely to occur. Nonetheless, if you have any reason to suspect an overdose, call your doctor, emergency medical services (EMS), or the nearest poison control center.

▼ INTERACTIONS

DRUG INTERACTIONS
Saquinavir should not be used at the same time as triazolam, midazolam, or ergot-amine/belladonna alkaloids. Consult your doctor if you are taking any other drug, especially rifampin, rifabutin, or nevirapine. Some drugs, such as ketoconazole, delavirdine, ritonavir, and nelfinavir, are used in combination with saquinavir because they increase its blood levels and, possibly, its effectiveness.

FOOD INTERACTIONS
Fatty foods and grapefruit juice enhance the body's absorption of saquinavir. Food may reduce side effects.

DISEASE INTERACTIONS
Consult your doctor if you have any other medical condition. Use of saquinavir may cause complications in patients with liver disease, because this organ works to remove the medication from the body.

SIDE EFFECTS

SERIOUS
High blood sugar (diabetes) has occurred in patients taking drugs of this class, although a cause-and-effect relationship has not been established. Contact your doctor if you develop increased thirst or excessive urination. Other side effects include psychosis, thoughts of suicide, and lung disease.

COMMON
Burning, prickling, numbness, or tingling sensations in various parts of the body; confusion; seizures; headache; loss of muscle coordination; diarrhea; abdominal discomfort; nausea; skin rash; increased skin sensitivity to light; general weakness.

LESS COMMON
Loss of appetite, kidney stones, urinary tract bleeding, hair loss, swelling of the eyelid, nail problems, night sweats, small bumplike growths on the skin, impotence, anxiety attack, leg cramps.

SCOPOLAMINE OPHTHALMIC

BRAND NAME

Isopto Hyoscine

Available in: Ophthalmic solution
Available OTC? No **As Generic?** No
Drug Class: Eye muscle relaxant, pupil enlarger

▼ USAGE INFORMATION

WHY IT'S PRESCRIBED
Used for eye examinations, before and after eye surgery, and to treat certain eye conditions, including uveitis (inflammation of the uvea, or the central portion of the eye) and posterior synechiae (a potentially blinding eye disorder).

HOW IT WORKS
Scopolamine relaxes the muscles that control the lens and pupil. This prevents the lens from focusing and widens the pupil to allow the doctor to view the interior structures of the eye. It immobilizes tiny structures within the eye, which prevents scarring of eye tissue and may alleviate pain somewhat.

▼ DOSAGE GUIDELINES

RANGE AND FREQUENCY
Uveitis: 1 drop up to 4 times a day for adults and children, depending on the severity of the condition and the size and weight of the patient. Posterior synechiae: 1 drop every 10 minutes for 3 doses for adults. Use in children must be determined by your pediatrician.

ONSET OF EFFECT
In less than 1 hour.

DURATION OF ACTION
Up to 1 week.

DIETARY ADVICE
No special restrictions.

STORAGE
Store in a tightly sealed container away from heat, moisture, and direct light. Keep refrigerated, but do not allow it to freeze.

MISSED DOSE
Apply it as soon as you remember. If it is near the time for the next dose, skip the missed dose and resume your regular dosage schedule. Do not double the next dose.

STOPPING THE DRUG
Use it as prescribed for the full treatment period, even if you feel better before the scheduled end of therapy.

PROLONGED USE
Prolonged use may produce eye irritation, including redness, swelling, oozing of fluid, or skin inflammation. Call your doctor if such symptoms persist for more than 7 days.

▼ PRECAUTIONS

Over 60: Adverse reactions may be more likely and more severe in older patients.

Driving and Hazardous Work: Do not drive or engage in hazardous work until you determine how the medicine affects your vision. Extreme caution should be observed for activities that require sharp vision for close objects (less than an arm's length away).

Alcohol: No special warnings.

Pregnancy: Adequate studies have not been done. Tell your doctor if you are pregnant or plan to become pregnant.

Breast Feeding: Use extreme caution. Ophthalmic scopolamine is absorbed systemically and passes into breast milk in small amounts. Breast-fed infants may exhibit a rapid pulse, fever, or dry skin.

Infants and Children: Infants and children with blond hair or blue eyes may be more sensitive to ophthalmic scopolamine and may have an increased risk of side effects. Use with extreme caution.

Special Concerns: To use the eye drops, first wash your hands. Tilt your head back. Gently apply pressure to the inside corner of the eyelid and with the index finger of the same hand, pull downward on the lower eyelid to make a space. Drop the medicine into this space and close your eye. Apply pressure for 1 or 2 minutes while keeping the eye closed without blinking. Wash your hands again. Make certain that the tip of the dropper does not touch your eye, finger, or any other surface.

OVERDOSE
Symptoms: Drowsiness, hallucinations, memory problems, dry mouth, dry skin, restlessness, palpitations, dizziness and disorientation, delirium.

What to Do: Call your doctor, emergency medical services (EMS), or the nearest poison control center immediately.

▼ INTERACTIONS

DRUG INTERACTIONS
If absorbed into the body, it may interact with the following: anticholinergics; certain antiglaucoma agents, such as demecarium, echothiophate, or pilocarpine; antimyasthenics; potassium citrate or supplements; or medications producing central nervous system depression, such as antiemetic agents, phenothiazines, or barbiturates.

FOOD INTERACTIONS
No known food interactions.

DISEASE INTERACTIONS
Consult your doctor for advice if you have glaucoma or another eye problem; or if a child has Down syndrome, spastic paralysis, or brain damage.

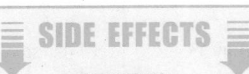

SIDE EFFECTS

SERIOUS
If absorbed into the bloodstream: Clumsiness or unsteadiness, flushing or redness of face, confusion or unusual behavior, hallucinations, slurred speech, fever, unusual tiredness or weakness, dizziness, rapid or irregular heartbeat, unusually dry skin, skin rash, dry mouth, swollen stomach (in infants). Seek medical assistance immediately.

COMMON
Blurred vision, increased sensitivity to light.

LESS COMMON
Eye irritation not present or not as severe as before use, swelling of eyelids.

SCOPOLAMINE SYSTEMIC

BRAND NAME

Transderm-Scop

Available in: Transdermal patch, injection
Available OTC? No   **As Generic?** Yes
Drug Class: Anticholinergic; antispasmodic

▼ USAGE INFORMATION

WHY IT'S PRESCRIBED
To treat urinary, stomach, or intestinal cramps, or motion sickness.

HOW IT WORKS
Acetylcholine is a naturally occurring chemical in the body involved in the activity of nerves, muscles, glands, and other physiological processes. Scopolamine interferes with the action of acetylcholine, leading to a variety of effects, including the drying of secretions (saliva, perspiration), relief of intestinal muscle spasm, and changing the size of the pupils. Scopolamine may relieve nausea, vomiting, and motion sickness by acting on nerves affecting balance in the inner ear.

▼ DOSAGE GUIDELINES

RANGE AND FREQUENCY
To treat urinary problems or intestinal problems— Injection: 10 to 20 mg, 3 or 4 times a day. The dose may be changed by your doctor. To treat motion sickness— Transdermal patch: Apply a 1.5 mg patch behind the ear at least 4 to 12 hours before travel. Use of scopolamine in children is not recommended.

ONSET OF EFFECT
Injection: Within 30 minutes. Transdermal patch: Unknown.

DURATION OF ACTION
Injection: 4 hours. Transdermal patch: Up to 72 hours.

DIETARY ADVICE
No special restrictions.

STORAGE
Store in a tightly sealed container away from heat and direct light.

MISSED DOSE
Take it as soon as you remember. However, if it is near the time for the next dose, skip the missed dose and resume your regular dosage schedule. Do not double the next dose.

STOPPING THE DRUG
The decision to stop taking the drug should be made by your doctor.

PROLONGED USE
See your doctor regularly for tests and examinations if you take this medicine for a prolonged period.

▼ PRECAUTIONS

Over 60: Adverse reactions may be more likely and more severe in older patients.

Driving and Hazardous Work: Do not drive or engage in hazardous work until you determine how the medicine affects you.

Alcohol: Avoid alcohol.

Pregnancy: Adequate human studies have not been completed. Before taking scopolamine, tell your doctor if you are pregnant or plan to become pregnant.

Breast Feeding: Scopolamine may pass into breast milk; caution is advised. Consult your doctor for specific advice.

Infants and Children: Adverse reactions may be more common and more severe in children and infants. Consult your doctor for specific advice.

Special Concerns: Do not touch the adhesive area of the patch. Wash hands thoroughly before and after application. If patch is dislodged, place a new patch behind the other ear. Do not reapply a dislodged patch. If you use the patch for more than 72 hours, you may experience nausea, vomiting, headache, or dizziness.

OVERDOSE
Symptoms: Dry mouth, dilated pupils, delirium, disorientation, memory disturbances, dizziness, restlessness, hallucinations, drowsiness.

What to Do: Call your doctor, emergency medical services (EMS), or the nearest poison control center immediately.

▼ INTERACTIONS

DRUG INTERACTIONS
Consult your doctor for specific advice if you are taking antacids, diarrhea medicines, digoxin, ketoconazole, central nervous system depressants (such as antihistamines, sleep aids, or tranquilizers), other cholinergics, tricyclic antidepressants, potassium chloride.

FOOD INTERACTIONS
No known food interactions.

DISEASE INTERACTIONS
Caution is advised when taking scopolamine. Consult your doctor if you have a history of bleeding disorders, colitis, severe mouth dryness, enlarged prostate, fever, glaucoma, heart disease, hiatal hernia, high blood pressure, any intestinal problem, lung disease, myasthenia gravis, toxemia of pregnancy, urinary tract blockage, difficulty urinating, kidney or liver disease, or an overactive thyroid; or if a child has brain damage, Down syndrome, or spastic paralysis.

⇊ SIDE EFFECTS ⇊

SERIOUS
Confusion, lightheadedness, dizziness, skin rash or hives, fainting, eye pain. Call your doctor immediately.

COMMON
Constipation; dryness of mouth, nose, throat, or skin; decreased sweating.

LESS COMMON
Blurred vision, decreased breast milk flow, unusual fatigue, difficulty swallowing, drowsiness, false sense of well-being, headache, increased sensitivity of eyes to light, loss of memory, difficulty with urination, nausea, vomiting, bloated feeling, irritation at injection site, insomnia.

SELEGILINE HYDROCHLORIDE (L-DEPRENYL)

Available in: Tablets
Available OTC? No   **As Generic?** Yes
Drug Class: Antiparkinsonism drug

▼ USAGE INFORMATION

WHY IT'S PRESCRIBED
To treat Parkinson's disease, in conjunction with levodopa/carbidopa. Also used to treat Parkinson-like syndromes, which may occur following infection of or injury to the central nervous system (brain and spinal cord), because of damage to blood vessels in the brain, or after exposure to certain toxins. Without levodopa/carbidopa, this drug has no known benefit.

HOW IT WORKS
When used with levodopa/carbidopa, selegiline allows more levodopa/carbidopa to be available for use in the body by inhibiting a nervous system enzyme called monoamine oxidase (MAO). MAO, which is found in the brain and intestinal tract, acts to break down certain chemicals that play a role in the initiation and control of muscle movement.

▼ DOSAGE GUIDELINES

RANGE AND FREQUENCY
Adults: 5 mg twice daily. Children: This drug should not be used by children.

ONSET OF EFFECT
Approximately 1 to 2 hours.

DURATION OF ACTION
Approximately 4 hours.

DIETARY ADVICE
On rare occasions, patients taking the recommended dose of selegiline have had reactions with foods that contain tyramines. (See Food Interactions for more information.)

STORAGE
Store in a tightly sealed container away from heat, moisture, and direct light.

MISSED DOSE
Take it as soon as you remember, unless the time for your next scheduled dose is within the next 2 hours. If so, skip the missed dose and resume your regular dosage schedule. Do not double the next dose.

STOPPING THE DRUG
Consult with your physician before stopping this drug. The dose should be tapered gradually—from 2 tablets to a single tablet for 7 days—before the drug is completely discontinued.

PROLONGED USE
Selegiline may be taken for prolonged periods. There are no known untoward effects specifically associated with long-term use.

▼ PRECAUTIONS

Over 60: Adverse reactions may be more likely and more severe in older people. The medication should be used with caution by patients in this age group.

Driving and Hazardous Work: This drug may cause confusion or drowsiness. Do not drive or engage in hazardous work until you determine how it affects you.

Alcohol: Avoid alcohol.

Pregnancy: Adequate human studies have not been done to determine the safety of this drug during pregnancy. It should not be used by pregnant women.

Breast Feeding: The extent to which selegiline passes through breast milk is unknown. It should therefore be avoided by nursing mothers.

Infants and Children: This drug has not been tested in infants and children; safety and effectiveness have not been established. It should therefore not be used by patients in this age group.

OVERDOSE
Symptoms: Dizziness, fainting, confusion, delirium, abdominal pain.

What to Do: Call your doctor, emergency medical services

(EMS), or the nearest poison control center immediately.

▼ INTERACTIONS

DRUG INTERACTIONS
Other drugs may interact with selegiline. Consult your doctor for specific advice if you are taking meperidine hydrochloride or other opioid (narcotic) analgesics, or MAO inhibitor antidepressants such as phenelzine sulfate or tranylcypromine sulfate.

FOOD INTERACTIONS
Consult your doctor before eating tyramine-rich foods, which include aged cheeses, avocados, banana skins, bean curd, bologna and other processed lunch meats, chicken livers, chocolate, figs, canned or dried fish, pickled herring, meat extracts, pepperoni, raisins, raspberries, unpasteurized beer, Chianti, sherry, vermouth, red wines in general, and caffeine-rich beverages or foods.

DISEASE INTERACTIONS
Caution is advised when taking selegiline hydrochloride. Consult your doctor if you have any of the following: a change in your mental state, significant heart disease, peptic ulcer disease, or wheezing or feelings of tightness or pressure in the chest.

≡ SIDE EFFECTS ≡

SERIOUS
Dizziness, low blood pressure (causing dizziness, lightheadedness, fainting, or confusion), involuntary muscle movements, heart rhythm abnormalities.

COMMON
Nausea, dry mouth.

LESS COMMON
Palpitations, drowsiness.

SENNA

Available in: Tablets, granules, oral solution, syrup
Available OTC? Yes **As Generic?** No
Drug Class: Laxative

▼ USAGE INFORMATION

WHY IT'S PRESCRIBED
For short-term treatment of constipation.

HOW IT WORKS
Senna stimulates water and electrolyte (mineral salt) secretion in the intestine to induce defecation.

▼ DOSAGE GUIDELINES

RANGE AND FREQUENCY
Adults and teenagers: 2 tablets, or 1 teaspoon of granules, or 10 to 15 ml of syrup. Children ages 6 to 12: 1 tablet or ½ teaspoon of granules. The medicine should be given at bedtime.

ONSET OF EFFECT
Within 6 to 10 hours.

DURATION OF ACTION
Variable.

DIETARY ADVICE
Each dose of senna should be taken on an empty stomach with a full glass (8 oz) of water or fruit juice.

STORAGE
Store in a tightly sealed container away from heat, moisture, and direct light.

MISSED DOSE
Take it as soon as you remember. If it is near the time for the next dose, skip the missed dose and resume your regular dosage schedule. Do not double the next dose.

STOPPING THE DRUG
Take senna as prescribed for the full treatment period. However, you may stop taking the drug if you are feeling better before the scheduled end of therapy.

PROLONGED USE
If regular bowel movement does not resume in 1 week, discontinue use of senna and consult your doctor.

▼ PRECAUTIONS

Over 60:
Adverse reactions may be more likely and more severe in older patients.

Driving and Hazardous Work:
Do not drive or engage in hazardous work until you determine how the medicine affects you.

Alcohol:
Avoid alcohol.

Pregnancy:
Senna may cause unwanted effects during pregnancy if not used properly. Consult your doctor.

Breast Feeding:
Senna may pass into breast milk; caution is advised. Consult your doctor for advice.

Infants and Children:
Senna is not recommended for use by children under the age of 6 unless it has been prescribed by a doctor.

Special Concerns:
You should increase your intake of foods containing vitamin D, such as milk products, and maintain an adequate intake of foods containing folic acid, such as fresh vegetables, fruits, whole grains, and liver, while taking senna. Senna is one of the most effective laxatives for relieving constipation caused by narcotic analgesics like morphine and codeine.

OVERDOSE

Symptoms: Sudden vomiting, nausea, diarrhea, or cramping.

What to Do: An overdose of senna is unlikely to be life-threatening. However, if someone takes a much larger dose than prescribed, call your doctor, emergency medical services (EMS), or the nearest poison control center immediately.

▼ INTERACTIONS

DRUG INTERACTIONS
Do not take any other medicine within 2 hours of taking senna. Consult your doctor for specific advice if you are taking anticoagulants, digitalis drugs, ciprofloxacin, etidronate, sodium polystyrene sulfonate, or oral tetracyclines.

FOOD INTERACTIONS
No known food interactions.

DISEASE INTERACTIONS
Caution is advised when taking senna. Consult your doctor if you have a history of any of the following: appendicitis, rectal bleeding of unknown cause, colostomy, intestinal blockage, ileostomy, diabetes, heart disease, high blood pressure, kidney disease, or difficulty swallowing.

⧨ SIDE EFFECTS ⧨

SERIOUS
Confusion, irregular heartbeat, muscle cramps, pink-to-red or yellow-to-brown coloration of urine and stools, unusual tiredness or weakness, laxative dependence. Call your doctor immediately.

COMMON
Belching, cramping, diarrhea, nausea.

LESS COMMON
No less-common side effects have been reported.

SERTRALINE HYDROCHLORIDE

Available in: Capsules, tablets
Available OTC? No   **As Generic?** No
Drug Class: Selective serotonin reuptake inhibitor (SSRI) antidepressant

▼ USAGE INFORMATION

WHY IT'S PRESCRIBED
To treat symptoms of major depression, obsessive-compulsive disorder, and panic disorder.

HOW IT WORKS
Sertraline affects levels of serotonin, a brain chemical that is thought to be linked to mood, emotions, and mental state.

▼ DOSAGE GUIDELINES

RANGE AND FREQUENCY
Adults: To start, 50 mg once a day, in the morning or evening. Dose may be gradually increased by your doctor to 200 mg a day. Older adults: To start, 12.5 to 25 mg once a day. Dose may be gradually increased by your doctor to 200 mg a day. Children ages 6 to 12: To start, 25 mg once a day. Children ages 13 to 17: To start, 50 mg once a day. Dose may be gradually increased by your pediatrician.

ONSET OF EFFECT
1 to 4 weeks.

DURATION OF ACTION
Unknown.

DIETARY ADVICE
No special restrictions.

STORAGE
Store in a tightly sealed container away from heat, moisture and direct light.

MISSED DOSE
Take it as soon as you remember. If it is near the time for the next dose, skip the missed dose and resume your regular dosage schedule. Do not double the next dose.

STOPPING THE DRUG
Take it as prescribed for the full treatment period. When it is time to stop therapy, your dosage will be tapered gradually by your doctor.

PROLONGED USE
Usual course of therapy lasts 6 months to 1 year; some patients benefit from additional therapy.

▼ PRECAUTIONS

Over 60: No special problems have been reported.

Driving and Hazardous Work: Use caution when driving or engaging in hazardous work until you determine how the medicine affects you.

Alcohol: Avoid alcohol.

Pregnancy: Adequate studies of sertraline use during pregnancy have not been done. Before you take sertraline, tell your doctor if you are currently pregnant or plan to become pregnant.

Breast Feeding: It is not known whether sertraline passes into breast milk; caution is advised. Consult your doctor for specific advice.

Infants and Children: The safety and effectiveness of the use of sertraline in children under age 6 have not been established.

Special Concerns: Take sertraline at least 6 hours before bedtime to prevent insomnia, unless it causes drowsiness.

OVERDOSE
Symptoms: Sleepiness, nausea, vomiting, rapid heartbeat, anxiety, dilated pupils.

What to Do: Call your doctor, emergency medical services (EMS), or the nearest poison control center immediately.

▼ INTERACTIONS

DRUG INTERACTIONS
Sertraline and MAO inhibitors should not be used within 14 days of each other. Very serious side effects such as myoclonus (uncontrolled muscle spasms), hyperthermia (excessive rise in body temperature), and extreme stiffness may result. The following drugs may also interact with sertraline; consult your doctor for advice if you are taking cimetidine, digitoxin, warfarin, sumatriptan, naratriptan, zolmitriptan, oral antidiabetic agents (such as tolbutamide), tricyclic antidepressants, or any prescription or over-the-counter drugs that depress the central nervous system (including antihistamines, barbiturates, sedatives, cough medicines, and decongestants).

FOOD INTERACTIONS
No known food interactions.

DISEASE INTERACTIONS
Consult your doctor if you have a history of alcohol or drug abuse. Use of sertraline may cause complications in patients with liver or kidney disease, since these organs work together to remove the medication from the body.

 SIDE EFFECTS

SERIOUS
Skin rash, hives, or itching; unusually fast speech, fever, extreme agitation. Call your doctor immediately.

COMMON
Insomnia, diarrhea, sexual dysfunction, decrease in appetite, weight loss, drowsiness, headache, dry mouth, stomach cramps, abdominal pain, gas, trembling, fatigue, loss of initiative.

LESS COMMON
Anxiety, agitation, increased appetite, blurred or altered vision, constipation, heartbeat irregularities, flushing, unusual feeling of warmth, vomiting.

SIBUTRAMINE HYDROCHLORIDE MONOHYDRATE

Available in: Capsules
Available OTC? No   **As Generic?** No
Drug Class: Inhibitor of neurotransmitter reuptake

▼ USAGE INFORMATION

WHY IT'S PRESCRIBED
To aid in the medical management of obesity in conjunction with a carefully supervised diet and exercise program. The drug is only recommended for overweight people with a body mass index (BMI) greater than 30 or greater than 27 in people with other risk factors, such as diabetes or high blood pressure.

HOW IT WORKS
Sibutramine affects the appetite control center in the brain by inhibiting the reuptake of neurotransmitters like serotonin. The resulting increase in their availability suppresses appetite.

▼ DOSAGE GUIDELINES

RANGE AND FREQUENCY
To start, 10 mg once a day. Dose may be increased up to 15 mg once a day.

ONSET OF EFFECT
Significant weight changes may take several weeks or months to develop.

DURATION OF ACTION
When taking sibutramine regularly, most people lose weight within the first six months. Weight loss is maintained for the duration of therapy.

DIETARY ADVICE
Can be taken with a meal or on an empty stomach.

STORAGE
Store in a tightly sealed container away from heat, moisture, and direct light.

MISSED DOSE
If you miss a dose one day, do not double the dose the next day. Resume your regular dosage schedule.

STOPPING THE DRUG
The decision to stop taking the drug should be made in consultation with your doctor.

PROLONGED USE
The safety and effectiveness have not been determined beyond 1 year of use.

▼ PRECAUTIONS

Over 60: No specific studies have been done on older patients.

Driving and Hazardous Work: Do not drive or engage in hazardous work until you determine how the medicine affects you.

Alcohol: Sibutramine may increase the sedative effects of alcohol. Consult you doctor for specific advice.

Pregnancy: Sibutramine should not be used by pregnant women. Before taking sibutramine, tell your doctor if you are pregnant or plan to become pregnant.

Breast Feeding: Sibutramine should not be used by nursing mothers.

Infants and Children: Children under the age of 16 should not use sibutramine.

Special Concerns: Although no serious adverse reactions have been reported with sibutramine (at the time of publication), other diet drugs have been associated with an increased risk of potentially grave cardiovascular and cardiopulmonary problems. If you experience any unusual or disturbing adverse effects, stop taking sibutramine and call your doctor immediately.

OVERDOSE
Symptoms: No cases of overdose have been reported.

What to Do: If someone takes a much larger dose than prescribed or a child swallows the drug, call your doctor, emergency medical services (EMS), or the nearest poison control immediately.

▼ INTERACTIONS

DRUG INTERACTIONS
You should not take sibutramine if you take MAO inhibitors, other weight loss medications, medications for depression, migraine medications, dihydroergotamine, meperidine, fentanyl, pentazocine, dextromethorphan (found in many cough medicines), lithium, or tryptophan. Sibutramine may interact with ketoconazole, erythromycin, over-the-counter cough and cold medications, allergy medicines, and decongestants. Consult your doctor for specific advice.

FOOD INTERACTIONS
No known food interactions.

DISEASE INTERACTIONS
You should not take sibutramine if you have coronary artery disease, angina, cardiac arrhythmia, history of heart attack, congestive heart failure, history of stroke, anorexia nervosa, history of seizures, or narrow angle glaucoma. Sibutramine can substantially raise blood pressure in some patients. Use of sibutramine may cause complications in patients with liver or kidney disease, since these organs work together to remove the medication from the body. Consult your doctor if you have a history of migraines, mental depression, Parkinson's disease, thyroid disorders, osteoporosis, gallbladder disease, a major eating disorder (anorexia nervosa or bulimia nervosa), or any other medical problem.

 SIDE EFFECTS

SERIOUS
No serious side effects have yet been reported. However, if you experience symptoms, such as shortness of breath or chest pain, that were not present before taking the medication, call your doctor.

COMMON
Dry mouth, constipation, insomnia.

LESS COMMON
Headache, increased sweating, increased blood pressure and heart rate.

SILDENAFIL CITRATE

Available in: Tablets
Available OTC? No   **As Generic?** No
Drug Class: Phosphodiesterase type 5 inhibitor

▼ USAGE INFORMATION

WHY IT'S PRESCRIBED
To treat erectile dysfunction (impotence), which may occur in association with atherosclerosis, vascular disease or other circulatory problems, diabetes, kidney disease, hormonal abnormalities, neurological disease or injury, severe depression or other psychological difficulties.

HOW IT WORKS
Sildenafil selectively inhibits the action of an enzyme (phosphodiesterase type 5) that breaks down a substance that relaxes smooth muscles and permits blood flow that engorges the columns of erectile tissue in the penis. Unlike other treatments for erectile dysfunction, which produce erections with or without sexual arousal, sildenafil allows the patient to respond naturally to sexual stimulation.

▼ DOSAGE GUIDELINES

RANGE AND FREQUENCY
The recommended dose for most patients is 50 mg, taken approximately 1 hour before sexual activity. The dose may be increased to no more than 100 mg, or decreased to 25 mg. Your doctor will help to determine the correct dose. Do not take the drug more than once in a 24-hour period.

ONSET OF EFFECT
Within 30 minutes to 4 hours.

DURATION OF ACTION
Unknown.

DIETARY ADVICE
No special recommendations.

STORAGE
Store in a tightly sealed container away from heat, moisture, and direct light.

MISSED DOSE
Not applicable.

STOPPING THE DRUG
Not applicable.

PROLONGED USE
Sildenafil treats but does not cure erectile dysfunction. Patients must continue using sildenafil to maintain its benefit; lifelong therapy may be warranted.

▼ PRECAUTIONS

Over 60: No special problems are expected.

Driving and Hazardous Work: This drug should not impair your ability to perform such tasks safely.

Alcohol: No special precautions are necessary. However, alcohol is known to decrease sexual function.

Pregnancy: Not applicable; sildenafil is not approved for use by women.

Breast Feeding: Not applicable; sildenafil is not approved for use by women.

Infants and Children: Not applicable; sildenafil is not to be used by children.

Special Concerns: Sildenafil does not offer any protection against sexually transmitted diseases. Appropriate measures (for example, using condoms) should be taken to ensure adequate protection against sexually transmitted diseases, including infection with the human immunodeficiency virus (HIV). Sildenafil should be taken only by men who have been clinically evaluated for and diagnosed with erectile dysfunction by a doctor.

OVERDOSE
Symptoms: No cases of overdose have been reported.

What to Do: An overdose with sildenafil is unlikely. If someone takes a much larger dose than prescribed, call your doctor.

▼ INTERACTIONS

DRUG INTERACTIONS
Sildenafil can enhance the action of nitrates (such as nitroglycerin, which is used to treat episodes of angina), causing potentially dangerous decreases in blood pressure. Therefore, sildenafil should not be used by patients taking nitrates of any kind. Use of sildenafil in conjunction with other erectile-dysfunction medications is not recommended. Consult your doctor if you are taking protease inhibitors, such as ritonavir and saquinavir, which may affect levels of sildenafil in the blood.

FOOD INTERACTIONS
No known food interactions.

DISEASE INTERACTIONS
Caution is advised when taking sildenafil. Consult your doctor if you have a history of any of the following: high or very low blood pressure; structural deformity of the penis; a bleeding disorder; heart attack, stroke, or life-threatening arrhythmia within the past six months; heart failure; coronary heart disease; retinitis pigmentosa; peptic ulcer; sickle cell anemia; multiple myeloma; or leukemia.

≡ SIDE EFFECTS ≡

SERIOUS
Rarely, a painful or prolonged erection (lasting more than 4 hours) may occur. If erection does not resolve on its own in a reasonable amount of time, seek medical help promptly. If prolonged erection does resolve, consult your doctor for specific guidelines. Serious cardiovascular events, such as heart attack, cardiac arrhythmias, cerebral hemorrhage, and transient ischemic attack, have been reported following the use of sildenafil. However, it is unclear whether these events are due to sildenafil, the presence of preexisting cardiovascular risk factors, to sexual activity, or a combination of these factors.

COMMON
Headache, flushing, indigestion. Such side effects are generally mild to moderate and usually short-lived.

LESS COMMON
Nasal congestion, vision abnormalities, bloodshot or burning eyes, diarrhea, blood in the urine.

SIMETHICONE

Available in: Tablets, chewable tablets, capsules, drops
Available OTC? Yes   **As Generic?** Yes
Drug Class: Antacid; antiflatulant

▼ USAGE INFORMATION

WHY IT'S PRESCRIBED
To relieve pain caused by excess gas in stomach and intestines. It may also be employed in a clinical setting to decrease gas before diagnostic radiography of the stomach or intestines, or prior to endoscopy.

HOW IT WORKS
Simethicone disperses and prevents the formation of gas bubbles in the gastrointestinal tract.

▼ DOSAGE GUIDELINES

RANGE AND FREQUENCY
Tablets or capsules: 60 to 125 mg, 4 times a day, after meals and at bedtime. Chewable tablets: 40 to 125 mg, 4 times a day after meals and at bedtime, or 150 mg, 3 times a day after meals. Drops: 40 to 95 mg, 4 times a day after meals and at bedtime. The liquid form should be taken by mouth even if it comes in a dropper bottle. The dose should not exceed 500 mg a day for all forms unless your doctor advises otherwise.

ONSET OF EFFECT
Immediate.

DURATION OF ACTION
Unknown.

DIETARY ADVICE
This medicine should be taken after meals and at bedtime for optimal results.

STORAGE
Store in a tightly sealed container away from heat, moisture, and direct light. Store the liquid form at room temperature.

MISSED DOSE
Take it as soon as you remember. However, if it is near the time for the next dose, skip the missed dose and resume your regular dosage schedule. Do not double the next dose.

STOPPING THE DRUG
Take simethicone as prescribed for the full treatment period. However, you may stop taking the drug if you are feeling better before the scheduled end of therapy.

PROLONGED USE
Consult your doctor if you take simethicone for a prolonged period.

▼ PRECAUTIONS

Over 60: There is no specific information comparing use of simethicone in older persons with use in younger persons. However, no special problems are expected.

Driving and Hazardous Work: The use of simethicone should not impair your ability to perform such tasks safely.

Alcohol: No special problems are expected.

Pregnancy: Simethicone is not absorbed into the body and is not expected to cause problems during pregnancy.

Breast Feeding: Simethicone has not been reported to cause problems in nursing babies.

Infants and Children: Use of simethicone for the treatment of infant colic is not recommended because of limited information on its safety in infants. Simethicone should not be dispensed to children unless a doctor instructs otherwise.

Special Concerns: If you take the chewable tablets, chew them thoroughly before swallowing for more complete and faster results. Shake the liquid form well before using. You should change position frequently and walk about to help eliminate gas. Tell your doctor if you are on a low-sodium, low-sugar or other special diet. You should exercise regularly and develop regular bowel habits. Do not smoke before meals.

OVERDOSE
Symptoms: No specific ones have been reported.

What to Do: An overdose of simethicone is not life-threatening. However, if someone takes a much larger dose than recommended, call your doctor or the nearest poison control center.

▼ INTERACTIONS

DRUG INTERACTIONS
None known.

FOOD INTERACTIONS
Avoid any foods that increase gas formation. Chew your food slowly and thoroughly. Avoid carbonated drinks.

DISEASE INTERACTIONS
None known.

≡ SIDE EFFECTS ≡

SERIOUS
No serious side effects have been reported.

COMMON
Expulsion of excess gas, causing belching and flatulence.

LESS COMMON
No less-common side effects have been reported.

SIMVASTATIN

Available in: Tablets
Available OTC? No **As Generic?** No
Drug Class: Antilipidemic (cholesterol-lowering agent)

▼ USAGE INFORMATION

WHY IT'S PRESCRIBED
To treat high cholesterol. Also used to reduce the risk of stroke or transient ischemic attack ("mini-stroke") in patients with high cholesterol and coronary artery disease. Usually prescribed after first lines of treatment—including diet, weight loss, and exercise—fail to reduce total and low-density lipoprotein (LDL) cholesterol to acceptable levels.

HOW IT WORKS
Simvastatin blocks the action of an enzyme required for the manufacture of cholesterol, thereby interfering with its formation. By lowering the amount of cholesterol in the liver cells, simvastatin increases the formation of receptors for LDL, and thereby reduces blood levels of total and LDL cholesterol. In addition to lowering LDL cholesterol, simvastatin also modestly reduces triglyceride levels and raises HDL (the so-called good) cholesterol.

▼ DOSAGE GUIDELINES

RANGE AND FREQUENCY
Initial dose is 10 to 40 mg once a day. It may be increased to a maximum of 80 mg per day. Simvastatin is most effective when taken in the evening.

ONSET OF EFFECT
2 to 4 weeks.

DURATION OF ACTION
The effect persists for the duration of therapy.

DIETARY ADVICE
Cholesterol-lowering drugs are only one part of a total program that should include regular exercise and a healthy diet. The American Heart Association publishes a "Healthy Heart" diet, which is recommended.

STORAGE
Store in a tightly sealed container away from heat and direct light.

MISSED DOSE
Take it as soon as you remember. Take your next dose at the proper time and resume your regular dosage schedule. Do not double the next dose.

STOPPING THE DRUG
The decision to stop taking the drug should be made in consultation with your doctor. Once the medication is discontinued, blood cholesterol is likely to return to original elevated levels.

PROLONGED USE
Side effects are more likely with prolonged use. As you continue with simvastatin, your doctor will periodically order blood tests to evaluate liver function.

▼ PRECAUTIONS

Over 60: No special problems are expected in older patients.

Driving and Hazardous Work: The use of simvastatin should not impair your ability to perform such tasks safely.

Alcohol: No special precautions are necessary.

Pregnancy: Should not be used during pregnancy or by women who plan to become pregnant in the near future.

Breast Feeding: This drug is not recommended for women who are nursing.

Infants and Children: The long-term effects of simvastatin in children have not been determined. It is rarely used in children; consult your pediatrician.

Special Concerns: Important elements of treatment for high cholesterol include proper diet, weight loss, regular moderate exercise, and the avoidance of certain medications that may increase cholesterol levels. Because simvastatin has potential side effects, it is important that you maintain a recommended healthy diet and cooperate with other treatments your physician may suggest.

OVERDOSE
Symptoms: No specific ones have been reported; overdose is unlikely.

What to Do: Emergency instructions not applicable.

▼ INTERACTIONS

DRUG INTERACTIONS
Consult your doctor if you are taking cyclosporine, gemfibrozil, niacin, antibiotics, especially erythromycin, HIV protease inhibitors, or medications for fungus infections. All of these drugs may increase the risk of myositis (muscle inflammation) when taken with simvastatin and may lead to kidney failure.

FOOD INTERACTIONS
No known food interactions.

DISEASE INTERACTIONS
Consult your doctor if you have liver, kidney, or muscle disease, or a medical history involving organ transplant or recent surgery.

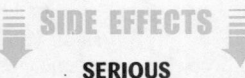
SIDE EFFECTS

SERIOUS
Fever, unusual or unexplained muscle aches and tenderness. Call your doctor right away.

COMMON
Side effects occur in only 1% to 2% of patients. They may include constipation or diarrhea, dizziness or lightheadedness, bloating or gas, heartburn, nausea, skin rash, stomach pain, rise in liver enzymes.

LESS COMMON
Insomnia.

SODIUM BICARBONATE

Available in: Effervescent powder, powder, tablets
Available OTC? Yes   **As Generic?** Yes
Drug Class: Antacid

▼ USAGE INFORMATION

WHY IT'S PRESCRIBED
To relieve heartburn, sour stomach, or acid indigestion. It may also be prescribed to treat metabolic acidosis (excess acid buildup in the body fluids), to prevent urinary stones, and as part of the treatment of gout.

HOW IT WORKS
Sodium bicarbonate neutralizes stomach acid and reduces the action of pepsin, a digestive enzyme. This provides symptomatic relief from excess stomach acid. Also, the bicarbonate is a base, meaning it can help correct the pH balance (reduce the acidity) of blood and urine.

▼ DOSAGE GUIDELINES

RANGE AND FREQUENCY
Effervescent powder— For heartburn or sour stomach: 3.9 to 10 g (1 to 2½ teaspoons) in a glass of cold water. Usually not more than 19.5 g a day (5 teaspoons). Children ages 6 to 12: 1 to 1.9 g (¼ to ½ teaspoon) in a glass of cold water. Powder—

For heartburn or sour stomach: ½ teaspoon in a glass of water every 2 hours. Dose may be changed if needed. To make the urine less acidic: 1 teaspoon (1.9 g) in a glass of water every 4 hours; usually not more than 4 teaspoons a day. Dose may be changed by your doctor. Tablets— For heartburn or sour stomach: 325 mg to 2 g, 1 to 4 times a day. Children ages 6 to 12: 520 mg. Dose may be repeated in 30 minutes. To make the urine less acidic— To start, 4 g; then 1 to 2 g every 4 hours. Maximum adult dose usually not more than 16 g a day. Children: 23 to 230 mg per 2.2 lbs (1 kg) of body weight a day. Dose may be changed if needed.

ONSET OF EFFECT
Rapid when used as an antacid for heartburn and sour stomach.

DURATION OF ACTION
Unknown.

DIETARY ADVICE
Sodium bicarbonate should be taken after meals. Be sure to account for the large

amount of sodium in this medication if you are on a salt-restricted diet.

STORAGE
Store in a tightly sealed container away from heat, moisture, and direct light.

MISSED DOSE
Take it as soon as you remember. If it is near the time for the next dose, skip the missed dose and resume your regular dosage schedule. Do not double the next dose.

STOPPING THE DRUG
Take as directed if taking it by prescription.

PROLONGED USE
Do not take sodium bicarbonate for more than 2 weeks or on a routine basis without consulting your physician.

▼ PRECAUTIONS

Over 60: See Dietary Advice.

Driving and Hazardous Work: No special precautions are necessary.

Alcohol: Avoid alcohol.

Pregnancy: No problems have been reported.

Breast Feeding: No problems have been reported.

Infants and Children: Use and dosage for infants and children under 6 years of age should be determined by your doctor.

OVERDOSE
Symptoms: See Serious Side Effects.

What to Do: An overdose of sodium bicarbonate is unlikely to be life-threatening. However, if someone takes a much larger dose than recommended, call your doctor, emergency medical services (EMS), or the nearest poison control center immediately.

▼ INTERACTIONS

DRUG INTERACTIONS
Do not take any other over-the-counter medications containing sodium bicarbonate such as Alka-Seltzer. Consult your doctor for specific advice if you are taking ketoconazole, tetracyclines, mecamylamine, methenamine, urinary acidifiers, amphetamines, anticholinergics, quinidine, citrates, enteric-coated medications, ephedrine, flecainide, fluoroquinolones, iron, lithium, methotrexate, mexiletine, sucralfate, or salicylates.

FOOD INTERACTIONS
Do not take sodium bicarbonate with milk or milk products.

DISEASE INTERACTIONS
Do not take sodium bicarbonate if you have any sign of appendicitis (stomach pain, bloating, nausea, and vomiting). If you have kidney problems, use sodium bicarbonate only on advice of your doctor. Consult your doctor if you have intestinal or rectal bleeding, edema (swelling of the hands or feet), heart, liver, or kidney disease, hypertension, urination problems, or toxemia of pregnancy.

SIDE EFFECTS

SERIOUS
Frequent urge to urinate, nervousness or restlessness, mental or mood changes, muscle twitching or pain, nausea or vomiting, slow breathing, continuing headache, loss of appetite, swelling of feet or lower legs, unpleasant taste, unusual fatigue. Call your doctor immediately.

COMMON
No common side effects have been reported.

LESS COMMON
Stomach cramps, increased thirst.

SODIUM PHOSPHATE/SODIUM BIPHOSPHATE

BRAND NAMES

Fleet, Fleet Phospho-Soda

Available in: Oral solution, effervescent powder, enema
Available OTC? Yes **As Generic?** Yes
Drug Class: Hyperosmotic laxative

▼ USAGE INFORMATION

WHY IT'S PRESCRIBED
To treat short-term constipation or for rapid emptying of the colon prior to bowel or rectal examination.

HOW IT WORKS
This medication attracts and retains water in the intestine, increasing peristalsis (bowel activity) and the urge to defecate.

▼ DOSAGE GUIDELINES

RANGE AND FREQUENCY
Oral— Adults and teenagers: 20 to 30 ml (4 to 6 teaspoons) mixed with ½ glass cool water. Children ages 10 to 12: 10 ml (2 teaspoons). Children ages 6 to 10: 5 ml (1 teaspoon). Enema— Adults and teenagers: 118 ml (contents of 1 disposable adult enema) given rectally. Children over 2: ½ adult dose (contents of 1 disposable pediatric enema).

ONSET OF EFFECT
30 minutes to 3 hours after oral administration, 3 to 5 minutes after enema.

DURATION OF ACTION
Variable with oral use; upon evacuation with enema.

DIETARY ADVICE
Sodium phosphate/sodium biphosphate should not be used with food. The unpleasant taste that may occur when you take the medicine can be lessened by taking it with citrus fruit juice or a citrus-flavored soft drink.

STORAGE
Store in a tightly sealed container away from heat and direct light.

MISSED DOSE
Oral forms: If you are taking this laxative on a fixed schedule, take the missed dose as soon as you remember. If it is near the time for the next dose, skip the missed dose and resume your regular dosage schedule. Do not double the next dose. Enema: Not applicable.

STOPPING THE DRUG
Take it as prescribed for the full treatment period. However, you may stop taking the drug if you feel better before the scheduled end of therapy.

PROLONGED USE
Do not use any laxative for longer than 2 weeks without consulting your doctor.

▼ PRECAUTIONS

Over 60: Adverse reactions may be more likely and more severe in older patients.

Driving and Hazardous Work: Do not drive or engage in hazardous work until you determine how the medicine affects you.

Alcohol: Avoid alcohol.

Pregnancy: This laxative contains a large amount of sodium, which may have unwanted effects during pregnancy, such as higher blood pressure. If you have to take a laxative during pregnancy, consult your doctor for specific advice.

Breast Feeding: Sodium phosphate may pass into breast milk; caution is advised. Consult your doctor for specific advice.

Infants and Children: Do not give sodium phosphate/sodium biphosphate to children under the age of 6 without consulting your doctor.

Special Concerns: Chilling the oral form of the medication or taking it with ice or following it with citrus fruit juice or citrus-flavored carbonated beverages may make it more palatable. Remember that chronic use of sodium phosphate or any laxative can lead to laxative dependence. You should consume adequate amounts of bulk (fiber) in your diet, such as bran, whole-grain cereals, fruit, and vegetables. This laxative should be taken on a schedule that does not interfere with activities or sleep; it produces watery stools within 3 to 6 hours. It should not be taken within 2 hours of taking other medications.

OVERDOSE
Symptoms: Excessive bowel activity, dehydration causing low blood pressure and abnormal heartbeat, metabolic acidosis, blood chemistry abnormalities.

What to Do: An overdose of sodium phosphate/sodium biphosphate is unlikely to be life-threatening. However, if someone takes a much larger dose than prescribed, call your doctor, emergency medical services (EMS), or the nearest poison control center immediately.

▼ INTERACTIONS

DRUG INTERACTIONS
Consult your doctor for advice if you are taking anticoagulants, digitalis drugs, ciprofloxacin, etidronate, sodium polystyrene sulfonate, or oral tetracyclines.

FOOD INTERACTIONS
No known food interactions.

DISEASE INTERACTIONS
Consult your doctor if you have a history of appendicitis, rectal bleeding of unknown cause, colostomy, intestinal blockage, ileostomy, diabetes, heart disease, high blood pressure, kidney disease, or swallowing difficulties.

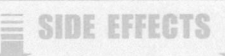

SIDE EFFECTS

SERIOUS
Confusion, dizziness or lightheadedness, irregular heartbeat, muscle cramps, unusual tiredness or weakness. Call your doctor immediately.

COMMON
Cramping, diarrhea, gas, increased thirst.

LESS COMMON
No less-common side effects have been reported.

SODIUM POLYSTYRENE SULFONATE

Available in: Powder for suspension, suspension
Available OTC? No   **As Generic?** Yes
Drug Class: Potassium-removing resin

▼ USAGE INFORMATION

WHY IT'S PRESCRIBED
To treat abnormally high blood levels of potassium (hyperkalemia) caused by acute kidney failure.

HOW IT WORKS
Sodium polystyrene sulfonate is a resin that lowers potassium levels by exchanging sodium present in the medication with potassium present in the body. This process occurs within the intestines.

▼ DOSAGE GUIDELINES

RANGE AND FREQUENCY
The powder for suspension and the suspension can be taken either orally or rectally. Adults— Oral: 15 g (4 level tablespoons of powder), 1 to 4 times a day; may be increased to 40 g, 4 times a day. Rectal: 25 to 100 g as needed, given as an enema or in a dialysis bag. Children— Oral: 1 g per 2.2 lbs (1 kg) of body weight, as needed. Rectal: 1 g per 2.2 lbs, as needed, given as an enema or in a dialysis bag. Oral dosage is preferred because the drug should remain in the intestine for at least 6 hours.

ONSET OF EFFECT
Unknown.

DURATION OF ACTION
Unknown.

DIETARY ADVICE
The oral medication should not be mixed with orange juice (orange juice is high in potassium).

STORAGE
Store in a tightly sealed container away from heat, moisture, and direct light. Liquid form can be refrigerated, but do not allow it to freeze.

MISSED DOSE
Take it as soon as you remember. However, if it is near the time for the next dose, skip the missed dose and resume your regular dosage schedule. Do not double the next dose.

STOPPING THE DRUG
The decision to stop taking the drug should be made in consultation with your doctor.

PROLONGED USE
See your doctor regularly for tests and examinations if you must take this medication for a prolonged period.

▼ PRECAUTIONS

Over 60: Side effects, especially fecal impaction, may be more likely in older patients.

Driving and Hazardous Work: Do not drive or engage in hazardous work until you determine how the medicine affects you.

Alcohol: Avoid alcohol.

Pregnancy: Adequate studies of the use of sodium polystyrene sulfonate during pregnancy have not been done. Before taking it, consult your doctor if you are pregnant or plan to become pregnant.

Breast Feeding: It is not known whether sodium polystyrene sulfonate passes into breast milk; consult your doctor for advice.

Infants and Children: No special problems are expected.

Special Concerns: If you are taking the suspension made from the powder, shake it well before using. Do not use mineral oil when administering this drug rectally. The suspension should be used within 24 hours of preparation.

OVERDOSE
Symptoms: Severe nausea, vomiting, fecal impaction, swelling of hands, feet, or lower legs, decreased urination, severe muscle fatigue, confusion.

What to Do: Call your doctor, emergency medical services (EMS), or the nearest poison control center immediately.

▼ INTERACTIONS

DRUG INTERACTIONS
The following drugs may interact with sodium polystyrene sulfonate. Consult your doctor for specific advice if you are taking antacids, digitalis drugs, laxatives, diuretics, potassium supplements, or any other prescription or over-the-counter medication.

FOOD INTERACTIONS
Orange juice can increase blood levels of potassium.

DISEASE INTERACTIONS
Caution is advised when taking sodium polystyrene sulfonate. Consult your doctor for advice if you have a history of congestive heart failure, severe high blood pressure, or severe edema (swelling of body tissues caused by fluid retention).

 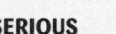
SIDE EFFECTS

SERIOUS
Severe stomach pain with nausea and vomiting (fecal impaction); heartbeat irregularities; abdominal and muscle cramps; weight gain; irritability, difficulty thinking; confusion; decreased urination; severe muscle fatigue; swelling of hands, feet, or lower legs. Call your doctor immediately.

COMMON
Loss of appetite, constipation, nausea, vomiting.

LESS COMMON
There are no less-common side effects associated with sodium polystyrene sulfonate.

SOMATREM

Available in: Injection
Available OTC? No   **As Generic?** No
Drug Class: Growth hormone

▼ USAGE INFORMATION

WHY IT'S PRESCRIBED
To replace growth hormone if it is not produced sufficiently by the pituitary gland.

HOW IT WORKS
Somatrem stimulates growth in the same manner as natural growth hormone.

▼ DOSAGE GUIDELINES

RANGE AND FREQUENCY
0.136 mg per lb of body weight weekly, in multiple doses as determined by your doctor.

ONSET OF EFFECT
Within 1 hour.

DURATION OF ACTION
12 to 48 hours.

DIETARY ADVICE
None.

STORAGE
Keep the liquid refrigerated, but do not allow it to freeze. Use it within 7 days.

MISSED DOSE
Take it as soon as you remember. If it is near the time for the next dose, skip the missed dose and resume your regular dosage schedule. Do not double the next dose.

STOPPING THE DRUG
The decision to stop taking the drug should be made by your doctor.

PROLONGED USE
After 2 years of use, growth rate generally decreases. If this occurs, the patient should be checked for compliance with therapy or the presence of other medical problems or the presence of antibodies to the medicine. Prolonged use of somatrem may cause a condition known as "acromegaly" (overgrowth of face, hands, and feet, organ enlargement, diabetes, atherosclerosis, high blood pressure, and carpal tunnel syndrome), resulting from excess quantities of pituitary hormone.

▼ PRECAUTIONS

Over 60:
Somatrem can be used to replace deficient growth hormone levels in people of any age. Though not approved for this use, growth hormone has been administered to elderly patients to increase muscle strength. Such use can result in edema (swelling of tissues due to excess fluid retention) and high blood pressure.

Driving and Hazardous Work:
The use of somatrem should not impair the ability to perform such tasks safely.

Alcohol:
No special precautions are necessary.

Pregnancy:
It is unknown whether somatrem causes fetal harm; the drug should be used by pregnant women only if absolutely necessary. Consult your doctor for specific advice.

Breast Feeding:
It is unknown whether somatrem passes into breast milk or causes harm to a nursing infant; the drug should be used by nursing mothers only if clearly needed. Consult your doctor.

Infants and Children:
Somatrem should not be given to a child whose bone ends (epiphyses) have closed, signaling the end of bone growth.

Special Concerns:
If somatrem is given to adults or children with normal growth hormone production, serious unwanted effects may occur, such as diabetes, high blood pressure, atherosclerosis, and abnormal growth of bone and internal organs including the heart, kidneys, and liver. If growth with somatrem is not satisfactory, some patients may be given low doses of sex hormones to improve their response to the medication. Annual tests of bone age are recommended. Periodic tests of thyroid function should be done, since low thyroid function interferes with the response to human growth hormone. If low growth hormone production is due to a lesion in the cranium, the lesion should be monitored at frequent intervals. If somatrem is injected into muscle, the needle used for injections should be at least 1 inch long to ensure that the medicine reaches the muscle.

OVERDOSE
Symptoms: No specific ones have been reported.

What to Do: An overdose of somatrem is unlikely to be life-threatening. However, if someone receives a much larger dose than prescribed, call your doctor, emergency medical services (EMS), or local poison control center immediately.

▼ INTERACTIONS

DRUG INTERACTIONS
Consult your doctor for specific advice if you (or your child) are also taking the following drugs that may interact with somatrem: anabolic steroids, estrogens, androgens, thyroid hormones, corticosteroids, or corticotropin.

FOOD INTERACTIONS
No known food interactions.

DISEASE INTERACTIONS
Caution is advised when taking somatrem. Consult your doctor if you have low thyroid function or any malignancy (cancerous growth).

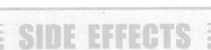

SIDE EFFECTS

SERIOUS
Pain and swelling at the site of injection, pain in hip or knee (possibly causing a limp), skin rash or itching. Call your doctor right away.

COMMON
No common side effects are associated with somatrem.

LESS COMMON
No uncommon side effects are associated with somatrem.

SOMATROPIN

Available in: Injection
Available OTC? No   **As Generic?** No
Drug Class: Growth hormone

▼ USAGE INFORMATION

WHY IT'S PRESCRIBED
To replace growth hormone if it is not produced sufficiently by the pituitary gland.

HOW IT WORKS
Somatropin stimulates growth in the same manner as natural growth hormone.

▼ DOSAGE GUIDELINES

RANGE AND FREQUENCY
Adults: To start, not more than 0.006 mg per kg (2.2 lbs) of body weight given daily as an injection under the skin. The dosage may be increased by your doctor to no more than 0.025 mg per kg in patients under 35 years and 0.0125 mg per kg in patients over 35 years. Children: Up to 0.3 mg per kg weekly, divided into daily injections under the skin as determined by the doctor.

ONSET OF EFFECT
Within 1 hour.

DURATION OF ACTION
12 to 48 hours.

DIETARY ADVICE
No special restrictions.

STORAGE
Keep the liquid refrigerated, but do not allow it to freeze. Use it within 7 days.

MISSED DOSE
Take it as soon as you remember. If it is near the time for the next dose, skip the missed dose and resume your regular dosage schedule. Do not double the next dose.

STOPPING THE DRUG
The decision to stop taking the drug should be made by your doctor.

PROLONGED USE
After 2 years of use, growth rate generally decreases. If this occurs, the patient should be checked for compliance with therapy or the presence of other medical problems or the presence of antibodies to the medicine. Prolonged use of somatropin may cause a condition known as "acromegaly" (overgrowth of face, hands, and feet, organ enlargement, diabetes, atherosclerosis, high blood pressure, and carpal tunnel syndrome), resulting from excess quantities of pituitary hormone.

▼ PRECAUTIONS

Over 60: Somatropin can be used to replace deficient growth hormone levels in people of any age. Though not approved for this use, growth hormone has been administered to elderly patients to increase muscle strength. Such use can result in edema (swelling of tissues due to excess fluid retention) and high blood pressure.

Driving and Hazardous Work: The use of somatropin should not impair the ability to perform such tasks safely.

Alcohol: No special precautions are necessary.

Pregnancy: It is unknown whether somatropin causes fetal harm; the drug should be used by pregnant women only if absolutely necessary. Consult your doctor for specific advice.

Breast Feeding: It is not known whether somatropin passes into breast milk or causes harm to a nursing infant; the drug should be used by nursing mothers only if clearly needed. Consult your doctor.

Infants and Children: Somatropin should not be given to a child whose bone ends (epiphyses) have closed, signaling the end of bone growth.

Special Concerns: If somatropin is given to adults or children with normal growth hormone production, serious unwanted effects may occur, such as diabetes, high blood pressure, atherosclerosis, and abnormal growth of bone and internal organs including the heart, kidneys, and liver. If growth is not satisfactory, some patients may be given low doses of sex hormones to improve their response to somatropin. Annual tests of bone age are recommended. Periodic tests of thyroid function should be done, since low thyroid function interferes with response to human growth hormone. If low growth hormone production is due to a lesion in the cranium, the lesion should be monitored frequently. If somatropin is injected into muscle, the needle used for injections should be at least 1 inch long.

OVERDOSE
Symptoms: None.

What to Do: An overdose is unlikely to be life-threatening. However, if someone receives a much larger dose than prescribed, seek medical assistance immediately.

▼ INTERACTIONS

DRUG INTERACTIONS
Consult your doctor for specific advice if you (or your child) are also taking the following drugs that may interact with somatropin: anabolic steroids, estrogens, androgens, thyroid hormones, corticosteroids, or corticotropin.

FOOD INTERACTIONS
No known food interactions.

DISEASE INTERACTIONS
Consult your doctor if you have low thyroid function or any malignancy (cancerous growth).

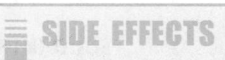

SIDE EFFECTS

SERIOUS
Pain and swelling at the site of injection, pain in hip or knee (possibly causing a limp), skin rash or itching. Call your doctor right away.

COMMON
No common side effects are associated with somatropin.

LESS COMMON
No uncommon side effects are associated with somatropin.

SOTALOL HYDROCHLORIDE

Available in: Tablets
Available OTC? No   **As Generic?** No
Drug Class: Beta-blocker; antiarrhythmic

BRAND NAME
Betapace

▼ USAGE INFORMATION

WHY IT'S PRESCRIBED
This drug is used only to treat or prevent life-threatening heart rhythm disturbances (cardiac arrhythmias). It requires close monitoring by a physician.

HOW IT WORKS
Beta-blockers such as sotalol work by preventing—or blocking—nerve impulses from exerting an accelerating or intensifying effect on specific parts of the body, especially the blood vessels and heart. In this way, sotalol slows and stabilizes heartbeat.

▼ DOSAGE GUIDELINES

RANGE AND FREQUENCY
Adults: 80 mg, 2 times a day. The dosage may be increased to 320 mg a day in 2 or 3 divided doses.

ONSET OF EFFECT
Unknown.

DURATION OF ACTION
Up to 12 hours.

DIETARY ADVICE
Should be taken on an empty stomach, 1 hour before or 2 hours after meals.

STORAGE
Store in a tightly sealed container away from heat and direct light.

MISSED DOSE
Take it as soon as you remember. However, if it is near the time for the next dose, skip the missed dose and resume your regular dosage schedule. Do not double the next dose.

STOPPING THE DRUG
Do not discontinue the drug abruptly, as this may cause serious health problems.

Dosage must be gradually tapered in accordance with your doctor's instructions.

PROLONGED USE
Your doctor should check your progress in regular visits if you take sotalol for a prolonged period.

▼ PRECAUTIONS

Over 60: Adverse reactions may be more likely and more severe. Resistance to cold temperatures may be decreased in older patients.

Driving and Hazardous Work: Do not drive or engage in hazardous work until you determine how the medicine affects you.

Alcohol: Avoid alcohol.

Pregnancy: Before taking sotalol, tell your doctor if you are pregnant or plan to become pregnant.

Breast Feeding: Sotalol passes into breast milk; consult your doctor about its use during nursing.

Infants and Children: Dosage for infants and children must be determined by your pediatrician.

Special Concerns: To avoid dizziness and fainting, take extra care during exercise or hot weather. Check your pulse regularly while taking sotalol. If it is slower than your usual rate, or less than 50 beats per minute, check with your doctor; a slow pulse rate may indicate circulation problems.

OVERDOSE
Symptoms: Unusually slow or rapid heartbeat, confusion, severe dizziness or fainting, poor circulation in the hands (bluish skin), breathing difficulty.

What to Do: Call your doctor, emergency medical services (EMS), or the nearest poison control center immediately.

▼ INTERACTIONS

DRUG INTERACTIONS
Consult your doctor for specific advice if you are taking amphetamines, oral antidiabetic agents, asthma medication (such as aminophylline or theophylline), calcium channel blockers, clonidine, guanabenz, halothane, immunotherapy for allergies (allergy shots), insulin, MAO inhibitors, reserpine, other beta-blockers, or any over-the-counter drug.

FOOD INTERACTIONS
No known food interactions.

DISEASE INTERACTIONS
People with the following conditions should consult their doctor before using sotalol: allergies or asthma; diabetes mellitus; heart or blood vessel disease (including congestive heart failure and peripheral vascular disease); hyperthyroidism; irregular (slow) heartbeat; a history of mental depression; myasthenia gravis; psoriasis; respiratory problems such as bronchitis or emphysema; kidney or liver disease.

≡ SIDE EFFECTS ≡

SERIOUS
Severe, occasionally life-threatening arrhythmias, shortness of breath, wheezing; irregular or slow heartbeat (50 beats per minute or less); pain or feelings of tightness or pressure in the chest; swelling of the ankles, feet, and lower legs; mental depression. If you experience such symptoms, stop taking sotalol and call your doctor immediately.

COMMON
Dizziness or lightheadedness, especially when rising suddenly to a standing position; rapid heartbeat or palpitations; decreased sexual ability; unusual fatigue, weakness, or drowsiness; insomnia. Notify your doctor.

LESS COMMON
Anxiety, irritability, nervousness; constipation; diarrhea; dry, sore eyes; itching; nausea or vomiting; nightmares or intensely vivid dreams; numbness, tingling, or other unusual sensations in the fingers, toes, or scalp. Call your doctor if such symptoms persist.

SPARFLOXACIN

BRAND NAME

Zagam

Available in: Tablets
Available OTC? No **As Generic?** No
Drug Class: Fluoroquinolone antibiotic

▼ USAGE INFORMATION

WHY IT'S PRESCRIBED
To treat pneumonia, chronic bronchitis, and other bacterial infections.

HOW IT WORKS
Sparfloxacin inhibits the activity of a bacterial enzyme (gyrase) that is necessary for proper DNA formation and replication. This fights infection by preventing bacteria cells from reproducing.

▼ DOSAGE GUIDELINES

RANGE AND FREQUENCY
Adults: 400 mg in 1 dose on the first day, then take 200 mg, once a day for 9 days. For patients with kidney impairment, 400 mg to start, wait 2 days, then take 200 mg every other day for 9 days.

ONSET OF EFFECT
Varies depending on the infection being treated.

DURATION OF ACTION
Unknown.

DIETARY ADVICE
Drink plenty of fluids.

STORAGE
Store in a tightly sealed container away from heat and direct light.

MISSED DOSE
Take it as soon as you remember. If it is near the time for the next dose, skip the missed dose and resume your regular dosage schedule. Do not double the next dose.

STOPPING THE DRUG
It is very important to take this drug as prescribed for the full treatment period, even if you begin to feel better before the scheduled end of therapy (unless you experience intolerable side effects, including increased sensitivity to sunlight, in which case, discontinue taking the drug and call your doctor).

PROLONGED USE
See your doctor regularly for tests and examinations if you must take this medicine for a prolonged period.

▼ PRECAUTIONS

Over 60: No special problems are expected.

Driving and Hazardous Work: Do not drive or engage in hazardous work until you determine how the medicine affects you.

Alcohol: It is advisable to abstain from alcohol when fighting an infection.

Pregnancy: In some animal tests, sparfloxacin has caused birth defects. Adequate studies in humans have not been done. It should be used during pregnancy only if the potential benefit justifies the risk. Before you take sparfloxacin, tell your doctor if you are pregnant or plan to become pregnant.

Breast Feeding: Sparfloxacin passes into breast milk and may cause serious side effects in the nursing infant; use of the drug is discouraged when nursing.

Infants and Children: Not recommended for use by persons under age 18, as it has been shown to interfere with bone development.

Special Concerns: If this drug causes increased sensitivity to sunlight, stop taking the medicine and try to avoid exposure to sunlight for the next week; also wear protective clothing and use a sunblock.

Sparfloxacin should not be taken by a patient whose work makes it impossible to avoid exposure to sunlight. It is important to drink plenty of fluids while taking this antibiotic.

OVERDOSE
Symptoms: No specific ones have been reported.

What to Do: If you have any reason to suspect an overdose, call your doctor, emergency medical services (EMS), or the nearest poison control center.

▼ INTERACTIONS

DRUG INTERACTIONS
The following drugs may interact with sparfloxacin. Consult your doctor for specific advice if you are taking aminophylline, antacids, didanosine, iron supplements, sucralfate, or zinc salts. Also tell your doctor if you are taking any other prescription or over-the-counter drug.

FOOD INTERACTIONS
No known food interactions.

DISEASE INTERACTIONS
Caution is advised when taking sparfloxacin. Consult your doctor if you have any other medical condition. Use of sparfloxacin can cause complications in patients with kidney disease, since this organ works to remove the medication from the body.

≡ SIDE EFFECTS ≡

SERIOUS
Serious reactions to sparfloxacin are rare and include seizures, mental confusion, hallucinations, agitation, nightmares, depression, shortness of breath, unusual swelling in the face or extremities, and loss of consciousness. Also skin burning, redness, blisters, rash, or itching on exposure to sunlight; increased risk of tendinitis or tendon rupture. Call your doctor immediately.

COMMON
Increased sensitivity to sunlight (and increased risk of sunburn) for days following therapy.

LESS COMMON
Diarrhea, nausea and vomiting, stomach pain and upset, gas, headache, dizziness, restlessness, insomnia, changes in taste perception, drowsiness, itching, dry mouth, unusual body aches or pains.

SPIRONOLACTONE

Available in: Tablets
Available OTC? No   **As Generic?** Yes
Drug Class: Potassium-sparing diuretic

▼ USAGE INFORMATION

WHY IT'S PRESCRIBED
As adjunctive (supplementary) treatment with other diuretics to increase excretion of sodium and water in the urine while conserving potassium. Spironolactone may be used on its own in patients with liver disease or primary hyperaldosteronism, a life-threatening disorder that occurs when the adrenal glands secrete too much of the hormone aldosterone.

HOW IT WORKS
Spironolactone blocks the effect of aldosterone in the kidneys to increase excretion of sodium and water in the urine while conserving potassium. In conjunction with thiazide or loop diuretics, it reduces the overall fluid volume in the body, which helps to control symptoms of liver disease, heart disease, and kidney disease.

▼ DOSAGE GUIDELINES

RANGE AND FREQUENCY
Adults: 100 to 400 mg a day in 2 to 4 doses. Children: 1 to 3 mg per 2.2 lbs (1 kg) of body weight, in 1 to 4 doses a day.

ONSET OF EFFECT
1 to 2 days.

DURATION OF ACTION
2 to 3 days.

DIETARY ADVICE
Take it with meals to enhance absorption.

STORAGE
Store in a tightly sealed container away from heat and direct light.

MISSED DOSE
Take it as soon as you remember. If it is near the time for the next dose, skip the missed dose and resume your regular dosage schedule. Do not double the next dose.

STOPPING THE DRUG
The decision to stop taking the drug should be made by your doctor.

PROLONGED USE
You should see your doctor periodically for tests if you take this medicine for a prolonged period.

≣ SIDE EFFECTS ≣

SERIOUS
Skin rash or itching, shortness of breath, cough or hoarseness, fever or chills, pain in lower back or side, painful or difficult urination. Call your doctor immediately.

COMMON
Nausea, vomiting, diarrhea.

LESS COMMON
Dizziness, headache, sweating, decreased sexual ability, breast tenderness, breast enlargement in men, increased hair growth in females, irregular menstrual periods.

▼ PRECAUTIONS

Over 60: No special precautions are warranted.

Driving and Hazardous Work: The use of spironolactone should not impair your ability to perform such tasks safely.

Alcohol: No special warnings.

Pregnancy: This drug has not been shown to cause birth defects in animals; human tests have not been done. In any case, spironolactone is not usually prescribed during pregnancy.

Breast Feeding: Spironolactone passes into breast milk but has not been reported to cause problems. Consult your doctor for advice about its use while nursing.

Infants and Children: No special problems are expected.

OVERDOSE
Symptoms: Acute electrolyte imbalance causing central nervous system disturbances.

What to Do: An overdose of spironolactone is unlikely to be life-threatening. However, if someone takes a much larger dose than prescribed, call your doctor, emergency medical services (EMS), or the nearest poison control.

▼ INTERACTIONS

DRUG INTERACTIONS
Consult your doctor for specific advice if you are taking cyclosporine, potassium-containing medicines or supplements, digoxin, or lithium. Also, since angiotensin-converting enzyme (ACE) inhibitors block aldosterone production, spironolactone is not useful in patients taking this type of medication.

FOOD INTERACTIONS
Avoid consuming large servings of high-potassium foods, which include bananas, melons, prunes, citrus fruits and juices (and most fruits in general), avocados, potatoes, nuts, baked beans, brussels sprouts, and skim milk.

DISEASE INTERACTIONS
Caution is advised when taking spironolactone. Consult your doctor if you have any of the following: kidney stones, menstrual problems, breast enlargement, liver disease, or kidney disease.

SPIRONOLACTONE/HYDROCHLOROTHIAZIDE

BRAND NAMES

Aldactazide, Spirozide

Available in: Tablets
Available OTC? No **As Generic?** Yes
Drug Class: Diuretic combination

▼ USAGE INFORMATION

WHY IT'S PRESCRIBED
To treat edema (swelling of body tissues resulting from excess salt and water retention) and to control high blood pressure.

HOW IT WORKS
Spironolactone, a potassium-sparing diuretic, blocks the effect of aldosterone—a hormone that regulates sodium and potassium levels in the body—in the kidneys to increase excretion of sodium and water in the urine while conserving potassium. Hydrochlorothiazide, a thiazide diuretic, increases the excretion of sodium and water in the urine. By reducing the overall fluid volume in the body, diuretics reduce pressure within the blood vessels.

▼ DOSAGE GUIDELINES

RANGE AND FREQUENCY
Adults: 1 to 4 tablets a day, usually taken as a single dose.

ONSET OF EFFECT
Within 2 hours.

DURATION OF ACTION
24 hours.

DIETARY ADVICE
Take it in the morning after breakfast.

STORAGE
Store in a tightly sealed container away from heat, moisture, and direct light.

MISSED DOSE
Take it as soon as you remember. However, if it is near the time for the next dose, skip the missed dose and resume your regular dosage schedule. Do not double the next dose.

STOPPING THE DRUG
Take it as prescribed for the full treatment period. The decision to stop taking the drug should be made in consultation with your physician.

PROLONGED USE
See your doctor regularly for tests and examinations if you must take this medication for a prolonged period. If you are taking this medication for high blood pressure, lifelong therapy may be necessary.

▼ PRECAUTIONS

Over 60: No special problems are expected.

Driving and Hazardous Work: The use of this drug should not impair your ability to perform such tasks safely.

Alcohol: No special precautions are necessary.

Pregnancy: This medication should not be taken during pregnancy unless recommended by your physician. Other diuretics are preferred.

Breast Feeding: Spironolactone and hydrochlorothiazide pass into breast milk; avoid or discontinue usage during the first month of breast feeding.

Infants and Children: This drug is seldom prescribed for children and infants.

Special Concerns: If you are taking this medicine to control high blood pressure, you should also follow your doctor's advice on weight control, diet, and exercise. Avoid exposure to sunlight until you determine how the medicine affects you. Spironolactone sometimes causes enlarged breasts in men and irregular menstrual periods in women.

OVERDOSE
Symptoms: Acute electrolyte imbalance causing central nervous system disturbances, fainting, lethargy, dizziness, drowsiness, confusion, gastrointestinal irritation.

What to Do: Call your doctor, emergency medical services (EMS), or the nearest poison control center immediately.

▼ INTERACTIONS

DRUG INTERACTIONS
Consult your doctor for specific advice if you are taking ACE inhibitors, cyclosporine, any potassium-containing medicines or supplements, cholestyramine, colestipol, digitalis drugs, or lithium.

FOOD INTERACTIONS
Avoid potassium-rich foods and beverages, such as apple, orange, or other citrus fruit juices.

DISEASE INTERACTIONS
Consult your doctor if you have diabetes mellitus, a history of gout or kidney stones, heart or blood vessel disease, systemic lupus erythematosus, liver disease, kidney disease, or pancreatitis.

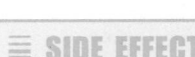
SIDE EFFECTS

SERIOUS
Skin rash, hives, palpitations, lightheadedness, unusual bleeding. Call your doctor immediately.

COMMON
Fluid depletion leading to dizziness, especially when rising from a sitting or lying position.

LESS COMMON
Gout, increased blood sugar levels, breast enlargement in men, decreased sexual ability, increased sensitivity of the skin to sunlight.

STAVUDINE (D4T)

Available in: Capsules
Available OTC? No   **As Generic?** No
Drug Class: Antiviral

▼ USAGE INFORMATION

WHY IT'S PRESCRIBED
To treat HIV (human immunodeficiency virus) infection. While not a cure for HIV infection, this drug may suppress the replication of the virus and delay the progression of the disease.

HOW IT WORKS
Stavudine (d4T) interferes with the activity of enzymes needed for the replication of DNA in viral cells, thus preventing the virus from reproducing.

▼ DOSAGE GUIDELINES

RANGE AND FREQUENCY
Adults and teenagers weighing 132 lbs or more: 40 mg, 2 times a day. Adults and teenagers weighing up to 132 lbs: 30 mg, 2 times a day. Doses of 20 mg, 2 times a day, are sometimes used in patients with advanced HIV disease or mild peripheral neuropathy. Stavudine is usually given in combination with other antiretroviral drugs.

ONSET OF EFFECT
Unknown. With most antiretroviral drugs, an early response can be seen within the first few days of therapy, but the maximum effect may take 12 to 16 weeks.

DURATION OF ACTION
Unknown. Effects of the drug may be prolonged if stavudine is used in combination with other effective drugs and the virus is maximally suppressed.

DIETARY ADVICE
Drink plenty of fluids.

STORAGE
Store in a tightly sealed container away from heat and direct light.

MISSED DOSE
Take it as soon as you remember. However, if it is near the time for the next dose, skip the missed dose and resume your regular dosage schedule. Do not double the next dose.

STOPPING THE DRUG
The decision to stop taking the drug should be made in consultation with your physician.

PROLONGED USE
See your doctor regularly for tests and examinations if you must take this medicine for a prolonged period.

▼ PRECAUTIONS

Over 60: No special studies have been done on older patients. A lower dose may be warranted, especially if kidney function is impaired.

Driving and Hazardous Work: Do not drive or engage in hazardous work until you determine how the medicine affects you.

Alcohol: Avoid alcohol if liver function is impaired.

Pregnancy: Stavudine has been shown to cause birth defects in animals. Human studies have not been done. Nevertheless, stavudine is increasingly being used in combination with other antiretroviral drugs to treat pregnant HIV-infected women.

Breast Feeding: It is unknown whether stavudine passes into breast milk; however, women infected with HIV should not breast-feed, to avoid transmitting the virus to an uninfected child.

Infants and Children: It is not known whether stavudine causes different or more severe side effects in infants and children than it does in older persons.

Special Concerns: Use of stavudine does not reduce the risk of passing the AIDS virus to others. Take appropriate preventive measures.

OVERDOSE
Symptoms: No cases of overdose have been reported.

What to Do: An overdose of stavudine is unlikely to occur. Nonetheless, if you have any reason to suspect an overdose, call your doctor, emergency medical services (EMS), or the nearest poison control center.

▼ INTERACTIONS

DRUG INTERACTIONS
Consult your doctor for advice if you are taking any other prescription or over-the-counter medication, especially chloramphenicol, cisplatin, dapsone, didanosine, ethambutol, ethionamide, hydralazine, isoniazid, lithium, metronidazole, nitrofurantoin, phenytoin, vincristine, or zalcitabine.

FOOD INTERACTIONS
No known food interactions.

DISEASE INTERACTIONS
Caution is advised when taking stavudine. Consult your doctor if you have pancreatitis or peripheral neuropathy. Use of stavudine may cause complications in patients with kidney or liver disease, because these organs work to remove the drug from the body.

SIDE EFFECTS

SERIOUS
Burning, tingling, pain, or numbness in hands or feet. Also fever, muscle aches, joint pain, skin rash, nausea, vomiting, severe abdominal pain, unusual fatigue. Call your doctor immediately.

COMMON
No common side effects are associated with the use of stavudine.

LESS COMMON
Diarrhea, insomnia, headache, loss of appetite, general weakness and loss of energy.

SUCRALFATE

Available in: Oral suspension, tablets
Available OTC? No   **As Generic?** Yes
Drug Class: Antiulcer/antireflux agent

▼ USAGE INFORMATION

WHY IT'S PRESCRIBED
To treat and prevent ulcers of the duodenum, the first portion of the small intestine located just after the stomach in the digestive tract.

HOW IT WORKS
Sucralfate coats the surface of an ulcer, protecting the tissue from irritation by stomach acids, digestive enzymes, bile salts, and other substances that are present in the stomach and duodenum.

▼ DOSAGE GUIDELINES

RANGE AND FREQUENCY
Suspension— 1 g, 4 times a day, 1 hour before each meal and at bedtime, or 2 g, 2 times a day, upon waking and at bedtime. Tablets— To treat ulcer: 1 g, 4 times a day, 1 hour before each meal and at bedtime. To prevent the recurrence of duodenal ulcers: 1 g, 2 times a day on an empty stomach.

ONSET OF EFFECT
Unknown.

DURATION OF ACTION
Up to 6 hours.

DIETARY ADVICE
This medication should be taken without food and with an 8 oz glass of water.

STORAGE
Store in a tightly sealed container away from heat and direct light. Do not refrigerate the liquid form; also keep it from freezing.

MISSED DOSE
Take it as soon as you remember. If it is near the time for the next dose, skip the missed dose and resume your regular dosage schedule. Do not double the next dose.

STOPPING THE DRUG
Take the drug as prescribed for the full treatment period, even if you begin to feel better before the scheduled end of therapy.

PROLONGED USE
You should see your doctor regularly for tests and examinations if you take this drug for a prolonged period.

▼ PRECAUTIONS

Over 60: There is no specific information about the use of sucralfate in older persons. It is not expected to produce side effects different from those in younger persons.

Driving and Hazardous Work: Do not drive or engage in hazardous work until you determine how the medicine affects you.

Alcohol: Avoid alcohol while using this drug.

Pregnancy: Sucralfate has not caused birth defects in animals. Human studies have not been done. Before you use sucralfate, tell your doctor if you are pregnant or plan to become pregnant.

Breast Feeding: Sucralfate may pass into breast milk but has not been shown to cause problems in nursing babies. Consult your doctor for specific advice.

Infants and Children: In limited trials sucralfate has not been shown to cause problems in children. The dose must be determined by your pediatrician.

Special Concerns: Take other medications at least 2 hours before or after taking sucralfate. Do not take antacids within 30 minutes of taking sucralfate. Regular exercise and intake of dietary fiber along with plenty of fluid can help to prevent drug-induced constipation.

OVERDOSE
Symptoms: No specific ones have been reported.

What to Do: An overdose of sucralfate is unlikely to be life-threatening. However, if someone takes a much larger dose than prescribed, call your doctor, emergency medical services (EMS), or the nearest poison control center.

▼ INTERACTIONS

DRUG INTERACTIONS
Consult your doctor for specific advice if you are taking ciprofloxacin, digoxin, norfloxacin, ofloxacin, phenytoin, theophylline, or any antacid or other drug that contains aluminum. Consult your doctor or pharmacist for advice if you are taking any over-the-counter drug.

FOOD INTERACTIONS
No known food interactions.

DISEASE INTERACTIONS
Caution is advised when taking sucralfate. Consult your doctor if you have a history of gastrointestinal tract obstruction or kidney failure.

≡ SIDE EFFECTS ≡

SERIOUS
Drowsiness, seizures. Call your doctor immediately.

COMMON
Constipation.

LESS COMMON
Backache, diarrhea, dizziness or lightheadedness, dry mouth, indigestion, nausea, stomach pain or cramps, skin rash, hives, or itching.

SULFACETAMIDE

Available in: Ophthalmic solution, ointment
Available OTC? No   **As Generic?** Yes
Drug Class: Anti-infective

▼ USAGE INFORMATION

WHY IT'S PRESCRIBED
To treat bacterial conjunctivitis (inflammation of the mucous membranes that line the inner surface of the eyelids and whites of the eyes) and other eye infections.

HOW IT WORKS
Sulfacetamide inhibits the spread of bacteria by preventing the synthesis of folic acid, which is necessary for bacterial growth and multiplication.

▼ DOSAGE GUIDELINES

RANGE AND FREQUENCY
Adults and teenagers— Solution: 1 drop, 4 to 6 times per day. Ointment: Apply 3 to 4 times per day. Infants and children— Both the use and dosage must be determined by your doctor.

ONSET OF EFFECT
Unknown.

DURATION OF ACTION
Unknown.

DIETARY ADVICE
This medication can be used without regard to diet.

STORAGE
Store in a tightly sealed container away from heat, moisture, and direct light. Do not allow it to freeze.

MISSED DOSE
Apply it as soon as you remember. If it is near the time for the next dose, skip the missed dose and resume your regular dosage schedule. Do not double the next dose.

STOPPING THE DRUG
Use this drug as prescribed for the full treatment period, even if you begin to feel better before the scheduled end of therapy.

PROLONGED USE
You should see your doctor regularly for tests and examinations if you use this drug for a prolonged period.

▼ PRECAUTIONS

Over 60: No special problems are expected.

Driving and Hazardous Work: The use of sulfacetamide should not impair your ability to perform such tasks safely.

Alcohol: No special precautions are necessary.

Pregnancy: Sulfacetamide has not been shown to cause problems during pregnancy. Before you take sulfacetamide, tell your doctor if you are pregnant or plan to become pregnant.

Breast Feeding: Sulfacetamide has not been reported to cause problems in nursing babies. Consult your doctor for advice.

Infants and Children: This drug is not recommended for use by infants under the age of 2 months.

Special Concerns: To use the eye drops or the ointment, first wash your hands. Tilt your head back. Gently apply pressure to the inside corner of the eyelid and with the index finger of the same hand, pull downward on the lower eyelid to make a space. Drop the medicine or put a short strip of ointment (about ⅓ inch long) into this space and close your eye. Apply pressure for 1 or 2 minutes while keeping the eye closed without blinking. Then wash your hands again. Make sure the tip of the dropper or the applicator does not touch your eye, finger, or any other surface. If your symptoms do not improve in a few days or if they become worse, check with your doctor.

OVERDOSE
Symptoms: No specific ones have been reported.

What to Do: An overdose of sulfacetamide is unlikely to be life-threatening. If a large volume enters the eye, flush with water. If someone accidentally ingests the medicine, call your doctor, emergency medical services (EMS), or the nearest poison control.

▼ INTERACTIONS

DRUG INTERACTIONS
Other drugs may interact with sulfacetamide. Consult your doctor for specific advice if you are taking eye preparations containing silver, such as silver nitrate.

FOOD INTERACTIONS
No known food interactions.

DISEASE INTERACTIONS
Caution is advised when taking sulfacetamide. Consult your doctor if you have any other medical condition.

SIDE EFFECTS

SERIOUS
No serious side effects have been reported.

COMMON
Eye itching, redness, swelling, and other signs of irritation not present before use of the medicine. Stop using the medication and call your doctor.

LESS COMMON
No less-common side effects have been reported.

SULFASALAZINE

BRAND NAMES

Azaline, Azulfidine,
Azulfidine EN-Tabs

Available in: Tablets, enteric-coated tablets
Available OTC? No   **As Generic?** Yes
Drug Class: Anti-infective/sulfa drug; anti-inflammatory agent

▼ USAGE INFORMATION

WHY IT'S PRESCRIBED
To prevent and treat inflammatory bowel disease (ulcerative colitis, Crohn's disease).

HOW IT WORKS
The exact mechanism of action is unknown. One explanation is that it acts as an anti-inflammatory in the bowel. It also has antibiotic properties that may be important in changing the bacteria in the bowel.

▼ DOSAGE GUIDELINES

RANGE AND FREQUENCY
Adults and teenagers: To start, 500 to 1,000 mg, 3 or 4 times a day. The dose may be decreased to 500 mg, 4 times a day, to reduce the incidence of gastrointestinal side effects. Children age 2 and over: To start, 3 to 4.55 mg per lb of body weight.

ONSET OF EFFECT
Unknown.

DURATION OF ACTION
Unknown.

DIETARY ADVICE
Take it with or immediately following meals. Take each dose with a full glass of water, and consume several additional glasses of water during the day to reduce the chance of side effects.

STORAGE
Store in a tightly sealed container away from heat, moisture, and direct light.

MISSED DOSE
Take it as soon as you remember. If it is near the time for the next dose, skip the missed dose and resume your regular dosage schedule. Do not double the next dose.

STOPPING THE DRUG
Take it as prescribed for the full treatment period.

PROLONGED USE
Sulfasalazine can be used for as long as it is needed; see your doctor for periodic evaluation if prolonged use is necessary.

▼ PRECAUTIONS

Over 60: No special problems are expected.

Driving and Hazardous Work: Do not drive or engage in hazardous work until you determine how the medicine affects you.

Alcohol: No special precautions are necessary.

Pregnancy: Adequate studies of use during pregnancy have not been done, although no problems have been reported. Consult your doctor for specific advice.

Breast Feeding: Small amounts of sulfasalazine pass into breast milk; use of this drug is not recommended while nursing, unless benefits clearly outweigh potential risks. Consult your doctor for advice.

Infants and Children: Not recommended for use by children under age 2.

Special Concerns: Since some patients experience sensitivity to sunlight, take preventive measures when starting therapy: use sunscreens, wear protective clothing, and avoid exposure to the sun. Be careful when brushing or flossing your teeth, because sulfasalazine can increase the risk of mouth infections. The drug

may also turn skin, urine, or contact lenses yellow.

OVERDOSE
Symptoms: Nausea, vomiting, stomach upset, blood in urine, decreased urine volume, low back pain; in more serious cases, extreme drowsiness or seizures.

What to Do: Call your doctor, emergency medical services (EMS), or the nearest poison control center immediately.

▼ INTERACTIONS

DRUG INTERACTIONS
Consult your doctor for specific advice if you are taking acetaminophen, acetohydroxamic acid, alfentanil, amiodarone, aminophylline, anabolic steroids, androgens, antithyroid drugs, anticoagulants, oral antidiabetics, caffeine, carbamazepine, carmustine, chloramphenicol, chloroquine, oral contraceptives, dantrolene, dapsone, daunorubicin, disulfiram, divalproex, estrogens, etretinate, gold salts, hydroxychloroquine, methotrexate, mercaptopurine, methyldopa, naltrexone, oral contraceptives, phenothiazine, phenytoin, plicamycin, primaquine, procainamide, quinidine, quinine, sulfoxone, or vitamin K.

FOOD INTERACTIONS
No known food interactions.

DISEASE INTERACTIONS
Consult your doctor if you have anemia, another blood problem, G6PD deficiency, kidney disease, liver disease, intestinal or urinary obstruction, or porphyria.

≣ SIDE EFFECTS ≣

SERIOUS
Aching joints and muscles; pain in back, legs or stomach; bloody diarrhea; blue fingernails, lips, or skin; chest pain; cough; breathing difficulty; swallowing difficulty; fever; sore throat; general discomfort; loss of appetite; paleness of skin or redness, peeling, blistering, or loosening of skin; unusual bleeding or bruising; unusual fatigue; yellow discoloration of eyes or skin; increased sensitivity to sunlight. Call your physician immediately.

COMMON
Stomach or abdominal discomfort and cramps, diarrhea, loss of appetite, nausea, vomiting. Call your doctor; these symptoms may be alleviated by lowering the dosage.

LESS COMMON
No less-common side effects have been reported.

SULFINPYRAZONE

BRAND NAME

Anturane

Available in: Capsules, tablets
Available OTC? No   **As Generic?** Yes
Drug Class: Antigout drug

▼ USAGE INFORMATION

WHY IT'S PRESCRIBED
To treat chronic (recurring) gout or gouty arthritis by preventing attacks. (It should not be used for treating acute gout attacks in progress.)

HOW IT WORKS
Gout occurs when too much uric acid builds up in the blood. This leads to the formation of uric-acid-based crystals that are deposited in the joints, causing inflammation and leading to the sharp, excruciating pain of a gout attack. Sulfinpyrazone promotes excretion of excess uric acid from the body and so eases or prevents gout attacks. It also slows the body's removal of antibiotics, thus increasing their levels in the blood and prolonging their duration of action.

▼ DOSAGE GUIDELINES

RANGE AND FREQUENCY
200 to 400 mg a day in 2 doses to start; can be increased to as much as 800 mg a day in 2 doses.

ONSET OF EFFECT
It may take months before this medicine begins to prevent gout attacks.

DURATION OF ACTION
6 to 8 hours.

DIETARY ADVICE
Sulfinpyrazone may be taken with meals or milk to reduce stomach upset.

STORAGE
Store in a tightly sealed container away from heat and direct light.

MISSED DOSE
Take it as soon as you remember. However, if it is near the time for the next dose, skip the missed dose and resume your regular dosage schedule. Do not double the next dose.

STOPPING THE DRUG
The decision to stop taking the drug should be made by your doctor.

PROLONGED USE
You should see your doctor regularly for tests and examinations if you take this drug for a prolonged period.

▼ PRECAUTIONS

Over 60: No special problems are expected.

Driving and Hazardous Work: The use of this drug should not impair your ability to perform such tasks safely.

Alcohol: Avoid alcohol.

Pregnancy: Sulfinpyrazone has not been reported to cause problems during pregnancy. Before you take sulfinpyrazone, tell your doctor if you are pregnant or plan to become pregnant.

Breast Feeding: Sulfinpyrazone may pass into breast milk; caution is advised. Consult your doctor for advice.

Infants and Children: There is no specific information on the use of sulfinpyrazone in children, since it is generally prescribed only for adults.

Special Concerns: Your doctor may advise you to drink 10 to 12 full glasses of fluid every day while you take sulfinpyrazone to help prevent the formation of uric acid kidney stones. Sulfinpyrazone will not relieve a gout attack that has already started. You may also be prescribed another medicine for gout while you take this drug.

OVERDOSE
Symptoms: Nausea, vomiting, diarrhea, stomach pain, clumsiness or unsteadiness, seizures, difficulty breathing, loss of consciousness.

What to Do: Call your doctor, emergency medical services (EMS), or the nearest poison control center immediately.

▼ INTERACTIONS

DRUG INTERACTIONS
Consult your physician for specific advice if you are taking anticoagulants, carbenicillin, cefamandole, cefoperazone, cefotetan, dipyridamole, divalproex, heparin, medicine for pain or inflammation, moxalactam, pentoxifylline, plicamycin, ticarcillin, valproic acid, any cancer medicine, aspirin or other salicylates, or nitrofurantoin.

FOOD INTERACTIONS
None are likely, but a low-purine diet is recommended to reduce the risk of gout attacks. Foods high in purines include anchovies, sardines, legumes, poultry, sweet-breads, liver, kidneys, and other organ meats.

DISEASE INTERACTIONS
Consult your physician if you have any of the following: blood disease, cancer being treated by drugs or radiation, kidney stones or any other kidney disease, stomach ulcer, or any other stomach or intestinal problem.

≡ SIDE EFFECTS ≡

SERIOUS
Shortness of breath, breathing difficulty, tightness in chest, sores, ulcers, or white spots on lips or in mouth, sore throat and fever with or without chills, swollen or painful glands, unusual bleeding or bruising. Call your doctor immediately.

COMMON
Pain in lower back or side, painful or bloody urination.

LESS COMMON
Skin rash; bloody or black stools; high blood pressure; tiny bright red spots on skin; sudden decrease in urine; swelling of face, fingers, feet, or lower legs; unusual fatigue; vomiting of blood or dark material; weight gain.

SULFISOXAZOLE OPHTHALMIC

Available in: Ophthalmic solution, ointment
Available OTC? No   **As Generic?** No
Drug Class: Anti-infective

▼ USAGE INFORMATION

WHY IT'S PRESCRIBED
To treat bacterial conjunctivitis (inflammation of the mucous membranes that line the inner surface of the eyelids and whites of the eyes) and other eye infections.

HOW IT WORKS
Sulfisoxazole inhibits the spread of bacteria by preventing the synthesis of folic acid, which is necessary for bacterial growth and multiplication.

▼ DOSAGE GUIDELINES

RANGE AND FREQUENCY
Solution, adults and children 2 months of age and older: 1 drop 4 times a day. Ointment, adults and children: 3 times a day and at bedtime. All forms, infants up to 2 months of age: Use and dosage must be determined by your doctor.

ONSET OF EFFECT
Unknown.

DURATION OF ACTION
Unknown.

DIETARY ADVICE
This medication can be used without regard to diet.

STORAGE
Store in a tightly sealed container away from heat, moisture, and direct light. Do not allow it to freeze.

MISSED DOSE
Apply it as soon as you remember. If it is near the time for the next dose, skip the missed dose and resume your regular dosage schedule. Do not double the next dose.

STOPPING THE DRUG
Use this drug as prescribed for the full treatment period, even if you begin to feel better before the scheduled end of therapy.

PROLONGED USE
You should see your doctor regularly for tests and examinations if you use this drug for a prolonged period.

▼ PRECAUTIONS

Over 60: No special problems are expected.

Driving and Hazardous Work: The use of ophthalmic sulfisoxazole solution should not impair your ability to perform such tasks safely. The use of the ointment, however, may temporarily but significantly blur vision and may interfere with your ability to drive or perform other sight-dependent tasks.

Alcohol: No special precautions are necessary.

Pregnancy: Ophthalmic sulfisoxazole has not been shown to cause problems during pregnancy. Before you take it, tell your physician if you are pregnant or plan to become pregnant.

Breast Feeding: Ophthalmic sulfisoxazole has not been reported to cause problems in nursing babies. Consult your doctor for advice.

Infants and Children: Use and dosage for infants under the age of 2 months must be determined by your doctor.

Special Concerns: To use the eye drops or the ointment, first wash your hands. Tilt your head back. Gently apply pressure to the inside corner of the eyelid and with the index finger of the same hand, pull downward on the lower eyelid to make a space. Drop the medicine or put a short strip of ointment (about ⅓ inch long) into this space and close your eye. Apply gentle pressure for 1 or 2 minutes while keeping the eye closed without blinking. Then wash your hands again. Make sure the tip of the dropper or the applicator does not touch your eye, finger, or any other surface. If your symptoms do not improve in a few days or if they become worse, check with your doctor.

OVERDOSE
Symptoms: No specific ones have been reported.

What to Do: An overdose of ophthalmic sulfisoxazole is unlikely to be life-threatening. If a large volume enters the eye, flush with water. If someone accidentally ingests the medicine, call your doctor, emergency medical services (EMS), or the nearest poison control center immediately.

▼ INTERACTIONS

DRUG INTERACTIONS
Other drugs may interact with ophthalmic sulfisoxazole. Consult your doctor for specific advice if you are taking eye preparations containing silver, such as silver nitrate.

FOOD INTERACTIONS
No known food interactions.

DISEASE INTERACTIONS
Caution is advised when taking ophthalmic sulfisoxazole. Consult your doctor if you have any other medical condition.

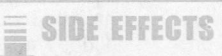
SIDE EFFECTS

SERIOUS
No serious side effects have been reported.

COMMON
Eye itching, redness, swelling, and other signs of irritation not present before use of the medicine. If this occurs, stop using the medication and call your doctor.

LESS COMMON
No less-common side effects have been reported.

SULFISOXAZOLE SYSTEMIC

Available in: Oral suspension, syrup, tablets
Available OTC? No   **As Generic?** Yes
Drug Class: Anti-infective

▼ USAGE INFORMATION

WHY IT'S PRESCRIBED
To treat bacterial infections, such as middle ear infections or urinary tract infections. It is also used, in combination with other medications, to treat malaria.

HOW IT WORKS
Sulfisoxazole kills bacterial cells by preventing them from utilizing folic acid, a vitamin essential to cell growth and reproduction.

▼ DOSAGE GUIDELINES

RANGE AND FREQUENCY
Adults and teenagers: To start, 2,000 to 4,000 mg for first dose. Then 750 to 1,500 mg, 6 times a day, or 1,000 to 2,000 mg, 4 times a day. Children over 2 months of age: To start, 34 mg per lb of body weight. Then 11.4 mg per lb, 6 times a day, or 37.5 mg per lb, 4 times a day.

ONSET OF EFFECT
Unknown.

DURATION OF ACTION
Unknown.

DIETARY ADVICE
Take it with or immediately after meals. Each dose should be taken with a full glass of water, and several additional glasses of water should be consumed daily to decrease the chance of side effects.

STORAGE
Store in a tightly sealed container away from heat, moisture, and direct light.

MISSED DOSE
Take it as soon as you remember. If it is near the time for the next dose, skip the missed dose and resume your regular dosage schedule. Do not double the next dose.

STOPPING THE DRUG
Take it as prescribed for the full treatment period, even if you feel better before the scheduled end of therapy.

PROLONGED USE
See your doctor regularly for tests and examinations if you take it for a prolonged period.

▼ PRECAUTIONS

Over 60: Adverse reactions may be more likely and more severe in older patients.

Driving and Hazardous Work: Do not drive or engage in hazardous work until you determine how the medicine affects you.

Alcohol: No special precautions are necessary.

Pregnancy: Adequate human studies have not been done. Before taking sulfisoxazole, tell your doctor if you are pregnant or plan to become pregnant.

Breast Feeding: Sulfisoxazole passes into breast milk; avoid or discontinue use while breast feeding.

Infants and Children: Not recommended for use by infants under the age of 2 months.

Special Concerns: Since some patients experience sensitivity to sunlight, take preventive measures when starting therapy: use sunscreens, wear protective clothing, and avoid exposure to the sun. Be careful when brushing or flossing your teeth, because sulfisoxazole can increase the risk of mouth infections. If your symptoms do not improve or become worse in a few days, consult your doctor.

OVERDOSE
Symptoms: Loss of appetite, nausea, vomiting, dizziness, headache, drowsiness, loss of consciousness, blood in the urine, decreased urination, low back pain, yellow discoloration of the eyes or skin.

What to Do: Call your doctor, emergency medical services (EMS), or the nearest poison control center immediately.

▼ INTERACTIONS

DRUG INTERACTIONS
Consult your doctor for specific advice if you are taking acetaminophen, acetohydroxamic acid, amiodarone, anabolic steroids, androgens, antithyroid drugs, anticoagulants, oral antidiabetics, carbamazepine, carmustine, chloroquine, oral contraceptives, dantrolene, dapsone, daunorubicin, disulfiram, divalproex, estrogens, etretinate, gold salts, hydroxychloroquine, methenamine, methotrexate, mercaptopurine, methyldopa, naltrexone, oral contraceptives, phenothiazines, phenytoin, plicamycin, primaquine, procainamide, quinidine, quinine, sulfoxone, or vitamin K.

FOOD INTERACTIONS
No known food interactions.

DISEASE INTERACTIONS
Consult your doctor if you have anemia, another blood problem, G6PD deficiency, kidney disease, liver disease, or porphyria.

≡ SIDE EFFECTS ≡

SERIOUS
Itching; skin rash; aching joints and muscles; difficulty swallowing; pale skin or reddened, blistered, and peeling skin; sore throat and fever; unusual bleeding or bruising; unusual fatigue; yellow discoloration of the eyes or skin; pain in stomach or abdomen; bloody urine; greatly increased or decreased urine output; pain or burning while urinating; unusual thirst; lower back pain; mood or mental changes; swelling in the neck; increased sensitivity to sunlight. Call your doctor right away.

COMMON
Dizziness, diarrhea, headache, loss of appetite, nausea, vomiting, fatigue. Call your doctor. These symptoms may be alleviated by lowering the dosage.

LESS COMMON
No less-common side effects have been reported.

SULFUR TOPICAL

Available in: Cream, lotion, ointment, bar soap
Available OTC? Yes   **As Generic?** Yes
Drug Class: Acne drug

▼ USAGE INFORMATION

WHY IT'S PRESCRIBED
To treat skin conditions including acne, seborrheic dermatitis, and scabies.

HOW IT WORKS
Topical sulfur is lethal to various strains of bacteria (which are a primary cause of acne), fungus, parasites, and other types of microorganisms. It also promotes softening, dissolution, and peeling of hard, scaly, roughened, or irregular surface skin.

▼ DOSAGE GUIDELINES

RANGE AND FREQUENCY
For acne, lotion, cream, or bar soap: Use on skin as needed. To use the soap, work up a rich lather using warm water. Wash the affected area, rinse thoroughly, apply again and rub in gently for a few minutes. Remove excess lather with a towel or tissue, without rinsing. Lotion: Apply 2 or 3 times a day. Ointment: Apply the 0.5% ointment as needed. Wash the affected area with soap and water and dry thoroughly before application. For seborrheic dermatitis: Use 1 or 2 times a day as directed on the package instructions. For scabies: Apply the 6% ointment every night for 3 nights. The ointment should be applied to the entire body from the neck down. You may bathe before each application and should bathe 24 hours after the last application.

ONSET OF EFFECT
Unknown.

DURATION OF ACTION
Unknown.

DIETARY ADVICE
Topical sulfur can be used without regard to diet.

STORAGE
Store in a tightly sealed container away from heat and direct light. Keep the cream, lotion, and ointment forms from freezing.

MISSED DOSE
Resume your regular dosage schedule with the next application. Do not double the next dose.

STOPPING THE DRUG
If you are using sulfur by prescription, the decision to stop taking the drug should be made by your doctor. If you are using it without prescription, you may stop taking the drug when your skin has cleared; however, it is likely that the condition will recur.

PROLONGED USE
If prescribed, do not use sulfur for longer than your doctor recommends.

▼ PRECAUTIONS

Over 60: No special precautions required.

Driving and Hazardous Work: No special precautions are necessary.

Alcohol: No special precautions are necessary.

Pregnancy: Sulfur has not been shown to cause birth defects or other problems during pregnancy. Before you use sulfur, tell your doctor if you are pregnant or plan to become pregnant.

Breast Feeding: Topical sulfur has not been reported to cause problems in nursing infants. Consult your doctor for specific advice.

Infants and Children: Use and dosage for children must be determined by your pediatrician.

Special Concerns: Anyone with a history of allergy to sulfur and other ingredients in the medication should not use this product. Keep sulfur away from the eyes. If you accidentally get some of the medicine in your eyes, flush them thoroughly with water.

OVERDOSE
Symptoms: Excessive application of topical sulfur may lead to more-severe irritation of the skin.

What to Do: If topical sulfur is accidentally ingested, call your doctor, emergency medical services (EMS), or the nearest poison control center immediately.

▼ INTERACTIONS

DRUG INTERACTIONS
Consult your doctor for specific advice if you are using abrasive soaps or cleansers; alcohol-containing preparations; any other acne agent; any preparation containing a peeling agent such as benzoyl peroxide, salicylic acid, alpha hydroxy acids, sulfur, or vitamin A; or soaps, medicated cosmetics, or other cosmetics that dry the skin. Also tell your doctor if you are using any other prescription or over-the-counter drug for a skin condition.

FOOD INTERACTIONS
No known food interactions.

DISEASE INTERACTIONS
You should not use sulfur if you have had a prior allergic reaction to it.

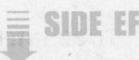
SIDE EFFECTS

SERIOUS
No serious side effects have been reported.

COMMON
Mild redness and peeling of skin.

LESS COMMON
Skin irritation or allergy with redness, peeling, burning, stinging, itching, or rash. Contact your doctor.

SULINDAC

BRAND NAMES

Apo-Sulin, Clinoril, Novo-Sundac

Available in: Tablets
Available OTC? No   **As Generic?** Yes
Drug Class: Nonsteroidal anti-inflammatory drug (NSAID)

▼ USAGE INFORMATION

WHY IT'S PRESCRIBED
To treat mild to moderate pain and inflammation caused by tendinitis, arthritis, bursitis, gout, soft tissue injuries, migraine and other vascular headaches, menstrual cramps, and other conditions. When patients fail to respond to one NSAID, another may be tried. The greatest effectiveness often requires trial and error of several different NSAIDs.

HOW IT WORKS
NSAIDs work by interfering with the formation of prostaglandins, naturally occurring substances in the body that cause inflammation and make nerves more sensitive to pain impulses. NSAIDs also have other modes of action that are less well understood.

▼ DOSAGE GUIDELINES

RANGE AND FREQUENCY
Adults: 150 mg, 2 times a day, up to a maximum dose of 200 mg, 2 times a day. For children's dose, consult your pediatrician.

ONSET OF EFFECT
Initial effect occurs within several hours; full effect occurs in several days.

DURATION OF ACTION
Varies.

DIETARY ADVICE
Take with food; maintain your usual food and fluid intake.

STORAGE
Store in a tightly sealed container away from heat, moisture, and direct light.

MISSED DOSE
Take it as soon as you remember. If it is near the time for the next dose, skip the missed dose and resume your regular dosage schedule. Do not double the next dose.

STOPPING THE DRUG
The decision to stop taking the drug should be made in consultation with your doctor.

PROLONGED USE
Prolonged use can cause gastrointestinal problems, including ulceration and bleeding, kidney dysfunction, and liver inflammation. Consult your doctor about the need for medical examinations and laboratory tests.

▼ PRECAUTIONS

Over 60: Because of the potentially greater consequences of gastrointestinal side effects, the dose of NSAIDs for older patients, especially those over age 70, is often cut in half.

Driving and Hazardous Work: Avoid such activities until you determine how the medicine affects you.

Alcohol: Avoid alcohol when using this medication because it increases the risk of stomach irritation.

Pregnancy: Avoid or discontinue this drug if you are pregnant or are planning to become pregnant.

Breast Feeding: Sulindac passes into breast milk; avoid use while nursing.

Infants and Children: May be used in exceptional circumstances; consult your doctor.

Special Concerns: Because NSAIDs can interfere with blood coagulation, this drug should be stopped at least 3 days prior to any surgery.

OVERDOSE
Symptoms: Severe nausea, vomiting, headache, confusion, seizures.

What to Do: Call your doctor, emergency medical services (EMS), or the nearest poison control center immediately.

▼ INTERACTIONS

DRUG INTERACTIONS
Do not take this drug with aspirin or any other NSAIDs without your doctor's approval. In addition, consult your doctor if you are taking antihypertensives, steroids, anticoagulants, antibiotics, itraconazole or ketoconazole, plicamycin, penicillamine, valproic acid, phenytoin, cyclosporine, digitalis drugs, lithium, methotrexate, probenecid, triamterene, or zidovudine.

FOOD INTERACTIONS
No known food interactions.

DISEASE INTERACTIONS
Caution is advised when taking sulindac. Consult your doctor if you have any of the following: bleeding problems, inflammation or ulcers of the stomach and intestines, diabetes mellitus, systemic lupus erythematosus (SLE, lupus), anemia, asthma, epilepsy, Parkinson's disease, kidney stones, or a history of heart disease or alcohol abuse. Use of sulindac may cause complications in patients with liver or kidney disease, since these organs work together to remove the medication from the body.

 SIDE EFFECTS

SERIOUS
Shortness of breath or wheezing, with or without swelling of legs or other signs of heart failure; chest pain; peptic ulcer disease with vomiting of blood; black, tarry stools; decreasing kidney function. Call your doctor immediately.

COMMON
Nausea, vomiting, heartburn, diarrhea, constipation, headache, dizziness, sleepiness.

LESS COMMON
Ulcers or sores in mouth, depression, rashes or blistering of skin, ringing sound in the ears, unusual tingling or numbness of the hands or feet, seizures, blurred vision. Also elevated potassium levels, decreased blood counts; such problems can be detected by your doctor.

SUMATRIPTAN SUCCINATE

Available in: Tablets, injection, nasal spray
Available OTC? No   **As Generic?** No
Drug Class: Antimigraine/antiheadache drug

▼ USAGE INFORMATION

WHY IT'S PRESCRIBED
To treat severe, acute migraine headaches (sumatriptan is not effective against any other kinds of pain or headache). Because of the risk of side effects, sumatriptan is generally used only when other treatments prove ineffective.

HOW IT WORKS
Sumatriptan appears to activate chemical messengers that cause blood vessels in the brain to constrict, thus lessening the effects of a migraine. It not only relieves the pain, but also nausea, vomiting, sensitivity to sound and light, and other symptoms associated with migraines.

▼ DOSAGE GUIDELINES

RANGE AND FREQUENCY
Tablets— A single dose of 25 to 100 mg taken with fluid is generally effective. If the head-ache returns or there is only partial relief, additional single doses of up to 50 mg may be given at intervals of least 2 hours, but no more than 200 mg should be taken in a 24-hour period. Injection— Initial dose: 6 mg. Additional doses: Another 6 mg injection separated by at least one hour. Nasal spray— A single dose of 5, 10, or 20 mg into one nostril. A 10-mg dose may be achieved by administering a 5-mg dose in each nostril. If the headache returns or there is only partial relief, an additional single dose of up to 20 mg may be given at an interval of least 2 hours, but no more than 40 mg should be taken in a 24-hour period.

ONSET OF EFFECT
Tablets: Within 30 minutes. Injection: Within 10 to 20 minutes. Nasal spray: Within 15 to 30 minutes.

DURATION OF ACTION
Unknown, but peak effect occurs within 1 to 4 hours.

DIETARY ADVICE
The medication can be taken with or without food.

STORAGE
Keep away from heat and direct light; do not allow solution to freeze.

MISSED DOSE
Not applicable, since the drug is taken only when necessary.

STOPPING THE DRUG
Consult your doctor before discontinuing sumatriptan.

PROLONGED USE
Consult your doctor if you have used sumatriptan for three migraine episodes and have not had relief, there is no improvement in symptoms after several weeks of use, or migraines increase in severity or frequency.

▼ PRECAUTIONS

Over 60: No special problems are expected.

Driving and Hazardous Work: Sumatriptan may cause drowsiness or dizziness. Do not drive or engage in hazardous work until you determine how the medication affects you.

Alcohol: No special warnings, although alcohol may trigger or exacerbate migraines.

Pregnancy: Do not use this drug while pregnant.

Breast Feeding: Do not use this drug while nursing.

Infants and Children: Sumatriptan is not recommended for children.

Special Concerns: Rare but serious heart-related problems may occur after sumatriptan use. Anyone at risk for unrecognized coronary artery disease—such as postmenopausal women, men over age 40, or those with heart disease risk factors—should have the first dose of sumatriptan administered in a doctor's office. It should not be used by anyone with any symptoms of active heart disease (chest pain or tightness, shortness of breath).

OVERDOSE
Symptoms: No overdoses have been reported.

What to Do: Although overdose is unlikely, if you take a much larger dose than prescribed, call your doctor, emergency medical services (EMS), or the nearest poison control center immediately.

▼ INTERACTIONS

DRUG INTERACTIONS
Do not take sumatriptan within 24 hours of taking any other migraine drug. Consult your doctor for advice if you are taking antidepressants, selective serotonin reuptake inhibitors (SSRIs), or lithium.

FOOD INTERACTIONS
See Dietary Advice.

DISEASE INTERACTIONS
You should not take sumatriptan if you have a history of coronary artery disease, especially angina, heart attack, Prinzmetal's angina, or uncontrolled hypertension. It should be used with caution in patients with liver disease or severe kidney dysfunction.

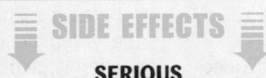

SIDE EFFECTS

SERIOUS
Chest pain (mild to severe) or feeling of heaviness or pressure in the chest; wheezing or shortness of breath, and rapid, shallow, or irregular breathing; puffiness or swelling of the eyelids, face or, lips; hives; intense itching.

COMMON
Pain, burning, or redness at injection site; a general feeling of warmth or heat; a feeling of numbness, tightness, or tingling; mild pain of the jaw, mouth, tongue, throat, nose, or sinuses; dizziness; drowsiness; feeling cold or weak; feeling flushed or lightheaded; muscle aches, cramps, or stiffness; nausea or vomiting.

LESS COMMON
Mild chest pain, heaviness or pressure in the chest or neck, anxiety, feeling tired or ill, vision changes.

TACRINE

Available in: Capsules
Available OTC? No **As Generic?** No
Drug Class: Psychotherapeutic; antidementia agent

▼ USAGE INFORMATION

WHY IT'S PRESCRIBED
To treat mild to moderate Alzheimer's disease.

HOW IT WORKS
Tacrine prevents the breakdown of acetylcholine, a brain chemical crucial to memory. Acetylcholine deficiency is thought to result in memory loss associated with Alzheimer's disease.

▼ DOSAGE GUIDELINES

RANGE AND FREQUENCY
To start, 10 mg, 4 times a day. The dose may be raised to 40 mg, 4 times a day.

ONSET OF EFFECT
Unknown.

DURATION OF ACTION
Unknown.

DIETARY ADVICE
Best taken on an empty stomach, at least 1 hour before or 2 hours after eating. Tacrine can be taken with food to minimize stomach upset, but this will decrease the absorption and effectiveness of the drug.

STORAGE
Store in a tightly sealed container away from heat, moisture, and direct light.

MISSED DOSE
Take it as soon as you remember, unless the time for your next scheduled dose is within the next 2 hours. If so, do not take the missed dose. Take your next scheduled dose at the proper time and resume your regular dosage schedule. Do not double the next dose.

STOPPING THE DRUG
The decision to stop taking the drug should be made in consultation with your doctor.

PROLONGED USE
You should see your doctor regularly for tests and examinations if you must take this drug for a prolonged period.

≡ SIDE EFFECTS ≡

SERIOUS
Clumsiness or unsteadiness, severe vomiting, rapid or pounding heartbeat, slow heartbeat, seizures, elevated liver function tests (detectable by your doctor). Call your doctor right away.

COMMON
Nausea and vomiting, stomach pain or cramps, indigestion, muscle aches or pains, headache, dizziness, loss of appetite, diarrhea.

LESS COMMON
Belching, general feeling of discomfort or illness, rapid breathing, flushed skin, increased urination, increased sweating, watering of the eyes and mouth, insomnia, runny nose, swelling of the feet or lower legs.

▼ PRECAUTIONS

Over 60: No special problems are expected.

Driving and Hazardous Work: Do not drive or engage in hazardous work until you determine how the medicine affects you.

Alcohol: Avoid alcohol.

Pregnancy: Adequate studies on the use of tacrine during pregnancy have not been done. Consult your doctor for specific advice.

Breast Feeding: Tacrine may pass into breast milk and be harmful to the nursing infant; do not use the drug while nursing.

Infants and Children: Tacrine is not intended for use by infants and children.

Special Concerns: Have your blood tested every other week for at least 16 weeks when you start taking tacrine, to see if it is affecting your liver. Do not smoke tobacco products while taking tacrine. Smoking will decrease the effects of tacrine.

OVERDOSE
Symptoms: Sweating and watering of mouth, seizures, increased muscle weakness, low blood pressure, severe nausea or vomiting, fast and weak pulse, large pupils, irregular breathing, slow heartbeat.

What to Do: Call your doctor, emergency medical services (EMS), or the nearest poison control center immediately.

▼ INTERACTIONS

DRUG INTERACTIONS
The following drugs may interact with tacrine. Consult your doctor for advice if you are taking: cimetidine, medicine for inflammation or pain, or theophylline.

FOOD INTERACTIONS
No known food interactions.

DISEASE INTERACTIONS
Caution is advised when taking tacrine. Consult your doctor if you have any of the following: asthma, epilepsy or a history of seizures, heart problems, intestinal blockage, stomach or duodenal ulcer, liver disease, Parkinson's disease, urinary problems, brain disease, or history of a head injury that involved a loss of consciousness.

TACROLIMUS (FK506)

Available in: Capsules, injection
Available OTC? No   **As Generic?** No
Drug Class: Immunosuppressant

▼ USAGE INFORMATION

WHY IT'S PRESCRIBED
To slow down or reduce the natural tendency of the immune system to reject liver or kidney transplants.

HOW IT WORKS
Tacrolimus suppresses the immune system's reaction against foreign tissue by inhibiting the activity of white blood cells, a major component of the immune system's arsenal.

▼ DOSAGE GUIDELINES

RANGE AND FREQUENCY
Adults— Capsules: 0.1 to 0.2 mg per 2.2 lbs (1 kg) of body weight daily in 2 divided doses every 12 hours. Injection: Dosage to be determined by your doctor. Children— 0.15 to 0.2 mg per 2.2 lbs of body weight daily in capsules on a schedule similar to that of adults.

ONSET OF EFFECT
Unknown.

DURATION OF ACTION
Unknown.

DIETARY ADVICE
The oral medication is most effective on an empty stomach; take it 30 minutes before or 2 hours after a meal. It can be taken with a full glass of water to lessen stomach upset. Do not take tacrolimus with grapefruit juice.

STORAGE
Capsules: Store in a tightly sealed container away from heat, moisture, and direct light. Injection: Not applicable; administered only at a health care facility.

MISSED DOSE
Capsules: Take it as soon as you remember. If it is near the time for the next dose, skip the missed dose and resume your regular dosage schedule. Do not double the next dose. Injection: Not applicable; administered by health care professional.

STOPPING THE DRUG
The decision to stop taking the drug should be made by your doctor.

PROLONGED USE
See your doctor regularly for tests and examinations if you take this medication for a prolonged period.

▼ PRECAUTIONS

Over 60: Adverse reactions may be more likely and more severe in older patients.

Driving and Hazardous Work: Do not drive or engage in hazardous work until you determine how the medicine affects you.

Alcohol: Avoid alcohol.

Pregnancy: Very high doses of tacrolimus have caused birth defects in animals. Human studies have not been done. Before you take tacrolimus, tell your doctor if you are pregnant or plan to become pregnant.

Breast Feeding: Tacrolimus passes into breast milk; discontinue breast feeding while taking the drug.

Infants and Children: No special problems have been observed, even though children may actually require higher doses than adults.

Special Concerns: In some cases, tacrolimus has been shown to cause diabetes. Consult your doctor right away if you develop symptoms of increased hunger, thirst, and urination while taking this drug.

OVERDOSE
Symptoms: No acute effects have been reported.

What to Do: Call your doctor, emergency medical services (EMS), or the nearest poison control center immediately.

▼ INTERACTIONS

DRUG INTERACTIONS
Tacrolimus should not be taken within 24 hours of receiving cyclosporine. Avoid live vaccines. Consult your doctor for specific advice if you are taking bromocriptine, cimetidine, clarithromycin, danazol, erythromycin, antifungal drugs, methylprednisolone, metoclopramide, calcium channel blockers, carbamazepine, phenobarbital, phenytoin, rifabutin, rifampin, other immunosuppressants, some vaccinations, aminoglycosides, amphotericin B, or cisplatin.

FOOD INTERACTIONS
Do not take tacrolimus with grapefruit juice.

DISEASE INTERACTIONS
Caution is advised when taking tacrolimus. Consult your doctor if you have a history of high blood pressure, heart problems, kidney disease, or liver disease.

 SIDE EFFECTS

SERIOUS
Increased bleeding, increased bruising, fluid buildup in lungs causing fever, chest pain, difficulty breathing, and cough. Call your doctor immediately.

COMMON
Headache; fever; weakness; tremor; high blood pressure, causing headache and blurred vision; diarrhea; nausea; decreased urination; high blood sugar levels, causing increased thirst, hunger, and urination.

LESS COMMON
Insomnia, swelling of feet or lower legs, numbness or tingling sensations, constipation, loss of appetite, abdominal pain, abdominal swelling due to fluid buildup, painful urination, back pain, electrolyte imbalance causing nausea, diarrhea, muscle weakness, and fatigue.

TAMOXIFEN CITRATE

BRAND NAME

Nolvadex

Available in: Tablets
Available OTC? No   **As Generic?** No
Drug Class: Antiestrogen; antineoplastic (anticancer) agent

▼ USAGE INFORMATION

WHY IT'S PRESCRIBED
To treat breast cancer in wo-men and men; to help reduce the incidence of breast can-cer in women at high risk.

HOW IT WORKS
Tamoxifen blocks the effects of the hormone estrogen on certain organs in the body. Because the growth of some types of breast cancer is stim-ulated by estrogen, tamoxifen interferes with the growth of such tumors.

▼ DOSAGE GUIDELINES

RANGE AND FREQUENCY
For treatment and prevention: 20 mg a day.

ONSET OF EFFECT
Several weeks.

DURATION OF ACTION
Several weeks.

DIETARY ADVICE
It is recommended that tamoxifen be taken after breakfast and after dinner. Swallow the tablet whole with a glass of water.

STORAGE
Store in a tightly sealed con-tainer away from heat, mois-ture, and direct light.

MISSED DOSE
Take it as soon as you remember and resume your regular dosage schedule.

STOPPING THE DRUG
The decision to stop taking the drug should be made by your doctor.

PROLONGED USE
See your doctor regularly for tests and examinations if you take this drug for a prolonged period. Tamoxifen does not prevent all breast cancers, so women taking the drug for prevention should continue to have regular breast exams and mammograms.

▼ PRECAUTIONS

Over 60: No different side effects or problems are expected in older patients.

Driving and Hazardous Work: No special precautions.

Alcohol: No special problems are expected, but you should consult your doctor.

Pregnancy: Tamoxifen may cause miscarriage, birth defects, fetal death, and unex-pected vaginal bleeding, and so should not be taken during pregnancy. Avoid becoming pregnant for at least two months after stopping tamox-ifen. Notify your doctor and stop taking tamoxifen immedi-ately if pregnancy occurs.

Breast Feeding: Tamoxifen may pass into breast milk; do not nurse while taking it.

Infants and Children: Tamox-ifen is not prescribed for infants and children.

Special Concerns: Women should have regular gyneco-logical examinations while tak-ing tamoxifen and for months or years after discontinuing it, since the medication may increase the long-term risk of uterine cancer. Tamoxifen may change or stop a woman's normal menstrual cycle; how-ever, she may still be fertile. A reliable birth control method other than oral contraceptives (barrier method) should therefore be used while tak-ing this drug. Tamoxifen for breast cancer risk reduction has not been studied in women under the age of 35. Risk factors for breast cancer include: early age at first menstruation, late age at first pregnancy, no pregnancies, breast cancer in a first-degree relative, history of previous breast biopsies, or high-risk changes seen on a biopsy.

OVERDOSE
Symptoms: Nausea, vomiting, irregular heartbeat, tremor, dizziness, seizures, exagger-ated reflexes.

What to Do: Call your doctor, emergency medical services (EMS), or the nearest poison control center immediately.

▼ INTERACTIONS

DRUG INTERACTIONS
You should not take tamox-ifen to prevent breast cancer if you are taking anticoagu-lants. Consult your doctor if you are taking antacids, cimetidine, famotidine, ranit-idine, birth control pills.

FOOD INTERACTIONS
No known food interactions.

DISEASE INTERACTIONS
Consult your doctor if you have a medical history that includes any of the following: cataracts or other vision dis-turbances, high blood levels of cholesterol or triglycerides, blood clots, low white blood cell and/or platelet counts. Tamoxifen should not be taken to prevent breast can-cer by women with a history of deep vein thrombosis or pulmonary embolism.

SIDE EFFECTS

SERIOUS
Endometrial cancer (menstrual irregularities, abnormal nonmenstrual vaginal bleeding, changes in vaginal dis-charge, pelvic pain or pressure); deep vein thrombosis and pulmonary embolism (pain or swelling in legs, shortness of breath, sudden chest pain, coughing up blood); cataracts; new breast lumps; confusion, weakness, or drowsiness; yellowish tinge to eyes or skin. Call your doctor promptly.

COMMON
Hot flashes, weight gain.

LESS COMMON
Bone pain, headache, nausea or vomiting, skin dryness or rash, changes in menstrual period, vaginal discharge, itch-ing in genital area of women, depression, erectile dysfunc-tion (impotence) or decreased sexual interest in men. Other side effects include high blood calcium levels and liver dys-function; such problems can be detected by your doctor.

TAMSULOSIN HYDROCHLORIDE

Available in: Capsules
Available OTC? No **As Generic?** No
Drug Class: BPH therapy agent

▼ USAGE INFORMATION

WHY IT'S PRESCRIBED
To treat symptoms of urinary difficulty that occur with benign prostatic hyperplasia (BPH)—a noncancerous enlargement of the prostate gland. BPH is extremely common among men over the age of 50.

HOW IT WORKS
By blocking a specific (alpha) receptor, tamsulosin relaxes muscle tissue in the prostate and the opening of the bladder. Note that tamsulosin will not shrink the prostate; symptoms may worsen and surgery may eventually be required. Unlike other alpha receptor blockers used to treat BPH, tamsulosin is not used to treat hypertension.

▼ DOSAGE GUIDELINES

RANGE AND FREQUENCY
0.4 mg once a day. It should be taken 30 minutes following the same meal each day. If patients fail to respond to the 0.4-mg dose after 2 to 4 weeks of therapy, they may increase the dose to 0.8 mg once a day.

ONSET OF EFFECT
Unknown.

DURATION OF ACTION
Unknown.

DIETARY ADVICE
There are no dietary restrictions. However, tamsulosin should be taken 30 minutes after the same meal every day. Do not chew, crush, or open the capsules.

STORAGE
Store in a tightly sealed container away from heat, moisture, and direct light.

MISSED DOSE
If therapy is discontinued or interrupted for several days at either the 0.4-mg dose or the 0.8-mg dose, therapy should be started again with the 0.4-mg once-daily dose.

STOPPING THE DRUG
Take tamsulosin as prescribed for the full treatment period.

PROLONGED USE
If you take this drug for a prolonged period, see your doctor regularly so that changes in prostate size can be monitored.

▼ PRECAUTIONS

Over 60: No special problems are expected.

Driving and Hazardous Work: Tamsulosin may impair mental functioning, causing drowsiness, lightheadedness, or dizziness, especially when you take the medication for the first time. Caution is advised; for 24 hours after the initial dose, avoid driving or other activities requiring mental alertness. Effects should diminish after several doses.

Alcohol: May increase effects of dizziness or fainting; drink in moderation.

Pregnancy: Tamsulosin is not indicated for use by women.

Breast Feeding: Tamsulosin is not indicated for use by women.

Infants and Children: Tamsulosin is not indicated for use by children.

Special Concerns: The first dose is likely to cause dizziness or lightheadedness. Take the drug at night and get out of bed slowly the next day. Be cautious while exercising and during hot weather. Tell your primary-care physician if you are planning to have surgery requiring general anesthesia, including dental surgery. Do not chew, crush, or open the capsules.

OVERDOSE
Symptoms: An overdose is unlikely to occur. Possible symptoms after an excessive dose may include severe headache or orthostatic hypotension (see Less Common Side Effects).

What to Do: If someone takes a much larger dose than prescribed, keep the patient lying down and call your doctor, emergency medical services (EMS), or the nearest poison control center immediately.

▼ INTERACTIONS

DRUG INTERACTIONS
Tamsulosin should not be used in conjunction with other BPH therapy agents. Consult your doctor if you are taking either cimetidine or warfarin, which may interact with tamsulosin.

FOOD INTERACTIONS
None reported.

DISEASE INTERACTIONS
None reported.

≣ SIDE EFFECTS ≣

SERIOUS
No serious side effects have been reported.

COMMON
Headache, increased susceptibility to infection, joint pain, back pain, muscle pain, dizziness, runny nose, diarrhea, abnormal ejaculation.

LESS COMMON
Mild chest pain, drowsiness, insomnia, decreased libido, sore throat, cough, sinus infection, nausea, mouth pain, vision problems. The drug may also promote orthostatic hypotension (episodes of low blood pressure most likely to occur when getting up quickly from a seated or lying position), which produces symptoms of lightheadedness, dizziness, confusion, or fainting.

TAZAROTENE

Available in: Topical gel
Available OTC? No   **As Generic?** No
Drug Class: Retinoid

▼ USAGE INFORMATION

WHY IT'S PRESCRIBED
To treat psoriasis. Tazarotene is also used to treat mild to moderate acne.

HOW IT WORKS
The exact way in which tazarotene works is unknown. It appears to establish a more normal pattern of growth and shedding of skin cells.

▼ DOSAGE GUIDELINES

RANGE AND FREQUENCY
For psoriasis: Apply to the affected area once a day, in the evening, using enough to cover the lesion with a thin film. Be sure the area is clean and dry before applying. For acne: Apply once a day in the evening. First gently wash and dry your face, then spread a thin film on the area of skin where acne appears. Avoid applying tazarotene near the eyes, eyelids, and mouth.

ONSET OF EFFECT
1 to 4 weeks.

DURATION OF ACTION
Unknown.

DIETARY ADVICE
Tazarotene can be used without regard to diet.

STORAGE
Store in a tightly sealed container away from heat, moisture, and direct light.

MISSED DOSE
If you fail to apply the drug on one day, return to your regular schedule the next day; do not apply an extra amount in an attempt to compensate for the missed dose.

STOPPING THE DRUG
In the treatment of psoriasis, you should apply it for the full treatment period as prescribed by your doctor. For acne, apply the drug for up to 12 weeks as directed by your doctor.

PROLONGED USE
Side effects are more likely with prolonged use.

▼ PRECAUTIONS

Over 60:
No special problems are expected.

Driving and Hazardous Work:
The use of tazarotene should not impair your ability to perform such tasks safely.

Alcohol:
No special precautions are necessary.

Pregnancy:
Tazarotene should not be used if you are pregnant or plan to become pregnant. Adequate birth-control methods should be practiced when tazarotene is used in women of child-bearing age.

Breast Feeding:
Tazarotene may pass into breast milk; caution is advised. Consult your doctor for specific advice.

Infants and Children:
Not recommended for use by children under age 12.

Special Concerns:
If tazarotene comes in contact with your eyes, flush your eyes with large amounts of cool water. If eye irritation persists, contact your doctor. Wash your hands after applying the medication. Do not cover the treated area with tight-fitting clothing or bandages. If the drug causes increased sensitivity to sunlight, wear protective clothing, use a sunblock, and try to avoid exposure to direct sunlight. Avoid sunlamps completely. Caution is advised for all patients with fair skin or who are particularly sensitive to sunlight. Weather extremes, such as wind or cold, may be more irritating to the skin while you use this drug.

When tazarotene is used to treat psoriasis, avoid applying it to normal-appearing areas of skin.

OVERDOSE
Symptoms: Excessive use of tazarotene may lead to skin redness, peeling, or discomfort.

What to Do: An overdose is unlikely to occur. If someone accidentally ingests tazarotene, call your doctor.

▼ INTERACTIONS

DRUG INTERACTIONS
Consult your doctor for advice if you are taking any of the following drugs that may interact with tazarotene: vitamin A supplements; other skin medications, creams, or lotions; drugs that increase your sensitivity to sunlight (such as thiazide diuretics, tetracyclines, fluoroquinolone antibiotics, phenothiazines, or sulfonamides); or products, such as astringents or medicated soaps, that dry the skin.

FOOD INTERACTIONS
No known food interactions.

DISEASE INTERACTIONS
You should not use tazarotene if you have eczema or other chronic skin diseases, or a recent sunburn.

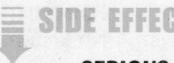

SIDE EFFECTS

SERIOUS
No serious side effects have been reported.

COMMON
Common side effects are limited to the skin. When used for psoriasis: Itching, redness, burning, stinging, worsening of psoriasis, irritation, skin pain. When used for acne: Peeling, burning, stinging, dry skin, redness, itching.

LESS COMMON
When used for psoriasis: Skin rash, peeling or scaling, increased risk of dermatitis caused by external irritants, skin inflammation, cracking, bleeding, dry skin. When used for acne: Skin pain, irritation, cracking, swelling of treated area, skin discoloration.

TELMISARTAN

BRAND NAME

Micardis

Available in: Tablets
Available OTC? No   **As Generic?** No
Drug Class: Antihypertensive/angiotensin II antagonist

▼ USAGE INFORMATION

WHY IT'S PRESCRIBED
To control high blood pressure. This drug appears to have the same benefits as the class of antihypertensive drugs known as "ACE inhibitors," without producing the common side effect (experienced by as many as 30% of patients) of a dry cough. Telmisartan may be used by itself or in conjunction with other antihypertensive drugs.

HOW IT WORKS
Telmisartan blocks the effects of angiotensin II, a naturally occurring substance that causes blood vessels to narrow. Telmisartan causes the blood vessels to dilate, thereby lowering blood pressure and decreasing the workload of the heart.

▼ DOSAGE GUIDELINES

RANGE AND FREQUENCY
To start, 40 mg once a day when used as the only drug to treat hypertension. Usual maintenance dose is 20 to 80 mg daily.

ONSET OF EFFECT
Within 2 weeks.

DURATION OF ACTION
Up to 24 hours.

DIETARY ADVICE
No special restrictions, unless your doctor has advised a low-sodium diet or other dietary modifications to help you control your blood pressure.

STORAGE
Store in a tightly sealed container away from heat, moisture, and direct light.

MISSED DOSE
Take it as soon as you remember. If it is near the time for the next dose, skip the missed dose and resume your regular dosage schedule. Do not double the next dose.

STOPPING THE DRUG
Take it as prescribed for the full treatment period. The decision to stop taking the drug should be made in consultation with your physician.

PROLONGED USE
Lifelong therapy may be necessary. However, if you do change certain health habits (for example, increasing exercise or losing weight), a reduced dose may be possible under a doctor's supervision.

▼ PRECAUTIONS

Over 60: No special problems are expected.

Driving and Hazardous Work: Do not drive or engage in hazardous work until you determine how the medicine affects you.

Alcohol: No special precautions are necessary.

Pregnancy: Telmisartan should not be used by pregnant women. Discontinue taking the drug as soon as possible when pregnancy is detected and discuss treatment alternatives with your doctor.

Breast Feeding: Telmisartan may pass into breast milk; caution is advised. Consult your doctor for advice.

Infants and Children: The safety and effectiveness of use in children have not been established.

Special Concerns: Telmisartan may cause excessively low blood pressure with dizziness or lightheadedness, which is most noticeable when you change position. This may lead to fainting, falls, and injury. Sit or lie down immediately if you feel dizzy or lightheaded. This side effect may be worsened by alcohol, hot weather, dehydration, salt depletion from diuretic use, fever, prolonged standing, prolonged sitting, or exercise.

OVERDOSE
Symptoms: Few cases of overdose have been reported. However, if you take a much larger dose than prescribed, you may experience fainting, dizziness, or a weak pulse that might be very slow or very fast.

What to Do: Call your doctor, emergency medical services (EMS), or the nearest poison control center immediately.

▼ INTERACTIONS

DRUG INTERACTIONS
No clinically significant drug interactions have yet been observed with telmisartan. Consult your doctor for specific advice if you are taking digoxin or any other medication, especially other drugs for high blood pressure. Telmisartan can be taken together with diuretics or other medications for high blood pressure, if your doctor approves.

FOOD INTERACTIONS
No known food interactions.

DISEASE INTERACTIONS
Patients with moderate to severe liver or kidney disease are advised to exercise caution when taking telmisartan.

 SIDE EFFECTS

SERIOUS
No serious side effects are associated with the use of telmisartan. (In clinical trials, the incidence of adverse effects was not significantly greater with the medication than with a placebo.)

COMMON
No common side effects are associated with the use of telmisartan.

LESS COMMON
Headache, dizziness, back pain, upper respiratory tract infection, sore throat, and nasal congestion.

TEMAZEPAM

Available in: Capsules, tablets
Available OTC? No **As Generic?** Yes
Drug Class: Benzodiazepine tranquilizer

▼ USAGE INFORMATION

WHY IT'S PRESCRIBED
To treat insomnia.

HOW IT WORKS
In general, temazepam produces mild sedation by depressing activity in the central nervous system. In particular, temazepam appears to enhance the effect of gamma-aminobutyric acid (GABA), a natural chemical that inhibits the firing of neurons and dampens the transmission of nerve signals, thus decreasing nervous excitation.

▼ DOSAGE GUIDELINES

RANGE AND FREQUENCY
Adults: 15 mg, taken at bedtime. Older adults: To start, 7.5 mg, taken at bedtime. The dose may be increased. Use and dose for children under 18 must be determined by your doctor.

ONSET OF EFFECT
Unknown.

DURATION OF ACTION
Unknown. It may take more than 2 hours.

DIETARY ADVICE
Take it 30 minutes before bedtime with a full glass of water. Temazepam can be taken with food to prevent gastrointestinal upset.

STORAGE
Store in a tightly sealed container away from heat and direct light.

MISSED DOSE
Take it as soon as you remember, unless it is late at night. Do not take the medicine unless your schedule allows a full night's sleep.

STOPPING THE DRUG
Discontinuing the drug abruptly may produce withdrawal symptoms (sleep disruption, nervousness, irritability, diarrhea, abdominal cramps, muscle aches, memory impairment). The dosage should be reduced gradually according to your doctor's instructions.

PROLONGED USE
This medication may slowly lose its effectiveness, and adverse reactions are more likely to occur with prolonged use. You should see your doctor for periodic evaluation if you must take it for an extended time.

▼ PRECAUTIONS

Over 60: Adverse reactions may be more likely and more severe. A lower dose may be warranted.

Driving and Hazardous Work: Do not drive or engage in hazardous work until you determine how the medicine affects you.

Alcohol: Avoid alcohol.

Pregnancy: Use during pregnancy should be avoided if possible. Be sure to tell your doctor if you are pregnant or plan to become pregnant.

Breast Feeding: Temazepam passes into breast milk; do not take it while nursing.

Infants and Children: Safety and effectiveness have not been established for children under age 18.

Special Concerns: Temazepam use can lead to psychological or physical dependence if the drug is not taken in strict accordance with your doctor's instructions. Never take more than the prescribed daily dose.

OVERDOSE
Symptoms: Extreme drowsiness, confusion, slurred speech, slow reflexes, poor coordination, staggering gait, tremor, slowed breathing, loss of consciousness.

What to Do: Call your doctor, emergency medical services (EMS), or the nearest poison control center immediately.

▼ INTERACTIONS

DRUG INTERACTIONS
Consult your physician for advice if you are taking any drugs that depress the central nervous system; these include antihistamines, antidepressants or other psychiatric medications, barbiturates, sedatives, cough medicines, decongestants, and painkillers. Be sure your doctor knows about any over-the-counter drug you may take.

FOOD INTERACTIONS
None reported.

DISEASE INTERACTIONS
Consult your doctor if you have a history of alcohol or drug abuse, stroke or other brain disease, any chronic lung disease, glaucoma, hyperactivity, depression or other mental illness, myasthenia gravis, sleep apnea, epilepsy, porphyria, kidney disease, or liver disease.

SIDE EFFECTS

SERIOUS
Difficulty concentrating, outbursts of anger, other behavior problems, depression, convulsions, hallucinations, low blood pressure (causing faintness or confusion), memory impairment, muscle weakness, skin rash or itching, sore throat, fever and chills, sores or ulcers in throat or mouth, unusual bruising or bleeding, extreme fatigue, yellowish tinge to eyes or skin. Call your doctor immediately.

COMMON
Loss of coordination, unsteady gait, dizziness, lightheadedness, drowsiness, slurred speech.

LESS COMMON
Stomach cramps or pain, vision disturbances, change in sexual desire or ability, constipation or diarrhea, dry mouth or watering mouth, false sense of well-being, rapid or pounding heartbeat, headache, muscle spasms, nausea and vomiting, urinary problems, trembling.

TERAZOSIN

Available in: Tablets, capsules
Available OTC? No **As Generic?** Yes
Drug Class: Antihypertensive; BPH therapy agent

▼ USAGE INFORMATION

WHY IT'S PRESCRIBED
To lower and control high blood pressure (hypertension). It is also used to treat symptoms of urinary difficulty that occur with benign prostatic hyperplasia (BPH).

HOW IT WORKS
Terazosin helps to control hypertension by relaxing blood vessels and permitting them to expand, decreasing blood pressure in the process. When used for BPH, it helps relax the muscles in the prostate gland and the opening of the bladder, improving the passage of urine.

▼ DOSAGE GUIDELINES

RANGE AND FREQUENCY
For high blood pressure: Initially, 1 mg taken at bedtime, then 1 to 5 mg once daily. For children, the dose and frequency must be determined by your pediatrician. For BPH: Initially, 1 mg taken at bedtime, then 5 to 10 mg once daily.

ONSET OF EFFECT
Within 15 minutes, with peak blood pressure effect within 2 to 3 hours. When the drug is used to treat urinary difficulty associated with BPH, the full effect may not be seen for 4 to 6 weeks.

DURATION OF ACTION
24 hours.

DIETARY ADVICE
Terazosin can be taken before, with, or after meals.

STORAGE
Store in a tightly sealed container away from heat, moisture, and direct light.

MISSED DOSE
Take it as soon as possible the same day. If it is the next day, skip the missed dose. Do not double the dose. Resume your regular dosage schedule.

STOPPING THE DRUG
Do not discontinue taking the medication suddenly, even if you start to experience unpleasant side effects. Consult your physician. If terazosin is discontinued for several days, you may need to start therapy over, using the initial dosing regimen.

PROLONGED USE
When taking the medication for hypertension, blood pressure measurement is recommended at regular intervals.

▼ PRECAUTIONS

Over 60: Older persons are generally more sensitive to terazosin and more likely to experience adverse side effects, especially when getting up from a lying or seated position. Rise slowly to minimize symptoms.

Driving and Hazardous Work: Terazosin may impair mental ability, causing drowsiness, lightheadedness, or dizziness, especially when you take the medication for the first time. Caution is advised; for 24 hours after the initial dose, avoid driving or other activities requiring mental alertness. Effects should diminish after several doses.

Alcohol: May increase effects of dizziness or fainting; drink in strict moderation, if at all.

Pregnancy: Well-controlled studies have not been done. Consult your physician if you are pregnant or plan to become pregnant.

Breast Feeding: It is not known whether terazosin passes into breast milk. Consult your physician for specific advice.

Infants and Children: Adequate studies of terazosin use in this age group have not been performed. Discuss the risks and benefits with your pediatrician.

Special Concerns: Be sure to notify your doctor if you are taking nonprescription medications for asthma, colds, cough, allergy, or appetite suppression. These drugs can increase blood pressure and cause other complications if they are taken with terazosin.

OVERDOSE
Symptoms: Extremely low blood pressure (hypotension), with accompanying fatigue, weakness, head-ache, palpitations, fainting, or dizziness.

What to Do: Call your doctor, emergency medical services (EMS), or the nearest poison control center immediately.

▼ INTERACTIONS

DRUG INTERACTIONS
Several drugs may interact with terazosin, including anti-inflammatory medications, especially indomethacin, which can cause fluid and sodium retention, and estrogen, which can reduce the antihypertensive effects of the drug. Consult your doctor.

FOOD INTERACTIONS
None are expected.

DISEASE INTERACTIONS
Consult your physician if you have kidney disease, severe heart disease, or chest pain caused by angina pectoris. Terazosin may aggravate these conditions.

≡ SIDE EFFECTS ≡

SERIOUS
No serious side effects have been reported.

COMMON
Dizziness.

LESS COMMON
Chest pain; lightheadedness or fainting, especially when getting up quickly from a seated or lying position. Such symptoms are typically more common when you first take the medication, and generally diminish over time. These symptoms tend to recur when the dosage is increased. Take it at bedtime to minimize such problems.

TERBINAFINE HYDROCHLORIDE

Available in: Tablets, topical cream, topical gel, topical solution
Available OTC? Yes **As Generic?** No
Drug Class: Antifungal

▼ USAGE INFORMATION

WHY IT'S PRESCRIBED
The tablets are used only to treat fungal infections of the fingernails and toenails (tinea unguium). The topical forms are used to treat fungal infections of the skin, such as tinea versicolor, tinea corporis (ringworm), tinea cruris (jock itch), and tinea pedis (athlete's foot).

HOW IT WORKS
Terbinafine inhibits an enzyme essential for the production of substances vital for the reproduction and survival of some types of fungal organisms.

▼ DOSAGE GUIDELINES

RANGE AND FREQUENCY
Tablets: 250 mg once a day for 6 weeks for fingernail fungus; 250 mg once a day for 12 weeks for toenail fungus. Cream: Apply a thin film of medicine to the affected area 1 to 2 times a day for ringworm or jock itch; 2 times a day for athlete's foot. Apply the cream for at least 1 week, but no longer than 4 weeks. Gel: Apply enough terbinafine to cover the affected area once a day for 1 week. Solution: Apply twice a day for 1 week for tinea versicolor and athlete's foot. Apply once a day for 1 week for ringworm or jock itch.

ONSET OF EFFECT
Variable.

DURATION OF ACTION
Unknown.

DIETARY ADVICE
Terbinafine can be taken or applied without regard to meals.

STORAGE
Store in a tightly sealed container away from heat, moisture, and direct light. Do not allow the topical forms to freeze.

MISSED DOSE
It is important to not miss any doses. Take or apply as soon as you remember. If you do not remember until the next day, skip the missed dose and resume your regular dosage schedule. Do not double the next dose or use excessive amounts of the topical forms.

STOPPING THE DRUG
Take terbinafine tablets as prescribed for the full treatment period.

PROLONGED USE
Side effects are more likely to occur with prolonged use. Tests of liver function are recommended if the tablets are used for longer than 6 weeks.

▼ PRECAUTIONS

Over 60: No special advice.

Driving and Hazardous Work: No special precautions.

Alcohol: No special warnings.

Pregnancy: Terbinafine tablets are not recommended for pregnant women.

Breast Feeding: Avoid use of the tablets while nursing.

Infants and Children: Terbinafine is not recommended for children under the age of 18.

Special Concerns: Wash your hands before and after applying the topical forms. Avoid allowing topical terbinafine to come into contact with the eyes, nose, and mouth. If using terbinafine for ringworm, wear loose-fitting, well-ventilated clothing and avoid excess heat and humidity. It is also recommended to use a bland, absorbent powder like talcum once or twice a day after the cream has been applied and absorbed by the skin. If using the drug for jock itch, do not wear underwear that is tight or made from synthetic materials; wear loose-fitting cotton underwear. If using terbinafine for athlete's foot, dry your feet carefully after bathing and wear clean cotton socks with sandals or well-ventilated shoes. Before applying, wash the affected area with soap and warm water and dry thoroughly.

OVERDOSE
Symptoms: Tablets: nausea, vomiting, abdominal pain, dizziness, rash, frequent urination, and headache.

What to Do: Call your doctor as soon as possible.

▼ INTERACTIONS

DRUG INTERACTIONS
Consult your doctor if you are taking rifampin, cimetidine, or any other preparation that is to be applied to the same area of skin as topical terbinafine.

FOOD INTERACTIONS
No known food interactions.

DISEASE INTERACTIONS
Terbinafine tablets may cause complications in patients with liver or kidney disease, since these organs work together to remove the drug from the body. Consult your doctor if you have a history of alcohol abuse (a potential cause of liver disease).

≡ SIDE EFFECTS ≡

SERIOUS
Serious side effects with terbinafine are rare. However, terbinafine tablets may cause liver dysfunction; severe skin reactions, such as Stevens-Johnson syndrome; severe blood disorders, potentially resulting in increased susceptibility to infection, uncontrolled bleeding or other problems; or severe allergic reactions. Seek emergency medical assistance immediately.

COMMON
Headache, diarrhea, rash, stomach pain, indigestion, nausea.

LESS COMMON
Tablets may cause flatulence, itching, skin eruptions, loss of taste, weakness, fatigue, vomiting, joint and muscle pain, or hair loss. Topical forms may cause redness, itching, burning, blistering, swelling, oozing, or other signs of skin irritation not present before using the drug.

TERBUTALINE SULFATE

Available in: Inhalation aerosol, tablets
Available OTC? No   **As Generic?** Yes
Drug Class: Bronchodilator/sympathomimetic

▼ USAGE INFORMATION

WHY IT'S PRESCRIBED
Terbutaline is used to dilate air passages in the lungs that have become narrowed as a result of disease or inflammation. It is used in the treatment of asthma and chronic obstructive pulmonary disease (COPD).

HOW IT WORKS
Terbutaline widens constricted airways in the lungs by relaxing the smooth muscles that surround bronchial passages.

▼ DOSAGE GUIDELINES

RANGE AND FREQUENCY
Use when needed to relieve breathing difficulty. Inhalation aerosol— Adults and children age 12 and older: 1 to 2 inhalations every 4 to 6 hours. Wait 1 minute between first and second inhalations. Infants and children under 12 years of age: Not recommended. Tablets— Adults and children age 12 and older: 2.5 to 5 mg taken 3 times a day, ideally at 6-hour intervals. Children under 12 years of age: Consult a pediatrician.

ONSET OF EFFECT
Inhalation: Within 5 minutes. Oral: 1 to 2 hours.

DURATION OF ACTION
3 to 6 hours for the inhalation; up to 8 hours for tablets.

DIETARY ADVICE
Maintain your usual food and fluid intake.

STORAGE
Store in a tightly sealed container away from heat and direct light. Do not refrigerate inhalation solutions.

MISSED DOSE
Skip the missed dose and resume your regular dosage schedule. Do not double the next dose.

STOPPING THE DRUG
It may not be necessary to finish the recommended course of therapy. Consult your doctor.

PROLONGED USE
Therapy with this medication may require months or years. Excessive use may result in temporary loss of the drug's effectiveness.

▼ PRECAUTIONS

Over 60: Adverse reactions may be more likely and more severe.

Driving and Hazardous Work: Avoid such activities until you determine how the medicine affects you.

Alcohol: No special precautions are necessary.

Pregnancy: Adequate studies have not been done; the benefits must be weighed against potential risks. Consult your doctor for advice.

Breast Feeding: It is not known if terbutaline passes into breast milk. Mothers who wish to breast-feed while taking this drug should discuss the matter with their doctor.

Infants and Children: Use of the inhalation aerosol is not recommended in children younger than 12.

Special Concerns: Pay heed to any asthma attack or other breathing problem that does not improve after your usual nebulizer treatment or usual number of puffs. Seek help immediately if you feel your lungs are persistently constricted, if you are using more than the recommended number of treatments or puffs per day, or if you feel a recent attack is somehow different from others.

OVERDOSE
Symptoms: Chest pain or heaviness; irregular, racing, fluttering, or pounding heartbeat; dizziness or lightheadedness; fainting; severe weakness; severe headache.

What to Do: Call your doctor, emergency medical services (EMS), or the nearest poison control center immediately.

▼ INTERACTIONS

DRUG INTERACTIONS
Consult your doctor for specific advice if you are taking a beta-blocker, ergotamine or ergotamine-like medications, antidepressants, digitalis drugs, or an MAO inhibitor.

FOOD INTERACTIONS
No known food interactions.

DISEASE INTERACTIONS
Consult your doctor if you have a history of substance abuse (especially cocaine), seizures, brain damage, heart disease, heartbeat irregularities, high blood pressure, anxiety disorders, or a thyroid condition.

SIDE EFFECTS

SERIOUS
Inhaled form: May become ineffective if used too often, resulting in more-severe breathing difficulty that does not improve. Signs include persistent wheezing, coughing, or shortness of breath; confusion; bluish color to lips or fingernails; inability to speak. Ingested form: Chest pain or heaviness; irregular, racing, fluttering, or pounding heartbeat; lightheadedness; fainting; severe weakness; severe headache.

COMMON
Insomnia, dry mouth, sore throat, anxiety, nervousness, restlessness.

LESS COMMON
Trembling, sweating, headache, nausea or vomiting, flushing or redness to cheeks or other skin surfaces, muscle aches, cramps, or twitching, unpleasant or unusual taste in the mouth.

TERCONAZOLE

BRAND NAMES

Terazol 3, Terazol 7

Available in: Cream, suppositories
Available OTC? No   **As Generic?** No
Drug Class: Antifungal

▼ USAGE INFORMATION

WHY IT'S PRESCRIBED
To treat candidiasis, a fungal infection of the vagina.

HOW IT WORKS
Terconazole prevents fungal organisms from producing vital substances required for growth and function. This drug is effective only for infections caused by fungal organisms. It will not work for bacterial or viral infections.

▼ DOSAGE GUIDELINES

RANGE AND FREQUENCY
Cream— 0.4% cream: 20 mg (1 applicator) inserted in the vagina at bedtime for 7 nights. 0.8% cream: 40 mg (1 applicator) inserted in the vagina at bedtime for 3 nights. Suppositories— 80 mg (1 suppository) inserted in the vagina at bedtime for 3 nights. Wash your hands before and after insertion or application.

ONSET OF EFFECT
Unknown.

DURATION OF ACTION
Unknown.

DIETARY ADVICE
Terconazole can be taken without regard to diet.

STORAGE
Store in a tightly sealed container away from heat, moisture, and direct light. Do not refrigerate or freeze.

MISSED DOSE
Take it as soon as you remember. However, if it is near the time for the next dose, skip the missed dose and resume your regular dosage schedule. Do not double the next dose.

STOPPING THE DRUG
Take it as prescribed for the full treatment period, even if you begin to feel better before the scheduled end of therapy.

PROLONGED USE
If your symptoms do not improve after a few days, or if they become worse, consult your doctor.

▼ PRECAUTIONS

Over 60: Adverse reactions may be more likely and more severe in older patients.

Driving and Hazardous Work: The use of terconazole should not impair your ability to perform such tasks safely.

Alcohol: No special precautions are necessary.

Pregnancy: Studies on the use of terconazole during the first 3 months (trimester) of pregnancy have not been done. No adverse effects from using terconazole during the second or third trimesters have been reported.

Breast Feeding: Terconazole may pass into breast milk; caution is advised. Consult your doctor for advice.

Infants and Children: Studies of the use of terconazole in infants and children have not been done.

Special Concerns: Sanitary napkins should be used to prevent staining of clothing. The affected area should be kept cool and dry. The patient should wear loose-fitting cotton clothing and freshly laundered cotton underwear or pantyhose with a cotton crotch. Avoid underwear made from nonventilating materials. Do not sit for a long time in a wet bathing suit. Avoid feminine hygiene sprays. Wash daily with unscented soap and dry thoroughly with a clean towel. Tampons should not be used during therapy. The patient's sexual partner should wear a condom during intercourse and should consult a doctor if penile redness, itching, or discomfort occur. Do not stop using this medicine during your menstrual period. After urination or a bowel movement, cleanse by wiping the area from front to back to prevent reinfection.

OVERDOSE
Symptoms: An overdose with terconazole is unlikely.

What to Do: Emergency instructions not applicable.

▼ INTERACTIONS

DRUG INTERACTIONS
Other drugs may interact with terconazole. Consult your doctor for specific advice if you are taking any other prescription or over-the-counter medication.

FOOD INTERACTIONS
No known food interactions.

DISEASE INTERACTIONS
Consult your doctor for advice if you have any other medical condition.

≡ SIDE EFFECTS ≡

SERIOUS
Vaginal burning, itching, discharge, or irritation not present prior to treatment. Call your doctor immediately.

COMMON
No common side effects have been reported.

LESS COMMON
Headache, stomach cramps or pain, irritation or burning of sexual partner's penis.

TESTOLACTONE

Available in: Tablets
Available OTC? No   **As Generic?** No
Drug Class: Antineoplastic (anticancer) agent

▼ USAGE INFORMATION

WHY IT'S PRESCRIBED
To treat some cases of advanced breast cancer in either postmenopausal women or premenopausal women in whom ovarian function has been terminated. It is not recommended for treatment of breast cancer in men.

HOW IT WORKS
Testolactone is chemically similar to the hormone testosterone. The mechanism by which testolactone inhibits breast cancer growth is unclear. The growth of some types of breast cancer is stimulated by the hormone estrogen; testolactone is thought to interfere with the synthesis of estrogen and thus slow the growth of such types of breast cancer.

▼ DOSAGE GUIDELINES

RANGE AND FREQUENCY
The dosage should be 250 mg, 4 times a day, for at least 3 months.

ONSET OF EFFECT
6 to 12 weeks.

DURATION OF ACTION
Unknown.

DIETARY ADVICE
Testolactone can be taken with or between meals. Be sure to get plenty of fluids.

STORAGE
Store in a tightly sealed container away from heat and direct light.

MISSED DOSE
Take it as soon as you remember. If it is close to the next dose, skip the missed dose and resume your regular dosage schedule. Do not double the next dose. If you miss more than 1 dose, consult your doctor.

STOPPING THE DRUG
The decision to stop taking the drug should be made by your doctor.

PROLONGED USE
You should see your doctor regularly for tests and examinations if you must take this drug for a prolonged period.

SIDE EFFECTS

SERIOUS
No serious side effects have been reported.

COMMON
No common side effects have been reported.

LESS COMMON
Skin rash; increased blood pressure; numbness or tingling of fingers, toes, or face; diarrhea; loss of appetite; nausea or vomiting; pain or swelling in feet or lower legs; swelling or redness of the tongue; hair loss; aching and swelling of arms and legs; high blood calcium levels, causing confusion, increased thirst, and constipation.

▼ PRECAUTIONS

Over 60: There is no specific information comparing the use of testolactone in the elderly with use in other age groups. However, no special problems or side effects are expected in older patients.

Driving and Hazardous Work: The use of testolactone should not impair your ability to perform such tasks safely.

Alcohol: Avoid alcohol.

Pregnancy: Large doses of testolactone have been shown to cause birth defects and other problems in animal studies. Human studies have not been done. Before you take testolactone, tell your doctor if you are pregnant or plan to become pregnant. If you become pregnant while taking testolactone, tell your doctor immediately.

Breast Feeding: Testolactone may pass into breast milk; caution is advised. Consult your doctor for advice.

Infants and Children: Safety and effectiveness of testolactone in infants and children have not been determined.

Special Concerns: If you vomit shortly after taking a dose of testolactone, check with your doctor to learn whether you should take the dose again or wait for the next dose. Testolactone may cause an excess buildup of calcium in the body, which can produce unwanted or even dangerous side effects. Therefore, drink large amounts of fluids while taking testolactone to rid your body of excess calcium. Your doctor may want to check blood calcium levels regularly while you take testolactone.

OVERDOSE
Symptoms: No specific ones have been reported.

What to Do: An overdose of testolactone is unlikely to be life-threatening. However, if someone takes a much larger dose than prescribed, call your doctor, emergency medical services (EMS), or the nearest poison control center.

▼ INTERACTIONS

DRUG INTERACTIONS
Consult your doctor for specific advice if you are taking anticoagulants, such as warfarin. Testolactone may boost the anticlotting effect of such drugs, leading to uncontrolled internal or external bleeding.

FOOD INTERACTIONS
No known food interactions.

DISEASE INTERACTIONS
Caution is advised when taking testolactone. Consult your doctor if you have a medical history that includes heart or kidney disease.

TESTOSTERONE

Available in: Injection, skin patch
Available OTC? No   **As Generic?** Yes
Drug Class: Male hormone (androgen)

▼ USAGE INFORMATION

WHY IT'S PRESCRIBED
To replace the hormone when the body does not produce enough; to stimulate puberty in boys with delayed onset of puberty; to increase libido in women (prescribed in combination with estrogen; brand name: Estratest).

HOW IT WORKS
Testosterone supplementation replaces the natural testosterone normally produced by the body.

▼ DOSAGE GUIDELINES

RANGE AND FREQUENCY
For hormone replacement in men: 100 mg weekly intramuscular injection or 200 mg injection every 2 weeks. For delayed puberty in boys: Up to 100 mg injection once a month for 4 to 6 months. For all purposes— Scrotal patch: One new patch applied to scrotal skin in the morning. Nonscrotal patch: 2 to 3 patches a day applied to skin on the arm, back, or upper buttocks.

ONSET OF EFFECT
Blood levels of testosterone peak 5 to 12 hours with the skin patch and in 24 hours with intramuscular injection. Some long-term effects, such as improved sexual function, may occur after a few weeks of therapy. Other effects (such as those affecting body composition and maturation) may take months to years.

DURATION OF ACTION
Unknown.

DIETARY ADVICE
Testosterone can be taken without regard to diet.

≡ SIDE EFFECTS ≡

SERIOUS
In men: Prolonged, possibly painful erection (which may cause permanent damage to the tissues of the penis and result in the inability to achieve further erections), frequent headache, increased thirst, increased urination, nausea or vomiting, swollen feet or legs, unusual bleeding, unusual fatigue, rapid weight gain, hives, significant changes in emotions. Call your doctor immediately. In women: Enlarged clitoris, deepening of voice, male-pattern baldness. Such side effects are rare; call your doctor immediately if any occur.

COMMON
In men: Enlarged, sore breasts, frequent erections, acne, frequent urination. The skin patch may cause itching. In women: Acne, decreased breast size, excessive hair growth, irregular menstrual periods.

LESS COMMON
No less-common minor side effects are associated with testosterone.

STORAGE
Store skin patch in a tightly sealed container away from heat and direct light.

MISSED DOSE
Take it as soon as you remember. If it is near the time for the next dose, skip the missed dose and resume your regular dosage schedule. Do not double the next dose.

STOPPING THE DRUG
The decision to stop taking the drug should be made by your doctor.

PROLONGED USE
You should see your doctor regularly if you are required to use this hormone for a prolonged period.

▼ PRECAUTIONS

Over 60: Increased risk of causing dormant prostate cancer to grow in men. Repeated examinations should be done, using a blood test for prostate specific antigen (PSA) and a digital rectal examination by your doctor.

Driving and Hazardous Work: Do not drive or engage in hazardous work until you determine how the medicine affects you.

Alcohol: Moderate alcohol consumption is acceptable while taking this drug.

Pregnancy: Testosterone should not be taken during pregnancy.

Breast Feeding: Testosterone passes into breast milk and may be harmful; do not use it while breast feeding.

Infants and Children: Not recommended for use by children under the age of puberty.

Special Concerns: The scrotal skin patch should be applied to a shaved area of the scrotum. Men who have experienced skin irritation using a nonscrotal patch can apply triamcinolone cream (0.1%) prior to placement.

OVERDOSE
Symptoms: No specific ones have been reported.

What to Do: An overdose of testosterone is unlikely to be life-threatening. However, if someone takes a much larger dose than prescribed, call your doctor.

▼ INTERACTIONS

DRUG INTERACTIONS
Consult your doctor if you are taking anabolic steroids, anticoagulants (blood thinners, such as warfarin), or an oral contraceptive.

FOOD INTERACTIONS
No known food interactions.

DISEASE INTERACTIONS
Consult your doctor if you have a history of breast cancer (men or women), prostate cancer, diabetes, edema (swelling due to fluid retention), kidney disease, liver disease, enlarged prostate, or cardiovascular disease.

TETANUS TOXOID

Available in: Injection
Available OTC? No   **As Generic?** No
Drug Class: Vaccine

▼ USAGE INFORMATION

WHY IT'S PRESCRIBED
To prevent, but not to treat, tetanus (lockjaw).

HOW IT WORKS
Tetanus toxoid stimulates the body's immune system to produce protective antibodies against tetanus.

▼ DOSAGE GUIDELINES

RANGE AND FREQUENCY
Depending on the type of vaccine being administered, injections are given in the upper arm or midthigh, either into a muscle or under the skin. For adults, children, and infants 6 weeks of age and older: An initial dose at first visit, a second dose 8 weeks later. Depending on the vaccine being used, a third dose may be given 8 weeks after the second dose, and a fourth dose 6 to 12 months later (usually at 15 to 18 months of age in infants). Booster shots should be administered every 10 years. If you sustain a wound that is unclean or difficult to clean, you may need an emergency booster injection if more than 5 years have elapsed since your last booster shot.

ONSET OF EFFECT
Most patients develop immunity following the second dose.

DURATION OF ACTION
Up to 10 years.

DIETARY ADVICE
It may be administered without regard to diet.

STORAGE
Not applicable; the immunizations are administered only at a health care facility.

MISSED DOSE
If you miss a scheduled vaccination, contact your doctor to reschedule it.

STOPPING THE DRUG
Follow the full immunization schedule unless a medical problem arises that rules out receiving a vaccination.

PROLONGED USE
No special problems are expected.

▼ PRECAUTIONS

Over 60: Tetanus toxoid should not cause different or more severe side effects in older patients than in younger persons. Vaccine may be slightly less effective. Two-thirds of all tetanus cases in the past few years have been in people age 50 and older.

Driving and Hazardous Work: The administration of tetanus toxoid should not impair your ability to perform such tasks safely.

Alcohol: No special precautions are necessary.

Pregnancy: Adequate studies have not been done. However, if the mother is immune to tetanus, tetanus antibodies from the mother can protect the child from tetanus infection at birth.

Breast Feeding: Tetanus toxoid has not been shown to cause problems during breast feeding.

Infants and Children: Not recommended for use by children less than 6 weeks old.

Special Concerns: Regardless of immunization status, dirty wounds should always be properly cleaned and treated.

OVERDOSE
Symptoms: No specific ones have been reported.

What to Do: If any unexplained symptoms arise after receiving an immunization, call your doctor, emergency medical services (EMS), or the nearest poison control center.

▼ INTERACTIONS

DRUG INTERACTIONS
Other drugs may interact with tetanus toxoid. Consult your doctor for advice if you are taking any prescription or over-the-counter medication.

FOOD INTERACTIONS
No known food interactions.

DISEASE INTERACTIONS
Consult your doctor if you have had a severe reaction or a high fever following a previous injection; or if you have pneumonia, bronchitis, or another illness affecting the lungs; any severe illness that is causing fever; or neurological disorders or a history of seizures.

≣ SIDE EFFECTS ≣

SERIOUS
Serious allergic reaction involving difficulty swallowing or breathing; reddened skin, especially around the ears; itching, particularly of the hands or feet; hives; unusual and severe fatigue; and swollen face, eyes, or nasal passages. Call your doctor immediately.

COMMON
Hard lump or redness at site of injection.

LESS COMMON
Fever, chills, unusual fatigue, irritability. Also skin rash, pain, itching, swelling, or tenderness at site of injection.

TETRACYCLINE HYDROCHLORIDE

Available in: Capsules, tablets, liquid, topical forms, ophthalmic forms, injection
Available OTC? No   **As Generic?** Yes
Drug Class: Tetracycline antibiotic

▼ USAGE INFORMATION

WHY IT'S PRESCRIBED
To treat infections caused by bacteria or protozoa (tiny single-celled organisms); also, to treat acne.

HOW IT WORKS
Tetracycline kills bacteria and protozoa by inhibiting the manufacture of specific proteins needed by the organisms to survive.

▼ DOSAGE GUIDELINES

RANGE AND FREQUENCY
Oral forms (capsules, tablets, liquid), for bacterial and protozoal infections: 500 to 2,000 mg, 1 to 4 times a day, as determined by your doctor. Topical forms (cream, topical ointment, topical solution), for acne or skin infections: Apply 1 or 2 times a day to affected areas. Ophthalmic forms (ophthalmic ointment, ophthalmic solution) for eye infections: Apply once every 2 to 12 hours as determined by your doctor.

ONSET OF EFFECT
Unknown.

DURATION OF ACTION
Unknown.

DIETARY ADVICE
Oral forms are best taken on an empty stomach with a full glass of water.

STORAGE
Store in a tightly sealed container away from heat and direct light. Refrigerate liquid forms but do not freeze.

MISSED DOSE
Take it as soon as you remember. If it is near the time for the next dose, skip the missed dose and resume your regular dosage schedule. Do not double the next dose.

STOPPING THE DRUG
Take as prescribed for the full treatment period, even if you begin to feel better before the scheduled end of therapy.

PROLONGED USE
May increase susceptibility to infections by microorganisms resistant to antibiotics.

▼ PRECAUTIONS

Over 60: It is not known whether tetracycline causes different or more severe adverse reactions in older patients than it does in younger persons.

Driving and Hazardous Work: Do not drive or engage in hazardous work until you determine how the medicine affects you.

Alcohol: It is advisable to abstain from alcohol when fighting an infection.

Pregnancy: Tetracycline should not be used during pregnancy.

Breast Feeding: Tetracycline passes into breast milk and may be harmful to the nursing infant. The patient must choose between using the drug or breast feeding.

Infants and Children: Tetracycline should be used by children younger than 8 years of age only if other antibiotics are unlikely to be effective, since it can cause permanent tooth staining.

Special Concerns: If tetracycline causes increased sensitivity of your skin to sunlight, wear protective clothing, use a sunscreen with an SPF (sun protection factor) of 15 or higher, and try to avoid direct exposure to sunlight, especially between 10 am and 3 pm. Before having surgery, tell the doctor or dentist in charge that you are taking tetracycline. If you use makeup, it is best to apply only water-based cosmetics and to keep the amount to a minimum during tetracycline therapy for the skin. Tetracycline can reduce the effectiveness of oral contraceptives. You should use a different method of birth control while taking this antibiotic. Absorption of tetracycline may be altered if you take antacids.

OVERDOSE

Symptoms: Severe nausea, vomiting, diarrhea, difficulty swallowing.

What to Do: An overdose is unlikely to be life-threatening. However, if someone takes a much larger dose than prescribed, call your doctor, emergency medical services (EMS), or the nearest poison control center immediately.

▼ INTERACTIONS

DRUG INTERACTIONS
Consult your physician for advice if you are taking antacids, calcium supplements, cholestyramine, choline and magnesium salicylates, medicines containing iron, laxatives containing magnesium, or oral contraceptives.

FOOD INTERACTIONS
Avoid dairy products while taking tetracycline.

DISEASE INTERACTIONS
Consult your doctor if you have a history of kidney disease or liver disease.

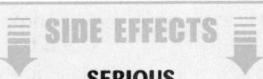

SIDE EFFECTS

SERIOUS
Increased frequency of urination, increased thirst, unusual fatigue, discoloration of skin and mucous membranes. Call your doctor immediately.

COMMON
Stomach cramps and discomfort, diarrhea, nausea, vomiting, increased sensitivity of skin to sunlight, itching in genital or rectal area, sore mouth or tongue, dizziness, lightheadedness, or unsteadiness.

LESS COMMON
No less-common side effects have been reported.

THEOPHYLLINE

Available in: Tablets, capsules, extended release forms, elixir, syrup, oral solution
Available OTC? No   **As Generic?** Yes
Drug Class: Bronchodilator/xanthine

▼ USAGE INFORMATION

WHY IT'S PRESCRIBED
Theophylline is used to reduce the frequency and severity of breathing problems in people with asthma, emphysema, bronchitis, and other lung disorders.

HOW IT WORKS
An asthma attack occurs when the smooth muscles in the bronchial passages of the lungs go into a spasm (bronchospasm). Theophylline relaxes these muscles, helping to widen the constricted airways and restore normal breathing.

▼ DOSAGE GUIDELINES

RANGE AND FREQUENCY
Adults not currently taking any theophylline medications: Your physician will prescribe a "loading dose," which is based on your weight and taken only once. This is followed by a daily maintenance dose, usually 300 to 600 mg per day, taken in 1 or 2 doses. Patients given extended-release capsules: After the loading dose, take one-half of the total daily dose at 12-hour intervals, unless otherwise directed by your doctor. Adults currently taking theophylline: Dose is determined by blood level of theophylline. Children: Consult a pediatrician.

ONSET OF EFFECT
Variable.

DURATION OF ACTION
Variable.

DIETARY ADVICE
Avoid large amounts of caffeine-containing foods or beverages, including colas. Otherwise, maintain your usual food and fluid intake.

STORAGE
Store in a tightly sealed container away from heat and direct light. Keep away from moisture and extremes in temperature.

MISSED DOSE
Take it as soon as you remember. If it is near the time for the next dose, skip the missed dose and resume your regular dosage schedule. Do not double the next dose.

STOPPING THE DRUG
The decision to stop taking the drug should be made by your doctor.

PROLONGED USE
Therapy with this medication may require months or years.

▼ PRECAUTIONS

Over 60: Adverse reactions may be more likely and more severe in older patients.

Driving and Hazardous Work: Do not drive or engage in hazardous work until you determine how the medicine affects you.

Alcohol: Avoid alcohol.

Pregnancy: Discuss the relative risks with your doctor. Generally, this drug should be used only if necessary and if a substitute cannot be prescribed.

Breast Feeding: Theophylline passes into breast milk and may be toxic to nursing infants; avoid or discontinue use while breast feeding.

Infants and Children: Theophylline has been used in children of all ages. Consult your pediatrician for specific dosages. Theophylline elixir contains alcohol and should not be used by children.

Special Concerns: You will need periodic blood tests to determine theophylline levels. Do not switch between different brands of theophylline, and especially do not switch between extended-release forms and other forms without notifying your doctor. Inform your doctor if you have stopped smoking; tobacco affects the level of theophylline in the blood.

OVERDOSE

Symptoms: Abdominal pain; disorientation, extreme anxiety, or unusual behavior; bloody vomiting; twitching, trembling, or shaking; seizures; rapid, pounding, or irregular heartbeat; lightheadedness, dizziness, or fainting.

What to Do: Call your doctor, emergency medical services (EMS), or the nearest poison control center immediately.

▼ INTERACTIONS

DRUG INTERACTIONS
Consult your doctor for specific advice if you are taking beta-blockers, cimetidine, ciprofloxacin, clarithromycin, enoxacin, erythromycin, fluvoxamine, mexiletine, pentoxifylline, propranolol, tacrine, thiabendazole, ticlopidine, troleandomycin; moricizine, phenytoin, or rifampin.

FOOD INTERACTIONS
Your doctor may suggest that you restrict caffeine intake.

DISEASE INTERACTIONS
Consult your doctor if you have a history of convulsions, heart failure, liver disease, or underactive thyroid.

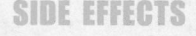
SIDE EFFECTS

SERIOUS
Vomiting, trembling, confusion, rapid, irregular, or pounding pulse, chest pain, dizziness, convulsions, skin rashes.

COMMON
Restlessness, insomnia, loss of appetite, nervousness, irritability, nausea.

LESS COMMON
Heartburn, diarrhea.

THIABENDAZOLE

Available in: Oral suspension, chewable tablets
Available OTC? No   **As Generic?** No
Drug Class: Anthelmintic

▼ USAGE INFORMATION

WHY IT'S PRESCRIBED
To treat infections caused by worms, primarily strongyloidiasis (threadworms). It may also be used to treat cutaneous larva migrans (creeping eruption), trichinosis, and visceral larva migrans, although less toxic drugs are available.

HOW IT WORKS
The exact way in which thiabendazole works is unknown. It appears to interfere with the metabolic or energy-producing processes of worms, including the uptake of glucose (sugar).

▼ DOSAGE GUIDELINES

RANGE AND FREQUENCY
Adults and children: 25 mg per 2.2 lbs (1 kg) of body weight twice a day (up to a maximum of 3,000 mg per day) for 2 to 5 days. Consult your doctor for specific dose. The oral suspension can be used topically for cutaneous larva migrans.

ONSET OF EFFECT
Unknown.

DURATION OF ACTION
Unknown.

DIETARY ADVICE
Take it after meals to reduce stomach upset and some of the common side effects.

STORAGE
Store in a tightly sealed container away from heat, moisture, and direct light. Keep the oral suspension from freezing.

MISSED DOSE
Take it as soon as you remember. If it is near the time for the next dose, skip the missed dose and resume your regular dosage schedule. Do not double the next dose.

STOPPING THE DRUG
Take it as prescribed for the full treatment period, even if you feel better before the scheduled end of therapy.

PROLONGED USE
Thiabendazole is generally prescribed for short-term therapy (2 to 5 days). If your condition shows no signs of improvement or worsens within this time, consult your doctor. Another treatment regimen may be prescribed.

▼ PRECAUTIONS

Over 60: Adverse reactions may be more likely and more severe in older patients.

Driving and Hazardous Work: Do not drive or engage in hazardous work while undergoing treatment.

Alcohol: No special precautions are necessary.

Pregnancy: Do not take thiabendazole while pregnant. Consult your doctor for advice if you are pregnant or plan to become pregnant.

Breast Feeding: Thiabendazole may pass into breast milk. Breast feeding may need to be discontinued while you take the drug. Consult your doctor for advice.

Infants and Children: Use and dosage for infants weighing less than 30 pounds should be determined by your doctor.

Special Concerns: To prevent reinfection with trichinosis, all pork, pork-containing products, and game meat should be cooked until the center is no longer pink. To prevent reinfection with cutaneous larva migrans or visceral larva migrans, keep your dogs or cats away from beaches and bathing areas, deworm them regularly, and keep children's sandboxes covered when not in use. Note that approximately half of all patients who take thiabendazole experience at least one side effect.

OVERDOSE
Symptoms: Sporadic vision disturbances, changes in mental state.

What to Do: An overdose of thiabendazole is unlikely to be life-threatening. However, if someone takes a much larger dose than prescribed, call your doctor, emergency medical services (EMS), or the nearest poison control center.

▼ INTERACTIONS

DRUG INTERACTIONS
Consult your doctor for specific advice if you are taking theophylline. Also tell your doctor if you are taking any other prescription or over-the-counter medicine. If you have trichinosis, your doctor may also prescribe a corticosteroid to help reduce inflammation from the pork worm larvae; it is important to take the corticosteroid and thiabendazole together.

FOOD INTERACTIONS
No known food interactions.

DISEASE INTERACTIONS
Use of thiabendazole may cause complications in patients with liver disease, since this organ removes the drug from the body.

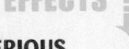

SIDE EFFECTS

SERIOUS
Severe nausea and vomiting, confusion, skin rash or itching, severe diarrhea, hallucinations, delirium, disorientation, loss of appetite, irritability, tingling or numbness of hands or feet, decreased pulse or blood pressure. Call your physician immediately.

COMMON
Dry eyes or mouth, dizziness, drowsiness, buzzing or ringing in ears, headache, asparaguslike odor from urine.

LESS COMMON
Elevated liver enzymes, temporary decrease in white blood cell count (these effects are detectable by your doctor); fever, flushing of the face, swelling.

THIOGUANINE

Available in: Tablets
Available OTC? No   **As Generic?** Yes
Drug Class: Antimetabolite; antineoplastic (anticancer) agent

▼ USAGE INFORMATION

WHY IT'S PRESCRIBED
To treat some forms of leukemia.

HOW IT WORKS
It kills cancer cells by interfering with the activity of their genetic material, which prevents the cells from reproducing. It may also affect the growth and development of other cells in the body, resulting in unpleasant side effects.

▼ DOSAGE GUIDELINES

RANGE AND FREQUENCY
2 mg per 2.2 lbs (1 kg) of body weight per day, usually in 1 dose. The dose can be increased to 3 mg per 2.2 lbs per day if there is no response after 3 weeks.

ONSET OF EFFECT
Unknown.

DURATION OF ACTION
Unknown.

DIETARY ADVICE
Maintain adequate food and fluid intake. Calorie, protein, and vitamin needs increase in patients with cancer. Good nutrition is essential to cope with chemotherapy.

STORAGE
Store in a tightly sealed container away from heat and direct light.

MISSED DOSE
If you miss a dose, skip the missed dose and resume your regular dosage schedule. Do not double the next dose.

STOPPING THE DRUG
The decision to stop taking the drug should be made in consultation with your doctor.

PROLONGED USE
You should see your doctor regularly for tests and examinations if you take this drug for a prolonged period.

▼ PRECAUTIONS

Over 60: No special problems are expected.

Driving and Hazardous Work: Do not drive or engage in hazardous work until you determine how the medicine affects you.

Alcohol: Consult your doctor about drinking alcohol while taking this drug.

Pregnancy: Thioguanine can cause birth defects if either the father or mother takes it. It is best to use some kind of birth control while taking thioguanine. Consult your doctor for specific advice if you are pregnant or plan to become pregnant.

Breast Feeding: Thioguanine may pass into breast milk; avoid or discontinue use while nursing.

Infants and Children: No special problems are expected.

Special Concerns: While taking thioguanine, do not receive any immunizations without consulting your doctor. Avoid people with infections and those who have recently had oral polio vaccine. Be careful when using a toothbrush, dental floss, or toothpick. Check with your doctor before having any dental work done. If you are going to have surgery, tell the doctor or dentist in charge that you are taking thioguanine. Do not touch your eyes or the inside of your nose unless you have just washed your hands. Be careful not to cut yourself when using sharp objects such as a razor. Avoid contact sports and other activities where bruising could occur. If you vomit shortly after taking a dose of thioguanine, consult your doctor about taking the dose again.

OVERDOSE
Symptoms: Nausea, vomiting, general malaise, high blood pressure.

What to Do: Call your doctor, emergency medical services (EMS), or the nearest poison control center immediately.

▼ INTERACTIONS

DRUG INTERACTIONS
Consult your doctor for specific advice if you are taking antithyroid agents, azathioprine, chloramphenicol, colchicine, flucytosine, interferon, plicamycin, zidovudine, probenecid, or sulfinpyrazone.

FOOD INTERACTIONS
No known food interactions.

DISEASE INTERACTIONS
Caution is advised when taking thioguanine. Consult your doctor if you have any of the following: chickenpox, shingles, gout, kidney stones, kidney disease, liver disease, or any infection.

≡ SIDE EFFECTS ≡

SERIOUS
Black, tarry, or bloody stools; blood-tinged (pink or maroon) urine; cough or hoarseness; fever and chills; lower back or flank pain; painful, difficult urination; tiny bright red spots on skin; bleeding from gums, nose, or other unusual places; easy bruising, shortness of breath. These side effects may mean that normal blood cells and special blood-clotting cells have been affected, or that normal immune cells have been affected and an infection is developing somewhere in your body. See your doctor immediately if any of these occur. Some of these side effects may occur after you stop taking thioguanine; notify your doctor if they do.

COMMON
No common side effects have been reported.

LESS COMMON
Diarrhea, loss of appetite, nausea and vomiting, skin rash or itching.

THIORIDAZINE HYDROCHLORIDE

Available in: Oral solution, oral suspension, tablets
Available OTC? No   **As Generic?** Yes
Drug Class: Neuroleptic; antipsychotic

▼ USAGE INFORMATION

WHY IT'S PRESCRIBED
To treat moderate to severe psychiatric conditions including schizophrenia, manic states, and drug-induced psychosis. It is also used to treat extreme behavior problems in children (including infantile autism), to ease the symptoms of Tourette's syndrome, and to reduce nausea and vomiting associated with chemotherapy for cancer.

HOW IT WORKS
Thioridazine blocks receptors of dopamine (a chemical that aids in the transmission of nerve impulses) in the central nervous system. Presumably, this produces a tranquilizing and antipsychotic effect.

▼ DOSAGE GUIDELINES

RANGE AND FREQUENCY
Adults: Initially, 25 to 100 mg, 3 times a day. Your doctor may increase the dose as needed and tolerated, not to exceed 800 mg a day.

ONSET OF EFFECT
Sedation may occur within minutes, but onset of antipsychotic effect may take hours to occur or may not occur until days or weeks after the beginning of therapy.

DURATION OF ACTION
12 to 24 hours, but effects may persist for several days.

DIETARY ADVICE
Should be taken with food and a full glass of water.

STORAGE
Store in a tightly sealed container away from heat and direct light. Do not allow liquid forms to freeze.

MISSED DOSE
Take it as soon as you remember. If it is near the time for the next dose, skip the missed dose and resume your regular dosage schedule. Do not double the next dose.

STOPPING THE DRUG
The decision to stop taking the drug should be made in consultation with your doctor. Gradual reduction of doses may be required if you have taken this medication for an extended period.

PROLONGED USE
See your doctor regularly for tests and examinations if you must take this medicine for a prolonged period.

▼ PRECAUTIONS

Over 60: Adverse reactions are more likely and more severe in older patients.

Driving and Hazardous Work: Do not drive or engage in hazardous work until you learn how this medication affects you.

Alcohol: Avoid alcohol.

Pregnancy: Avoid using thioridazine if you are pregnant or plan to become pregnant.

Breast Feeding: Either avoid taking the drug if possible or refrain from breast feeding.

Infants and Children: Adverse reactions may be more likely and more severe in children.

Special Concerns: Avoid prolonged exposure to high temperatures or hot climates. Drink plenty of fluids and stay cool in the summertime. Avoid overexposure to sunlight until you determine if the medication heightens your skin's sensitivity to ultraviolet light.

OVERDOSE
Symptoms: Extreme drowsiness or paradoxical restlessness or agitation, heart rhythm irregularities or palpitations, dry mouth, seizures, stiffness or impaired muscle control, loss of consciousness.

What to Do: Call your doctor, emergency medical services (EMS), or the nearest poison control center immediately.

▼ INTERACTIONS

DRUG INTERACTIONS
Consult your doctor for specific advice if you are taking anticholinergics; anticonvulsants; antidepressants; antihistamines; antihypertensives; bupropion; central nervous system depressants, such as barbiturates; clozapine; dronabinol; ethinamate; fluoxetine; guanethidine; guanfacine; lithium; methyldopa; carbamazepine; rifampin; or trihexyphenidyl.

FOOD INTERACTIONS
No known food interactions.

DISEASE INTERACTIONS
Consult your doctor if you have Parkinson's disease or any movement disorder, glaucoma, epilepsy, liver disease, or kidney disease.

SIDE EFFECTS

SERIOUS
Rapid heartbeat, profuse sweating, seizures, difficulty breathing, neck stiffness, swelling of the tongue, difficulty swallowing. Also a rare condition can develop called neuroleptic malignant syndrome, characterized by stiffness or spasms of the muscles, high fever, and confusion or disorientation. Call your doctor immediately.

COMMON
Dizziness or faintness, drowsiness, constipation, decreased sweating, dry mouth, nasal congestion, shaking or trembling of the hands, stiffness, stooped posture.

LESS COMMON
Menstrual irregularities, sexual dysfunction, unusual milk secretion, breast pain or swelling, unexpected weight gain, difficult urination.

THIOTHIXENE

BRAND NAMES

Navane, Thiothixene HCl
Intensol

Available in: Capsules, solution, injection
Available OTC? No **As Generic?** Yes
Drug Class: Neuroleptic; antipsychotic

▼ USAGE INFORMATION

WHY IT'S PRESCRIBED
To treat psychotic conditions (severe mental disorders marked by distorted thoughts, perceptions, and emotions), such as schizophrenia.

HOW IT WORKS
Thiothixene blocks receptors of dopamine (a chemical that allows the transmission of nerve impulses) in the central nervous system. Presumably, this produces a tranquilizing or antipsychotic effect.

▼ DOSAGE GUIDELINES

RANGE AND FREQUENCY
Oral forms: Initial dose is 2 mg, 3 times a day, or 5 mg, 2 times a day. The dose may be increased up to 60 mg a day. Injection: 4 mg injected into a muscle, 2 to 4 times a day. The dose may be increased up to 30 mg a day.

ONSET OF EFFECT
Sedation may occur within minutes, but onset of antipsychotic effect may take hours to occur or may not occur until days or weeks after the beginning of therapy.

DURATION OF ACTION
12 to 24 hours, but effects may persist for several days.

DIETARY ADVICE
This drug may be taken without regard to diet.

STORAGE
Store in a tightly sealed container away from heat and direct light. Do not allow liquid forms to freeze.

MISSED DOSE
Take it as soon as you remember. However, if it is within 2 hours of the next dose, skip the missed dose and resume your regular dosage schedule. Do not double the next dose.

STOPPING THE DRUG
The decision to stop taking the drug should be made in consultation with your doctor.

PROLONGED USE
Prolonged use may lead to tardive dyskinesia (involuntary movements of the jaw, lips, tongue, and, in rare cases, the arms, legs, hands, or body). Consult your doctor about the need for follow-up evaluations and tests if you must take this drug for an extended period.

▼ PRECAUTIONS

Over 60: Adverse reactions are more likely and more severe in older patients.

Driving and Hazardous Work: Do not drive or engage in hazardous work until you determine how the medicine affects you.

Alcohol: Avoid alcohol.

Pregnancy: Adequate studies have not been done. Before you take thiothixene, tell your doctor if you are pregnant or plan to become pregnant.

Breast Feeding: It is unknown if thiothixene passes into breast milk; consult your doctor for advice.

Infants and Children: Thiothixene is not commonly prescribed for patients under the age of 12.

Special Concerns: Avoid prolonged exposure to high temperatures or hot climates. Drink plenty of fluids and stay cool in the summertime. Avoid overexposure to sun-

light until you determine if the drug heightens your skin's sensitivity to ultraviolet light.

OVERDOSE
Symptoms: Severe breathing difficulty, severe dizziness, extreme fatigue or sedation, muscle spasms, stiffness, or twitching, constricted pupils, unusual excitability.

What to Do: Call your doctor, emergency medical services (EMS), or the nearest poison control center immediately.

▼ INTERACTIONS

DRUG INTERACTIONS
Other drugs may interact with thiothixene. Consult your doctor for advice if you are taking anticholinergics; anticonvulsants; antidepressants; antihistamines; antihypertensives; bupropion; central nervous system depressants, such as barbiturates; clozapine; dronabinol; ethinamate; fluoxetine; guanethidine; guanfacine; lithium; methyldopa; carbamazepine; rifampin; or trihexyphenidyl.

FOOD INTERACTIONS
No known food interactions.

DISEASE INTERACTIONS
Consult your doctor if you have Parkinson's disease or any movement disorder, glaucoma, epilepsy, liver disease, or kidney disease.

SIDE EFFECTS

SERIOUS
Rapid heartbeat, profuse sweating, seizures, difficulty breathing, neck stiffness, swelling of the tongue, difficulty swallowing. Also a rare condition can develop called neuroleptic malignant syndrome, characterized by stiffness or spasms of the muscles, high fever, and confusion or disorientation. Call your doctor immediately.

COMMON
Nausea, reduced perspiration, dry mouth, blurred vision, drowsiness, shaking of the hands, muscle stiffness, stooped posture.

LESS COMMON
Difficult urination, menstrual irregularities, breast pain or swelling, unexpected weight gain, uncontrolled movements of the tongue, fever, chills, sore throat, unusual bruising or bleeding, heart palpitations, skin rash, itching, increased sensitivity of the skin to sunlight.

TIAGABINE HYDROCHLORIDE

Available in: Tablets
Available OTC? No   **As Generic?** No
Drug Class: Anticonvulsant

▼ USAGE INFORMATION

WHY IT'S PRESCRIBED
Used in combination with one or more anticonvulsant drugs to control partial seizures (those which begin with an abnormal burst of electrical activity in a small portion of the brain).

HOW IT WORKS
Although its precise mechanism of action is unknown, tiagabine is thought to increase the activity of an inhibiting neurotransmitter that depresses brain activity and suppresses the abnormal firing of neurons that causes seizures.

▼ DOSAGE GUIDELINES

RANGE AND FREQUENCY
Teenagers: For the first week, 4 mg once a day. At the beginning of the second week, the total daily dose may be increased by 4 mg. The total daily dose may be further adjusted by 4 to 8 mg on a weekly basis, up to 32 mg a day in 2 to 4 divided doses. Adults: For the first week, 4 mg once a day. The total daily dose may be further adjusted by 4 to 8 mg on a weekly basis, up to 56 mg a day in 2 to 4 divided doses.

ONSET OF EFFECT
Unknown.

DURATION OF ACTION
Unknown.

DIETARY ADVICE
Tiagabine should be taken with meals.

STORAGE
Store in a tightly sealed container away from heat, moisture, and direct light.

MISSED DOSE
Take it as soon as you remember. If it is near the time for the next dose, skip the missed dose and resume your regular dosage schedule. Do not double the next dose.

STOPPING THE DRUG
The decision to stop taking the drug should be made by your doctor. Never stop this drug abruptly because this may cause seizures. The dose is typically tapered over a period of weeks.

PROLONGED USE
Side effects are more likely with prolonged use.

▼ PRECAUTIONS

Over 60: Adverse reactions may be more likely and more severe.

Driving and Hazardous Work: Do not drive or engage in hazardous work until you determine how the medicine affects you.

Alcohol: May contribute to excessive drowsiness.

Pregnancy: Adequate human studies have not been done. Before taking tiagabine, tell your doctor if you are or are planning to become pregnant. Discuss with your doctor the relative risks and benefits of using this drug while pregnant.

Breast Feeding: Tiagabine may pass into breast milk; caution is advised. Consult your doctor for specific advice.

Infants and Children: Not recommended for use by children under age 12.

Special Concerns: Your doctor may want you to wear a medical alert bracelet or carry an identification card saying that you are taking this drug.

OVERDOSE
Symptoms: Few cases of overdose have been reported. In clinical trials, the most common symptoms following overdose have been drowsiness, agitation, confusion, speech problems, hostility, mental depression, weakness, and muscle spasms.

What to Do: Call your doctor, emergency medical services (EMS), or the nearest poison control center immediately.

▼ INTERACTIONS

DRUG INTERACTIONS
There are no significant drug interactions.

FOOD INTERACTIONS
No known food interactions.

DISEASE INTERACTIONS
A lower dose or longer dosing intervals may be warranted in patients with impaired liver function.

 SIDE EFFECTS

SERIOUS
No serious side effects are associated with the use of tiagabine.

COMMON
Dizziness, fatigue, lack of energy, drowsiness, nausea, nervousness, irritability, tremor.

LESS COMMON
Abdominal pain, diarrhea, vomiting, general pain, increased appetite, mouth sores, joint aches, insomnia, speech difficulties, clumsiness or incoordination, difficulty concentrating, amnesia, mental depression, emotional instability, hostility or agitation, confusion, abnormal eye movements, sore throat, numbness, prickling or tingling sensations, rash, flulike symptoms.

TICLOPIDINE HYDROCHLORIDE

Available in: Tablets
Available OTC? No **As Generic?** No
Drug Class: Antiplatelet drug

▼ USAGE INFORMATION

WHY IT'S PRESCRIBED
To reduce the chance of stroke in patients who have had a stroke or have high risk factors for stroke. While beneficial in this regard, ticlopidine is potentially a very dangerous medication prescribed only when all other therapeutic measures have failed.

HOW IT WORKS
Blood clots are a primary cause of stroke and heart attack. Ticlopidine prevents platelets from clumping clumping together to form blood clots, thus reducing the risk of stroke.

▼ DOSAGE GUIDELINES

RANGE AND FREQUENCY
250 mg, 2 times a day.

ONSET OF EFFECT
Within 2 days.

DURATION OF ACTION
1 to 2 weeks.

DIETARY ADVICE
Should be taken with food.

STORAGE
Store in a tightly sealed container away from heat and direct light.

MISSED DOSE
Take it as soon as you remember. If it is near the time for the next dose, skip the missed dose and resume your regular dosage schedule. Do not double the next dose.

STOPPING THE DRUG
The decision to stop taking the drug should be made by your doctor.

PROLONGED USE
You should see your doctor regularly for blood cell counts and physical examinations if you must take this medication for a prolonged period.

▼ PRECAUTIONS

Over 60: No special problems are expected.

Driving and Hazardous Work: Do not drive or engage in hazardous work until you determine how the medicine affects you.

Alcohol: Avoid alcohol.

Pregnancy: In animal studies, ticlopidine has caused harmful effects; human studies have not been done. Before you take ticlopidine, be sure to tell your doctor if you are currently pregnant or plan to become pregnant.

Breast Feeding: It is not known whether ticlopidine passes into breast milk; caution is advised. Consult your doctor for specific advice.

Infants and Children: There are no studies of ticlopidine use in children.

Special Concerns: Be sure to tell all of your doctors, dentists, and pharmacists that you are taking ticlopidine. You may have to stop taking the drug 10 days to 2 weeks before an operation or dental work. Ticlopidine can cause serious bleeding, especially after an injury. Ask your doctor whether there are activities you should avoid while taking this drug. Frequent blood tests, every 1 or 2 weeks, should be done during the first 6 months of ticlopidine therapy.

OVERDOSE
Symptoms: Uncontrolled bleeding, fever, infection.

What to Do: Discontinue the medication and call your doctor, emergency medical services (EMS), or the nearest poison control right away.

▼ INTERACTIONS

DRUG INTERACTIONS
Consult your doctor for specific advice if you are taking anticoagulants, carbenicillin, dipyridamole, divalproex, heparin, medicine for pain or inflammation, pentoxifylline, plicamycin, sulfinpyrazone, ticarcillin, or valproic acid.

FOOD INTERACTIONS
No known food interactions.

DISEASE INTERACTIONS
Caution is advised when taking ticlopidine. Consult your doctor if you have a history of any of the following: a blood clotting problem, severe liver disease, stomach ulcers, any blood disease, or severe kidney disease.

≣ SIDE EFFECTS ≣

SERIOUS
Bleeding that is difficult to stop, bruising, increased susceptibility to infection, sores, ulcers or white spots in the mouth, severe abdominal or stomach pain, back pain, peeling or loosening of the skin or lips or mucous membranes, bloody or tarry stools, blood in urine, coughing up blood, dizziness, fever or chills, severe headache, loss of coordination, pinpoint red spots on skin, thickened or scaly skin, difficulty speaking, unusually heavy menstrual flow, vomiting of blood or dark material. Call your doctor immediately.

COMMON
Skin rash, mild stomach pain, diarrhea, indigestion, nausea.

LESS COMMON
Gas or bloating, dizziness, vomiting.

TILUDRONATE DISODIUM

Available in: Tablets
Available OTC? No   **As Generic?** No
Drug Class: Bisphosphonate inhibitor of bone resorption

▼ USAGE INFORMATION

WHY IT'S PRESCRIBED
To treat Paget's disease, a disorder characterized by rapid breakdown and reformation of bone, which can lead to fragility and malformation of bones. Treatment is indicated if serum alkaline phosphatase (as measured in blood tests) is at least two times normal, or if the patient has symptoms or is at risk for complications.

HOW IT WORKS
Healthy bones are continuously remodeled (broken down and then reformed); the minerals and other components of bones are reabsorbed by one set of cells (osteoclasts) and replaced by another set of cells to form new bone. Tiludronate suppresses the activity of osteoclasts; consequently, the breakdown of bone tissue occurs more slowly than the laying down of new bone. As a result, bone density and strength are preserved.

▼ DOSAGE GUIDELINES

RANGE AND FREQUENCY
400 mg a day for 3 months.

ONSET OF EFFECT
Unknown.

DURATION OF ACTION
Unknown.

DIETARY ADVICE
Take it with a full glass of plain water. Taking tiludronate with food or beverages (including mineral water) other than plain water is likely to reduce the absorption of the drug from the intestine. Take the tablets at least 2 hours before or after eating. Maintain adequate vitamin D and calcium intake; however, vitamin or mineral supplements should also be taken at least 2 hours before or after taking the drug.

STORAGE
Store in a tightly sealed container away from heat, moisture, and direct light. Do not remove from the foil strips until they are to be used.

MISSED DOSE
If you miss a dose on one day, do not double the dose the next day. Resume your regular dosage schedule.

STOPPING THE DRUG
Take it as prescribed for the full treatment period. The decision to stop taking the drug should be made in consultation with your physician.

PROLONGED USE
Tiludronate is generally prescribed for a 3-month course of therapy. Adequate studies on the safety and effectiveness of tiludronate beyond this period of time have not been done.

▼ PRECAUTIONS

Over 60: No special problems are expected.

Driving and Hazardous Work: The use of tiludronate should not impair your ability to perform such tasks safely.

Alcohol: No special precautions are necessary.

Pregnancy: Adequate human studies have not been done. Discuss with your doctor the relative risks and benefits of using this drug while pregnant.

Breast Feeding: Tiludronate may pass into breast milk; caution is advised. Consult your doctor for specific advice.

Infants and Children: Not recommended for use by children under age 18.

OVERDOSE
Symptoms: No cases of overdose have been reported.

What to Do: An overdose with tiludronate is unlikely. If someone takes a much larger dose than prescribed, call your doctor.

▼ INTERACTIONS

DRUG INTERACTIONS
Calcium supplements, aspirin, and indomethacin should not be taken within 2 hours before or after taking tiludronate. Aluminum- or magnesium-containing antacids, if needed, should be taken at least 2 hours after taking tiludronate.

FOOD INTERACTIONS
No known food interactions, although tiludronate works best when taken on an empty stomach.

DISEASE INTERACTIONS
Patients with severe kidney disease should not take tiludronate.

 SIDE EFFECTS

SERIOUS
No serious side effects have been reported.

COMMON
Diarrhea, nausea, stomach upset, indigestion.

LESS COMMON
Mild chest pain, swelling of the ankles, numbness, rash, vomiting, flatulence, increased susceptibility to infection, runny nose, sinus infection, cataract, conjunctivitis, glaucoma, dental problems.

TIMOLOL MALEATE OPHTHALMIC

BRAND NAMES

Timoptic, Timoptic in Ocudose

Available in: Ophthalmic solution
Available OTC? No **As Generic?** No
Drug Class: Antiglaucoma drug; ophthalmic beta-blocker

▼ USAGE INFORMATION

WHY IT'S PRESCRIBED
To treat glaucoma.

HOW IT WORKS
Glaucoma, a sight-threatening disorder, occurs when aqueous humor (the fluid inside the eye) cannot drain properly, causing an increase in pressure within the eyeball (intraocular pressure). This can damage the optic nerve and lead to a gradually progressive loss of vision. Timolol decreases the production of aqueous humor, thereby reducing intraocular pressure.

▼ DOSAGE GUIDELINES

RANGE AND FREQUENCY
Adults and older children: 1 drop 1 or 2 times a day. Younger children and infants: Use and dosage must be determined by your doctor.

ONSET OF EFFECT
Within 30 minutes.

DURATION OF ACTION
12 to 24 hours.

DIETARY ADVICE
This medication can be used without regard to diet.

STORAGE
Store in a tightly sealed container away from heat, moisture, and direct light. Do not allow it to freeze.

MISSED DOSE
Apply it as soon as you remember. If it is near the time for the next dose, skip the missed dose and resume your regular dosage schedule. Do not double the next dose.

STOPPING THE DRUG
The decision to stop using the drug should be made by your doctor.

PROLONGED USE
You should see your doctor regularly for tests and examinations as part of glaucoma follow up if you take this drug for a prolonged period.

▼ PRECAUTIONS

Over 60: Adverse reactions may be more likely and more severe in older patients.

Driving and Hazardous Work: Do not drive or engage in hazardous work until you determine how the medicine affects your vision.

Alcohol: Use alcohol with caution.

Pregnancy: Timolol has not caused birth defects in animals. Human studies have not been completed. Before you take timolol, tell your doctor if you are pregnant or plan to become pregnant.

Breast Feeding: Timolol may pass into breast milk; caution is advised. Consult your doctor for advice.

Infants and Children: Adverse reactions may be more likely and more severe in infants.

Special Concerns: To use the eye drops, first wash your hands. Tilt your head back. Gently apply pressure to the inside corner of the eyelid and with the index finger of the same hand, pull downward on the lower eyelid to make a space. Drop the medicine into this space and close your eye. Apply pressure for 1 or 2 minutes while keeping the eye closed without blinking. Then wash your hands again. Make sure the tip of the dropper does not touch your eye, finger, or any other surface. Timolol may make your eyes more sensitive to bright light. If this occurs, wear sunglasses or avoid bright light as necessary. Before you have any surgery, dental treatment, or emergency treatment, tell the doctor or dentist in charge that you are using timolol.

OVERDOSE
Symptoms: Nervousness, chest pain, irregular or pounding heartbeat, hallucinations, wheezing, mental confusion.

What to Do: If a large volume enters the eye, flush with water. If someone accidentally ingests the medicine, call your doctor, emergency medical services (EMS), or the nearest poison control center.

▼ INTERACTIONS

DRUG INTERACTIONS
It is not recommended to use two ophthalmic beta-blockers at the same time. Special caution is warranted in people taking antidiabetic drugs, as timolol may mask symptoms of low blood sugar. Consult your doctor for specific advice if you are taking any other prescription or over-the-counter medication.

FOOD INTERACTIONS
No known food interactions.

DISEASE INTERACTIONS
Caution is advised when taking timolol. Consult your doctor if you have any of the following: asthma, emphysema or another lung disease, low blood sugar, heart disease, blood vessel disease, or an overactive thyroid. In diabetes, timolol can affect blood sugar levels or mask symptoms of low blood sugar.

≡ SIDE EFFECTS ≡

SERIOUS
Palpitations, trouble breathing, dizziness and weakness caused by low blood pressure. Call your doctor right away.

COMMON
Stinging or irritation of the eye when drops are applied, tearing.

LESS COMMON
Decreased night vision; eyebrow pain; crusted eyelashes; dry eyes; increased sensitivity of eyes to light; redness, stinging, burning, watering, or other irritation of the eye; droopy eyelid; eye inflammation.

TIMOLOL MALEATE ORAL

Available in: Tablets
Available OTC? No   **As Generic?** Yes
Drug Class: Beta-blocker

▼ USAGE INFORMATION

WHY IT'S PRESCRIBED
To treat high blood pressure; to prevent recurrence of and lower mortality from heart attack; to prevent migraine headaches.

HOW IT WORKS
Beta-blockers such as timolol work by preventing—or blocking—nerve impulses from exerting an accelerating or intensifying effect on specific parts of the body, especially blood vessels and the heart. This slows the heart and widens the vessels, thus lowering blood pressure. By relaxing blood vessels in the brain, timolol also helps prevent migraines.

▼ DOSAGE GUIDELINES

RANGE AND FREQUENCY
For high blood pressure: 10 mg, 2 times a day; may be increased to a maximum of 60 mg per day. After heart attack: 10 mg, 2 times a day. Migraine headache prevention: 10 mg, 2 times a day; may be increased to 30 mg per day.

ONSET OF EFFECT
Within 15 to 30 minutes.

DURATION OF ACTION
Up to 12 hours.

DIETARY ADVICE
Timolol can be taken with meals to minimize the risk of stomach upset.

STORAGE
Store in a tightly sealed container away from heat and direct light.

MISSED DOSE
Take it as soon as you remember. If it is near the time for the next dose, skip the missed dose and resume your regular dosage schedule. Do not double the next dose.

STOPPING THE DRUG
Do not discontinue the drug suddenly, as this may cause serious health problems. The dosage must be gradually tapered in accordance with your physician's instructions.

PROLONGED USE
Lifelong therapy with timolol may be necessary. Visit your doctor regularly if you take it for a prolonged period.

▼ PRECAUTIONS

Over 60: Adverse reactions may be more likely and more severe. Resistance to cold temperatures may be decreased in older patients.

Driving and Hazardous Work: Do not drive or engage in hazardous work until you determine how the medicine affects you.

Alcohol: Avoid alcohol.

Pregnancy: Discuss with your doctor the relative risks and benefits of using this drug while pregnant.

Breast Feeding: Timolol passes into breast milk; consult your doctor about its use while nursing.

Infants and Children: The dosage must be determined by your pediatrician.

Special Concerns: Take extra care during exercise or hot weather to avoid dizziness and fainting. Check your pulse regularly while taking timolol. If it is slower than your usual rate or less than 50 beats a minute, check with your doctor.

OVERDOSE

Symptoms: Unusually slow or rapid heartbeat, severe dizziness or fainting, poor circulation in the hands (bluish skin), breathing difficulty, seizures.

What to Do: Call your doctor, emergency medical services (EMS), or the nearest poison control center immediately.

▼ INTERACTIONS

DRUG INTERACTIONS
Consult your doctor if you are taking amphetamines, oral antidiabetic agents, asthma medication (such as aminophylline or theophylline), calcium channel blockers, clonidine, guanabenz, halothane, immunotherapy for allergies (allergy shots), insulin, MAO inhibitors, reserpine, other beta-blockers, or any over-the-counter drug.

FOOD INTERACTIONS
No known food interactions.

DISEASE INTERACTIONS
Timolol should be used with caution in people with diabetes, especially insulin-dependent diabetes, since the drug may mask symptoms of hypoglycemia. People with the following conditions should consult their doctor before using timolol: allergies or asthma, heart or blood vessel disease (including congestive heart failure and peripheral vascular disease), hyperthyroidism, irregular (slow) heartbeat, myasthenia gravis, psoriasis, respiratory problems such as bronchitis or emphysema, kidney or liver disease, or a history of mental depression.

≡ SIDE EFFECTS ≡

SERIOUS
Shortness of breath, wheezing; irregular or slow heartbeat (50 beats per minute or less); pain or feelings of tightness or pressure in the chest; swelling of the ankles, feet, and lower legs; mental depression. If you experience any such symptoms, stop taking timolol and contact your doctor right away.

COMMON
Dizziness or lightheadedness, especially when rising suddenly to a standing position; decreased sexual ability; unusual fatigue, weakness, or drowsiness; insomnia.

LESS COMMON
Anxiety, irritability, nervousness; constipation; diarrhea; dry, sore eyes; itching; nausea or vomiting; nightmares or intensely vivid dreams; numbness, tingling, or other unusual sensations in the fingers, toes, or scalp.

TIOCONAZOLE

Available in: Vaginal ointment
Available OTC? Yes   **As Generic?** No
Drug Class: Antifungal

▼ USAGE INFORMATION

WHY IT'S PRESCRIBED
To treat fungal (yeast) infections of the vagina.

HOW IT WORKS
Tioconazole prevents the growth and function of some fungal organisms by interfering with the production of substances needed to preserve the cell membrane. This drug is effective only for infections caused by fungal organisms. It will not work for bacterial or viral infections.

▼ DOSAGE GUIDELINES

RANGE AND FREQUENCY
A single 300 mg (1 applicatorful) dose of ointment, inserted with an applicator into the vagina at bedtime.

ONSET OF EFFECT
Some relief may be felt within 1 day. Complete relief of symptoms generally occurs within 7 days.

DURATION OF ACTION
Unknown.

DIETARY ADVICE
Tioconazole may be used without regard to diet.

STORAGE
Store in a tightly sealed container away from heat, moisture, and direct light. Do not allow it to freeze.

MISSED DOSE
Not applicable. Tioconazole is usually effective with a single, one-time use.

STOPPING THE DRUG
Tioconazole is generally used on a one-time basis. If needed, a second dose may be applied 1 to 2 weeks following the first dose.

PROLONGED USE
Tioconazole is for short-term use only.

▼ PRECAUTIONS

Over 60: No special problems are expected.

Driving and Hazardous Work: This drug should not impair your ability to perform such tasks safely.

Alcohol: No special warnings.

Pregnancy: Adequate studies on the use of tioconazole during pregnancy have not been done; however, there are no reports of adverse effects while using it. Consult your doctor.

Breast Feeding: No problems are expected. Consult your doctor before using this medicine while nursing.

Infants and Children: No studies have been done on the use of tioconazole in children. Consult your pediatrician for specific advice.

Special Concerns: Tioconazole may be used with oral contraceptives and antibiotic therapy. Sanitary napkins should be used to prevent staining of clothing. The affected area should be kept cool and dry. The patient should wear loose-fitting cotton clothing and freshly laundered cotton underwear or pantyhose with a cotton crotch. Avoid underwear made from nonventilating materials. Do not sit for a long time in a wet bathing suit. Avoid feminine hygiene sprays. Wash daily with unscented soap and dry thoroughly with a clean towel. Tampons should not be used during therapy. Do not have sex for 3 days after treatment and wait an additional 3 days before relying upon a condom or diaphragm, since the medication may weaken latex. After this time, the patient's sexual partner should wear a condom during intercourse and should consult a doctor if penile redness, itching, or discomfort occurs. You may use this medicine during your menstrual period. After urination or a bowel movement, cleanse by wiping the area from front to back to prevent reinfection.

OVERDOSE
Symptoms: An overdose with tioconazole is unlikely.

What to Do: If someone should swallow a large amount of the medicine, call your doctor.

▼ INTERACTIONS

DRUG INTERACTIONS
Tell your doctor if you are using any other vaginal prescription or over-the-counter medication.

FOOD INTERACTIONS
No food interactions have been reported.

DISEASE INTERACTIONS
No disease interactions have been reported.

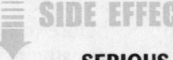

SIDE EFFECTS

SERIOUS
Vaginal itching, burning, discharge, or irritation not present prior to treatment. Call your doctor as soon as possible.

COMMON
No common side effects have been reported.

LESS COMMON
Headache, stomach cramps or pain, irritation or burning of sexual partner's penis.

TIZANIDINE HYDROCHLORIDE

Available in: Tablets
Available OTC? No   **As Generic?** No
Drug Class: Muscle relaxant

▼ USAGE INFORMATION

WHY IT'S PRESCRIBED
To relieve the muscle spasticity and cramping associated with multiple sclerosis and spinal cord injury.

HOW IT WORKS
Tizanidine is a short-acting drug that temporarily inhibits nerve activity that causes spasticity. Because of the risk of side effects, it should be taken only at times of the day when reduced spasticity is most important.

▼ DOSAGE GUIDELINES

RANGE AND FREQUENCY
Initial dose is 4 mg, every 6 to 8 hours. This may be increased as needed in 2 to 4 mg increments to 8 mg every 6 to 8 hours (not exceeding 3 doses in 24 hours), until a satisfactory therapeutic effect is achieved. Maximum dose is 36 mg a day.

ONSET OF EFFECT
Within 1 hour.

DURATION OF ACTION
Up to 6 hours.

DIETARY ADVICE
It can be taken with or between meals. Dry mouth is a common complaint with such drugs; maintain adequate fluid intake and suck on ice chips if desired.

STORAGE
Store in a tightly sealed container away from heat and direct light.

MISSED DOSE
Take it as soon as you remember. If it is near the time for the next dose, skip the missed dose and resume your regular dosage schedule. Do not double the next dose.

STOPPING THE DRUG
The decision to stop taking the drug should be made by your doctor.

PROLONGED USE
You should see your doctor regularly for tests and examinations if you must take this drug for a prolonged period.

▼ PRECAUTIONS

Over 60: Adverse reactions may be more likely and more severe in older patients.

Driving and Hazardous Work: Do not drive or engage in hazardous work until you determine how the medicine affects you.

Alcohol: Avoid alcohol.

Pregnancy: In some animal studies, large doses of tizanidine have been shown to cause problems. Human studies have not been done. This drug should be used during pregnancy only if clearly needed. Consult your doctor for advice.

Breast Feeding: Tizanidine may pass into breast milk; caution is advised. Consult your doctor for advice.

Infants and Children: There is no specific information about the use of tizanidine in infants and children.

Special Concerns: Tizanidine is a newly introduced medication, and it is possible that side effects not found in early studies may occur with widespread use. Patients should be alert for the signs of significantly lowered blood pressure (dizziness, faintness, disorientation). In clinical trials of tizanidine, a small number of patients experienced hallucinations that continued after treatment was stopped. Dose-related eye damage (retinal degeneration and corneal opacities) was detected in some animal studies but has not been seen in human clinical trials.

OVERDOSE

Symptoms: Loss of consciousness and respiratory depression have been noted thus far in limited experience with the drug. Other symptoms may occur.

What to Do: If apparent overdose occurs, call your doctor, emergency medical services (EMS), or the nearest poison control center immediately.

▼ INTERACTIONS

DRUG INTERACTIONS
Consult your doctor for specific advice if you are taking oral contraceptives or any other prescription or over-the-counter medication, especially those that produce sedation as a side effect, such as benzodiazepine tranquilizers and baclofen, or medications that are used for lowering high blood pressure.

FOOD INTERACTIONS
No known food interactions.

DISEASE INTERACTIONS
Caution is advised when taking tizanidine. Consult your doctor if you have any other medical condition. Tizanidine may cause complications in patients with kidney disease, since the kidneys are involved in the removal of the drug from the body.

 SIDE EFFECTS

SERIOUS
Liver damage causing nausea, vomiting, loss of appetite, and yellowish tinge to eyes and skin (jaundice). Call your doctor immediately.

COMMON
Drowsiness; dry mouth; dizziness; slowed heartbeat; very low blood pressure, causing lightheadedness when arising from a sitting or lying position.

LESS COMMON
Infection, constipation, rapid heartbeat, vomiting, speech problems, blurred vision, frequent urination, flu syndrome, nervousness, movement difficulties, inflamed mucous membranes, nasal inflammation.

TOBRAMYCIN

BRAND NAMES

Nebcin, Tobi, Tobrex

Available in: Injection, ophthalmic solution and ointment, inhalation
Available OTC? No   **As Generic?** Yes
Drug Class: Aminoglycoside antibiotic

▼ USAGE INFORMATION

WHY IT'S PRESCRIBED
To treat bacterial infections including those of the bones and joints, central nervous system, the abdominal cavity, eyes, skin and soft tissue, urinary tract, and the blood. Tobramycin is also used in the management of lung infections in patients with cystic fibrosis.

HOW IT WORKS
Tobramycin interferes with bacteria's genetic material—specifically its RNA, which is necessary in the manufacture of proteins. Without the ability to manufacture protein, the bacteria cannot survive.

▼ DOSAGE GUIDELINES

RANGE AND FREQUENCY
Most infections— Injection: Dosage depends on the weight of the patient and the infection being treated. Mild eye infections— Adults and teenagers: 1 drop of solution in the affected eye every 4 hours or a thin strip of oint-ment applied every 8 to 12 hours. Severe eye infections— Apply the solution or ointment every 3 to 4 hours until improvement occurs, then adjust the frequency of doses as directed by your doctor. Lung infections in those with cystic fibrosis— Injection: Initially, 10 mg per 2.2 lbs (1 kg) of body weight a day in 4 divided doses. Inhalation: 300 mg 2 times a day for 28 days. Stop therapy for 28 days, and then resume therapy for the next 28 days. Inhalations should be taken as close to 12 hours apart as possible and not less than 6 hours apart.

ONSET OF EFFECT
Variable.

DURATION OF ACTION
Variable.

DIETARY ADVICE
Drink plenty of fluids.

STORAGE
Store in a tightly sealed container away from heat and direct light. Refrigerate the inhalation form.

≡ SIDE EFFECTS ≡

SERIOUS
Loss of balance, dizziness; ringing, buzzing, or feeling of fullness in the ears, any loss of hearing; increased thirst, greatly decreased or increased amount of urine or frequency of urination, loss of appetite, nausea or vomiting; muscle twitching or seizures; skin rash, itching, redness, or swelling (especially around the eye or eyelid) not present prior to treatment. Call your doctor immediately.

COMMON
Ophthalmic ointment: Temporary blurred vision immediately following administration.

LESS COMMON
Ophthalmic forms: Stinging or burning of the eyes.

MISSED DOSE
Take it as soon as you remember. If it is near the time (within 6 hours for the inhalation) for the next dose, skip the missed dose and resume your regular dosage schedule. Do not double the next dose.

STOPPING THE DRUG
Take as prescribed for the full treatment period.

PROLONGED USE
Periodic kidney function tests may be needed. Consult your doctor if your condition does not improve after 7 days, or 1 to 3 days for eye infections.

▼ PRECAUTIONS

Over 60: Adverse reactions may be more likely and more severe.

Driving and Hazardous Work: Avoid such activities until you determine how the medicine affects you.

Alcohol: Avoid alcohol.

Pregnancy: Discuss with your doctor the relative risks and benefits of using this drug while pregnant. Some studies show that injectable tobramycin may cause damage to the infant's hearing, sense of balance, and kidneys. However, this medication may be necessary for the mother.

Breast Feeding: Tobramycin may pass into breast milk; caution is advised.

Infants and Children: Tobramycin may be used by infants and children with proper doses.

Special Concerns: To use the drops or the ointment, first wash your hands. Tilt your head back. Gently apply pressure to the inside corner of the eyelid and with the index finger of the same hand, pull downward on the lower eyelid to make a space. Drop the medicine or put a short strip of ointment (about ⅓ inch long) into this space and close your eye. Apply pressure for 1 or 2 minutes while keeping the eye closed. Wash hands again. Make sure the tip of the dropper or applicator does not touch your eye, finger, or any other surface.

OVERDOSE
Symptoms: Injection: Blood in the urine, decreased urine output, swelling of the ankles or other body parts, impaired muscle control, breathing difficulty. Ophthalmic forms: Eye pain and redness, increased tear production, swelling and itching of the eyes or eyelids. Inhalation: None reported.

What to Do: Seek medical attention immediately.

▼ INTERACTIONS

DRUG INTERACTIONS
Consult your doctor if you are taking any other aminoglycoside, capreomycin, methoxyflurane, polymyxins, cyclosporine, dornase alfa, or vancomycin.

FOOD INTERACTIONS
No known food interactions.

DISEASE INTERACTIONS
Consult your doctor for specific advice if you have loss of hearing or balance, kidney disease, Parkinson's disease, or myasthenia gravis.

TOCAINIDE HYDROCHLORIDE

Available in: Tablets
Available OTC? No   **As Generic?** No
Drug Class: Antiarrhythmic

▼ USAGE INFORMATION

WHY IT'S PRESCRIBED
To correct irregular heartbeats (cardiac arrhythmias). This drug is used only to treat severe, life-threatening heart rhythm disorders, since it has been shown to cause serious adverse side effects in some patients.

HOW IT WORKS
Tocainide slows nerve impulses in the heart and reduces the sensitivity of heart tissue to certain nerve impulses, thus stabilizing heartbeat.

▼ DOSAGE GUIDELINES

RANGE AND FREQUENCY
To start, 400 mg every 8 hours. The dose may be increased to 600 mg, 3 times a day. It is best to take doses at equally spaced intervals. Early adverse effects may be decreased by administering the medication in smaller, more frequent doses.

ONSET OF EFFECT
Within 2 hours.

DURATION OF ACTION
Approximately 8 to 11 hours.

DIETARY ADVICE
Tocainide can be taken with food or milk to avoid gastrointestinal upset.

STORAGE
Store in a tightly sealed container in a dry place away from heat and direct light.

MISSED DOSE
Take it as soon as you remember. However, if it is near the time for the next dose, skip the missed dose and resume your regular dosage schedule. Do not double the next dose.

STOPPING THE DRUG
Take tocainide as prescribed for the full treatment period, even if you begin to feel better before the scheduled end of therapy. The decision to stop taking the drug should be made by your doctor.

PROLONGED USE
Lifelong therapy may be necessary. See your doctor regularly for examinations and diagnostic tests if you must take this medicine for a prolonged period.

▼ PRECAUTIONS

Over 60: Adverse reactions may be more likely and more severe in older patients.

Driving and Hazardous Work: Avoid such activities until you determine how the medicine affects you.

Alcohol: Avoid alcohol.

Pregnancy: Animal studies have shown that high doses of tocainide can cause fetal deaths. No defects or other problems have been found in humans. Before you take tocainide, tell your doctor if you are pregnant or plan to become pregnant.

Breast Feeding: Tocainide may pass into breast milk; caution is advised. Consult your doctor for advice.

Infants and Children: Studies of tocainide in infants and children have not been done. Use and dose must be determined by your pediatrician.

Special Concerns: Before having any kind of surgery, tell the doctor or dentist in charge that you are taking tocainide. Your doctor may require weekly blood tests for the first 3 weeks of treatment and frequently after that. Tell your doctor if you have any unusual allergic reaction to tocainide or to an anesthetic.

▼ OVERDOSE

Symptoms: Tremors, seizures, heartbeat irregularities, nausea, vomiting, weakness, cardiac arrest.

What to Do: Call your doctor, emergency medical services (EMS), or the nearest poison control center immediately.

▼ INTERACTIONS

DRUG INTERACTIONS
Consult your doctor for specific advice if you are taking rifampin, beta-blockers, or any other prescription or over-the-counter medication.

FOOD INTERACTIONS
No known food interactions.

DISEASE INTERACTIONS
Caution is advised when taking tocainide. Avoid this medication if you have congestive heart failure. Use of tocainide may cause complications in patients with liver or kidney disease, since these organs work together to remove the medication from the body.

SIDE EFFECTS

SERIOUS
Fainting; rapid or irregular heartbeats (palpitations); trembling or shaking; severe rash, blisters, peeling or scaling of skin; cough or shortness of breath; fever or chills; unusually slow heartbeat; mouth sores; unusual bleeding or bruising, loss of appetite, unusual anxiety; jaundice (yellowish tinge to skin or whites of eyes); profuse sweating. Call your doctor immediately.

COMMON
Dizziness or lightheadedness, loss of appetite, nausea.

LESS COMMON
Mental confusion, blurred vision, headache, anxiety or irritability, skin rash, sweating, vomiting, numbness or tingling of fingers and toes.

TOLAZAMIDE

Available in: Tablets
Available OTC? No   **As Generic?** Yes
Drug Class: Antidiabetic agent/sulfonylurea

▼ USAGE INFORMATION

WHY IT'S PRESCRIBED
To help control blood sugar in patients with non-insulin-dependent (type 2) diabetes.

HOW IT WORKS
Tolazamide stimulates insulin release from the pancreas and reduces glucose output by the liver.

▼ DOSAGE GUIDELINES

RANGE AND FREQUENCY
Adults: 100 to 250 mg once a day to start. It can be increased to 1,000 mg per day. If more than 500 mg per day, tablets are usually taken in 2 doses. Children: The dose must be determined by your doctor.

ONSET OF EFFECT
Within 4 to 6 hours.

DURATION OF ACTION
12 to 24 hours.

DIETARY ADVICE
If 1 dose daily, take it before breakfast. If 2 doses, take one before breakfast and one before dinner.

STORAGE
Store in a tightly sealed container away from heat and direct light.

MISSED DOSE
Take it as soon as you remember. If it is near the time for the next dose, skip the missed dose and resume your regular dosage schedule. Do not double the next dose.

STOPPING THE DRUG
The decision to stop taking the drug should be made by your doctor.

PROLONGED USE
At some point, tolazamide may stop working effectively and your blood sugar may go up. Consult your doctor about the need for periodic examinations and blood tests.

▼ PRECAUTIONS

Over 60: Adverse reactions may be more likely and more severe in older patients.

Driving and Hazardous Work: Do not drive or engage in hazardous work until you determine how the medicine affects you.

Alcohol: Alcohol should be avoided while taking this medication.

Pregnancy: Before you take tolazamide, tell your doctor if you are pregnant or plan to become pregnant. This medicine is rarely used during pregnancy (insulin is the treatment of choice for pregnant diabetic women).

Breast Feeding: Tolbutamide may pass into breast milk; caution is advised. Consult your doctor for advice.

Infants and Children: Non-insulin-dependent (type 2) diabetes is rare in infants and children.

Special Concerns: Be sure to carry a card or medical ID bracelet saying that you have this type of diabetes. Follow your prescribed diet closely. Consult your doctor about exercises you should do. Be sure you take your daily dose of tolazamide even when you become ill. You may have to be switched temporarily to insulin. Test your blood sugar level at least every 4 hours when you are ill. Keep some source of quick-acting sugar readily available to handle episodes of low blood sugar.

OVERDOSE
Symptoms: Tingling of lips and tongue, lethargy, confusion, nausea, nervousness, sweating, tremors, hunger, convulsions, loss of consciousness. (Most symptoms of overdose are due to serious hypoglycemia.)

What to Do: Call your doctor, emergency medical services (EMS), or the nearest poison control center immediately.

▼ INTERACTIONS

DRUG INTERACTIONS
Consult your doctor for specific advice if you are taking anticoagulants, antifungal agents, aspirin, chloramphenicol, cimetidine, ciprofloxacin, quinidine, ranitidine, asparaginase, corticosteroids, lithium, asthma medicine, allergy drugs, beta-blockers, cyclosporine, guanethidine, MAO inhibitors, octreotide, pentamidine, or anticonvulsants.

FOOD INTERACTIONS
Be careful to follow the low-sugar diet prescribed for you by your doctor.

DISEASE INTERACTIONS
Consult your physician if you have any of the following: diarrhea, heart disease, hyperthyroidism, or underactive adrenal or pituitary gland. Use of tolazamide may cause complications in patients with liver or kidney disease, since these organs work together to remove the medication from the body.

≡ SIDE EFFECTS ≡

SERIOUS
Convulsions; fainting; low blood sugar, causing anxious feeling; blurred vision; cold sweats; confusion; drowsiness; excessive hunger; rapid heartbeat; headache; nausea; nervousness; restless sleep; shortness of breath; unusual weight gain; unusual bleeding or bruising. Call your doctor at once. Other serious but less common side effects include bone marrow suppression, hemolytic anemia, and elevation of liver-associated enzymes; these problems can be detected by your doctor.

COMMON
Changes in taste, constipation or diarrhea, more frequent urination, headache, heartburn, increased or decreased appetite, nausea, stomach pain or fullness, vomiting.

LESS COMMON
Increased sensitivity of skin to the sun.

TOLBUTAMIDE

BRAND NAMES
Orinase, Tol-Tab

Available in: Tablets
Available OTC? No   **As Generic?** Yes
Drug Class: Antidiabetic agent/sulfonylurea

▼ USAGE INFORMATION

WHY IT'S PRESCRIBED
To help control blood sugar in patients with non-insulin-dependent (type 2) diabetes.

HOW IT WORKS
Tolbutamide stimulates insulin release from the pancreas and reduces glucose output by the liver.

▼ DOSAGE GUIDELINES

RANGE AND FREQUENCY
Adults: 1,000 to 2,000 mg per day to start, in 2 divided doses. It can be increased to 3,000 mg (3 g) a day, although little additional benefit is derived from more than 2 g a day. Children: The dose must be set by a pediatrician.

ONSET OF EFFECT
Within 1 hour.

DURATION OF ACTION
6 to 12 hours.

DIETARY ADVICE
Tolbutamide should be taken 30 minutes before the morning and evening meals.

STORAGE
Store in a tightly sealed container away from heat and direct light.

MISSED DOSE
Take it as soon as you remember. If it is near the time for the next dose, skip the missed dose and resume your regular dosage schedule. Do not double the next dose.

STOPPING THE DRUG
The decision to stop taking the drug should be made by your doctor.

PROLONGED USE
At some point, tolbutamide may stop working effectively and your blood sugar may rise unexpectedly. Consult your doctor about the need for periodic examinations and blood tests.

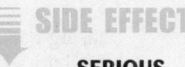

SIDE EFFECTS

SERIOUS
Seizures, fainting, low blood sugar causing anxious feeling, blurred vision, cold sweats, confusion, drowsiness, excessive hunger, fast heartbeat, headache, nausea, nervousness, restless sleep, shortness of breath, unusual weight gain, unusual bleeding or bruising. Call your doctor at once. Other serious but less common side effects include bone marrow suppression, hemolytic anemia, and elevation of liver-associated enzymes; these problems can be detected by your doctor.

COMMON
Changes in taste, constipation or diarrhea, more frequent urination, headache, heartburn, increased or decreased appetite, nausea, stomach pain or fullness, vomiting.

LESS COMMON
Increased sensitivity of skin to the sun.

▼ PRECAUTIONS

Over 60: Adverse reactions may be more likely and more severe in older patients.

Driving and Hazardous Work: Avoid such activities until you determine how the medicine affects you.

Alcohol: Avoid alcohol.

Pregnancy: Before you take tolbutamide, tell your doctor if you are pregnant or plan to become pregnant. This medicine is rarely used during pregnancy.

Breast Feeding: Tolbutamide may pass into breast milk; caution is advised. Consult your doctor for advice.

Infants and Children: The safety and effectiveness have not been established for young patients.

Special Concerns: Be sure to carry a card or medical ID bracelet saying that you have this type of diabetes. Follow your prescribed diet closely. Consult your doctor about exercises you should do. Be sure you take your daily dose of tolbutamide even when you become ill. You may have to be switched temporarily to insulin. Test your blood sugar level at least every 4 hours when you are ill.

OVERDOSE
Symptoms: Tingling of lips and tongue, lethargy, confusion, nausea, nervousness, sweating, tremors, hunger, convulsions, loss of consciousness. (Most symptoms of overdose are due to serious hypoglycemia.)

What to Do: Call your doctor, emergency medical services (EMS), or the nearest poison control center immediately.

▼ INTERACTIONS

DRUG INTERACTIONS
Consult your doctor if you are taking anticoagulants, antifungal agents, aspirin, chloramphenicol, cimetidine, ciprofloxacin, quinidine, ranitidine, antiseizure medication, asparaginase, corticosteroids, lithium, asthma medicine, allergy medicine, beta-blockers, cyclosporine, guanethidine, MAO inhibitors, octreotide, or pentamidine.

FOOD INTERACTIONS
Be careful to follow the low-sugar diet as prescribed.

DISEASE INTERACTIONS
Caution is advised when taking tolbutamide. Consult your doctor if you have any of the following: diarrhea, heart disease, overactive thyroid, or underactive adrenal or pituitary gland. Use of tolbutamide may cause complications in patients who have liver or kidney disease, since these organs work together to remove the medication from the body.

TOLCAPONE

Available in: Tablets
Available OTC? No   **As Generic?** No
Drug Class: Antiparkinsonism drug/COMT inhibitor

▼ USAGE INFORMATION

WHY IT'S PRESCRIBED
To treat Parkinson's disease in conjunction with standard levodopa/carbidopa therapy. It should only be used by patients who are experiencing symptom fluctuations and are not responding satisfactorily or those who are inappropriate candidates for other adjunctive therapies.

HOW IT WORKS
When used with levodopa/carbidopa, tolcapone sustains higher levels of levodopa in the blood. Tolcapone is believed to increase blood levels of levodopa by blocking the action of catechol-O-methyltransferase (COMT), one of the enzymes responsible for breaking down levodopa, before it reaches its receptors in the brain. Levodopa raises the amount of dopamine available in the brain; dopamine plays an essential role in smooth movement of muscles and is deficient in patients with Parkinson's disease.

▼ DOSAGE GUIDELINES

RANGE AND FREQUENCY
Initial dose: 100 mg, 3 times a day in conjunction with levodopa/carbidopa. The first dose of the day should be taken together with levodopa/carbidopa and the remaining doses should be taken 6 and 12 hours later. The dose can be increased to 200 mg 3 times a day if the anticipated increase in benefit is justified. Many patients may need to reduce their daily dose of levodopa.

ONSET OF EFFECT
Unknown.

DURATION OF ACTION
Unknown.

SIDE EFFECTS

SERIOUS
Liver damage is a significant serious side effect. Symptoms include persistent nausea, fatigue, lethargy, loss of appetite, jaundice, dark urine, itchiness, and abdominal pain on the right side. Call your doctor immediately. Dizziness, lightheadedness, or fainting, especially when rising from a sitting or lying position, owing to a sudden drop in blood pressure (orthostatic hypotension).

COMMON
Impaired movement, nausea, sleep difficulties, quirky involuntary movements that contort the body, excessive dreaming, loss of appetite, muscle cramps, drowsiness, diarrhea, confusion, headaches, hallucinations, vomiting.

LESS COMMON
Constipation, increased susceptibility to upper respiratory tract infection, increased incidence of falling, increased sweating, dry mouth, abdominal pain, discolored urine.

DIETARY ADVICE
Tolcapone can be taken without regard to meals.

STORAGE
Store in a tightly sealed container away from heat, moisture, and direct light.

MISSED DOSE
Take it as soon as you remember. If it is near the time for the next dose, skip the missed dose and resume your regular dosage schedule. Do not double the next dose.

STOPPING THE DRUG
Take it as prescribed for the full treatment period. The decision to stop taking the drug should be made in consultation with your physician.

PROLONGED USE
Liver function tests are strongly recommended just prior to treatment, every 2 weeks for the first year of therapy, every 4 weeks for the next 6 months, and then every 8 weeks thereafter.

▼ PRECAUTIONS

Over 60: Adverse reactions may be more likely and more severe in older patients.

Driving and Hazardous Work: Avoid such activities until you determine how the medicine affects you.

Alcohol: Avoid alcohol.

Pregnancy: Before taking tolcapone, tell your doctor if you are or are planning to become pregnant. Discuss with your doctor the relative risks and benefits of using this drug.

Breast Feeding: Tolcapone may pass into breast milk; caution is advised. Consult your doctor for advice.

Infants and Children: Not applicable.

Special Concerns: If tolcapone does does not provide significant benefit within three weeks of the initiation of treatment, therapy should be discontinued.

OVERDOSE
Symptoms: An overdose with tolcapone is unlikely. However, nausea, vomiting, and dizziness or fainting may occur with an excessive dose.

What to Do: If someone takes a much larger dose than prescribed, call your doctor, emergency medical services (EMS), or the nearest poison control immediately.

▼ INTERACTIONS

DRUG INTERACTIONS
Consult your doctor if you are taking desipramine, MAO inhibitor antidepressants (such as phenelzine sulfate or tranylcypromine sulfate, but not selegiline), or antihypertensive drugs.

FOOD INTERACTIONS
No known food interactions.

DISEASE INTERACTIONS
Do not use tolcapone if you have liver disease or have had a prior reaction to tolcapone. Caution is advised for patients with low blood pressure or severe kidney dysfunction.

TOLMETIN SODIUM

Available in: Tablets, capsules
Available OTC? No   **As Generic?** Yes
Drug Class: Nonsteroidal anti-inflammatory drug (NSAID)

▼ USAGE INFORMATION

WHY IT'S PRESCRIBED
To treat mild to moderate pain and inflammation caused by tendinitis, arthritis, bursitis, gout, soft tissue injuries, migraine and other vascular headaches, menstrual cramps, and other conditions. When patients fail to respond to one NSAID, another may be tried. The greatest effectiveness often requires trial and error of several different NSAIDs.

HOW IT WORKS
NSAIDs work by interfering with the formation of prostaglandins, naturally occurring substances in the body that cause inflammation and make nerves more sensitive to pain impulses. NSAIDs also have other modes of action that are less well understood.

▼ DOSAGE GUIDELINES

RANGE AND FREQUENCY
Adults: 400 mg, 3 times a day. Maximum dose is 1,800 mg a day. Children: Consult your pediatrician.

ONSET OF EFFECT
From 30 minutes to several hours or longer.

DURATION OF ACTION
Varies.

DIETARY ADVICE
Take with food; maintain your usual food and fluid intake.

STORAGE
Store in a tightly sealed container away from heat, moisture, and direct light.

MISSED DOSE
Take it as soon as you remember. If it is near the time for the next dose, skip the missed dose and resume your regular dosage schedule. Do not double the next dose.

STOPPING THE DRUG
The decision to stop taking the drug should be made in consultation with your physician.

PROLONGED USE
Prolonged use can cause gastrointestinal problems, including ulceration and bleeding, kidney dysfunction, and liver inflammation. Consult your doctor about the need for medical examinations and laboratory tests.

▼ PRECAUTIONS

Over 60: Because of the potentially greater consequences of gastrointestinal side effects, the dose of NSAIDs for older patients, especially those over age 70, is often cut in half.

Driving and Hazardous Work: Avoid such activities until you determine how the medicine affects you.

Alcohol: Avoid alcohol when using this medication because it increases the risk of stomach irritation.

Pregnancy: Avoid or discontinue this drug if you are pregnant or are planning to become pregnant.

Breast Feeding: Tolmetin passes into breast milk; avoid use while nursing.

Infants and Children: May be used in exceptional circumstances; consult your doctor.

Special Concerns: Because NSAIDs can interfere with blood coagulation, this drug should be stopped at least 3 days prior to any surgery.

OVERDOSE
Symptoms: Severe nausea, vomiting, headache, confusion, seizures.

What to Do: Call your doctor, emergency medical services (EMS), or the nearest poison control center immediately.

▼ INTERACTIONS

DRUG INTERACTIONS
Do not take this drug with aspirin or any other NSAIDs without your doctor's approval. In addition, consult your doctor if you are taking antihypertensives, steroids, anticoagulants, antibiotics, itraconazole or ketoconazole, plicamycin, penicillamine, valproic acid, phenytoin, cyclosporine, digitalis drugs, lithium, methotrexate, probenecid, triamterene, or zidovudine.

FOOD INTERACTIONS
No known food interactions.

DISEASE INTERACTIONS
Consult your doctor if you have any of the following: bleeding problems, inflammation or ulcers of the stomach and intestines, diabetes mellitus, systemic lupus erythematosus (SLE, lupus), anemia, asthma, epilepsy, Parkinson's disease, kidney stones, or a history of heart disease or alcohol abuse. Use of tolmetin may cause complications in patients with liver or kidney disease, since these organs work together to remove the medication from the body.

SIDE EFFECTS

SERIOUS
Shortness of breath or wheezing, with or without swelling of legs or other signs of heart failure; chest pain; peptic ulcer disease with vomiting of blood; black, tarry stools; decreasing kidney function. Call your doctor immediately.

COMMON
Nausea, vomiting, heartburn, diarrhea, constipation, headache, dizziness, sleepiness.

LESS COMMON
Ulcers or sores in mouth, depression, rashes or blistering of skin, ringing sound in the ears, unusual tingling or numbness of the hands or feet, seizures, blurred vision. Also elevated potassium levels, decreased blood counts; such problems can be detected by your doctor.

TOLNAFTATE

Available in: Cream, gel, powder, solution
Available OTC? Yes   **As Generic?** Yes
Drug Class: Topical antifungal

▼ USAGE INFORMATION

WHY IT'S PRESCRIBED
To treat a variety of fungal
infections of the skin, including tinea corporis (ringworm),
tinea cruris (jock itch), and
tinea pedis (athlete's foot).

HOW IT WORKS
Tolnaftate prevents fungi from
manufacturing vital sub-
stances required for growth
and function. This medication
is effective only for infections
caused by ringworm fungal
organisms. It will not work for
bacterial or viral infections.

▼ DOSAGE GUIDELINES

RANGE AND FREQUENCY
Apply to the affected area 2
times a day. All forms should
be used immediately after the
affected area is washed and
dried. Wash your hands
before and after application.

ONSET OF EFFECT
Unknown.

DURATION OF ACTION
Unknown.

DIETARY ADVICE
No special restrictions.

STORAGE
Store in a tightly sealed container away from heat, moisture, and direct light.

MISSED DOSE
Apply it as soon as you
remember. If it is near the
time for the next dose, skip
the missed dose and resume
your regular dosage schedule.
Do not double the next dose.

STOPPING THE DRUG
Use of tolnaftate should continue for 2 weeks beyond the
time that symptoms disap-
pear. This helps to ensure
eradication of the fungus.

PROLONGED USE
You should consult your
doctor if symptoms do not
improve within 10 days of
beginning therapy.

▼ PRECAUTIONS

Over 60: No special problems are expected.

**Driving and Hazardous
Work:** The use of tolnaftate
should not impair your ability
to perform such tasks safely.

Alcohol: No special warnings.

Pregnancy: Tolnaftate has not
been shown in studies to
cause problems when used
during pregnancy.

Breast Feeding: Tolnaftate
may pass into breast milk, but
no problems have been
reported. Consult your doctor
for specific advice.

Infants and Children: Tolnaftate should be used by children under the age of 2 years
only under a doctor's close
supervision.

Special Concerns: Do not
allow tolnaftate to come into
contact with your eyes. If
your skin condition does not
improve or instead gets worse
after 10 days of treatment,
consult your doctor. Tolnaftate should not be used alone
to treat fungal infections of
the hair or nails; your doctor
will prescribe an additional
medication. If you are using
tolnaftate for an infection of
the feet, be sure to wear well-
fitting and well-ventilated
shoes and to change your
shoes and socks every day.
Do not cover the treated area
of skin with bandages unless
your doctor instructs you to
do so.

OVERDOSE
Symptoms: None are known;
no cases of overdose have
been reported.

What to Do: An overdose of
tolnaftate is unlikely to occur.
However, if someone acci-
dentally ingests some of the
medication, call your doctor,
emergency medical services
(EMS), or the nearest poison
control center immediately.

▼ INTERACTIONS

DRUG INTERACTIONS
Some drugs may interact
adversely with tolnaftate. Consult your doctor for specific
advice if you are taking any
other prescription or over-
the-counter medication that
is applied to the same area
of skin being treated by
tolnaftate.

FOOD INTERACTIONS
No known food interactions.

DISEASE INTERACTIONS
Caution is advised when taking tolnaftate. Consult your
doctor for specific advice if
you have a history of any
other skin condition.

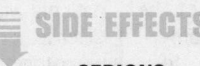
SIDE EFFECTS

SERIOUS
Skin irritation that was not present before use of tolnaftate.
Call your doctor immediately.

COMMON
No common side effects are associated with the use of
tolnaftate.

LESS COMMON
No less-common side effects are associated with the use
of tolnaftate.

TOLTERODINE TARTRATE

Available in: Tablets
Available OTC? No   **As Generic?** No
Drug Class: Anticholinergic

▼ USAGE INFORMATION

WHY IT'S PRESCRIBED
To treat overactive bladder with symptoms of urinary frequency, urgency, or urge incontinence.

HOW IT WORKS
Tolterodine decreases the urge to urinate by blocking nerve receptors that trigger contractions of the bladder.

▼ DOSAGE GUIDELINES

RANGE AND FREQUENCY
Adults: 2 mg, twice a day. Dose may be lowered by your doctor to 1 mg, twice a day, depending upon response to the medication. Adults with impaired liver function: no more than 1 mg, twice a day.

ONSET OF EFFECT
Unknown.

DURATION OF ACTION
Unknown.

DIETARY ADVICE
Tolterodine can be taken without regard to diet.

STORAGE
Store in a tightly sealed container away from heat, moisture, and direct light.

MISSED DOSE
Take it as soon as you remember. If it is near the time for the next dose, skip the missed dose and resume your regular dosage schedule. Do not double the next dose.

STOPPING THE DRUG
The decision to stop taking the drug should be made in consultation with your physician.

PROLONGED USE
See your doctor periodically if you must take this drug for a prolonged period.

▼ PRECAUTIONS

Over 60: No special problems are expected.

Driving and Hazardous Work: The use of tolterodine should not impair your ability to perform such tasks safely.

Alcohol: No special problems are expected.

Pregnancy: No human studies have been done. Before taking tolterodine, tell your doctor if you are pregnant or plan to become pregnant.

Breast Feeding: Tolterodine may pass into breast milk; avoid use while nursing. Consult your doctor for specific advice.

Infants and Children: Not recommended for use by children under the age of 18.

OVERDOSE
Symptoms: Drowsiness, mental confusion, dizziness, loss of coordination, dry mouth.

What to Do: Few cases of overdose have been reported. However, if someone takes a much larger dose than prescribed, call your doctor, emergency medical services (EMS), or the nearest poison control center immediately.

▼ INTERACTIONS

DRUG INTERACTIONS
The following drugs may interact with tolterodine. Consult your doctor for specific advice if you are taking fluoxetine, macrolide antibiotics, or antifungal drugs.

FOOD INTERACTIONS
No known food interactions.

DISEASE INTERACTIONS
You should not take tolterodine if you have urinary retention, gastric retention, or uncontrolled narrow-angle glaucoma. Tolterodine should be used with caution in patients with liver or kidney disease, since these organs work together to remove the medication from the body.

SIDE EFFECTS

SERIOUS
Chest pain. Consult your doctor immediately.

COMMON
Headache, constipation, indigestion, dry eye, dry mouth.

LESS COMMON
Numbness, tingling or prickling sensation, abdominal pain, flatulence, nausea or vomiting, bronchitis, cough, dry skin, nervousness, drowsiness, blurred vision.

TOPIRAMATE

Available in: Tablets, capsules
Available OTC? No   **As Generic?** No
Drug Class: Anticonvulsant

▼ USAGE INFORMATION

WHY IT'S PRESCRIBED
To help control certain types of seizures in the treatment of epilepsy and other disorders. It is often used in conjunction with other anticonvulsant drugs after they have failed to be effective on their own.

HOW IT WORKS
Topiramate appears to block the uncontrolled firing of neurons that causes seizures, but its precise mechanism of action is unknown.

▼ DOSAGE GUIDELINES

RANGE AND FREQUENCY
Adults: 100 to 400 mg a day, in 2 divided doses. Some patients require higher doses. Initially, a low dose is prescribed; it may then be gradually increased by your doctor. Children ages 2 to 16: 5 to 9 mg per 2.2 lbs (1 kg) a day, in 2 divided doses. As with adults, dosage may be adjusted by your doctor.

ONSET OF EFFECT
Several hours.

DURATION OF ACTION
Maximum effectiveness lasts 24 hours or longer; effectiveness then gradually decreases.

DIETARY ADVICE
Take it with food or milk to minimize stomach upset. Because of their bitter taste, tablets should be swallowed whole. Capsules may be swallowed whole or opened and the contents sprinkled on one teaspoon of soft food to make the drug more palatable. It should be swallowed immediately, without chewing.

STORAGE
Store in a tightly sealed container away from heat, moisture, and direct light.

MISSED DOSE
Take it as soon as you remember. If it is near the time for the next dose, skip the missed dose and resume your regular dosage schedule. Do not double the next dose unless so advised by your doctor.

STOPPING THE DRUG
Never stop this drug abruptly, because seizures may ensue. The dose is typically tapered over a period of weeks to months under your doctor's supervision.

PROLONGED USE
This drug may be taken on a long-term basis. See your doctor regularly for tests.

▼ PRECAUTIONS

Over 60: Older patients may require lower doses to minimize side effects.

Driving and Hazardous Work: Avoid such activities until you determine how this medication affects you.

Alcohol: May contribute to excessive drowsiness.

Pregnancy: Human studies with this drug have not been done, but other anticonvulsants are known to increase the risk of birth defects. However, seizures during pregnancy can also increase the risks to the fetus. Discuss with your doctor the potential risks and benefits of using this drug during pregnancy. Folate supplementation is advised starting 1 to 2 months before conception and throughout pregnancy.

Breast Feeding: Topiramate may pass into breast milk, although at low levels. Consult your doctor for advice.

Infants and Children: Special caution is advised in children. Use of the drug in children has been limited.

Special Concerns: Because this drug may predispose to the formation of kidney stones, you should drink plenty of fluids while taking it. Your doctor may suggest that you carry an ID card or bracelet saying that you are taking this medication.

OVERDOSE
Symptoms: No specific symptoms of overdose have been reported.

What to Do: Call your doctor, emergency medical services (EMS), or the nearest poison control center immediately.

▼ INTERACTIONS

DRUG INTERACTIONS
Topiramate interacts with a number of other drugs, including other anticonvulsants; carbonic anhydrase inhibitors, such as acetazolamide or dichlorphenamide; and digoxin. This drug can interfere with oral contraceptives, leading to contraceptive failure.

FOOD INTERACTIONS
No known food interactions.

DISEASE INTERACTIONS
Special caution is advised if you have liver disease or kidney disease, including a history of kidney stones or hemodialysis.

SIDE EFFECTS

SERIOUS
Intense pain in the kidney area (the lower back or flanks) may be a sign of kidney stones, which occur with greater frequency in those taking topiramate.

COMMON
Drowsiness, fatigue, dizziness, anxiety, loss of coordination, unusual eye movements, tingling sensations, confusion, speech problems, depression, poor concentration or attention, mood changes, memory impairment, poor appetite, weight loss, tremor.

LESS COMMON
Back pain, nausea and vomiting, indigestion, dry mouth, abdominal pain, constipation, muscle aches, hearing difficulty, menstrual irregularities, sinus infections, double vision. Many additional side effects can occur; consult your doctor if you are concerned about any adverse or unusual reactions you experience while taking this drug.

TOREMIFENE CITRATE

Available in: Tablets
Available OTC? No   **As Generic?** No
Drug Class: Antiestrogen; antineoplastic (anticancer) agent

▼ USAGE INFORMATION

WHY IT'S PRESCRIBED
To treat metastatic breast cancer in postmenopausal women.

HOW IT WORKS
Toremifene blocks the effects of the hormone estrogen by interfering with the binding of estrogen to its receptors on estrogen-sensitive cells. The growth of some breast tumors is stimulated by estrogens; toremifene may therefore slow the growth of such tumors.

▼ DOSAGE GUIDELINES

RANGE AND FREQUENCY
60 mg once a day.

ONSET OF EFFECT
Unknown.

DURATION OF ACTION
Unknown.

DIETARY ADVICE
Toremifene can be taken without regard to meals. Maintain adequate food and fluid intake, since calorie, protein, and vitamin needs increase in patients with cancer.

STORAGE
Store in a tightly sealed container away from heat, moisture, and direct light.

MISSED DOSE
Toremifene is prescribed for once-daily use only. If you are unable to take the medication on a particular day, simply resume your regular dosage schedule the following day. Do not double the next dose.

STOPPING THE DRUG
You may need to remain on this medication for an extended period, and you should take toremifene exactly as prescribed throughout the course of treatment. The decision to stop taking the drug should be made in consultation with your physician. Do not stop taking toremifene on your own.

PROLONGED USE
There is no standard duration of therapy with toremifene, although you can expect to remain on it for at least several weeks in order to determine if it is effective. Your doctor will decide whether your response to the drug is satisfactory or not, and will recommend continuation or discontinuation of therapy.

▼ PRECAUTIONS

Over 60: No special problems are expected.

Driving and Hazardous Work: The use of toremifene should not impair your ability to perform such tasks safely.

Alcohol: No special precautions are necessary.

Pregnancy: Toremifene must not be used in pregnant women. Although toremifene is not generally prescribed for premenopausal women, it is important that patients be sure they are not pregnant before starting treatment with this drug.

Breast Feeding: Use of this drug is not recommended while nursing; the benefits must clearly outweigh potential risks. Consult your doctor for advice.

Infants and Children: Use of toremifene is not approved for infants and children.

Special Concerns: Patients with cancer are very often weakened by their illness, by poor nutrition, and by the effects of chemotherapy, radiation, and surgery. Such patients are more likely to experience undesirable side effects of a medication. In addition, these side effects may be more pronounced. Follow all medication directions carefully. Some women with metastases to bone may develop musculoskeletal pain and elevated levels of blood calcium during the first week of treatment.

OVERDOSE
Symptoms: No cases of overdose have been reported.

What to Do: An overdose is unlikely; however, if you have any reason to suspect that one has occurred, call emergency medical services (EMS) to receive evaluation and treatment in the closest emergency facility.

▼ INTERACTIONS

DRUG INTERACTIONS
Consult your doctor for specific advice if you are taking thiazide diuretics or warfarin, which may interact with toremifene.

FOOD INTERACTIONS
No known food interactions.

DISEASE INTERACTIONS
Toremifene should not be used in women with a history of thromboembolic disease. Long-term treatment is not generally advised in women with preexisting endometrial hyperplasia.

≡ SIDE EFFECTS ≡

SERIOUS
Vaginal bleeding, cataracts or other eye problems.

COMMON
Hot flashes, sweating, nausea, vaginal discharge, dizziness.

LESS COMMON
Swelling in the extremities, vomiting.

TORSEMIDE

Available in: Tablets, injection
Available OTC? No   **As Generic?** No
Drug Class: Loop diuretic

▼ USAGE INFORMATION

WHY IT'S PRESCRIBED
To reduce fluid (salt and water) accumulation that leads to edema (swelling of body tissues) and breathlessness in patients with heart disease, liver disease, and kidney disease. Torsemide is also sometimes prescribed to help control high blood pressure.

HOW IT WORKS
Loop diuretics work on a specific portion of the kidney (the loop of Henle) to increase the excretion of water and sodium (and other salts) in the urine.

▼ DOSAGE GUIDELINES

RANGE AND FREQUENCY
For high blood pressure—Tablets: 5 to 10 mg once a day. The dose may be increased as determined by your doctor. For eliminating excess body water (edema)—Tablets: 5 to 60 mg once a day. Injection: 5 to 20 mg, injected once a day. The dose may be increased.

ONSET OF EFFECT
For injection, 10 minutes; for tablets, 1 hour.

DURATION OF ACTION
6 to 8 hours.

DIETARY ADVICE
Take it with or after meals to reduce stomach irritation.

STORAGE
Store in a tightly sealed container away from heat and direct light.

MISSED DOSE
Take it as soon as you remember. If it is near the time for the next dose, skip the missed dose and resume your regular dosage schedule. Do not double the next dose.

STOPPING THE DRUG
The decision to stop taking the drug should be made by your doctor.

PROLONGED USE
See your doctor regularly if you must take this medicine for a prolonged period.

▼ PRECAUTIONS

Over 60: No special precautions are warranted.

Driving and Hazardous Work: The use of this drug should not impair your ability to perform such tasks safely.

Alcohol: No special precautions are necessary.

Pregnancy: Human studies have not been done. Consult your doctor about taking torsemide during pregnancy.

Breast Feeding: Torsemide may pass into breast milk; caution is advised. Consult your doctor for advice.

Infants and Children: There is no specific information on the use of torsemide in infants and children. Use and dose must be determined by a pediatrician.

Special Concerns: If you take torsemide for high blood pressure, follow your doctor's advice on diet and weight control. This medicine may cause your body to lose potassium. Consult your doctor about eating potassium-rich foods or taking a supplement.

OVERDOSE
Symptoms: Dehydration, palpitations or heartbeat irregularities, weakness, dizziness, confusion, vomiting, cramps, loss of consciousness.

What to Do: Call your doctor, emergency medical services (EMS), or the nearest poison control center immediately.

▼ INTERACTIONS

DRUG INTERACTIONS
Consult your doctor for specific advice if you are taking any ACE inhibitor, antibiotics, amphotericin B, carmustine, cisplatin, corticosteroids, corticotropin, cyclosporine, deferoxamine, dichlorphenamide, digitalis drugs, lithium, methazolamide, methotrexate, penicillamine, gold salts, pentamidine, streptozocin, tiopronin, or vitamin B12.

FOOD INTERACTIONS
No known food interactions.

DISEASE INTERACTIONS
Caution is advised when taking torsemide. Consult your doctor for advice if you have diabetes, gout, or a hearing problem, or have had a recent heart attack.

☰ SIDE EFFECTS ☰

SERIOUS
Skin rash, hives, intense itching, swelling of the mouth and throat, breathing difficulty, heart rhythm irregularities, light-headedness, unusual bleeding or bruising, black or tarry stools. Call your doctor immediately.

COMMON
Muscle cramps or pain. Potassium depletion may lead to heart palpitations and weakness. Fluid depletion may lead to dizziness, especially upon arising from a sitting or lying position, as well as thirst, dry mouth, and constipation.

LESS COMMON
Buzzing or ringing in ears, loss of hearing (particularly after intravenous treatment or with very high doses), diarrhea, loss of appetite, gout, increased blood sugar (a problem for diabetic patients).

TRAMADOL HYDROCHLORIDE

Available in: Tablets
Available OTC? No   **As Generic?** No
Drug Class: Analgesic

▼ USAGE INFORMATION

WHY IT'S PRESCRIBED
To help manage moderate to somewhat severe pain, such as that which occurs following joint surgery and certain gynecological procedures (for example, cesarean section).

HOW IT WORKS
Tramadol acts on the central nervous system to block the transmission of pain signals. It works similarly to narcotic analgesics, and while not a narcotic, it can be habit-forming, leading to mental and physical drug dependence.

▼ DOSAGE GUIDELINES

RANGE AND FREQUENCY
1 or 2 tablets (50 mg each) every 6 hours as needed. For severe pain, your doctor may prescribe 2 tablets for the first dose.

ONSET OF EFFECT
Usually within 1 hour, with a peak effect at 2 hours.

DURATION OF ACTION
6 to 7 hours.

DIETARY ADVICE
Tramadol can be taken with or without food.

STORAGE
Store in a tightly sealed container away from heat and direct light.

MISSED DOSE
Take it as soon as you remember. However, if it is near the time for the next dose, skip the missed dose and resume your regular dosage schedule. Do not double the next dose.

STOPPING THE DRUG
The decision to stop taking the drug should be made by your doctor.

PROLONGED USE
You should see your doctor regularly for tests and examinations if you take this drug for a prolonged period.

▼ PRECAUTIONS

Over 60: Tramadol stays longer in the body of older patients than younger ones; your doctor may adjust the dose accordingly.

Driving and Hazardous Work: Do not drive or engage in hazardous work until you determine how the medicine affects you.

Alcohol: Do not consume alcohol while taking this medication since it may compound the drug's sedative effect on the central nervous system.

Pregnancy: Tramadol has caused birth defects and other problems in animals. Human studies have not been done. Before you take tramadol, tell your doctor if you are pregnant or are planning to become pregnant.

Breast Feeding: Tramadol passes into breast milk; avoid or discontinue use while breast feeding.

Infants and Children: Safety and effectiveness have not been established for the use of tramadol in children under 16 years old.

Special Concerns: Before undergoing any kind of surgery, including dental surgery, be sure your doctor or dentist knows that you are taking tramadol.

OVERDOSE
Symptoms: Breathing difficulty, seizures, vomiting.

What to Do: Call your doctor, emergency medical services (EMS), or the nearest poison control center immediately.

▼ INTERACTIONS

DRUG INTERACTIONS
Consult your doctor for specific advice if you are taking carbamazepine, anesthetics, MAO inhibitors, or any drugs known to depress the central nervous system, including antihistamines, sedatives, tranquilizers, sleeping pills, other prescription pain medicines, barbiturates, medications for seizures, or muscle relaxants.

FOOD INTERACTIONS
No known food interactions.

DISEASE INTERACTIONS
Caution is advised when taking tramadol. Consult your doctor if you have severe abdominal or stomach conditions, or a history of alcohol abuse, drug abuse, head injury, or seizure disorders. Use of tramadol may cause complications in patients with liver or kidney disease, since these organs work together to remove the medication from the body.

≣ SIDE EFFECTS ≣

SERIOUS
Blurred vision, difficulty urinating, frequent urge to urinate, blisters under the skin, change in walking balance, dizziness or lightheadedness when getting up, fainting, fast heartbeat, memory loss, hallucinations, shortness of breath. Also numbness, tingling, pain, or weakness in hands or feet; redness, swelling, and itching of skin; trembling and shaking of hands or feet; trouble performing routine tasks. Call your doctor immediately.

COMMON
Dizziness, vertigo, headache, drowsiness, nausea, vomiting, constipation.

LESS COMMON
Weakness, lack of energy, anxiety, confusion, euphoria, nervousness, insomnia, visual disturbances, stomach upset, dry mouth, diarrhea, abdominal pain, loss of appetite, gas, menopausal symptoms, sweating, muscle spasm, rash.

TRANDOLAPRIL

Available in: Tablet
Available OTC? No   **As Generic?** No
Drug Class: Angiotensin-converting enzyme (ACE) inhibitor

▼ USAGE INFORMATION

WHY IT'S PRESCRIBED
To control high blood pressure; to treat congestive heart failure; to treat patients with left ventricular dysfunction (damage to the pumping chamber of the heart); and to minimize further kidney damage in diabetics with mild kidney disease.

HOW IT WORKS
Angiotensin-converting enzyme (ACE) inhibitors block an enzyme that produces angiotensin, a naturally occurring substance that causes blood vessels to constrict and stimulates production of the adrenal hormone, aldosterone, which promotes sodium retention in the body. As a result, ACE inhibitors relax blood vessels (causing them to widen) and reduces sodium retention, which lowers blood pressure and so decreases the workload of the heart.

▼ DOSAGE GUIDELINES

RANGE AND FREQUENCY
To start, 1 mg once a day, except black patients, who should start with 2 mg once a day. Doses may be increased to a maximum of 8 mg a day.

ONSET OF EFFECT
Within 4 hours.

DURATION OF ACTION
Up to 24 hours.

DIETARY ADVICE
Take it on an empty stomach, about 1 hour before mealtime. Follow your doctor's dietary advice (such as low-salt or low-cholesterol restrictions) to improve control over hypertension and heart disease. Avoid high-potassium foods like bananas and citrus fruits and juices, unless you are also taking drugs that lower potassium levels.

STORAGE
Store in a tightly sealed container away from heat, moisture, and direct light.

MISSED DOSE
Take it as soon as you remember. If it is near the time for the next dose, skip the missed dose and resume your regular dosage schedule. Do not double the next dose.

STOPPING THE DRUG
Do not stop taking this drug abruptly, as this may cause potentially serious health problems. Dosage should be reduced gradually, according to your doctor's instructions.

PROLONGED USE
See your doctor regularly for examinations and tests if you must take this medicine for a prolonged period. Remember that trandolapril helps control high blood pressure but does not cure it.

▼ PRECAUTIONS

Over 60: Some elderly patients may be more sensitive to the effects of this drug; smaller doses may be warranted.

Driving and Hazardous Work: Exercise caution until you determine how the medicine affects you.

Alcohol: Consume alcohol only in moderation since it may increase the effect of the drug and cause an excessive drop in blood pressure.

Pregnancy: Not recommended, especially during the last 2 trimesters (final 6 months) of pregnancy. If you become pregnant, notify your doctor as soon as possible.

Breast Feeding: Trace amounts of trandolapril can be found in breast milk; however, adverse effects in infants have not been documented. Consult your doctor.

Infants and Children: The safety and effectiveness of trandolapril in children 18 and under have not been established.

OVERDOSE
Symptoms: No specific ones have been reported.

What to Do: While overdose is unlikely, call your doctor, emergency medical services (EMS), or the nearest poison control center immediately if you suspect that someone has taken a much larger dose than prescribed.

▼ INTERACTIONS

DRUG INTERACTIONS
Consult your doctor if you are taking diuretics (especially potassium-sparing diuretics), potassium supplements or drugs containing potassium, lithium, anticoagulants, anti-inflammatory drugs, any over-the-counter drugs (especially cold remedies and diet pills).

FOOD INTERACTIONS
Avoid low-salt milk and salt substitutes. Many of these products contain potassium.

DISEASE INTERACTIONS
Consult your doctor if you have lupus or if you have had a prior allergic reaction to ACE inhibitors. Trandolapril should be used with caution by patients with severe kidney disease or renal artery stenosis (narrowing of one or both of the arteries that supply blood to the kidneys).

  SIDE EFFECTS

SERIOUS
Fever and chills; sore throat and hoarseness; sudden difficulty breathing or swallowing; swelling of the face, mouth, or extremities; impaired kidney function (ankle swelling, decreased urination); confusion; yellow discoloration of the eyes or skin (indicating liver disorder); intense itching; chest pain or palpitations; abdominal pain. Serious side effects are very rare; contact your doctor immediately.

COMMON
Dry, persistent cough.

LESS COMMON
Dizziness or fainting; skin rash; numbness or tingling in the hands, feet, or lips; unusual fatigue or muscle weakness; nausea; drowsiness; loss of taste; headache.

TRANDOLAPRIL/VERAPAMIL HYDROCHLORIDE

Available in: Tablets
Available OTC? No   **As Generic?** No
Drug Class: ACE inhibitor/calcium channel blocker combination

BRAND NAME

Tarka

▼ USAGE INFORMATION

WHY IT'S PRESCRIBED
To control high blood pressure (hypertension).

HOW IT WORKS
Angiotensin-converting enzyme (ACE) inhibitors, such as trandolapril, block an enzyme that produces angiotensin, a naturally occurring substance that causes blood vessels to constrict and stimulates production of the adrenal hormone, aldosterone, which promotes sodium retention in the body. As a result, ACE inhibitors relax blood vessels (causing them to widen) and reduces sodium retention. Verapamil, a calcium channel blocker, interferes with the movement of calcium into heart muscle cells and the smooth muscle cells in the walls of the arteries. As a result of the combined action of trandolapril and verapamil, blood vessels relax, which lowers blood pressure and thereby decreases the workload of the heart.

▼ DOSAGE GUIDELINES

RANGE AND FREQUENCY
From 1 to 4 mg of trandolapril and 120 to 480 micrograms (mcg) of verapamil per day. Tablets containing both active ingredients are taken either once a day or in 2 divided doses.

ONSET OF EFFECT
Within 15 hours.

DURATION OF ACTION
Unknown.

DIETARY ADVICE
Best taken without food. Can be taken with grapefruit juice.

STORAGE
Store in a tightly sealed container away from heat, moisture, and direct light.

MISSED DOSE
Take it as soon as you remember. If it is near the time for the next dose, skip the missed dose and resume your regular dosage schedule. Do not double the next dose.

STOPPING THE DRUG
The decision to stop taking the drug should be made by your doctor.

PROLONGED USE
See your doctor periodically for tests and examinations if you must take this medication for a prolonged period.

▼ PRECAUTIONS

Over 60: No special problems are expected.

Driving and Hazardous Work: Avoid such activities until you determine how the medicine affects you.

Alcohol: Consume alcohol only in moderation since it may increase the effect of the drug and cause an excessive drop in blood pressure.

Pregnancy: This drug should not be used during pregnancy and is especially dangerous to the unborn child during the final 6 months (second and third trimesters). Consult your doctor if you are pregnant or plan to become pregnant.

Breast Feeding: Trandolapril with verapamil passes into breast milk; avoid use while nursing or discontinue breast feeding.

Infants and Children: The safety and effectiveness of trandolapril with verapamil use by children have not been established.

Special Concerns: Trandolapril with verapamil is not recommended as the first line of therapy when hypertension is diagnosed. It may be prescribed after other drugs have proved unsatisfactory. Before you undergo surgery, tell the doctor or dentist in charge that you are taking this drug.

OVERDOSE
Symptoms: No cases have been reported. Symptoms might include extreme dizziness, fainting, or confusion.

What to Do: If someone takes a much larger dose than prescribed, seek medical assistance right away.

▼ INTERACTIONS

DRUG INTERACTIONS
Consult your doctor if you are taking digitalis, lithium, cimetidine, beta-blockers, antiarrhythmic drugs, anticonvulsants, cyclosporine, or theophylline.

FOOD INTERACTIONS
No known food interactions.

DISEASE INTERACTIONS
Consult your doctor if you have congestive heart failure (CHF), heart rhythm irregularities, or any other medical condition. This drug should be used with caution by patients with severe kidney disease or renal artery stenosis (narrowing of one or both of the arteries that supply blood to the kidneys).

≡ SIDE EFFECTS ≡

SERIOUS
Serious side effects are very rare; they include fever and chills; sore throat and hoarseness; sudden difficulty breathing or swallowing; swelling of the face, mouth, or extremities; worsening kidney function (ankle swelling, decreased urination); confusion; jaundice (yellowish tinge to eyes or skin, indicating liver problems); intense itching; chest pain or heart palpitations; abdominal pain; irregular or slow heartbeats; low blood pressure (causing dizziness or faintness). Call your doctor immediately.

COMMON
Mild swelling of arms and legs (edema), fatigue, mild headache, dizziness, constipation, cough, flushed skin.

LESS COMMON
Fainting, dry mouth, diarrhea, gas, nausea, vomiting, rectal pain, gout, neck pain, joint swelling, nervousness, insomnia, drowsiness, skin rash, increased eye pressure, impotence, hot flashes.

TRANYLCYPROMINE SULFATE

Available in: Tablets
Available OTC? No **As Generic?** No
Drug Class: Monoamine oxidase (MAO) inhibitor antidepressant

▼ USAGE INFORMATION

WHY IT'S PRESCRIBED
To treat symptoms of major mental depression.

HOW IT WORKS
Tranylcypromine inhibits the activity of monoamine oxidase, an enzyme that renders certain brain chemicals (epinephrine, norepinephrine, and dopamine) inactive. Consequently, this drug increases the availability of these chemicals in the nervous system; this is thought to have an antidepressant effect.

▼ DOSAGE GUIDELINES

RANGE AND FREQUENCY
Adults: To start, 10 mg, 3 times a day; this may be increased to 60 mg a day. Older adults: To start, 10 mg, 2 times a day; this may be increased to 40 mg a day.

ONSET OF EFFECT
48 hours; it may take up to 3 weeks for full effect.

DURATION OF ACTION
Up to 10 days after stopping treatment.

DIETARY ADVICE
See Food Interactions.

STORAGE
Store in a tightly sealed container away from heat, moisture, and direct light.

MISSED DOSE
Take it as soon as you remember. However, if it is near the time for the next dose, skip the missed dose and resume your regular dosage schedule. Do not double the next dose.

STOPPING THE DRUG
Take it as prescribed for the full treatment period. The decision to stop taking the drug should be made in consultation with your physician.

PROLONGED USE
The usual course of therapy lasts 6 months to 1 year; some patients benefit from additional therapy.

▼ PRECAUTIONS

Over 60: Adverse reactions may be more likely and more severe in older patients. A lower dose may be warranted.

Driving and Hazardous Work: Use caution until you determine how the medicine affects you.

Alcohol: Avoid alcohol.

Pregnancy: Use during pregnancy may increase the risk of birth defects.

Breast Feeding: Tranylcypromine may pass into breast milk; caution is advised. Consult your doctor for specific advice.

Infants and Children: This medication is not recommended for children age 16 and under.

Special Concerns: Before having any surgery, emergency treatment, or dental treatment, tell the doctor or dentist in charge that you are taking tranylcypromine. Your doctor may advise you to carry a card saying that you use tranylcypromine.

OVERDOSE

Symptoms: Profound anxiety, confusion, seizures, cold, clammy skin, severe drowsiness, irregular pulse, hallucinations, severe headache, fainting, stiff muscles, sweating, breathing difficulty.

What to Do: Call your doctor, emergency medical services (EMS), or the nearest poison control center immediately.

▼ INTERACTIONS

DRUG INTERACTIONS
Consult your doctor for specific advice if you are taking or have recently taken amphetamines, blood pressure medications, diet pills, cyclobenzaprine, fluoxetine, levodopa, maprotiline, asthma medication, cold or allergy medicine, meperidine, methylphenidate, another MAO inhibitor, paroxetine, sertraline, a tricyclic antidepressant, an oral diabetes drug, insulin, bupropion, buspirone, carbamazepine, a central nervous system depressant, dextromethorphan, trazodone, or tryptophan.

FOOD INTERACTIONS
Do not eat foods with a high tyramine content, such as cheeses; yeast or meat extracts; pickled or smoked meat, poultry, or fish; processed meats like bologna, salami, and pepperoni; and sauerkraut. Do not drink alcohol-free or reduced-alcohol beer and wine. Do not drink beverages or eat food with a high caffeine content, such as coffee and chocolate.

DISEASE INTERACTIONS
Consult your physician if you have any of the following: a history of alcohol abuse, angina, frequent headaches, asthma, bronchitis, diabetes mellitus, epilepsy, heart disease or a recent heart attack, blood vessel disease, liver disease, Parkinson's disease, a recent stroke, kidney disease, an overactive thyroid, or pheochromocytoma.

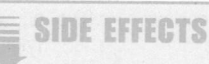 SIDE EFFECTS

SERIOUS
Severe chest pain, dilated pupils, irregular heartbeat, sensitivity of eyes to light, sweating or fever, nausea and vomiting, stiff neck, extreme dizziness. Call your doctor immediately.

COMMON
Blurring of vision; decreased urination; sexual dysfunction; mild dizziness or lightheadedness; mild headache; appetite changes, including cravings for sweets; weight gain; increase in sweating; muscle twitching during sleep; restlessness; shakiness; fatigue; insomnia.

LESS COMMON
Chills, constipation, decrease in appetite, dry mouth.

TRAZODONE

Available in: Tablets
Available OTC? No   **As Generic?** Yes
Drug Class: Antidepressant

▼ USAGE INFORMATION

WHY IT'S PRESCRIBED
To treat symptoms of major depression. It may be taken with selective serotonin reuptake inhibitor (SSRI) antidepressants such as fluoxetine, sertraline, and paroxetine when these drugs cause insomnia.

HOW IT WORKS
Trazodone helps to balance levels of serotonin, a brain chemical that is profoundly linked to mood, emotions, and mental state.

▼ DOSAGE GUIDELINES

RANGE AND FREQUENCY
Adults: To start, 50 mg, 3 times a day, or 75 mg, 2 times a day, or 100 mg at bedtime. The dose may be gradually increased by your doctor to 400 mg a day. Older adults: To start, 25 mg, 3 times a day, or 50 mg at bedtime. The dose may be increased by your doctor.

ONSET OF EFFECT
1 to 4 weeks.

DURATION OF ACTION
Unknown.

DIETARY ADVICE
It can be taken with a meal or light snack to reduce the chance of dizziness and to increase the absorption of the drug by the body.

STORAGE
Store in a tightly sealed container away from heat, moisture, and direct light.

MISSED DOSE
Take it as soon as you remember, unless the time for your next scheduled dose is within the next 4 hours. If so, do not take the missed dose. Take your next scheduled dose at the proper time and resume your regular dosage schedule. Do not double the next dose.

STOPPING THE DRUG
Take as prescribed for the full treatment period, even if you begin to feel better before the scheduled end of therapy. The decision to stop taking the drug should be made in consultation with your doctor.

PROLONGED USE
The usual course of therapy lasts for 6 months to 1 year; some patients benefit from additional therapy beyond that period.

≡ SIDE EFFECTS ≡

SERIOUS
Muscle twitching, confusion. Call your doctor immediately.

COMMON
Drowsiness, dry mouth, dizziness, lightheadedness, unpleasant taste in mouth, nausea and vomiting, headache.

LESS COMMON
Blurred vision, muscle pains, diarrhea, constipation, unusual fatigue.

▼ PRECAUTIONS

Over 60: Adverse reactions may be more likely and more severe in older patients. Lower doses may be needed.

Driving and Hazardous Work: Use caution when driving or engaging in hazardous work until you determine how the medicine affects you. Drowsiness may occur.

Alcohol: Avoid alcohol.

Pregnancy: Adequate studies of trazodone use during pregnancy have not been done. Before you take trazodone, tell your doctor if you are pregnant or plan to become pregnant.

Breast Feeding: Trazodone passes into breast milk; caution is advised. Consult your doctor for specific advice.

Infants and Children: The safety and effectiveness have not been established for infants and children.

OVERDOSE
Symptoms: Severe nausea and vomiting, loss of coordination, drowsiness.

What to Do: Call your doctor, emergency medical services (EMS), or the nearest poison control center immediately.

▼ INTERACTIONS

DRUG INTERACTIONS
The following drugs may interact with trazodone. Consult your doctor for specific advice if you are taking high blood pressure medication, central nervous system depressants (including cold and allergy drugs, narcotic pain relievers, and muscle relaxants), fluoxetine, or tricyclic antidepressants.

FOOD INTERACTIONS
No known food interactions.

DISEASE INTERACTIONS
Caution is advised when taking trazodone. Consult your doctor if you have a history of alcohol abuse or any heart condition. Use of trazodone may cause complications in patients with liver or kidney disease, since these organs work together to remove the medication from the body.

TRETINOIN

Available in: Cream, gel, liquid
Available OTC? No **As Generic?** Yes
Drug Class: Acne drug

▼ USAGE INFORMATION

WHY IT'S PRESCRIBED
Tretinoin is used to treat mild to moderate acne.

HOW IT WORKS
Although the exact mechanism of action is unknown, tretinoin appears to affect skin cells so that they are shed in a more normal fashion, therefore "unplugging" blackheads and whiteheads (comedones), the initial changes in acne formation.

▼ DOSAGE GUIDELINES

RANGE AND FREQUENCY
Adults: Apply once daily at bedtime.

ONSET OF EFFECT
Variable, usually within 2 to 6 weeks after starting therapy.

DURATION OF ACTION
The effect of tretinoin typically persists for as long as the drug is being used.

DIETARY ADVICE
No special restrictions.

STORAGE
Store in a tightly sealed container away from heat and direct light. Keep away from moisture and extremes in temperature. The gel form of this medication is flammable; keep away from heat and open flame.

MISSED DOSE
This drug is applied once every 24 hours, at night. If you miss a day, resume your regular dosage schedule the next day. There is no need to apply extra medication with the next dose to compensate for the missed dose.

STOPPING THE DRUG
Use as prescribed for the full treatment period, even if you show signs of improvement before the scheduled end of therapy.

PROLONGED USE
Therapy with this medication is frequently prolonged.

▼ PRECAUTIONS

Over 60: No special problems are expected.

Driving and Hazardous Work: No special precautions are necessary.

Alcohol: No special precautions are necessary.

Pregnancy: Avoid or discontinue tretinoin if you are pregnant or trying to become pregnant.

Breast Feeding: Tretinoin may pass into breast milk; caution is advised. Consult your doctor for advice.

Infants and Children: Not recommended for use on children.

Special Concerns: Persons with a history of allergy to tretinoin or any other ingredients in the medication should not use the product. Do not apply large amounts of tretinoin to your skin in expectation of better or faster results. This will only lead to unnecessary irritation of affected skin and surrounding areas. Sunburned skin is more susceptible to irritation from tretinoin, and application should be avoided. Avoid excessive exposure to sunlight or use of sunlamps. Keep this medication away from your eyes, mouth, and nostrils. Severe irritation and redness may result. Do not apply tretinoin to inflamed skin. If your skin becomes reddened and painful while using tretinoin, discontinue use of the medication and call your doctor. If you are using cosmetics, gently cleanse skin to be treated before applying the medication.

OVERDOSE
Symptoms: Excessive application of tretinoin may lead to severe irritation of the skin.

What to Do: If tretinoin is ingested, call your doctor, emergency medical services (EMS), or the nearest poison control center.

▼ INTERACTIONS

DRUG INTERACTIONS
Consult your doctor for specific advice if you are taking other acne medications that are applied to the same area of skin, including prescription and nonprescription treatments containing sulfur, resorcinol, alpha hydroxy acids, or salicylic acid; medicated soaps, abrasives, cleansers, or cosmetics; topical preparations with a high concentration of alcohol, astringents, extract of lime, or spices; and medications used for a drying effect.

FOOD INTERACTIONS
No known food interactions.

DISEASE INTERACTIONS
Caution is advised when using tretinoin. Consult your doctor if you have eczema.

SIDE EFFECTS

SERIOUS
No serious side effects are associated with regular applications of tretinoin when used as directed.

COMMON
Mild redness and peeling, or excessive dryness, at the site of application.

LESS COMMON
Irritation or allergy, with severe redness, swelling, blistering, pain, rash, or crusting at sites of application; changes in pigment (either lightening or darkening of skin color). These problems generally improve when the medication is stopped or reduced in dosage or frequency of application. Consult your doctor.

TRIAMCINOLONE INHALANT AND NASAL

BRAND NAMES

Azmacort, Nasacort

Available in: Nasal spray, oral inhalation
Available OTC? No   **As Generic?** No
Drug Class: Respiratory corticosteroid

▼ USAGE INFORMATION

WHY IT'S PRESCRIBED
Oral inhalation: To treat bronchial asthma. Nasal spray: To treat allergic rhinitis (seasonal or perennial allergies such as hay fever), and to prevent recurrence of nasal polyps after surgical removal.

HOW IT WORKS
Respiratory corticosteroids such as triamcinolone primarily reduce or prevent inflammation of the lining of the airways (the underlying cause of asthma), reduce the allergic response to inhaled allergens, and inhibit the secretion of mucus within the airways.

▼ DOSAGE GUIDELINES

RANGE AND FREQUENCY
Adults and children ages 12 and older– Oral inhalation: 2 inhalations of 100 micrograms (mcg) each, 3 or 4 times a day. Maximum dose is 16 inhalations a day. In some patients maintenance can be achieved when the total daily dose is given 2 times a day. Nasal spray: 2 sprays (55 mcg each) in each nostril once a day. It can be increased to 440 mcg per day in 1 or up to 4 doses. After relief is achieved, it can be decreased to as little as 1 spray (55 mcg) in each nostril once a day.

ONSET OF EFFECT
Usually within 1 week; it may take 3 weeks for the full effect to occur.

DURATION OF ACTION
Several days.

DIETARY ADVICE
No special restrictions.

STORAGE
Store in a tightly sealed container away from heat and direct light.

MISSED DOSE
Take it as soon as you remember. However, if it is near the time for the next dose, skip the missed dose and resume your regular dosage schedule. Do not double the next dose.

STOPPING THE DRUG
The decision to stop taking the drug should be made in consultation with your doctor.

PROLONGED USE
Consult your doctor about the need for regular periodic medical tests and examinations if you must take this drug for a prolonged period.

▼ PRECAUTIONS

Over 60: No special problems are expected with older patients.

Driving and Hazardous Work: The use of triamcinolone should not impair your ability to perform such tasks safely.

Alcohol: No special precautions are necessary.

Pregnancy: Inhaled or nasal steroids have not been reported to cause birth defects if taken during pregnancy. Before using such drugs, tell your doctor if you are or are planning to become pregnant.

Breast Feeding: Triamcinolone may pass into breast milk; caution is advised. Consult your doctor for advice.

Infants and Children: No special problems are expected in children, but the lowest possible dose should be used.

Special Concerns: Inhaled steroids will not help an asthma attack in progress. Inhaled steroids can lower resistance to yeast infections of the mouth, throat, or voice box. To prevent yeast infections, gargle or rinse your mouth with water after each use; do not swallow the water. Know how to use the spray properly; read and follow the directions that come with the device. Before you have surgery, tell the doctor or dentist that you are using a steroid.

OVERDOSE
Symptoms: No specific ones have been reported.

What to Do: Call your doctor, emergency medical services (EMS), or the nearest poison control center if you have any reason to suspect an overdose.

▼ INTERACTIONS

DRUG INTERACTIONS
Consult your physician for advice if you are taking systemic corticosteroids, other inhaled corticosteroids, or any drugs that suppress the immune system.

FOOD INTERACTIONS
No known food interactions.

DISEASE INTERACTIONS
Consult your physician if you have any of the following: nasal septal ulcers, ocular herpes simplex, or any fungal, bacterial, or systemic viral infection. If you are exposed to chickenpox or measles, tell your doctor at once.

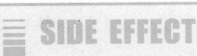

SIDE EFFECTS

SERIOUS
No serious side effects have been reported.

COMMON
Oral inhalation: Sore throat, white patches in mouth or throat, hoarseness. Nasal spray: Nosebleeds or bloody nasal secretions, nasal burning or irritation, sore throat.

LESS COMMON
Eye pain, watering eyes, gradual decrease of vision, stomach pain and digestive disturbances.

TRIAMCINOLONE SYSTEMIC

Available in: Syrup, tablets, injection
Available OTC? No   **As Generic?** Yes
Drug Class: Corticosteroid

▼ USAGE INFORMATION

WHY IT'S PRESCRIBED
To treat numerous conditions that involve inflammation (a response by body tissues, producing redness, warmth, swelling, and pain). Such conditions include arthritis, allergic reactions, asthma, some skin diseases, multiple sclerosis flare-ups, and other autoimmune diseases. Also prescribed to treat deficiency of natural steroid hormones.

HOW IT WORKS
This hormone mimics the effects of the body's natural corticosteroids. It depresses the synthesis, release, and activity of inflammation-producing body chemicals. It also suppresses the activity of the immune system.

▼ DOSAGE GUIDELINES

RANGE AND FREQUENCY
Adults and teenagers: 4 to 60 mg a day in 1 or several doses. Children's doses depend on size and body weight and should be determined by your doctor.

ONSET OF EFFECT
Variable.

DURATION OF ACTION
Variable.

DIETARY ADVICE
It can be taken with food or milk to minimize stomach upset. Your doctor may recommend a special diet.

STORAGE
Store in a tightly sealed container away from heat, moisture, and direct light. Do not freeze the liquid form.

MISSED DOSE
If you take several doses a day and it is close to the next dose, double the next dose. If you take 1 dose a day and you do not remember until the next day, skip the missed dose and do not double the next dose.

STOPPING THE DRUG
The decision to stop taking the drug should be made by your doctor.

PROLONGED USE
Long-term use may lead to cataracts, diabetes, hypertension, or osteoporosis; see your doctor for regular visits.

▼ PRECAUTIONS

Over 60: Adverse reactions may be more likely and more severe in older patients.

Driving and Hazardous Work: Avoid such activities until you determine how the medicine affects you.

Alcohol: May cause stomach problems; avoid it unless your physician approves occasional moderate drinking.

Pregnancy: Overuse during pregnancy can impair growth and development of the child.

Breast Feeding: Do not use this drug while nursing.

Infants and Children: Triamcinolone may retard the development of bone and other tissues.

Special Concerns: This drug can lower your resistance to infection. Avoid immunizations with live vaccines. Patients undergoing long-term therapy should wear a medical-alert bracelet. Call your doctor right away if you develop a fever.

OVERDOSE

Symptoms: Fever, muscle or joint pain, nausea, dizziness, fainting, difficulty breathing.

Prolonged overuse: Moon-face, obesity, unusual hair growth, acne, loss of sexual function, muscle wasting.

What to Do: Call your doctor, emergency medical services (EMS), or the nearest poison control center immediately.

▼ INTERACTIONS

DRUG INTERACTIONS
Consult your doctor for specific advice if you are taking aminoglutethimide, antacids, barbiturates, carbamazepine, griseofulvin, mitotane, phenylbutazone, phenytoin, primidone, rifampin, injectable amphotericin B, oral antidiabetes agents, insulin, digitalis, diuretics, or medications containing potassium or sodium.

FOOD INTERACTIONS
Avoid excess sodium.

DISEASE INTERACTIONS
Consult your doctor if you have a history of bone disease, chicken pox, measles, gastrointestinal disorders, diabetes, recent serious infection, glaucoma, heart disease, hypertension, liver or kidney disorders, high blood cholesterol, thyroid problems, myasthenia gravis, or lupus.

≡ SIDE EFFECTS ≡

SERIOUS
Vision problems, frequent urination, increased thirst, rectal bleeding, blistering skin, confusion, hallucinations, paranoia, euphoria, depression, mood swings, redness and swelling at injection site. Call your doctor immediately.

COMMON
Increased appetite, indigestion, nervousness, insomnia, greater susceptibility to infections, increased blood pressure, slowed wound healing, weight gain, easy bruising, fluid retention.

LESS COMMON
Change in skin color, dizziness, headache, increased sweating, unusual growth of body or facial hair, increased blood sugar, peptic ulcers, adrenal insufficiency, muscle weakness, cataracts, glaucoma, osteoporosis.

TRIAMCINOLONE TOPICAL

Available in: Cream, lotion, ointment, aerosol, dental paste
Available OTC? No   **As Generic?** Yes
Drug Class: Topical corticosteroid

▼ USAGE INFORMATION

WHY IT'S PRESCRIBED
To treat rashes and inflammation of the skin. It is also used for treatment of inflammatory conditions within the mouth.

HOW IT WORKS
Topical triamcinolone appears to interfere with the formation of natural substances within the body that are directly responsible for the process of inflammation, which produces swelling, redness, and pain.

▼ DOSAGE GUIDELINES

RANGE AND FREQUENCY
Cream (0.025%, 0.1%, and 0.5% strength)– Adults: Apply 2 to 3 times daily. Children: 1 to 2 times daily (0.025%); once daily for all others (0.1% and 0.5%). Lotion (0.025% and 0.1% strength)– Adults: Apply 2 to 4 times daily. Children: 1 to 2 times daily (0.025%); once daily for all others (0.1%). Ointment (0.025%, 0.1%, and 0.5% strength)– Adults: Apply 2 to 4 times daily. Children: 1 to 2 times daily (0.025%); once daily for all others (0.1% and 0.5%). Aerosol (0.015% strength)– Adults: Apply 3 or 4 times daily. Children: 1 or 2 times daily. Dental paste (0.1% strength)– Adults: Apply to affected areas of the mouth 2 to 3 times daily after meals and at bedtime. Children: Consult a pediatrician.

ONSET OF EFFECT
Soon after application. However, recognizable changes in your condition may take several days or more to develop.

DURATION OF ACTION
Unknown.

DIETARY ADVICE
No special restrictions.

STORAGE
Store in a tightly sealed container away from heat and direct light.

MISSED DOSE
Apply it as soon as you remember. If it is near the time for the next dose, skip the missed dose and resume your regular dosage schedule.

STOPPING THE DRUG
Take as prescribed for the full treatment period, even if you begin to feel better before the scheduled end of therapy.

PROLONGED USE
Avoid prolonged use, particularly near the eyes, on the face, genital, or rectal areas, or in the folds of the skin.

▼ PRECAUTIONS

Over 60: Side effects may be more likely and more severe in elderly patients.

Driving and Hazardous Work: No special warnings.

Alcohol: No special warnings.

Pregnancy: This drug should not be used for prolonged periods by pregnant women or by women trying to become pregnant.

Breast Feeding: Although problems have not been documented, caution is advised. Do not apply to breasts prior to nursing. Consult your doctor for specific advice.

Infants and Children: Should not be used for more than 2 weeks in children and adolescents, unless otherwise directed by your doctor. Do not use tight-fitting diapers or plastic pants on children when treating skin irritation in the diaper area.

Special Concerns: Wash your hands thoroughly after application. Do not wrap the treated area with bandages or tight-fitting clothing unless otherwise instructed by your doctor.

OVERDOSE
Symptoms: None known.

What to Do: An overdose of a topical corticosteroid is unlikely to be life-threatening. However, in case of accidental ingestion or an apparent overdose, call your doctor, emergency medical services (EMS), or the nearest poison control center right away.

▼ INTERACTIONS

DRUG INTERACTIONS
Do not mix topical triamcinolone with other products, especially alcohol-containing preparations (which include colognes, aftershave, and many moisturizer lotions), since this may cause dryness and irritation, or increase the risk of an allergic reaction.

FOOD INTERACTIONS
Potassium supplements may decrease this drug's effects. Avoid foods high in sodium.

DISEASE INTERACTIONS
Caution is advised when taking this drug. Consult your doctor if you have any of the following: cataracts; diabetes mellitus; glaucoma; infection, sores, or ulcerations of the skin; infection at another site in your body; tuberculosis.

 SIDE EFFECTS

SERIOUS
Serious side effects from the use of topical triamcinolone are very rare.

COMMON
Burning, itching, irritation, redness, dryness, acne, stinging and cracking of skin, and numbness or tingling in the extremities have been reported in 0.5% to 1% of patients, although the risk is increased when the medication is used with bandages or other occlusive dressings.

LESS COMMON
Blistering and pus near hair follicles, unusual bleeding or easy bruising, darkening or prominence of small surface veins, increased susceptibility to infection.

TRIAMTERENE

Available in: Capsules
Available OTC? No **As Generic?** No
Drug Class: Potassium-sparing diuretic

▼ USAGE INFORMATION

WHY IT'S PRESCRIBED
Used as an adjunctive, supplementary treatment with other diuretics to conserve potassium while promoting the excretion of sodium and water. In conjunction with thiazide or loop diuretics, triamterene reduces the overall fluid volume in the body and so helps to control symptoms of heart disease, kidney disease, and liver disease.

HOW IT WORKS
Triamterene promotes the excretion of sodium and excess water by altering kidney enzymes that control urine production. Unlike most other types of diuretics, triamterene promotes fluid and salt loss but does not deplete normal levels of potassium.

▼ DOSAGE GUIDELINES

RANGE AND FREQUENCY
Adults: 25 to 100 mg a day. Dose may be increased to no more than 300 mg a day. Children: 0.9 to 1.82 mg per lb of body weight, once a day or once every other day. Dose may be increased.

ONSET OF EFFECT
Within 2 to 4 hours.

DURATION OF ACTION
From 7 to 9 hours.

DIETARY ADVICE
Triamterene should be taken after meals, though it can be taken with food or a full glass of milk to minimize the risk of stomach upset.

STORAGE
Store in a tightly sealed container away from heat, moisture, and direct light.

MISSED DOSE
Take it as soon as you remember. However, if it is near the time for the next dose, skip the missed dose and resume your regular dosage schedule. Do not double the next dose.

STOPPING THE DRUG
The decision to stop taking the drug should be made by your doctor.

PROLONGED USE
See your doctor regularly for tests and examinations if you must take this drug for a prolonged period.

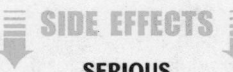

SIDE EFFECTS

SERIOUS
Skin rash, hives, lightheadedness, unusual bleeding. Call your doctor immediately.

COMMON
No common side effects have been reported.

LESS COMMON
Dizziness, nausea, vomiting, stomach cramps, diarrhea, headache, increased sensitivity of skin to sunlight.

▼ PRECAUTIONS

Over 60: Adverse reactions may be more likely and more severe in older patients. In particular, signs of excess potassium levels are more likely to occur in older patients.

Driving and Hazardous Work: The use of triamterene should not impair your ability to perform such tasks safely.

Alcohol: No special precautions are necessary.

Pregnancy: Adequate human studies have not been done. Before taking triamterene, tell your doctor if you are pregnant or plan to become pregnant.

Breast Feeding: Triamterene passes into breast milk; caution is advised. Consult your doctor for specific advice.

Infants and Children: No special problems are expected.

Special Concerns: Avoid exposure to the sun until you determine how the medicine affects you. Before having any kind of surgery, tell the doctor or dentist in charge that you are taking triamterene.

OVERDOSE
Symptoms: Dizziness or faintness, nausea, vomiting, confusion, heartbeat irregularities, nervousness, numbness or tingling in hands, feet, or lips, weak or heavy legs, unusual fatigue or tiredness.

What to Do: Call your doctor, emergency medical services (EMS), or the nearest poison control center immediately.

▼ INTERACTIONS

DRUG INTERACTIONS
Other drugs may interact with triamterene. Consult your doctor for specific advice if you are taking ACE inhibitors, cyclosporine, potassium-containing medicines or supplements, digoxin, or lithium.

FOOD INTERACTIONS
Avoid foods and beverages high in potassium, such as some salt substitutes, bananas, and citrus juices.

DISEASE INTERACTIONS
Consult your doctor if you have a history of gout or kidney stones. Use of triamterene may cause complications in patients with liver or kidney disease, since these organs work together to remove the medication from the body.

TRIAZOLAM

Available in: Tablets
Available OTC? No   **As Generic?** Yes
Drug Class: Benzodiazepine tranquilizer

▼ USAGE INFORMATION

WHY IT'S PRESCRIBED
To treat insomnia.

HOW IT WORKS
In general, triazolam produces mild sedation by depressing activity in the central nervous system (brain and spinal cord). In particular, triazolam appears to enhance the effect of gamma-aminobutyric acid (GABA), a natural chemical that inhibits the firing of neurons and dampens the transmission of nerve signals, thus decreasing nervous excitation.

▼ DOSAGE GUIDELINES

RANGE AND FREQUENCY
Adults: 0.125 to 0.250 mg at bedtime. Use and dose for children under 18 must be determined by your doctor.

ONSET OF EFFECT
Unknown.

DURATION OF ACTION
Unknown.

DIETARY ADVICE
Take with a full glass of water. Can be taken with food to lessen stomach upset.

STORAGE
Store in a tightly sealed container away from heat and direct light.

MISSED DOSE
Take it as soon as you remember, unless it is late at night. Do not take the medicine unless your schedule allows a full night's sleep.

STOPPING THE DRUG
Stopping the drug abruptly may produce withdrawal symptoms (sleep disruption, nervousness, irritability, diarrhea, abdominal cramps, muscle aches, memory impairment). Dose should be reduced gradually according to your doctor's instructions.

PROLONGED USE
Triazolam may slowly lose its effectiveness, and adverse reactions are more likely to occur with prolonged use. You should see your doctor for periodic evaluation if you must take it for an extended time.

▼ PRECAUTIONS

Over 60: Adverse reactions may be more likely and more severe. A lower dose may be warranted.

Driving and Hazardous Work: Triazolam can impair mental alertness and physical coordination. Adjust your activities accordingly.

Alcohol: Avoid alcohol.

Pregnancy: Use during pregnancy should be avoided if possible. Be sure to tell your doctor if you are pregnant or plan to become pregnant.

Breast Feeding: Triazolam passes into breast milk; do not take it while nursing.

Infants and Children: Safety and effectiveness have not been established for children under age 18.

Special Concerns: Triazolam use can lead to psychological or physical dependence if it is not taken in strict accordance with your doctor's instructions. Never take more than the prescribed daily dose.

OVERDOSE
Symptoms: Extreme drowsiness, confusion, slurred speech, slow reflexes, poor coordination, staggering gait, tremor, slowed breathing, loss of consciousness.

What to Do: Call your doctor, emergency medical services (EMS), or the nearest poison control center immediately.

▼ INTERACTIONS

DRUG INTERACTIONS
Other drugs may interact with triazolam. Consult your doctor for specific advice if you are taking any drugs that depress the central nervous system; these include antihistamines, antidepressants or other psychiatric medications, barbiturates, sedatives, cough medicines, decongestants, and pain-killers. Be sure your physician knows about any over-the-counter medication you may take.

FOOD INTERACTIONS
None reported.

DISEASE INTERACTIONS
Caution is advised when taking triazolam. Consult your doctor if you have a history of alcohol or drug abuse, stroke or other brain disease, any chronic lung disease, glaucoma, hyperactivity, depression or other mental illness, myasthenia gravis, sleep apnea, epilepsy, porphyria, kidney disease, or liver disease.

SIDE EFFECTS

SERIOUS
Difficulty concentrating, outbursts of anger, other behavior problems, depression, convulsions, hallucinations, low blood pressure (causing faintness or confusion), memory impairment, muscle weakness, skin rash or itching, sore throat, fever and chills, sores or ulcers in throat or mouth, unusual bruising or bleeding, extreme fatigue, yellowish tinge to eyes or skin. Call your doctor immediately.

COMMON
Loss of coordination, unsteady gait, dizziness, lightheadedness, drowsiness, slurred speech.

LESS COMMON
Stomach cramps or pain, vision disturbances, change in sexual desire or ability, constipation or diarrhea, dry mouth or watering mouth, false sense of well-being, rapid or pounding heartbeat, headache, muscle spasms, nausea and vomiting, urinary problems, trembling, unusual fatigue.

TRIFLUOPERAZINE HYDROCHLORIDE

Available in: Oral solution, tablets, injection
Available OTC? No **As Generic?** Yes
Drug Class: Neuroleptic; antipsychotic

▼ USAGE INFORMATION

WHY IT'S PRESCRIBED
To treat psychotic conditions (severe mental disorders characterized by distorted thoughts, perceptions, and emotions), such as schizophrenia.

HOW IT WORKS
Trifluoperazine appears to block receptors of dopamine (a chemical that aids in the transmission of nerve impulses) in the central nervous system. Presumably, this produces a tranquilizing and antipsychotic effect.

▼ DOSAGE GUIDELINES

RANGE AND FREQUENCY
Usual adult dose: Initially, 2 to 5 mg, 2 times a day. Your doctor may increase the dose if necessary (and if side effects are tolerated) up to a maximum of 40 mg a day.

ONSET OF EFFECT
Sedation may occur within minutes, but onset of antipsychotic effect may take hours to occur or may not occur until days or weeks after the beginning of therapy.

DURATION OF ACTION
12 to 24 hours, but effects may persist for several days.

DIETARY ADVICE
Can be taken with food or a full glass of milk or water.

STORAGE
Store in a tightly sealed container away from heat and direct light.

MISSED DOSE
Take it as soon as you remember. However, if it is near the time for the next dose, skip the missed dose and resume your regular dosage schedule. Do not double the next dose.

STOPPING THE DRUG
The decision to stop taking the drug should be made in consultation with your doctor. Gradual reduction of doses may be required if you have taken this medication for an extended period.

PROLONGED USE
Prolonged use may lead to tardive dyskinesia (involuntary movements of the jaw, lips, tongue, and, in rare cases, the arms, legs, hands, or body). Consult your doctor about the need for follow-up evaluations and tests if you must take this drug for an extended period.

▼ PRECAUTIONS

Over 60: Adverse reactions are more common in elderly patients. A lower dose may be warranted.

Driving and Hazardous Work: Do not drive or engage in hazardous work until you determine how the medicine affects you.

Alcohol: Avoid alcohol.

Pregnancy: Avoid using this drug during pregnancy.

Breast Feeding: Either avoid taking the drug if possible or refrain from breast feeding.

Infants and Children: Adverse reactions may be more likely and more severe in children.

Special Concerns: Avoid prolonged exposure to high temperatures or hot climates. Drink plenty of fluids and stay cool in the summertime. Also, avoid overexposure to sunlight until you determine if the drug heightens your skin's sensitivity to ultraviolet light.

OVERDOSE
Symptoms: Extreme drowsiness or paradoxical restlessness or agitation, heart rhythm irregularities or palpitations, dry mouth, seizures, stiffness or impaired mental control, loss of consciousness.

What to Do: Call your doctor, emergency medical services (EMS), or the nearest poison control center immediately.

▼ INTERACTIONS

DRUG INTERACTIONS
Consult your physician for specific advice if you are taking amantadine, high blood pressure medication, bromocriptine, deferoxamine, diuretics, levobunolol, heart medication, metipranolol, nabilone, other psychiatric drugs, pentamidine, pimozide, promethazine, trimeprazine, a thyroid agent, central nervous system depressants, epinephrine, lithium, levodopa, methyldopa, metoclopramide, metyrosine, pemoline, a rauwolfia alkaloid, or metrizamide.

FOOD INTERACTIONS
No known food interactions.

DISEASE INTERACTIONS
Consult your doctor if you have Parkinson's disease or any movement disorder, glaucoma, epilepsy, liver disease, or kidney disease.

SIDE EFFECTS

SERIOUS
Rapid heartbeat, profuse sweating, seizures, difficulty breathing, neck stiffness, swelling of the tongue, difficulty swallowing. Also a rare condition can develop called neuroleptic malignant syndrome, characterized by stiffness or spasms of the muscles, high fever, and confusion or disorientation. Call your doctor immediately.

COMMON
Nausea, reduced perspiration, dry mouth, blurred vision, drowsiness, shaking of the hands, muscle stiffness, stooped posture.

LESS COMMON
Difficult urination, menstrual irregularities, breast pain or swelling, unexpected weight gain, uncontrolled movements of the tongue, fever, chills, sore throat, unusual bruising or bleeding, heart palpitations, skin rash, itching, increased sensitivity of the skin to sunlight.

TRIHEXYPHENIDYL HYDROCHLORIDE

Available in: Tablets, sustained-release capsules, elixir
Available OTC? No **As Generic?** Yes
Drug Class: Antiparkinsonism drug

▼ USAGE INFORMATION

WHY IT'S PRESCRIBED
To treat Parkinson's disease and the Parkinson-like symptoms induced by certain central nervous system drugs. Such symptoms include slowed movement, stiffness and muscle rigidity, tremor, and loss of balance. Trihexyphenidyl is also used to treat Parkinson-like syndromes that can occur as a result of injury to or infection of the central nervous system, damage to blood vessels in the brain, or exposure to certain toxins.

HOW IT WORKS
The exact mechanism of action of trihexyphenidyl is unknown, although it is thought to increase the availability of dopamine, a brain chemical that is critical in the initiation and smooth control of voluntary muscle movement.

▼ DOSAGE GUIDELINES

RANGE AND FREQUENCY
Adults: To start, 2 mg, 3 times a day. The dose is gradually increased until the desired therapeutic response is achieved. The usual maximum maintenance dose is 5 mg, 3 times a day. Once a maintenance dosage is established, your physician may switch you to sustained-release capsules (sequels), which can be taken less frequently (once or twice a day). Children: The dosage for children has not been established; consult your pediatrician for advice.

ONSET OF EFFECT
Usually within 1 hour.

DURATION OF ACTION
The effect may last for at least 24 hours.

DIETARY ADVICE
No special restrictions.

STORAGE
Store in a tightly sealed container away from heat, moisture, and direct light.

MISSED DOSE
Take it as soon as you remember, unless the time for your next scheduled dose is within the next 2 hours. If so, skip the missed dose and resume your regular dosage schedule. Do not double the next dose.

STOPPING THE DRUG
The decision to stop taking the drug should be made in consultation with your doctor. The dosage is typically tapered gradually over the course of 7 days.

PROLONGED USE
The prolonged use of trihexyphenidyl may cause glaucoma (elevated pressure within the eye, and a leading cause of blindness) or increase its severity. Arrange for regular check-ups with your eye doctor to have your eye pressure monitored.

▼ PRECAUTIONS

Over 60: Adverse reactions may be more likely and more severe in older patients. Lower doses may be needed.

Driving and Hazardous Work: Avoid such activities until you determine how the medicine affects you.

Alcohol: Avoid alcohol.

Pregnancy: This drug should not be used by pregnant women.

Breast Feeding: Trihexyphenidyl passes into breast milk; this drug should not be used by nursing mothers.

Infants and Children: Very low doses may be used by children; consult your pediatrician. The drug is not recommended for use by children under age 10.

Special Concerns: Your eye doctor should regularly monitor your intraocular pressure to check for glaucoma. Consult your doctor to determine the best schedule for regular physical examinations.

OVERDOSE
Symptoms: Clumsiness, confusion, delirium, inability to urinate, seizures.

What to Do: Call your doctor, emergency medical services (EMS), or the nearest poison control center immediately.

▼ INTERACTIONS

DRUG INTERACTIONS
Consult your doctor for specific advice if you are taking any of the following: other drugs for Parkinson's disease (such as levodopa), medications that depress the central nervous system (such as alcohol, barbiturates, or other sleep-inducing drugs), or MAO inhibitor antidepressants (such as phenelzine sulfate or tranylcypromine sulfate).

FOOD INTERACTIONS
No known food interactions.

DISEASE INTERACTIONS
Caution is advised when taking trihexyphenidyl. Consult your doctor for specific advice if you have glaucoma, prostate disease, or enlarged prostate (benign prostatic hyperplasia).

 SIDE EFFECTS

SERIOUS
Confusion, hallucinations, blurred vision, glaucoma. Call your doctor at once.

COMMON
Dry mouth, nausea.

LESS COMMON
Difficult urination.

TRIMETHOBENZAMIDE HYDROCHLORIDE

BRAND NAMES

Arrestin, Benzacot, Bio-Gan, Stemetic, T-Gen, Tebamide, Tegamide, Ticon, Tigan, Tiject-20, Triban, Tribenzagan

Available in: Capsules, injection, suppositories
Available OTC? No   **As Generic?** Yes
Drug Class: Antiemetic

▼ USAGE INFORMATION

WHY IT'S PRESCRIBED
To treat nausea, vomiting, and motion sickness.

HOW IT WORKS
Trimethobenzamide acts on the brain center that controls vomiting.

▼ DOSAGE GUIDELINES

RANGE AND FREQUENCY
Capsules— Adults and children 12 years and older: 250 mg, 3 or 4 times a day, as needed. Children weighing 30 to 90 lbs: 6.8 mg per lb of body weight, not to exceed 200 mg, 3 or 4 times a day. Injection— Adults and children 12 years and older: 200 mg into a muscle, 3 or 4 times a day. Suppositories— Adults and children 12 years and older: 200 mg, 3 or 4 times a day. Children 30 to 90 lbs: ½ to 1 suppository (100 to 200 mg), 3 or 4 times a day. Children under 30 lbs: ½ suppository (100 mg), 3 or 4 times a day.

ONSET OF EFFECT
Capsules: 10 to 20 minutes.

Injection: 15 to 35 minutes.
Suppositories: Variable.

DURATION OF ACTION
Capsules: 3 to 4 hours.
Injection: 2 to 3 hours.
Suppositories: Variable.

DIETARY ADVICE
Capsules can be opened and the contents mixed with food if so desired.

STORAGE
Store in a tightly sealed container away from heat, moisture, and direct light. Suppositories should be refrigerated.

MISSED DOSE
Take it as soon as you remember. If it is near the time for the next dose, skip the missed dose and resume your regular dosage schedule. Do not double the next dose.

STOPPING THE DRUG
The decision to stop taking the drug should be made by your doctor.

PROLONGED USE
See your doctor regularly for tests and examinations if you take trimethobenzamide for a prolonged period. Using more than the recommended dosage or taking it more often than directed can increase the possibility of side effects.

▼ PRECAUTIONS

Over 60: No special problems are expected.

Driving and Hazardous Work: Do not drive or engage in hazardous work until you determine how the medicine affects you.

Alcohol: Avoid alcohol.

Pregnancy: Adequate human studies have not been completed. Before taking trimethobenzamide, tell your doctor if you are pregnant or plan to become pregnant.

Breast Feeding: Trimethobenzamide may pass into breast milk; caution is advised. Consult your doctor for advice.

Infants and Children: Trimethobenzamide should be used in infants and children only under the direction of your doctor. Some side effects may be more severe in children. Do not use the injectable form in children. Do not use the suppository form in either premature or newborn infants.

Special Concerns: When used for motion sickness, trimethobenzamide should be taken 30 minutes before exposure to motion. If the suppository is too soft to insert, chill it with running water or refrigerate it for 30 minutes. To reduce irritation and pain around the area of the injection, inject the medicine deeply into the outer area of the buttocks.

OVERDOSE
Symptoms: Seizures, unconsciousness.

What to Do: Call your doctor, emergency medical services (EMS), or the nearest poison control center immediately.

▼ INTERACTIONS

DRUG INTERACTIONS
Consult your doctor for specific advice if you are taking aspirin, phenobarbital, tricyclic antidepressants, or other central nervous system depressants such as tranquilizers, sleeping pills, or cold and allergy drugs.

FOOD INTERACTIONS
No known food interactions.

DISEASE INTERACTIONS
Caution is advised when taking trimethobenzamide. Consult your doctor if you have a high fever, severe vomiting, dehydration, or an intestinal infection, or if a child has Reye's syndrome.

SIDE EFFECTS

SERIOUS
Seizures, yellow discoloration of the eyes and skin, skin rash, body spasms, convulsions, mental depression, shakiness or tremors, sore throat and fever, unusual fatigue, severe or continuing vomiting. Call your doctor immediately.

COMMON
Drowsiness.

LESS COMMON
Dizziness, lightheadedness, muscle cramps, fainting, blurred vision, diarrhea, headache.

TRIMETHOPRIM/SULFAMETHOXAZOLE

Available in: Tablets, injection
Available OTC? No   **As Generic?** Yes
Drug Class: Anti-infective

▼ USAGE INFORMATION

WHY IT'S PRESCRIBED
To treat urinary tract infections, ear infections, chronic bronchitis, Pneumocystis carinii pneumonia (a lung infection commonly seen in patients with compromised immune systems), traveler's diarrhea, and other types of diarrheal disease.

HOW IT WORKS
This medication is a combination of two active ingredients. Both trimethoprim and sulfamethoxazole kill or inhibit growth of bacteria by disrupting their ability to make necessary proteins.

▼ DOSAGE GUIDELINES

RANGE AND FREQUENCY
For common bacterial infections– Adults: The usual dose is 1 double strength (DS) tablet 2 times a day. Duration of therapy depends on the type of infection and will be determined by your doctor. For alternative dosages and for treatment of children, consult your pediatrician, as dosages can vary considerably depending on age, weight, and kidney function.

ONSET OF EFFECT
Unknown.

DURATION OF ACTION
Unknown.

DIETARY ADVICE
Tablets should be taken with a full glass of water and can be taken with food to lessen stomach upset.

STORAGE
Store in a tightly sealed container away from heat and direct light.

MISSED DOSE
Take it as soon as you remember. However, if it is near the time for the next dose, skip the missed dose and resume your regular dosage schedule. Do not double the next dose.

STOPPING THE DRUG
Take the drug as prescribed for the full treatment period, even if you begin to feel better before the scheduled end of therapy.

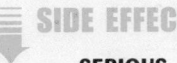
SIDE EFFECTS

SERIOUS
Skin rash, sore throat, fever, joint pain, shortness of breath, pale skin, reddish spots on skin, unusual bleeding or bruising. Call your doctor immediately.

COMMON
Nausea, vomiting, loss of appetite, allergic skin reactions, itching, hives.

LESS COMMON
Abdominal pain, diarrhea, seizures, dizziness, ringing in ears, headache, hallucinations, depression, unusual sensitivity to sunlight.

PROLONGED USE
See your doctor regularly for tests and examinations if you must take this medicine for a prolonged period.

▼ PRECAUTIONS

Over 60: Adverse reactions may be more likely and more severe in older patients.

Driving and Hazardous Work: Do not drive or engage in hazardous work until you determine how the medicine affects you.

Alcohol: No special problems are expected, although it is generally advisable to abstain from alcohol when fighting an infection.

Pregnancy: Trimethoprim with sulfamethoxazole has caused birth defects in animals. Human studies have not been done. It should be used during pregnancy only if the benefits clearly outweigh the possible risks. Before you take this medication, tell your doctor if you are pregnant or plan to become pregnant.

Breast Feeding: Trimethoprim with sulfamethoxazole passes into breast milk; avoid or discontinue use while nursing.

Infants and Children: This medication is not recommended for use by children under the age of 2 months.

Special Concerns: Since some patients experience increased sensitivity to sunlight, take preventive measures: use sunscreens, wear protective clothing, and avoid exposure to the sun. Patients with acquired immunodeficiency syndrome (AIDS) may have a higher incidence of side effects, especially rash. Nonetheless, trimethoprim with sulfamethoxazole remains valuable for treating a number of problems associated with this disease.

OVERDOSE
Symptoms: Loss of appetite, nausea, vomiting, dizziness, headache, drowsiness, depression, confusion, altered mental status, fever, blood in urine, yellow skin or eyes.

What to Do: Call your doctor, emergency medical services (EMS), or the nearest poison control center immediately.

▼ INTERACTIONS

DRUG INTERACTIONS
The following drugs may interact with trimethoprim with sulfamethoxazole. Consult your doctor for specific advice if you are taking cyclosporine, methotrexate, phenytoin, procainamide, sulfonylureas, or warfarin.

FOOD INTERACTIONS
No known food interactions.

DISEASE INTERACTIONS
Use of sulfamethoxazole may cause complications in patients with liver or kidney disease, since these organs work together to remove the medication from the body. This drug can also cause complications in patients with certain types of anemia. Consult your doctor for specific advice if you have any other medical condition.

TRIPROLIDINE HYDROCHLORIDE

Available in: Syrup
Available OTC? Yes **As Generic?** Yes
Drug Class: Antihistamine

▼ USAGE INFORMATION

WHY IT'S PRESCRIBED
To relieve symptoms of hay fever and other allergies.

HOW IT WORKS
Triprolidine blocks the effects of histamine, a naturally occurring substance that causes swelling, itching, sneezing, watery eyes, hives, and other symptoms of allergic reaction.

▼ DOSAGE GUIDELINES

RANGE AND FREQUENCY
Adults and children age 12 and over: 2.5 mg every 4 to 6 hours. The maximum dose is 10 mg per day. Children ages 6 to 12: 1.25 mg (1 teaspoon) every 4 to 6 hours. The maximum dose is 5 mg per day. Children ages 4 to 6: 0.938 mg (¾ teaspoon) every 4 to 6 hours. The maximum dose is 3.744 mg per day. Children ages 2 to 4: 0.625 mg (½ teaspoon) every 4 to 6 hours. The maximum dose is 2.5 mg per day. Children ages 4 months to 2 years: 0.313 mg (¼ teaspoon) every 4 to 6 hours. The maximum dose is 1.25 mg per day.

ONSET OF EFFECT
15 to 60 minutes.

DURATION OF ACTION
4 to 6 hours.

DIETARY ADVICE
Take with food or milk to reduce stomach upset.

STORAGE
Store in a tightly sealed container away from heat and direct light. Do not allow the drug to freeze.

MISSED DOSE
Take it as soon as you remember. If it is near the time for the next dose, skip the missed dose and resume your regular dosage schedule. Do not double the next dose.

STOPPING THE DRUG
The decision to stop taking the drug should be made by your doctor.

PROLONGED USE
Tolerance, or decreased responsiveness to the drug, usually does not develop with prolonged use. If it does, consult your doctor.

▼ PRECAUTIONS

Over 60: Adverse reactions may be more likely and more severe in older patients.

Driving and Hazardous Work: Do not drive or engage in hazardous work until you determine how the medicine affects you.

Alcohol: Avoid alcohol.

Pregnancy: Before you take triprolidine, tell your doctor if you are pregnant or plan to become pregnant.

Breast Feeding: Triprolidine passes into breast milk; avoid or discontinue use while nursing. Flow of breast milk may be reduced.

Infants and Children: Adverse effects may be more likely and more severe in children.

Special Concerns: Stop taking triprolidine 4 days before you have an allergy skin test. Drink water frequently or use ice chips, sugarless candy, or sugarless gum if dry mouth occurs. Coffee or tea may reduce the common side effect of drowsiness.

OVERDOSE
Symptoms: Central nervous system depression or, paradoxically, nervous system stimulation; very low blood pressure; breathing difficulty; seizures; loss of consciousness; severe dryness of the mouth, nose, or throat.

What to Do: Call your doctor, emergency medical services (EMS), or the nearest poison control center immediately.

▼ INTERACTIONS

DRUG INTERACTIONS
Consult your doctor for specific advice if you are taking anticholinergics, clarithromycin, erythromycin, itraconazole, ketoconazole, bepridil, disopyramide, maprotiline, phenothiazines, pimozide, procainamide, quinidine, tricyclic antidepressants, central nervous system depressants, MAO inhibitors, or quinine.

FOOD INTERACTIONS
No known food interactions.

DISEASE INTERACTIONS
Caution is advised when taking triprolidine. Consult your doctor if you have an enlarged prostate, urinary tract blockage, difficult urination, or glaucoma. Use of triprolidine may cause complications in patients with liver disease, since this organ works to remove the medication from the body.

SIDE EFFECTS

SERIOUS
Sore throat and fever, unusual tiredness or weakness, unusual bleeding or bruising. Call your doctor immediately.

COMMON
Drowsiness, thickening of mucus.

LESS COMMON
Blurred vision; rapid heartbeat; skin rash; stomach upset; nervousness; increased sensitivity of skin to sunlight; confusion; difficult or painful urination; dizziness; dry mouth, nose, or throat; loss of appetite; nightmares; ringing or buzzing in ears; restlessness; irritability.

TROVAFLOXACIN

BRAND NAME

Trovan

Available in: Tablets, injection
Available OTC? No   **As Generic?** No
Drug Class: Antibiotic

▼ USAGE INFORMATION

WHY IT'S PRESCRIBED
To treat a number of serious bacterial infections, such as pneumonia, gynecological infections, and complicated skin infections, especially when acquired in a hospital or nursing home. Your doctor will determine if this drug is appropriate for your condition.

HOW IT WORKS
Trovafloxacin inhibits the activity of two bacterial enzymes, including DNA gyrase, that are necessary for proper DNA formation and replication. This fights infection by preventing bacteria cells from reproducing.

▼ DOSAGE GUIDELINES

RANGE AND FREQUENCY
The dosage varies, depending on the site and type of infection. Daily doses of the tablets range from 100 to 200 mg for periods of 3 to 14 days. Your doctor will determine the correct dosage for your specific condition. Intravenous doses, when necessary, are administered by a health care professional.

ONSET OF EFFECT
Unknown.

DURATION OF ACTION
Unknown.

DIETARY ADVICE
Trovafloxacin can be taken without regard to meals.

STORAGE
Tablets: Store in a tightly sealed container away from heat, moisture, and direct light. Injection: Not applicable; injectable dose is administered only at a health care facility.

MISSED DOSE
Tablet: Take it as soon as you remember. If you miss the dose one day, resume your regular dosage schedule. Do not double the next dose. Injection: Consult your doctor.

STOPPING THE DRUG
Take it as prescribed for the full treatment period, even if you begin to feel better before the scheduled end of therapy. The decision to stop taking the drug should be made by your doctor.

PROLONGED USE
Trovafloxacin is generally prescribed only for short-term use and should not be used for more than 14 days.

▼ PRECAUTIONS

Over 60: No special problems are expected.

Driving and Hazardous Work: Do not drive or engage in hazardous work until you determine how the medicine affects you.

Alcohol: It is advisable to abstain from alcohol when fighting an infection.

Pregnancy: Adequate human studies have not been done. Before taking trovafloxacin, discuss with your doctor the relative risks and benefits of using this drug.

Breast Feeding: Trovafloxacin passes into breast milk; extreme caution is advised. Consult your doctor for advice.

Infants and Children: Not recommended for use by children under the age of 18.

Special Concerns: Take trovafloxacin with food or at bedtime to reduce the likelihood of dizziness. If trovafloxacin causes heightened sensitivity to sunlight, stop taking the drug and try to avoid exposure to sunlight for the next 5 days; also wear protective clothing and use a sunblock.

OVERDOSE
Symptoms: An overdose with trovafloxacin is unlikely to occur.

What to Do: If someone takes a much larger dose than prescribed, call your doctor, emergency medical services (EMS), or the nearest poison control immediately.

▼ INTERACTIONS

DRUG INTERACTIONS
Trovafloxacin should be taken at least 2 hours before or after taking certain antacids, sucralfate, citric acid buffered with sodium citrate, or vitamin or mineral supplements containing iron.

FOOD INTERACTIONS
No known food interactions.

DISEASE INTERACTIONS
Trovafloxacin should not be used at all in patients with liver disease or those who have had an allergic reaction to quinolone antibiotics in the past. The drug should be used with caution in those with a history of seizures or any nervous system disorders that may increase the risk of seizures. Be sure to inform your doctor if you have any other medical condition.

SIDE EFFECTS

SERIOUS
Serious reactions are rare. The most serious potential side effect is liver toxicity, which can cause jaundice (characterized by yellowish discoloration of the skin and eyes), nausea, vomiting, abdominal pain, fatigue, loss of appetite, and dark urine. Liver failure has led to a small number of deaths and liver transplants. Other serious side effects may include chest pain; heart rhythm irregularities; diarrhea; anaphylaxis (a severe allergic reaction marked by sudden swelling of the lips, tongue, face, or throat; breathing difficulty; skin rash, itching, or hives); seizures; and confusion or other mental disturbances, such as restlessness, nightmares, and insomnia. Call your doctor immediately.

COMMON
Dizziness, lightheadedness, nausea, headache.

LESS COMMON
Vomiting, abdominal pain, yeast infection (females), itching, increased sensitivity to sunlight.

UNDECYLENIC ACID

Available in: Aerosol foam, aerosol powder, cream, ointment, powder, solution
Available OTC? Yes   **As Generic?** Yes
Drug Class: Topical antifungal

▼ USAGE INFORMATION

WHY IT'S PRESCRIBED
To treat fungal infections of the skin. (Note: Undecylenic acid has generally been replaced by newer and more effective topical antifungal medications; however, your physician may find it worthwhile to prescribe undecylenic acid under certain circumstances—for example, if you have a history of allergic reaction to other antifungal preparations.)

HOW IT WORKS
Undecylenic acid prevents the growth and reproduction of fungus cells.

▼ DOSAGE GUIDELINES

RANGE AND FREQUENCY
Aerosol foam, aerosol powder, ointment, powder, or solution: Apply to the affected area of the skin 2 times a day. The aerosol powder and aerosol spray form of the medicine should be sprayed on the affected area from a distance of 4 to 6 inches. The powder may also be sprayed in socks and shoes. If the powder is used on the feet, sprinkle it between the toes, on the feet, and in shoes and socks. Cream: Apply to the affected area of the skin as often as necessary.

ONSET OF EFFECT
Unknown.

DURATION OF ACTION
Unknown.

DIETARY ADVICE
No special restrictions.

STORAGE
Store in a tightly sealed container away from heat and direct light. Keep aerosol, cream, ointment, and liquid solution forms of undecylenic acid from freezing. Do not puncture, rupture, or incinerate the aerosol container.

MISSED DOSE
Apply a missed dose as soon as you remember. If it is close to the next dose, skip the missed dose and resume your regular dosage schedule. Do not apply a double dose.

STOPPING THE DRUG
Take as prescribed for the full treatment period, even if you begin to feel better before the scheduled end of therapy. Discontinuing the drug prematurely may result in an even worse fungal infection later (known as rebound infection). In general, keep using this medication for two weeks after burning, itching, and other symptoms have cleared up.

PROLONGED USE
If your skin problem does not improve or becomes worse after 4 weeks of treatment, consult your doctor.

▼ PRECAUTIONS

Over 60: There is no specific information comparing use of undecylenic acid in older persons with use in other age groups.

Driving and Hazardous Work: No special precautions are necessary.

Alcohol: No special precautions are necessary.

Pregnancy: Undecylenic acid has not been shown to cause birth defects or other problems in humans.

Breast Feeding: Undecylenic acid may pass into breast milk; caution is advised. Consult your doctor for specific advice.

Infants and Children: Not recommended for use on children under age 2.

Special Concerns: Keep this medicine away from the eyes, nose, and mouth. To help prevent reinfection, the powder or spray form of undecylenic acid may be used every day after bathing and careful drying. Do not use on pus-producing sores or on badly broken skin.

OVERDOSE
Symptoms: No specific ones have been reported.

What to Do: An overdose of undecylenic acid is unlikely. However, if someone accidentally ingests the drug, call your doctor, emergency medical services (EMS), or the nearest poison control center.

▼ INTERACTIONS

DRUG INTERACTIONS
Consult your doctor for specific advice if you are taking any other topical prescription or over-the-counter medication that is to be applied to the same area of the skin.

FOOD INTERACTIONS
No known food interactions.

DISEASE INTERACTIONS
Caution is advised when taking undecylenic acid. Consult your doctor if you have any other medical condition that affects the skin.

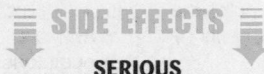

SIDE EFFECTS

SERIOUS
No serious side effects have been reported.

COMMON
No common side effects have been reported.

LESS COMMON
Skin irritation that was not present before use of this medicine. Call your doctor promptly.

URACIL MUSTARD

Available in: Capsules
Available OTC? No   **As Generic?** Yes
Drug Class: Alkylating agent

▼ USAGE INFORMATION

WHY IT'S PRESCRIBED
To treat leukemia, Hodgkin's disease and other lymphomas (a type of cancer affecting the lymphatic system), poly-cythemia vera (a blood disease characterized by the overproduction of some types of blood cells), and mycosis fungoides (a rare type of skin cancer that affects the lymphatic system).

HOW IT WORKS
Uracil mustard kills cancer cells by interfering with the activity of their genetic material, thus preventing the cells from reproducing. The drug may also affect the growth and development of healthy cells in the body, resulting in unpleasant side effects.

▼ DOSAGE GUIDELINES

RANGE AND FREQUENCY
Initial weekly dose of 0.15 mg per 2.2 lbs (1 kg) of body weight for at least 4 weeks to provide an adequate trial period. Dosage and duration of treatment can then be altered to meet the needs of individual patients.

ONSET OF EFFECT
Unknown.

DURATION OF ACTION
Unknown.

DIETARY ADVICE
Best taken at bedtime to mini-mize stomach upset.

STORAGE
Store in a tightly sealed container away from heat and direct light.

MISSED DOSE
Take it as soon as you remember. If it is near the time for the next dose, skip the missed dose and resume your regular dosage schedule. Do not double the next dose.

STOPPING THE DRUG
The decision to stop taking the drug should be made by your doctor.

PROLONGED USE
You should see your doctor regularly for tests and examinations if you must take this medication for a prolonged period of time.

▼ PRECAUTIONS

Over 60: No special problems are expected.

Driving and Hazardous Work: The use of this medication should not impair your ability to perform such tasks safely.

Alcohol: Avoid alcohol.

Pregnancy: Uracil mustard can cause birth defects if taken by either the father or the mother. Persons of child-bearing years should take steps to prevent pregnancy when taking it.

Breast Feeding: Not recommended during therapy.

Infants and Children: Although there is no specific information about the use of uracil mustard in infants and children, it is not expected to cause different side effects than it does in adults.

Special Concerns: Do not receive any immunizations without your doctor's approval while taking uracil mustard. Avoid persons who have recently had oral polio vaccine and those with any infection. Check with your doctor before having any dental work done. Consult your doctor or dentist about appropriate ways to clean your teeth to avoid injury. Be careful not to cut yourself when using sharp objects such as a safety razor or nail cutters. Avoid activities and contact sports where bruising or injury could occur. If you vomit shortly after taking a dose of uracil mustard, check with your doctor. You may be told to take the dose again. After completing a different regimen of chemotherapy or radiation, a period of 2 to 3 weeks is recommended before starting uracil mustard because of the risk of bone marrow damage.

OVERDOSE
Symptoms: Vomiting, severe nausea, severe diarrhea, unusual weakness, hemorrhaging.

What to Do: Call your doctor, emergency medical services (EMS), or the nearest poison control center immediately.

▼ INTERACTIONS

DRUG INTERACTIONS
Consult your doctor for advice if you are taking amphotericin B, antithyroid agents, azathioprine, chloramphenicol, colchicine, flucyto-sine, interferon, plicamycin, probenecid, sulfinpyrazone, or zidovudine. Also consult your doctor if you are taking any over-the-counter drugs.

FOOD INTERACTIONS
None are known.

DISEASE INTERACTIONS
Caution is advised when taking uracil mustard. Consult your doctor if you have chickenpox, shingles, any infection, gout, kidney disease, or liver disease.

SIDE EFFECTS

SERIOUS
Black, tarry, or bloody stools; blood in urine; fever and chills; cough or hoarseness; pain in lower back or side; difficult or painful urination; red spots on skin; unusual bleeding or bruising; joint pain; sores on lips or in mouth; swollen feet or lower legs; yellow tinge to eyes or skin (jaundice). Call your doctor immediately. Some of these side effects may recur after you stop taking uracil mustard. Consult your doctor if they do.

COMMON
Diarrhea, nausea or vomiting, temporary hair loss.

LESS COMMON
Darkening of the skin, irritability, depression, nervousness, skin rash and itching.

URSODIOL

BRAND NAMES

Actigall, Urso

Available in: Capsules, tablets
Available OTC? No   **As Generic?** Yes
Drug Class: Antigallstone agent

▼ USAGE INFORMATION

WHY IT'S PRESCRIBED
To treat gallstones as an alternative to surgical removal of the gallbladder (cholecystectomy). Ursodiol works only when gallstones are composed entirely of cholesterol, and works best when the gallstones are small.

HOW IT WORKS
Ursodiol is a natural bile acid that safely dissolves cholesterol gallstones over a period of months or years. The time required to dissolve a stone is proportional to the stone's size. Multiple stones usually dissolve more easily than a single large stone.

▼ DOSAGE GUIDELINES

RANGE AND FREQUENCY
Adults and teenagers: 3.6 to 4.5 mg per lb of body weight a day, divided into 2 or 3 equal doses.

ONSET OF EFFECT
Variable. It may take 6 months to 2 years for gallstones to dissolve.

DURATION OF ACTION
For as long as the medication is taken.

DIETARY ADVICE
Ursodiol should be taken with or immediately after meals.

STORAGE
Store in a tightly sealed container away from heat, moisture, and direct light.

MISSED DOSE
Take as soon as you remember or double the next dose.

STOPPING THE DRUG
Take it as prescribed for the full treatment period.

PROLONGED USE
You should see your doctor regularly for tests and examinations if you take this medicine for a prolonged period. Liver function tests (AST and ALT) should be done periodically. Ultrasound imaging should be done every 6 months for the first year of therapy to monitor the response to ursodiol. It may take 6 months to 2 years to dissolve gallstones, depending on their size and composition. Ursodiol treatment is not likely to be effective if gallstones are not partially dissolved after 12 months of therapy. Ursodiol should be continued for at least 3 months after the gallstones have dissolved.

▼ PRECAUTIONS

Over 60: No special precautions are needed.

Driving and Hazardous Work: The use of ursodiol should not impair your ability to perform such tasks safely.

Alcohol: No special precautions are necessary.

Pregnancy: Adequate human studies have not been done. Before taking ursodiol, tell your doctor if you are or are planning to become pregnant.

Breast Feeding: It is not known whether ursodiol passes into breast milk; caution is advised. Consult your doctor for specific advice.

Infants and Children: Ursodiol is not expected to cause different or more severe side effects in children than it does in older persons.

Special Concerns: If you experience severe pain in the abdomen or stomach, particularly on the upper right side, or nausea and vomiting, call your doctor immediately. These symptoms may indicate the presence of other medical problems or that your gallbladder condition requires immediate care. Gallstones recur after 5 years in about half of those patients whose stones were successfully dissolved by ursodiol.

OVERDOSE
Symptoms: An overdose with ursodiol is unlikely.

What to Do: If someone takes a much larger dose than prescribed, call your doctor, emergency medical services (EMS), or the nearest poison control right away.

▼ INTERACTIONS

DRUG INTERACTIONS
Other drugs may interact with ursodiol. Cholestyramine, colestipol, and antacids that contain aluminum can prevent the absorption of ursodiol from the intestine. Estrogen and oral contraceptives may interfere with the action of this medication.

FOOD INTERACTIONS
No known food interactions.

DISEASE INTERACTIONS
Ursodiol treatment is usually inappropriate when complications of gallstone disease, such as obstruction of the bile duct, cholecystitis (inflammation of the gallbladder) or pancreatitis (inflammation of the pancreas) are present. These conditions may require gallbladder surgery, because benefits from ursodiol would take too long to achieve.

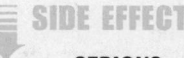

SIDE EFFECTS

SERIOUS
No serious side effects have been reported.

COMMON
No common side effects have been reported.

LESS COMMON
Diarrhea.

VALACYCLOVIR HYDROCHLORIDE

Available in: Tablets
Available OTC? No **As Generic?** No
Drug Class: Antiviral

▼ USAGE INFORMATION

WHY IT'S PRESCRIBED
To treat the symptoms of shingles (herpes zoster). Also used for the treatment and suppression of genital herpes.

HOW IT WORKS
Valacyclovir is converted in the body to acyclovir, which interferes with the activity of enzymes needed for the replication of viral DNA in cells, thus preventing the virus from multiplying. Although it cannot cure herpes infections, it can relieve symptoms and speed the healing of herpes lesions. It may also reduce the duration of any lingering pain (postherpetic neuralgia).

▼ DOSAGE GUIDELINES

RANGE AND FREQUENCY
For shingles: Adults: 1 gram (g), 3 times a day for 7 days. To treat initial episodes of genital herpes: 1 g, 2 times a day for 10 days. To treat recurrent genital herpes: 500 mg, 2 times a day for 5 days. For suppression of chronic recurrent genital herpes: 1 g, once a day. In patients with a history of 9 or fewer recurrences per year: 500 mg, once a day.

ONSET OF EFFECT
Within 30 minutes.

DURATION OF ACTION
Unknown.

DIETARY ADVICE
No special restrictions.

STORAGE
Store in a tightly sealed container away from heat, moisture, and direct light.

MISSED DOSE
Take it as soon as you remember. If it is near the time for the next dose, skip the missed dose and resume your regular dosage schedule. Do not double the next dose.

STOPPING THE DRUG
The decision to stop taking the drug should be made with your doctor.

PROLONGED USE
Usual course of therapy lasts 7 to 10 days. If for any reason you must take it for a longer period, see your doctor for regular tests and exams.

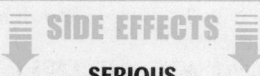

SIDE EFFECTS

SERIOUS
A rare but serious bleeding disorder marked by symptoms such as bruising, pinpoint red spots on the skin, and blood in the urine has been reported in a few patients with severely weakened immune systems.

COMMON
Headache, nausea.

LESS COMMON
Constipation or diarrhea, loss of appetite, dizziness, stomach pain, vomiting, unusual fatigue.

▼ PRECAUTIONS

Over 60: No special problems are expected, although a smaller dose may be warranted for those with a history of impaired renal (kidney) function.

Driving and Hazardous Work: Exercise caution until you determine how the medication affects you.

Alcohol: No special warnings.

Pregnancy: Human studies of valacyclovir in pregnancy have not been done, but birth defects or other problems have not been reported. Before you take valacyclovir, tell your doctor if you are pregnant or plan to become pregnant.

Breast Feeding: Valacyclovir may pass into breast milk. It is unknown if this poses any risks to the nursing infant; no problems have been reported. Consult your doctor for advice.

Infants and Children: The safety and effectiveness of this drug in children have not been established.

Special Concerns: Keep the body areas affected by shingles or herpes clean and dry, and wear comfortable, loose-fitting clothes to avoid irritation. Start taking valacyclovir as soon as possible after the symptoms appear, ideally within 72 hours. Do not take valacyclovir if you have ever had an allergic reaction to antiviral drugs.

OVERDOSE
Symptoms: No cases of overdose of valacyclovir have been reported. If an overdose were to occur, symptoms would likely be those of acute kidney failure, which include blood in the urine, passing only small amounts of urine, swelling of the ankles, hands, face, or other areas, shortness of breath, itching, fever, and flank pain.

What to Do: Seek medical assistance right away.

▼ INTERACTIONS

DRUG INTERACTIONS
Consult your doctor if you are taking any other prescription or over-the-counter medication, especially cimetidine or probenecid. These drugs slow the kidney's removal of valacyclovir, increasing the possibility of adverse side effects.

FOOD INTERACTIONS
No known food interactions.

DISEASE INTERACTIONS
Caution is advised when taking valacyclovir. Use of valacyclovir may cause complications in patients with kidney disease, since this organ works to remove the drug from the body. Consult your doctor if you have a weakened immune system; for example, if you are infected with the human immunodeficiency virus (HIV), or are taking immunosuppressant drugs to prevent organ rejection following a kidney or bone marrow transplant. Use of valacyclovir by patients with weakened immune systems can cause extreme side effects that may be fatal.

VALPROIC ACID (VALPROATE; DIVALPROEX SODIUM)

Available in: Capsules, syrup
Available OTC? No   **As Generic?** Yes
Drug Class: Anticonvulsant

BRAND NAMES

Depakene, Depakene Syrup, Depakote, Depakote Sprinkle

▼ USAGE INFORMATION

WHY IT'S PRESCRIBED
To control certain types of seizures in the treatment of epilepsy and other disorders. Also used to treat acute mania in the treatment of bipolar disorder.

HOW IT WORKS
Valproic acid is thought to depress the activity of certain parts of the brain and suppress the abnormal firing of neurons that causes seizures.

▼ DOSAGE GUIDELINES

RANGE AND FREQUENCY
Adults and children: 7 to 27 mg per lb of body weight, in 3 or 4 divided doses. Higher doses may be required. A low dose is used to start; it may be gradually increased by your doctor to achieve maximum therapeutic benefit with a minimum of side effects.

ONSET OF EFFECT
Within several hours.

DURATION OF ACTION
Maximum effect lasts for 12 hours or longer. Effectiveness then gradually decreases.

DIETARY ADVICE
Take it with food to minimize stomach upset. The syrup can be taken with liquids, but avoid carbonated beverages because the combination can irritate the mouth and throat.

STORAGE
Store in a tightly sealed container away from heat, moisture, and direct light. Do not allow the syrup to freeze.

MISSED DOSE
Take it as soon as you remember. If it is almost time for the next dose, skip the missed dose and resume your regular dosage schedule. Do not double the next dose without doctor's approval.

STOPPING THE DRUG
Abruptly stopping this drug may cause seizures. Your doctor will taper the dose over a period of weeks.

PROLONGED USE
See your doctor regularly for tests if you must take this drug for a prolonged period.

▼ PRECAUTIONS

Over 60: Older patients may require lower doses to minimize side effects.

Driving and Hazardous Work: This drug may cause drowsiness or dizziness. Do not drive or engage in hazardous work until you determine how it affects you.

Alcohol: May contribute to excessive drowsiness.

Pregnancy: Valproic acid is associated with an increased risk of birth defects when taken during pregnancy. However, seizures during pregnancy can also increase the risks to the fetus. Discuss with your doctor the potential risks and benefits of using this drug during pregnancy. Folate supplementation is recommended starting 1 to 2 months before conception and throughout pregnancy.

Breast Feeding: Valproic acid passes into breast milk, although at low levels. Consult your doctor for specific advice before nursing.

Infants and Children: Adverse reactions may be more likely and more severe in children.

Special Concerns: The generic version of this drug is not recommended. Your doctor may advise you to wear a medical bracelet or carry an identification card saying that you are taking this drug.

OVERDOSE
Symptoms: Restlessness, sleepiness, hallucinations, trembling arms and hands, loss of consciousness.

What to Do: Call your doctor, emergency medical services (EMS), or the nearest poison control center immediately.

▼ INTERACTIONS

DRUG INTERACTIONS
Valproic acid can interact with many drugs, including other anticonvulsants (carbamazepine, clonazepam, ethosuximide, felbamate, lamotrigine, phenobarbital, phenytoin, primidone), antacids, aspirin and other NSAIDs, barbiturates, cholestyramine, haloperidol, heparin, isoniazid, loxapine, MAO inhibitors, maprotiline, phenobarbital, tricyclic antidepressants, and warfarin.

FOOD INTERACTIONS
No known food interactions.

DISEASE INTERACTIONS
Special caution is advised if you have a history of blood disease, brain disease, or kidney or liver disease.

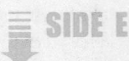
SIDE EFFECTS

SERIOUS
Severe abdominal pain and vomiting, muscle weakness and lethargy, yellow discoloration of the skin or eyes, facial swelling, abnormal bleeding or bruising, or seizures may be a sign of liver failure or other potentially fatal complications. Call your doctor immediately.

COMMON
Nausea and vomiting, heartburn, diarrhea, cramps, loss of appetite and weight loss, increased appetite and weight gain, hair loss, tremor, dizziness, clumsiness or unsteadiness, confusion, sedation.

LESS COMMON
Drowsiness, restlessness, constipation, unusual excitability, skin rash, headache, blurred or double vision, irritability or other changes in mental state. There are numerous additional side effects; consult your doctor if you are concerned about any adverse or unusual reactions.

VALSARTAN

Available in: Capsules
Available OTC? No   **As Generic?** No
Drug Class: Antihypertensive/angiotensin II antagonist

▼ USAGE INFORMATION

WHY IT'S PRESCRIBED
To control high blood pressure. This drug appears to have the same benefits as the class of antihypertensive drugs known as ACE inhibitors, without producing the common side effect (experienced by as many as 30% of patients) of a dry cough. Valsartan may be used by itself or in conjunction with other antihypertensive medications.

HOW IT WORKS
Valsartan blocks the effects of angiotensin II, a naturally occurring substance that causes blood vessels to narrow. Valsartan causes the blood vessels to dilate, thereby lowering blood pressure and decreasing the workload of the heart.

▼ DOSAGE GUIDELINES

RANGE AND FREQUENCY
To start, 80 mg once a day. It may be increased by your doctor to a maximum dose of 320 mg per day.

ONSET OF EFFECT
Within 2 to 4 weeks.

DURATION OF ACTION
Unknown.

DIETARY ADVICE
Follow a healthy diet (low-salt, low-fat, low-cholesterol) as advised by your doctor to help control blood pressure and prevent heart disease.

STORAGE
Store in a tightly sealed container away from heat, moisture, and direct light.

MISSED DOSE
Take it as soon as you remember. If it is near the time for the next dose, skip the missed dose and resume your regular dosage schedule. Do not double the next dose.

STOPPING THE DRUG
Take it as prescribed for the full treatment period. The decision to stop taking the drug should be made in consultation with your physician.

PROLONGED USE
Lifelong therapy may be necessary. However, if you do change certain health habits (for example, increasing exercise or losing weight), a reduced dose may be possible under a doctor's supervision.

▼ PRECAUTIONS

Over 60: No special problems are expected.

Driving and Hazardous Work: Do not drive or engage in hazardous work until you determine how the medicine affects you.

Alcohol: No special precautions are necessary.

Pregnancy: In certain ways valsartan is similar to a class of drugs that have caused damage to the unborn child when taken in the second or third trimester of pregnancy. Because safer, more effective medications can lower blood pressure during pregnancy, and because adequate studies on the use of valsartan during pregnancy have not been done, women who are pregnant or planning to become pregnant should not take it.

Breast Feeding: Valsartan may pass into breast milk; caution is advised. Consult your doctor for advice.

Infants and Children: The safety and effectiveness of use in children have not been established.

Special Concerns: Valsartan may cause dizziness or light-headedness, which is most noticeable when you change position. This may lead to fainting, falls, and injury. Sit or lie down immediately if you feel dizzy or lightheaded. This side effect may be worsened by alcohol, hot weather, dehydration, fever, prolonged standing, prolonged sitting, or exercise.

OVERDOSE
Symptoms: Fainting, dizziness, weak pulse that might be very slow or very fast, nausea, vomiting, confusion, chest pain.

What to Do: An overdose of valsartan is unlikely to be life-threatening. However, if someone takes a much larger dose than prescribed, call your doctor, emergency medical services (EMS), or the nearest poison control center immediately.

▼ INTERACTIONS

DRUG INTERACTIONS
No drug interactions have yet been observed with valsartan. Consult your doctor for specific advice if you are taking any other medication, including other drugs for high blood pressure. Valsartan can be taken together with diuretics or other medications for high blood pressure, if your doctor approves.

FOOD INTERACTIONS
No known food interactions.

DISEASE INTERACTIONS
Caution is advised when taking valsartan. Use of valsartan may cause complications in patients with liver or kidney disease, since these organs work together to remove the medication from the body.

SIDE EFFECTS

SERIOUS
No serious side effects have been reported.

COMMON
No common side effects have been reported.

LESS COMMON
Headache, dizziness, upper respiratory infection, cough, diarrhea, rhinitis, sinusitis, nausea, viral infection, abdominal pain, fatigue, edema, joint pains, heart palpitations, skin rash, constipation, dry mouth, gas, anxiety, insomnia, erectile dysfunction (impotence) in men.

VALSARTAN/HYDROCHLOROTHIAZIDE

Available in: Tablets
Available OTC? No   **As Generic?** No
Drug Class: Antihypertensive/angiotensin II antagonist; thiazide diuretic

▼ USAGE INFORMATION

WHY IT'S PRESCRIBED
To control high blood pressure (hypertension). Valsartan appears to have the same benefits as the class of antihypertensive drugs known as "ACE inhibitors," without producing the common side effect (experienced by as many as 30% of patients) of a dry cough. This drug combination is not used as initial treatment for hypertension.

HOW IT WORKS
This drug combines an angiotensin II antagonist (valsartan) and a thiazide diuretic (hydrochlorothiazide). Valsartan blocks the effects of angiotensin II, a naturally occurring substance that causes blood vessels to narrow. Valsartan causes the blood vessels to dilate, thereby lowering blood pressure and decreasing the workload of the heart. Hydrochlorothiazide (HCTZ) increases the excretion of salt and water in the urine. By reducing the overall fluid volume in the body, it decreases blood volume and so reduces pressure within the blood vessels.

▼ DOSAGE GUIDELINES

RANGE AND FREQUENCY
To start, 1 tablet containing 80 mg valsartan and 12.5 mg HCTZ once a day. The dose may be increased by your doctor to a maximum of 4 of these tablets or 2 tablets containing 160 mg valsartan and 12.5 mg HCTZ once a day.

ONSET OF EFFECT
Valsartan component: 2 to 4 weeks. HCTZ component: 2 to 4 hours.

DURATION OF ACTION
Valsartan component: Unknown. HCTZ component: 6 to 12 hours.

DIETARY ADVICE
It can be be taken with food to avoid stomach upset.

STORAGE
Store in a tightly sealed container away from heat, moisture, and direct light.

MISSED DOSE
If you miss a dose on one day, do not double the dose the next day.

STOPPING THE DRUG
The decision to stop taking it should be made in consultation with your doctor.

PROLONGED USE
Lifelong therapy may be necessary.

▼ PRECAUTIONS

Over 60: No special problems are expected.

Driving and Hazardous Work: Exercise caution until you determine how the medicine affects you.

Alcohol: No special precautions are necessary.

Pregnancy: Because safer, more effective medications can lower blood pressure during pregnancy, and because adequate studies have not been done on the use of this drug during pregnancy, women who are pregnant or planning to become pregnant should not take this medication unless recommended by your doctor.

Breast Feeding: Because of the potential for side effects on the infant, discuss with your doctor the relative risks and benefits of using this drug while nursing.

Infants and Children: The safety and effectiveness of use in children have not been established.

Special Concerns: The drug may cause dizziness or lightheadedness, which is most noticeable when you change position. This may lead to fainting, falls, and injury. Sit or lie down immediately if you feel dizzy or lightheaded. This side effect may be worsened by alcohol, hot weather, dehydration, fever, prolonged standing or sitting, or exercise. This medicine may cause your body to lose potassium. However, do not eat potassium-rich foods, salt substitutes, or take a potassium supplement without consulting your doctor.

OVERDOSE
Symptoms: Few cases of overdose have been reported. Symptoms may include fainting, lethargy, dizziness, drowsiness, weak pulse that might be very slow or very fast, nausea, vomiting, confusion, chest pain.

What to Do: Call your doctor, emergency medical services (EMS), or the nearest poison control center immediately.

▼ INTERACTIONS

DRUG INTERACTIONS
Consult your doctor for specific advice if you are taking anticoagulants, cholestyramine, colestipol, drugs for diabetes, nonsteroidal anti-inflammatory drugs, digitalis drugs, or lithium.

FOOD INTERACTIONS
No known food interactions.

DISEASE INTERACTIONS
Consult your doctor if you have any of the following: diabetes, gout, lupus, pancreatitis, heart disease, blood vessel disease. This medication should be used with caution in patients with moderate to severe liver or kidney disease.

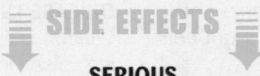

SIDE EFFECTS

SERIOUS
No serious side effects have been associated with the use of this medication.

COMMON
Dizziness, fatigue.

LESS COMMON
Viral infection, sore throat, coughing, diarrhea.

VANCOMYCIN

Available in: Capsules, oral solution, injection
Available OTC? No **As Generic?** Yes
Drug Class: Antibiotic

▼ USAGE INFORMATION

WHY IT'S PRESCRIBED
To treat severe bacterial infections such as colitis (infection and inflammation of the colon); also used prior to surgical or dental procedures to prevent heart valve infection in susceptible patients (for example, those with a history of rheumatic fever or heart valve replacement) who are allergic to penicillin.

HOW IT WORKS
Vancomycin kills and inhibits the growth of bacteria by interrupting their formation of cell walls.

▼ DOSAGE GUIDELINES

RANGE AND FREQUENCY
To treat bacterial infections—Oral forms: Adults and teenagers: 125 to 500 mg, 4 times a day for 5 to 10 days. Children: 4.5 mg per lb of body weight (up to 125 mg), 4 times a day for 5 to 10 days. Injection: Adults and teenagers: 1,000 mg twice a day or 500 mg, 4 times a day. Children: 4.5 mg per lb, 4 times a day or 9.1 mg per lb, 2 times a day. Infants over 1 week: 6.8 mg per lb to start, then 4.5 mg per lb, 3 times a day. Newborns up to 1 week: 6.8 mg per lb to start, then 4.5 mg per lb, 2 times a day. To prevent heart valve infection— Injection: Adults and teenagers: 1,000 mg 1 hour before surgery or dental work, then 1,000 mg, 8 hours later. Children: 9.1 mg per lb of body weight 1 hour before surgery or dental work, then 9.1 mg per lb, 8 hours later.

ONSET OF EFFECT
Unknown.

DURATION OF ACTION
Unknown.

DIETARY ADVICE
No special restrictions.

STORAGE
Store the medicine in a tightly sealed container away from heat, moisture, and direct light. Refrigerate any liquid form but do not allow it to freeze.

MISSED DOSE
Take it as soon as you remember. If it is near the time for the next dose, skip the missed dose and resume your regular dosage schedule. Do not double the next dose.

STOPPING THE DRUG
Take it as prescribed for the full treatment period, even if you feel better before the scheduled end of therapy.

PROLONGED USE
If your symptoms do not improve or instead become worse after a few days, consult your doctor.

▼ PRECAUTIONS

Over 60: Adverse reactions may be more likely and more severe in older patients.

Driving and Hazardous Work: No special precautions are necessary.

Alcohol: No special problems are expected, although it is generally advisable to avoid alcohol when recovering from an infection.

Pregnancy: Adequate studies of the use of vancomycin during pregnancy have not been done, although no problems are expected. Before using vancomycin, consult your doctor if you are pregnant or plan to become pregnant.

Breast Feeding: Vancomycin passes into breast milk; caution is advised. Consult your doctor for specific advice.

Infants and Children: Consult your doctor about the relative risks and benefits of using vancomycin for children.

Special Concerns: If you take vancomycin for diarrhea caused by other antibiotics, do not take any other diarrhea medicine without consulting your doctor.

OVERDOSE
Symptoms: Hearing loss, ringing in ears, dizziness.

What to Do: Call your doctor, emergency medical services (EMS), or the nearest poison control center immediately.

▼ INTERACTIONS

DRUG INTERACTIONS
Other drugs may interact with vancomycin. Consult your doctor for specific advice if you are taking cholestyramine, colestipol (with oral forms of vancomycin), aminoglycosides, amphotericin B, bacitracin, bumetanide, capreomycin, cisplatin, cyclosporine, ethacrynic acid, furosemide, paromomycin, polymixins, or streptozocin.

FOOD INTERACTIONS
No known food interactions.

DISEASE INTERACTIONS
Consult your doctor if you have a history of kidney disease, inflammatory bowel disease, or hearing loss.

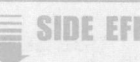

SIDE EFFECTS

SERIOUS
Skin rash (with oral forms); change in the frequency or amount of urination; breathing difficulty; drowsiness; unusual thirst; loss of appetite; weakness; hearing loss; ringing or buzzing in ears; chills or fever; fast heartbeat; fainting; nausea or vomiting; itching; redness of face, neck, upper back, and arms; tingling; unpleasant taste. Call your doctor immediately.

COMMON
Bitter or unpleasant taste, mouth irritation.

LESS COMMON
There are no less-common side effects associated with the use of vancomycin.

VASOPRESSIN (8-ARGININE-VASOPRESSIN)

Available in: Injection, nasal spray
Available OTC? No   **As Generic?** No
Drug Class: Antidiuretic hormone

▼ USAGE INFORMATION

WHY IT'S PRESCRIBED
To treat diabetes insipidus, a relatively rare disorder characterized by excessive loss of water in the urine, potentially leading to dehydration. Vasopressin is generally prescribed for short-term use only and has largely been replaced by a long-lasting analog known as DDAVP (desmopressin acetate).

HOW IT WORKS
Vasopressin is a hormone involved in kidney function. It helps the kidneys to reabsorb water from urine before it is excreted, thereby maintaining proper fluid and electrolyte balance in the body.

▼ DOSAGE GUIDELINES

RANGE AND FREQUENCY
Subcutaneous (under the skin) injection— Adults: 5 to 10 units, 2 or 3 times a day.

Children: 2.5 to 10 units, 3 or 4 times a day. Nasal spray— Adults or children: Spray into nostril as directed by your doctor.

ONSET OF EFFECT
Within 1 hour.

DURATION OF ACTION
From 6 to 8 hours.

DIETARY ADVICE
It can be taken with or between meals. Take it with 1 or 2 glasses of water to prevent nausea, skin whitening, and abdominal cramps.

STORAGE
Store in a tightly sealed container away from heat and direct light.

MISSED DOSE
Take it as soon as you remember. If it is near the time for the next dose, skip the missed dose and resume your regular dosage schedule. Do not double the next dose.

STOPPING THE DRUG
The decision to stop taking the drug should be made by your doctor.

PROLONGED USE
No apparent problems are associated with prolonged use of vasopressin.

▼ PRECAUTIONS

Over 60: Adverse reactions may be more likely and more severe in older patients.

Driving and Hazardous Work: Do not drive or engage in hazardous work until you determine how the medicine affects you.

Alcohol: Drink alcohol only in moderation.

Pregnancy: Vasopressin has not been shown to cause birth defects or other problems in humans. Animal and human studies have not been done. Before you take the drug, tell your doctor if you are pregnant or are planning to become pregnant.

Breast Feeding: Vasopressin has not been shown to cause problems in nursing babies. Consult your doctor about its use if you are breast feeding.

Infants and Children: Adverse reactions may be more likely and more severe in children under age 18.

Special Concerns: Electrocardiograms and laboratory tests of fluid status should be done periodically while you take vasopressin. Tell your doctor if you are allergic to any preservative or dye. Vaso-

pressin may worsen the effect of migraine headaches.

OVERDOSE
Symptoms: Drowsiness, listlessness, headache, confusion, inability to urinate, unexpected weight gain or fluid retention.

What to Do: An overdose of vasopressin is unlikely to be life-threatening, but it can cause excessive retention of water (water intoxication) and spasm of the blood vessels. If someone takes a much larger dose than prescribed, call your doctor, emergency medical services (EMS), or poison control center immediately.

▼ INTERACTIONS

DRUG INTERACTIONS
Consult your doctor for advice if you are taking carbamazepine, chlorpropamide, demeclocycline, ethanol, fludrocortisone, heparin, lithium, norepinephrine, or tricyclic antidepressants.

FOOD INTERACTIONS
No known food interactions.

DISEASE INTERACTIONS
Consult your doctor if you have a history of any of the following: seizures, migraine headaches, asthma, heart disease, blood vessel disease, heart failure, or kidney disease.

≡ SIDE EFFECTS ≡

SERIOUS
Allergic response characterized by wheezing; rash; hives; itching; swelling of face, lips, hands, or feet; closing of throat; breathing difficulty; and slow or irregular pulse; drowsiness; water intoxication, causing listlessness; headache; confusion; weight gain; seizures; loss of consciousness. Call your doctor immediately.

COMMON
No common side effects are associated with the use of vasopressin.

LESS COMMON
Tremor, dizziness, chest pain, abdominal cramps, nausea, vomiting, diarrhea, inability to urinate, pale skin around mouth, profuse or unusual sweating, uterine cramps. Such symptoms are generally associated only with excessively large doses.

VENLAFAXINE

Available in: Tablets, extended-release capsules
Available OTC? No   **As Generic?** No
Drug Class: Antidepressant

▼ USAGE INFORMATION

WHY IT'S PRESCRIBED
To treat symptoms of major depression and generalized anxiety disorder (GAD).

HOW IT WORKS
Venlafaxine helps to balance levels of serotonin and norepinephrine, brain chemicals that are profoundly linked to mood, emotions, and mental state.

▼ DOSAGE GUIDELINES

RANGE AND FREQUENCY
Tablets: Adults: 75 mg a day in 2 or 3 divided doses. The dose may be gradually increased by your doctor to 375 mg a day. Extended-release capsules: To start, 75 mg, once a day. The dose may be increased by up to 75 mg at a time at intervals of not less than 4 days, up to a maximum dose of 225 mg a day.

ONSET OF EFFECT
2 weeks or more.

DURATION OF ACTION
Unknown.

DIETARY ADVICE
Venlafaxine should be taken with meals.

STORAGE
Store in a tightly sealed container away from heat, moisture, and direct light.

MISSED DOSE
Tablets: Take it as soon as you remember, unless the time for your next scheduled dose is within the next 2 hours. If so, skip the missed dose, take the next scheduled dose, and resume your regular schedule. Do not double the next dose. Extended-release capsules: If you miss a dose on one day, do not double the dose the next day.

STOPPING THE DRUG
Take as prescribed for the full treatment period

PROLONGED USE
See your doctor regularly for tests and examinations if you must take this medicine for a prolonged period.

▼ PRECAUTIONS

Over 60: No special problems are expected.

Driving and Hazardous Work: Do not drive or engage in hazardous work until you determine how the medicine affects you.

Alcohol: Avoid alcohol.

Pregnancy: Adequate studies of venlafaxine use during pregnancy have not been done. Before you take venlafaxine, tell your doctor if you are pregnant or plan to become pregnant.

Breast Feeding: It is not known whether venlafaxine passes into breast milk; caution is advised. Consult your doctor for specific advice.

Infants and Children: The safety and effectiveness of venlafaxine use by children have not been established.

Special Concerns: Venlafaxine can cause an elevation in blood pressure. Therefore, blood pressure should be monitored regularly, especially in the first several months of therapy.

**OVERDOSE
Symptoms:** Extreme drowsiness or fatigue.

What to Do: Call your doctor, emergency medical services (EMS), or the nearest poison control center immediately.

▼ INTERACTIONS

DRUG INTERACTIONS
Venlafaxine and MAO inhibitors should not be used within 14 days of each other. Serious side effects such as myoclonus (uncontrolled muscle spasms), hyperthermia (excessive rise in body temperature), and extreme stiffness may result. Consult your doctor for specific advice if you are taking any other prescription or over-the-counter medication.

FOOD INTERACTIONS
No known food interactions.

DISEASE INTERACTIONS
Consult your physician if you have a history of any of the following: high or low blood pressure, alcohol or drug abuse, heart disease, or seizures. Use of venlafaxine may cause complications in patients with liver or kidney disease, since these organs work together to remove the medication from the body.

≡ SIDE EFFECTS ≡

SERIOUS
Headache, changes in or blurred vision, decreased sexual ability or desire, difficulty urinating, itching, skin rash, chest pain, heartbeat irregularities, changes in moods or mental state, extreme drowsiness or fatigue. Call your physician immediately.

COMMON
Fatigue, dizziness or drowsiness, anxiety, dry mouth, changed sense of taste, loss of appetite, nausea, vomiting, chills, diarrhea, constipation, prickly sensation of skin, heartburn, increased sweating, runny nose, stomach gas or pain, insomnia, unusual dreams, weight loss.

LESS COMMON
Frequent yawning, twitching.

VERAPAMIL HYDROCHLORIDE

Available in: Extended-release capsules, tablets, injection
Available OTC? No   **As Generic?** Yes
Drug Class: Calcium channel blocker

▼ USAGE INFORMATION

WHY IT'S PRESCRIBED
To treat high blood pressure (hypertension), angina pectoris (chest pain associated with heart disease), and heartbeat irregularities (cardiac arrhythmias).

HOW IT WORKS
Verapamil interferes with the movement of calcium into heart muscle cells and the smooth muscle cells in the walls of the arteries. This action relaxes blood vessels (causing them to widen), which lowers blood pressure, increases the blood supply to the heart, and decreases the heart's overall workload.

▼ DOSAGE GUIDELINES

RANGE AND FREQUENCY
Adults: 40 to 160 mg, 3 times a day. Your doctor may increase dose as necessary, up to a maximum of 480 mg per day. Extended-release capsules: 200 to 480 mg once a day. Extended-release tablets: 120 mg once a day to 240 mg every 12 hours.

Children: The dose will be determined by a pediatrician.

ONSET OF EFFECT
Oral forms: 1 to 2 hours. Injection: 1 to 5 minutes.

DURATION OF ACTION
Extended-release capsules: 24 hours. Tablets: 8 to 10 hours. Injection: 1 to 6 hours.

DIETARY ADVICE
Take oral forms with food.

STORAGE
Store in a tightly sealed container away from heat and direct light.

MISSED DOSE
Take it as soon as you remember. If it is near the time for the next dose, skip the missed dose and resume your regular dosage schedule. Do not double the next dose.

STOPPING THE DRUG
Do not stop taking this drug suddenly, as this may cause potentially serious health problems. If therapy is to be discontinued, dosage should be reduced gradually, according to doctor's instructions.

PROLONGED USE
Lifetime therapy with verapamil may be necessary; regular medical exams and tests are important in such cases.

▼ PRECAUTIONS

Over 60: Adverse reactions may be more likely and more severe in older patients.

Driving and Hazardous Work: Do not drive or engage in hazardous work until you determine how the medicine affects you.

Alcohol: Avoid alcohol.

Pregnancy: Large doses of verapamil have been shown to cause birth defects in animals; human studies have not been done. Before you take verapamil, tell your doctor if you are pregnant or plan to become pregnant.

Breast Feeding: Verapamil passes into breast milk but has not been reported to cause problems; caution is advised. Consult your doctor for advice.

Infants and Children: Oral doses for children 1 to 15 years old must be determined by your pediatrician.

Special Concerns: In addition to taking verapamil, be sure to follow all special instructions on weight control and diet. Your doctor will tell you which specific factors are most important for you. Check with your doctor before making changes in your diet. Extended-release forms should not be crushed or chewed.

OVERDOSE

Symptoms: Extremely slow heartbeat and heart palpitations; dizziness or fainting (due to excessively low blood pressure).

What to Do: Call your doctor, emergency medical services (EMS), or the nearest poison control center immediately.

▼ INTERACTIONS

DRUG INTERACTIONS
Consult your physician for specific advice if you are taking acetazolamide, amphotericin B, corticosteroids, dichlorphenamide, diuretics, methazolamide, beta-blockers, carbamazepine, cyclosporine, lithium, procainamide, quinidine, digitalis, disopyramide or the following eye medicines: betaxolol, levobunolol, metipranolol, or timolol.

FOOD INTERACTIONS
Avoid foods high in sodium.

DISEASE INTERACTIONS
Caution is advised when taking verapamil. Consult your doctor if you have any of the following: abnormal heart rhythm or other disorders of the heart and blood vessels, mental depression, or Parkinson's disease. Verapamil may cause complications in patients with liver or kidney disease, since these organs work together to remove the medication from the body.

≡ SIDE EFFECTS ≡

SERIOUS
Breathing difficulty, coughing, or wheezing; irregular or pounding heartbeat; chest pain; extreme dizziness; fainting. Call your doctor immediately.

COMMON
Headache; dizziness; constipation; flushing and a feeling of warmth; swelling in the feet, ankles, or calves; heart palpitations.

LESS COMMON
Diarrhea, nausea, unusual fatigue and weakness, skin rash, increased urination, ringing in the ears.

VITAMIN A (RETINOL)

Available in: Capsules, oral solution, tablets
Available OTC? Yes **As Generic?** Yes
Drug Class: Vitamin

▼ USAGE INFORMATION

WHY IT'S PRESCRIBED
To treat vitamin A deficiency. Most Americans get sufficient amounts of vitamin A from their diet. Most vitamin A is obtained from the conversion of dietary beta-carotene to vitamin A in the intestine. Foods rich in beta-carotene include yellow-orange fruits and vegetables; dark-green leafy vegetables, such as spinach and lettuce; liver; and fortified milk and margarine. Supplementation may be necessary with certain medical conditions such as long-term chronic illness, liver disorders, intestinal malabsorption associated with chronic diarrhea or pancreatic disease, and surgical removal of the stomach. Vitamin A deficiency can cause night blindness, dry eyes, eye infections, and skin problems.

HOW IT WORKS
Vitamin A plays an essential role in night vision and proper growth and maintenance of the skin, bones, and reproductive organs.

▼ DOSAGE GUIDELINES

RANGE AND FREQUENCY
For severe vitamin A deficiency: 100,000 International Units (IU) daily for 3 days, followed by 25,000 to 50,000 IU daily for 2 weeks, then 10,000 to 20,000 IU daily for 2 months. To prevent vitamin deficiency (recommended daily allowance)— Adults: 3,330 IU daily for men, 2,665 IU daily for women. Children ages 7 to 10: 2,330 IU daily. Children ages 4 to 6: 1,665 IU daily. Children ages 1 to 3: 1,330 IU daily. Infants: 1,250 IU daily.

ONSET OF EFFECT
Unknown.

DURATION OF ACTION
Unknown.

DIETARY ADVICE
Absorption of vitamin A requires some fat in the diet.

STORAGE
Store in a tightly sealed container away from heat, moisture, and direct light.

MISSED DOSE
Take it as soon as you remember.

STOPPING THE DRUG
If you are taking vitamin A because of a deficiency, take it as prescribed for the full treatment period.

PROLONGED USE
Prolonged use of high doses may cause serious toxicity (see Overdose).

▼ PRECAUTIONS

Over 60: Adverse reactions associated with high-dose, long-term use may be more likely and more severe in older patients.

Driving and Hazardous Work: The use of recommended doses of vitamin A should not impair your ability to perform such tasks safely.

Alcohol: No special precautions are necessary.

Pregnancy: Adequate vitamin A intake is essential during pregnancy. However, vitamin A overdose (more than 6,000 IU daily) can cause birth defects or slow or reduce growth in the fetus.

Breast Feeding: Vitamin A passes into breast milk; caution is advised. Ingesting too much vitamin A during breast feeding can be harmful to the nursing infant.

Infants and Children: Children are more sensitive to side effects from high doses of vitamin A.

Special Concerns: Vitamin A can be highly toxic (see Overdose) when taken in high doses. Take only as directed.

OVERDOSE
Symptoms: Acute overdose: Bleeding from gums, sore mouth, confusion or unusual excitement, diarrhea, drowsiness or dizziness, double vision, severe headache, irritability, peeling skin, especially on lips and palms, severe vomiting. Chronic overdose (with prolonged overuse): Drying or cracking of skin or lips, bone or joint pain, fever, general feeling of discomfort, increased sensitivity of skin to sunlight, increased urination, loss of appetite, hair loss, stomach pain, unusual fatigue, yellow-orange patches on soles of feet, palms of hands, or skin around the nose and lips.

What to Do: For an acute overdose, call your doctor, emergency medical services (EMS), or the nearest poison control center immediately. For symptoms of chronic overdose, contact your doctor.

▼ INTERACTIONS

DRUG INTERACTIONS
Consult your doctor for specific advice if you are taking etretinate or isotretinoin.

FOOD INTERACTIONS
No known food interactions.

DISEASE INTERACTIONS
Consult your doctor if you have a history of alcohol abuse, liver disease, or kidney disease.

≡ SIDE EFFECTS ≡

SERIOUS
No serious side effects occur with recommended doses of vitamin A (see Overdose).

COMMON
No common side effects occur with recommended doses of vitamin A.

LESS COMMON
No less-common side effects occur with recommended doses of vitamin A.

VITAMIN B1 (THIAMINE)

Available in: Tablets, injection
Available OTC? Yes **As Generic?** Yes
Drug Class: Vitamin

▼ USAGE INFORMATION

WHY IT'S PRESCRIBED
To prevent and treat a vitamin B1 deficiency. Vitamin B1 deficiency can lead to either beriberi, which affects many body tissues, including the heart and nervous system (symptoms include constipation, loss of appetite, pain or tingling in arms and legs, emaciation, paralysis, heart failure, and mental deficits), or a severe brain disorder known as Wernicke's encephalopathy.

HOW IT WORKS
Thiamine is one of the B-complex vitamins, which are essential for normal metabolism and for the health and proper functioning of the cardiovascular and nervous systems. Thiamine is required for the formation of a factor needed for the function of enzymes involved in the metabolism of carbohydrates.

▼ DOSAGE GUIDELINES

RANGE AND FREQUENCY
Recommended daily allowance– Infants, birth to 3 years: 0.4 mg per day. Children ages 4 to 6: 0.9 mg. Children ages 7 to 10: 1 mg. Males ages 11 to 14: 1.3 mg. Males ages 15 to 50: 1.5 mg. Males ages 51 and over: 1.2 mg. Women ages 11 to 50: 1.1 mg. Women ages 51 and over: 1 mg. Pregnant women: 1.5 mg. Breast-feeding women: 1.6 mg. To treat beriberi– Adults and teenagers: 5 to 10 mg, 3 times a day. Children: 10 mg a day.

ONSET OF EFFECT
Unknown.

DURATION OF ACTION
Unknown.

DIETARY ADVICE
Take it with or between meals.

STORAGE
Store in a tightly sealed container away from heat, moisture, and direct light.

MISSED DOSE
Take it as soon as you remember.

STOPPING THE DRUG
If thiamine is being taken to treat beriberi, the decision to stop taking the drug should be made by your doctor.

≋ SIDE EFFECTS ≋

SERIOUS
There are no serious side effects associated with the use of thiamine (except in very rare cases pertaining to high doses administered by injection, which occur exclusively in a hospital setting).

COMMON
No common side effects have been reported.

LESS COMMON
No less-common side effects have been reported.

PROLONGED USE
No problems are expected.

▼ PRECAUTIONS

Over 60: No problems have been reported in older persons, who are more likely to have low blood levels of thiamine and thus require a supplement.

Driving and Hazardous Work: No special precautions are necessary.

Alcohol: No special precautions are necessary.

Pregnancy: A thiamine-containing vitamin supplement may be recommended, but taking large amounts of a supplement during pregnancy may be harmful to the mother or fetus. Consult your doctor for advice.

Breast Feeding: Taking large amounts of a dietary supplement while breast feeding may be harmful to the infant. Consult your doctor for specific advice. If thiamine deficiency occurs during breast feeding, both the mother and the nursing infant should be treated.

Infants and Children: No problems reported in infants and children with the intake of recommended daily allowances.

Special Concerns: Good nutritional habits are necessary to avoid vitamin deficiency. Thiamine-rich foods include pork, organ meats, green leafy vegetables, legumes, sweet corn, corn meal, egg yolks, brown rice, yeast, whole grains, berries, and nuts. Supplements of more than 15 mg taken 3 times a day are poorly absorbed from the intestine.

OVERDOSE
Symptoms: No cases of thiamine overdose have been reported.

What to Do: Emergency instructions not applicable.

▼ INTERACTIONS

DRUG INTERACTIONS
Consult your doctor for specific advice if you are taking any prescription or over-the-counter medication.

FOOD INTERACTIONS
No known food interactions.

DISEASE INTERACTIONS
Thiamine deficiency is most likely to occur in people on extremely low-calorie diets or those suffering from gastrointestinal disease (leading to chronic malabsorption), cirrhosis, or alcoholism. A clinically significant deficiency can occur after a few weeks of a diet with little or no thiamine.

VITAMIN B2 (RIBOFLAVIN)

Available in: Tablets, sugar-free tablets
Available OTC? Yes   **As Generic?** Yes
Drug Class: Dietary supplement

▼ USAGE INFORMATION

WHY IT'S PRESCRIBED
To treat vitamin B2 deficiency. Riboflavin must be included in the nutrients administered to patients receiving all their nutrition intravenously. A riboflavin deficiency may have symptoms that include sensitivity of eyes to light; itching and burning eyes; itching and peeling skin on the nose and scrotum; and sores at the corners of the mouth and on the tongue. Riboflavin requirements may be increased in people suffering from severe burns, chronic diarrhea, cirrhosis of the liver, alcoholism, cancer, or in those who have undergone surgical removal of the stomach.

HOW IT WORKS
Riboflavin is one of the B-complex vitamins, which are essential for normal metabolism and for the health and proper functioning of the cardiovascular and nervous systems. Specifically, body cells convert riboflavin into two products essential to the activity of enzymes that break down carbohydrates, proteins, and fats, and that enable oxygen to be used by the body's cells.

▼ DOSAGE GUIDELINES

RANGE AND FREQUENCY
Recommended intakes—Adult and teenage males: 1.4 to 1.8 mg daily. Adult and teenage females: 1.2 to 1.3 mg daily. Children ages 7 to 10: 1.2 mg daily. Children ages 4 to 6: 1.1 mg daily. Infants from birth to 3: 0.4 to 0.8 mg daily. Pregnant women: 1.6 mg daily. Breast-feeding women: 1.7 to 1.8 mg daily. Sufficient vitamin B2 is usually provided by adequate diets.

ONSET OF EFFECT
Unknown.

DURATION OF ACTION
Unknown.

DIETARY ADVICE
Avoid alcohol; it reduces the absorption of riboflavin from the intestine.

STORAGE
Store in a tightly sealed container away from heat, moisture, and direct light.

MISSED DOSE
Take it as soon as you remember. No problems are expected as a result of missing a dose.

≡ SIDE EFFECTS ≡

SERIOUS
No serious side effects have been reported.

COMMON
Urine may appear bright yellow when riboflavin is taken in high doses.

LESS COMMON
No less-common side effects have been reported.

STOPPING THE DRUG
If riboflavin is prescribed for a vitamin deficiency, take it as prescribed for the full treatment period.

PROLONGED USE
No special problems are expected.

▼ PRECAUTIONS

Over 60: No special problems are expected.

Driving and Hazardous Work: No special precautions are necessary.

Alcohol: Alcohol may reduce the absorption of vitamin B2 from the intestine.

Pregnancy: No known problems. Riboflavin requirements are increased slightly during pregnancy.

Breast Feeding: Recommended intake of riboflavin and other vitamins is increased during breast feeding. Taking excessive amounts while breast feeding may be harmful to the nursing baby. Consult your doctor for specific advice.

Infants and Children: No problems are expected.

Special Concerns: Riboflavin supplements may cause a harmless yellow discoloration of the urine. Severe weight-reducing diets may reduce riboflavin intake below recommended amounts, and require supplementation or increased intake of riboflavin-rich foods like eggs, organ meats, whole-grain cereals and breads, green leafy vegetables, mushrooms, avocados, legumes (such as kidney beans), cashews, chestnuts, milk, and cheeses.

OVERDOSE
Symptoms: No specific ones have been reported.

What to Do: Emergency instructions not applicable.

▼ INTERACTIONS

DRUG INTERACTIONS
Consult your doctor for specific advice if you are taking propantheline, phenothiazines, tricyclic antidepressants, or probenecid.

FOOD INTERACTIONS
None expected.

DISEASE INTERACTIONS
None expected.

VITAMIN B3 (NIACIN)

Available in: Tablets, extended-release tablets
Available OTC? Yes **As Generic?** Yes
Drug Class: Dietary supplement; antilipidemic (lipid-lowering) agent

▼ USAGE INFORMATION

WHY IT'S PRESCRIBED
As a dietary supplement: To prevent or treat niacin deficiency (pellagra). Symptoms include dermatitis, diarrhea, and dementia. (Healthy people eating a well-rounded diet do not develop niacin deficiency.) As an antilipidemic: Large doses of niacin are used to lower total and LDL cholesterol and triglyceride levels. It is the most effective drug currently available to increase HDL cholesterol levels.

HOW IT WORKS
Niacin is required for the proper action of enzymes involved in energy metabolism. It lowers blood lipids by partially blocking the release of fatty acids from adipose (fat) tissue and reducing the liver's production of the triglyceride-carrying lipoprotein, very-low-density lipoprotein (VLDL).

▼ DOSAGE GUIDELINES

RANGE AND FREQUENCY
Tablets— Recommended daily allowances for niacin are 5 to 15 mg a day for children; 15 to 20 mg a day for adolescent and adult men; and 13 to 15 mg a day for adolescent and adult women. To treat pellagra: 250 to 500 mg a day. As an antilipidemic: 500 to 4,500 mg a day in divided doses with meals. Extended-release tablets— As an antilipidemic: All doses are taken once a day at bedtime following a low-fat snack. Week 1: 375 mg. Week 2: 500 mg. Week 3: 750 mg. Weeks 4 to 7: 1,000 mg. After week 7, your doctor will evaluate your response to your dose.

ONSET OF EFFECT
2 to 4 weeks.

DURATION OF ACTION
As long as it is taken.

DIETARY ADVICE
A well-balanced diet will prevent niacin deficiency.

STORAGE
Avoid heat and direct light.

MISSED DOSE
Skip the missed dose and resume you regular dosage schedule. Do not double the next dose.

STOPPING THE DRUG
If you take this vitamin as an antilipidemic, do not stop unless so instructed by your doctor. Once niacin is stopped, lipids will increase to pretreatment levels.

PROLONGED USE
Side effects are more likely with prolonged use.

▼ PRECAUTIONS

Over 60: Possible increase in side effects and risk of developing diabetes.

Driving and Hazardous Work: No special precautions are necessary.

Alcohol: Niacin deficiency is more common in alcoholics because of their poor diets. Alcohol can increase blood triglycerides in people with blood lipid abnormalities. Alcohol also increases the likelihood of flushing reactions.

Pregnancy: Pregnancy increases dietary niacin needs to 17 to 20 mg a day. If taken as an antilipidemic, niacin therapy should be discontinued unless the doctor believes benefits clearly outweigh possible risks.

Breast Feeding: Breast feeding increases dietary niacin needs to 20 mg a day. There is no evidence of danger to the infant from niacin as an antilipidemic, but your doctor should reconsider whether continued therapy is absolutely necessary.

Infants and Children: Safety has not been established for treatment of lipid problems.

Special Concerns: Periodic tests to assess liver function, blood glucose, and uric acid levels are needed.

OVERDOSE
Symptoms: Flushing, abdominal pain, nausea, vomiting.

What to Do: Call your doctor.

▼ INTERACTIONS

DRUG INTERACTIONS
Niacin combined with HMG-CoA reductase inhibitors (lipid-lowering drugs known as statins) can cause myositis (muscle inflammation) with muscle pain and tenderness. Severe myositis can damage kidneys and lead to kidney failure. The drugs must be stopped immediately if symptoms of myositis occur.

FOOD INTERACTIONS
Flushing may be worse when niacin is taken with hot foods or drinks.

DISEASE INTERACTIONS
Niacin should not be used by those with a history of gout or peptic ulcer. It should be used with caution by people with diabetes, borderline high glucose levels, or any evidence of liver abnormalities.

SIDE EFFECTS

SERIOUS
Liver toxicity leading to jaundice (yellow discoloration of skin and eyes) and fatigue (more common with slow-release forms of niacin); gastrointestinal irritation, causing nausea, vomiting, and abdominal pain; peptic ulcer; increased uric acid levels, leading to gout attacks; elevated blood glucose levels.

COMMON
Itching, flushing, sweating, and dizziness, often within 20 to 40 minutes after taking niacin. These symptoms can usually be reduced or eliminated by taking an aspirin 30 minutes before the niacin. They tend to diminish or disappear with prolonged use. Slow-release forms reduce these side effects. Nausea and vomiting may also occur.

LESS COMMON
Dry skin, headaches, eye problems.

VITAMIN B6 (PYRIDOXINE)

Available in: Tablets
Available OTC? Yes   **As Generic?** Yes
Drug Class: Dietary supplement

▼ USAGE INFORMATION

WHY IT'S PRESCRIBED
To treat or prevent vitamin B6 deficiency, which can cause anemia, dermatitis, nervous system problems, and painful cracking at the outer sides of the mouth. Deficiency does not occur in healthy people eating a well-balanced diet. However, several genetic abnormalities may lead to a requirement for higher doses of vitamin B6 than can be obtained from the diet. Supplements may also be necessary in people with alcoholism, an overactive thyroid, or intestinal diseases associated with nutritional malabsorption.

HOW IT WORKS
Vitamin B6 is used to manufacture a substance required for the proper action of enzymes involved in the metabolism of carbohydrates, fats, and proteins.

▼ DOSAGE GUIDELINES

RANGE AND FREQUENCY
Recommended daily allowances for vitamin B6 are 0.3 to 1 mg from birth to age 3; 1.1 mg from age 4 to 7; 1.4 mg from age 7 to 10; 1.7 to 2 mg in adolescent and adult males; and 1.4 to 1.6 mg in adolescent and adult females. For vitamin B6 deficiency or an inherited abnormality causing increased vitamin B6 requirements, consult your doctor.

ONSET OF EFFECT
Unknown.

DURATION OF ACTION
As long as the vitamin is taken.

DIETARY ADVICE
Eat a well-balanced diet. Foods rich in vitamin B6 include egg yolks, meats, bananas, and whole grain cereals.

STORAGE
Store in a cool, dry place.

MISSED DOSE
Take the next regularly scheduled dose.

STOPPING THE DRUG
If the vitamin was prescribed for a deficiency, consult your doctor before stopping.

PROLONGED USE
No problems are expected with recommended doses of vitamin B6.

▼ PRECAUTIONS

Over 60: No special problems are expected with recommended doses.

Driving and Hazardous Work: No special precautions are necessary.

Alcohol: Alcoholism can lead to a vitamin B6 deficiency. Conversely, those who are being treated for vitamin B6 deficiency should abstain from alcohol.

Pregnancy: Vitamin B6 requirements increase during pregnancy to 2.2 mg per day. Very large doses may cause vitamin B6 dependency in the newborn child.

Breast Feeding: Vitamin B6 requirements increase during breast feeding to 2.1 mg per day.

Infants and Children: No problems are expected with recommended doses.

OVERDOSE
Symptoms: Overdose is extremely rare. Two cases that caused central nervous system toxicity (see Serious Side Effects) have been reported.

What to Do: Although an overdose is highly unlikely to occur, call your doctor right away if you have any reason to suspect that one has occurred.

▼ INTERACTIONS

DRUG INTERACTIONS
Vitamin B6 is used in the treatment of toxicity associated with the drugs cycloserine and isoniazid. Other drugs that may increase the daily requirement for vitamin B6 include ethionamide, hydralazine, penicillamine, immunosuppressants, and estrogen.

FOOD INTERACTIONS
No food interactions have been reported.

DISEASE INTERACTIONS
No disease interactions have been reported.

≡ SIDE EFFECTS ≡

SERIOUS
When taken for several months, high doses of vitamin B6 (2 to 6 grams daily) may cause reversible nerve damage; symptoms include numbness, tingling, or prickling in the feet; loss of manual dexterity; and unsteady gait.

COMMON
No common side effects are associated with recommended doses.

LESS COMMON
No less-common side effects are associated with recommended doses.

VITAMIN B12 (CYANOCOBALAMIN)

Available in: Tablets, extended-release tablets, injection, nasal gel
Available OTC? Yes   **As Generic?** Yes
Drug Class: Dietary supplement

▼ USAGE INFORMATION

WHY IT'S PRESCRIBED
Cyanocobalamin is a synthetic form of vitamin B12, prescribed to correct vitamin B12 deficiency and to remedy the associated medical conditions (anemia and nerve damage) that may result from such a deficiency. B12 deficiency can occur for a number of reasons, including a diet lacking in animal protein, pernicious anemia, intestinal malabsorption, surgical removal of portions of the stomach or small intestine, the effects of certain drugs (including colchicine, neomycin, and PAS), or because an individual is unable to keep up with an increase in the daily requirements of the vitamin (as occurs during pregnancy or during periods of great physical stress).

HOW IT WORKS
Vitamin B12 is essential for the proper production of blood platelets and red and white blood cells, the manufacture of vital substances needed for cell function, and the metabolism of nutrients necessary for cell growth.

▼ DOSAGE GUIDELINES

RANGE AND FREQUENCY
Recommended daily allowances (RDA)— Adults and teenagers: 2 micrograms (mcg). Pregnant or breast-feeding women: 2.2 mcg. Children ages 7 to 10: 1.4 mcg. Children ages 4 to 6: 1 mcg. From birth to 3 years of age: 0.3 to 0.7 mcg. (Extended-release tablets are not recommended for children.) To treat severe vitamin B12 deficiency— The dose will be determined by your doctor based on individual criteria. Patients with pernicious anemia or loss of intestinal function require the injection form of vitamin B12. As an alternative to the injection, patients may use the nasal gel with a dose of 500 mcg, once a week.

ONSET OF EFFECT
Immediate.

DURATION OF ACTION
For as long as the supplement is taken.

DIETARY ADVICE
Eat a healthy, well-balanced diet. Foods rich in vitamin B12 include animal protein (such as beef, lamb, and veal), clams and oysters, liver, fish, milk, and egg yolks.

STORAGE
Store in a tightly sealed container away from heat, moisture, and direct light.

MISSED DOSE
Take the next regularly scheduled dose.

STOPPING THE DRUG
If the vitamin was prescribed for a deficiency, consult your doctor before stopping.

PROLONGED USE
Therapy may require weeks or months. Lifelong therapy is necessary for pernicious anemia or following certain types of gastrointestinal surgery. No problems are expected with prolonged use when the vitamin is taken as directed.

▼ PRECAUTIONS

Over 60: No special problems are expected with recommended doses.

Driving and Hazardous Work: No special precautions are necessary.

Alcohol: Alcoholism can lead to pancreatic insufficiency and vitamin B12 malabsorption.

Pregnancy: Vitamin B12 requirements increase during pregnancy to 2.2 mcg daily.

Breast Feeding: Vitamin B12 requirements increase during breast feeding to 2.2 mcg per day.

Infants and Children: No problems are expected with recommended doses.

Special Concerns: Vitamin B12 deficiency is highly unlikely to occur in healthy people who are able to consume a normal, balanced diet. However, nutritional supplements should be considered for those who are ill or weakened by radiation therapy, chemotherapy, or any other condition that interferes with normal food and fluid intake. Vitamin supplements are not a substitute for a healthy, balanced diet.

OVERDOSE
Symptoms: Overdose is extremely rare.

What to Do: Although an overdose is highly unlikely, call your doctor right away if you have any reason to suspect that one has occurred.

▼ INTERACTIONS

DRUG INTERACTIONS
Consult your doctor for specific advice if you are taking analgesics, antibiotics, colchicine, folic acid, or other vitamin supplements.

FOOD INTERACTIONS
No known food interactions.

DISEASE INTERACTIONS
Consult your doctor if you have Leber's disease (a very rare eye disease).

SIDE EFFECTS

SERIOUS
Breathing difficulty; fever; hives; rash; swelling of face, mouth, lips, throat, or tongue. These may be signs of a rare but potentially serious allergic reaction. Seek medical assistance immediately.

COMMON
No common side effects have been reported with recommended doses.

LESS COMMON
Mild allergic reaction, diarrhea, itching.

VITAMIN C (ASCORBIC ACID)

Available in: Tablets, capsules
Available OTC? Yes   **As Generic?** Yes
Drug Class: Dietary supplement

▼ USAGE INFORMATION

WHY IT'S PRESCRIBED
To prevent or treat vitamin C deficiency, which causes scurvy, a disorder characterized by bleeding into the skin, swollen and bleeding gums, poor wound healing, muscle weakness, and fatigue. Deficiency does not occur in healthy people eating a well-balanced diet. Vitamin C requirements may be increased in those with AIDS, alcoholism, overactive thyroid, chronic infection, and intestinal diseases associated with nutritional malabsorption.

HOW IT WORKS
Vitamin C is required for the body's synthesis of collagen (tissue that constitutes the tendons, ligaments, and other inelastic fibers), for the metabolism of a variety of body substances, and to maintain structural and functional integrity of cell walls and small blood vessels.

▼ DOSAGE GUIDELINES

RANGE AND FREQUENCY
Recommended daily allowances for vitamin C are as follows: 30 to 40 mg from birth to 3 years of age; 45 mg from age 4 to 10; 50 to 60 mg in adolescents and adults; 100 mg in smokers.

ONSET OF EFFECT
Unknown.

DURATION OF ACTION
As long as it is taken.

DIETARY ADVICE
Eat a well-balanced diet to avoid vitamin C deficiency. Foods rich in vitamin C include citrus fruits and juices, green vegetables, and tomatoes.

STORAGE
Store in tightly sealed container away from heat, moisture, and direct light.

MISSED DOSE
No problems are expected. Take the next dose at the regularly scheduled time and do not double the next dose.

STOPPING THE DRUG
If vitamin C is taken for a deficiency or because of a disorder associated with a need for a higher intake of the vitamin, consult your doctor before stopping.

PROLONGED USE
No problems are expected with prolonged use.

▼ PRECAUTIONS

Over 60: No special problems are expected.

Driving and Hazardous Work: No special precautions are necessary.

Alcohol: Alcoholism may lead to vitamin C deficiency.

Pregnancy: Vitamin C requirements increase during pregnancy to 70 mg per day. Very large doses during pregnancy may harm the fetus.

Breast Feeding: Vitamin C requirements increase during breast feeding to 90 to 95 mg per day. Vitamin C does enter breast milk, but so far no problems have been reported from taking the recommended amounts of it.

Infants and Children: No problems are associated with recommended doses.

Special Concerns: Use of large doses of vitamin C is commonplace for the prevention of colds, cancer, and other disorders. Studies have shown that blood levels of the vitamin do not increase further when vitamin C doses exceed 250 to 500 mg per day. High doses of vitamin C may cause kidney stones in people with a prior history of the disorder or those with kidney disease treated with hemodialysis.

OVERDOSE
Symptoms: No specific ones have been reported.

What to Do: Emergency instructions not applicable.

▼ INTERACTIONS

DRUG INTERACTIONS
None reported with recommended doses.

FOOD INTERACTIONS
No known food interactions. However, it is worth noting that vitamin C can improve the body's absorption of iron, specifically nonheme iron (the type of iron found in foods derived from plant sources).

DISEASE INTERACTIONS
None reported.

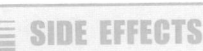

SIDE EFFECTS

SERIOUS
Occasionally, kidney stones may develop (especially with doses greater than 1 g per day over a prolonged period of time), causing back, side, or flank pain.

COMMON
No common side effects are associated with recommended doses.

LESS COMMON
High doses may cause diarrhea, flushing and redness of the skin, nausea and vomiting, or headache.

VITAMIN D

Available in: Capsules, oral solution, tablets
Available OTC? Yes   **As Generic?** Yes
Drug Class: Dietary supplement

▼ USAGE INFORMATION

WHY IT'S PRESCRIBED
Vitamin D is necessary for good health, and especially to maintain strong, healthy bones. It is derived from dietary sources, plus the body manufactures its own vitamin D upon exposure to sunlight. Vitamin D deficiency is thus rare among Americans, but some people—notably, those who are bedridden, have poor or highly restricted (vegan or macrobiotic) diets, or who cannot get adequate nutrition due to intestinal malabsorption—require supplementation. Supplements may also be prescribed for people with chronically low blood levels of calcium, and for alcoholics, dark-skinned people (who manufacture smaller amounts of vitamin D on their own), pregnant women, and nursing infants who get inadequate exposure to sunlight. Vitamin D supplements are also often recommended to increase calcium absorption and prevent osteoporosis in post-menopausal women.

HOW IT WORKS
Vitamin D promotes the absorption of calcium from the intestine and the utilization of calcium and phosphorus in the body. This ensures that levels of these minerals are high enough to support the constant breakdown and rebuilding of bone tissue, and to supply cells with the calcium needed to perform essential functions. Some tablets contain both vitamin D and calcium.

▼ DOSAGE GUIDELINES

RANGE AND FREQUENCY
Recommended daily allowances— Adults and teenagers: 200 to 400 international units (IU). Infants and children up to age 12: 300 to 400 IU. Pregnant or breast-feeding women: 400 IU. Vitamin D supplementation for deficiency or other medical condition— Same as above or higher, as determined by your doctor.

ONSET OF EFFECT
Within 12 to 24 hours; maximum effect: 10 to 14 days.

DURATION OF ACTION
As long as vitamin is taken.

DIETARY ADVICE
The best sources of vitamin D are fish and vitamin D fortified milk.

STORAGE
Store in a tightly sealed container away from heat and direct light.

MISSED DOSE
When vitamin D is used as a dietary supplement, no problems are expected if you miss a dose. When it is prescribed to treat a specific medical condition, take the missed dose as soon as you remember. If it is near the time for the next dose, skip the missed dose and resume your regular dosage schedule. Do not double the next dose.

STOPPING THE DRUG
Do not stop taking the supplement without first consulting your doctor.

PROLONGED USE
Your doctor will take periodic blood tests to check levels of calcium and phosphorus if you are taking vitamin D for the treatment of low blood calcium levels.

▼ PRECAUTIONS

Over 60: No special problems are expected.

Driving and Hazardous Work: No special precautions are necessary.

Alcohol: No special warnings.

Pregnancy: Daily requirements for vitamin D increase during pregnancy.

Breast Feeding: Trace amounts pass into breast milk; however, no problems have been reported. Vitamin D intake should in fact be increased while nursing.

Infants and Children: Infants who get little exposure to the sun and are totally breast-fed, especially those with dark-skinned mothers, may require vitamin D supplementation. Problems have not been reported with recommended amounts; however, prolonged excess doses may stunt a child's growth.

OVERDOSE
Symptoms: Early symptoms: Constipation (especially in children), diarrhea, dry mouth, increased thirst and frequency of urination, persistent headache, loss of appetite, metallic taste, nausea and vomiting, unusual fatigue. Advanced symptoms: Bone and muscle pain, irregular heartbeat, persistent itching, extreme drowsiness, mental changes. Severe vitamin D toxicity may be fatal.

What to Do: See your doctor at once.

▼ INTERACTIONS

DRUG INTERACTIONS
Consult your doctor for specific advice if you are taking calcium-containing preparations, magnesium-containing antacids, or thiazide diuretics.

FOOD INTERACTIONS
No known food interactions.

DISEASE INTERACTIONS
Consult your doctor if you have high blood levels of calcium (hypercalcemia), a history of heart or blood vessel disease, pancreatitis, or impaired kidney function.

SIDE EFFECTS

SERIOUS
Serious side effects are associated with excessively high doses (see Overdose).

COMMON
No side effects are expected with recommended doses.

LESS COMMON
No side effects are expected with recommended doses.

VITAMIN E (TOCOPHEROL)

Available in: Capsules
Available OTC? Yes   **As Generic?** Yes
Drug Class: Dietary supplement

▼ USAGE INFORMATION

WHY IT'S PRESCRIBED
For the prevention and treatment of vitamin E deficiency. Vitamin E deficiency is extremely rare and does not occur in healthy individuals eating a well-balanced diet. However, a deficiency of vitamin E can result from any disorder that causes poor absorption of fat from the intestine. Vitamin E is an antioxidant that is often prescribed to prevent the oxidation of low-density lipoprotein in an effort to prevent atherosclerosis (buildup of fatty plaques within the arteries), the underlying cause of coronary heart disease. The value of vitamin E supplements for this purpose is unproven.

HOW IT WORKS
Although considered an essential vitamin, the exact function of vitamin E remains unknown. It does help to prevent oxidation of the fatty acids present in the membranes of all cells (that is, it has antioxidant properties).

▼ DOSAGE GUIDELINES

RANGE AND FREQUENCY
Daily vitamin E requirements are small, ranging from 5 international units (IU) at birth to 20 IU in breast-feeding women. Large doses (100 IU) are given when deficiency results from intestinal malabsorption. The usual doses prescribed for protection against coronary heart disease range from 400 to 800 IU per day.

ONSET OF EFFECT
Unknown.

DURATION OF ACTION
Unknown.

DIETARY ADVICE
Eat a well-balanced diet. Foods rich in vitamin E include vegetable oils, whole grains, and leafy green vegetables. Cooking and storage may cause significant losses of vitamin E.

STORAGE
Store in a tightly sealed container away from heat, moisture, and direct light.

MISSED DOSE
No problems are expected. Take the next dose at the regularly scheduled time and do not double the next dose.

STOPPING THE DRUG
If prescribed for a deficiency, do not stop taking vitamin E without consulting your doctor first. There is no evidence that stopping vitamin E when it is taken to prevent coronary heart disease is harmful.

PROLONGED USE
No problems are associated with prolonged use.

▼ PRECAUTIONS

Over 60: No problems are expected at recommended doses.

Driving and Hazardous Work: No special precautions are necessary.

Alcohol: No special precautions are necessary.

Pregnancy: No problems are expected with recommended doses.

Breast Feeding: Vitamin E enters breast milk, but no problems have been reported with recommended doses.

Infants and Children: No problems have been documented at recommended doses.

OVERDOSE
Symptoms: No cases of vitamin E overdose have been reported.

What to Do: Emergency instructions not applicable.

▼ INTERACTIONS

DRUG INTERACTIONS
Consumption of large doses of vitamin E in combination with anticoagulants (such as warfarin) might lead to uncontrolled bleeding.

FOOD INTERACTIONS
Absorption of vitamin E from the intestine requires the consumption of some dietary fat.

DISEASE INTERACTIONS
No disease interactions have been reported.

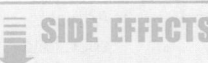
SIDE EFFECTS

SERIOUS
No serious side effects are associated with recommended doses.

COMMON
No common side effects are associated with recommended doses.

LESS COMMON
Large doses (greater than 400 IU per day) have been associated with diarrhea, nausea, headache, blurred vision, dizziness, and fatigue. Doses greater than 800 IU per day have been reported to increase the danger of bleeding, especially in people deficient in vitamin K.

VITAMIN K (PHYTONADIONE; MENADIOL)

Available in: Tablets, injection
Available OTC? No   **As Generic?** No
Drug Class: Dietary supplement

▼ USAGE INFORMATION

WHY IT'S PRESCRIBED

Vitamin K is used to prevent or treat bleeding disorders resulting from reduced formation of proteins needed for blood coagulation. The need may be due either to vitamin K deficiency or impairment of its function by anticoagulant drugs such as warfarin, salicylates, and some antibiotics. Vitamin K does not overcome the anticoagulant effects of heparin. Because vitamin K is normally made by bacteria in the intestine, dietary deficiency is rare. Bile salts are needed for absorption of vitamin K from the intestine, so absorption may be poor when obstruction of the bile ducts prevents entry of bile salts into the intestine. In newborns, the American Academy of Pediatrics recommends administration of phytonadione at birth to prevent bleeding disorders that can occur because adequate amounts of vitamin K may fail to cross the placenta from the mother to the fetus, and newborns have no bacteria in their intestines at birth. In people receiving all nutrition by injection for long periods, intramuscular injections of vitamin K are needed.

HOW IT WORKS

Vitamin K is necessary before a number of blood coagulation factors can become active in preventing or stopping bleeding.

▼ DOSAGE GUIDELINES

RANGE AND FREQUENCY

Oral doses— Menadiol sodium phosphate: Adults: For obstruction of bile duct: 5 mg a day. For problems related to use of antibacterials or salicylates: 5 to 10 mg a day. Children: 5 mg a day. Phytonadione: Adults: 2.5 to 10 mg (but up to 25 mg) if needed; can be repeated after 12 to 48 hours. Injections— Menadiol sodium phosphate: Adults: 5 to 15 mg once or twice a day. Children: 5 to 10 mg once or twice a day. Phytonadione: Adolescents and adults: 2.5 to 25 mg; can be repeated if necessary. Children: 5 to 10 mg. Infants: 1 to 2 mg. During long-term total intravenous nutrition: Adults: 5 to 10 mg a week. Children: 2 to 5 mg a week.

ONSET OF EFFECT

Oral phytonadione: 6 to 12 hours. Injected phytonadione: 1 to 2 hours. Injected menadiol sodium phosphate: 8 to 24 hours.

DURATION OF ACTION

12 to 24 hours.

DIETARY ADVICE

No interactions. The best dietary sources of vitamin K are leafy green vegetables, meats, and dairy products.

STORAGE

Store in a cool dry place away from light. Avoid allowing injectable forms to freeze.

MISSED DOSE

Take as soon as remembered unless close to next dose. Do not double the next dose.

STOPPING THE DRUG

Do not stop taking vitamin K unless instructed to do so by your doctor.

PROLONGED USE

Prolonged use is uncommon; no problems are expected at recommended doses.

▼ PRECAUTIONS

Over 60: No information is available.

Driving and Hazardous Work: No special precautions are necessary.

Alcohol: No special warnings.

Pregnancy: No information is available.

Breast Feeding: No problems have been reported.

Infants and Children: Caution is required with vitamin K injections in newborns because of the risk of anemia and liver toxicity.

Special Concerns: The smallest effective dose should be given to overcome bleeding due to an overdose of anticoagulant. Too large a dose may delay the subsequent action of the anticoagulant. Laboratory tests of clotting function (prothrombin time) are needed to determine the proper dose of vitamin K.

OVERDOSE

Symptoms: No specific ones have been reported.

What to Do: Emergency instructions not applicable.

▼ INTERACTIONS

DRUG INTERACTIONS

Antacids, antibiotics, and sucralfate can decrease vitamin K absorption. Vitamin K can interfere with the action of drugs like salicylates and anticoagulants. Other drugs may interact with vitamin K; consult your doctor if you are taking any prescription or over-the-counter drug.

FOOD INTERACTIONS

None reported.

DISEASE INTERACTIONS

Caution is advised in people with liver disease.

SIDE EFFECTS

SERIOUS

Menadiol has been associated with anemia and jaundice (yellow discoloration of the eyes and skin) in some newborns because their liver function is still poorly developed. Unless high doses are used, the risk is less with phytonadione.

COMMON

No common side effects are associated with recommended doses.

LESS COMMON

Flushing of the face, reactions at injection site.

WARFARIN

BRAND NAMES

Coumadin, Panwarfin, Sofarin

Available in: Tablets, injection
Available OTC? No   **As Generic?** Yes
Drug Class: Anticoagulant

▼ USAGE INFORMATION

WHY IT'S PRESCRIBED
To prevent blood clot forma-tion in patients suffering from heart, lung, and blood vessel disorders that could lead to heart attack, stroke, or other problems.

HOW IT WORKS
Warfarin blocks the action of vitamin K, a compound nec-essary for blood clotting.

▼ DOSAGE GUIDELINES

RANGE AND FREQUENCY
Adults: To start, 10 to 15 mg daily, taken once a day. Long-term, usually 2 to 10 mg per day, taken once a day. Children: The dose must be determined by a pediatrician. It should be taken at the same time every day.

ONSET OF EFFECT
36 to 48 hours.

DURATION OF ACTION
24 to 96 hours.

DIETARY ADVICE
Warfarin can be taken with liquid or food.

STORAGE
Store in a tightly sealed con-tainer away from heat and direct light.

MISSED DOSE
If you miss a dose, take it as soon as you remember, unless it is almost time for the next dose. In that case, skip the missed dose and go back to your regular schedule. Do not double the next dose.

STOPPING THE DRUG
Take it as prescribed for the full treatment period, even if you begin to feel better before the scheduled end of therapy. The decision to stop taking the drug should be made by your doctor.

PROLONGED USE
Regular tests of prothrombin time (a simple test that mea-sures the time it takes for one stage of blood coagulation to occur) are needed when tak-ing this drug. Your doctor

may also take stool and urine samples periodically to check for the presence of blood.

▼ PRECAUTIONS

Over 60: Adverse reactions may be more likely and more severe in older patients.

Driving and Hazardous Work: Avoid if you have blurred vision or feel dizzy. Avoid activities that could cause injury.

Alcohol: Use with caution. Alcohol can increase or decrease the effect of war-farin. Usually, consume no more than one drink a day.

Pregnancy: Warfarin may cause birth defects. Do not use during pregnancy.

Breast Feeding: Warfarin passes into breast milk. Do not use while nursing.

Infants and Children: Not recommended for children under 18.

OVERDOSE
Symptoms: Bleeding gums, uncontrolled nosebleeds, blood in the urine or stools.

What to Do: Discontinue the medication and call your doc-tor, emergency medical ser-vices (EMS), or the nearest poison control right away.

▼ INTERACTIONS

DRUG INTERACTIONS
Consult your doctor for spe-cific advice if you are taking steroid drugs, acetaminophen, allopurinol, aminogluthemide,

antibiotics, antiarrhythmic heart drugs, androgens, antacids, antifungal drugs, antihistamines, aspirin, anti-diabetic drugs, disulfiram, a nonsteroidal anti-inflammatory drug (NSAID), barbiturates, benzodiazepine tranquilizers, calcium supplements, chlor-amphenicol, or any choles-terol-lowering drugs.

FOOD INTERACTIONS
Avoid green, leafy vegetables and other foods that are rich in vitamin K (liver, broccoli, cauliflower, kale, spinach, and cabbage). Intake of too much vitamin K can override the anticlotting effect of warfarin and render the drug useless. Conversely, certain sub-stances can interfere with the absorption of vitamin K so much that normal, healthy clotting (necessary for wounds to heal) is impaired. Megadoses of vitamin E can do this, as can fish oil supple-ments and foods high in omega-3 fatty acids. These substances can enhance the effect of anticlotting drugs so much that a tendency to hemorrhage may result.

DISEASE INTERACTIONS
Consult your doctor about taking warfarin if you have high blood pressure, diabetes, serious liver or kidney dis-ease, or a severe allergy.

SIDE EFFECTS

SERIOUS
Allergic reaction (marked by wheezing; breathing difficulty; hives; or swelling of lips, tongue, and throat); bleeding into skin and soft tissue; abnormal bleeding from nose, gas-trointestinal tract, urinary tract, or uterus; severe infection; excessive or unexpected menstrual bleeding; black vomit; bruises or purple marks on skin. Consult your doctor immediately.

COMMON
No common side effects have been reported.

LESS COMMON
Loss of appetite, unusual weight loss, nausea, vomiting, skin rash, diarrhea, cramping.

YOHIMBINE

Available in: Tablets
Available OTC? Yes   **As Generic?** Yes
Drug Class: Alpha-adrenergic blocking agent

▼ USAGE INFORMATION

WHY IT'S PRESCRIBED
To aid in the treatment of male erectile dysfunction (impotence).

HOW IT WORKS
The exact way in which yohimbine works has not been determined. It is believed to block certain chemical receptors that cause constriction of blood vessels. In doing so, yohimbine theoretically improves blood flow into (and inhibits blood flow out of) the spongy columns of tissue in the penis involved in the mechanics of erection. Yohimbine may also have a mild stimulant effect and may promote the release of brain chemicals that control mood, relaxation, and sex drive, among other functions.

▼ DOSAGE GUIDELINES

RANGE AND FREQUENCY
Adult males: 5.4 mg, 3 times a day.

ONSET OF EFFECT
Within 2 to 3 weeks in most cases.

DURATION OF ACTION
Unknown.

DIETARY ADVICE
No special restrictions.

STORAGE
Store in a tightly sealed container away from heat, moisture, and direct light. Do not refrigerate medication or allow it to freeze.

MISSED DOSE
Take it as soon as you remember. If it is near the time for the next dose, skip the missed dose and resume your regular dosage schedule. Do not double the next dose.

STOPPING THE DRUG
The decision to stop taking the drug should be made in consultation with your doctor.

PROLONGED USE
See your doctor regularly for tests and examinations if you take this drug for a prolonged period of time.

▼ PRECAUTIONS

Over 60:
No special problems are expected.

Driving and Hazardous Work: Do not drive or engage in hazardous work until you determine how the medicine affects you.

Alcohol: No special restrictions; however, excess alcohol consumption may impair sexual function.

Pregnancy: Yohimbine is generally not prescribed for women and should not be used during pregnancy.

Breast Feeding: Not applicable to female patients.

Infants and Children: Not applicable to children.

Special Concerns: This drug should be used only by men who have been diagnosed with and are being medically treated for erectile dysfunction.

OVERDOSE
Symptoms: Agitation, restlessness, dizziness, heart palpitations.

What to Do: An overdose with yohimbine is unlikely. However, if someone takes a much larger dose than prescribed, call your doctor, emergency medical services (EMS), or the nearest poison control center.

▼ INTERACTIONS

DRUG INTERACTIONS
Consult your doctor for specific advice if you are taking antidepressants (especially MAO inhibitors) or any other mood-modifying medications, including selective serotonin reuptake inhibitors (SSRIs), such as fluoxetine. Before you take yohimbine, tell your doctor if you are taking any other prescription or over-the-counter drugs, especially cold remedies or weight-loss aids.

FOOD INTERACTIONS
Since yohimbine is a mild MAO inhibitor, it should not be taken with any food or drink containing tyramines, including cheese, chocolate, beer, aged meats, and nuts, and particularly not with the amino acids tyrosine or phenylalanine. A dangerous rise in blood pressure may result.

DISEASE INTERACTIONS
Caution is advised when taking yohimbine. Consult your doctor if you have a history of angina pectoris, mental depression or any other psychiatric illness, heart disease, high blood pressure, or impaired kidney function. Use of yohimbine may cause complications in patients with liver disease, since this organ works to remove the medication from the body.

≡ SIDE EFFECTS ≡

SERIOUS
Rapid heartbeat; increased blood pressure, possibly causing symptoms, such as persistent headaches or ringing in the ears. Call your doctor immediately.

COMMON
No common side effects have been reported.

LESS COMMON
Headache, dizziness, irritability, nervousness, restlessness, flushing of skin, shakiness, increased sweating.

ZAFIRLUKAST

Available in: Tablets
Available OTC? No   **As Generic?** No
Drug Class: Leukotriene receptor antagonist

▼ USAGE INFORMATION

WHY IT'S PRESCRIBED
To prevent the symptoms of asthma on a maintenance basis and to prevent bronchospasm (contraction of the smooth muscle tissue surrounding the airways, which results in narrowing and obstruction of the air passages). Zafirlukast may be used in conjunction with other asthma treatments.

HOW IT WORKS
Zafirlukast blocks cell receptors for leukotrienes, chemicals that cause inflammation and constriction of the bronchial airways. Unlike bronchodilators, which relieve the acute symptoms of an asthma attack, zafirlukast is prescribed to be taken regularly when no symptoms are present, to reduce the chronic inflammation of the airways that underlies asthma. This prevents symptomatic asthma attacks.

▼ DOSAGE GUIDELINES

RANGE AND FREQUENCY
Adults and teenagers: 20 mg twice a day. Children ages 7 to 11: 10 mg twice a day. Doses are usually taken in the morning and evening, on an empty stomach (at least 1 hour before or 2 hours after eating).

ONSET OF EFFECT
Within 1 week.

DURATION OF ACTION
Unknown.

DIETARY ADVICE
Zafirlukast should be taken 1 hour before or 2 hours after meals. Taking with a high-fat or high-protein meal reduces its availability in the body by 40%.

STORAGE
Store in a tightly sealed container away from heat and direct light.

MISSED DOSE
Take it as soon as you remember. If it is near the time for the next dose, skip the missed dose and resume your regular dosage schedule. Do not double the next dose.

STOPPING THE DRUG
The decision to stop taking the drug should be made by your doctor.

PROLONGED USE
No problems are expected. It is important to take zafirlukast every day, even during symptom-free periods.

▼ PRECAUTIONS

Over 60: In clinical trials, mild or moderate infections, primarily of the respiratory tract, occurred more often than expected in older patients. The rate of infection was proportional to the dose of zafirlukast taken. Other adverse reactions were no more likely or more severe in older patients than in younger persons.

Driving and Hazardous Work: Do not drive or engage in hazardous work until you determine how the medication affects you.

Alcohol: No special warnings.

Pregnancy: In some animal studies, zafirlukast caused birth defects and other problems. Human studies have not been done. Before you take zafirlukast, tell your doctor if you are pregnant or plan to become pregnant.

Breast Feeding: Zafirlukast passes into breast milk; do not use it while nursing.

Infants and Children: The safety and effectiveness of zafirlukast in children under the age of 7 have not been established.

Special Concerns: Zafirlukast has no effect on an asthma attack already in progress. In very rare cases, the drug may cause Churg-Strauss syndrome, a tissue disorder that strikes adult asthma patients and, if untreated, can destroy organs. Early symptoms include fever, muscle aches, and weight loss.

OVERDOSE
Symptoms: None.

What to Do: Call your doctor if you suspect an overdose.

▼ INTERACTIONS

DRUG INTERACTIONS
Consult your doctor for specific advice if you are taking aspirin, carbamazepine, cyclosporine, felodipine, isradipine, nicardipine, nifedipine, nimodipine, carbamazepine, phenytoin, tolbutamide, erythromycin, terfenadine, theophylline, or warfarin. Patients who are taking warfarin or any other anticoagulant should have their prothrombin time monitored closely, and appropriate changes made in the anticoagulant dosage, when they start taking zafirlukast. Before you take zafirlukast, tell your doctor if you are allergic to any prescription or over-the-counter medicine.

FOOD INTERACTIONS
No known food interactions.

DISEASE INTERACTIONS
Consult your doctor if you have any other medical condition. Use of zafirlukast can cause complications in patients with liver disease, since this organ works to remove the medication from the body.

SIDE EFFECTS

SERIOUS
Burning or prickling sensation, skin rash. A rare side effect with high doses is liver dysfunction (symptoms include abdominal pain, nausea, fatigue, lethargy, itching, yellow discoloration of the eyes or skin, and flulike symptoms). Call your doctor immediately.

COMMON
Headache.

LESS COMMON
Weakness, abdominal pain, back pain, diarrhea, dizziness, mouth ulcers, nausea, vomiting.

ZALCITABINE (DIDEOXYCYTIDINE; DDC)

Available in: Tablets
Available OTC? No   **As Generic?** No
Drug Class: Antiviral

▼ USAGE INFORMATION

WHY IT'S PRESCRIBED
To treat HIV (human immu-nodeficiency virus) infection, usually in combination with other antiretroviral drugs. While not a cure for HIV, such medications may sup-press the replication of the virus and delay the progres-sion of the disease.

HOW IT WORKS
Zalcitabine (ddC) interferes with the activity of enzymes needed for the replication of DNA in viral cells, thus preventing the virus from reproducing.

▼ DOSAGE GUIDELINES

RANGE AND FREQUENCY
Adults and teenagers: 0.75 mg, 3 times a day in combi-nation with other antiretroviral drugs. Children: Dose must be determined by your doctor.

ONSET OF EFFECT
Unknown. With most anti-retroviral drugs, an early response can be seen within the first few days of therapy, but the maximum effect may take 12 to 16 weeks.

DURATION OF ACTION
Unknown. Effects of the drug may be prolonged if zal-citabine is used in combina-tion with other effective drugs and the virus is maximally suppressed.

DIETARY ADVICE
No special restrictions.

STORAGE
Store in a tightly sealed con-tainer away from heat and direct light.

MISSED DOSE
Take it as soon as you remember. If it is near the time for the next dose, skip the missed dose and resume your regular dosage schedule. Do not double the next dose.

STOPPING THE DRUG
The decision to stop taking the drug should be made in consultation with your physician.

PROLONGED USE
See your doctor regularly for tests and examinations if you must take this medicine for a prolonged period.

▼ PRECAUTIONS

Over 60: No special studies have been done on older patients. A lower dose may be warranted, especially if kidney function is impaired.

Driving and Hazardous Work: Do not drive or engage in hazardous work until you determine how the medicine affects you.

Alcohol: Avoid alcohol if liver function is impaired.

Pregnancy: Zalcitabine has been shown to cause birth defects in animals. Human studies have not been done. Nevertheless, zalcitabine is increasingly being used in combination with other antiretroviral drugs to treat pregnant HIV-infected women.

Breast Feeding: It is unknown whether zalcitabine passes into breast milk; how-ever, women infected with HIV should not breast feed, to avoid transmitting the virus to an uninfected child.

Infants and Children: It is not known whether zal-citabine causes different or more severe side effects in children than it does in older persons. Use it for young patients only under close medical supervision.

Special Concerns: Use of zal-citabine does not reduce the risk of passing HIV to other persons. Take appropriate preventive measures.

OVERDOSE
Symptoms: Rash; fever; numbness, tingling, or prick-

ling sensation in the arms and legs.

What to Do: An overdose of zalcitabine is unlikely to occur. Nonetheless, if you have any reason to suspect an overdose, call your doctor, emergency medical services (EMS), or the nearest poison control center.

▼ INTERACTIONS

DRUG INTERACTIONS
Consult your doctor for spe-cific advice if you are taking asparaginase, azathioprine, estrogens, furosemide, methyldopa, pentamidine, sul-fonamides, sulindac, tetracy-clines, thiazide diuretics, valproic acid, injected amino-glycosides, amphotericin B, foscarnet, antacids, chloram-phenicol, cisplatin, dapsone, didanosine, ethambutol, ethionamide, hydralazine, iso-niazid, lithium, metronidazole, nitrous oxide, phenytoin, stavudine, vincristine, cimetidine, probenecid, or nitrofurantoin.

FOOD INTERACTIONS
No known food interactions.

DISEASE INTERACTIONS
Consult your doctor if you have a history of pancreatitis, peripheral neuropathy, or high levels of cholesterol or triglycerides in the blood. Use of zalcitabine may cause complications in patients who have kidney or liver disease, because these organs work to remove the medication from the body.

⟱ SIDE EFFECTS ⟱

SERIOUS
Burning, tingling, pain, or numbness in hands or feet, fever, muscle pain, joint pain, skin rash, ulcers in mouth and throat, nausea, vomiting, fever, sore throat, yellow dis-coloration of eyes or skin. Call your doctor immediately.

COMMON
No common side effects have been reported.

LESS COMMON
Diarrhea, headache.

ZALEPLON

Available in: Capsules
Available OTC? No   **As Generic?** No
Drug Class: Sedative/hypnotic

▼ USAGE INFORMATION

WHY IT'S PRESCRIBED
For the short-term treatment of insomnia.

HOW IT WORKS
By depressing activity in the central nervous system (the brain and spinal cord), zaleplon causes drowsiness and mild sedation. Because the drug is metabolized quickly compared with similar medications, zaleplon is associated with a lower incidence of side effects, such as daytime drowsiness.

▼ DOSAGE GUIDELINES

RANGE AND FREQUENCY
The appropriate dosage will be determined by your doctor. The recommended dosage for adults: 10 mg. Debilitated patients and people over 60: 5 mg. Zaleplon should only be taken at bedtime or after the patient has gone to bed and has difficulty falling asleep.

ONSET OF EFFECT
Within 1 hour.

DURATION OF ACTION
About 4 hours.

DIETARY ADVICE
Do not take following a high-fat, heavy meal. The absorption of zaleplon may be slowed and reduce the drug's effectiveness.

STORAGE
Store in a tightly sealed container away from heat, moisture, and direct light.

MISSED DOSE
If the medication was not taken at bedtime and you are unable to fall asleep, the drug may be used unless it is within 4 hours of when you need to be awake.

STOPPING THE DRUG
The decision to stop taking the drug should be made in consultation with your doctor.

PROLONGED USE
Zaleplon is usually prescribed only for short-term therapy (lasting several days or up to 4 weeks). See your doctor for periodic evaluation if you must take this drug for a longer time. Persistent insomnia may be a sign of an underlying medical problem.

▼ PRECAUTIONS

Over 60: Adverse reactions may be more likely in older patients. Smaller doses usually are prescribed.

Driving and Hazardous Work: Avoid such activities until you determine how this medication affects you.

Alcohol: Avoid alcohol.

Pregnancy: In large doses zaleplon has been shown to slow the progress of fetal development in animals. Human studies have not been done. Zaleplon is not recommended for use by pregnant women. Before you take zaleplon, be sure to tell your doctor if you are pregnant or plan to become pregnant.

Breast Feeding: Zaleplon passes into breast milk, but its effect on the nursing infant is unknown. Women who are nursing should not take this medication.

Infants and Children: Safety and effectiveness have not been established for patients under age 18.

Special Concerns: When you stop taking zaleplon, you may have trouble falling asleep for the first few nights.

OVERDOSE
Symptoms: Severe drowsiness, breathing difficulty, severe clumsiness or unsteadiness, severe dizziness, severe nausea and vomiting, slow heartbeat, vision problems.

What to Do: Call your doctor, emergency medical services (EMS), or the nearest poison control center immediately.

▼ INTERACTIONS

DRUG INTERACTIONS
Other drugs may interact with zaleplon. Consult your doctor for specific advice if you are taking rifampin, phenytoin, carbamazepine, phenobarbital or other drugs that depress the central nervous system; these include antihistamines, other psychiatric medications, barbiturates, sedatives, cough medicines, decongestants, and painkillers. Be sure your doctor knows about any over-the-counter medication you may take.

FOOD INTERACTIONS
No known food interactions.

DISEASE INTERACTIONS
Caution is advised when taking zaleplon. Consult your doctor if you have a history of alcohol abuse or drug dependence, chronic respiratory disease (including asthma, bronchitis, or emphysema), mental depression, or sleep apnea. Use of zaleplon may cause complications in patients with liver disease, since this organ works to remove the medication from the body.

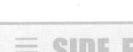 SIDE EFFECTS

SERIOUS
Hallucinations, abnormal thoughts or behavior, confusion or disorientation, unsteadiness, dizziness, lightheadedness, unusual nervousness, agitation, difficulty breathing. Call your doctor immediately.

COMMON
Daytime drowsiness, general pain or discomfort, memory problems, headache.

LESS COMMON
Abdominal pain, weakness, fever.

ZANAMIVIR

Available in: Inhalant
Available OTC? No   **As Generic?** No
Drug Class: Antiviral

▼ USAGE INFORMATION

WHY IT'S PRESCRIBED
To treat influenza type A or B. Zanamivir can reduce the severity of symptoms and shorten the duration of flu episodes.

HOW IT WORKS
Zanamivir is believed to interfere with the synthesis of the viral enzyme neuraminidase, which is needed in order for the virus to infect cells in the respiratory tract and elsewhere in the body. The drug affects only certain susceptible strains of the influenza type A or B viruses.

▼ DOSAGE GUIDELINES

RANGE AND FREQUENCY
Adults and teenagers: 2 inhalations (one 5-mg blister per inhalation) every 12 hours for 5 days. On the first day of treatment, however, 2 doses should be taken whenever possible provided there is at least 2 hours between doses. On subsequent days, follow the above dosage schedule. Treatment should be initiated within 2 days after the onset of signs or symptoms of the flu.

ONSET OF EFFECT
Unknown.

DURATION OF ACTION
Unknown.

DIETARY ADVICE
No special restrictions.

STORAGE
Store in a tightly sealed container away from heat and direct light.

MISSED DOSE
Take it as soon as you remember. If it is near the time for the next dose, skip the missed dose and resume your regular dosage schedule. Do not double the next dose.

STOPPING THE DRUG
It is important to take zanamivir for the full treatment period as prescribed. Do not stop taking the drug before the scheduled end of therapy even if you begin to feel better, as this may lead to a relapse.

PROLONGED USE
If your symptoms do not improve or if they become worse in a few days, you should consult your doctor.

⇩ SIDE EFFECTS ⇩

SERIOUS
There are no serious side effects are associated with the use of zanamivir.

COMMON
There are no common side effects associated with the use of zanamivir.

LESS COMMON
Dizziness.

▼ PRECAUTIONS

Over 60: No special problems are expected.

Driving and Hazardous Work: Avoid such activities until you determine how the medicine affects you.

Alcohol: No special warnings.

Pregnancy: Adequate studies on the use of zanamivir during pregnancy have not been completed. Discuss with your doctor the relative risks and benefits of using this drug while pregnant.

Breast Feeding: Zanamivir may pass into breast milk, although it is unknown if this poses any risks to the nursing infant. Consult your doctor for specific advice.

Infants and Children: Zanamivir is not recommended for children under the age of 12.

Special Concerns: Zanamivir should be administered using the Diskhaler device. See your doctor for instructions and a demonstration of the proper use of this device.

OVERDOSE
Symptoms: None reported.

What to Do: If you have any reason to suspect an overdose, call your doctor, emergency medical services (EMS), or the nearest poison control center.

▼ INTERACTIONS

DRUG INTERACTIONS
No known drug interactions.

FOOD INTERACTIONS
No known food interactions.

DISEASE INTERACTIONS
Consult your doctor if you have any respiratory illness, such as chronic obstructive pulmonary disease or asthma.

ZIDOVUDINE (AZT)

Available in: Capsules, syrup, injection
Available OTC? No   **As Generic?** No
Drug Class: Antiviral

▼ USAGE INFORMATION

WHY IT'S PRESCRIBED
To treat HIV infection in combination with other drugs and to prevent passage of the virus from pregnant women to their babies. While not a cure for HIV, this drug may suppress the replication of the virus and delay the progression of the disease. Also used to treat HIV-related dementia and HIV-related thrombocytopenia (low platelet count).

HOW IT WORKS
Zidovudine (AZT) interferes with the activity of enzymes needed for the replication of DNA in viral cells, thus preventing the human immuno-deficiency virus (HIV) from reproducing.

▼ DOSAGE GUIDELINES

RANGE AND FREQUENCY
For HIV infection— Adults and teenagers: Capsules: 200 mg, 3 times a day, or 300 mg, 2 times a day. Injection (given until oral dose can be taken): Adults and teenagers: 0.9 mg per lb of body weight injected slowly into a vein every 4 hours (6 times a day). To prevent the transmission of HIV to newborns— For pregnant women: Capsules: 100 mg, 5 times a day from 14th week of pregnancy to delivery. Injection: 0.9 mg per lb of body weight for first hour of delivery, followed by 0.45 mg per lb until baby is delivered. For newborns: Syrup: 0.9 mg per lb of body weight starting within 12 hours of birth and continuing for 6 weeks. Higher doses (up to 1,200 mg per day) are sometimes use to treat HIV-related dementia or thrombocytopenia.

ONSET OF EFFECT
Unknown. With most anti-retroviral drugs, an early response can be seen within the first few days of therapy, but the maximum effect may take 12 to 16 weeks.

DURATION OF ACTION
Unknown. Effects of the drug may be prolonged if zidovudine is used in combination with other effective drugs and the virus is maximally suppressed.

⬇ SIDE EFFECTS ⬇

SERIOUS
Anemia (low red blood cell count), causing paleness, fatigue, or shortness of breath; fever. If such symptoms occur, call your doctor right away.

COMMON
Headaches, nausea, muscle aches, insomnia, mood swings, stomach upset, loss of appetite.

LESS COMMON
Bands of discoloration on the fingernails; hepatitis (liver inflammation, which may cause yellowish discoloration of skin and eyes).

DIETARY ADVICE
Take with food to minimize side effects.

STORAGE
Store in a tightly sealed container away from heat and direct light.

MISSED DOSE
Take it as soon as you remember. If it is near the time for the next dose, skip the missed dose and resume your regular dosage schedule. Do not double the next dose.

STOPPING THE DRUG
The decision to stop taking the drug should be made in consultation with your doctor.

PROLONGED USE
See your doctor regularly for tests and examinations as long as you take this drug.

▼ PRECAUTIONS

Over 60: No special studies have been done on older patients. A lower dose may be warranted, especially if kidney function is impaired.

Driving and Hazardous Work: Do not drive or engage in hazardous work until you determine how the medicine affects you.

Alcohol: Avoid alcohol if liver function is impaired.

Pregnancy: Zidovudine can decrease the risk of passing the AIDS virus to the unborn child; in animal studies it has not caused birth defects.

Breast Feeding: Women who are infected with HIV should not breast feed, to avoid transmitting the virus to an uninfected child.

Infants and Children: Use and dose in infants and children must be established by your doctor.

Special Concerns: Use of zidovudine does not eliminate the risk of passing HIV to other persons. You should take appropriate preventive measures.

OVERDOSE
Symptoms: Sudden nausea and vomiting; headache, dizziness, or drowsiness.

What to Do: Seek medical assistance right away.

▼ INTERACTIONS

DRUG INTERACTIONS
Consult your doctor for specific advice if you are taking amphotericin B (by injection), anticancer agents, thyroid drugs, azathioprine, chloramphenicol, colchicine, cyclophosphamide, flucytosine, ganciclovir, interferon, mercaptopurine, methotrexate, plicamycin, clarithromycin, or probenecid. Also consult your doctor for specific advice if you are taking any other prescription or over-the-counter medication.

FOOD INTERACTIONS
Zidovudine may be better tolerated if taken with food.

DISEASE INTERACTIONS
Caution is advised when taking zidovudine. Consult your doctor if you have anemia or another blood problem or liver disease.

ZILEUTON

Available in: Tablets
Available OTC? No **As Generic?** No
Drug Class: Selective 5-lipoxygenase inhibitor

▼ USAGE INFORMATION

WHY IT'S PRESCRIBED
To prevent and treat chronic asthma. Zileuton will not relieve a chronic asthma attack once it has started.

HOW IT WORKS
Zileuton blocks the activity of a specific enzyme needed in the manufacture of certain substances known as leukotrienes, which are known to contribute to allergic and inflammatory reactions, and appear to play a role in the development of inflammatory diseases, including asthma and rheumatoid arthritis.

▼ DOSAGE GUIDELINES

RANGE AND FREQUENCY
Adults and teenagers: 600 mg, 4 times a day.

ONSET OF EFFECT
Within 1 to 2 hours. Several days or weeks may be required for the full effect in preventing asthma attacks.

DURATION OF ACTION
Unknown.

DIETARY ADVICE
Zileuton can be taken with meals and at bedtime, without regard to diet.

STORAGE
Store in a tightly sealed container away from heat, moisture, and direct light.

MISSED DOSE
Take it as soon as you remember. If it is near the time for the next dose, skip the missed dose and resume your regular dosage schedule. Do not double the next dose.

STOPPING THE DRUG
Take it as prescribed for the full treatment period, even if you feel better before the scheduled end of therapy.

PROLONGED USE
See your doctor regularly for examinations and tests, especially of liver function, if you must take zileuton for a prolonged period.

▼ PRECAUTIONS

Over 60: No special problems are expected.

Driving and Hazardous Work: Do not drive or engage in hazardous work until you determine how the medicine affects you.

Alcohol: Avoid alcohol.

Pregnancy: Adequate studies have not been done. Before taking zileuton, tell your doctor if you are pregnant or plan to become pregnant, and discuss the relative risks and benefits of using this drug.

Breast Feeding: Zileuton may pass into breast milk and be harmful to the nursing infant; avoid or discontinue using the drug while nursing or discontinue breast feeding.

Infants and Children: The safety and effectiveness of zileuton for children under the age of 12 have not been determined.

Special Concerns: Liver function should be tested before you start taking zileuton. While taking the drug, you should continue to take any other asthma medications that your doctor has prescribed. Tell your doctor if your use of short-acting bronchodilators increases when you start taking zileuton. It may indicate a worsening of your asthma that may require a change in dosage.

OVERDOSE
Symptoms: None are known; no cases of overdose have been reported.

What to Do: An overdose is unlikely to occur. However, if someone takes a much larger dose than prescribed, call your doctor, emergency medical services (EMS), or the nearest poison control center.

▼ INTERACTIONS

DRUG INTERACTIONS
Other drugs may interact with zileuton. Consult your doctor for specific advice if you are taking warfarin, propranolol, terfenadine, theophylline, calcium channel blockers, cyclosporine, cisapride, and astemizole. Before you start taking zileuton, tell your doctor if you regularly take any other prescription or over-the-counter medication.

FOOD INTERACTIONS
No known food interactions.

DISEASE INTERACTIONS
Caution is advised when taking zileuton. Consult your doctor if you have hepatitis or jaundice. Use of zileuton may cause complications in patients with liver disease, since this organ works to remove the medication from the body.

SIDE EFFECTS

SERIOUS
Liver problems, causing nausea, fatigue, lethargy, skin rash or itching, yellow discoloration of the eyes or skin, flulike symptoms, urine that is darker than normal. Call your doctor immediately.

COMMON
Headache, general pain, abdominal pain, nausea, indigestion, muscle soreness, weakness.

LESS COMMON
Joint pain, chest pain, inflammation of the tissues surrounding the eye (conjunctivitis), constipation, dizziness, fever, gas, insomnia or sleepiness, neck pain, nervousness, urinary tract infection, vomiting.

ZINC OXIDE

Available in: Cream, ointment
Available OTC? Yes   **As Generic?** Yes
Drug Class: Sunscreen

▼ USAGE INFORMATION

WHY IT'S PRESCRIBED
To prevent sunburn.

HOW IT WORKS
Zinc oxide blocks ultraviolet radiation in sunlight from reaching the skin.

▼ DOSAGE GUIDELINES

RANGE AND FREQUENCY
Apply as needed before exposure to sunlight. A sunscreen should be applied uniformly to all exposed skin surfaces, including the lips.

ONSET OF EFFECT
Immediate.

DURATION OF ACTION
Keeps working until removed or worn off from perspiration or swimming.

DIETARY ADVICE
Zinc oxide can be used without regard to diet.

STORAGE
Store in a tightly sealed container away from heat and direct light.

MISSED DOSE
If you forget to apply zinc oxide before exposure to sunlight, apply as soon as you remember.

STOPPING THE DRUG
No special warnings.

PROLONGED USE
No problems are expected.

▼ PRECAUTIONS

Over 60: Studies suggest that frequent use of sunscreens like zinc oxide may increase the risk of vitamin D deficiency, which may promote osteoporosis or bone fractures later in life. Oral vitamin D supplements and consumption of foods rich in vitamin D may be recommended.

Driving and Hazardous Work: The use of zinc oxide should not impair your ability to perform such tasks safely.

Alcohol: No special precautions are necessary.

Pregnancy: No problems have been reported.

Breast Feeding: No problems have been reported.

Infants and Children: Zinc oxide should not be used on children (especially infants under 6 months of age) who have shown signs of allergic skin reaction (hypersensitivity). Otherwise, it is safe for use in children. To prevent accidental ingestion, do not allow small children to apply sunscreens themselves. In general, children should be kept out of the sun during peak daylight hours (from 10 am to 2 pm) and physically protected from direct sun exposure with clothing and other physical barriers (such as a beach umbrella). Infants over 6 months of age should be protected by a sunscreen with an SPF (sun protection factor) of 15 or higher. Older children should regularly use a sunscreen with an SPF of 15 or higher to protect against excess and repeated exposure to solar ultraviolet radiation, which can lead to skin cancer and other skin damage later in life.

Special Concerns: Zinc oxide sunscreen should be applied liberally before exposure to sunlight and reapplied every 1 to 2 hours, especially after swimming or heavy perspiration and after eating and drinking. Contact of zinc oxide with the eyes should be avoided. If skin rash or irritation develops, consult your doctor. Keep sun exposure to a minimum during peak daylight hours (10 am to 2 pm), when the sun's rays are strongest. Extra precautions should be taken around reflective surfaces, such as sand, water, and concrete.

OVERDOSE
Symptoms: No specific ones have been reported.

What to Do: Not applicable. However, if someone accidentally ingests zinc oxide, call a doctor, emergency medical services (EMS), or the nearest poison control center.

▼ INTERACTIONS

DRUG INTERACTIONS
Consult your doctor for specific advice if you are using any other topical medications or skin preparations.

FOOD INTERACTIONS
No known food interactions.

DISEASE INTERACTIONS
Consult your doctor for advice if you have a history of any of the following: dermatitis (skin inflammation), herpes labialis (herpes simplex of the mouth and face), lichen planus (a rare nonmalignant skin condition causing chronic itching and a distinctive skin eruption), systemic lupus erythematosus (lupus), photosensitivity (heightened sensitivity to sunlight), phytophotodermatitis (dermatitis caused by contact with certain plants followed by exposure to sunlight), polymorphous light eruption (skin lesions occurring after exposure to sunlight), or xeroderma pigmentosum (a rare genetic disorder causing extreme sensitivity to ultraviolet light, skin lesions including malignancies, and serious eye problems).

≡ SIDE EFFECTS ≡

SERIOUS
Acne, folliculitis (burning, pain, inflammation, and itching in hairy regions of the skin; pus in hair follicles), and skin rash may occur with zinc oxide and other physical sunscreens that block the pores. Notify your doctor if you experience such side effects.

COMMON
No common side effects have been reported.

LESS COMMON
No less-common side effects have been reported.

ZINC SULFATE OPHTHALMIC

Available in: Ophthalmic solution
Available OTC? Yes **As Generic?** Yes
Drug Class: Ophthalmic astringent/analgesic

▼ USAGE INFORMATION

WHY IT'S PRESCRIBED
For the temporary relief of discomfort and redness from minor eye irritation. It is prescribed in combination with other drugs such as phenylephrine, naphazoline, and tetrahydrozoline.

HOW IT WORKS
The mineral zinc is an integral component in the proper functioning of several important enzymes involved in wound healing and the general maintenance and proper hydration of certain body tissues. Zinc sulfate ophthalmic solution has a mild astringent effect (that is, it causes tissues to contract when applied topically), which can help to shrink the tiny blood vessels in the whites of the eye (sclera) and so relieve redness and irritation.

▼ DOSAGE GUIDELINES

RANGE AND FREQUENCY
Instill 1 to 2 drops in the affected eye(s) up to 4 times a day.

ONSET OF EFFECT
Rapid.

DURATION OF ACTION
Up to several hours.

DIETARY ADVICE
No special restrictions.

STORAGE
Store in a tightly sealed container away from heat and direct light. Do not allow the solution to freeze.

MISSED DOSE
Instill the missed dose as soon as possible unless it is near the time for the next dose. In that case, skip the missed dose and go back to your regular schedule. Do not double the next dose.

STOPPING THE DRUG
You may stop applying this drug, or resume using it after discontinuing, as comfort dictates. No complications are expected.

PROLONGED USE
Eye drops containing zinc sulfate should generally not be used for self-medication for more than 3 days. If relief is not achieved in this time, or if redness and irritation persist or worsen, discontinue using it and contact your doctor or ophthalmologist right away.

▼ PRECAUTIONS

Over 60: No special problems are expected.

Driving and Hazardous Work: The use of this medication should not affect your ability to perform such tasks safely.

Alcohol: No special precautions are necessary.

Pregnancy: No problems are expected; however, if you are pregnant or plan to become pregnant and you have any concerns about the safe use of this or any other medication, consult your doctor.

Breast Feeding: Adequate studies on the use of ophthalmic zinc sulfate during breast feeding have not been done; however, no adverse consequences have been reported. Consult your doctor for specific advice.

Infants and Children: No specific information is available on the use of this medication by children.

Special Concerns: Contact your ophthalmologist or general practitioner right away if you experience eye pain, changes in vision, or if eye irritation persists for more than 72 hours. To use the eye drops, first wash your hands. Tilt your head back. Gently apply pressure to the inside corner of the lower eyelid and with the index finger of the same hand, pull downward on the eyelid to make a space. Drop the medicine into this space and close your eye. Apply pressure for 1 or 2 minutes while keeping the eye closed without blinking. Then wash your hands again. Make sure that the tip of the dropper does not touch your eye, finger, or any other surface.

OVERDOSE
Symptoms: No cases of overdose have been reported.

What to Do: An overdose is unlikely to occur; in case of accidental ingestion, call your doctor, emergency medical services (EMS), or the nearest poison control right away.

▼ INTERACTIONS

DRUG INTERACTIONS
No drug interactions have been reported, although phenylephrine, naphazoline, and tetrahydrozoline (other medications prescribed in combination with zinc sulfate ophthalmic solution) may adversely affect the action of certain glaucoma drops. Consult your doctor first before taking any other prescription or over-the-counter eye medications.

FOOD INTERACTIONS
No known food interactions.

DISEASE INTERACTIONS
If you have glaucoma, do not use this medication without consulting your doctor first. It is not an over-the-counter substitute for antibiotic or anti-inflammatory drops. Consult your doctor for specific advice if you have any other eye disorders or a history of allergic reaction to any other ophthalmic preparations.

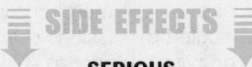
SIDE EFFECTS

SERIOUS
No serious side effects have been reported.

COMMON
Overuse of this drug may cause increased eye irritation and redness.

LESS COMMON
No less-common side effects have been reported.

ZINC SULFATE SYSTEMIC

Available in: Capsules, tablets, extended-release tablets, injection
Available OTC? Yes   **As Generic?** Yes
Drug Class: Dietary supplement

▼ USAGE INFORMATION

WHY IT'S PRESCRIBED
To prevent or treat zinc deficiency. Zinc deficiency does not occur in healthy people who eat a proper, balanced diet. Conditions associated with zinc deficiency include alcoholism, eating disorders, and intestinal problems that result from malabsorption.

HOW IT WORKS
Zinc is essential to numerous physiological processes, including the function of many enzymes in the body. Deficiency may lead to poor night vision, slow healing of wounds, poor sexual development and function in males, poor appetite (perhaps owing to a decrease in the sense of taste and smell), a reduced ability to ward off infections, diarrhea, dermatitis, and, in children, retarded growth.

▼ DOSAGE GUIDELINES

RANGE AND FREQUENCY
Recommended daily allowances are as follows: 5 to 10 mg a day for children from birth to age 3; 10 mg a day for children ages 4 to 10; 15 mg a day for adolescent and adult males; 12 mg a day for adolescent and adult females; 15 mg a day for pregnant women; and 16 to 19 mg a day for breast-feeding women.

ONSET OF EFFECT
Unknown.

DURATION OF ACTION
Unknown.

DIETARY ADVICE
Most effective if taken 1 hour before or 2 hours after meals. It can be taken with food if stomach upset occurs.

STORAGE
Store in a tightly sealed container away from heat, moisture, and direct light.

MISSED DOSE
No cause for concern.

STOPPING THE DRUG
If you are taking zinc sulfate by prescription, the decision to stop should be made by your doctor.

PROLONGED USE
You should see your doctor regularly for tests and examinations if you take zinc sulfate for a prolonged period.

▼ PRECAUTIONS

Over 60: Zinc deficiency is more likely to occur in older persons; no special problems are expected from zinc supplementation.

Driving and Hazardous Work: The use of zinc sulfate should not impair your ability to perform such tasks safely.

Alcohol: Excessive alcohol intake can increase the likelihood of zinc deficiency.

Pregnancy: There are no known problems with recommended doses, but taking large amounts of zinc during pregnancy may be harmful to the fetus.

Breast Feeding: No problems have been reported with recommended doses.

Infants and Children: Problems have not been reported in infants and children receiving the recommended daily intake of zinc sulfate.

Special Concerns: Injectable zinc sulfate should be given under the supervision of a health care professional. Zinc is found in peas, beans, seafood such as oysters and herring, and in lean red meats. It is also found in whole grains, but consuming large amounts of whole grains can decrease the amount of zinc absorbed from the intestine. Be aware that food stored in uncoated tin cans may have less zinc available for absorption.

OVERDOSE
Symptoms: Chest pain, vomiting, yellowish tinge to eyes or skin, dehydration, shortness of breath, restlessness, profuse sweating, dizziness.

What to Do: Call your doctor, emergency medical services (EMS), or the nearest poison control center immediately.

▼ INTERACTIONS

DRUG INTERACTIONS
Consult your doctor for specific advice if you are taking copper supplements or oral tetracyclines.

FOOD INTERACTIONS
Some foods can interfere with absorption of zinc sulfate into your body. Avoid taking zinc sulfate within 2 hours of eating bran, whole-wheat breads and cereals, and other fiber-rich foods, or phosphorus-containing foods such as milk and poultry.

DISEASE INTERACTIONS
Consult your doctor if you have a copper deficiency or any other medical condition. Zinc supplements make a copper deficiency worse.

▬ SIDE EFFECTS ▬

SERIOUS
Side effects are rare and occur only with large doses. Zinc itself may cause indigestion, heartburn, and nausea from irritation of the stomach. By interfering with the absorption of copper, zinc may interfere with the production of white and red blood cells, leading to infections, sores, or ulcers in the mouth or throat, and weakness due to anemia. Call your doctor if such symptoms occur.

COMMON
No common side effects have been reported.

LESS COMMON
No less-common side effects have been reported.

ZOLMITRIPTAN

Available in: Tablets
Available OTC? No   **As Generic?** No
Drug Class: Antimigraine/antiheadache drug

▼ USAGE INFORMATION

WHY IT'S PRESCRIBED
To treat severe, acute migraine headaches. Zolmitriptan is not intended as a migraine preventive or for use against any other kinds of pain or headache, including basilar and hemiplegic migraines. Your doctor will determine whether this medication is appropriate in your particular case.

HOW IT WORKS
The exact mechanism of zolmitriptan's action is unknown.

▼ DOSAGE GUIDELINES

RANGE AND FREQUENCY
A single dose ranging from half of a 2.5-mg tablet to one 5-mg tablet is generally effective. If the migraine returns or there is only partial relief, the dose may be repeated once after 2 hours, but no more than 10 mg should be taken in a 24-hour period. Since individual response to zolmitriptan may vary, your

doctor will determine the appropriate dosage. A general recommendation is to take one 2.5-mg tablet as the initial dose.

ONSET OF EFFECT
Within 2 hours.

DURATION OF ACTION
Up to 24 hours.

DIETARY ADVICE
The medication can be taken with or without food.

STORAGE
Store in a tightly sealed container away from heat, moisture, and direct light.

MISSED DOSE
Not applicable, since the drug is taken only when necessary.

STOPPING THE DRUG
Consult your doctor before discontinuing zolmitriptan.

PROLONGED USE
No special problems are expected. Patients at risk for heart disease should undergo periodic medical tests and evaluation.

⇊ SIDE EFFECTS ⇊

SERIOUS
Serious side effects with zolmitriptan are rare. However, zolmitriptan may cause a heart attack; chest pain or tightness; sudden or severe abdominal pain; shortness of breath; wheezing; heartbeat irregularities; swelling of eyelids, face, or lips; skin rash; or hives. Call your doctor immediately.

COMMON
Hot flashes or chills, numbness, prickling or tingling sensations, dry mouth, dizziness, drowsiness, weakness.

LESS COMMON
Indigestion, nausea, muscle ache.

▼ PRECAUTIONS

Over 60: Zolmitriptan is not recommended for use in older patients.

Driving and Hazardous Work: Do not drive or engage in dangerous work until you determine how the medication affects you.

Alcohol: No special warnings, although alcohol may trigger or exacerbate migraine headaches.

Pregnancy: Do not use zolmitriptan without first consulting your doctor if you are pregnant or suspect you might be pregnant.

Breast Feeding: Zolmitriptan may pass into breast milk; consult your doctor.

Infants and Children: The safety and effectiveness in patients under age 18 have not been established.

Special Concerns: Serious, but rare, heart-related problems may occur after using zolmitriptan. Anyone at risk for unrecognized coronary artery disease—such as postmenopausal women, men over the age of 40, or those with known risk factors for heart disease (hypertension, high blood cholesterol levels, obesity, diabetes, strong family history of heart disease, or cigarette smoking)—should have the first dose of zolmitriptan administered in a doctor's office. Zolmitriptan should not be used by anyone with any symptoms of active heart disease (chest pain or tightness, shortness of breath).

OVERDOSE
Symptoms: Increase in blood pressure resulting in lightheadedness, tension in the neck, fatigue, and loss of coordination.

What to Do: An overdose with zolmitriptan is unlikely. If someone takes a much larger dose than prescribed, call your doctor, emergency medical services (EMS), or the nearest poison control center immediately.

▼ INTERACTIONS

DRUG INTERACTIONS
Do not take zolmitriptan within 24 hours of taking naratriptan, sumatriptan, rizatriptan, ergotamine-containing medication, dihydroergotamine mesylate, or methysergide mesylate. Zolmitriptan and MAO inhibitors, such as phenelzine, tranylcypromine, procarbazine, and selegiline, should not be used within 14 days of each other. Zolmitriptan should be used with caution in patients taking SSRIs (selective serotonin reuptake inhibitors), which include fluoxetine, fluvoxamine, paroxetine, and sertraline.

FOOD INTERACTIONS
See Dietary Advice.

DISEASE INTERACTIONS
You should not take zolmitriptan if you have a history of angina, heart disease, stroke, uncontrolled hypertension, heartbeat irregularities, or peripheral vascular disease. Zolmitriptan should be used with caution in patients with liver disease or severely impaired kidney function.

ZOLPIDEM TARTRATE

Available in: Tablets
Available OTC? No   **As Generic?** No
Drug Class: Sedative/hypnotic

▼ USAGE INFORMATION

WHY IT'S PRESCRIBED
For the short-term treatment of insomnia.

HOW IT WORKS
Zolpidem depresses activity in the central nervous system (the brain and spinal cord), which causes drowsiness and mild sedation.

▼ DOSAGE GUIDELINES

RANGE AND FREQUENCY
Adults: 10 mg at bedtime. Patients over 60: 5 mg at bedtime.

ONSET OF EFFECT
Within minutes.

DURATION OF ACTION
2 to 4 hours.

DIETARY ADVICE
Zolpidem may be taken without regard to diet, although it generally works faster on an empty stomach.

STORAGE
Store in a tightly sealed container away from heat and direct light.

MISSED DOSE
Take it as soon as you remember unless it is late at night. Do not take the drug unless your schedule permits 7 or 8 hours of sleep.

STOPPING THE DRUG
The decision to stop taking the drug should be made in consultation with your doctor. Discontinuing the drug abruptly may produce withdrawal symptoms (sleep disruption, nervousness, irritability, diarrhea, abdominal cramps, muscle aches, memory impairment). The dosage should be reduced gradually according to your doctor's instructions.

PROLONGED USE
Zolpidem is usually prescribed only for short-term therapy (lasting several days or up to 2 weeks). See your doctor for periodic evaluation if you must take this drug for a longer time. Persistent insomnia may be a sign of an underlying medical problem.

▼ PRECAUTIONS

Over 60: Adverse reactions may be more likely and more severe in older patients. Smaller doses usually are prescribed.

Driving and Hazardous Work: Zolpidem may impair mental alertness and physical coordination. Adjust your activities accordingly.

Alcohol: Avoid alcohol.

Pregnancy: In large doses zolpidem has been shown to slow the progress of fetal development in animals. Human studies have not been done. Before you take zolpidem, be sure to tell your doctor if you are pregnant or plan to become pregnant.

Breast Feeding: Zolpidem passes into breast milk, but its effect on the nursing infant is unknown. Consult your doctor for advice.

Infants and Children: Safety and effectiveness have not been established for patients under age 18.

Special Concerns: When you stop taking zolpidem, you may have trouble falling asleep for the first few nights.

OVERDOSE
Symptoms: Severe drowsiness, breathing difficulty, severe clumsiness or unsteadiness, severe dizziness, severe nausea and vomiting, slow heartbeat, vision problems.

What to Do: Call your doctor, emergency medical services (EMS), or the nearest poison control center immediately.

▼ INTERACTIONS

DRUG INTERACTIONS
Other drugs may interact with zolpidem. Consult your doctor for specific advice if you are taking tricyclic antidepressants (such as amitriptyline, clomipramine, doxepin, or nortriptyline) or other drugs that depress the central nervous system; these include antihistamines, other psychiatric medications, barbiturates, sedatives, cough medicines, decongestants, and painkillers. Be sure your doctor knows about any over-the-counter medication you may take.

FOOD INTERACTIONS
No known food interactions.

DISEASE INTERACTIONS
Caution is advised when taking zolpidem. Consult your doctor if you have a history of alcohol abuse or drug dependence, chronic respiratory disease (including asthma, bronchitis, or emphysema), mental depression, or sleep apnea. Use of zolpidem may cause complications in patients with liver or kidney disease, since these organs work together to remove the medication from the body.

SIDE EFFECTS

SERIOUS
Hallucinations, abnormal thoughts or behavior, confusion or disorientation, unsteadiness, dizziness, lightheadedness, unusual nervousness, agitation, difficulty breathing. Call your doctor immediately.

COMMON
Daytime drowsiness, diarrhea, general pain or discomfort, memory problems, nausea, bizarre or unusually vivid dreams, vomiting.

LESS COMMON
Stomach discomfort, agitation, feelings of panic, convulsions, muscle cramps, nausea, vomiting, unusual fatigue, uncontrolled weeping, worsening of emotional problems, vision problems, dry mouth.

GLOSSARY OF DRUG TERMS

▼

ACE inhibitor: An abbreviation for angiotensin-converting enzyme inhibitor, a type of *antihypertensive* drug. ACE inhibitors prevent the formation of angiotensin II, a naturally occurring substance that constricts blood vessels, thus causing blood pressure to rise.

active ingredient: The chemical component of a drug preparation that exerts the desired therapeutic effects. The active ingredient is commonly what we think of as the "drug." Drugs contain *inactive ingredients* as well, such as the binders and colorings added to a pill to hold it together and give it its characteristic color.

addiction: A term used to describe physical dependence on a drug; psychological factors may also play a role in addiction.

adverse reaction: A harmful and unintended response to a drug.

agonist: A drug or other compound that stimulates activity in specific cells, setting into motion particular chemical reactions and bodily processes.

allergic drug reaction: An exaggerated immune response to a drug, which can result in hives, itching, or, in serious cases, shock and breathing difficulty. People who are allergic to one drug, such as penicillin, may be allergic to chemically related drugs in the same drug class.

aminoglycoside: One of a group of chemically related *antibiotics* that is used to treat a variety of infections.

amphetamine: One of a group of drugs, chemically related to the generic

parent drug amphetamine, that stimulates the central nervous system.

analgesic: An agent that relieves pain. Examples include *narcotics*, *nonsteroidal anti-inflammatory drugs* (which have properties in addition to pain relief), and miscellaneous pain-relievers, such as capsaicin and acetaminophen.

anaphylaxis: An acute allergic reaction to a drug or venom, as from a bee sting, that may be marked by swollen airways and severe breathing difficulty.

androgen: A male sex hormone, such as testosterone, that is administered for certain endocrine disorders, for cancer, and a few other conditions.

anesthetic: A drug that eliminates the sensation of pain.

angiotensin-converting enzyme inhibitor: See *ACE inhibitor*.

anorectic: A drug that suppresses appetite. Some drugs suppress appetite as a *side effect*.

antacid: A drug that counteracts stomach acids. Antacids are used to relieve indigestion, heartburn, peptic ulcers, and a few other gastrointestinal disorders.

antagonist: A drug or other compound that inhibits chemical activity in specific cells, suppressing particular physiological reactions and bodily processes.

antianginal: A drug, such as a *nitrate*, that relieves the chest pain caused by insufficient flow of heart blood, a characteristic of angina.

antianxiety agent: A psychiatric drug, also called an anxiolytic, that relieves anxiety. These drugs also help to relax muscles and to treat insomnia.

antiarrhythmic: A drug used to correct heart rhythm abnormalities.

antiasthmatic: A drug used in the treatment of asthma.

antibacterial: A drug used specifically to combat bacterial infections, as opposed to infections caused by other microorganisms, such as fungi and viruses. Also commonly referred to as an *antibiotic*.

antibiotic: A drug that kills or inhibits the growth of infectious bacteria or other germs. Some antibiotics are naturally produced by bacteria, fungi, and other microorganisms; others are synthetic (man-made).

antibody: A protein produced by the immune system that normally acts to neutralize or eliminate foreign substances in the body. A *drug allergy* is associated with an overactive response of an antibody to a particular drug.

anticancer agent: A drug used to combat cancer.

anticlotting agent: A general term describing a drug that inhibits the clotting of blood. These drugs are sometimes referred to as *anticoagulants*.

anticoagulant: A drug that blocks the activity of certain blood clotting factors that promote the formation of fibrin, a protein essential in the formation of blood clots. Anticoagulant drugs can either impede the formation of a clot or prevent an already formed clot from breaking away, traveling to a narrow blood vessel, and stopping circulation in a critical organ.

anticonvulsant: A drug used to control seizures or convulsions, typically those brought on by epilepsy.

antidementia drug: A drug that slows the progression of Alzheimer's disease and related forms of mental deterioration.

antidepressant: A drug that elevates mood and relieves depression. Types of antidepressants include *tricyclic antidepressants*, *monoamine oxidase (MAO) inhibitors*, and *selective serotonin reuptake inhibitors*.

antidiabetic agent: A drug used to treat diabetes mellitus.

antidiarrheal agent: A drug that relieves diarrhea.

antidote: A compound that counteracts *poisoning*.

antiemetic: A drug used to stop or prevent vomiting.

antifungal: A drug that combats fungal infections, such as athlete's foot or nail fungus. *Topical* antifungals are applied externally to the skin, hair, or nails. *Systemic* antifungals are taken orally or by injection; typically they help to fight fungal infections affecting the bloodstream or other internal organs or tissues.

antiglaucoma agent: A drug used to treat glaucoma, the buildup of excessive pressure in the eye, which is a common cause of blindness in older people.

antigout agent: A type of drug that relieves gout (a painful arthritic condition of the joints) by limiting the buildup of the metabolic waste product, uric acid, in the body.

antihistamine: A drug that blocks the actions of *histamine*. Such drugs relieve allergies, hay fever, cold symptoms, hives, rashes, itching, and motion sickness.

antihypertensive: A drug that lowers blood pressure in people who have dangerously high blood pressure (hypertension).

antihypotensive: A drug that elevates blood pressure in people who have dangerously low blood pressure (hypotension).

anti-infective: A drug used to treat infections, including those caused by bacteria (*antibacterials*), fungi (*antifungals*), viruses (*antivirals*), parasites (*antiparasitics*), and other disease-causing microorganisms.

anti-inflammatory: A drug used to reduce the swelling, redness, or pain caused by inflammation, an immune reaction to injury that can occur either inside the body (for example, arthritic joints) or on a localized external area (for example, skin rash). Some anti-inflammatory drugs are *steroids* (compounds with a particular chemical structure that include the *hormones*); others are nonsteroidal (see *NSAIDs*).

antimalarial: An *antiparasitic* drug used specifically to treat or prevent malaria, a mosquito-borne illness caused by the plasmodia parasite.

antimanic drug: A medication that relieves the mental and physical hyperactivity and incapacitating mania and mood elevation that are characteristic of manic-depressive illness (bipolar disorder).

antimicrobial agent: A general term for a drug used to treat infections due to microorganisms, such as bacteria, fungi, and viruses. This group of drugs includes *anti-infectives*, *antibiotics*, *antifungals*, and *antivirals*.

antimigraine drug: A drug that relieves or prevents migraine headaches.

antinauseant: A medication that relieves or prevents the queasy sensations of nausea.

antineoplastic agent: A drug used against cancer.

antiobesity agent: A drug that works to promote weight loss through any of various mechanisms. Some of the antiobesity drugs are *serotonergics*.

antiparasitic: A drug used to treat infestations of parasites, including worms and amoebas.

antiparkinsonism agent: A drug used to relieve the trembling and rigidity of Parkinson's disease and related disorders. These drugs are also called antiparkinsonian agents.

antiplatelet agent: A drug that reduces the tendency of blood cells known as platelets to clump together and form clots where the normal flow of blood is disrupted. For example, blood flow may be impaired by fatty deposits in the coronary arteries of someone who has heart disease, predisposing that person to a heart attack. Aspirin, taken in low doses, is the most widely prescribed antiplatelet drug.

antiproliferative: A drug that suppresses the excess proliferation of skin cells that occurs in certain skin disorders, such as psoriasis.

antipruritic: A drug that is used to relieve itching.

antipsoriatic: A drug used to treat psoriasis, a chronic skin and joint condition marked by scaly red patches. In some cases, this medication is also used for arthritis.

antipsychotic: A drug used to treat severe psychiatric disorders, such as schizophrenia and others that cause hallucinations or delusions.

antipyretic: A drug used to reduce fever (elevated body temperature).

antireflux agent: A drug that alleviates gastroesophageal reflux (commonly known as heartburn).

antirheumatic: A drug used to treat rheumatoid arthritis, a persistent form of arthritis marked by pain and inflammation of the joints.

antiseptic: A drug or other substance that arrests the growth and action of bacteria and other microorganisms. Also called a germicide.

antispasmodic: A drug used to reduce involuntary muscle spasms, such as those that can occur in the gastrointestinal tract or bladder.

antitubercular agent: A type of drug used in the treatment and prevention of tuberculosis.

antitussive: A cough suppressant.

antiurolithic: A drug used in the treatment of kidney stones, a relatively common disorder that is marked by the formation of small, hard pellets in the urinary tract.

antiviral: A drug used to combat infections caused by viruses, such as AIDS.

anxiolytic: See *antianxiety agent.*

aplastic anemia: A rare but potentially fatal side effect of certain drugs characterized by suppression of the bone marrow, resulting in the inability to produce adequate amounts of essential blood components.

autonomic nervous system: The part of the nervous system that controls smooth muscle (the type that surrounds blood vessels and other structures), heart muscle, and many of the body's so-called involuntary actions, such as glandular secretions, motion of the gastrointestinal tract, and contraction or dilation of blood vessels. Many drugs, such as some used for hypertension, act through the autonomic nervous system. Because this system has such wide-ranging effects, drugs that affect it typically produce a wide variety of adverse side effects in addition to their desired therapeutic actions.

azalide: A type of *antibiotic* used to fight infections.

barbiturate: One of a class of related drugs that are used as *hypnotics, sedatives,* and *antispasmodics* to induce sleep, relieve anxiety, and relax muscles. Examples include phenobarbital and amobarbital; most end in the suffix "-ital."

behavior modifier: A drug that can facilitate a behavior change, such as stopping excessive drinking or quitting smoking.

benzodiazepine: One of a class of related *antianxiety* drugs used as tranquilizers. Examples include diazepam and triazolam; most end in the suffix "-epam" or "-olam."

beta-blocker: A drug that inhibits chemical activity in specialized nervous system structures called beta receptors, which are found in the heart, the airways, and other areas. Beta-blockers are commonly used as *antihypertensive* drugs; they lower blood pressure by slowing the heart rate and reducing the force of the heartbeat. They are also sometimes used to treat angina, abnormal heart rhythm, anxiety, glaucoma, and other disorders.

bioavailability: A scientific term for the amount of drug that is absorbed into the body and available to exert therapeutic effects.

bioequivalent: A scientific term for drugs that have equivalent chemical properties, so that equal amounts of each drug are delivered to the body in a similar time frame. Generic drugs, for example, are bioequivalent to brand name drugs.

bone resorption inhibitor: A drug that suppresses the normal breakdown of bone. These drugs are useful for treating high blood calcium levels (hypercalcemia) or bone disorders such as Paget's disease.

brand name: The name chosen by a drug manufacturer to market a drug. Prozac, for example, is the brand name for the antidepressant drug with the *generic name* fluoxetine.

brand name drug: A drug that is sold under a registered *brand name.*

broad-spectrum antibiotic: An antibiotic that is active against a wide range of infectious bacteria.

bronchodilator: A drug that causes the bronchial air passages to expand, making breathing easier. Used primarily in the treatment of asthma and related conditions.

calcium channel blocker: A type of antihypertensive drug that induces the muscle surrounding blood vessels to relax by decreasing the movement of calcium ions through the muscle cell membranes, thus causing the blood vessels to dilate and blood pressure to fall.

caplets: Capsule-shaped tablets that are generally easier to swallow than round pills.

carbonic anhydrase inhibitor: An *antiglaucoma* drug, such as acetazolamide, that works by blocking the activity of carbonic anhydrase, an enzyme that is involved in the production of the fluid that fills the interior of the eye.

cardiac glycoside: See *digitalis drug*.

catecholamine: One of a group of chemical messengers that have widespread effects on the body, such as speeding up the heart, raising blood pressure, and increasing respiration. Man-made catecholamines have been prepared as drugs, primarily for use in emergency situations.

centrally acting: A drug or other agent that works via the *central nervous system* to produce its desired therapeutic effects.

central nervous system (CNS): The part of the nervous system consisting of the brain and spinal cord.

cephalosporin: One of a group of chemically related *antibiotics*, originally derived from a fungus and since enhanced with the production of man-made versions, that are widely used against a variety of infections.

chelating agent: A drug, such as penicillamine, that binds with metals, reducing their concentration in body tissues. Toxic levels of metals can build up in cases of lead poisoning or in such conditions as Wilson's disease, a hereditary disorder marked by the buildup of copper in the body.

chemotherapy: The use of drugs to combat cancer or other conditions.

clearance: The rate at which a drug is eliminated by the kidneys.

contraceptive: A drug or device used to prevent pregnancy.

contraindication: A disease or condition that either completely precludes the use of a certain drug or means that the drug should be used with special caution.

corticosteroid: A type of anti-inflammatory drug that mimics the actions of powerful naturally occurring substances called *steroids*, which are released by the adrenal glands and have numerous and widespread effects on the body. Cortico-steroids are available in many forms, including *inhalant, ophthalmic, otic, topical,* and *systemic* preparations. They are used to treat asthma, allergies, skin inflammations, inflammatory bowel disease, some forms of cancer, and other disorders.

cytotoxic drug: A drug that works by killing rapidly dividing cells, typically those associated with cancer.

decongestant: A drug that relieves nasal or sinus congestion due to colds or allergies.

dependence: Addiction to a drug, or the need to continue to use a drug because of psychological or physical factors. *Narcotics*, for example, commonly lead to dependence.

desensitization: A medical treatment for drug allergy that aims to improve tolerance to a drug by the administration of a series of slightly increasing doses.

digitalis drug: A type of drug that slows the heartbeat and increases the force with which the heart beats, thereby improving the pumping action of the heart and relieving the symptoms of congestive heart failure. Also known as a cardiac glycoside.

diuretic: A drug that alters kidney function to draw water from the body and increase the total output of urine.

divided doses: Individual doses of a drug given at intervals spaced throughout the day, rather than as a single daily dose.

drug allergy: An allergic reaction to a specific drug, such as penicillin, or to a drug component. Responses can range from mild (for example, a skin rash) to severe (shock and difficulty breathing). Anyone with a drug allergy should avoid use of it and chemically related drugs in the future and be sure to inform his doctor, dentist, and other health-care personnel of any history of allergies.

drug class: A group of drugs that have similar chemical structures and actions on or within the body. There are many different classes of drugs. Although members of a drug class have similar properties, there are variations among them that may make one particular drug preferable for a specific disorder or patient than other drugs in that class.

drug fever: An adverse drug reaction marked by elevated body temperature, resulting from an allergic reaction or other causes.

drug interaction: Reciprocal activity or influence between two or more drugs that may alter the effects of one or all of the drugs involved. Drug interactions vary widely. They may increase—or decrease—the amount of active drug, the effectiveness of a drug, and the likelihood of adverse side effects. Responses to an interaction can range from clinically inapparent or mild to life-threatening.

drug rash: A skin rash resulting from an allergic reaction to a particular medication, usually appearing during the first few days after taking it. Drug rashes can occur with either *topical* or *systemic* preparations.

electrolyte: A chemical, such as calcium, potassium, or sodium, dissolved in blood or cellular fluids, that acts as a vital messenger for many bodily processes. Electrolytes are essential, for example, in maintaining heart rhythm and kidney function. Certain drugs can disrupt electrolyte levels.

elixir: A form of liquid medication that consists of a drug mixed in a flavored alcohol solution.

emollient: A drug preparation or other substance that soothes and softens the skin, lips, or *mucous membranes.*

estrogen: A female sex hormone, produced by the ovaries, that has multiple effects, including stimulating the reproductive cycle and the development of female secondary sex characteristics. Various forms of estrogen are used as drugs to treat menopause, breast cancer, and other conditions.

estrogen replacement therapy: The use of supplemental *estrogen*, one of the female sex hormones produced by the ovaries, to relieve the adverse effects of menopause.

expectorant: A type of drug commonly used in cough preparations that promotes the discharge and expulsion of mucus or phlegm from the throat and airways.

Food and Drug Administration (FDA): The U.S. governmental agency that regulates and monitors food and drug safety. Its functions include ruling on the safety of new drugs before they become available to the public, reclassification of drugs from prescription to *OTC* status, regulating food and drug labeling, and establishing safe limits for additives.

food interactions: An action between a specific food and a drug, which may influence the amount of drug available for therapeutic effects. Because of food interactions, some drugs should not be taken with meals in general, or with specific foods in particular.

g or gm: An abbreviation for *gram.*

generic drug: A copycat version of a brand name drug. Generic drugs are chemically equivalent to brand name drugs but cost loss. Generics, which cannot be marketed until the exclusive patent for the brand name drug has expired (usually after about 20 years), are normally sold simply under the drug's *generic name.*

generic name: The scientific name for a drug. Generic names, as opposed to *brand names*, are nonproprietary and are recognized worldwide.

gram (g): A metric measure of weight, sometimes used in drug dosages. There are about 454 grams in a pound.

growth hormone: A naturally occurring chemical secreted by the pituitary gland that promotes growth by acting through a number of intermediaries on numerous body tissues. Synthetic versions of the hormone are available as drugs and are usually administered long-term by injection to children. Also called somatotropic hormone or somatotropin.

habituation: A term used to describe psychological dependence on a drug.

histamine: A compound produced by cells in the stomach, skin, respiratory tract, and elsewhere. Histamine aids digestion by triggering stomach acid secretion. It also plays a central role in allergic reactions, causing inflammation, hives, itching, and constriction of the airways.

histamine (H1) blocker: A type of *antihistamine* used to treat hay fever and other allergies.

histamine (H2) blocker: A drug that binds to a specialized receptor in the stomach wall termed an H2 receptor, thereby preventing the release of *histamine*. In the digestive tract, histamine triggers stomach acid secretion. The drugs in this group are commonly used to treat heartburn, ulcers, and other digestive disorders.

hormone: Chemicals, secreted by various body organs, that are typically carried by the bloodstream and exert their effects on distant cells and tissues. Some hormones have been synthesized and are used as drugs to promote growth, regulate the menstrual cycle, combat cancer, and treat other conditions.

hypersensitivity: An exaggerated response to a drug, or a drug-related allergic reaction.

hypnotic: A drug that is used primarily to induce sleep (for example, a *benzodiazepine*).

hypoglycemic agent: A drug that lowers blood sugar levels, commonly used in the treatment of diabetes.

immunization: Stimulation of the immune system to produce antibodies against a specific disease, thereby conferring protection against it, through the oral or injectable administration of a *vaccine*, a *toxoid*, or cells or blood serum from infected persons. The term is sometimes used interchangeably with *vaccination*.

immunosuppressant: A drug that suppresses the immune system. Such an effect may be desirable to prevent the immune system from rejecting a new organ following a transplant, and sometimes in the treatment of cancer, rheumatoid arthritis, or other serious conditions.

implant: A capsule implanted under the skin that slowly releases a drug into the body for an extended period.

inactive ingredient: A substance, such as a coloring, flavoring, binder, gelatin capsule coating, or preservative, that does not have any therapeutic effects but that is combined with an active drug compound during the manufacturing process to make a medication. Most manufacturers list the inactive ingredients alphabetically on the ingredients list.

indication: The disorder, condition, disease, or symptom for which a drug is prescribed or approved for use by the Food and Drug Administration.

inhalant: A drug preparation that is inhaled through the mouth or nose.

interferon: A naturally occurring substance that activates the body's immune response. Interferons have been synthesized for use as anti-cancer agents and also as drugs for various other purposes.

intramuscular: Into the muscle. Some medications or vaccines are formulated as solutions that are to be injected into a muscle, often the buttock or thigh. The drug is then absorbed from the muscle.

intravenous: Into the vein. Many drugs are formulated as solutions that are to be injected or slowly dripped into a vein, where they gain immediate access to the bloodstream. The drug is then carried by the blood to other parts of the body.

jaundice: A liver disorder, marked by yellow discoloration of the skin and eyes that may be the result of a drug allergy, adverse drug reaction that affects the liver, or a liver disease.

keratolytic: A medication used to treat certain skin conditions, such as acne, that causes the layer of dead skin on the skin's uppermost surface to peel off.

kg: An abbreviation for *kilogram*.

kilogram (kg): A metric unit of weight equal to about 2.2 pounds. Some drug doses are prescribed per kg of body weight.

laxative: One of a group of drugs that relieves constipation by adding bulk to stools (bulk-forming laxative), softening stools (stool softener), lubricating the gastrointestinal tract (lubricant), or increasing intestinal tract motility (stimulant).

lipid-lowering drug: A medication that lowers harmful blood cholesterol levels and helps to reduce the risk of heart disease. Also called a cholesterol-lowering drug.

local: An effect that is felt within a restricted portion or area of the body. Drugs that tend to act locally—including most *topical* agents applied to the skin, *inhalants* that act on the airways, and *ophthalmic* preparations applied to the eyes—generally produce less serious *side effects* than *systemic* drugs, which act on multiple sites throughout the body.

loop diuretic: One of a class of *diuretic* drugs commonly prescribed for the treatment of high blood pressure. Loop diuretics act on the part of the kidneys known as the loop of Henle to block the reabsorption of sodium and water by the bloodstream, thus leading to an increase in the ouput of urine.

macrolide: One of a group of *antibiotics* that are active against various infectious microorganisms and that share a characteristic chemical ring structure.

MAO inhibitor: See *monoamine oxidase inhibitor*.

mast-cell stabilizer: A drug, such as cromolyn sodium, that prevents the release of *histamine* from specialized cells (mast cells) in the respiratory passages, thus reducing inflammation of the airways. They are commonly used in the treatment of asthma.

mcg: An abbreviation for *microgram*.

mEq: An abbreviation for *milliequivalent*.

metered-dose inhaler: A device, commonly used by patients with asthma, that converts liquid medicine into an aerosol spray. The spray can then be breathed in through the mouth, delivering a standard dose of medication to the airways.

mg: An abbreviation for *milligram*.

microgram (mcg): A metric measure of weight, equal to one-millionth of a *gram*, that is sometimes used in drug dosages.

milliequivalent (mEq): A chemical unit of measure that is sometimes used to indicate dosages of vitamins and other drugs.

milligram (mg): A metric measure of weight, equal to one-thousandth of a *gram*, that is commonly used in drug dosages.

milliliter (ml): A metric measure of volume, equal to one-thousandth of a liter, that is sometimes used in dosing recommendations for liquid medications. There are about 5 ml in a teaspoon.

mineral: An inorganic substance, found in the earth's crust, that plays a crucial role in the human body for enzyme synthesis, regulation of heart rhythm, bone formation, digestion, and other metabolic processes. Humans constantly replenish their mineral supply with food and water.

miotic: A drug that causes constriction of the pupils (miosis). Some miotics, such as pilocarpine, are used as *antiglaucoma agents* because they increase the outflow of fluid from within the eye and thereby decrease inner eye pressure.

ml: An abbreviation for *milliliter*.

monoamine oxidase (MAO) inhibitor: An *antidepressant* drug that elevates mood by blocking the actions of the nervous system enzyme, monoamine oxidase, thereby increasing levels of specialized substances called monoamines in the brain.

mucolytic: A drug that is used in the treatment of coughs to break up and thin excessive mucus secretions.

mucous membrane: The pink and shiny skin-like layers that line the lips, mouth, vagina, eyelids, stomach, gastrointestinal and urinary tracts, and other cavities and passages in the body. The mucous membranes secrete the thick and slippery fluid called mucus, which lubricates and protects these tissues. Some drugs are formulated as *topical* preparations for application specifically to the mucous membranes.

narcotic: A drug that acts on the *central nervous system* and that is used primarily to diminish pain but which has numerous effects on the body, including drowsiness and mental clouding (without loss of consciousness), slowed breathing, and decreased motility of the gastrointestinal tract. Also sometimes called an opiate or opioid.

nebulizer: A device that uses compressed air to convert liquid medications into aerosolized mists that can then be inhaled through the mouth or nose. Also known as a metered-dose inhaler.

nephrotoxicity: A scientific term for the kidney damage that can occur as a side effect of certain drugs (for example, *aminoglycoside antibiotics*) or *toxins*.

neuropathy: An adverse side effect of certain drugs that is caused by damage to nerves and marked by burning, tingling, pain, or numbness in the fingers, toes, limbs, or other areas.

neurotoxicity: A scientific term for the nerve damage that can occur as a side effect of certain drugs or *toxins*.

nitrates: A group of *antianginal* drugs that dilate the heart's blood vessels, making it easier for blood to flow through them.

nonsteroidal anti-inflammatory drug: See *NSAID*.

NSAID: An abbreviation for nonsteroidal anti-inflammatory drug, which reduces pain and inflammation in such conditions as arthritis by blocking the production of specialized *hormone*-like chemicals called *prostaglandins*.

off-label use: A common—and legitimate—practice in which a doctor prescribes one or more drugs for a disease, symptom, or condition that has not been specifically approved by the *FDA*. Once a drug has been approved for one *indication*, doctors are then free to prescribe it for other purposes.

ointment: A semisolid drug preparation, usually having a greasy or fatty base and typically applied to the skin.

ophthalmic: A drug that has been formulated for administration onto or around the eye.

opiate or opioid: A morphine-like pain-relieving drug chemically related to opium. See *narcotic*.

oral agent: A drug in solid (such as a pill or capsule) or liquid form that is meant to be ingested by swallowing.

orthostatic hypotension: Low blood pressure, which occurs as a side effect of certain *antihypertensive* agents and other drugs, causing symptoms such as faintness, dizziness, or loss of balance, especially when sitting or standing up quickly.

OTC: A common abbreviation for *over-the-counter* drugs.

otic: A drug that has been formulated for administration into or on the surface of the ear.

ototoxicity: A scientific term for the damage to structures in the ear and loss of hearing that can occur as a side effect of certain drugs (for example, *aminoglycoside antibiotics*) or *toxins*.

over-the-counter (OTC): A drug that can be sold without a prescription—for example, at a corner pharmacy, supermarket, or convenience store. An increasing number of drugs that were formerly available only by prescription are now available OTC, typically in a lower dose than that of the prescription version.

overdose: Excessive accumulation of a drug in the body, resulting in toxic levels that can be dangerous. Accidental overdose is of particular concern in children, older adults, and those with kidney, liver, or other diseases that may impair their ability to process and excrete a drug. Intentional overdose is a concern in depressed patients attempting suicide.

parenteral: A drug that is intended to be administered by a route other than the gastrointestinal tract, such as by injection into the muscles (*intramuscular*) or veins (*intravenous*).

parkinsonism: A relatively common side effect of certain drugs that results in symptoms resembling those of Parkinson's disease, including a rigid, mask-like facial expression; trembling in the hands, arms, or legs; and a rigid posture and gait.

penicillin: One of a group of *antibiotics* (first mass-produced for clinical use in the 1940s) that are widely used against a range of infections. Many

derivatives of penicillin, such as ampicillin and ticarcillin, have since been synthesized; their names end with the suffix "-illin" and they are a common cause of *drug allergy*.

peripherally acting: A drug or other agent that works on or near the surface or periphery of the body, often via the *peripheral nervous system*.

peripheral nervous sytem: The part of the nervous system outside of the brain and spinal cord, such as the nerves leading to the hands or feet.

pharmacist: A professional who is licensed to dispense *prescription* medicines.

photosensitivity: An adverse *side effect* of certain medications marked by a decreased tolerance to the sun's ultraviolet rays, resulting in a tendency for exposed skin to sunburn easily.

pioneer drug: The first version of a new, *brand name* drug.

poisoning: A massive *overdose* of a drug or toxin that can have life-threatening consequences.

potassium-sparing diuretic: A mild *diuretic* drug commonly prescribed for the treatment of high blood pressure. Such drugs act on the kidneys to block the reabsorption of sodium and water by the bloodstream, leading to an increase in the volume of urine. Potassium-sparing diuretics help to prevent excessive loss of the electrolyte potassium, a common problem with other types of diuretics.

prescription: An instruction by a physician that directs a pharmacist to dispense a particular drug in a specific formulation and dose. Prescription medications, unlike *over-the-counter*

drugs, require an M.D.'s approval, usually in written form.

priapism: A medical term for a condition marked by prolonged and painful erection of the penis, resulting from an obstructed outflow of blood. Priapism may occur as a rare side effect of certain drugs.

progestin: A general term for progesterone, a female *hormone* produced by the ovaries that helps to regulate menstruation. Synthetic versions of progestin have been prepared as drugs for use as *contraceptives* and in the treatment of menopause, certain cancers, abnormal uterine bleeding, and other conditions.

prostaglandin: One of a group of chemicals, occurring naturally in the body, that produce a wide range of effects, such as inducing inflammation, stimulating uterine contractions during labor, and protecting the stomach's lining. Some drugs, such as misoprostol, are man-made prostaglandins. Other drugs, such as *NSAIDs*, counteract the effects of certain prostaglandins.

protease inhibitor: A drug that blocks production of a key enzyme, protease, that is needed by the AIDS virus to replicate itself.

retinoid: A man-made derivative of vitamin A used to treat acne, skin wrinkling, and other skin conditions. Drugs that are retinoids include acitretin, tretinoin, and isotretinoin.

Reye or Reye's syndrome: A rare but potentially fatal condition in children and teenagers marked by liver degeneration and swelling of the brain, thought to be related to the administration of aspirin to children under age 16 who have chicken pox, the flu, or flu-like viral illnesses.

sedative: A drug that has a calming effect, used primarily to reduce anxiety or nervousness.

selective serotonin reuptake inhibitor (SSRI): One of a newer class of *antidepressant* drugs that elevates mood by increasing the levels of a specialized chemical in the brain called serotonin.

serotonergic: A drug that increases the supply of a nervous system chemical in the brain called serotonin. Some serotonergics are used as *antiobesity agents* because they help make the patient feel full.

serotonin-blocker: A drug that blocks activity of the nervous system chemical serotonin in the brain. This effect may help to stimulate appetite or relieve certain types of headache.

side effect: A secondary, and usually adverse, effect of a drug. Side effects are known and predictable responses to a specific drug, though usually only a small minority of patients taking the drug will be affected by them.

soft tissue: A general term for internal body parts other than bones and joints, such as muscles, ligaments, and the tissue underlying the skin. Soft tissue can become infected by bacteria and other microorganisms. A number of *anti-infectives* are used to treat such infections.

solution: A mixture of one or more drugs, dissolved in a liquid.

spacer: A device commonly used in conjunction with a *metered-dose inhaler* that attaches to the inhaler's mouthpiece and that acts as a reservoir to hold the air-borne medicine. It helps to assure that a standard dose of medication is delivered to airways.

SPF: An abbreviation for Sun Protection Factor, which indicates the relative ability of a sunscreen to block out ultraviolet rays. Experts recommend using an SPF of at least 15, which will allow a person to remain in the sun without burning 15 times longer, on average, than if no sunscreen were applied.

SSRI: See *selective serotonin reuptake inhibitor.*

stability: The chemical properties of a drug that assure it will not decompose readily during storage, so that it will remain potent and effective through the expiration date.

statin: One of a group of drugs that lowers harmful cholesterol levels by inhibiting a critical enzyme needed for the manufacture of cholesterol in the liver. Also known as an HMG-CoA reductase inhibitor.

steroid: A naturally-occurring compound or drug that has far-ranging effects on numerous body processes. Some steroids are *hormones*—either sex hormones (for example, testosterone) or adrenal gland hormones (for example, prednisone). The terms steroid and *corticosteroid* are often used interchangably.

stool softener: A type of *laxative* that softens the consistency of fecal matter, thus easing the passage of bowel movements.

sulfa drug: One of a class of synthetic bacteria-inhibiting *antibiotics* that is related to the chemical compound sulfanilamide.

sulfonylurea: One of a class of chemically related and commonly used oral diabetes drugs that reduces and controls levels of blood sugar.

superinfection: A dangerous *side effect* of certain *antibiotics* that is marked by the emergence of a secondary infection during the course of antibiotic therapy. It can occur when antibiotics alter the normal balance of microbes in the respiratory, gastrointestinal, or urinary tracts, allowing certain potentially hazardous microorganisms to predominate and flourish.

suspension: A form of liquid medication, often cloudy in appearance, consisting of powdered medicine mixed into water or another fluid.

sympatholytic: An *antihypertensive* drug that acts on the *peripheral nervous system* to block nerve signals that trigger the constriction of blood vessels, thus causing the blood vessels to dilate and blood pressure to decline. Drugs that are sympatholytic include the *beta-blockers* and other medications used for treating high blood pressure.

sympathomimetic: A drug that acts on the nervous system and stimulates the involuntary activities of the organs, glands, muscles, and other structures in the body. Examples include albuterol and isoproterenol, which dilate the respiratory passages and help to relieve asthma.

syrup: A form of liquid medication consisting of a drug dissolved in a concentrated sugar solution.

systemic: Affecting the body in general, as opposed to a limited *local* area. Drugs taken orally or injected *intravenously*, for example, are sometimes referred to as systemic medications, since they are widely distributed throughout the body by the bloodstream. In contrast, most medications applied *topically* to the skin, or dropped into the ears or eyes would generally be considered non-systemic, or local, preparations.

tardive dyskinesia: A medical term for an irreversible nervous condition, marked by unusual involuntary movements of the mouth, tongue, neck, lips, and sometimes fingers, that can occur after prolonged treatment with potent *antipsychotic* drugs.

tetracycline: A type of *antibiotic* that is used against various infections.

thiazide: A type of *diuretic* drug commonly prescribed for the treatment of high blood pressure. These drugs act on the kidneys to block the reabsorption of sodium and water by the bloodstream, leading to an increase in the volume and output of urine.

thrombolytic agent: A drug that dissolves blood clots, or thrombi. These medications are typically given in a hospital by *intravenous* injection—for example, to clear a blood clot that is blocking a coronary artery and causing a heart attack.

tolerance: The body's adaptation to a drug, so that the drug's effects are lessened with continued use. Tolerance may work beneficially; for example, a *side effect* may become much less pronounced with continued use of a drug. On the other hand, drugs such as painkillers may become less effective as tolerance develops, and higher and higher doses may be required.

topical: Designed to be applied to and to act locally on a restricted area of the body, such as the application of a *cream* medication to the skin, an *ointment* to the eyelid, or an *anesthetic* injection to the gums. Topical drug preparations generally have fewer *side effects* than systemic drugs, which are distributed widely throughout the body.

toxin: A poisonous substance that has adverse effects on the body. Some toxins are produced by disease-causing bacteria or by certain plants (for example, mushrooms) or animals (such as snakes). Affected persons are sometimes inoculated with antitoxins, which neutralize the effects of toxins.

toxoid: A substance derived from bacteria and used for some forms of *vaccination* that is capable of combatting or neutralizing the toxic effects of certain infectious microorganisms.

tranquilizer: An *antianxiety* drug that is used to induce sedation and relieve nervous tension.

transdermal patch: A drug-containing adhesive bandage that is worn on the skin and slowly releases medication.

tricyclic antidepressant: A common type of *antidepressant* medication characterized by a three-ring chemical structure that increases the activity of specialized substances called catecholamines in the brain.

tyramines: Substances found in certain foods and drinks, including aged cheeses, salami, soy sauce, beer, and red wines, that can cause a dangerous elevation of blood pressure in patients taking *MAO inhibitors*.

uricosuric drug: A drug that prevents recurrent gout attacks by promoting the excretion of uric acid in the urine.

vaccination: The oral or injectable administration of killed or inactivated microorganisms (*vaccines*) for the purpose of conferring immunity against a particular disease. The term is sometimes used interchangeably with *immunization*.

vaccine: A preparation of dead or inactivated bacteria, viruses, or *toxins* that stimulates the immune system to produce long-term *antibodies* against a particular infectious microorganism.

vasodilator: A drug that causes the blood vessels to widen (dilate), increasing blood flow through them.

vitamin: An organic substance that plays an essential role in regulating cell functions. Most vitamins must be ingested, because the body cannot manufacture them.

xanthine: A drug that opens bronchial air passages and makes breathing easier in patients with asthma and related conditions. Examples include aminophylline and theophylline.

CERTIFIED POISON CONTROL CENTERS

▼

A poison control center can provide valuable instruction in the event of a potential drug overdose or other emergency involving an ingested substance. The places below, listed by state, are all certified by the American Association of Poison Control Centers. Each is staffed 24 hours a day by trained pharmacists and nurses who can answer questions about what to do in the event of a possible drug overdose or poisoning with a toxic substance. Many of the toll-free 800 numbers are usable only when calling within that state. In addition to the centers listed here, many other hospitals and medical centers provide emergency services within a local area. Keep your area numbers handy in the event of an emergency. In addition, keep a bottle of ipecac syrup on hand, in case you are told to "induce vomiting," as well as a supply of activated charcoal.

Alabama
Alabama Poison Center, Tuscaloosa
(800) 462-0800

Regional Poison Control Center, Birmingham
(800) 292-6678 (AL only)
(205) 939-9201; (205) 933-4050

Arizona
Arizona Poison and Drug Information Center, Tucson
(800) 362-0101 (AZ only)
(520) 626-6016

Samaritan Regional Poison Center, Phoenix
(800) 362-0101 (AZ only)
(602) 253-3334

California
Central California Regional Poison Control Center, Fresno
(800) 346-5922
(209) 445-1222

San Diego Regional Poison Center
(800) 876-4766 (619 area code only)
(619) 543-6000

San Francisco Bay Area Regional Poison Control Center
(800) 523-2222

Santa Clara Valley Regional Poison Center, San Jose
(800) 662-9886 (CA only)
(408) 885-6000

University of California at Davis Medical Center, Regional Poison Control Center, Sacramento

(800) 342-9293 (Northern CA only)
(916) 734-3692

Colorado
Rocky Mountain Poison and Drug Center, Denver
(800) 332-3073 (CO only)
(303) 629-1123
(303) 739-1127 (TTY)

Connecticut
Connecticut Regional Poison Center, Farmington
(800) 343-2722 (CT only)
(203) 679-3056

Delaware
The Poison Control Center, Philadelphia
800-722-7112
(215) 386-2100

District of Columbia
National Capital Poison Center, Washington, D.C.
(202) 625-3333
(202) 362-8563 (TTY)

Florida
Florida Poison Information Center– Jacksonville
(800) 282-3171 (FL only)
(904) 549-4465

Florida Poison Information and Toxicology Resource Center, Tampa General Hospital
(800) 282-3171 (FL only)
(813) 256-4444

Georgia
Georgia Poison Center, Atlanta

(800) 282-5846 (GA only)
(404) 616-9000

Indiana
Indiana Poison Center, Indianapolis
(800) 382-9097 (IN only)
(317) 929-2323

Kentucky
Kentucky Regional Poison Center of Kosair's Children's Hospital, Louisville
(800) 722-5725 (KY only)
(502) 589-8222

Louisiana
Lousiana Drug and Poison Information Center, Monroe
(800) 256-9822 (LA only)
(318) 362-5393

Maryland
Maryland Poison Center, Baltimore
(800) 492-2414 (MD only)
(410) 528-7701

Massachusetts
Massachusetts Poison Control System, Boston
(800) 682-9211
(617) 232-2120
(617) 735-6089 (TDD)

Michigan
Poison Control Center, Children's Hospital of Michigan, Detroit
(800) 764-7661
(313) 745-5711

Minnesota
Hennepin Regional Poison Center, Minneapolis

(612) 347-3141
(612) 337-7387 (Petline)
(612) 337-7474 (TDD)

Minnesota Regional Poison Center,
Minneapolis
(612) 221-2113

Missouri
Cardinal Glennon Children's Hospital
Regional Poison Center, St. Louis
(800) 366-8888
(800) 392-9111
(314) 772-5200

Montana
Rocky Mountain Poison and Drug
Center, Denver, CO
(800) 525-5042 (MT only)
(303) 629-1123
(303) 739-1127 (TTY)

Nebraska
The Poison Center, Omaha
(800) 955-9119 (NE & WY only)
(402) 390-5555

Nevada
Rocky Mountain Poison and Drug
Center, Denver, CO
(800) 446-6179 (NV only)
(303) 629-1123
(303) 739-1127 (TTY)

New Jersey
New Jersey Poison Information and
Education System
(800) POISON-1 (800-764-7661)

New Mexico
New Mexico Poison and Drug
Information Center, Albuquerque
(800) 432-6866 (NM only)
(505) 843-2551

New York
Finger Lakes Regional Poison Center,
Rochester
(800) 333-0542
(716) 275-5151

Hudson Valley Poison Center, North
Tarrytown
(800) 336-6997
(914) 336-3030

Long Island Regional Poison Control
Center, Mineola
(516) 542-2323

New York City Poison Control Center
(212) 340-4494
(212) POISONS (764-7667)
(212) 689-9014 (TDD)

North Carolina
Carolinas Poison Center, Charlotte
(800) 84-TOXIN (800-848-6946)
(704) 355-4000

Ohio
Central Ohio Poison Center, Columbus
(800) 682-7625
(614) 228-1323
(614) 228-2272 (TTY)

Cincinnati Drug & Poison Information
Center and Regional Poison Control
System
(800) 872-5111 (OH only)
(513) 558-5111

Oregon
Oregon Poison Center, Portland
(800) 452-7165 (OR only)
(503) 494-8968

Pennsylvania
Central Pennsylvania Poison Center,
Hershey Medical Center
(800) 521-6110
(717) 531-6111

The Poison Control Center, Philadelphia
(800) 722-7112
(215) 386-2100

Pittsburgh Poison Center
(412) 681-6669

Rhode Island
Rhode Island Poison Center, Providence
(401) 444-5727

Tennessee
Middle Tennessee Poison Center,
Nashville
(800) 288-9999
(615) 936-2034

Texas
North Texas Poison Center, Dallas
(800) POISON-1 (800-746-7661)

Texas Poison Control Network
at Galveston
(800) 764-1420 (TX only)
(409) 765-1420 (Galveston)
(713) 654-1701 (Houston)

Utah
Utah Poison Control Center,
Salt Lake City
(800) 456-7707 (UT only)
(801) 581-2151

Virginia
Blue Ridge Poison Center,
Charlottesville
(800) 451-1428
(804) 924-5543

Washington
Washington Poison Center, Seattle
(800) 732-6985 (WA only)
(206) 526-2121
(800) 572-0638 (TDD: WA only)
(206) 517-2394 (TDD)

West Virginia
West Virginia Poison Center, Charleston
(800) 642-3625 (WV only)
(304) 348-4211

Wyoming
The Poison Center, Omaha, NE
(800) 955-9119 (NE & WY only)

There are hundreds of health information organizations in this country. They offer a range of services, from sending literature on a specific disorder or providing updates on the latest drugs and treatments to making referrals to physicians, hospitals, or local support groups. Some focus on a single disease or area of health; others operate on a national level and offer general advice on a wide range of health issues.

Which type of group or organization is right for you depends on your particular needs. When looking for additional informa-

tion or support, a good place to start is with your doctor, who may be able to recommend specific groups for you to contact. You can also refer to the list of major national health information organizations below. Many have toll-free phone numbers or fax lines. Others can be contacted via computer (World Wide Web) or e-mail. This is a limited listing. There are many more associations that offer valuable patient support. If one organization doesn't have the information you need, a staff member may be able to refer you to another one that does.

Agency for Health Care Policy and Research (AHCPR)
P.O. Box 8547
Silver Spring, MD 20907-8547
(800) 358-9295
Fax: (301) 594-2800
Internet site: http://text.nlm.nih.gov
An information clearinghouse sponsored by the U.S. Department of Health and Human Services. Offers publications on back pain, HIV infection, living with heart disease, and many other topics.

American Academy of Pediatrics
P.O. Box 927
Elk Grove Village, IL 60009-0927
Internet site: http://www.aap.org
Offers publications on antibiotics, safety, first aid, and other topics.

American Cancer Society (ACS)
1599 Clifton Road, NE
Atlanta, GA 30329-4251
(404) 320-3333
Internet site: http://www.cancer.org
A national voluntary organization offering information on the management of all types of cancer. Makes referrals to local self-help organizations.

American Cancer Society
Response Line
(800) 227-2345
Provides publications and information about cancer and its treatment.

American Diabetes Assocation
1660 Duke Street
Alexandria, VA 22314
(800) ADA-DISC (232-3472)
(703) 549-1500
Fax: (703) 683-2890
Internet site: http://www.diabetes.org
Provides information and public education programs on diabetes.

American Dietetic Association
216 West Jackson Boulevard, Suite 800
Chicago, IL 60606-6995
(800) 366-1655 Nutrition Hotline
Internet site: http://www.eatright.org
Provides recorded nutritional messages from registered dietitians. The organization also answers food and nutrition questions and makes referrals to registered dietitians.

American Heart Association
P.O. Box 3049
Syracuse, NY 13220-3049
(800) 242-8721
Internet site: http://www.amhrt.org
A national organization with many local branches, offering pamphlets and public education programs on all aspects of cardiovascular health. Check your telephone book for a branch near you.

American Self-Help Clearinghouse
St. Clare's Riverside Medical Center
25 Pocono Road
Denville, NJ 07834
(201) 625-7101
A voluntary agency that makes referrals to more than 700 national self-help groups. Also provides information on how to start your own local self-help group.

Arthritis Foundation
P.O. Box 7669
Atlanta, GA 30357-0669
(800) 283-7800
Fax: (404) 872-0457
E-mail: help@arthritis.org
Internet site: http://www.arthritis.org
Makes referrals to local chapters and provides information on the causes and treatment of rheumatoid arthritis, osteoarthritis, and other musculoskeletal disorders. Also supports research to find cures and provides services to improve quality of life for people with arthritis.

Cancer Information Service
Office of Cancer Communications
National Cancer Institute
Building 31, Room 10A16
9000 Rockville Pike
Bethesda, MD 20892
(800) 4-CANCER (422-6237)
A hotline of the National Cancer Institute, offering information on cancer, smoking cessation, and other topics.

CDC National Aids Hotline
(800) 342-AIDS (342-2437)
Sponsored by the Centers for Disease Control and Prevention. Offers publications and referrals to thousands of community-based organizations that deal with AIDS and HIV infection.

CDC National STD Hotline
(800) 227-8922
Sponsored by the Centers for Disease Control and Prevention. Provides detailed information on 22 different sexually transmitted diseases.

CDC Travel Health Line
(404) 332-4559
Fax-on-command: (404) 332-4565
Internet site:
http://www.cdc.gov/travel/travel.html
Detailed health advice tailored to your specific international travel destination.

Centers for Disease Control and Prevention (CDC)
Office of Public Affairs
1600 Clifton Road, NE
Atlanta, GA 30333
(404) 639-3286
Internet site: http://www.cdc.gov
A U.S. government agency dealing with issues of public health, including AIDS and other infectious diseases, environmental concerns, and occupational safety.

Consumer Health Information Research Institute (CHIRI)
300 East Pinkhill Road
Independence, MO 64057
(816) 228-4595
A nonprofit organization that answers consumer questions on health-related fraud and quackery.

Food and Drug Administration (FDA)
5600 Fishers Lane
Rockville, MD 20857
(301) 443-1240
Internet site: http://www.fda.gov
The U.S. government agency that aims to protect consumers against impure and unsafe foods, drugs, and cosmetics. Answers questions, listens to complaints, and makes referrals to other appropriate agencies. Offers FDA publications on drug labeling, safe use of medications, food and nutrition, and other topics.

National Cancer Institute
National Institutes of Health
9000 Rockville Pike
Bethesda, MD 20892
(301) 496-5615
CancerFax: (301) 402-5874
Internet site: http://www.nci.nih.gov
A branch of the National Institutes of Health that provides information on dozens of types of cancers.

National Eye Institute
Box 20/20
Bethesda, MD 20892-2510
(301) 496-5248 General Information
(800) 869-2020 Publications List
Internet site: http://www.nei.nih.gov
A branch of the National Institutes of Health that provides information on various eye ailments.

National Heart, Lung, and Blood Institute
Education Programs
Information Center
P.O. Box 30105
Bethesda, MD 20824-0105
(301) 251-1222
Internet site: http://www.nhlbi.nih.gov
A branch of the National Institutes of Health that provides written material on cardiovascular and respiratory health.

National Institute of Allergy and Infectious Diseases
Department of Health and Human Services
Building 31, Room 7A-32
9000 Rockville Pike
Bethesda, MD 20892
(301) 496-5717
Internet site: http://www.niaid.nih.gov
Provides information on pollen allergies, dust allergies, sexually transmitted diseases, and other topics.

National Institute of Arthritis and Musculoskeletal and Skin Diseases (NIAMS)
1 AMS Circle
Bethesda, MD 20892-3675
(301) 495-4484
Internet site: http://www.nih.gov/niams/
A branch of the National Institutes of Health, offering information on arthritis, osteoporosis, various skin diseases, and other topics.

National Institute of Child Health and Human Development
(301) 496-3454
Internet site: http://www.nih.gov/nichd/
A branch of the National Institutes of Health that provides information on issues of child health and development.

National Institute of Diabetes and Digestive and Kidney Disorders (NIDDK)
(301) 496-5877
Internet site: http://www.niddk.nih.gov/
A branch of the National Institutes of Health that offers information on diabetes, digestive disorders, endocrine and metabolic disorders, kidney disease, nutrition and obesity, and urologic disease.

National Institute on Aging Information Center
P.O. Box 8059
Gaithersburg, MD 20898-8057
(800) 222-2225
Internet site: http://www.nih.gov/nia/
A branch of the National Institutes of Health that provides information and publications on arthritis, accident prevention, incontinence, cancer, menopause, osteoporosis, nutrition, heart disease, and other topics of interest to older adults.

National Institutes of Health
900 Rockville Pike
Bethesda, MD 20892
(301) 496-4461
Fax: (301) 496-0017
Internet site: http://www.nih.gov
The principal medical research arm of the U.S. government. Call for referral to an appropriate federal agency.

National Institute of Mental Health (NIMH)
NIMH Public Affairs Office
5600 Fishers Lane
Room 7C-02
Rockville, MD 20857
(301) 443-4513
Internet site: http:/www.nimh.gov/
Makes referrals to local mental health associations and offers publications on depression, bipolar disorder, anxiety, phobias, panic disorder, Alzheimer's disease, and other conditions.

National Library of Medicine
Public Health Service
National Institutes of Health
National Library of Medicine
Bethesda, MD 20894
(301) 496-6308
(800) 272-4787
Internet site: http://www.nlm.nih.gov/
One of the world's largest health science libraries. Open to the public. Offers reference services to general consumers.

National Self-Help Clearinghouse (NSHC)
25 West 43rd Street
Room 620
New York, NY 10036
(212) 642-2944
Provides referral services to local self-help groups and organizations.

Office on Women's Health
Room 730B
Humphrey Building
200 Independence Avenue, SW
Washington, DC 20201
(202) 690-7650
Fax: (202) 690-7172
A branch of the U.S. Public Health Service. Provides general fact sheets on various issues in women's health.

ACKNOWLEDGMENTS

MEDICAL CONSULTANTS

*Chief of Medical
Advisory Board*
Simeon Margolis, M.D., Ph.D.
*Professor of Medicine and
Biological Chemistry
Johns Hopkins
School of Medicine*

Franklin Adkinson, M.D.
Asthma and Allergy Medicine

Frank Anania, M.D.
*Gastroenterology and
Hepatology*

Lawrence Appel, M.D.
Internal Medicine

Paul Auwaerter, M.D.
*Internal Medicine and
Infectious Disease*

William Bell, M.D.
Hematology

Ivan Borrello, M.D.
Oncology

Steven Brant, M.D.
Gastroenterology

Richard Chaisson, M.D.
Infectious Disease

Lawrence Cheskin, M.D.
Gastroenterology and Nutrition

Bernard Cohen, M.D.
Dermatology

David Cromwell, M.D.
Gastroenterology

E. Claire Dees, M.D.
Oncology

Phillip Dennis, M.D.
Oncology

Adrian Dobs, M.D.
Endocrinology

Christopher Earley, M.D.
Neurology

David Essayan, M.D.
Allergy and Immunology

John Flynn, M.D.
*Internal Medicine and
Rheumatology*

Joel Gallant, M.D.
Infectious Disease (HIV/AIDS)

Mary Lawrence Harris, M.D.
Gastroenterology

Bradley Hinz, M.D.
Ophthalmology

Thomas Inglesby, M.D.
*Internal Medicine and
Infectious Disease*

Suzanne Jan de Beur, M.D.
Endocrinology

Christopher Karp, M.D.
Parasitology

Beth Kirkpatrick, M.D.
Infectious Disease

Susan Koch, M.D.
Dermatology

Alan Krasner, M.D.
Endocrinology

Julie Krop, M.D.
Endocrinology and Metabolism

Ralph Kuncl, M.D.
Neurology

John Lawrence, M.D.
Cardiovascular Medicine

Linda Lee, M.D.
Gastroenterology

Ronald Lesser, M.D.
Neurology

John Lipsey, M.D.
Psychiatry

Dan Martin, M.D.
*Internal Medicine and
Rheumatology*

William Moss, M.D.
Immunology

Patrick Murphy, M.D.
Infectious Disease

Philip Norman, M.D.
Allergy and Immunology

Steve O'Connell, M.D.
Ophthalmology

Paul O'Donnell, M.D.
Oncology

Peter Pak, M.D.
Cardiology

Marco Pappagallo, M.D.
*Neurology (Chronic Pain
Management)*

Wendy Post, M.D.
Cardiovascular Medicine

Charles Pound, M.D.
Urology

Thomas Preziosi, M.D.
Neurology

Peter Rabins, M.D.
Neuropsychiatry

Stuart Ray, M.D.
*Internal Medicine and
Infectious Disease*

Jon Resar, M.D.
Cardiovascular Medicine

Beryl Rosenstein, M.D.
Pulmonary Medicine

Walter Royal, M.D.
Neurology and Virology

Christopher Saudek, M.D.
Endocrinology and Metabolism

Eduardo Sotomayor, M.D.
Oncology

Jerry Spivak, M.D.
Hematology

Timothy Sterling, M.D.
Infectious Disease

Francisco Tausk, M.D.
Dermatology

Peter Terry, M.D.
Asthma and Allergy Medicine

Chloe Thio, M.D.
Infectious Disease

Jason Thompson, M.D.
Nephrology

Thomas Traill, M.D.
Cardiovascular Medicine

Glenn Treisman, M.D.
Psychiatry

John Ulatowski, M.D.
Neurology

Edward Wallach, M.D.
Obstetrics and Gynecology

Gary Wand, M.D.
Endocrinology

James Weiss, M.D.
Cardiovascular Medicine

James Weisz, M.D.
Ophthalmology

Elizabeth Whitmore, M.D.
Dermatology

CONTRIBUTORS

Digital Photography
Katz Digital Technologies

Pharmacological Resources
Deborah Wible and the staff
of the Department of Pharmacy, Beth Israel Medical
Center, New York City

GENERIC names appear in capital letters.   "C" before page number refers to color pill locator.

881

GENERIC names appear in capital letters.   "C" before page number refers to color pill locator.

883

GENERIC names appear in capital letters. "C" before page number refers to color pill locator.

885

GENERIC names appear in capital letters.   "C" before page number refers to color pill locator.

GENERIC names appear in capital letters. "C" before page number refers to color pill locator.

GENERIC names appear in capital letters.   "C" before page number refers to color pill locator.

GENERIC names appear in capital letters. "C" before page number refers to color pill locator.

GENERIC names appear in capital letters.   "C" before page number refers to color pill locator.

895

Soda Mint, 758
SODIUM BICARBONATE, 758, C-93
Sodium P.A.S., 129
SODIUM PHOSPHATE/ SODIUM BIPHOSPHATE, 759
SODIUM POLYSTYRENE SULFONATE, 760
Sodium Sulamyd, 769
Sofarin, 853
Soft tissue injuries, 26
Solaneed, 843
Solatene, 170
Solfoton, 665
Solu-Medrol, 562
Solurex, 298
Soma, 214
SOMATREM, 761
SOMATROPIN, 762
Sominex, 318, C-71
Sominex Formula 2, 318
Somophyllin, 792
Sonata, 857, C-70
Sorbitrate, 475, C-72
Sore throat, 63
Soriatane, 111
SOTALOL HYDROCHLORIDE, 763, C-87
Spacers, 9
SPARFLOXACIN, 764, C-98
Spaslin, 154
Spasmoject, 308
Spasmolin, 154
Spasmophen, 154
Spasquid, 154
Spec-T Sore Throat Anesthetic, 166
Spectazole, 335
Spectro-Chlor, 239
Spectro-Homatropine, 428
Spectro-Pentolate, 283
Spectro-Sporin, 604
Spectro-Sulf, 769
Spectrobid, 160
SPIRONOLACTONE, 765, C-96
SPIRONOLACTONE/HYDRO- CHLOROTHIAZIDE, 766
Spirozide, 766
Sporanox, 481, C-84
Sprains, 15
SPS, 760
SSRIs (selective serotonin reuptake inhibitors), 48, 49
St. Joseph Adult Chewable, C-82
St. Joseph Cough Suppressant for Children, 301
Stadol NS, 200
Stagesic, 432
Statins, 23

STAVUDINE (D4T), 767
Stelazine, 826
Stelazine Concentrate, 826
Stemetic, 828
Sterapred, 691
Steri-Units Sulfacetamide, 769
Steroids, 26-27, 32, 35, 38, 43, 44, 52
Stilbestrol, 311
Stilbetin, 311
Stimate, 295
Stings, insect, 15, 54, 63
Stomach upset, 8, 10, 14, 29-30, 53
Stool softeners, 30
Stopping a drug, 16, 17
Storage of drugs, 14-16, 17
Storz-Dexa, 297
Storzolamide, 108
Stoxil, 442
Strains, 15
Strep throat, 63
Stress incontinence, 32
Stri-Dex Maximum Strength, 167
Strifon Forte DSC, 251
Strong Iodine (generic), 467
Stulex, 326
Subcutaneous injections, 9, 10
Sublingual drugs, 10
SUCRALFATE, 768, C-73
Sudafed, 712, C-78
Sudafed 12 Hour, C-86
Sufedrin, 712
SULBACTAM SODIUM/ AMPICILLIN SODIUM, 142
Sulf-10, 769
Sulfa drugs, 18, 51
SULFACETAMIDE, 769
Sulfair, 769
Sulfalax, 326
Sulfamethoprim, 829
SULFAMETHOXAZOLE/ TRIMETHOPRIM, 829, C-98
Sulfamide, 769
SULFASALAZINE, 770, C-69
Sulfimycin, 350
SULFINPYRAZONE, 771, C-96
SULFISOXAZOLE OPH- THALMIC, 772
SULFISOXAZOLE SYSTEMIC, 773
SULFISOXAZOLE/ERYTHRO- MYCIN ETHYLSUCCINATE, 350
Sulfonylureas, 38
SULFUR TOPICAL, 774
SULINDAC, 775, C-69
Sulpho-Lac, 774

Sulten-10, 769
SUMATRIPTAN SUCCINATE, 776, C-91
Sumycin, 791
Sun protection, 15, 63
Sunkist, 849
Supac, 107
Superchar, 236
Suppap, 104
Supplements, herbal, 20
Suprax, 225, C-99
Surfak, 326, C-80
Susano, 154
SusPhrine, 346
Sustained-release drugs, 8, 10
Sustaire, 792
Sustiva, 336, C-84
Swallowing pills, 8
Syllact, 714
Symadine, 125
Symmetrel, 125
Sympatholytics, 22
Synacort, 436
Synarel, 593
Synkayvite (menadiol), 852
Synthroid, 509
Syphilis, 41, 63
Systemic drugs, 10

T

T-Cypionate, 789
T-Diet, 667
T-Gen, 828
T-Gesic, 432
T-Phyl, 792
T-Quil, 302
T/Derm Tar Emollient, 271
T/Gel Therapeutic Shampoo, 271
TACE, 246
TACRINE, 777, C-83
TACROLIMUS (FK506), 778
Tagamet, 255, C-65
Tagamet HB, 255, C-88
Tagamet HB 200, 255
Talwin, 655
Tambocor, 381, C-72
Tamiflu, 632
TAMOXIFEN CITRATE, 779, C-93
Tampering, package, 11
TAMSULOSIN HYDROCHLO- RIDE, 780, C-84
Tapanol, 104
Tapazole, 557, C-90
Taraphilic, 271

Tarbonis, 271
Tarka, 817
Tarpaste 'Doak', 271
Tasmar, 808
Tavist, 261
Tavist-1, 261
Tavist-1 12 Hour, C-87
Tavist-D, 261
Taxol, 643
TAZAROTENE, 781
Tazorac, 781
Tebamide, 828
Teczem, 339
Tega-Vert, 317
Tegamide, 828
Tegretol, 212, C-77, C-96
Tegretol-XR, 212
Tegrin, 271
Teladar, 172
Teldrin, 247
TELMISARTAN, 782, C-89
TEMAZEPAM, 783, C-71
Tempra Quicklets Junior Strength, C-73
Tencet, 194
Tendinitis, 26
Tenex, 423
Tenoretic, 149, C-95
Tenormin, 148
Tenuate, 310
Tenuate Dospan, C-100
Tequin, 405, C-99
Terazol 3, 787
Terazol 7, 787
TERAZOSIN, 784, C-85
TERBINAFINE HYDROCHLO- RIDE, 785, C-98
TERBUTALINE SULFATE, 786, C-87, C-94
TERCONAZOLE, 787
Tersa-Tar Soapless Tar Shampoo, 271
Teslac, 788, C-95
Testoderm, 789
Testoject, 789
TESTOLACTONE, 788, C-95
TESTOSTERONE, 789
Tetanus, 63
TETANUS TOXOID, 790
Tetanus Toxoid Adsorbed, 790
Tetanus Toxoid Fluid, 790
TETRACYCLINE HYDROCHLO- RIDE, 791, C-83
Tetracyn, 791
Texacort, 436
Thalitone, 250
Theo-24, 792
Theo-Dur, 792, C-88, C-99
Theo-Time, 792

GENERIC names appear in capital letters.   "C" before page number refers to color pill locator.

897

GENERIC names appear in capital letters.   "C" before page number refers to color pill locator.

899